NUTRITIONAL REQUIREMENTS OF MAN: A CONSPECTUS OF RESEARCH

by M. Isabel Irwin, Ph.D.,

In collaboration with Jean Bowering,
James A. Halsted, D. Mark Hegsted,
Bobbie K. Hutchins, Eldon W. Kienholz,
Karl S. Mason, Mildred S. Rodriguez,
Ann Macpherson Sanchez, and J. Cecil
Smith, Jr.

The Nutrition Foundation, Inc.

New York, Washington
1980

NUTRITIONAL REQUIREMENTS OF MAN: A CONSPECTUS
OF RESEARCH
© Copyright 1971-79, by the Journal of Nutrition

Published by
The Nutrition Foundation, Inc.
Office of Education and Public Affairs
888 Seventeenth Street, N.W.
Washington, D.C. 20006

Printed in the United States of America

Library of Congress Catalog Card Number 80-50451
ISBN 0-935368-23-X

Foreword

THE SCIENTIST today faces a formidable task in keeping abreast of the proliferating, emerging knowledge appearing in the literature in his or her specialty. The task poses even greater difficulties if the literature of research many decades earlier must be identified and evaluated.

The Food and Nutrition Board of the National Research Council has highlighted a serious problem in recommending optimal nutrient intakes:

"The starting point for developing nutrient allowances is the scientific evidence of nutrient requirements . . . Unfortunately, experiments on man are costly, they must be of long duration, certain types of experiments are not possible for ethical reasons, and, even under the best conditions, only a small number of subjects can be studied in a single experiment. Thus, requirement estimates must often be derived from limited information."

The human nutrition research program of the U.S. Department of Agriculture undertook the arduous task of reviewing the world's literature to assess the research base for current dietary recommendations for specific nutrients, and identifying those areas in which information is scarce and where further research is urgently needed. These major studies, some done under contract, led to a series of "conspectuses" on human nutrient requirements. Each appeared originally as a special supplement in the *Journal of Nutrition*.

This project to uncover and bring together past work on human needs for specific nutrients began when I was Director of the Human Nutrition Research Division in the U.S. Department of Agriculture. Dr. M. Isabel Irwin brought her perseverance and dedication, as well as her critical scientific and editorial talents to the task; she provided the leadership for the review series until her untimely death. Fortunately, the USDA continued the prestigious series of conspectuses.

Until now, there has been no single source where one could go to find out the status of research in this area — what has been done and what is currently known about specific nutritional needs of man. With this publication, the Nutrition Foundation, in cooperation with the American Institute of Nutrition, has brought together in a single volume the nine conspectuses which originally appeared in the *Journal of Nutrition's* series on the Nutritional Requirements of Man. The information reflects the data base on the nutritional needs of healthy people of all ages and provides a scope both national and international. This volume will be important and pertinent to research planning and to nutrition program implementation. Much of the nutritional investigation with humans may be expected to come from medical researchers; frequently their exposure is to a different part of the scientific literature than the experimental nutritionist. This publication should meet a major need for the clinical researcher, for teachers and students of nutrition, and for the graduate student, post-doctoral fellow, or clinician planning to conduct research on nutrient requirements of humans. Nutrition educators will find a wealth of information in the chapters that follow.

Grateful acknowledgment is made to the Nutrition Foundation and to the American Institute of Nutrition for assistance in bringing about this publication.

Willis A. Gortner

Contents

A CONSPECTUS OF RESEARCH
ON
PROTEIN REQUIREMENTS OF MAN

by

M. ISABEL IRWIN

Human Nutrition Research Division
Agricultural Research Service
United States Department of Agriculture
Beltsville, Maryland 20705

and

D. MARK HEGSTED

Department of Nutrition
Harvard School of Public Health
Boston, Massachusetts 02115

THE JOURNAL OF NUTRITION

VOLUME 101, NUMBER 3, MARCH 1971

(Pages 385-430)

TABLE OF CONTENTS

INTRODUCTION

Biological research often reveals more problems than it solves. A review of the nutrition literature supports this conclusion. Many of the problems now under active investigation have been studied for over 100 years. Because older studies become buried in the literature and are unknown to current investigators, there is a tendency to "re-search" the same problems, sometimes without obvious improvements in experimental design or techniques. This tendency becomes worrisome as the volume of literature increases. Means must be sought to make past work known and the citations pertinent to it available to present investigators. In this way, the quality of new research proposals can be evaluated more adequately and new or improved research techniques and designs can be appreciated. One method for bringing the past work to light is a broad review of the past literature. The purpose of this review is to summarize the studies relating to protein requirements that have been conducted with human subjects, primarily to indicate the research basis for current dietary recommendations and the areas in which further research would be most useful.

The interpretation of findings, current and past, is a different matter. The significance of results may vary from one investigator to another, depending upon the individual's perspective and the current scientific climate surrounding each area of investigation. The same findings may be interpreted quite differently at different times by different investigators. Thus, a definitive assessment of the significance of past research is not a reasonable expectation. In a broad review of literature, therefore, it may not be possible or desirable for a single investigator to attempt a scientific evaluation of the real significance of the findings that have been presented. The primary objective of this paper is to provide a listing and description of the studies and the conclusions drawn. Some personal comments and evaluation can be made, however, and are included.

Human protein requirements have been studied for over 100 years. The earliest studies, in which food consumption data were collected, were used as a basis for recommendations on protein intakes necessary for health. Although it is commonly believed that such studies overestimated protein needs, the same approach has been used in more recent years. Later studies were designed to estimate the minimal protein needs to maintain life functions. This minimum intake was presumably insufficient to allow for growth or repair of tissue. In other studies, therefore, requirements for growth and anabolism of tissue were investigated. Recognition that proteins are of unequal nutritive value has complicated the establishment of reasonable estimates of requirements under various physiological and environmental conditions.

EARLY STUDIES

Studies on adequate protein intakes

Food consumption, determined either by family purchase records or individual ad libitum intake records, was the basis for the early estimates of protein requirements. The assumption was made that what healthy people customarily ate was an estimate of what they needed. Standards developed on this basis were high; for example, Voit's and Atwater's standards of 118 and 125 g protein/day, respectively, for an adult man (1, 2). When urinary and fecal nitrogen excretion as well as ad libitum food intake was measured, somewhat lower

Received for publication June 25, 1970.

recommendations resulted. Smith (3), for instance, suggested an intake of about 80 g protein/day (200 grains nitrogen) and Nakahama (4) recommended 85 g protein/day for an adult man.

Numerous studies, contemporary to these studies and in the years that followed them, indicated that nitrogen balance could be maintained with much lower intakes even with the vegetarian diets apparently popular at that time. In many of these studies the nitrogen intake was calculated rather than determined by analysis. In others, the fecal losses were not determined. In some, the experimental periods were very short — 1 to 3 days — with no stabilization periods; and in some, the size and age of the subject were not recorded.

In 1898, Atwater and Langworthy (5) tabulated data from more than 2,000 determinations carried out in metabolic studies with human subjects. In these studies, nitrogen intake and outgo had been studied as they were affected by dietary constituents, fasting, water consumption, various types of therapy, disease, etc. In obtaining 49 of the determinations, attempts had been made to estimate the protein intake required "by persons of various occupations and under various conditions." Many of these studies showed that the Voit standard was much too high; some observed that, with sufficient energy provided by fat and carbohydrate, an adult man of approximately 70 kg weight could be maintained in nitrogen equilibrium with as little as 30 to 40 g protein/day (6).

In spite of considerable experimental evidence for lower protein requirements, Voit's standard was regarded as generally correct for ordinary living conditions. Then Chittenden (7), using long periods of observation with 24 healthy adult males engaged in activities ranging from sedentary to very active, demonstrated clearly that the Voit protein standard could be cut at least in half for the normal healthy adult. His work, however, did not seek to discover the minimum amount of protein required by healthy men.

Studies on the "protein minimum"

The evidence that people could be maintained in health with protein intakes considerably lower than the customary intake aroused interest in the minimum protein or nitrogen requirement of man.

Rubner (8) had demonstrated earlier that protein, fat, and carbohydrate could all be used as sources of energy. Protein, however, had another unique function, that of providing material for the repair of nitrogenous tissue. Voit (9) considered the minimum nitrogen requirement to be two-and-one-half to three times that which would cover nitrogenous losses under conditions of fasting. Siven (10) demonstrated that he could maintain his subject in nitrogen equilibrium on intakes lower than the fasting nitrogen excretion. But he did not claim to have found the minimum nitrogen requirement. Then Landergren (11) proposed that the minimum protein or nitrogen intake would be that which would cover the minimum nitrogen losses when sufficient energy for maintenance was provided by fat and carbohydrate. To test this hypothesis, he studied urinary nitrogen output on diets very low in nitrogen with calories supplied by carbohydrate, fat, or both. He did not succeed in determining the "protein minimum." He did conclude, however, that, calorie for calorie, carbohydrate had about twice as much protein-sparing effect as fat — thus entering another dispute that was engaging the physiologists of that time.

The metabolic studies that had been carried out with animals during the last quarter of the nineteenth century had made it clear that some food proteins were more useful than others. In human studies, various protein-containing foods were fed in order to determine the minimum amount required to maintain nitrogen equilibrium. Steck (12), for instance, in experiments on himself found that equilibrium could be maintained if meat, egg albumin, and casein were fed in small amounts that would supply nitrogen just equivalent to the endogenous nitrogen loss. Hindhede (13, 14), studying potato protein and bread protein, attempted to determine the lowest protein intake consistent with nitrogen equilibrium as a measure of protein quality.

Rubner (15, 16) in reviewing Hindhede's work and that of others declared that the "protein minimum" was a variable quantity, because it depended on the needs of the cells at the specific time of ingestion.

The amount of accompanying energy-yielding nutrients, particularly carbohydrate, also would influence the level of protein intake at which equilibrium could be maintained. With dogs he had found that the minimum protein requirement should provide 4 to 5% of the total dietary energy. His observations with humans indicated that a similar relationship probably was true for them.

Sherman (17) who, with his co-workers, had been studying human nutritional requirements and the ability of cereal foods to meet these requirements, tabulated the results of 109 experiments (67 balance studies with 29 men and 42 balance studies with eight women). These 109 experiments were ones in which Sherman believed that the minimum protein requirement had been most accurately determined. The average minimum protein requirement calculated from the data of all 109 experiments was 0.635 g/kilogram body weight or 44.4 g/day per 70-kg man. When protein intake was expressed in terms of body weight, there was no significant difference between the needs of men and women. Observing that there was a wide range of values for minimum protein requirement in the data (21 to 65 g/day), Sherman, omitting the most divergent data, recalculated the mean requirement using data from 94 of the 109 studies. This calculation yielded a mean value of 0.61 g protein/kilogram or 42.8 g/day for a 70-kg man based on data covering 34 subjects. The range of values represented by this mean was 29 to 56 g/70 kg. Upon a second rejection of extreme values, Sherman calculated from data obtained with 24 subjects a mean of 0.58 g/kg or 40.6 g/day per 70-kg man (with a range of 30 to 50 g/ 70 kg). His paper does not reveal whether he used any biometric criteria when reducing the size of his sample.

Having observed that as his selection of data became more critical, the mean protein requirement became lower, Sherman decided that there would probably be a smaller error in estimating the average protein requirement at 0.6 g/kg (42 g/70 kg) than at any higher figure. He noted that the results of the longest and most carefully controlled experiments all fell below this level. He also noted that 0.6 g protein/kilo-

gram would supply approximately 6% of the commonly accepted calorie requirement for moderately active adults (40 kcal/kg). This relationship agrees reasonably well with that found by Rubner with dogs (minimum protein calories equal 4 to 5% of the total dietary calories). Rubner's dogs had been fed meat, whereas many of Sherman's data were obtained with humans eating vegetarian or predominantly cereal diets.

From his own studies (17–19), Sherman reported that one man (80 kg) and two women (54 and 67 kg) were maintained in nitrogen equilibrium with daily intakes of 6.0, 4.36, 4.5, 5.0, and 5.8 g nitrogen/ day when 10% of the protein was supplied by milk and the rest mainly by wheat, corn, or oats. Sherman concluded from these results that 0.5 g mixed protein/kilogram body weight is probably enough for maintenance. He suggested that a standard allowance of 1 g protein/kilogram body weight would provide a margin of safety of 50 to 100% in meeting the requirement for adult maintenance. And thus a new "standard" was born.

STUDIES ON REQUIREMENTS TO COVER MINIMUM NITROGEN LOSSES
(APPENDIX TABLE 1)

Endogenous (urinary) nitrogen

During this time, protein research was gradually shifting from a search for the "protein minimum" to a search for the proteins that would meet the "endogenous" or maintenance protein needs of the body most economically. Refinements on Thomas' (20) biological value were proposed by Mitchell (21). This method, developed with rats as subjects, described a protein in terms of the proportion of absorbed nitrogen retained in the body. It required that the fecal and urinary nitrogen excretion be determined when the subjects were eating an essentially nitrogen-free diet and then again when the protein under study was included in the diet. The determination of the endogenous or maintenance nitrogen excretion is an undertaking which is difficult with human subjects. In some laboratories, therefore, the search began for a value that would represent the minimum nitrogen excretion and that could be used in other studies. Martin and Robison (22) ate an almost nitrogen-free diet for two 7-day periods and determined that their endogenous nitrogen excretion was 38 and 35 mg/kilogram body weight. Smith (23) in a 24-day study with a young man eating an almost nitrogen-free diet obtained a urinary nitrogen excretion of 1.58 g on the last day (24.2 mg/kg body weight). Smith believed that this was the "absolute minimum endogenous nitrogen metabolism." Deuel et al. (24), however, in 1928 obtained an even smaller excretion of 24.1 mg/kg after the "protein stores" had been exhausted following thyroxine administration.

More recently, Young and Scrimshaw (37) reported data obtained with eight young men eating an essentially protein-free diet (6 mg N/kg per day) for 7 to 10 days. After a steady-state urinary nitrogen excretion was achieved in 4 to 7 days, the mean daily urinary nitrogen excretion was 36.6 ± 3.0 mg/kilogram body weight. Calloway and Margen (37a) obtained a similar endogenous urinary excretion (38 mg N/kg) in a closely controlled study with 13 men. Thus, in five studies with a total of 25 men, the endogenous urinary nitrogen excretion estimations have varied between 24 and 38 mg/kilogram body weight.

Another approach to determining endogenous nitrogen excretion was to relate it to some other physiological parameter. Terroine and Sorg-Matter (25) examined the relationship of endogenous nitrogen excretion to basal energy requirements. Their studies with various animals led them to conclude that there is a constant relationship between minimal nitrogen output and basal energy metabolism that holds for homeotherms of widely differing sizes. In these studies, however, they designated the sum of fecal and urinary nitrogen excretions with a nitrogen-free diet as "endogenous nitrogen excretion." Smuts (26) suggested that the endogenous nitrogen excretion might be more accurately measured in urinary excretion alone rather than in a combination of urinary and fecal nitrogen. With five species — mouse, rat, guinea pig, rabbit, and pig — he obtained data indicating that 2 mg nitrogen are excreted for each basal kilocalorie. Further calculations showed that this relationship

would yield values for human requirements agreeing reasonably well with the value of 0.6 g protein/kilogram body weight calculated by Sherman (17). Smuts, therefore, concluded that the relationship of 2 mg nitrogen/basal kilocalorie could be used in computing the human maintenance protein requirement. In studies conducted with human subjects, however, lower values have been obtained. The values obtained in six studies with a total of 39 men (24, 27, 28, 37, 37a) ranged from 1.3 to 1.6 mg nitrogen/kcal. Two studies with a total of 15 women (28, 29) yielded values of 1.19 and 1.42 mg nitrogen/kcal. In a study with 11 infants, Fomon et al. (30) reported mean endogenous nitrogen excretions of 0.6 mg/kcal (7 infants) and 0.8 mg/kcal (4 infants). They suggested that the infants' previous protein intake appeared to influence the endogenous nitrogen excretion.

Other parameters have been associated with maintenance protein requirement and endogenous nitrogen excretion. Hegsted et al. (31), for instance, studied the nitrogen balances of 26 adults eating controlled diets in which the level and kind of protein were manipulated. Intake at nitrogen equilibrium was calculated by regression. Their data indicated that maintenance protein requirement was more closely related to body surface area ($r = 0.71$) than to body weight ($r = 0.61$). With an all-plant protein diet the minimum protein requirement was approximately 2.9 g nitrogen (18 g protein) per square meter. Indian workers (32) found a slightly higher requirement (3.55 g N/m²) with five men eating an all-plant protein diet.

In the study of Young and Scrimshaw (37) body cell mass estimated in eight men from determinations of total body ^{40}K was significantly correlated with endogenous urinary nitrogen excretion (79.4 ± 4 mg N/kg body cell mass). When the number of subjects was increased to 49 men[1] a similar relationship was observed. The coefficients of variation (C) in the unpublished work, however, indicated that there was less variation in the data when urinary nitrogen excretion was expressed in terms

[1] Hussein, M., V. R. Young and N. S. Scrimshaw 1968 Variations in endogenous nitrogen excretion in young men. Federation Proc. 27: 485 (abstr.).

of body weight ($C = 13.7\%$) than in terms of either basal metabolism ($C = 17.6\%$) or lean body mass ($C = 16.1\%$). Calloway and Margen (37a) also found a somewhat lower coefficient of variation when endogenous urinary nitrogen was expressed in terms of body weight ($C = 18\%$) than when it was expressed in terms of basal metabolism ($C = 25\%$) or lean body mass ($C = 23\%$). In their study, however, they found that endogenous urinary nitrogen was correlated, albeit poorly ($r = 0.712$) with lean body mass (estimated from body density and total body water) but not at all with body weight ($r = 0.450$) or basal metabolic rate ($r = 0.399$).

Regardless of the accuracy of the relationship by which it is calculated, endogenous urinary nitrogen is not a complete measure of minimum protein requirement. Additional protein is needed to cover losses in feces, skin and sweat, and to cover increments in growing tissue (hair, nails) in adults. Studies on the extent of these losses and their significance as compared to the urinary nitrogen loss have produced conflicting data.

Metabolic (fecal) nitrogen

Fecal nitrogen losses are made up of two parts, a) the nondigested portion of the food nitrogen and b) the metabolic nitrogen which is not related to the digestibility of the dietary protein. How to distinguish between the two parts has been a subject of controversy.

Rubner (33) believed that he could distinguish between metabolic nitrogen and the nitrogen of undigested protein by the relative solubility of the former in acid alcohol and chloral hydrate.

Hindhede (13), in calculating "true digestibility" of protein, subtracted 1 g nitrogen from the total fecal nitrogen excretion. This was the amount which he said he had found in previous studies to represent metabolic fecal nitrogen. Reifenstein (34) reported that, in his clinical practice, he had found that fecal nitrogen excretion remained constant at about 1.28 g/day when protein intake was varied over a fairly wide range. Similarly, McCance and his associates (35, 36) observed little change in fecal nitrogen when diets containing different levels of wheat protein were fed. They con-

cluded that all of the fecal nitrogen observed in their studies was endogenous in origin.

Hegsted et al. (31) measured fecal nitrogen excretion where diets of similar composition were fed at different levels of nitrogen intake to six adults. By regression they calculated the mean metabolic fecal nitrogen excretion to be 0.395 g/day. Data obtained at Massachusetts Institute of Technology (MIT) by Young and Scrimshaw (37) with eight young men eating an essentially protein-free diet, yielded a mean metabolic nitrogen excretion value of 9.0 ± 1.1 mg nitrogen/kilogram body weight. Calloway and Margen (37a), with 13 men eating a protein-free diet, observed a mean fecal nitrogen excretion of 0.96 ± 0.14 g nitrogen/day. They found that fecal nitrogen was not significantly associated with body weight ($r = 0.227$) or basal metabolic rate ($r = -0.551$) and only poorly correlated with height ($r = 0.688$). Hegsted's data when recalculated on the basis of body weight yield a mean value of 6 to 7 mg/kg — a value that agrees reasonably well with the MIT data but is lower than that obtained in the Calloway study (14 mg/kg). All three estimations are much lower than those (38, 39) calculated by regression in studies with 81 young children recovering from protein–calorie malnutrition (30 and 33 mg N/kg). The differences between the values for adults and for children may be a reflection on the health status of the subjects.

Evidence obtained with animals (40–42), however, and that indicated above, suggest that metabolic fecal nitrogen is not a useful constant and that nitrogen excretion from the gut depends upon the diet fed. The separation of metabolic nitrogen from undigested food nitrogen may be of some value in attempting to explain why proteins vary in nutritional quality. It is not particularly pertinent in estimating human protein requirements.

Skin and sweat losses

That sweat contains nitrogenous substances has been known at least since 1852 when Favre (43) reported finding about 4.4 mg urea/100 ml perspiration. The early studies on the quantitative loss of nitrogen through the skin usually involved only one or two subjects under incompletely controlled conditions (44, 45). The nitrogen excretions determined in these studies varied from 0.013 g nitrogen/day (45) for one man at rest to 1.362 g nitrogen/day for a man doing light work in the tropics (45). Benedict (46) observed that skin losses increased with increasing activity (up to 0.22 g N/hour in his studies). Observing a mean loss of 0.071 g nitrogen/day through the skin of resting men maintained in a respiration chamber, he suggested that even the resting losses excreted under nonsweating conditions were large enough to warrant consideration particularly when protein intake was low. A similar conclusion was reached by Hawawini and Schreier (47). They studied seventeen 5- to 13-week-old infants for 4-day periods and found that 3 to 5% of the total nitrogen excretion was lost through the skin. Greater losses than the resting losses observed by Benedict were those of 12 sedentary African men (254 ± 22.9 mg N/24 hours) studied by Darke (48) and of two men engaged in light activity (254 to 420 mg N/day) studied by Freyberg and Grant (49). Both of these studies were conducted under "nonsweating" conditions. Neither food intake nor activity was closely controlled.

While it is obvious that the skin losses would be proportionately greater with smaller protein intake, it is not clear whether quality or quantity of protein intake influences the nitrogen excretion through the skin. No reports have been found in the literature on the effect of quality of protein on skin losses of nitrogen. The early evidence on the effect of quantity of protein was contradictory (50–53).

Recently Sirbu et al. (54) in a carefully controlled study with 20 young men confined to controlled environmental conditions, controlled diets and controlled activity for periods of 60, 88 and 43 days demonstrated a significantly higher mean cutaneous nitrogen excretion (under "nonsweating" conditions) with an intake of 76 g protein/day than with intakes of 24 and 4 g protein/day. The excretion of nitrogen through the skin was closely correlated with the blood urea nitrogen levels. Other studies (55, 56) have demonstrated a similar relationship.

Sirbu et al. (54) studied hair and nail nitrogen loss as well as skin and sweat loss. The loss of nitrogen through hair and nails was not affected by dietary protein intake. They found an average loss of 24 mg nitrogen/day from hair (head hair and whiskers) and nails. The loss, added to the skin and sweat loss of 119 mg nitrogen/day (dietary intake = 76 g protein) gave a total integumental loss of 143 mg nitrogen/day (about 0.9 g protein). This total is considerably less than that of Voit (57) who found integumental losses (epidermis, hair, and nails) of 179 mg nitrogen/square meter body surface per day under nonsweating conditions. It is also much less than the value of 360 mg/day found by Mitchell and Hamilton (53) with young men during exposures to a "comfortable" environment, or that of 250 mg/m² reported by Kraut and Müller-Wecker (58) for six men. The latter team also reported a value of 120 mg/m² for seven women.

The length of the Sirbu studies suggests that acclimatization may have been responsible, at least in part, for the lower skin losses of nitrogen. Ashworth and Harrower (59) recently reported data which they suggested indicate that, with acclimatization to high temperatures, nitrogen loss in sweat is reduced. They argued that if people in actual practice did lose nitrogen at the rate found by Consolazio et al. (60) or Mitchell and Hamilton (53) (3 to 5 g N/day) in controlled environment studies at high temperatures, they would not be able to maintain nitrogen balance in the tropics with their customary protein intake of about 60 g/day. Ashworth and Harrower attempted to determine the nitrogen losses in sweat of acclimatized people engaged in fairly strenuous but "natural" work in a hot climate. Insensible water loss under conditions of minimal sweating and gross sweat loss under conditions of heavy sweating were both measured by changes in body weight during the collection period. The gross sweat rates and "net sweat" rates (gross sweat minus insensible water loss) of the subjects were similar to but slightly higher (mean 516 g/hour and 430 g/hour) than the mean sweat rate of 406 g/hour determined with Consolazio's subjects at 37.8° between days 13 and 16 of the Denver study. Ashworth's subjects, however, excreted much less nitrogen (0.20 and 0.21 mg N/g sweat) than Consolazio's men (0.53 mg N/g sweat). Nitrogen balances that included sweat losses were positive in the Ashworth study but were negative in the Consolazio study, although Ashworth's subjects had much lower nitrogen intakes (8.13 to 8.53 g N/day) than Consolazio's subjects (13.63 g N/day). This difference in response can quite conceivably be due to the effects of acclimatization. The higher nitrogen intake, presumably habitual, of the Consolazio subjects may have influenced their nitrogen excretions. Sweat used for analysis was collected from Consolazio's men by the arm-bag technique. This method was found in later studies in the same laboratory to give slightly higher nitrogen values than when total body sweat is used. On the other hand, collections made under laboratory conditions such as those used in Consolazio's study are likely to be more complete than those made under the "natural" working conditions under which Ashworth made her study.

The data obtained thus far suggest that skin losses of nitrogen are relatively unimportant for people living under comfortable atmospheric conditions. There is uncertainty about the importance of skin losses with high atmospheric temperatures. Nor is it clear whether there is an adaptation to different levels of protein intake. The answers to these questions may be of importance in tropical countries where protein intakes are low.

Nitrogen gas loss

High apparent nitrogen retentions without concomitant changes in body composition have puzzled many investigators. Costa et al. (61) proposed that the human body can produce nitrogen gas and that this unmeasured nitrogen loss might account for some of the discrepancy between true and apparent nitrogen retention. In support of their hypothesis, they reported data obtained with two men, each of whom was locked in a metabolic chamber after having eaten a high calorie, high protein diet for 4 to 14 days before the experiment. After the subject was locked in the unit, the chamber was flushed for 12 hours with a 80:20 helium–oxygen gas mixture. The subjects remained in the chamber for 17.5

and 36 hours after the flushing procedure. During the postflushing period the concentration of nitrogen rose significantly in the chamber. This was interpreted as indicating that nitrogen gas was being produced by the body. Because an outward leak developed during the experiment, the total amount of nitrogen produced was not measured. Studies with mice which preceded the human studies produced corroborating evidence. Costa et al. indicated that additional confirmation was being sought in studies using the ^{15}N isotope. Studies by Calloway et al. (62) indicated that nitrogen gas is produced by human intestinal microflora. The amount produced in their studies, however, was small and would not greatly influence nitrogen balance. If the Costa hypothesis were confirmed, additional work would be needed to determine the extent of nitrogen loss, the site of gas formation, and whether it is affected by kind and quantity of protein, by other nutrients, or by intestinal flora.

STUDIES ON OTHER FACTORS AFFECTING PROTEIN REQUIREMENTS

Muscular activity

Research on protein requirements for work had early beginnings. Von Leibig (63) held that protein, the main constituent of muscle, is metabolized during muscle contraction and therefore "determine(s) the continuance of force." This theory was effectively disproved in both animal and human studies (64–66). Some physiologists (67), however, observing an increase in urinary nitrogen excretion during activity, suggested that there might be a modest requirement for protein, not principally for energy, but for the maintenance of muscle. Other investigators (68) found no evidence for increased protein metabolism during work. Cathcart (69), after reviewing the early work back to 1855 concluded that the evidence supported the theory of enhanced protein metabolism, both anabolism and catabolism, with muscular activity. Several investigators supported this conclusion by providing evidence of increased urinary nitrogen excretion under conditions of controlled activity (70–73). Nocker (74) reported, however, that the endogenous nitrogen excretion of four men did not increase when they were required to march

20 km/day while eating a nitrogen-free diet. Cuthbertson et al. (75) suggested that the variable findings were largely due to the energy intake of the subjects. If the energy intake is inadequate, amino acids will be deaminated for energy production.

Recently, research on the effects of muscle activity (work, exercise, etc.) on protein metabolism has had three aspects, 1) the requirement of protein for activity, 2) the effect of protein (quality and quantity) on efficiency of work performance, and 3) the effect of lack of activity or immobilization on protein metabolism. Yoshimura (76) reported that anemia and hypoproteinemia appeared in young men receiving 60 g protein/day (which maintained nitrogen balance) when they were undergoing heavy muscular exercise. Bourges,[2] however, noted no changes in blood components when young men, exercising daily on a treadmill, were in slightly negative nitrogen balance with an intake of 0.71 g protein/kilogram body weight. With lower protein intakes there were significant decreases in serum protein, hemoglobin levels, and body cell mass. Egg was the main source of protein in the latter study, whereas animal protein (casein and fish) provided only 25% or less of the protein in the Japanese work (76).

The Japanese workers (76) and Gontzea et al. (77) agree that there is a higher protein requirement for subjects when they are training than when they are fully trained. The additional requirement is likely for the building of muscle tissue. Whether fully trained subjects need more than the maintenance requirement when they are engaged in muscular activity has not been determined.

Some investigators have suggested that dietary protein may influence muscular efficiency. The improvement in muscular efficiency with low protein diets noted by Chittenden (7) has been attributed by Pitts et al. (78) to the vigorous training program included in the study. Pitts found that with protein intakes ranging from 75 to 150 g/day, no significant differences in plasma protein levels or muscular efficiency were noted. In the same laboratory, Darling et al. (79) lowered protein intake by restricting high protein foods. Even with intakes as low as 50 g protein provided mainly by cereals and potatoes, no lowering of efficiency was noted.

In Germany, however, reduction of protein intake from 80 g to 70 g/day has been reported to result in decreased efficiency (80). From the same laboratory, reports were published of increased "muscle strength" when protein intake was raised from 55 to 110 g/day (81). In most of the studies, a change in protein quantity was accompanied by a change in protein quality. At the levels of protein fed, however, differences in protein quality would not be expected to be important. With vigorous physical activity, the total food and protein consumption will ordinarily rise markedly because energy must be supplied. Whether the protein needs for muscular activity may be limiting in areas where diets are relatively low in protein is as yet unknown.

Atrophy of muscle tissue during immobilization of a limb is commonly observed. Balance studies (82–84) show greater urinary nitrogen excretion during bed rest or immobilization than during moderate activity. Deitrick et al. (84) suggested from the observed ratios of sulfur to nitrogen in the urine that the increased nitrogen excretion was primarily from muscle tissue. With isotopic nitrogen, Schønheyder et al. (85) measured the turnover of nitrogen. Their calculation of nitrogen flow-rates from one postulated amino acid pool to another indicated that, during immobilization, the increased nitrogen excretion was due to reduced anabolism of tissue proteins with no change in their catabolic rate. Whether increasing protein intake will minimize the nitrogen loss or promote anabolism during immobilization may be of importance in therapeutics and also in planning for prolonged space flight.

In studies at the U.S. Air Force School of Aerospace Medicine (86), young men were confined to bed in a recumbent position but not restrained in plaster casts as in Deitrick's and Schønheyder's studies. Increased urinary nitrogen loss during the bed rest was observed. Some of the young men carried on programs of isometric exercises. Those taking the exercises suffered

[2] Bourges-Rodriguez, H. 1968 Heavy Dynamic Work and Protein Requirements in Man. A thesis submitted in partial fulfillment of the requirements for the degree of Doctor of Philosophy at the Massachusetts Institute of Technology, Cambridge, Mass.

less discomfort during reambulation than the more completely immobilized subjects, but there was no difference in the urinary nitrogen losses of the two groups. The recumbent position itself may have been responsible, at least in part, for the increased nitrogen losses observed or the kind and amount of exercise may not have been sufficient to prevent atrophy of some muscles.

Another aspect of the study by Lynch et al. (86) was the effect of atmospheric pressure. The men who underwent bed rest at a simulated 12,000 feet altitude had a smaller change in urinary nitrogen excretion than the men at 10,000 feet or at ground level.

Stress

Stress may take various forms — infection, injury (such as in surgery, fractures, or burns), nervous tension, or disruption of normal living patterns. The interaction of nutrition and infection has been reviewed thoroughly (87–89). While it seems obvious that the incidence of infection is higher among the poorly nourished than among the well nourished, it is difficult to separate the nutritional effects from other environmental factors such as sanitation and the lack of immunization programs. Studies conducted by INCAP (90–95) showed no improvement in the incidence of common communicable diseases of childhood, but some improvement in mortality rates and in incidence and duration of diarrheal disease when the diets of young Guatemalan children were supplemented with a protein-rich food mixture. The mortality and morbidity of both the supplemented and unsupplemented children, however, were much higher than those observed in developed countries. The growth rates of the Guatemalan children, on the other hand, were lower than those of children in developed countries. Though there appears to be ample evidence that severe protein depletion in animals affects antibody production, the data obtained with human subjects are conflicting (96–100). In general, they show little or no relationship between protein intake and antibody production or phagocytic activity. Because humans and other animals are born antibody-poor, dietary effects on antibody production might be expected to show up in early life more readily than

in adult years. Studies comparing the antibody production of malnourished children with that of well-nourished children (101, 102), however, have failed to show a difference. The findings of these studies may have been complicated by factors other than protein intake. Healthy infants, however, receiving 3 or 5 g protein/kilogram responded alike to diphtheria toxoid in a study by Dancis et al. (103), who concluded that if there is a difference in response due to protein intake, it must show up at intakes lower than 3 g protein/kilogram. In other studies with children with chicken pox or a mild viral infection (104, 105), increased urinary excretion of nitrogen was observed. There did not appear to be a change in nitrogen absorption. The observations were interpreted as indicating destruction of protoplasm. Whether the increased loss could be balanced by intake was not studied.

Some of the difficulties in studying protein and antibody responses in humans are obvious. To deplete a healthy subject of protein sufficiently to affect antibody production may not be possible and certainly is not ethical. To compare healthy subjects with patients who have been depleted because of wasting disease is not a truly valid comparison because of the uncontrollable complications which may be introduced by the disease. Furthermore, the antibody response of undernourished children may not be typical of the response of well-nourished children. As yet there do not appear to be any data available showing whether an allowance of protein over and above that which permits optimum growth in children is necessary to provide resistance to infection. It is likely that, with children as well as with adults, if sufficient protein is provided to meet the other vital needs of the body, the requirement for antibody formation will be met.

There is customarily an increased excretion of urinary nitrogen accompanying injury such as surgery or burns (106, 107). This urinary nitrogen, excreted mainly as urea, must represent the end products of tissue catabolism. Many observers believe that this catabolism is a reaction to stress (108, 109). Mašek (110) has reported increased nitrogen excretion during pain. Others (111–113), however, have reported data suggesting that, in uncomplicated surgery, calorie deficit is responsible for part of the nitrogen loss. Studies with rats (114) have indicated also that the level of protein intake prior to injury influences the amount of nitrogen lost. Effects of trauma were originally attributed to an adrenal response. Evidence in animals, however, indicates that such effects may be observed in adrenalectomized animals with adrenal hormone supplied from exogenous sources. The response, thus, appears to depend upon the presence of adrenal hormone but not upon differences in adrenal secretion (115).

In addition to the increased urinary nitrogen excretion which usually accompanies injury, there is an exudative loss of nitrogen that occurs with burns. Both Taylor and co-workers (116, 117) and Soroff et al. (118), studying the nitrogen losses of burned patients, concluded that high protein intakes were required. Taylor recommended 2 to 3 g protein/kilogram, whereas Soroff's data indicated high requirements of 20.7 to 25.5 g nitrogen/m^2 (about 3 to 4 g protein/kg) during the early burn period, gradually diminishing to 0.6 to 1.0 g/kg during 90 days. On the other hand, Troell and Wretlind (119) reported smaller protein levels (0.75 g/kg) to be adequate. All these investigators emphasized the need for high caloric intake in order to establish positive nitrogen balance.

Less well defined than the stress of infection or injury is the stress of nervous tension. The ability of an individual to adjust to stressful conditions may be effective in determining his metabolic response to the situation. A study with 26 MIT undergraduates (120) eating a controlled diet indicated that the freshmen were more responsive in terms of increased urinary nitrogen output than were the upperclassmen to the stress of academic examinations. The increases in urinary nitrogen excretion of the whole group varied from 4 to 18% of the baseline levels. This wide range in response suggests that for some individuals there may be an additional requirement for protein during mental stress. In the same laboratory other forms of stress — sleeplessness and reversal of diurnal activity patterns — were found to promote nitrogen excretion (121). The net nitrogen loss af-

ter 2 days of sleeplessness was 12% of the calculated basal nitrogen requirement. With reversal of diurnal activity, the nitrogen loss was 6% of the calculated basal requirement. Whether increased protein or caloric intake would compensate for these losses was not studied.

The effects of environmental stress — exposure to cold, heat, and high altitudes — have not been studied extensively under controlled conditions. Food consumption studies (122–124) indicated that high calorie, high protein diets (3400 to 4400 kcal, 100 to 135 g protein/day) are consumed by men working in frigid temperatures. Consolazio (125) suggested on the basis of his own observations and those of others (126, 127) that the increased caloric intake, provided sufficient clothing was available, was mainly due to the "hobbling" effect of the heavy clothing. Issekutz et al. (128) studied the nitrogen balance of lightly clad young men under varying conditions of protein intake, caloric intake, and environmental temperature. They concluded that negative nitrogen balances observed with low environmental temperatures were not caused solely by inadequate protein and caloric intakes. They suggested that the negative balances reflected a cold-induced hormone change. Whether the nitrogen losses could have been prevented by increasing the protein or calories or both was not reported.

Negative nitrogen balances of men working in a hot environment were reported by Gontzea et al. (129, 130). Eight men were studied, only four of whom had higher nitrogen losses at 35° than at 20°. The four men who had higher losses were those who expended more energy at their work. No comparison of nitrogen excretion with sedentary activity at 20° and 35° was made.

Some evidence is available for increased protein requirement at high altitudes. Consolazio et al. (131) and Surks (132) found negative nitrogen balances in young men eating diets supplying approximately 1 g protein/kilogram per day at elevations of 14,000 ft (4,300 m). Surks suggested that there may be some interference with thyroxine-stimulated protein synthesis at this altitude. Consolazio suggested, in addition, that the negative balance might be due to 1) an increased energy requirement, 2) an increased need for cardiovascular function and hyperventilation, and/or 3) an increased need for meeting environmental or psychological stress. If the first two of his suggestions are true, adding more calories to the diet should bring the subject into equilibrium. The diets used, however, were already high calorie diets in which protein provided approximately 11 to 12% of the energy.

The effect of another form of stress which has been studied in rats by Japanese workers is the effect of vibration (133, 134). The English summaries of these papers indicate contradictory results. No reports of such studies in human subjects have been found. With growing urbanization and increased mechanization, it is possible that some people may live or work under conditions of vibration that would produce stress.

Nitrogen reserves

Whether one believes that optimal nitrogen intake differs from minimal nitrogen intake may depend on one's concept of body nitrogen or protein reserves. There is disagreement in the literature, not only on the existence of such reserves, but also on the extent and form of the reserves if they do exist. Holt (135), for instance, questioned the existence of a "protein reserve." In support of his stand, he reported studies on rats in which high protein diets were found to be no more beneficial than moderate protein diets in protecting the animals from the effects of subsequent low protein intakes.

The concept of protein reserves originated with Voit (64) when he observed a lag in the urinary nitrogen excretion of dogs and cats when their protein intake was raised or lowered. The observations suggested to him that part of the body protein was a relatively mobile type, "circulating protein," which served as a reserve to protect tissue protein from being broken down when the food supply of protein was reduced. Voit's observations of a lag in nitrogen excretion in dogs and cats were confirmed later in human subjects (11, 22–24, 136, 137).

The nature of the labile protein or nitrogen reserves has been the subject of considerable discussion, some of which is probably not very productive. Animal studies (138, 139) make clear that the proteins of different tissues are depleted at varying rates when animals are fed protein-free diets. Wilson (137) concluded from measures of N/S ratios in the urine that the labile protein had a composition different from that of the more stable proteins. Basak (140) fed four adults a nitrogen-, sulfur-, and phosphorus-free diet and concluded from the N/S and N/P ratios in the urine that the labile nitrogen stores might be of nonprotein origin. The concept of rather large nonprotein nitrogenous stores has been suggested also by Cuthbertson et al. (141) and Fisher et al. (142) after observing relatively high apparent retention with high protein intakes but without concomitant changes in body composition. In view of the difficulties in accurately evaluating balance data, especially at high levels of intake, such conclusions must be viewed with suspicion although the true explanation is not apparent. Munro (143) has concluded that "it would appear most likely that labile body N takes the form of protein."

The data obtained in studies on human urinary nitrogen excretion with a nitrogen-free diet were used to estimate the proportion of total body nitrogen that may be considered labile. Munro (143) suggested that not more than 5% of the total body nitrogen is labile. Basak (140) calculated a labile proportion of about 6%. Recently, Young, Hussein, and Scrimshaw (144) studied nitrogen excretion of 22 young men, 10 of whom ate a "protein-free" diet (0.04 g protein/kg) and 12 of whom ate a low protein diet (0.1 g protein/kg) for 7 to 16 days. Nitrogen excretion declined rapidly and achieved a steady state in 3 to 9 days. Labile nitrogen was calculated as the nitrogen excreted above the steady state level during the days before steady state was achieved. The mean labile nitrogen of the 22 men was 0.70% ($\pm$0.24) of the total body nitrogen (the latter was estimated by measuring total body ^{40}K).

Using a similar method, Chan (145) in studies with infants, 7 to 26 months old, estimated the labile protein to be about 1.2% of the total body protein when the daily protein intake changed from 6.0 to 0.75 g protein/kilogram. When the intake changed from 1.5 to 0.75 g protein/kilogram, the labile protein was estimated to be 0.2% of the total body protein. The infants were recovering from malnutrition, but Chan reported finding no evidence of a relationship between amount of labile protein and degree of malnutrition. Chan concluded from the results of this study that labile protein does not represent reserve or storage protein but rather reflects a lag in metabolic adjustment to changes in protein intake.

Waterlow (146) has suggested that "it is misleading to regard labile protein as in any sense an entity." There must, however, be an optimum level of protein in various tissues even though the so-called reserves may be small. Munro (143) has suggested that, since liver is a repository of highly mobile protein and the maintenance of plasma albumin level is a function of the liver cells, a practical measure might be to determine the protein intake required to maintain plasma albumin levels.

Protein quality

Proteins from different sources differ in their usefulness as food. These differences, reflected in different requirements, are illustrated in a study with nine young women by Bricker et al. (29). The study yielded data from which daily requirements for the individual proteins under study were calculated as follows: (g/day) milk 22.4, white flour 38.7, soy flour 23.4, soy-white flour 27.5, mixed foods 25.4. Calculated on the basis of 70 kg body weight and including a rather large allowance for "adult growth," these values become 43.0, 74.4, 46.6, 54.3, and 49.5 g/day, respectively. The allowance for "adult growth" was used by Bricker et al. to cover unmeasured nitrogen losses, such as from the skin, estimated from data of Mitchell and Hamilton (53), as well as "a true retention of nitrogen in the growth of hair, epidermal tissues and structures and in changes in size and form of the body . . ." estimated from data of Grindley (147). The latter data showed an average daily nitrogen retention of 1.38 g by 23 young men eating 80 to 85 g protein/day over a period of 220 days. In a later study (148), young women were found to require 31.7 g protein/day or 3.1 g/m^2 when cereals pro-

vided 70% of the protein. This requirement included an allowance of 0.77 g nitrogen/m^2 for "adult growth." Lower values were found with an all-plant protein diet (62% from cereals) by Hegsted et al. (31) in a study with 26 adults. As noted earlier, they found a requirement of about 2.9 g nitrogen/m^2 (about 31.2 g protein/day). This requirement did not include an allowance for adult growth. When meat provided one-third of the protein, the requirement was found to be about 17% less than with the all-plant diet (about 2.4 g N/m^2 or 24.4 g protein/day). A similar requirement (25.4 g protein/day) was found when wheat germ provided one-third of the protein, whereas a requirement of 31.2 g protein/day was found when soy flour was substituted for meat or wheat germ.

Studies with rats begun by Osborne and Mendel (149) and continued with thoroughness in Rose's laboratory (150) demonstrated that some of the amino acid components were essential for maintenance of life and for growth, whereas others were not. The quality or usefulness of a protein was associated, therefore, with its essential amino acid or "essential nitrogen" content. How much "essential nitrogen" is needed, whether there is a need for additional "unessential" or nonspecific nitrogen after the essential nitrogen needs have been met, and whether the ratio in which the essential amino acids are found in a protein affects its usefulness, have been the subjects of research during the past 30 years.

Essential and nonessential nitrogen

Rose and Wixom (151) found that two young men could be maintained in positive balance with total nitrogen intakes of 3.5 g/day. At this level of intake, the essential amino acids provided 40% of the nitrogen; glycine provided most of the nonessential nitrogen. Whether nitrogen retention could have been maintained 1) with lower essential amino acid intake or 2) with a different source of nonessential nitrogen was not studied. Later studies (152–159) confirmed that man's requirement for nitrogen must be provided only in part by essential amino acids and that a considerable part of it may be provided by nonessential nitrogen. A question of economic importance is: how little of the total nitrogen may be provided by essential amino acids? Recent work indicates that the answer may depend a) on the source of essential amino acids, b) on the source of nonessential nitrogen, and c) on the total nitrogen intake.

a) *Source of essential amino acids.* A number of reports of studies using the "dilution technique" have shown that some proteins may be diluted more than others (154, 156, 157, 159–161). By this technique, the dietary protein is gradually replaced by isonitrogenous amounts of nonspecific nitrogen. Presumably proteins of high quality may be diluted to a greater extent than proteins of low quality without reducing their biological value. For instance, Kofrányi et al. (154, 160, 161) reported that egg protein and potato protein were required in similar amounts when each was fed as the sole source of nitrogen. When diluted, however, with nonessential nitrogen, egg could be diluted up to 60% but potato could not be diluted at all without lowering its biological value. Similarly milk could be diluted 10 to 15% and tuna could not be diluted at all. Kofrányi et al. pointed out that in egg, milk, and tuna, essential amino acids supplied similar amounts of nitrogen. The different performance of these three proteins, they suggested, indicated that neither the chemical score (162) nor the essential amino acid ratio (163) is an accurate measure of protein quality.

Similar studies in Scrimshaw's laboratory (156, 157, 159) have agreed in part with the Kofrányi studies but have disagreed on the extent to which milk protein may be diluted. In studies with 11 young men, urinary nitrogen did not change significantly when egg was diluted to 30% (25% of the total nitrogen supplied by essential amino acids). No change in response was shown by four men with 40% dilution of egg and by one man at the 50% dilution level. In addition, beef protein could be diluted by 25%. Milk protein, in contrast to Kofrányi's findings, was diluted to 20% and 25% without significant change in nitrogen excretion by some subjects. These differences between the findings of the two laboratories may be due to differences in techniques, differences among the subjects, and differences in criteria. The validity of such dilution studies,

of course, depends on the accuracy with which the original requirement of the protein was determined. If excess protein were fed, dilution could be more extensive.

b) *Source of nonessential nitrogen.* There are data to indicate that the sources of nonspecific nitrogen cannot be considered to be equivalent. Glycine, for instance, has been suspected of being less well utilized than some other nitrogen sources (164–166). Glycine mixed with diammonium citrate, however, has been found in some studies (165, 167, 168) to be as well utilized as a mixture of nonessential amino acids. In contrast, when the diluent in Scrimshaw's milk dilution study (157) was glycine plus diammonium citrate, the milk protein could be diluted by only 20%. When the diluent was nonessential amino acids in the proportion found in cow's milk, the milk protein could be diluted by 25%. Kies and Linkswiler (169) found that nitrogen retention was improved by the inclusion of four "semi-essential amino acids" (arginine, histidine, cystine, and tyrosine) in a diet in which essential amino acids, glycine, and diammonium citrate provided the nitrogen. Although the data are not definitive, it is logical to suspect that when most or all of the nonessential amino acids must be derived entirely by synthetic routes, the efficiency of the process may vary depending on the source of nitrogen.

c) *Total nitrogen intake.* Two approaches have been used in studying the effect of total nitrogen intake on the requirement for essential nitrogen: 1) the level of essential nitrogen has been held constant while the level of total nitrogen was varied and 2) the level of total nitrogen was held constant while the essential nitrogen was varied. Tuttle et al. (170), using the first approach with elderly men, found evidence of an increasing requirement for essential nitrogen with increasing total nitrogen intake. Swendseid et al. (153) using the second approach with young adults obtained equivocal results. Clark et al. (171) used the first approach and found that with an essential nitrogen intake equivalent to that in 20 g egg protein, the nitrogen retention of young adults improved as the total nitrogen intake rose to 9 g/day. With intakes of more than 9 g/day, no significant improvement in retention was noted.

When, however, the second approach was used (172) with total nitrogen intake held constant at either 6 or 9 g/day, nitrogen retention rose as the level of essential nitrogen intake was increased from 0.22 to 1.50 g/day.

The results of these studies, therefore, are inconclusive. Neither the lowest level of essential amino acids nor the lowest level of total nitrogen intake compatible with health has been clearly established. Young adults may be able, as Swendseid found, to adjust fairly readily to changes in nitrogen intake. Older people may not be as adaptable. It may be also that within a fairly wide range of nitrogen intake, the proportion of essential amino acids to total nitrogen (E/T_N ratio) is more effective in influencing nitrogen retention than the level of nitrogen intake per se.

Amino acid balance and ratios

Studies with animals demonstrated the need for balance among dietary essential amino acids before evidence of such a need was found in human studies (173–175). Hundley et al. (176) reported data which they interpreted as indicating the importance of amino acid balance in human diets. Specifically, in a study with four men, there was a highly significant decrease in nitrogen retention in one subject when his diet, containing 350 g of rice (total N intake = 5.07 g/day) and 3000 kcal, was supplemented with lysine and threonine. Similarly, another subject responded with a highly significant shift towards negative balance when his diet was supplemented with all eight essential amino acids. Conversely, Truswell and Brock (177) in a study with seven men eating a corn diet, observed a shift toward more positive nitrogen balance when lysine, tryptophan, and isoleucine were added to the diet. More recently, Clark et al. (178, 179) obtained data with young adults eating a diet in which the essential nitrogen was supplied by wheat and purified amino acids. The data obtained on nitrogen retention indicated that the dietary level of one amino acid helps to determine the most advantageous levels of others. The researchers concluded that for optimal utilization, the amino acids must be properly balanced, but that the adult human can "respond fa-

vorably to increasing quantities of essential amino acids even if they are not perfectly balanced."

An attempt to formulate the perfect balance was made by the FAO Committee on Protein Requirements (180). The Committee, considering what was then (1955) known of amino acid requirements, proposed a provisional amino acid pattern to be used as a standard of reference. The amount of each amino acid was expressed in relation to that of tryptophan which was taken as unity, or as milligrams/gram of nitrogen. Following the publication of this proposed reference pattern, a number of studies were initiated in which the dietary protein was supplemented with amino acids until it conformed to the FAO pattern. In the INCAP laboratories, young children (2 to 5 years old) were fed diets based on corn or wheat which were supplemented in this manner (181–185). The children's response measured in terms of nitrogen retention in these studies indicated that the proportion of methionine was too high in the reference pattern. Negative response to additions of tryptophan to a low protein diet (corn masa) indicated that the level of tryptophan in the FAO reference pattern was too high also.

In the studies by Bressani et al. (182–185), the lysine to tryptophan ratio found to be most efficient was 3:1 or 4:1. This is the ratio proposed in the FAO pattern. Fukui et al. (186, 187) provided lysine supplements to the diets of school children 10 to 11 years old. They reported that the lysine supplementation resulted in improved gains in growth and grip strength, and that the best ratio of lysine to tryptophan was 6:1.

In addition to studies in which various proteins were supplemented to match the FAO pattern, other studies were conducted in which the response to intakes of amino acids in the FAO pattern was compared with that to intakes of amino acids in the proportions found in human milk (188), cow's milk (189, 190), egg (191, 192), peanuts (189), oats (193), and wheat (194). Adult subjects were used in most of the studies. In the work on human milk (188), however, infants were studied. The results of these studies showed that, in the FAO pattern, the level of tryptophan was too high and the proportion of methionine in relation to tryptophan was too high. This was in agreement with the INCAP findings (181–185). Furthermore, the nitrogen retentions observed in these studies with the essential amino acids fed in the patterns found in human milk, cow's milk, egg, oats, and even wheat were higher than or equal to the retention with the FAO pattern. The FAO pattern, therefore, did not appear to have unique advantages over the pattern of amino acids in some of our commonly consumed foods.

Noting that the postabsorptive pattern of plasma amino acids remains fairly constant, Swendseid et al. (195) studied metabolic response to food amino acids fed in the plasma acid pattern. All four of the adult subjects studied retained less nitrogen with the "plasma pattern" than with the egg pattern.

Among other amino acid reference patterns that have been proposed is that of Swaminathan (196). In drawing up his "ideal pattern," Swaminathan took into consideration the then (1963) current knowledge on amino acid requirements. This included reports of research on infants and 11- to 12-year-old children that had not been available when the FAO pattern was proposed. Swaminathan's ideal pattern was designed principally to meet the needs of infants and children. Egg protein was calculated to be more capable of meeting the needs of adults than the "ideal amino acid mixture." So far, no reports of research studying the response of human subjects to this "ideal pattern" have been found in the literature since 1963.

STUDIES ON PROTEIN REQUIREMENTS FOR CERTAIN POPULATION GROUPS

Protein in excess of the maintenance requirement is needed when new tissue is being formed. Thus, growing children (Appendix table 2) and pregnant or lactating women (Appendix table 3) need protein to maintain their already existing cells and to provide material for the building of new ones. Whether older people need extra-maintenance levels of protein intake is not clearly indicated. With all age groups, more informative methods of study are needed.

Premature infants

The premature infant is a special type of baby, having missed 2 to 10 weeks of preparation which would help him cope with the world outside the uterus. The analyses of fetuses who have not survived to the end of the 10 lunar months gestation period show that approximately 62% of the nitrogen in a full-term infant's body is laid down in the last two lunar months of pregnancy (197). In order to lay down protein after premature birth at the same rate as he would have done in intrauterine life, the baby must receive a high protein diet. Young et al. (198) calculated that the premature infant should receive at least 4 g protein/kilogram in order to match the intrauterine growth rate. There is, however, some difference of opinion as to whether the premature infant should be encouraged to grow so fast. The high protein diets and the kind of protein fed have been thought by some to overload the infant's digestive and renal systems. Studies with human milk (199–201) indicated that the premature baby can utilize the protein as well as, if not better than, the full-term infant. Gordon et al. (202) found similar retentions with cow's milk and with human milk. Young (198) suggested, however, that cow's milk might be more difficult to assimilate than human milk by babies under conditions less well controlled than those used by Gordon in his studies. He suggested that casein hydrolysates might be advantageous under circumstances where the baby does not tolerate cow's milk.

Compared to other age groups, the number of premature infants whose protein requirements have been studied is large. Reports have appeared on about 12 or more studies involving more than 1500 infants (198, 202–212). The studies have examined both the minimum and maximum level of intake compatible with healthy development. The requirements determined in these studies have varied over a fairly wide range depending in part on the size of the baby. Cox and Filer (213), in reviewing the current knowledge suggested that the available data indicated intakes of from 2.25 to 5 g protein/day were satisfactory for good growth. The lower level is close to what might be provided by breast milk. Larger infants observed by Young et al. (198) could simulate intrauterine growth with fairly low protein intakes (2.7 g/kg) but smaller infants needed high protein, high calorie diets (in their studies 7.0 to 7.6 g protein, 128 to 154 kcal/kg).

The level of protein that will overtax the baby's renal system has not been clearly defined. Numerous investigators have reported higher nitrogen retention with high protein diets than with low protein diets (201, 202, 207). In the study by Snyderman et al. (207), the retained nitrogen with a high protein diet (9 g/kg) could not be wholly accounted for by cutaneous losses, blood nitrogen levels, or serum amino acid patterns. In other studies, however, high blood urea nitrogen (BUN) levels were found in babies receiving high protein diets (203, 208). In the study by Omans et al. (203), babies receiving over 5 g protein/kilogram had elevated BUN levels even at 4 to 6 months of age when they were eating a mixed diet. Furthermore, mortality and morbidity rates appeared to be higher in babies receiving 8 g protein/kilogram than in those receiving moderately high or moderate levels (5.4 and 3 g/kg). In another study (204), however, no appreciable differences in mortality or morbidity were found among babies receiving 2, 3, 4, or 8 g protein/kilogram. Growth rates alone may be a fairly gross parameter that is inadequate to measure the disadvantages of slightly suboptimal intakes or of excessive intakes. Although it is clear that artificial feeding as currently practiced (which often includes lower protein intakes than formerly) can be considered quite satisfactory, the problem of identifying the parameters that will most expeditiously define "optimum conditions" is and will remain difficult.

Another problem that has received some attention in the feeding of premature babies is the ability of protein from sources other than human and cow's milk to meet the infant's needs. Snyderman et al. (206) found that at least 3 g meat or fish protein were required to allow growth equivalent to that obtained with 2 g milk protein/kilogram. At least 5 g protein/kilogram were needed when the protein was provided by vegetable protein sources. The sources of the vegetable proteins were coconut protein isolates, cottonseed flour, peanut flour, sunflower seed flour, sesame seed flour, INCAP No. 8 (a mixture of corn masa, sesame flour, cottonseed flour, torula yeast, and leaf meal), a mixture of soy and rice protein, and a high protein cereal mix containing oat, soy, corn, cottonseed, and wheat protein. Of these, the soy and rice mixture and the high protein cereal gave the best performance. Swiss workers (209), on the other hand, have reported that a soya milk preparation was equivalent to human milk and modified cow's milk as judged by growth, serum proteins and minerals, hemoglobin, red cell count, and reticulocyte count in a group of premature and full-term infants.

Full-term infants

Most of the work with full-term infants has been done with babies less than 6 months old. Reports occur in the literature of about 11 studies with approximately 320 infants, 0 to 6 months of age (young infants) and of three studies with about 40 children, 6 to 24 months of age (older infants).

Young infants

His mother's milk was, in practice until recent times, and in theory still is, the diet of choice for the young infant. The high mortality rate due to "want of breast milk" (approximately 12,000 deaths between 1863 and 1876 in England) stimulated nineteenth century physicians to develop substitutes using cow's milk diluted to resemble breast milk (214, 215). Though some babies appeared to thrive with this "artificial food," breast-fed babies usually showed superior growth. We may suspect that artificial feeding had detrimental aspects, such as exposure to infection, not related to nutrition.

The breast milk versus cow's milk debate, however, has continued to the present day. Holt and Fales (216) observed that when cow's milk is substituted for breast milk, the protein intake must be doubled or tripled to elicit comparable growth. They attributed this difference in effect to the difference in amino acid content of the two milks. L. E. Holt, Jr. (217), in reviewing this part of his father's work, suggested that the inability of the baby to digest cow's milk casein may have been responsible for the difference in effect. He suggested further that the protein of processed milk (dried or evaporated) may be more available than that of raw milk, because it forms smaller and softer curds in the gastrointestinal tract. Evidence supporting this hypothesis had been provided by Jeans et al. (218, 219). The requirement for protein, when supplied by processed cow's milk, therefore, may be reduced to levels close to that of human milk. Reports by Widdowson (220) and Barness et al. (221) provide confirmatory evidence.

Estimates of the minimum requirement of young infants have been reported from three laboratories (30, 221, 222). The values suggested by Barness et al. (221) ($<$ 0.8 g protein/kg or approximately 120 mg N/kg) and by Kaye et al. (222) (100–110 mg N/kg) were obtained by feeding the least amount of protein that would maintain nitrogen equilibrium or slightly positive balance. Obligatory nitrogen losses (57 and 75 mg/kg) determined by Fomon et al. (30) with babies receiving a very low protein diet were much lower than those of Barness or Kaye. This observation suggests that the milk protein used in the latter two studies was not perfectly utilized.

Although the maintenance requirement is enough to keep a child alive, it is not enough to permit him to grow. Studies with breast-fed Chinese and African babies (223, 224) indicate that babies, for the first 3 or 4 months of life, grow normally on breast milk which usually contains about 1.2% protein. As the baby grows older, breast milk is not enough to support normal growth. Similar observations were made by Fomon (225) with eight infants fed cow's milk formulas adjusted to resemble breast milk. In Fomon's formula, 7% of the energy was provided by protein. As the children grew, their protein and energy intakes decreased from 2.0 g and 120 kcal/kg in the first 6 weeks to 1.4 g and 84 kcal/kg at 4 to 6 months. At about 3 to 4 months of age, some of the infants ceased to grow as fast as the normal rate.

In other studies, Fomon and his collaborators used "intermediate" and "high" levels of protein, 15% of the energy from protein (226) and 20% of the energy from protein (227), respectively. At both of these levels of protein intake, growth was similar to that observed with the lowest level (7% of the energy from protein). Nitrogen retention was higher but not proportionately higher as the level of protein intake was raised. It seems, therefore, from these studies that protein intakes higher than 2.0 to 2.5 g/kg did not measurably improve growth even though nitrogen retention was apparently increased.

Whether the apparent high nitrogen retentions were real is questionable. Fomon (227) calculated that if the nitrogen "retained" by one of his infants actually accumulated in the body, the total protein content of the body at 6 months of age would be about 24.6% of the body weight. This, as Fomon pointed out, is highly unlikely in view of analytical data obtained by Widdowson et al. (228); their data indicated that the newborn infant's body contains approximately 15% protein on a fat-free basis (12% of the wet weight), whereas the body of a reasonably well-nourished adult contains 19% protein (15 to 16% of the wet weight). Wallace (229) calculated that the human body achieves chemical maturity between 3 and 4 years of age and that most of the increase in proportion of protein occurs in the first year of life. This increase in protein content does not, however, as Fomon's data illustrate, account for all of the apparently retained nitrogen. One would expect that excess nitrogen would be eliminated eventually via the kidneys. Rominger and Meyer (230), however, found no evidence of greatly increased nitrogen excretion even after a 54-day period in which healthy infants were fed high protein diets. These observations cast doubt on the actuality of the apparent nitrogen retentions. Wallace's suggestion that nitrogen retentions unaccounted for by maturation, growth, and unmeasured losses are artifacts, has been disputed by Holt and Snyderman (231). They claim that in their carefully controlled studies, possible errors in estimation of intake and output could account for only a small part of the nitrogen retention. The significance of these apparent nitrogen retentions, therefore, remains as yet unknown and may vary from one study to another.

Another aspect of high nitrogen intakes by infants is found in the Fomon studies.

Mean hemoglobin levels found over the 6-month period were 10.2, 11.2 and 10.8 g/100 ml with the low, intermediate and high levels of protein, respectively. The slightly low mean values were attributed by Fomon to the rather frequent blood samples that were taken from the babies. The mean blood protein levels with the three diets were similar — 5.7, 5.3, and 6.2 g/100 ml. The blood urea nitrogen levels, however, rose with increased levels of protein intake. The means were 6.0, 8.9, and 21.8 mg nitrogen/100 ml with the low, intermediate, and high levels of dietary protein. Four determinations of urea nitrogen made on blood of infants less than 1 month old yielded a mean of 28.5 mg nitrogen/100 ml. Fomon stated that BUN levels of over 20 mg/100 ml are commonly found in infants receiving 20% of the dietary energy from protein.

The fact that growth was not improved in the Fomon studies by raising the level of protein intake suggests that the decline in growth rate observed in babies 4 to 6 months old by Su and Liang (223) and Sénécal (224) may have been due to calorie deficit. Studies by Rueda-Williamson and Rose (232) in Boston and by Horecny (233) in Bratislava support this hypothesis.

The substitution of cow's milk (whole, evaporated, dried), with its higher protein concentration, for human milk, however, has raised the possibility that the infant might be induced to develop faster, particularly in the neonatal stage, than is possible with a human milk diet. Goldman (234) fed 66 newborn babies formulas containing 4.6 to 3.8% protein from days 2 to 10 of life. The 4.6% protein formula was fed during the first 4 days, and the 3.8% protein mixture during the last 3 days of study. These 66 babies were compared with 36 others who received the routine hospital formulas containing approximately 2.3% protein. The high protein-fed babies had low initial weight losses and greater gains above birth weight during the 10 days than the routinely fed babies.

More recently, Slater (235) studied 13 breast-fed babies and nine formula-fed babies when they were 1 week old. The two groups were receiving similar levels of energy (about 96 kcal/kg/day) in their food. The bottle-fed babies (cow's milk) ingested and retained more nitrogen than the breast-fed babies. They also retained more potassium, phosphorus, calcium, and magnesium than the breast-fed babies. This greater retention of minerals, suggested Slater, may result in faster chemical maturation of the bones and soft tissues in bottle-fed babies than in breast-fed babies. Whether faster chemical maturation in babies is a desirable goal is not known at present. Nor is it known whether the apparent mineral retention was a true retention or the result of artifacts as has been suggested for nitrogen retention.

There is evidence also that the minerals which usually accompany a high protein diet may be detrimental. Johnston et al. (236) fed 31 infants, 9 to 75 days old, six different equicaloric formulas in which 8 to 25% of the energy was supplied by protein. When protein provided 8% of the calories, highest weight gains and lowest nitrogen retentions were observed. At three intermediate protein levels (13, 15, and 20% of the calories), no significant differences were noted in either weight gain or nitrogen retention. When protein provided 25% of the calories, lowest weight gains and highest nitrogen retentions were found. The infants did not tolerate the high protein diet (25% of the calories from protein) well. The investigators noted symptoms suggestive of azotemia or hyperelectrolytemia and secondary diminution of total body water with this diet. Indications that the difficulty lay in the total solute load presented to the kidneys rather than in the nitrogen level per se were found in infants fed a diet designed for premature infants. In this diet, protein supplied 24% of the calories but part of the protein was in the form of amino acid hydrolysates. The ash content was lower than in the high protein diet. The infants tolerated this diet well. Nitrogen retention was similar to that observed with the 25% protein-calorie diet, but weight gains were higher, and the relation of weight gain to nitrogen retention was higher, similar to that with the intermediate protein diets.

In Johnston's work, the metabolic studies were conducted in 3-day periods after the infant had been fed the diet under study for 2 weeks. The effects of long-term consumption of high protein diets by humans starting in infancy is a relatively unexplored field. Ross (237) has reported evidence, confirming previous work by McCay (238) obtained with rats, showing that high-protein high-calorie diets (overnutrition) predispose the animal to a short life and a high incidence of degenerative disease. These studies were run with rats from weaning until death and, therefore, their results may be less applicable to human infant studies than if Ross had attempted to modify the diet of suckling rats.

In Johnston's study also, part of the "protein" of the premature infants' diet was supplied not by intact protein but by amino acid hydrolysates. There is some evidence available (155) indicating that infants may be nourished adequately on lower protein intakes than those discussed heretofore providing that an adequate supply of nitrogen is furnished.

Recently, Snyderman et al. (239) reported the results of a study on plasma amino acid profiles as influenced by protein intake. Fifteen infants, 1 to 6 months of age, were fed cow's milk formulas providing 1.1, 1.3, 1.5, 1.7, and 9 g protein/kilogram body weight. Plasma aminograms determined on blood drawn 4 to 5 hours after a feeding were compared with plasma aminograms of blood similarly drawn from "normal" babies fed their customary cow's milk formula providing 3 to 3.5 g protein/kilogram. The aminograms of the infants fed formulas providing 1.1, 1.3, and 1.5 g protein/kilogram showed similar alterations from the "normal" aminogram. The concentrations of the branched-chain amino acids and of lysine and tyrosine were depressed, and the concentrations of glycine and serine were elevated. With the formula providing 9 g protein/kilogram, the concentrations of most amino acids, particularly of valine and methionine, were elevated. The aminograms of infants fed 1.7 g protein/kilogram were similar to the "normal" aminogram except for an elevated glycine concentration. This observation, Snyderman suggested, might indicate that the infant's protein requirement is close to 1.7 g/kg.

Snyderman also reported that the aminograms obtained after feeding intact protein were different from those obtained after feeding crystalline amino acids in amounts similar to those contained in the intact protein. For instance, with crystalline amino acids, the levels of the branched chain amino acids and also of alanine, proline, asparagine, and citrulline were lower, while the levels of threonine and serine were higher, than after feeding intact protein. The differences became obvious within 24 hours after switching from the intact protein to the crystalline amino acid formulas. This observation suggested to the investigators that the amino acids were absorbed at different rates when they were fed in crystalline form than when they were provided in intact protein.

Older infants

Dietary surveys show protein intake expressed in terms of body weight declining slightly as the child ages from 6 months to 2 years (232, 240). Chan and Waterlow (241) conducted controlled metabolic studies with 17 Jamaican infants 6 to 20 months old. They determined that the maintenance nitrogen requirement of the children was about 100 mg nitrogen/kilogram per day. This value is slightly less than, but comparable to, those determined for younger infants by Barness et al. (221) and Kaye et al. (222). Furthermore, Chan and Waterlow determined that an allowance of 200 mg nitrogen/kilogram per day (1.25 g protein/kg/day) was sufficient to maintain a desirable growth rate. The calorie intake of their infants was 120 kcal/kg. It should be pointed out that their infants, having just recovered from protein–calorie malnutrition, were growing faster than the normal rate (weight gains of 3 g/kg per day as compared to the average rate of 1.2 to 0.7 g/kg/day of children in the same age range). Chan and Waterlow concluded that if an intake of 200 mg nitrogen/kilogram was sufficient to allow growth at twice the normal rate, it should be enough to allow normal growth. Their work did not indicate whether less than 200 mg nitrogen would be sufficient. Their findings, however, were essentially in agreement with the requirement of 1.25 g protein/kilogram per day for 9- to 12-month-old children calculated from data on reported intakes by the Joint FAO/WHO Expert Group in 1965 (242).

Russian reports (243, 244) suggest higher requirements (3.5 to 4.0 g protein/kg). The Roubstein study (243), however, indicated that intakes of 2.5 to 2.8 g/kg were adequate for growth during summer. It is possible that caloric intakes were inadequate during the winter months when 3.5 to 3.6 g/kg were required to allow weight gains. The Moltschanova report (244) indicates that 4.0 g protein/kilogram were needed for "optimal" nitrogen retention. The abstract from which this information was obtained did not indicate whether growth had been measured.

Children of preschool age (2 to 5 years)

In 1917, Lucy Gillett (245) reviewed and compiled the existing data on protein intake and retention of children from birth to 18 years of age. She included only those data that were obtained with "healthy and moderately well-nourished children who, so far as can be judged, were growing normally at the time of observation." Dietary studies reviewed by her (246–249) showed that the average protein intake of healthy growing children, 2 to 5 years old, was 3.06 to 3.66 g/kg body weight. The metabolic studies reviewed (249–254) indicated that children of this age were in positive nitrogen balance with such protein intakes. Clearly, intakes of 3 to 4 g protein/kilogram were sufficient to allow growth and to permit nitrogen storage in these studies.

Some years later, Holt and Fales (216) reported on observations of food intake of over 100 healthy children, 1 to 17 years old. In their cases, the average protein intake varied from 4 g/kg at 1 year of age to 2.6 g/kg at 6 years of age. The intake then remained at this level until the end of the growth period. In the children's diets, protein supplied about 15% of the energy.

Although both compilations of data indicate protein intakes at which normal growth and nitrogen retention were allowed, neither indicates whether lower protein intakes might be equally efficacious or whether higher intakes might be more beneficial.

Since 1917, there have been reports of eight metabolic studies with a total of 44 preschool children (255–265). The results of these studies lack agreement. Protein requirements estimated for growth varied from 1 g/kg (255) to 4 g/kg (262–265). In one study (258), nitrogen retention without growth was observed in a 3.5-year-old and a diabetic 4-year-old child with daily intakes of 1.46 and 1.29 g protein/kilogram, respectively.

Some explanation for the lack of agreement among the various studies may be found in Porter's report (261). Three children, 2 to 5 years old, were studied for from 6 to 20 consecutive 3-day periods (18 to 60 days). An examination of the individual daily nitrogen retention values showed that they fluctuated up and down in a "wave-like" manner. Porter suggested that these fluctuations in nitrogen retention reflected fluctuations in the needs of the body for nitrogen. Statistical treatment of the data indicated that balance periods of 12 to 18 days were required to cover the range of variation in the retentions. If such fluctuations in need for nitrogen exist, then some of the lack of agreement in the literature on protein requirements may be due to the studies having been conducted at different stages of the cycle. In all of the studies discussed above, the dietary protein was reported to contain adequate amounts of animal protein, but no estimates of the biological value of the dietary proteins were reported.

Another factor which may have influenced the results is the caloric intake of the children. Hawks and her collaborators (262–265) fed children, 3 to 5 years old, diets providing 3 g protein/kilogram. When the calorie value of the diet was raised either by adding carbohydrate and fat or by increasing the protein level to 4 g/kilogram, better growth and higher nitrogen retention were observed. The investigators concluded, however, from the effects of protein and calorie intake on uric acid excretion that an intake of 3 g protein/kilogram is not sufficient for optimum growth but that 4 g/kg is a generous allowance.

Both Bartlett's study (255) and Porter's study (261) indicate a decreased requirement with age. The paucity of available data, however, particularly for the younger children (2 to 3 years old), prevents any conclusions being drawn even as to the range of the requirement throughout the preschool period. Beal's data (240) indicate that children 2 to 5 years old customarily eat 3.6 to 2.8 g protein/kilogram — values that agree very well with those compiled by Holt and Fales (216) 30 years earlier. There appears to be no logical reason why preschool children might require more protein per unit weight than older infants if the protein quality of the diets is similar. In normal children, under ordinary conditions with an adequate food supply, the protein intake will probably be determined by the calorie needs.

School children (6 to 12 years)

Early dietary studies with school-age children reviewed by Gillett (245) indicated that children, 6 years old, customarily ate about 3.23 g protein/kilogram per day (249, 266). This intake gradually declined to about 1.92 g/kg for 12-year-old children (246, 248, 249, 266–268). The metabolic studies reviewed by Gillett showed positive nitrogen balances with such intakes (249, 251–253, 266, 269–271). Holt and Fales (216) on the other hand, reporting on their observations of food intake of over 100 children, said that protein intake remained fairly constant at 2.6 g/kg for children from 6 years of age to the end of the growth period. Later, Koehne and Morrell (272) measured the food intake of 28 girls, 6 to 13 years old, over periods of 28 to 192 consecutive days. They found that protein consumption per kilogram body weight did fall from 2.68 at 6 to 7 years to 2.08 g at 11 to 12 years. In the children's diets, protein provided 14.0 to 14.4% of the energy.

Metabolic studies since 1921 have yielded a variety of results, possibly because the methods and objectives of the experiments varied. In all, about 250 children have been studied in 11 investigations (255, 256, 258, 273–279). Estimates of protein requirements resulting from these studies range from 0.7 g/kg (255) to 2.8 g/kg (274). In some of the studies, the results were confounded by inadequate calorie intake which was manifested in exaggerated protein requirements (256, 273). Maroney and Johnston (276) studied the caloric and protein requirements of 27 children, 4 to 14 years old, over a period of several months. There was considerable variation among the children in their caloric requirements for growth. When adequate energy was supplied, however, nitrogen retention was usually positive when protein supplied 15% of the calories.

Lower levels of protein were found to be adequate by Widdowson and McCance (280) in their study of 160 previously underfed children, 5 to 15 years old, in two German orphanages. The protein in the diet, supplied mainly by wheat flour and vegetables, provided 8 to 13% of the calories. The children gained in height and weight at rates faster than had been anticipated from reported observations on normal children.

The method for measuring growth may affect the estimation of protein requirements. In a study conducted over a period of 5 years, 36 girls, 7 to 10 years old, were observed in 59 balance periods 18 to 64 days long. Protein intake varied from 0.5 to 2.9 g/kg (279, 281, 282). Nitrogen retention was greatest in studies in which 2 to 3 g protein/kilogram were fed. Mean height gain and weight gain, however, were greatest with intakes of 1 to 2 protein/kilogram. With intakes of less than 1 g protein/kilogram, the mean height gain was lowest but the mean weight gain was similar to that found with intakes of 1 to 2 g protein/kilogram.

Other parameters in addition to nitrogen retention and growth have been used. Stearns et al. (277) used creatinine excretion per kilogram body weight as an indicator of growth of skeletal musculature. Using this method, they concluded that intakes of 3.0 to 3.5 g protein/kilogram for children, 1 to 4 years old, gradually declining to 2.5 g/kg for 10- to 11-year-olds are necessary to assure optimal growth and resistance to childhood diseases. Obviously the estimation of protein requirements depends greatly on the sensitivity of the criterion or combination of criteria used.

Adolescents (13 to 18 years)

Of all children, adolescents are the least studied in terms of their protein requirements. They have been included in large studies of food consumption, and a few dietary studies have been conducted to determine the protein intake of healthy adolescent boys and girls eating self-selected diets. Most of the metabolic studies, however, in which the protein requirement of adolescents was investigated have used non-normal subjects or have been designed essentially to study some other aspect of metabolism. No reports were found in the literature since 1917 of metabolic studies designed primarily to study the protein requirements of healthy boys and girls during their adolescent growth spurt. Criticism of the work prior to 1917 is that most of the few subjects studied were underweight, undernourished, or ill (283).

Although adolescence is customarily thought of as a developmental stage occurring approximately between the ages of 12 and 18 years, girls frequently begin to mature earlier, with the menarche usually occurring between the ages of 10 and 16 years. Presumably, for this reason, a number of the few studies reported on adolescents have included girls in the 10-, 11-, and 12-year-old range.

The very early work reviewed by Gillett (245) drew together data obtained in dietary studies on sixteen 13- to 18-year-old subjects by five investigators (248, 249, 266–268). These indicated protein intakes varying from 1.89 g/kg for the 13-year-olds (four subjects) to 2.39 g/kg for the 15-year-olds (three subjects). The data obtained in metabolic studies with a total of nine subjects (253, 271, 284–286) showed that positive balances were maintained with intakes of 1.72 to 2.50 g protein/kilogram in this age group. The data of Holt and Fales (216) on protein intake of over 100 children, 1 to 17 years of age, contain information on only five boys and four girls in the 13- to 18-year-old group. These data are sparse, but they show a tendency toward lowered intakes after the age of 15 years. Similar trends were noted many years later by Widdowson (287) in the data collected from 7-day food consumption records obtained from 1028 British children 1 to 18 years old. In her study, there were at least 20 boys and 20 girls in each age group.

In a longitudinal study by Burke et al. (288), the total protein intake of the boys progressively increased from 1 year until 18 years of age. The girls' intake, like that observed in the Widdowson study, in-

creased until the girls were 15 years old and then declined slightly. Similar observations were made by Eppright et al. (289) in a study of the nutrient intake of Iowa children.

The protein intake of the American children (288) was higher than that of the British children (287), particularly during the adolescent years. Both groups of children were reported to be healthy and growing normally. Wait and Roberts (283) in reviewing the available literature concluded that food intake data collected from underweight, malnourished, or convalescent children could not be used as true indicators of requirements for healthy children. Their own data collected from food intake records of 52 healthy girls, 10 to 17 years of age, eating self-chosen diets, showed average protein intakes of 2.0 g/kg at 10 and 11 years, 1.5 g/kg at 12 to 15 years, and 1.2 g/kg at 16 and 17 years. These intakes, they suggested, might be used as "tentative minimum standards" until more accurate data can be obtained.

In other similar studies of food intake records of apparently healthy adolescents, protein requirements of 2.5 g/kg for girls (290) and 1.9 g/kg for boys (291) were suggested. In Russia, requirements of 2 to 3 g/kg have been proposed (292, 293).

Some metabolic studies have been conducted with children who were diabetic (255), recuperating from scarlet fever (294), or tuberculin reactive (276). As might be expected a wide range of values (0.6 to 2.3 g protein/kg) resulted from these studies. Johnston (295), in reviewing his previous work with adolescent girls, noted a premenarchial and postmenarchial reduction in nitrogen retention. This decrease in retention was influenced in part by estrogens. To offset the increased loss and to maintain positive nitrogen balance, Johnston asserted that his previously proposed allowance of protein to provide 15% of the calories, when the calorie intake is adequate for growth (276), is minimal.

The qualifying statement in this proposed allowance "when the calorie intake is adequate for growth" is important. Heald and Hunt (296), in studies with obese children, have shown that the rapidly growing adolescent is extremely sensitive to calorie intake. They found that children who were retaining nitrogen at a given intake of protein and calories would go into negative balance when the energy content, but not the protein, of the diet was decreased. They also found that raising the protein intake while maintaining an inadequate calorie intake did not bring about positive nitrogen balance. Similar sensitivity to caloric changes had been noted earlier by Macy and Hunscher (297). In their study with ten 4- to 9-year-old children, growth was measured by weight gains. Increases of only 4 to 11 kcal/kg body weight in the daily energy intake were accompanied by weight gains for children who had previously been losing weight. Thus, what may appear to be a protein deficiency may be simply a calorie deficiency.

Among the metabolic studies with apparently healthy normal adolescents are those of Johnston and Schlaphoff (298) with six girls, 13 and 14 years old, of Hsu and Adolph (299) with 10 Chinese boys, 14 to 16 years old, and of Sakamoto (300) with one 16-year-old Japanese girl. The American (298) and Chinese (299) studies were principally on mineral metabolism (iron and calcium). Protein requirements were discussed in each report but the data obtained in each study did not support precise estimates.

The Sakamoto study (300) was essentially a study of protein requirements of laboring women. Three women were studied. One of them was an apparently normal, healthy 16-year-old girl. Though supporting data were not provided in the paper, Sakamoto concluded that the 16-year-old girl's minimal daily nitrogen requirement was 0.1126 g/kg (0.704 g protein/kg). To cover needs for labor (10 hours per day) her total nitrogen requirement was 0.113 to 0.143 g/kg (0.71 to 0.89 g protein/kg). There was no indication in the paper as to whether the subject was still growing.

Pregnant and lactating women

The determination of protein requirements during pregnancy and lactation originally was impeded by confusion caused by folklore and by data of dubious pertinence obtained from animal studies. Controlled studies have been conducted with small numbers of individuals for approximately

the last 80 years. In these studies, nitrogen retention has been the most commonly used index of the adequacy of protein intake by the pregnant or lactating woman. Comparison of the data obtained is difficult because 1) the women were at different stages of pregnancy or lactation when studied, 2) many of the balance studies were of short duration (3 to 10 days) and, therefore, possibly not representative of the entire period, 3) the diets frequently were not completely controlled and their nutrient contents frequently were calculated using food composition data from diverse sources.

Studies with large groups of subjects with less well controlled diets than those used in balance studies, or with uncontrolled but recorded food intakes, have been used also to study dietary effects on pregnancy and lactation. Such indices as the occurrence of various complications of pregnancy, anemia, duration and ease of labor, size and condition of the infant, ability of the mother to produce milk or enough milk for the child were recorded. There has been some agreement in the results of these studies but, on the other hand, there has been disagreement on the interpretation of the results.

In attempting to provide dietary guides, some investigators have examined the available literature on protein intakes during pregnancy and lactation and have made recommendations accordingly. These recommendations have in common the fact that they suggest increases over what is normally consumed in the nonpregnant state. They are sufficiently dissimilar to suggest that more precise indices are needed.

Pregnant women

The protein requirements of pregnancy have been investigated principally by a) nitrogen balance and b) dietary and clinical studies.

a) *Nitrogen balance.* Contrary to what, on the basis of animal studies, was believed to be true, Zacharjewski (301), in 1894, reported positive nitrogen retentions during the last 18 days before parturition. This observation was later confirmed by others (302–307). That a woman begins to retain nitrogen early in pregnancy was observed by Wilson (305) and that she apparently retains more than is accumulated in the fetus and adnexa was reported first by Hoffstrom (303) and later by others (306, 308, 309). Based on the work of previous investigators (302, 305, 310–315), Hunscher et al. (308) calculated that approximately 145 g of nitrogen (about 0.5 g N/day) are accumulated, during pregnancy, in the fetus, adnexa, and hypertrophied organs. A frequency distribution (308), based on nitrogen intake and retention values obtained from 917 daily balances reported in the literature, showed an average apparent retention of 2.28 g nitrogen/day. This is a fourfold increase over the calculated nitrogen content of the products of pregnancy.

The validity of such high retentions was questioned by Sandiford et al. (316) who found little support for it in their study with one woman. Furthermore, Coons et al. (306, 317–319), in studies with 15 pregnant women, observed that there was much variation in nitrogen storage between women and, from time to time, in any one woman. Their data and those of Hummel et al. (320) suggested that the pregravid nutritional status of the mother affected her storage of nitrogen during pregnancy. Another conclusion drawn by Coons et al. was that higher nitrogen intakes during pregnancy were associated with greater ease of lactation. Thomson's data (321) obtained in a study with 489 Aberdeen women were not in agreement with this conclusion.

Macy and Hunscher (322), summarizing the data from all preceding studies, suggested that the diet during pregnancy should provide 70 to 100 g protein/day. Higher intakes than these were suggested by Strauss (323), Holmes (324), and Heller (325) as being beneficial in preventing toxemia of pregnancy. The intakes suggested by these investigators ranged from 100 to 260 g protein/day.

Satisfactory results have, of course, been reported with lower levels. Some studies have indicated that with intakes in the region of 13 g nitrogen/day (81 g protein) (326, 327), women "store" nitrogen. In India, Jayalakshmi et al. (328), studying eight pregnant women, observed that nitrogen retention increased as protein intake rose from 60 to 84 g/day. Further increases in intake to 106 and 118 g/day resulted in slight increases in retention but also in gastrointestinal upsets. These investigators suggested that the "optimal" protein intake is 84 to 106 g/day from week 22 to 28 of pregnancy. They also calculated from their data that the minimum daily protein requirement for poor Indian women in pregnancy is about 0.9 g/kg. This is about twice the minimum daily requirement of 0.5 g/kg reported by others for normal Indian adults (32).

Another study conducted in India (329) was planned specifically to determine the maximum amount of dietary protein needed in the pregnant woman's diet to assure optimum health for her and her baby. The results of the study were inconclusive because nitrogen retention (the principal criterion used) continued to rise as the protein content of the diet rose from 70 to 93 to 110 to 115 g/day. Beyond the highest protein level, most of the 15 subjects found the diets intolerable because of their bulk.

The high retentions that have been reported, which cannot be accounted for as new tissue, make one skeptical of balance data as a measure of requirements or even of the amount of nitrogen retained. Hytten and Thomson (330) have suggested that it is doubtful whether any appreciable nitrogen storage, over that involved in the enlargement of the reproductive organs, takes place in the mother's body. The small number of subjects studied and the great variation from woman to woman and within the individual woman (319) also deter one from drawing conclusions on protein requirements from nitrogen balance studies. Werch et al. (331) measured the levels of various blood components of 54 pregnant women, all of whom had protein intakes lower than the then recommended allowance (85 g/day). Though the results were not conclusive, they were sufficiently promising to suggest to Werch that "careful correlation of the findings of a dietary interview with a chemical profile, including blood albumin, amylase, pseudocholinesterase determinations, and the A/G ratio," [3] might be a means for detecting protein deficiency. A similar procedure might prove more efficient and precise in determining

---

[3] A/G ratio = albumin/globulin ratio.

adequate protein intake than the more cumbersome nitrogen balance method.

b) *Dietary and clinical studies.* The basic data on requirements must come from performance such as an uneventful pregnancy; a delivery uncomplicated by anything attributable to nutrition; a viable, healthy infant; ability of the mother to provide sufficient milk for the child. These factors have been considered in several studies. The results have been inconclusive or contradictory. For instance, Ebbs et al. (332) and Burke et al. (333, 334) concluded from their studies of the dietary intake of 380 women in Toronto and 216 women in Boston that dietary quality and, in particular, level of dietary protein were closely related to the outcome of pregnancy. Women with good or excellent diets had fewer complications of pregnancy than those with poor diets. The effect of protein per se, however, was not studied in either of these investigations. The good diets had higher levels of protein than the poor diets, but other nutrients also were varied.

Dieckmann et al. (335) analyzed the food records kept by 602 women during pregnancy. They found no correlation between protein intake and toxemia, prematurity, duration of labor, or length and weight of the baby. Similar findings were reported by Williams and Fralen (336) who analyzed food intake records of 514 women.

The results of a Vanderbilt study (337) were interpreted as indicating that toxemia was not the result of, but rather a predisposing factor toward low protein intakes. In this study of 2046 women in the low to moderate income class, no correlations were found between dietary intake and clinical findings in pregnancy and childbirth.

In a study conducted by Thomson (321, 338, 339), the dietary intakes of 489 primaparae of Aberdeen were examined. The data showed that the intakes of most nutrients were highly correlated. This, Thomson suggested, indicated that, in data obtained by dietary survey, the intakes of single nutrients should not be interpreted as if they had been allowed to vary independently in the diet. For example, low protein diets were low calorie diets which were also low in calcium, thiamin, riboflavin and niacin. The data did not show

any significant relationship between the incidence of preeclampsia and low protein intake. Nor was the nature of the diet associated significantly with the incidence of delivery difficulties, fetal malformation, perinatal death, or failure to establish breast feeding. The mother's weight was more closely correlated with the baby's birthweight than was her dietary intake during pregnancy.

Burke et al. (334) suggested their data indicated that protein intakes less than 75 g/day during the latter part of pregnancy resulted in short, light infants. Dieckmann et al. (335) concluded from nitrogen "balances" (intake minus urinary excretion) obtained with 287 women that there was no "great advantage to a protein intake over 85 g/day." In more recent work, Iyenger (340), with Indian women of the poor socioeconomic class, compared birthweights of infants born of women whose customary diets (1400 kcal, 40 g protein/day) were supplemented to contain 2100 kcal and 60 g or 90 g protein/day during the last month of pregnancy, with birthweights of infants whose mothers had not received supplements. The birthweights of infants of the mothers with supplements were significantly higher than those of the infants of unsupplemented mothers. The birthweights of infants whose mothers had received 90 g protein were not significantly different from those whose mothers had received 60 g protein. The infants of the supplemented mothers had lower birthweights, however, than the weights reported for infants born to well-to-do mothers who had had adequate diets throughout pregnancy. How much of the effect of supplementation in this study was due to increased calories could not be evaluated.

Lactating women

The protein requirement of the lactating woman has been studied by attempting to determine the effect of the mother's protein intake on a) the amount and composition of the milk, b) nitrogen balance, and c) the growth of the infant.

a) *The amount and composition of the milk.* Hoobler's work (341) seems to be the first controlled study on the effects of diet on lactation. With three lactating women, he obtained data indicating that 14%

or more of the calories should be supplied by protein. The level of protein in the diet was related to the amount of milk secreted. The effect of level of dietary protein on the protein content of the milk was not clear. Similar conclusions were reached by Adair (342) and by Deem (343).

More recent studies in Nigeria (344) and in India (345–347) suggested that, at very low levels of protein intake (25 to 39 g/day), the level of dietary protein may affect the level of protein in the milk, whereas at higher levels of intake (60 to 90 g/day) only milk volume is affected.

Some of the work reviewed by Gopalan (348) indicates that other nitrogenous constituents of milk may be affected by the level of dietary protein intake. He reported that when the protein intake of eight lactating women was increased to 90 g/day (presumably from about 60 g) the creatine content of the milk was significantly reduced from what seemed to the investigators to be abnormally high levels. Creatinine levels, also high in the women's milk, were not lowered. The significance of these high levels of creatine and creatinine in milk and of the lowering of the creatine levels with increased protein intake is not known.

b) *Nitrogen balance.* Negative nitrogen balances commonly observed during the puerperium and in the early stages of lactation were believed by some (302, 305) to be the result of the involution of the uterus. Harding and Montgomery (349), however, from observations on four women (three lactating and one nonlactating) after normal labor, suggested that the initiation of lactation is accompanied by a nitrogen loss over and above that due to the involuting uterus. They suggested also that it might not be possible to attain nitrogen equilibrium with any protein intake in the early stages of lactation. The very low protein content of their diets (25 to 34 g/day) may have been at least partly responsible for their results.

The voluminous literature emanating from Macy, Hunscher, and their co-workers records painstaking research on nitrogen intake and losses during all stages of the reproductive cycle (308, 309, 350, 351). Though the three women on whom most of the observations were made could not really

be considered typical lactating women, data on changes in their food intake and nitrogen retention during the reproductive cycle provide useful guides on what one might expect in more typical women. These women were highly efficient milk producers who secreted large quantities (1.5 to 3 liters/day) over long periods. The calorie and protein intake necessary to sustain such production would probably not be required for the less herculean effort of producing 800 to 1000 ml/day. No apparent attempt was made to adjust the food intake above or below the levels selected by the women (the average intakes were 4300, 4600, and 3800 kcal and 160, 165, and 150 g protein/day). It is not possible to determine, therefore, whether the high calorie and protein intakes promoted the high milk production or whether, conversely, the natural aptitude for high milk production necessitated the high food intake. The studies showed, however, that a woman can go through a reproductive cycle without depleting her own body of nitrogen. Studies on the food consumption of the three women indicated that during lactation, protein intake was about 54% greater than during pregnancy. In the postlactation period (presumably a time of recuperation from the stress of lactation) the protein intake was about the same as during the latter half of pregnancy.

In spite of their high calorie and protein intakes, the two women who had the highest milk secretion lost weight during lactation. That they remained in positive nitrogen balance while losing weight suggests that the calorie intake rather than the protein intake was insufficient. The diets were providing 14 to 15% of the calories from protein of high quality.

Macy and Hunscher (322) reported the nitrogen intake of one healthy normal growing infant during the first 6 months of life to be 1.1 to 1.5 g nitrogen/day (approximately 7 to 9 g protein/day). Assuming, as did Rose (352) and McLester (353), an efficiency of about 50% in converting food protein to milk protein, the total requirement for lactation over the maintenance requirement would be less than 20 g protein/day. Using a similar method of calculation, Garry and Stiven (354), assuming a daily secretion of 1 liter of milk containing 2% protein, suggested a protein requirement of about 104 g/day during lactation. More realistically, Leitch and Duckworth (355) assumed a daily milk intake of 875 ml at 1 month to 1630 ml at 6 months for a normally growing infant, and a milk protein content of 1.15%. By their calculations the protein requirement during lactation would be 84 g/day at first, gradually increasing to 100 g at 6 months. Both teams of reviewers assumed a maintenance requirement of 64 g protein/day. Dieckmann and Swanson (356) and Williams (357), after reviewing the available literature, respectively proposed protein allowances of 90 g/day and 2 g/kg body weight/day. That some women can successfully lactate with protein intakes much lower than the foregoing recommendations was observed by Kaucher et al. (358) in a study of the food intake of 12 healthy lactating women. Furthermore, a study of Holemans et al. (359) on five lactating Basuku women during months 8 to 24 of lactation showed that these women could be maintained in positive nitrogen balance with daily intakes of about 1·g protein/kilogram body weight (a mean of 41.1 g protein/day). The women, when not lactating, usually had intakes of only about 25 g protein/day. The intake during the study, therefore, was an increase of approximately 64% over their usual nonlactating intake. The women's milk production, however, was low (293 to 323 ml/day). Holemans suggested that this low secretion might have been a result of, or a defense against, their low protein intake.

In India, six apparently normal lactating women were studied at three levels of protein intake (345, 346) — 61, 99, and 114 g/day. The diets provided 2900 to 3000 kcal. The three levels of protein were fed in consecutive 10-day periods. The increase in protein intakes from 61 to 99 g/day resulted in significantly higher protein retentions — from approximate equilibrium to distinctly positive balances. The additional increase to 114 g protein/day resulted in further small but not significant increases in retention. By calculating the regression coefficient of retention on intake, the investigators concluded that the minimum intake for equilibrium would be 0.24 g nitrogen/kilogram per day (about

1.5 g protein/kg per day). This is about 2.8 times greater than the minimum requirement of 0.087 g nitrogen/kilogram per day determined by Phansalkar and Patwardhan (32) for normal Indian men. It is an increase of about 67% over that estimated to be the minimum protein requirement of poor Indian women in pregnancy (328). Because an increase in intake beyond 99 g/day did not appreciably improve retention, an optimum intake of 100 g protein/day was suggested. This is equivalent to 2.2 g protein/kilogram for the average 45-kg Indian woman.

These studies were carried out with a small number of subjects whose customary protein intake is fairly low. The results may not be applicable, therefore, to populations accustomed to a generous protein allowance. Narasinga Rao (346) suggested that women in excellent nutritional status might have higher minimum nitrogen requirements than was determined here. It is noteworthy, however, that the optimum intake suggested by these studies is slightly higher than that recommended for North American women.

c) *The growth of the infant.* Gopalan (345), in India, studied the effect of the lactating mother's diet on the suckling's growth. Thirty women, whose customary protein intake was about 60 g/day, were divided into two groups. One group received a supplement of 30 g milk protein/day for 6 months. The other group served as controls. The average increases in body weight of the infants, measured every 2 weeks, were not significantly different between the two groups. It was noted previously that raising the protein intake of Indian lactating women above 60 g/day resulted in increased quantity of milk but not in increased protein content of the milk (345). If the infants were being fed to capacity when the mothers were eating 60 g protein/day, it is not likely that they would benefit merely by increasing the quantity of milk available. No reports have been found on the effect of infant growth when the protein intake of the mother was raised from customarily low levels.

The elderly

According to D. M. Watkin (360), "nutrition as it relates to aging in man is now an art. To dignify this relationship by calling it a science presumes not only much knowledge which does not exist, but also the means by which a scientist might integrate isolated data obtained in circumscribed studies in other species into the kaleidoscopic process operating between conception and death in man."

Nutrition studies with older people are scarce, and studies specific to protein requirements are even less numerous. It is difficult to decide who is an elderly or aged person. In the Medlars[4] age categories, those who are 65 years old or more are the aged. Yet, as Albanese et al. (361) pointed out, an individual may be "a tottering oldster at 60 or a youth at 80." In the studies available in the literature, persons as young as 41 years have been included in the older age bracket. A second problem is to find healthy individuals who are willing to be subjects in metabolic experiments. As age increases, the likelihood of physical and metabolic disorders increases. The result is that, in the studies on protein metabolism and requirement carried out on elderly people, few subjects have been free from all disorders and infirmities. The attempt is usually made to choose as subjects those whose infirmities are likely to affect the metabolic processes least.

Some early studies (362, 363) suggested that elderly people needed relatively high intakes of protein (1.6 to 2.1 g/kg) in order to maintain nitrogen equilibrium. In contrast, the indestructible Dr. C. Röse (364) who for 15 years or more ate a diet containing about 30 g protein/day was, at the age of 70 years, vigorously climbing mountains, exercising with a brake ergometer, and walking in the hot sun while maintaining positive nitrogen balance with an intake of 24 g protein/day.

Less spectacular but still evident divergence is to be found in the conclusions drawn from more recent work. Kountz et al. (365–368) concluded from a series of studies with 31 subjects, 50 to 86 years old, that the protein requirement of the elderly is greater than that of younger adults. Negative nitrogen balances persisted in the patients with protein intakes that normally assure positive balance in young adults. From studies with low protein intakes, Kountz et al. concluded that 0.7 g protein/kilogram was the minimum protein requirement for older people and 1.4 g/kg would be an appropriate recommended intake.

In contrast with the Kountz findings, Albanese et al. (361) found that nine women, 66 to 94 years old, were maintained in good health with mean self-chosen intakes of 0.6 to 0.8 g protein/kilogram. These observations led Albanese to conclude that the protein requirement of the elderly may be 20 to 30% lower than intakes recommended for young sedentary women. Subsequently, Albanese et al. (369) reported balance studies carried out with 20 healthy elderly women who maintained positive balance with a mean daily intake of about 0.9 g protein/kilogram.

Roberts et al. (370) concluded from a study with nine active women, 52 to 74 years old, that the protein requirement of elderly people is not substantially different from that of younger adults. A similar conclusion was drawn by Horwitt (371) from his studies over several years duration with older and younger men in a mental hospital. Taking a somewhat different approach, Silverstone et al. (372) found no significant difference between elderly men and middleaged men in their ability to adapt to changes in level of dietary protein. Adaptation was evaluated in terms of the amount of nitrogen "retained" or lost when the level of dietary protein was raised or lowered.

A major problem in studies with this age group is that most elderly people are not "normal" and suffer from a variety of infirmities which may or may not affect nutritional requirements. If healthy subjects are chosen for study, they may represent a special group who are relatively young physiologically and who certainly would be atypical of older people in general. If randomly selected subjects are studied, they presumably will be highly variable, and the diverse abnormalities from which they suffer may be more important than age itself in determining nutritional needs. As is generally appreciated, however, the aged constitute an increasingly large share of the population but nutritional studies with this group are limited.

---

[4] Medlars = medical literature analysis and retrieval system.

CONCLUSIONS

The determination of protein requirements remains elusive primarily because of the lack of precise and adequate methods for evaluating nutritional status with regard to protein. In most studies, requirements have been estimated by the use of nitrogen balance. Theoretically, it should be simple to determine the level of intake which allows maximum retention of nitrogen, assuming that this is an adequate measure of requirement. The literature, however, is replete with reports of nitrogen retentions which are not proportional to changes in body size or composition. In most studies, the more protein fed, the higher the apparent retentions, although few investigators have completed studies over a broad enough range of intakes to indicate the illogical nature of data obtained at high intakes. A variety of explanations has been offered. Macy (278) suggested that the body's efficiency might be such that it must retain about twice as much nitrogen as is calculated to be necessary for a desired weight gain; but this does not explain the fate of the retained nitrogen. Widdowson and McCance (280) suggested that the amount of protein in the cell may not be as fixed as is often supposed and that, within limits, an increase in nitrogen retention might be accompanied by a decrease in fluid content. Excessive losses through the skin, or more recently, losses as nitrogen gas (61) have been proposed. However, until explanatory data are actually available, the most logical explanation is that of Wallace (229) that these apparent retentions are due to technical errors. This explanation is supported by the conclusion of Duncan (373) that calcium balances in animals show similar false retentions and cannot be accounted for by carcass analysis. Unfortunately, there appears to be no approach toward estimating the actual size of the error. One might assume that the more carefully the balance trial is conducted, the smaller the errors would be, i.e., that those from a metabolic ward would be less subject to error than those of free living subjects. A review of the literature, however, provides few clues as to the accuracy of the studies reported. Investigators should at least be aware of the fact that most balance trials

in which different levels of intake of protein or other nutrients have been compared, often, if not always, have led to apparently highly questionable results. Conclusions must be tempered by this awareness.

The simplicity and logic of the balance trial have undoubtedly led to its widespread use and few alternatives are apparent. Changes in plasma protein levels, plasma urea levels, and the plasma aminogram may be very helpful. Unfortunately, the definition of "normal" or "desirable" levels, which may not be the same in common usage, will remain elusive. Real retentions of protein of appreciable magnitude must be related with changes in body size or tissue mass. Thus, measures of body composition, perhaps with ^{40}K, may be most useful if sufficient accuracy can be achieved. Long-term performance as judged by epidemiological studies, field trials, clinical practice, etc., will always be important. Laboratory conclusions which are inconsistent with such findings must be viewed with suspicion. Such data, however, are seldom uncomplicated and the important determinants may be difficult to identify. The interrelationship between protein and calories is a prime example. Even in many metabolic studies this interrelationship has not been sufficiently considered.

Adult men and women and premature infants are the age groups which have been studied most thoroughly. On the other hand, practically no data are available for adolescents, a group often presumed to be at high nutritional risk. Pregnancy in adolescence should impose unusual requirements. The aged are also a large and complicated group which has been little studied. Although age per se may be of little importance, the problems often associated with aging require special consideration from nutritional aspects.

Even in reasonably well studied groups the data often have been collected without consideration of or definition of the protein quality being fed. Since protein quality is a recognized determinant of protein requirements, estimates of protein requirements are obviously influenced by this factor but often to an unknown degree.

It may be possible to discern among the various national and international groups concerned with nutritional requirements and dietary recommendations a tendency toward uniformity of recommendations. This is to some extent encouraging but should not be construed to mean that the data upon which such recommendations are based are any better than they actually are. Such uniformity may be largely due to the limited amount of information available or the influence of a relatively few scientists.

Finally, it would seem to be incumbent upon those engaged in research to be sufficiently familiar with the literature to use their talents expeditiously and to explore those areas where information is lacking rather than to repeat unnecessarily studies that have already been reported.

ACKNOWLEDGMENTS

The authors wish to thank the personnel of the Francis A. Countway Library of Medicine, Boston, for their assistance and for putting the splendid facilities of the library at our disposal. The opportunity to work with such an extensive collection in such aesthetically pleasing surroundings made the literature search upon which this review is based a pleasant task.

We also thank Dr. Agnes M. Huber for assistance in translation; Miss Catherine E. Walsh and Mrs. Hilda K. MacMichael for stenographic and editorial assistance beyond the call of duty; and finally, Dr. W. A. Gortner for pushing, prodding, and for what is euphemistically called encouraging the first author towards the completion of the manuscript.

LITERATURE CITED

1. Voit, C. 1876 Über die Kost in öffentlichen Anstalten. Z. Biol. *12:* 1.

2. Atwater, W. O. 1903 The demands of the body for nourishment and dietary standards. 15th Ann. Rep. Storrs Agr. Exp. Sta., Storrs, Conn., p. 123.

3. Smith, E. 1865 Practical Dietary for Families, Schools, and the Labouring Classes. Walton and Maberly, London, p. 1.

4. Nakahama, T. 1888 Ueber den Eiweissbedarf des Erwachsenen mit Berücksichtigung der Beköstigung in Japan. Arch. Hyg. *8:* 78.

5. Atwater, W. O., and C. F. Langworthy 1898 A digest of metabolism experiments in which the balance of income and outgo was determined. USDA Off. Exp. Stat. Bull. 45 (rev. ed.), Washington, D. C.

6. Klemperer, G. 1889 Untersuchungen über Stoffwechsel und Ernährung in Krankheiten. Z. Klin. Med. *16:* 550.

7. Chittenden, R. H. 1904 Physiological Economy in Nutrition. Frederick A. Stokes Co., New York.

8. Rubner, M. 1885 Calorimetrische Untersuchungen. Z. Biol. *21:* 338.

9. Voit, C. 1881 Handbuch der Physiologie des Gesammtstoffwechsels und der Ernährung. Leipzig., p. 269. Cited by: Siven, V. O. 1900 Ueber das Stickstoffgleichgewicht beim erwachsenen Menschen. Skand. Arch. Physiol. *10:* 91.

10. Siven, V. O. 1900 Ueber das Stickstoffgleichgewicht beim erwachsenen Menschen. Skand. Arch. Physiol. *10:* 91.

11. Landergren, E. 1903 Untersuchungen über die Eiweissumsetzung des Menschen. Skand. Arch. Physiol. *14:* 112.

12. Steck, H. 1913 Über den Ort der Eiweisssynthese und die Erzielung des minimalen Stickstoffgleichgewichtes mit Eiweisskörpern verschiedener Zersetzlichkeit. Biochem. Z. *49:* 195.

13. Hindhede, M. 1913 Untersuchungen über die Verdaulichkeit einiger Brotsorten. Skand. Arch. Physiol. *28:* 165.

14. Hindhede, M. 1914 Das Eiweissminimum bei Brotkost. Skand. Arch. Physiol. *31:* 259.

15. Rubner, M. 1919 Hindhedes Untersuchungen über Eiweissminimum bei Brotkost. Arch. Physiol. *1919:* 124.

16. Rubner, M. 1919 Beitrage zur Lehre vom Eiweissstoffwechsel mit besonderer Berücksichtigung kohlehydratreicher Gemische. Arch. Physiol. *1919:* 24.

17. Sherman, H. C. 1920 Protein requirement of maintenance in man and the nutritive efficiency of bread protein. J. Biol. Chem. *41:* 97.

18. Sherman, H. C., and J. C. Winters 1918 Efficiency of maize protein in adult human nutrition. J. Biol. Chem. *35:* 301.

19. Sherman, H. C., J. C. Winters and V. Phillips 1919 Efficiency of oat protein in adult human maintenance. J. Biol. Chem. *39:* 53.

20. Thomas, K. 1909 Über die biologische Wertigkeit der Stickstoffsubstanzen in verschiedenen Nahrungsmitteln. Arch. Physiol. *1909:* 219.

21. Mitchell, H. H. 1924 A method of determining the biological value of food. J. Biol. Chem. *58:* 873.

22. Martin, C. J., and R. Robison 1922 The minimum nitrogen expenditure of man and the biological value of various proteins for human nutrition. Biochem. J. *16:* 407.

23. Smith, M. 1926 The minimum endogenous nitrogen metabolism. J. Biol. Chem. *68:* 15.

24. Deuel, H. J., Jr., I. Sandiford, K. Sandiford and W. M. Boothby 1928 A study of nitrogen minimum. The effect of sixty-three days of a protein-free diet on the nitrogen partition products in the urine and on the heat production. J. Biol. Chem. *76:* 391.

25. Terroine, E. F., and H. Sorg-Matter 1928 Influence de la température extérieure sur la

dépense azotée endogène des homéothermes. Arch. Int. Physiol. *30:* 115.

26. Smuts, D. B. 1935 The relation between the basal metabolism and the endogenous nitrogen metabolism with particular reference to the estimation of the maintenance requirement of protein. J. Nutr. *9:* 403.

27. Murlin, J. R., L. E. Edwards, E. E. Hawley and L. C. Clark 1946 Biological value of proteins in relation to the essential amino acids which they contain. I. The endogenous nitrogen of man. J. Nutr. *31:* 533.

28. Hawley, E. E., J. R. Murlin, E. S. Nasset and T. A. Szymanski (with M. Blackwood and J. A. Robinson) 1948 Biological values of six partially-purified proteins. J. Nutr. *36:* 153.

29. Bricker, M., H. H. Mitchell and G. M. Kinsman 1945 The protein requirements of adult human subjects in terms of the protein contained in individual foods and food combinations. J. Nutr. *30:* 269.

30. Fomon, S. J., E. M. DeMaeyer and G. M. Owen 1965 Urinary and fecal excretion of endogenous nitrogen by infants and children. J. Nutr. *85:* 235.

31. Hegsted, D. M., A. G. Tsongas, D. B. Abbott and F. J. Stare 1946 Protein requirements of adults. J. Lab. Clin. Med. *31:* 261.

32. Phansalkar, S. V., and V. N. Patwardhan 1956 Utilization of animal and vegetable proteins. Nitrogen balances at marginal protein intakes and the determination of minimum protein requirements for maintenance in young Indian men. Ind. J. Med. Res. *44:* 1.

33. Rubner, M. 1915 Der Kot nach gemischter Kost und sein Gehalt an pflanzlichen Zellmembranen. Arch. Physiol. *1915:* 145.

34. Reifenstein, E. C., Jr. 1944 Conference on metabolic aspects of convalescence including bone and wound healing. Transactions of the Eighth Meeting. Josiah Macy, Jr. Foundation, New York, p. 20.

35. McCance, R. A., and E. M. Widdowson 1947 The digestibility of English and Canadian wheats with special reference to the digestibility of wheat protein by man. J. Hyg. *45:* 59.

36. McCance, R. A., and C. M. Walsham 1949 The digestibility and absorption of the calories, proteins, purines, fat, and calcium in wholemeal wheaten bread. Brit. J. Nutr. *2:* 26.

37. Young, V. R., and N. S. Scrimshaw 1968 Endogenous nitrogen metabolism and plasma free amino acids in young adults given a "protein-free" diet. Brit. J. Nutr. *22:* 9.

37a. Calloway, D. H., and S. Margen 1971 Variation in endogenous nitrogen excretion and dietary nitrogen utilization as determinants of human protein requirement. J. Nutr. *101:* 205–216.

38. Holemans, K., and A. Lambrechts 1955 Nitrogen metabolism and fat absorption in malnutrition and in kwashiorkor. J. Nutr. *56:* 477.

39. Waterlow, J. C., and V. G. Wills 1960 Balance studies in malnourished Jamaican infants. 1. Absorption and retention of nitrogen and phosphorus. Brit. J. Nutr. *14:* 183.

40. Titus, H. W. 1927 The nitrogen metabolism of steers on rations containing alfalfa as the sole source of nitrogen. J. Agr. Res. *34:* 49.

41. Bosshardt, D. K., and R. H. Barnes 1946 The determination of metabolic fecal nitrogen and protein digestibility. J. Nutr. *31:* 13.

42. Schneider, B. H. 1935 The subdivision of the metabolic nitrogen in the feces of the rat, swine, and man. J. Biol. Chem. *109:* 249.

43. Favre, M. P. A. 1852 Recherches sur la composition chimique de la sueur chez l'homme. C. R. Acad. Sci. *2:* 721.

44. Cramer, E. 1890 Ueber die Beziehung der Kleidung zur Hautthätigkeit. Arch. Hyg. *10:* 231.

45. Eijkman, C. 1893 Verchow's Arch. Path. Anat. Physiol. *131:* 170. Cited by: Benedict, F. G. 1906 The cutaneous excretion of nitrogenous material. J. Biol. Chem. *1:* 263.

46. Benedict, F. G. 1906 The cutaneous excretion of nitrogenous material. J. Biol. Chem. *1:* 263.

47. Hawawini, E., and K. Schreier 1965 Die ernährungsphysiologische Bedeutung der Stickstoff- und Ionenverluste durch die Haut. Z. Kinderheilkunde *92:* 333.

48. Darke, S. J. 1960 The cutaneous loss of nitrogen compounds in African adults. Brit. J. Nutr. *14:* 115.

49. Freyberg, R. H., and R. L. Grant 1937 Loss of minerals through the skin of normal humans when sweating is avoided. J. Clin. Invest. *16:* 729.

50. Berry, E. 1916 Über die Abhängigkeit des Stickstoff- und Chlorgehaltes des Schweisses von der Diät. Biochem. Z. *72:* 284.

51. Bost, R. W., and P. Borgstrom 1926 Cutaneous excretion of nitrogenous material in New Orleans. Amer. J. Physiol. *79:* 242.

52. Cuthbertson, D. P., and W. S. W. Guthrie 1934 The effect of variations in protein and salt intake on nitrogen and chloride content of sweat. Biochem. J. *28:* 1444.

53. Mitchell, H. H., and T. S. Hamilton (with W. T. Haines) 1949 The dermal excretion under controlled environmental conditions of nitrogen and minerals in human subjects, with particular reference to calcium and iron. J. Biol. Chem. *178:* 345.

54. Sirbu, E. R., S. Margen and D. H. Calloway 1967 Effect of reduced protein intake on nitrogen loss from the human integument. Amer. J. Clin. Nutr. *20:* 1158.

55. Schwartz, I. L., J. H. Thaysen and V. P. Dole 1953 Urea excretion in human sweat as a tracer for movement of water within the secreting gland. J. Exp. Med. *97:* 429.

56. Komives, G. K., S. Robinson and J. T. Roberts 1966 Urea transfer across the sweat glands. J. Appl. Physiol. *21:* 1681.

57. Voit, E. 1930 Über die Grösse der Erneuerung der Harngebilde beim Menschen. Z. Biol. *90:* 508.

58. Kraut, H., and H. Müller-Wecker 1960 Die Stickstoffabgabe durch die menschliche Haut. Hoppe-Seyler's Z. Physiol. Chem. 320: 241.

59. Ashworth, A., and A. D. B. Harrower 1967 Protein requirements in tropical countries: nitrogen losses in sweat and their relation to nitrogen balance. Brit. J. Nutr. 21: 833.

60. Consolazio, C. F., R. H. Nelson, L. O. Matoush, R. S. Harding and J. E. Canham 1963 Nitrogen excretion in sweat and its relation to nitrogen balance requirements. J. Nutr. 79: 399.

61. Costa, G., L. Ullrich, F. Cantor and J. F. Holland 1968 Production of elemental nitrogen by certain mammals including man. Nature 218: 546.

62. Calloway, D. H., J. Colasito and R. D. Matthews 1966 Gases produced by human intestinal microflora. Nature 212: 1238.

63. von Leibig, J. 1846 Animal Chemistry, or Organic Chemistry in its Application to Physiology and Pathology, ed. 2, ed., Gregory William. London, Taylor and Walton, 1843; transl. from: Die Thier-Chemie oder die Organische Chemie in ihrer Anwendung auf Physiologie und Pathologie, ed. 3. F. Vieweg u. Sohn, Braunschweig, 1846. Cited by: Beach, E. F. 1948 Proteins in Nutrition (Historical), chapter 1 of: Proteins and Amino Acids in Nutrition, p. 13, ed., M. Sahyun. Reinhold Publishing Corp., New York.

64. Voit, C. 1866 Ueber die Verschiedenheiten der Eiweisszersetzung beim Hungern. Z. Biol. 2: 307.

65. von Pettenkofer, M., and C. Voit 1866 Untersuchungen über den Stoffverbrauch des normalen Menschen. Z. Biol. 2: 459.

66. Fick, A., and J. Wislicenus 1903 Gesammelte Schriften von Adolf Fick ueber die Entstehung der Muskelkraft. Physiologische Schriften, vol. 2, Würzburg. Cited by: Beach, E. F. 1948 Proteins in Nutrition (Historical), chapt. 1 of Proteins and Amino Acids in Nutrition, p. 24, ed., M. Sahyun. Reinhold Publishing Corp., New York.

67. North, W. 1883 The influence of bodily labour upon the discharge of nitrogen. Proc. Roy. Soc. (London) 36: 11.

68. Shaffer, P. A. 1908 Diminished muscular activity and protein metabolism. Amer. J. Physiol. 22: 445.

69. Cathcart, E. P. 1925 The influence of muscle work on protein metabolism. Physiol. Rev. 5: 225.

70. Cathcart, E. P., and W. A. Burnett 1926 The influence of muscle work on metabolism in varying conditions of diet. Proc. Roy. Soc. (London) B. 99: 405.

71. Garry, R. C. 1927 The static effort and excretion of uric acid. J. Physiol. 62: 364.

72. Wilson, H. E. C. 1932 The influence of muscular work on protein metabolism. J. Physiol. 75: 67.

73. Wilson, H. E. C. 1934 The effect of prolonged hard muscular work on sulphur and nitrogen metabolism. J. Physiol. 82: 184.

74. Nocker, J. 1951 Eiweiss-Stoffwechsel und Muskelarbeit. Deut. Z. Verdau. Stoffwechselkr. 11: 69. Cited in: Nutr. Abstr. Rev. 21: 393, 1951–52.

75. Cuthbertson, D. P., J. L. McGirr and H. N. Munro 1937 A study of the effect of overfeeding on the protein metabolism of man. 4. The effect of muscular work at different levels of energy intake, with particular reference to the timing of the work in relation to the taking of food. Biochem. J. 31: 2293.

76. Yoshimura, H. 1961 Adult protein requirements. Federation Proc. 20: 103.

77. Gontzea, I., P. Sutzesco and S. Dumitrache 1962 Influence de l'adaptation à l'effort sur le bilan azoté chez l'homme. Arch. Sci. Physiol. 16: 127.

78. Pitts, G. C., F. C. Consolazio and R. E. Johnson 1944 Dietary protein and physical fitness in temperate and hot environments. J. Nutr. 27: 497.

79. Darling, R. C., R. E. Johnson, G. C. Pitts, F. C. Consolazio and P. F. Robinson (with A. Kibler and M. Bartlett) 1944 Effects of variations in dietary protein on the physical well being of men doing manual work. J. Nutr. 28: 273.

80. Lehmann, G., and H. F. Michaelis 1948 Der Eiweissbedarf des Schwerarbeiters. 11. Messungen der Leistungsfähigkeit an Arbeitergruppen. Biochemische Z. 319: 247.

81. Kraut, H., and E. A. Müller 1950 Muskelkräfte und Eiweissration. Biochemische Z. 320: 302.

82. Cuthbertson, D. P. 1929 The influence of prolonged muscular rest on metabolism. Biochem. J. 23: 1328.

83. Keys, A. 1944 Effect of bed rest on nitrogen balance of normal individuals. Conference on Metabolic Aspects of Convalescence Including Bone and Wound Healing. Transactions of The Seventh Meeting. Josiah Macy, Jr. Foundation, Chicago, Ill., p. 90.

84. Deitrick, J. E., G. D. Whedon and E. Shorr (with V. Toscani and V. B. Davis) 1948 Effects of immobilization upon various metabolic and physiologic functions of normal men. Amer. J. Med. 4: 3.

85. Schønheyder, F., N. S. C. Heilskov and K. Olesen 1954 Isotopic studies on the mechanism of negative balance produced by immobilization. Scand. J. Clin. Lab. Invest. 6: 178.

86. Lynch, T. N., R. L. Jensen and P. M. Stevens 1967 Metabolic effects of prolonged bed rest: their modification by simulated altitude. Aerosp. Med. 38: 10.

87. Scrimshaw, N. S. 1959 Protein malnutrition and infection. Federation Proc. 18: 1207.

88. Scrimshaw, N. S. 1964 Ecological factors in nutritional disease. Amer. J. Clin. Nutr. 14: 112.

89. Scrimshaw, N. S., C. E. Taylor and J. E. Gordon 1968 Interactions of nutrition and infection. WHO Monograph Series No. 57. World Health Organization. Geneva, Switzerland.

90. Scrimshaw, N. S., M. A. Guzmán, J. J. Kevany, W. Ascoli, H. A. Bruch and J. E. Gordon 1967 Nutrition and infection field study in Guatemalan villages, 1959–1964. 2. Field reconnaissance, administrative and technical; study area; population characteristics; and organization for field activities. Arch. Environ. Health 14: 787.

91. Scrimshaw, N. S., W. Ascoli, J. J. Kevany, M. Flores, S. J. Iscaza and J. E. Gordon 1967 Nutrition and infection field study in Guatemalan villages 1959–1964. 3. Field procedure, collection of data and methods of measurement. Arch. Environ. Health 15: 6.

92. Ascoli, W., M. A. Guzmán, N. S. Scrimshaw and J. E. Gordon 1967 Nutrition and infection field study in Guatemalan villages 1959–1964. 4. Deaths of infants and preschool children. Arch. Environ. Health 15: 439.

93. Scrimshaw, N. S., M. A. Guzmán, M. Flores and J. E. Gordon 1968 Nutrition and infection field study in Guatemalan villages 1959–1964. 5. Disease incidence among preschool children under natural village conditions, with improved diet, and with medical and Public Health services. Arch. Environ. Health 16: 223.

94. Gordon, J. E., W. Ascoli, L. J. Mata, M. A. Guzmán and N. S. Scrimshaw 1968 Nutrition and infection field study in Guatemalan villages 1959–1964. 6. Acute diarrheal disease and nutritional disorders in general disease incidence. Arch. Environ. Health 16: 424.

95. Guzmán, M., N. S. Scrimshaw, H. A. Bruch and J. E. Gordon 1968 Nutrition and infection field study in Guatemalan villages 1959–1964. 7. Physical growth and development of preschool children. Arch. Environ. Health 17: 107.

96. Wohl, M. G., J. G. Reinhold and S. B. Rose 1949 Antibody response in patients with hypoproteinemia. Arch. Int. Med. 83: 402.

97. Bieler, M. M., E. E. Ecker and T. D. Spies 1947 Serum proteins in hypoproteinemia due to nutritional deficiency. J. Lab. Clin. Med. 32: 130.

98. Balch, H. H. 1950 Relation of nutritional deficiency in man to antibody production. J. Immunol. 64: 397.

99. Larson, D. L., and L. J. Tomlinson 1952 Quantitative antibody studies in man. II. The relation of the level of serum proteins to antibody production. J. Lab. Clin. Med. 39: 129.

100. Balch, H. H., and M. T. Spencer 1954 Phagocytosis by human leucocytes. II. Relation of nutritional deficiency in man to phagocytosis. J. Clin. Invest. 33: 1321.

101. Kahn, E., H. Stein and A. Zoutendyk 1957 Isohemagglutinins and immunity in malnutrition. Amer. J. Clin. Nutr. 5: 70.

102. Pretorius, P. J., and L. S. deVilliers 1962 Antibody response in children with protein malnutrition. Amer. J. Clin. Nutr. 10: 379.

103. Dancis, J., J. J. Osborn and J. F. Julia 1953 Studies of the immunology of the newborn infant. V. Effect of dietary protein on antibody production. Pediatrics 12: 395.

104. Wilson, D., R. Bressani and N. S. Scrimshaw 1961 Infection and nutritional status. I. The effect of chicken pox on nitrogen metabolism in children. Amer. J. Clin. Nutr. 9: 154.

105. Gandra, Y. R., and N. S. Scrimshaw 1961 Infection and nutritional status. II. Effect of mild virus infection induced by 17-D yellow fever vaccine on nitrogen metabolism in children. Amer. J. Clin. Nutr. 9: 159.

106. Moore, F. D. 1959 Metabolic Care of the Surgical Patient, chapt. 2, Convalescence in the healthy: Closed soft-tissue trauma of moderate severity. W. B. Saunders Co., Philadelphia, p. 25.

107. Peters, J. P. 1948 Effect of injury and disease on nitrogen metabolism. Amer. J. Med. 5: 100.

108. Cuthbertson, D. P. 1930 The disturbance of metabolism produced by bony and nonbony injury with notes on certain abnormal conditions of bone. Biochem. J. 24: 1244.

109. MacBeth, W. A. A. G., and G. R. Pope 1968 The effect of abdominal operation upon protein excretion in man. Lancet 1: 215.

110. Mašek, J. 1957 K vopsosu o potrebnosti čeloveka v belke. Vop. Pitan. 16 (2): 10. Cited in: Nutr. Abstr. Rev. 27: 1200, 1957.

111. Riegel, C., C. E. Koop, J. Drew, L. W. Stevens and J. E. Rhoads 1947 The nutritional requirements for nitrogen balance in surgical patients during the early post operative period. J. Clin. Invest. 26: 18.

112. Werner, S. C., D. V. Habif, H. T. Randall and J. S. Lockwood 1949 Postoperative nitrogen loss. A comparison of the effects of trauma and of caloric adjustment. Ann. Surg. 130: 688.

113. Abbott, W. E., H. Krieger and S. Levey 1958 Postoperative metabolic changes in relation to nutritional regimen. Lancet 1: 704.

114. Munro, H. N., and M. I. Chalmers 1945 Fracture metabolism at different levels of protein. Brit. J. Exp. Pathol. 26: 396.

115. Ingle, D. J., E. O. Ward and M. H. Kuizenga 1947 The relationship of the adrenal glands to changes in urinary non-protein nitrogen following multiple fractures in the force-fed rat. Amer. J. Physiol. 149: 510.

116. Taylor, F. H. L., S. M. Levenson, C. S. Davidson, N. C. Browder and C. C. Lund 1943 Problems of protein nutrition in burned patients. Ann. Surg. 118: 215.

117. Taylor, F. H. L. 1944 The nitrogen requirement of patients with thermal burns. J. Ind. Hyg. Toxicol. 26: 152.

118. Soroff, H. S., E. Pearson and C. P. Artz 1961 An estimation of the nitrogen requirements for equilibrium in burned patients. Surg. Gynecol. Obstet. 112: 159.

119. Troell, L., and A. Wretlind 1961 Protein and calorie requirements in burns. Acta Chir. Scand. 122: 15.

120. Scrimshaw, N. S., J. P. Habicht, M. L. Piché, B. Cholakos and G. Arroyave 1966 Protein metabolism of young men during uni-

versity examinations. Amer. J. Clin. Nutr. *18:* 321.

121. Scrimshaw, N. S., J. P. Habicht and J. Pellet 1966 Effects of sleep deprivation and reversal of diurnal activity on protein metabolism of young men. Amer. J. Clin. Nutr. *19:* 313.

122. Kark, R. M., R. R. M. Croome, J. Cawthorpe, D. M. Bell, A. Bryans, R. J. MacBeth, R. E. Johnson, F. C. Consolazio, J. L. Poulin, F. H. L. Taylor and R. C. Cogswell 1948 Observations on a mobile Arctic force. The health, physical fitness and nutrition of exercise "Musk Ox," February–May 1945. Appl. Physiol. *1:* 73.

123. Pedoya, C., and P. Gennesseaux 1958 L'aspect actual du problème alimentaire en climat très froid. Ann. Nutr. Aliment. *12:* 61. Cited in: Nutr. Abstr. Rev. *30:* 186, 1960.

124. Barja, I., M. E. Callejas, N. Contreras, I. Ugalde, I. Velasques, E. Vellegrán and G. Donoso 1962 Estudio sobre nutricion, alimentacion y aprovisionamiento de una base antartica. Nutr. Bromatol. Toxicol. *1:* 245.

125. Consolazio, C. F. 1963 The energy requirements of men living under extreme environmental conditions. World Rev. Nutr. Diet. *4:* 53.

126. Gray, E. LeB., C. F. Consolazio and R. M. Kark 1951 Nutritional requirements for men at work in cold, temperate and hot environments. J. Appl. Physiol. *4:* 270.

127. Belding, H. S., H. D. Russell, R. C. Darling and G. E. Folk 1945 The effect of moisture on clothing requirements in cold weather. Rep. No. 37 from the Harvard University Fatigue Laboratory to the Quartermaster General, Washington, D. C., p. 141.

128. Issekutz, B., Jr., K. Rodahl and N. C. Birkhead 1962 Effect of severe cold stress on the nitrogen balance of men under different dietary conditions. J. Nutr. *78:* 189.

129. Gontzea, J., P. Schutzescu and S. Dumitrache 1960 Untersuchungen über den Proteinbedarf des Menschen bei körperlicher Arbeit in heisser Umgebung. Int. Z. Angew. Physiol. Arbeitsphysiol. *18:* 248.

130. Goncja Ja., P. Sucesku and S. Dumitraki 1960 Vlijanie vysokoj témperatury okružajušČy sredy na potrebnost Čeloveka v belke (po dannym asotistogo balanso) v uslovijah myseČnoj nagruski. Vop. Pitan. *19* (6): 12. Cited in: Nutr. Abstr. Rev. *31:* 579, 1961.

131. Consolazio, C. F., L. O. Matoush, H. L. Johnson and T. A. Daws 1968 Protein and water balances of young adults during prolonged exposure to high altitudes (4,300 meters). Amer. J. Clin. Nutr. *21:* 154.

132. Surks, M. I. 1966 Metabolism of human serum albumin in man during acute exposure to high altitude (14,100 ft.). J. Clin. Invest. *45:* 1442.

133. Tadokoro, Y. 1963 Nutrition under abnormal environment. 1. Influence of vibration upon protein metabolism. Jap. J. Nutr. *21:* 148. Cited in: Nutr. Abstr. Rev. *35:* 705, 1965.

134. Tadokoro, Y. 1964 Nutrition under abnormal environment. 4. Influence of vibration and cold upon protein metabolism. Jap. J. Nutr. *22:* 5. Cited in: Nutr. Abstr. Rev. *35:* 705, 1965.

135. Holt, L. E., Jr., E. Halac and C. N. Kajdi 1962 The concept of protein stores and its implications in the diet. J. Amer. Med. Ass. *181:* 699.

136. Thomas, K. 1910 Über das physiologische Stickstoffminimum. Arch. Physiol. Suppl. 249.

137. Wilson, H. E. C. 1931 Studies on the physiology of protein retention. J. Physiol. *72:* 327.

138. Addis, T., L. J. Poo and W. Lew 1936 The quantities of protein lost by the various organs and tissues of the body during a fast. J. Biol. Chem. *115:* 111.

139. Addis, T., D. D. Lee, W. Lew and L. J. Poo 1940 The protein content of the organs and tissues at different levels of protein consumption. J. Nutr. *19:* 199.

140. Basak, M. N. 1958 The theory of endogenous metabolism in mammals. Indian J. Med. Res. *46:* 307.

141. Cuthbertson, D. P., A. McCutcheon and H. N. Munro 1937 A study of the effect of overfeeding on the protein metabolism of man. I. The effect of superimposing raw and boiled milks on a diet adequate for maintenance. II. The superimposition, on a diet adequate for maintenance, of beef (or soya flour) plus lactose plus butter, equivalent in carbohydrate and fat content to a litre of milk. J. Biochem. *31:* 681.

142. Fisher, H., M. K. Brush, P. Griminger and E. R. Sostman 1967 Nitrogen retention in adult man: a possible factor in protein requirements. Amer. J. Clin. Nutr. *20:* 927.

143. Munro, H. N. 1964 General aspects of the regulation of protein metabolism by diet and by hormones. In: Mammalian Protein Metabolism, vol. 1, eds., H. N. Munro and J. B. Allison. Academic Press, New York, p. 381.

144. Young, V. R., M. A. Hussein and N. S. Scrimshaw 1968 Estimate of loss of labile body nitrogen during acute protein deprivation in young adults. Nature *218:* 568.

145. Chan, H. 1968 Adaptation of urinary nitrogen excretion in infants to changes in protein intake. Brit. J. Nutr. *22:* 315.

146. Waterlow, J. C. 1968 Observations on the mechanism of adaptation to low protein intakes. Lancet *2:* 1091.

147. Grindley, H. S. 1912 Studies in nutrition. An investigation of the influence of saltpeter on the nutrition and health of man with reference to its occurrence in cured meats. In: The Experimental Data of the Biochemical Investigations, vol. 4. University of Illinois, 494 pp. Cited by: Bricker, M., H. H. Mitchell and G. M. Kinsman 1945 The protein requirements of adult human subjects in terms of the protein contained in individual food combinations. J. Nutr. *30:* 269.

148. Bricker, M. L., R. F. Shively, J. M. Smith, H. H. Mitchell and T. S. Hamilton 1949 The protein requirements of college women on high cereal diets with observations on the adequacy of short balance periods. J. Nutr. 37: 163.

149. Osborne, T. B., and L. B. Mendel 1914 Amino-acids in nutrition and growth. J. Biol. Chem. 17: 325.

150. Rose, W. C. 1938 The nutritive significance of amino acids. Physiol. Rev. 18: 109.

151. Rose, W. C., and R. L. Wixom 1955 The amino acid requirements of man. XVI. The role of the nitrogen intake. J. Biol. Chem. 217: 997.

152. Hoffman, W. S., and G. C. McNeil 1951 Nitrogen requirement of normal men on a diet of protein hydrolysate enriched with the limiting essential amino acids. J. Nutr. 44: 123.

153. Swendseid, M. E., R. J. Feeley, C. L. Harris and S. G. Tuttle 1959 Egg protein as a source of the essential amino acids. Requirement for nitrogen balance in young adults studied at two levels of nitrogen intake. J. Nutr. 68: 203.

154. Kofrányi, E., and H. Müller-Wecker 1961 Zur Bestimmung der biologischen Wertigkeit von Nahrungsproteinen. V. Der Einfluss des nichtessentiellen Stickstoffs auf die biologische Wertigkeit von Proteinen und die Wertigkeit von Kartoffelproteinen. Hoppe-Seyler's Z. Physiol. Chem. 325: 60.

155. Snyderman, S. E., L. E. Holt, Jr., J. Dancis, E. Roitman, A. Boyer and M. E. Balis 1962 "Unessential" nitrogen: a limiting factor for human growth. J. Nutr. 78: 57.

156. Scrimshaw, N. S., V. R. Young, R. Schwartz, M. L. Piche and J. B. Das 1966 Minimum dietary essential amino acid-to-total nitrogen ratio for whole egg protein fed to young men. J. Nutr. 89: 9.

157. Scrimshaw, N. S., V. R. Young, P. C. Huang, O. Thanangkul and B. V. Cholakos 1969 Partial dietary replacement of milk protein by nonspecific nitrogen in young men. J. Nutr. 98: 9.

158. Kies, C., E. Williams and H. M. Fox 1965 Determination of first limiting nitrogenous factor in corn protein for nitrogen retention in human adults. J. Nutr. 86: 350.

159. Huang, P. C., V. R. Young, B. Cholakos and N. S. Scrimshaw 1966 Determination of the minimum dietary essential amino acid-to-total nitrogen ratio for beef protein fed to young men. J. Nutr. 90: 416.

160. Kofrányi, E., and F. Jekat 1964 Zur Bestimmung der biologischen Wertigkeit von Nahrungsproteinen. IX. Der Ersatz von hochwertigem Eiweiss durch nichtessentiellen Stickstoff. Hoppe-Seyler's Z. Physiol. Chem. 338: 154.

161. Kofrányi, E., and F. Jekat 1964 Zur Bestimmung der biologischen Wertigkeit von Nahrungsproteinen. X. Vergleich der Bausteinanalysen mit dem Minimalbedarf gemischter Proteine für Menschen. Hoppe-Seyler's Z. Physiol. Chem. 338: 159.

162. Mitchell, H. H., and R. J. Block 1946 Some relationships between the amino acid contents of proteins and their nutritive values for the rat. J. Biol. Chem. 163: 599.

163. Oser, B. L. 1951 Method for integrating essential amino acid content in the nutritional evaluation of protein. J. Amer. Diet. Ass. 27: 396.

164. Lintzel, W., and W. Bertram 1938 Experimentelle Studien zur Theorie des Eiweissstoffwechsels. 1. Über die Verwertung von Glykokol beim Menschen. Biochemische Z. 297: 270.

165. Swendseid, M. E., C. L. Harris and S. G. Tuttle 1960 The effect of sources of nonessential nitrogen on nitrogen balance in young adults. J. Nutr. 71: 105.

166. Tuttle, S. G., S. H. Bassett, W. H. Griffith, D. B. Mulcare and M. E. Swendseid 1965 Further observations on the amino acid requirements of older men. I. Effects of nonessential nitrogen supplements fed with different amounts of essential amino acids. Amer. J. Clin. Nutr. 16: 225.

167. Rose, W. C., M. J. Coon and G. F. Lambert 1954 The amino acid requirements of man. VI. The role of the calorie intake. J. Biol. Chem. 210: 331.

168. Watts, J. H., B. Tolbert and W. L. Ruff 1964 Nitrogen balances for young adult males fed two sources of nonessential nitrogen at two levels of total nitrogen intake. Metabolism 13: 172.

169. Kies, C. V., and H. M. Linkswiler 1965 Effect on nitrogen retention of men of altering the intake of essential amino acids with total nitrogen held constant. J. Nutr. 85: 139.

170. Tuttle, S. G., M. E. Swendseid, D. Mulcare, W. H. Griffith and S. H. Bassett 1959 Essential amino acid requirements of older men in relation to total nitrogen intake. Metabolism 8: 61.

171. Clark, H. E., M. A. Kenney, A. F. Goodwin, K. Goyal and E. T. Mertz 1963 Effect of certain factors on nitrogen retention and lysine requirements of adult human subjects. IV. Total nitrogen intake. J. Nutr. 81: 223.

172. Clark, H. E., K. Fugate and P. E. Allen 1967 The effect of four multiples of a basic mixture of essential amino acids on nitrogen retention of adult human subjects. Amer. J. Clin. Nutr. 20: 233.

173. Salmon, W. D. 1954 The tryptophan requirement of the rat as affected by niacin and level of dietary nitrogen. Arch. Biochem. 51: 30. Cited by: Elvehjem, C. A., and A. E. Harper 1955 Importance of amino acid balance in nutrition. J. Amer. Med. Ass. 158: 655.

174. Harper, A. E., D. A. Benton, M. E. Winje and C. A. Elvehjem 1954 Antilipotropic effect of methionine in rats fed threonine-deficient diets containing choline. J. Biol. Chem. 209: 159. Cited by: Elvehjem, C. A., and A. E. Harper 1955 Importance of

amino acid balance in nutrition. J. Amer. Med. Ass. *158:* 655.

175. Sure, B. 1954 Relative nutritive values of protein in whole wheat and whole rye and effect of amino acid supplements. J. Agr. Food Chem. *2:* 1108. Cited by: Elvehjem, C. A., and A. E. Harper 1955 Importance of amino acid balance in nutrition. J. Amer. Med. Ass. *158:* 665.

176. Hundley, J. M., H. R. Sandstead, A. G. Sampson and G. D. Whedon 1957 Lysine, threonine, and other amino acids as supplements to rice diets in man: amino acid imbalance. Amer. J. Clin. Nutr. *5:* 316.

177. Truswell, A. S., and J. F. Brock 1961 Effects of amino acid supplements on the nutritive value of maize protein for human adults. Amer. J. Clin. Nutr. *9:* 715.

178. Clark, H. E., P. Myers, K. Goyal and J. Rinehart 1966 Influence of variable quantities of lysine, tryptophan and isoleucine on nitrogen retention of adult human subjects. Amer. J. Clin. Nutr. *18:* 91.

179. Clark, H. E., J. N. Boyd, S. M. Kolski and B. Shannon 1968 Nitrogen retention of adults given variable quantities and proportions of lysine. Amer. J. Clin. Nutr. *21:* 217.

180. Food and Agriculture Organization 1957 Protein Requirements. Report of the FAO Committee. FAO Nutrition Studies no. 16, Rome, Italy, Oct. 24–31, 1955.

181. Scrimshaw, N. S., R. Bressani, M. Béhar and F. Viteri 1958 Supplementation of cereal proteins with amino acids. I. Effect of amino acid supplementation of corn-masa at high levels of protein intake on the nitrogen retention of young children. J. Nutr. *66:* 485.

182. Bressani, R., N. S. Scrimshaw, M. Béhar and F. Viteri 1958 Supplementation of cereal proteins with amino acids. II. Effect of amino acid supplementation of corn-masa at intermediate levels of protein intake on the nitrogen retention of young children. J. Nutr. *66:* 501.

183. Bressani, R., D. L. Wilson, M. Béhar and N. S. Scrimshaw 1960 Supplementation of cereal proteins with amino acids. III. Effect of amino acid supplementation of wheat flour as measured by nitrogen retention of young children. J. Nutr. *70:* 176.

184. Bressani, R., D. Wilson, M. Béhar, M. Chung and N. S. Scrimshaw 1963 Supplementation of cereal proteins with amino acids. IV. Lysine supplementation of wheat flour fed to young children at different levels of protein intake in the presence and absence of other amino acids. J. Nutr. *79:* 333.

185. Bressani, R., D. Wilson, M. Chung, M. Béhar and N. S. Scrimshaw 1963 Supplementation of cereal proteins with amino acids. V. Effect of supplementing lime-treated corn with different levels of lysine, tryptophan, and isoleucine on the nitrogen retention of young children. J. Nutr. *80:* 80.

186. Fukui, T., H. Fukui and T. Sasaki 1960 Experiment of lysine supplementation in

school children feeding. Tokushima J. Exp. Med. *6:* 269.

187. Fukui, T., H. Fukui, T. Sasaki and T. Murakami 1961 Lysine supply to children of growing age. Tokushima J. Exp. Med. *8:* 1.

188. Snyderman, S. E., L. E. Holt, Jr., and A. Boyer 1960 A comparison of the pattern of human milk with the FAO pattern in human nutrition. J. Nutr. *72:* 404.

189. Kirk, M. C., N. Metheny and M. S. Reynolds 1962 Nitrogen balances of young women fed amino acids in the FAO reference pattern, the milk pattern, and the peanut pattern. J. Nutr. *77:* 448.

190. Watts, J. H., A. N. Mann, L. Bradley and D. J. Thompson 1964 Nitrogen balance of men over 65 fed the FAO and milk patterns of essential amino acids. J. Gerontol. *19:* 370.

191. Swendseid, M. E., J. H. Watts, C. L. Harris and S. G. Tuttle 1961 An evaluation of the FAO amino acid reference pattern in human nutrition. I. Studies with young men. J. Nutr. *75:* 295.

192. Swendseid, M. E., C. L. Harris and S. G. Tuttle 1962 An evaluation of the FAO amino acid reference pattern in human nutrition. II. Studies with young women. J. Nutr. *77:* 391.

193. Leverton, R. M., and D. Steel 1962 Nitrogen balances of young women fed the FAO reference pattern of amino acids and the oat pattern. J. Nutr. *78:* 10.

194. Watts, J. H., B. Tolbert and W. L. Ruff 1964 Nitrogen balances of young men fed selected amino acid patterns. I. FAO reference pattern, a modification of the FAO reference pattern and wheat flour pattern. Can. J. Biochem. *42:* 1437.

195. Swendseid, M. E., J. B. Hickson, J. Villalobos and S. G. Tuttle 1963 Nitrogen balance studies with subjects fed the essential amino acids in plasma pattern proportions. J. Nutr. *79:* 276.

196. Swaminathan, M. 1963 Amino acid and protein requirements of infants, children and adults. Indian J. Pediat. *30:* 189.

197. Swanson, W. W., and V. Iob 1939 The growth of fetus and infant as related to mineral intake during pregnancy. Amer. J. Obstet. Gynecol. *38:* 382.

198. Young, W. F., P. Poyner-Wall, H. C. Humphreys, E. Finch and I. Broadbent 1950 Protein requirements of infants. 3. The nutrition of premature infants. Arch. Dis. Childhood 25: 31.

199. Langstein, L., and A. Niemann 1910 Ein Beitrag zur Kenntnis der Stoffwechselvorgänge in den ersten vierzehn Lebenstagen normaler und frühgeborener Säuglinge. Jahrb. Kinderheilk. *71:* 604.

200. Rubner, M., and L. Langstein 1915 Energie- und Stoffwechsel zweier frühgeborener Säuglinge. Arch. Physiol. *39:* 39.

201. John, F. 1931 Über den Eiweissansatz bei Frühgeburten. Z. Kinderheilk. *51:* 794.

202. Gordon, H. H., S. Z. Levine, M. A. Wheatley and E. Marples 1937 Respiratory metabolism in infancy and in childhood. XX. The nitrogen metabolism in premature infants — comparative studies of human milk and cow's milk. Amer. J. Dis. Child. 54: 1030.

203. Omans, W. B., L. A. Barness, C. S. Rose and P. György 1961 Prolonged feeding studies in premature infants. J. Pediat. 59: 951.

204. Davidson, M., S. Z. Levine and C. H. Bauer 1967 Feeding studies in low-birth-weight infants. I. Relationships of dietary protein, fat, and electrolyte to rates of weight gain, clinical courses, and serum chemical concentrations. J. Pediat. 70: 695.

205. Plenert, W., B. Gassman and W. Heine 1965 Zur Frage des Eiweissbedarfs von Säuglingen. Ernährungsforschung 10: 611.

206. Snyderman, S. E., A. Boyer and L. E. Holt, Jr. 1961 Evaluation of protein foods in premature infants. N.A.S.–N.R.C. Publ. No. 843, Washington, D. C., p. 331.

207. Snyderman, S. E., A. Boyer, M. D. Kogut and L. E. Holt, Jr. 1969 The protein requirement of the premature infant. 1. The effect of protein intake on the retention of nitrogen. J. Pediat. 74: 872.

208. Nichols, M. M., and B. H. Danford 1966 Feeding premature infants: a comparison of effects on weight gain, blood, and urine of two formulas with varying protein and ash composition. Southern Med. J. 59: 1420.

209. Vest, M., A. Olafson and P. Schenker 1966 Eine neue Sojamilch als Nahrung für Frühgeborene und reife Säuglinge. Vergleich mit Frauenmilch und adaptierter Kuhmilch. Schweiz. Med. Wochenschr. 96: 762.

210. Kagan, B. M., J. H. Hess, E. Lundeen, K. Shafer, J. B. Parker and C. Stigall 1955 Feeding premature infants — a comparison of various milks. Pediatrics 15: 373.

211. Goldman, H. I., R. Freudenthal, B. Holland and S. Karelitz 1969 Clinical effects of two different levels of protein intake on low-birth-weight infants. J. Pediat. 74: 881.

212. Babson, S. G., and J. L. Bramhall 1969 Diet and growth in the premature infant. The effect of different dietary intakes of ash-electrolyte and protein on weight gain and linear growth. J. Pediat. 74: 890.

213. Cox, W. M., and L. J. Filer 1969 Protein intake for low-birth-weight infants. J. Pediat. 74: 1016.

214. Routh, C. H. F. 1876 Infant Feeding and its Influence on Life or the Causes and Prevention of Infant Mortality, ed. 3. J. and A. Churchill, London.

215. Meigs, A. V. 1896 Feeding in Early Infancy. W. B. Saunders Co., Philadelphia, 15 pp.

216. Holt, L. E., and H. L. Fales 1921 The food requirements of children. II. Protein requirements. Amer. J. Dis. Child. 22: 371.

217. Holt, L. E., Jr. 1959 The protein requirement of infants. J. Pediat. 54: 496.

218. Jeans, P. C., and G. Stearns 1933 Growth and retentions of calcium, phosphorus, and nitrogen of infants fed evaporated milk. Amer. J. Dis. Child. 46: 69.

219. Jeans, P. C., G. Stearns, J. B. McKinley, E. A. Goff and D. Stinger 1936 Factors possibly influencing the retention of calcium, phosphorus and nitrogen by infants given whole milk feedings. 1. The curding agent. J. Pediat. 8: 403.

220. Widdowson, E. M. 1965 Absorption and excretion of fat, nitrogen, and minerals from "filled" milks by babies one week old. Lancet 2: 1099.

221. Barness, L. A., D. Baker, P. Guilbert, F. E. Torres and P. György 1957 Nitrogen metabolism of infants fed human and cow's milk. J. Pediat. 51: 29.

222. Kaye, R., R. H. Caughey and W. W. McCrory 1954 Nitrogen balances on low nitrogen intakes in infants and the effects of gelatin supplementation with and without vitamin B_{12} and aureomycin. Pediatrics 14: 305.

223. Su, T. F., and C. J. Liang 1940 Growth and development of Chinese infants of Honan province. 1. Body weight, standing height and sitting height during the first year of life. Chinese Med. J. 58: 104.

224. Sénécal, J. 1959 Alimentation de l'enfant dans les pays tropicaux et subtropicaux. Courrier 9: 1.

225. Fomon, S. J. 1960 Comparative study of adequacy of protein from human milk and cow's milk in promoting nitrogen retention by normal full-term infants. Pediatrics 26: 51.

226. Fomon, S. J., and C. D. May 1958 Metabolic studies of normal full-term infants fed a prepared formula providing intermediate amounts of protein. Pediatrics 22: 1134.

227. Fomon, S. J. 1961 Nitrogen balance studies with normal full-term infants receiving high intakes of protein. Comparisons with previous studies employing lower intakes of protein. Pediatrics 28: 347.

228. Widdowson, E. M., R. A. McCance and C. M. Spray 1951 The chemical composition of the human body. Clin. Sci. 10: 113.

229. Wallace, W. M. 1959 Nitrogen content of the body and its relation to retention and loss of nitrogen. Federation Proc. 18: 1125.

230. Rominger, E., and H. Meyer 1931 Untersuchungen des Stickstoffumsatzes beim gesunden Säugling. Z. Kinderheilk. 50: 509.

231. Holt, L. E., Jr., and S. E. Snyderman 1965 Protein and amino acid requirements of infants and children. Nutr. Abstr. Rev. 35: 1.

232. Rueda-Williamson, R., and H. E. Rose 1962 Growth and nutrition of infants. The influence of diet and other factors on growth. Pediatrics 30: 639.

233. Horecny, J. 1956 Príspevok k metabolismu bielkovin u eutrofických kojencov. Csl. Gastroenterol. a vyz. 10: 309.

234. Goldman, T. H. 1942 Feeding the newborn high protein, low fat, low carbohydrate mixtures: a comparative, clinical two year study. Arch. Pediat. 59: 756.

235. Slater, J. E. 1961 Retentions of nitrogen and minerals by babies 1 week old. Brit. J. Nutr. 15: 83.

236. Johnston, J. A., M. J. Sweeney, R. C. Brown, J. W. Maroney and G. Manson 1961 The protein allowance in infancy and childhood. J. Pediat. 59: 47.

237. Ross, M. R. 1959 Protein, calories and life expectancy. Federation Proc. 18: 1190.

238. McCay, C. M. 1947 Effect of restricted feeding upon aging and chronic diseases in rats and dogs. Amer. J. Pub. Health 37: 521.

239. Snyderman, S. E., L. E. Holt, Jr., P. M. Norton, E. Roitman and S. V. Phansalkar 1968 The plasma aminogram. 1. Influence of the level of protein intake and a comparison of whole protein and amino acid diets. Pediat. Res. 2: 131.

240. Beal, V. A. 1953 Nutritional intake of children. 1. Calories, carbohydrate, fat and protein. J. Nutr. 50: 223.

241. Chan, H., and J. C. Waterlow 1966 The protein requirements of infants at the age of about 1 year. Brit. J. Nutr. 20: 775.

242. Food and Agriculture Organization 1965 Protein Requirements. Report of a Joint FAO/WHO Expert Group. FAO Nutrition Meetings Report Series no. 37, Rome, Italy.

243. Roubstein, L., L. Birger and R. Freid 1936 Influence de différentes rations albuminoïdes sur la croissance et le développement des enfants de 1½ à 2 années et demie. Bull. Biol. Med. Exp. U.R.S.S. 1: 235.

244. Moltschanova, O. P., I. M. Ivenskaja, E. R. Ryskina and J. K. Polteva 1936 Protein optimum and ratio of protein, fat and carbohydrate in the diet of children from 1½ to 3 years. Vop. Pitan. 5 (4): 103. Cited in: Nutr. Abstr. Rev. 6: 710, 1936–37.

245. Gillett, L. H. 1917 A survey of evidence regarding food allowances for healthy children. Pub. 115, Bureau of Food Supply. The New York Assoc. for Improving the Condition of the Poor. New York, 24 pp.

246. Hasse, H. 1882 Untersuchungen über die Ernährung von Kindern im Alter von 2 bis 11 Jahren. Z. Biol. 18: 553.

247. Hecht 1913 Rearing an imperial race. Cited by: Gillett, L. H. A survey of evidence regarding food allowance for healthy children. Pub. 115, Bureau of Food Supply. The New York Assoc. for Improving the Condition of the Poor. New York, 24 pp.

248. Herbst, O. 1898 Beiträge zur Kenntnis normaler Nahrungsmengen bei Kindern. Jahrb. Kinderheilk. 46: 245.

249. Sundstrom, S. 1907 Über die Ernährung bei freigewählter Kost. Skand. Arch. Physiol. 19: 78.

250. Bendix, B. 1894 Der Einfluss der Massage auf den Stoffwechsel des gesunden Menschen. Z. Klin. Med. 25: 301.

251. Camerer, W. 1878 Der Stoffwechsel eines Kindes im ersten Lebensjahre. Z. Biol. 14: 383.

252. Müller, E. 1907 Stoffwechselversuche an 32 Kindern im 3. bis 6. Lebensjahre mit besonderer Berücksichtigung des Kraft-

253. Siegert, F. 1908 Der Eiweissbedarf des Kindes. Arch. Exp. Pathol. Pharmacol. (Suppl. Band) 489.

254. Tunnicliffe, F. W. 1906 Concerning the behaviour in the body of certain organic and inorganic phosphorus compounds. Arch. Int. Pharmacodyn. Thér. 16: 207. Cited by: Gillett, L. H. 1917 A survey of evidence regarding food allowances for healthy children. Pub. 115 Bureau of Food Supply. The New York Assoc. for Improving the Condition of the Poor. New York, 24 pp.

255. Bartlett, W. M. 1926 Protein requirement as determined in diabetic children. Amer. J. Dis. Child. 32: 641.

256. Wang, C. C., J. E. Hawks and M. Kaucher 1928 Metabolism of undernourished children. VII. Effect of high and low protein diets on the nitrogen and caloric balance of undernourished children. Amer. J. Dis. Child. 36: 1161.

257. Kung, L.-C., and W.-Y. Fang 1935 A preliminary report on the nitrogen metabolism of preschool children. Chin. J. Physiol. 9: 375.

258. Parsons, J. P. 1930 Nitrogen metabolism of children with special reference to the protein requirements of children of preschool age. Amer. J. Dis. Child. 39: 1221.

259. Daniels, A. L., M. K. Hutton, E. M. Knott, O. E. Wright, G. J. Everson and F. Scoular 1935 A study of the protein needs of preschool children. J. Nutr. 9: 91.

260. Daniels, A. L. (with G. J. Everson, M. F. Deardorff, O. E. Wright and F. I. Scoular) 1941 Relation of calcium, phosphorus, and nitrogen retention to growth and osseous development. A long time study of three preschool boys. Amer. J. Dis. Child. 62: 279.

261. Porter, T. 1939 Metabolism of normal preschool children. 3. Variations in nitrogen storage on constant diets. J. Amer. Diet. Ass. 15: 427.

262. Hawks, J. E., M. M. Bray and M. Dye 1938 The influence of diet on the nitrogen balances of pre-school children. J. Nutr. 15: 125.

263. Hawks, J. E., J. M. Voorhees, M. M. Bray and M. Dye 1940 The influence of the nitrogen content of the diet on the calorie balance of pre-school children. J. Nutr. 19: 77.

264. Hawks, J. E., and G. Everson 1941 Influence of diet on the uric acid excretion of young children. Amer. J. Dis. Child. 66: 955.

265. Hawks, J. E., M. M. Bray, M. O. Wilde and M. Dye (with V. H. Wiltgren and A. Kirkpatrick) 1942 The interrelationship of calcium, phosphorus and nitrogen in the metabolism of pre-school children. J. Nutr. 24: 283.

266. Jaffa, M. E. 1899–1901 Nutrition investigations among fruitarians and Chinese at the California Agricultural Experiment Sta-

tion. U. S. Dept. Agri. Off. Exp. Sta. Bull. no. 107, p. 1.

267. Bryant, L. S. 1911 Recent experimental work on children's food needs. Diet. Hyg. Gaz. 27: 337.

268. Rubner, M. 1901 Der Energiewert der Kost des Menschen. Z. Biol. 24: 261.

269. Camerer, W. 1884 Der Stoffwechsel von fünf Kindern im Alter von 5 bis 15 Jahren. Z. Biol. 20: 566.

270. Camerer, W. 1896 Der Nahrungsbedarf von Kindern verschiedenen Lebensalters. Z. Biol. 33: 320.

271. Herbst, O. 1912 Beiträge zur Physiologie des Stoffwechsels im Knabenalter mit besonderer Berücksichtigung einiger Mineralstoffe. Jahrb. Kinderheilk. 76: 40.

272. Koehne, M., and E. Morrell 1934 Food requirements of girls from six to thirteen years of age. Amer. J. Dis. Child. 47: 548.

273. Ruotsalainen, A. 1921 Zur Kenntnis des Eiweissansatzes beim Kinde. Skand. Arch. Physiol. 41: 33.

274. Bjeloussoff, W. A. 1935 Protein optimum in the diet of school children. 1. Nitrogen retention at different levels of protein (chiefly plant) intake. Vop. Pitan. 4(4): 76 (Russian) Cited in: Nutr. Abstr. Rev. 5: 742, 1935–36.

275. Bronner, V. V., V. V. Kočegina and G. V. Zubrilina 1961 K voprosu o potrebnosti detej v belke i vitaminah C i B₂ v ustovijah školy-internata. Pediatrija No. 6: 21. Cited in: Nutr. Abstr. Rev. 32: 536, 1962.

276. Maroney, J. W., and J. A. Johnston 1937 Caloric and protein requirements and basal metabolism of children from four to fourteen years old. Amer. J. Dis. Child. 54: 29.

277. Stearns, G., K. L. Newman, J. B. McKinley and P. C. Jeans 1958 The protein requirement of children from one to ten years of age. Ann. N. Y. Acad. Sci. 69: 857.

278. Macy, I. G. 1942 Nutrition and Chemical Growth in Childhood, vol. 1, Evaluation. Charles C Thomas, Publisher, Springfield, Ill.

279. Technical Committee, Southern Regional Nutrition Research Project 1959 Metabolic patterns in preadolescent children. 1. Description of metabolic studies. Southern Coop. Series Bull. no. 64. 90 pp. (Available from Virginia Agr. Exp. Sta., Blacksburg, Va.)

280. Widdowson, E. M., and R. A. McCance 1954 Studies on the nutritive value of bread and on the effect of variations in the extractive rate of flour on the growth of undernourished children. Medical Research Council Special Report Series No. 287, 137 pp. H. M. Stationery Office, London.

281. James, W. H. 1960 Symposium on metabolic patterns in preadolescent children. Nitrogen balance. Federation Proc. 19: 1009.

282. Moyer, E. Z., and M. I. Irwin 1967 Basic data on metabolic patterns in 7- to 10-year-old girls in selected southern states. Home Economics Research Report no. 33. Agricul-

tural Research Service, U. S. Department of Agriculture, Washington, D. C.

283. Wait, B., and L. J. Roberts 1933 Studies in the food requirement of adolescent girls. 3. The protein intake of well-nourished girls 10 to 16 years of age. J. Amer. Diet. Ass. 8: 403.

284. Camerer, W. 1892 Stoffwechselversuche an meinen Kindern. Z. Biol. 11: 398.

285. Herbst, O. 1913 Calcium und Phosphor beim Wachstum am Ende der Kindheit. Z. Kinderheilk. 7: 161.

286. Hultgren, E. O. 1894 Nitrogen metabolism experiments. Pflügers Arch. 60: 205. Cited by: Gillett, L. H. 1917 A survey of evidence regarding food allowances for healthy children. Pub. 115, Bureau of Food Supply. The New York Assoc. for Improving the Condition of the Poor. New York, 24 pp.

287. Widdowson, E. M. 1947 A study of individual children's diets. Medical Research Council Special Report Series no. 257, 196 pp. H. M. Stationery Office, London.

288. Burke, B. S., R. R. Reed, A. S. van den Berg and H. C. Stuart 1959 Caloric and protein intakes of children between 1 and 18 years of age. Pediatrics 24: 922.

289. Eppright, E. S., V. D. Sidwell and P. P. Swanson 1954 Nutritive value of the diets of Iowa school children. J. Nutr. 54: 371.

290. Wang, C. C., C. Hogden and M. Wing 1936 Metabolism of adolescent girls. 2. Fat and protein metabolism. Amer. J. Dis. Child. 51: 1083.

291. Ward, M., I. Hawley, R. U. Thomas and H. Metz 1950 Nutritional status of children. 10. Feeding practices in child-caring agencies: Communal feeding of adolescent boys. J. Amer. Diet. Ass. 26: 421.

292. Moltschanova, O. P., V. A. Poroikova and V. Kotschegina (with M. L. Schkral) 1935 Nitrogen exchange of school children at different protein levels. Vop. Pitan. 4(3):1 (in Russian with German summary).

293. Bronner, V. V. 1965 K voprosu o potrebnosti v piščévyn veščestuah v uslovijah školy-internata. Vop. Pitan. 24(1):42.

294. Lesné E., and C. Richet fils 1926 Azoturie et azotémie basales chez l'enfant de 4 a 14 ans. C. R. Soc. Biol. 95: 1090.

295. Johnston, J. A. 1958 Protein requirements of adolescents. Ann. N. Y. Acad. Sci. 69: 881.

296. Heald, F. P., and S. M. Hunt 1965 Caloric dependency in obese adolescents as affected by degree of maturation. J. Pediat. 66: 1035.

297. Macy, I. G., and H. A. Hunscher 1951 Calories — a limiting factor in the growth of children. J. Nutr. 45: 189.

298. Johnston, F. A., and D. Schlaphoff 1951 Nitrogen retained by six adolescent girls from two levels of intake. J. Nutr. 45: 463.

299. Hsu, P. C., and W. H. Adolph 1940 Nitrogen, calcium, and phosphorus balances of adolescent boys. Chin. J. Physiol. 15: 317.

300. Sakamoto, J. 1922 Labour and nutrition. IV. On the general metabolism of several Japanese workwomen. J. Biochem. 2: 73.

301. Zacharjewsky, A. U. 1894 Ueber den Stickstoffwechsel während der letzten Tage der Schwangerschaft und der ersten Tage des Wochenbetts. Z. Biol. 30: 368.

302. Slemons, J. M. 1904 Metabolism during pregnancy, labor and the puerperium. Johns Hopkins Hosp. Rep. 12: 111.

303. Hoffstrom, K. A. 1910 Eine Stoffwechsel-untersuchung während der Schwangerschaft. Skand. Arch. Physiol. 23: 326.

304. Landsberg, E. 1914 Eiweiss- und Mineral-stoffwechseluntersuchungen bei der schwangeren Frau nebst Tierversuchen mit besonderer Berücksichtigung der Funktion endokriner Drüsen. Ein Versuch einer Darstellung der Stoffwechselveränderungen in der Gravidität auf allgemein-biologischer Basis. Z. Geburtsch. Gynaek. 76: 53.

305. Wilson, K. M. 1916 Nitrogen metabolism during pregnancy. Bull. Johns Hopkins Hospital 27: 121.

306. Coons, C. M., and K. Blunt 1930 The retention of nitrogen, calcium, phosphorus, and magnesium by pregnant women. J. Biol. Chem. 86: 1.

307. Macy, I. G., E. Donelson, M. L. Long and A. Graham 1931 Nitrogen, calcium and phosphorus balances in late gestation under a specified dietary régime. A record of one case. J. Amer. Diet. Ass. 6: 314.

308. Hunscher, H. A., E. Donelson, B. Nims, F. Kenyon and I. G. Macy 1933 Metabolism of women during the reproductive cycle. V. Nitrogen utilization. J. Biol. Chem. 99: 507.

309. Hunscher, H. A., F. C. Hummell, B. N. Erickson and I. G. Macy 1935 Metabolism of women during the reproductive cycle. VI. A case study of the continuous nitrogen utilization of a multipara during pregnancy, parturition, puerperium, and lactation. J. Nutr. 10: 579.

310. Fehling, H. 1877 Beiträge zur Physiologie des placenteren Stoffverkehrs. Archiv Gynäk. 11: 523.

311. Michel, C. 1899 Sur la composition chimique de l'embryo et du foetus humains aux différentes periodes de la grossesse. C. R. Soc. Biol. 51: 422.

312. Wehefritz, E. 1926 Kalkuntersuchungen an Placenten verschiedenen Alters. Archiv. Gynäk. 127: 106.

313. Higuchi, S. 1909 Ein Beitrag zur chemischen Zusammensetzung der Placenta. Biochem. Z. 15: 95.

314. Vonnegut, F. A. 1928 Systematische Fruchtwassermessungen in den verschiedenen Schwangerschaftsmonaten. Zentr. Gynäk. 52: 1306.

315. Uyeno, D. 1919 The physical properties and chemical composition of human amniotic fluid. J. Biol. Chem. 37: 77.

316. Sandiford, I., T. Wheeler and W. M. Boothby 1931 - Metabolic studies during pregnancy and menstruation. Amer. J. Physiol. 96: 191.

317. Coons, C. M. 1933 Dietary habits during pregnancy. J. Amer. Diet. Ass. 9: 95.

318. Coons, C. M., and G. B. Marshall 1934 Some factors influencing nitrogen economy during pregnancy. J. Nutr. 7: 67.

319. Coons, C. M., A. T. Schiefelbusch, G. B. Marshall and R. R. Coons 1935 Studies in metabolism during pregnancy. Exp. Sta. Bull. No. 223, Oklahoma Agricultural Experiment Station, Stillwater, Oklahoma.

320. Hummel, F. C., H. A. Hunscher, M. F. Bates, P. Bonner, I. G. Macy and J. A. Johnston 1937 A consideration of the nutritive state in the metabolism of women during pregnancy. J. Nutr. 13: 263.

321. Thomson, A. M. 1959 Diet in pregnancy. 3. Diet in relation to the course and outcome of pregnancy. Brit. J. Nutr. 13: 509.

322. Macy, I. G., and H. Hunscher 1934 An evaluation of maternal nitrogen and mineral needs during embryonic and infant development. Amer. J. Obstet. Gynecol. 27: 878.

323. Strauss, M. B. 1935 Observations on the etiology of the toxemia of pregnancy. The relationship of nutritional deficiency, hypoproteinemia and elevated venous pressure to water retention in pregnancy. Amer. J. Med. Sci. 190: 811.

324. Holmes, O. M. 1941 Protein diet in pregnancy. Western J. Surg. Obstet. Gynecol. 49: 56.

325. Heller, L. 1954–55 Stickstoffbilanzen in den letzten drei Schwangerschaftsmonaten. Arch. Gynäkol. 185: 566.

326. Freyberg, R. H., R. D. Reekie and C. Folsome 1938 A study of the water, sodium, and energy exchange during the latter part of pregnancy. Amer. J. Obstet. Gynecol. 36: 200.

327. Oberst, F. W., and E. D. Plass 1940 Calcium, phosphorus, and nitrogen metabolism in women during the second half of pregnancy and in early lactation. Amer. J. Obstet. Gynecol. 40: 399.

328. Jayalakshmi, V. T., P. S. Venkatachalam and C. Gopalan 1959 Nitrogen balance studies in pregnant women in South India. Indian J. Med. Res. 47: 86.

329. Hazari, K., M. P. John and A. Saran 1965 Protein metabolism in pregnancy. Indian J. Med. Res. 53: 884.

330. Hytten, F. E., and A. M. Thomson 1968 Maternal physiological adjustments. Biology of Gestation, vol. 1, The Maternal Organism, ed., N. S. Assali. Academic Press, New York, p. 449.

331. Werch, S. C., G. T. Lewis and J. H. Ferguson 1958 Can dietary protein deficiency be assessed biochemically? A study of fifty-four obstetric patients. Obstet. Gynecol. 11: 676.

332. Ebbs, J. H., F. F. Tisdall and W. A. Scott 1941 The influence of prenatal diet on the mother and child. J. Nutr. 22: 515.

333. Burke, B. S., V. A. Beal, S. B. Kirkwood and H. C. Stuart 1943 Nutrition studies during pregnancy. I. Problems, methods of study, and group studied. Amer. J. Obstet. Gynecol. 46: 38.

334. Burke, B. S., V. V. Harding and H. C. Stuart 1943 Nutrition studies during pregnancy. IV. Relation of protein content of mother's diet during pregnancy to birth length, birth weight, and condition of infant at birth. J. Pediat. 23: 506.

335. Dieckmann, W. J., D. F. Turner, E. J. Meiller, L. J. Savage, A. J. Hill, M. T. Straube, R. E. Pottinger and L. M. Rynkiewicz 1951 Observations on protein intake and the health of the mother and baby. I. Clinical and laboratory findings. J. Amer. Diet. Ass. 27: 1046.

336. Williams, P. F., and F. G. Fralen 1942 Nutrition study in pregnancy. Dietary analyses of seven-day food intake records of 514 pregnant women, comparison of actual food intakes with variously stated requirements, and relationship of food intake to various obstetric factors. Amer. J. Obstet. Gynecol. 43: 1.

337. McGanity, W. J., R. O. Cannon, E. B. Bridgforth, M. P. Martin, P. M. Densen, J. A. Newbill, G. S. McClellan, A. Christie, J. C. Peterson and W. J. Darby 1954 The Vanderbilt cooperative study of maternal and infant nutrition. VI. Relationship of obstetric performance to nutrition. Amer. J. Obstet. Gynecol. 67: 501.

338. Thomson, A. M. 1958 Diet in pregnancy. 1. Dietary survey technique and the nutritive value of diets taken by primagravidae. Brit. J. Nutr. 12: 446.

339. Thomson, A. M. 1959 Diet in pregnancy. 2. Assessment of the nutritive value of diets, especially in relation to differences between social classes. Brit. J. Nutr. 13: 190.

340. Iyenger, L. 1967 Effects of dietary supplements late in pregnancy on the expectant mother and her newborn. Indian J. Med. Res. 55: 85.

341. Hoobler, R. R. 1917 The effect on human milk production of diets containing various forms and quantities of protein. Amer. J. Dis. Child. 14: 105.

342. Adair, F. L. 1925 The influence of diet on lactation. Amer. J. Obstet. Gynecol. 9: 1.

343. Deem, H. E. 1931 Observations on the milk of New Zealand women. Arch. Dis. Child. 6: 53.

344. Bassir, O. 1959 Nutritional studies on breast milk of Nigerian women; supplementing the maternal diet with a protein-rich plant product. Trans. Roy. Soc. Trop. Med. Hyg. 53: 256.

345. Gopalan, C. 1958–59 Studies on lactation in poor Indian communities. J. Trop. Pediat. 4: 87.

346. Narasinga Rao, B. S., S. Pasricha and C. Gopalan 1958 Nitrogen balance studies in poor Indian women during lactation. Indian J. Med. Res. 46: 325.

347. Karmarkar, M. G., and C. V. Ramakrishnan 1960 Studies on human lactation. Relation between the dietary intake of lactating women and the chemical composition of milk with regard to principal and certain inorganic constituents. Acta Paediat. 49: 599.

348. Gopalan, C., and B. Belavady 1961 Nutrition and lactation. Federation Proc. 20(Suppl. 7): 177.

349. Harding, V. J., and R. C. Montgomery 1927 Metabolism in the puerperium. J. Biol. Chem. 73: 27.

350. Shukers, C. F., I. G. Macy, E. Donelson, B. Nims and H. A. Hunscher 1931 Food intake in pregnancy, lactation, and reproductive rest in the human mother. J. Nutr. 4: 399.

351. Shukers, C. F., I. G. Macy, B. Nims, E. Donelson and H. A. Hunscher 1932 A quantitative study of the dietary of the human mother, with respect to the nutrients secreted into breast milk. J. Nutr. 5: 127.

352. Rose, M. S. 1929 The Foundation of Nutrition. The MacMillan Co., New York, p. 452.

353. McLester, J. S. 1949 Nutrition and Diet in Health and Disease. W. B. Saunders Co., Philadelphia, p. 291.

354. Garry, R. C., and D. Stiven 1936 A review of recent work on dietary requirements in pregnancy and lactation, with an attempt to assess human requirements. Nutr. Abstr. Rev. 5: 855.

355. Leitch, I., and J. Duckworth 1937 The determination of the protein requirements of man. Nutr. Abstr. Rev. 7: 257.

356. Dieckmann, W. J., and W. W. Swanson 1937 Dietary requirements in pregnancy. Amer. J. Obstet. Gynecol. 38: 523.

357. Williams, P. F. 1945 Importance of adequate protein nutrition in pregnancy. J. Amer. Med. Ass. 127: 1052.

358. Kaucher, M., E. Z. Moyer, H. H. Williams and I. G. Macy 1946 Adequacy of the diet during lactation. J. Amer. Diet. Ass. 22: 594.

359. Holemans, K., A. Lambrechts, C. Huben and H. Martin 1959 Nitrogen, calcium, and phosphorus balances of the nursing African mother. (Evaluation of the minimal daily requirements.) J. Trop. Pediat. 5: 27.

360. Watkin, D. M. 1966 The impact of nutrition on the biochemistry of aging in man. World Rev. Nutr. Diet. 6: 124.

361. Albanese, A. A., R. A. Higgons, B. Vestal, L. Stephanson and M. Malsch 1952 Protein requirements of old age. Geriatrics 7: 109.

362. Fenger, S. 1904 Beiträge zur Kenntniss des Stoffwechsels im Greisenalter. Skand. Arch. Physiol. 16: 222.

363. Koch, E. 1911 Ein Beitrag zur Kenntnis des Nahrungsbedarfes bei alten Männern. Skand. Arch. Physiol. 25: 315.

364. Strieck, Fr. 1937–38 Metabolic studies in a man who lived for years on a minimum protein diet. Ann. Intern. Med. 11: 643.

365. Kountz, W. B., L. Hofstatter and P. Ackermann 1947 Nitrogen balance studies in elderly people. Geriatrics 2: 173.

366. Kountz, W. B., L. Hofstatter and P. Ackermann 1948 Nitrogen balance studies un-

der prolonged high nitrogen intake levels in elderly people. Geriatrics 3: 171.

367. Kountz, W. B., L. Hofstatter and P. G. Ackermann 1951 Nitrogen balance studies in four elderly men. J. Gerontol. 6: 20.

368. Kountz, W. B., P. G. Ackermann, T. Kheim and G. Toro 1953 Effects of increased protein intake in older people. Geriatrics 8: 63.

369. Albanese, A. A., R. A. Higgons, L. A. Orto and D. N. Zavattaro 1957 Protein and amino acid needs of the aged in health and convalescence. Geriatrics 12: 465.

370. Roberts, P. H., C. H. Kerr and M. A. Ohlson 1948 Nutritional status of older women. Nitrogen, calcium, and phosphorus retentions of nine women. J. Amer. Diet. Ass. 24: 292.

371. Horwitt, M. K. 1953 Dietary requirements of the aged. J. Amer. Diet. Ass. 29: 443.

372. Silverstone, Watkin and Shock 1966 Cited by: Watkin, D. M. The impact of nutrition on the biochemistry of aging in man. World Rev. Nutr. Diet. 6: 124.

373. Duncan, D. L. 1958 The interpretation of studies of calcium and phosphorus balance in ruminants. Nutr. Abstr. Rev. 28: 695.

APPENDIX TABLE 1

Studies on the quantitative determination of obligatory nitrogen losses

Kind of loss	Description of subjects	No. of studies	Results	References
Endogenous	25 men	4	24.1 to 37 mg/kg	22,23,24,37
(urinary)	39 men	5	1.32 to 1.6 mg/kcal	24,27,28,37
nitrogen	15 women	2	1.19, 1.42 mg/kcal	28,29
	11 infants	1	0.6, 0.8 mg/kcal	30
	8 men	1	79.4 mg/kg bcm[1]	37
	13 men	1	44 mg/kg lbm[2]	37a
Metabolic	19 adults	2	0.395, 0.96 g/day	31,37a
(fecal)	8 men	1	9.0 mg/kg	37
nitrogen	81 children	2	30, 33 mg/kg	38,39
	2 men (resting)	2	13, 17 mg/day	44,46
Skin and	40 men (sedentary)	4	143 to 415 mg/day	48,49,53,54
sweat	7 men	2	179, 250 mg/m^2	57,58
nitrogen	7 women	1	120 mg/m^2	58
	17 infants	1	3–5% of total N excretion	47
Hot environment				
Skin and				
sweat	8 men (in laboratory)	1	200 mg/hr	60
nitrogen	6 men (natural work)	1	0.49 g/6.5 hr	59

[1] bcm = body cell mass, estimated from total body ^{40}K.
[2] lbm = lean body mass, estimated from body density and total body water.

APPENDIX TABLE 2

Controlled studies on protein requirements of children since 1917

Subjects	No. of subjects	No. of studies	Principal criteria	Requirement suggested	References
Infants					
Premature	1597	12	growth	2 to 7 g/kg	198,202–212
Full-term					
Young, 0–6 mos.	322	13	growth	2 to 5 g/kg	220,221,224–227, 230,234–236
			N retention	<0.8 g/kg	30,221,222
			plasma aminogram	1.7 g/kg	239
Older, 6–24 mos.	41	3	growth	1.25 to 4 g/kg	241,243,244
Preschool children					
2–5 yr	44	8	growth	1 to 4 g/kg	255–265
			N retention	1.46, 1.29 g/kg	258
School-age children					
6–12 yr	243	11	growth	0.7 to 2.8 g/kg	255,256,258,273–279
			N retention	0.5 g/kg	279,281,282
			creatinine excretion	3.5 g/kg	277
Adolescents	0	0			

APPENDIX TABLE 3

Studies on protein requirements during pregnancy and lactation

Condition	Kind of study	No. of studies	No. of subjects	Suggested requirements	Reference
Pregnancy	Controlled or measured food intake, nitrogen balance	11	84	60 to 120 g/day	307,308,316,317,320, 325–329,340
				0.9 g/kg (minimum)	328
	Clinical and dietary surveys	7	5647	75 to 85 g/day	321,324,332–339
Lactation	Milk production	6	102	100 to 148 g/day	341,343–345,347,348
	Infant growth	1	30	—	345
	N balance	4	18	54 to 67% over the needs in pregnancy	308,309,322,346, 349–351,359

46

A CONSPECTUS OF RESEARCH

ON

AMINO ACID REQUIREMENTS OF MAN

by

M. ISABEL IRWIN

Human Nutrition Research Division
Agricultural Research Service
United States Department of Agriculture
Beltsville, Maryland 20705

and

D. MARK HEGSTED

Department of Nutrition
Harvard School of Public Health
Boston, Massachusetts 02115

THE JOURNAL OF NUTRITION

VOLUME 101, NUMBER 4, APRIL 1971

(Pages 539-566)

48

TABLE OF CONTENTS

Reprinted from THE JOURNAL OF NUTRITION
Vol. 101, No. 4, April 1971 © The American Institute of Nutrition 1971

INTRODUCTION

The discovery and identification of the individual amino acids began when Wollaston (1) isolated "cystic oxide," later renamed cystine, from a urinary calculus. In the following years other amino acids were isolated from various proteins. Studies on enzymatic digestion in vivo and in vitro revealed that amino acids were the end products of protein digestion (2). The suggestion that some amino acids might be indispensable while others are not was made by Blum (3). He had observed that protoalbuminoid, obtained from casein, supported dogs in nitrogen balance whereas heteroalbuminoid obtained from fibrin did not. He concluded that the difference in performance between the two albuminoids was due to the presence of tyrosine and indole groups in the one and their absence from the other. He suggested that tyrosine- and indole-supplying groups are indispensable whereas glycine (contained abundantly in heteroalbuminoid but in small quantities in protoalbuminoid) is not.

During the early part of the twentieth century, studies with animals suggested that other amino acids might also be essential, e.g., cystine (4), tryptophan (5), lysine (6). Clarification and quantification of the amino acid needs of animals followed during the succeeding decades. Reports of studies on which amino acids should be provided preformed in the diet of humans began to appear in the early part of the fifth decade of this century. Studies on quantitative requirements followed. The first studies and the majority of all the studies were carried out with young adult subjects (mainly of college age). Infants under 11 months have also been studied. More recently, reports on the amino acid requirements of boys 11 to 12 years of age and of elderly men have

appeared. No reports on the minimum needs of children between infancy and 11 years old or during puberty and adolescence have been located in the literature. The needs of postmenopausal women and women during pregnancy and lactation have received scant attention.

The criteria used to assess requirements have included nitrogen balance, urinary excretion of the amino acid under study or of its metabolites, and growth (in infants). The usefulness of plasma amino acid levels and ratios as indicators of requirement has been and is being explored. Of these criteria, nitrogen balance has been the most widely used. In the studies of Rose et al. with young men (7), the lowest level of amino acid intake that would allow positive nitrogen balance in all subjects was regarded as the minimum requirement. Twice the minimum was proposed as a safe allowance. In studies with young women (8–11), the lowest level of amino acid intake that would maintain all subjects in the "equilibrium zone" was regarded as the minimum requirement. The "equilibrium zone" was designated as a retention of $0 \pm 5\%$ of the intake. In other words, with an intake of 7 g nitrogen/day, a subject would be considered to be in equilibrium if his retention fell between -0.35 and $+0.35$ g nitrogen/day.

Two feeding approaches were used initially. They were to feed purified diets in which the nitrogen was provided by purified amino acids and nonprotein sources (12), and to feed a protein known to be low in the amino acid under study or a protein hydrolysate from which the amino acid in question had been removed (13). In later studies (8), diets containing natural foods of low nitrogen content to-

Received for publication September 17, 1970.

gether with a mixture of purified amino acids and sources of nonprotein nitrogen were used. In still other studies, measured amounts of the amino acid under study have been administered to fasted subjects and the subsequent urinary excretion of the amino acid has been measured (14).

In studies with infants (15) and in some studies with young men (16), formula-type diets which permit close control of the amounts and proportions of all other nutrients as well as the nitrogen-containing ones were used. Purified amino acids and nonprotein nitrogen sources provided the nitrogen in these diets.

In diets containing purified amino acids the proportion in which the amino acids were fed differed from one laboratory to another. Rose (7), for instance, initially incorporated the amino acids into the diet in the proportion of the minimum levels found necessary for growing rats. Leverton et al. (8), Jones et al. (9), Reynolds et al. (10), and Swendseid and Dunn (11) provided them in the proportion found in egg protein. Snyderman's group (15), studying the requirements of infants, provided the amino acids in the proportion found in breast milk.

In addition to actual experiments in which the investigators fed known amounts of amino acids and observed the subjects' reactions, other scientists have reviewed the literature on the minimum nitrogen requirement for equilibrium when proteins of well-documented amino acid composition have been fed. The levels of the amino acids in the minimum amounts of various proteins required to maintain equilibrium have been used to calculate the minimum amino acid requirement for maintenance (17).

In view of these divergent methods and criteria of response, disagreements in the published literature are not surprising. These disagreements have been not only on the amount of each amino acid actually required but also on which amino acids are essential (required to be furnished by sources outside the body). A consensus has been reached on which amino acids are apparently essential (isoleucine, leucine, lysine, methionine, phenylalanine, threonine, tryptophan, valine, for children and adults, and, in addition, histidine for in-

fants). The quantitative requirements are still not settled. Indeed, as indicated earlier, in some age groups their determination has not yet been attempted.

The review of the literature which is to follow will begin with the requirements of young adults because this is the group that has been studied most intensively, and because the results found with this age group have been used as comparative references in some of the work with other groups.

AMINO ACID REQUIREMENTS OF YOUNG ADULTS

Arginine was first cited as an essential amino acid by Holt and Albanese (13). They observed that three young men, eating diets deficient in arginine, maintained nitrogen equilibrium. After 9 days with the deficient diet, however, the seminal plasma of these young men contained abnormally low numbers of spermatozoa. The addition of arginine to the diet resulted in a "prompt rise in the sperm count." In 1954, Rose et al. (18) reported studies with three young men which led them to conclude that "arginine is not necessary for the maintenance of nitrogen equilibrium in adult man." In a subsequent report (19) from Rose's laboratory, evidence was given indicating normal to high spermatozoa counts and normal motility in the seminal plasma of two young men who had been deprived of arginine for 47 and 46 days. A third young man who was examined before and after 64 days of arginine deprivation had sperm counts of 140 million and 181 million per cubic centimeter. These data reinforced Rose's opinion on the nonessentiality of arginine.

Histidine, previously shown by Rose and his co-workers to be essential for rats and dogs, was reported in 1943 (20) by the same laboratory to be unnecessary for the maintenance of nitrogen equilibrium in young men. In the following year Albanese et al. (21) confirmed this observation in a study with three healthy men but reported that, with histidine deprivation, an abnormal metabolite which gave a green Jolles reaction appeared in the urine. This second observation suggested to them that histidine might not be completely unessential. In subsequent work, Rose et al. (19,

22, 23) confirmed their original observations but failed to find evidence of an unusual color reaction in the urine during histidine deprivation.

That histidine should be essential for human infants (24) but not for preadolescent children (25) or human adults is curious especially when it has been found to be essential for both young and adult rats (26). Studies with animals (27, 28) suggest that the histidyl imidazole ring, which is the point of attachment of the iron in heme to globin and myoglobin (29), is the essential portion of histidine. Furthermore, histidine is found in mammalian musculature as part of the dipeptide carnosine (β-alanylhistidine) (30–32). In the thigh muscle of rats, the concentration of carnosine increases until puberty. After that, although the total amount increases as the animal grows, the concentration gradually decreases.[1] If a similar phenomenon occurs in man, it may be that the amount of histidine provided by catabolism of hemoglobin and carnosine is sufficient to maintain nitrogen balance in the older child and adult for a fairly long time.

Such a possibility was suggested by Nasset and Gatewood (32a). In their study, they fed adult rats a "complete" amino acid mixture simulating the essential amino acid content of whole egg protein. When histidine was omitted from this mixture, negative nitrogen balances and a 17% decrease in hemoglobin levels were observed. The amount of histidine needed to maintain the rats in positive nitrogen balance was insufficient to maintain hemoglobin at the control levels. Nasset and Gatewood noted that in the study of Rose et al. (22), the hemoglobin level of one young man dropped from 15.2 to 14.7 g/100 ml and his nitrogen balance declined from 1.37 to 0.96 g/day when histidine was omitted from his diet for 8 days. Assuming that the subject contained 4.8 liters of blood and that his blood volume remained constant, Nasset and Gatewood calculated that approximately 240 mg of histidine/day could have been released by the hemoglobin that disappeared during the 8-day period. This amount of histidine, they suggested, on the basis of data obtained in their rat studies, might be sufficient to maintain

positive nitrogen balance. Recently, Josephson et al. (32b) in a study of intravenous amino acid feeding in chronic uremia, found in one patient that the addition of histidine to the essential amino acid feeding mixture resulted in increased nitrogen retention without an increase in the blood urea nitrogen level.

Recently, also, there has been a report (32c) of more direct evidence obtained by Giordano with uremic patients concerning the need for histidine in maintaining hemoglobin levels. These patients who were being treated with controlled low nitrogen diets (amino acid mixtures or low protein) were found to have consistently low serum histidine levels. Anemia was frequently observed also. When histidine was added to the amino acid diet, hemoglobin synthesis was increased, as indicated by increased uptake of radioisotope-labeled leucine by reticulocytes.

Additional evidence of the essentiality of histidine has been provided by Kofrányi et al. (33). In their studies, two young men ate diets containing essential amino acid mixtures in the patterns found in whole egg protein or potato protein. The nonessential nitrogen portions of the diets were diammonium citrate, sodium glutamate, glutamine, or a mixture of glycine, alanine, serine, proline, asparagine and glutamine. With both the whole egg pattern and the potato pattern, the activities of serum alanine aminotransferase (glutamic-pyruvic transaminase) and serum aspartate aminotransferase (glutamic-oxaloacetic transaminase) rose, indicating possible liver damage. When the experiments were terminated at 12 and 16 days, the enzyme activities continued to rise for several days. Normal activity levels were not regained for 20 to 30 days. When arginine and histidine were added to similar diets fed to another young man, no increases in transaminase activities were observed during 40 days with the "potato diet" and 54 days with the "whole egg diet." Whether both arginine and histidine

[1] Reddy, W. J. 1959 Studies on the Metabolic Role of Carnosine, its Biosynthesis and the Development of a Chromatographic Technique for its Measurement. A thesis submitted to the Faculty of the Harvard School of Public Health in partial fulfillment of the requirements for the degree of Doctor of Science in Hygiene in the field of nutrition. Boston, Massachusetts, December 31, 1959.

were needed could not be discerned from this study. According to Munro (34), "it is well known that arginine is synthesized by mammals in the liver." The synthesis of histidine is less clear. Munro has cited unpublished work of other investigators who found that human liver slices incubated with formate-^{14}C produced a labeled compound identified as histidine. This, Munro suggested, might indicate that "biosynthesis of histidine by man occurs in the liver." The results of Kofrányi et al., if confirmed, may indicate that, under some circumstances, man may require a supply of exogenously produced histidine or arginine, or both, in addition to that produced endogenously.

Another puzzling aspect of histidine metabolism is that it is excreted in the urine during normal pregnancy (35). Whether this histidine excretion during pregnancy is in any way associated with a requirement for histidine is not known.

Isoleucine was reported by Rose et al. (20, 23) to be essential for maintaining young men in nitrogen equilibrium. With four subjects, Rose et al. (36) found the minimal amounts of DL-isoleucine required to maintain positive nitrogen balance were 1.40, 1.40, 1.40 and 1.30 g/day. Furthermore they found that D-isoleucine was apparently not utilized, and if L-isoleucine alone were used, only half as much was required as was needed of the racemic mixture. The minimum requirements of L-isoleucine, therefore, they assumed were 0.70, 0.70, 0.70, and 0.65 g/day for the four young men studied. Recognizing that four subjects constitute a very small sample upon which to determine a requirement, Rose made a practice of choosing the highest value determined as the "tentative minimum" and twice this amount as a "safe allowance." The tentative minimum intake and the safe allowance of L-isoleucine were therefore suggested as 0.70 and 1.40 g/day, respectively.

Rose's studies were conducted with young men who ate a purified diet composed of amino acids, sources of nonessential nitrogen (glycine and urea), cornstarch, sucrose, butterfat, corn oil, minerals, and vitamins. In studies by Swendseid and Dunn (11), seven young women ate diets which contained some natural foods that were of low nitrogen content. Cornstarch, sucrose, and butter were the principal sources of energy. Most of the nitrogen was provided by glycine and purified L-amino acids and/or purified protein in amounts needed to simulate the essential amino acid content of whole egg protein. In these studies, the young women required from 250 to 450 mg L-isoleucine/day to be maintained in the "equilibrium zone" (retention = 0 ± 5% of the intake). In view of this wide range in the requirements of seven young women, the study by Linkswiler et al. (37) is of interest. In assessing the availability of isoleucine from corn with three young men and eight young women as subjects, the investigators found that the isoleucine requirement for both men and women appeared to be greater than 422 mg/day, regardless of whether the amino acid was fed in the purified form or in intact protein.

Leucine was reported by Rose et al. (20, 38) to be essential for maintaining human subjects in positive nitrogen balance. With five young men as subjects they attempted to determine its quantitative requirement (36). Unlike their data on isoleucine, the data obtained on leucine showed wide divergence. The requirements of five individual subjects ranged from 0.50 to 1.10 g L-leucine/day. Tests with D-leucine indicated that this isomer was not utilized to any practical extent. According to his practice, Rose selected the highest requirement found (1.10 g L-leucine/day) as the tentative minimum requirement and twice this amount (2.20 g/day) as a safe allowance. The requirement of young women for leucine was studied by Leverton et al. (39). In all, 13 young women were fed semipurified diets in which the essential amino acids were supplied in the proportions found in whole egg protein. Glycine or glycine plus diammonium citrate provided most of the nonessential nitrogen; cornstarch, sucrose, butterfat, and corn oil supplied most of the energy. The amount of leucine required to maintain the subjects in the equilibrium zone varied from 170 to 710 mg/day. All subjects but one were in equilibrium with 620 mg/day. The one exception was in negative balance with 460 mg and in positive balance with 710 mg; she was not studied with 620 mg/day.

The investigators suggested, therefore, that 620 mg/day may be regarded as the tentative leucine requirement for young women.

Lysine is one of the most studied of all the amino acids. Albanese et al. (40) were unable to maintain four young men and one young woman in positive nitrogen balance or in equilibrium when they were eating a diet in which the lysine had been destroyed. Hydrolyzed deaminated casein supplemented with tryptophan and cystine was the nitrogen source. Fats, starch, sugar, and fruits and vegetables of low protein content were the principal sources of energy. In a subsequent study with three of the same subjects, Albanese et al. (41) observed that during lysine deprivation the subjects complained of nausea, dizziness and hypersensitivity to metallic sounds. In addition, an increased output of nonketone organic acids in the urine was noted. These symptoms were relieved when lysine was added to the diet. These observations convinced Albanese and his co-workers that lysine is an essential amino acid. Rose (18, 42) reported studies with young men which confirmed Albanese's observations on the essentiality of lysine for maintenance of nitrogen equilibrium in human adults. Bricker et al. (43) also reported observations with one young woman indicating that nitrogen equilibrium could not be maintained when the lysine intake was deficient.

The quantitative requirement for lysine was investigated by Rose et al. (44) in studies with six young men. Using his customary procedures, they found that the minimum intake required to permit positive nitrogen balance varied from 0.4 to 0.8 g L-lysine/day. Their observations indicated the D-lysine is not utilized to any significant extent. Rose proposed that the tentative minimum requirement for L-lysine be set at 0.8 g/day with 1.6 g/day considered to be a safe allowance. Other observations made during these studies failed to reveal any symptoms which could be considered specific to lysine deficiency. Analysis of the urine of two young men during lysine feeding and lysine deprivation failed to show any significant change in the output of organic acids. Rose attributed the contradiction between his findings and those of Albanese to the differ-

ences in source of nitrogen in the diets used in the two laboratories.

Using a semisynthetic diet similar to that used by Leverton et al. (8) and by Swendseid et al. (11), Jones et al. (9), in studies with 14 women, 19 to 43 years old, found that intakes of 0.4 to 0.5 g L-lysine/day were necessary to maintain the subjects in nitrogen equilibrium. Because these intakes were similar to those found by Rose et al. (44) with young men as subjects, Jones et al. concluded that there was probably no sex difference in the requirement of lysine.

Neither Rose nor Jones found any correlation between lysine requirement and body size. Clark et al. (45), however, obtained data in a study with five young men and five young women that indicated significant relationships between lysine requirement and body weight, metabolic body size, surface area, and creatinine excretion. Regression coefficients calculated for these relationships were considered to be useful in determining the requirements of groups of people but not of individuals. In their studies, wheat flour and corn provided approximately half of the dietary nitrogen. Purified amino acids were added so that the quantities of essential amino acids approximated those of 20 g of whole egg. Diammonium citrate, glycine, and glutamic acid also were added to raise the total nitrogen intake to 9.0 g/day. Cornstarch, butterfat, and a few selected fruits were sources of additional calories. The subjects were maintained close to nitrogen equilibrium with lysine intakes that ranged from 500 to 900 mg/day. In a subsequent study (46), conducted with another group of five men and five women under the same experimental conditions as the first study, even wider ranges in requirements were observed. The lysine requirement of the ten men and ten women of both studies ranged from 400 to 1200 mg/day for the men and 300 to 700 mg/day for the women. The lysine requirement of all of the women and of all but one of the men could be met by an intake of 900 mg/day.

More recently, Fisher et al. (47) reported that five young women were maintained in positive nitrogen balance with dietary lysine intakes as low as 50 mg/day. Their diets provided 4.8 and 5.4 g nitrogen/day. Fisher suggested that the difference between his results and those of Jones (9) and Clark (45, 46) was likely due to the lower levels of essential amino acids (other than lysine) provided in his diets. Fisher's diets supplied the essential amino acids at twice the minimum levels suggested by Rose (48). In the other investigations (9, 45, 46), amounts simulating the essential amino acid content of 20 g of egg protein were fed.

Clark's data indicated that lysine requirement determined on the basis of nitrogen retention might be affected by various factors that could be modified in the experimental procedure. In subsequent studies, Clark and her team investigated the effect of some of these factors. These studies showed a) that negative nitrogen balances could occur even with adequate lysine intake when the calorie intake was reduced below what seemed to be a critical level specific for each individual (49), b) that nitrogen retention tested at three levels of lysine intake improved with time at each lysine level (50), c) that.the source of supplementary nonessential nitrogen might affect nitrogen retention but did not affect urinary lysine excretion (51), and d) that nitrogen retention was affected by both nitrogen intake and lysine intake but that there was apparently no significant relationship between nitrogen intake and the adequacy of lysine intake (52).

Methionine and the other sulfur-containing amino acids have also been studied extensively. Special properties as lactogogues were postulated for the sulfur-containing amino acids by Daggs (53). In 1942, Rose et al. (54) briefly reported studies that indicated that methionine is an indispensable amino acid for humans. The following year, Albanese et al. (55) reported the results of a study in which two men and one woman ate diets with protein supplied by hydrolyzed casein from which either methionine or cystine had been removed. The data showed that methionine was needed for maintaining the subjects in positive nitrogen balance. The data on cystine were inconclusive. Additional studies (56) confirmed the findings on methionine and showed that methionine alone could restore positive nitrogen balance in subjects who had previously been deprived of both cystine and methionine. Albanese, therefore, concluded that methionine, but not cystine, is essential for human adults.

Rose's detailed report on studies with two young men was published in 1950 (12). As in the preliminary report (54), methionine was shown to be essential for maintaining positive nitrogen balance. Subsequently he reported studies with six young men who required from 0.8 to 1.1 g of racemic methionine (57). D-Methionine appeared to be as useful as L-methionine. Rose therefore suggested 1.1 g of L- or DL-methionine as the tentative minimum requirement and 2.2 g of L- or DL-methionine as a safe allowance for man. In these studies amino acid mixtures devoid of cystine were used. From additional work, Rose and Wixom (58) concluded that L-cystine is capable of replacing 80 to 89% of the minimum methionine requirement.

In Rose's studies on quantitative requirements, the total nitrogen intake was about 10 g/day. The methionine safe allowance in relation to nitrogen intake was therefore approximately 220 mg methionine/g nitrogen. Later the FAO/WHO Expert Group on Protein Requirements (59) recommended an intake of 190 to 220 mg methionine and cystine/gram nitrogen intake as necessary for adequate human nutrition. Scrimshaw et al. (60) when studying essential amino acid to total nitrogen ratios with young men reported finding evidence to support this recommendation.

Albanese (61) and Rose et al. (57), using nitrogen balance as the basis for judgment, agreed that D-methionine appears to be as well utilized as DL-methionine. Camien et al. (62), however, studied urinary excretion of methionine by young men after oral administration of L- or DL-methionine. Their data indicated that about 25% of the ingested D-methionine was excreted in the urine whereas there was little change in the amount of the L-isomer excreted after its ingestion. They concluded, therefore, that the D-isomer is less efficiently utilized than the L-form.

Studies on women's requirement for sulfur-containing amino acids have been carried out by Swendseid et al. (63) and Reynolds et al. (10). In the Swendseid studies a semisynthetic diet containing low nitrogen foods was used. The dietary nitrogen was supplied by peanut protein (2 g N) plus essential L-amino acids (1 g N) simulating the essential amino acid composition of egg protein (3 g N). Glycine was used to raise the total nitrogen intake to levels found in preliminary work to be sufficient for nitrogen equilibrium. Methionine was added at the expense of glycine. Cornstarch, sucrose, and butter supplied energy. Of eight young women (21 to 30 years old), five were in equilibrium with intakes of 350 mg sulfur-containing amino acids (150 mg methionine, 200 mg cystine). The addition of 100 mg methionine (250 mg methionine, 200 mg cystine) brought two more subjects into equilibrium. The remaining one subject achieved equilibrium with an additional 100 mg methionine. Thus, with cystine held constant at 200 mg, the total sulfur-containing amino acid requirement, as studied, ranged from 350 to 550 mg. When the peanut flour in the diet was reduced by 50%, the cystine and methionine content was reduced to 175 mg. At this level (100 mg cystine, 75 mg methionine) three subjects were maintained in equilibrium.

Reynolds et al. (10) studied the response to varying levels and proportions of cystine and methionine in 20 women (18 to 64 years old) eating a diet similar to that used by Swendseid et al. (11). Their data also show a wide range of response. With 500 mg cystine, 240 to 290 mg methionine (740 to 790 mg sulfur amino acids) were required to maintain most of the 11 subjects studied in equilibrium. With 10 mg cystine and 290 mg methionine (300 mg sulfur amino acids) 9 of 13 subjects were in the equilibrium zone but only three were in positive balance. With 290 mg methionine and 260 mg cystine (550 mg sulfur-containing amino acids) all subjects were in positive balance. Reynolds concluded from these observations that total sulfur amino acid intakes of 300 mg were marginal and of 500 mg were adequate for women. The one subject who was 64 years old (the others were 18 to 36 years old) was in negative balance at all levels of intake ranging from 40 to 860 mg sulfur amino acids. Reynolds suggested that this might indicate a greater need in older people as compared to young adults.

The wide range of response shown in the Swendseid and Reynolds studies was shown also at higher levels by Clark and Woodward (64) in a study with six young men. As in studies previously cited (45) wheat flour provided a large portion of the dietary essential amino acids. When, by supplementation with L-methionine, the total sulfur-containing amino acid levels were raised from 1090 mg to 1240, 1390, and 1690 mg (equivalent to 1270, 1420, 1570, and 1870 mg of methionine), no significant differences in nitrogen retention occurred. That two of Clark's subjects were in negative balance at the lowest intake suggests that this level, though higher than that proposed as a tentative minimum by Rose, may have been less than adequate. The data also showed that methionine intake could be increased by at least 50% without toxic effects as indicated by nitrogen balance.

Phenylalanine was first reported to be essential for humans by Rose in 1943 as the result of studies (later reported in detail in 1951) with two healthy young men (20, 38). In Rose's studies L-phenylalanine was used. Albanese (61), by determining the urinary phenylalanine excretion after test doses of the L- and DL-forms, concluded that the D-isomer was not readily utilized by man. In quantitative studies, Rose et al. (65) observed that DL-phenylalanine was capable of replacing an equal weight of L-phenylalanine in maintaining positive nitrogen balance. When, however, D-phenylalanine was substituted for the L- or DL-form, negative nitrogen balance occurred. Rose concluded that the subjects could invert the D- to the L-form but the inversion was limited to about 0.50 g/day. The L-isomer, therefore, appears to be completely or almost completely replaced by the racemic form but not by the D-isomer. The six young men studied by Rose required daily L-phenylalanine intakes of 0.80 to 1.10 g. Rose, therefore, suggested the highest value (1.10 g/day) as the tentative minimum requirement and 2.20 g/day as a safe allowance. No relationship between phenylalanine requirement and body size was observed. The diets in these studies did not contain tyrosine. In subsequent experiments with two young men, Rose and Wixom (66) observed that tyrosine was capable of sparing phenylalanine to the extent of 70 to 75% of the minimal requirement.

In studies with ten young women eating a diet supplying 9.5 g nitrogen/day Leverton et al. (67) found that the amount of L-phenylalanine required to maintain the subjects in the equilibrium zone ranged between 120 and 220 mg/day when 900 mg of tyrosine were included in the diet. Another group of eight young women was maintained in equilibrium when 220 mg L-phenylalanine and 900 mg tyrosine were fed daily. A tentative minimum daily requirement of 220 mg L-phenylalanine in the presence of 900 mg tyrosine was therefore proposed. When tyrosine was omitted or reduced in quantity, more phenylalanine was required to maintain equilibrium. The sparing action of tyrosine on phenylalanine was therefore confirmed but no quantitative relationship was determined.

Tolbert and Watts (68) studied phenylalanine requirements and phenylalanine–tyrosine interrelationships with six young women. When no tyrosine was added to their semipurified diet supplying 10 g total nitrogen, the minimum phenylalanine requirement to assure positive nitrogen balance varied from 834 to 1184 mg/day. The highest value is fairly close to that determined with young men by Rose et al. (65) using the same criterion (positive nitrogen balance) and also reasonably close to that of Leverton et al. (67) using a different criterion (zone of equilibrium) when the tyrosine is converted to phenylalanine value (45 mg tyrosine = 41 mg phenylalanine). In another part of the study, Tolbert and Watts observed with three subjects that at least 70% of the phenylalanine requirement could be replaced by tyrosine.

Burrill and Schuck (69) studied phenylalanine requirements with and without tyrosine in nine young men and 13 young women. Their studies indicated that the replacement value of tyrosine was lower than that previously found by Rose and Wixon (66) and Tolbert and Watts (68), and that it depended slightly on the amount of tyrosine fed. Using a semipurified diet with the essential amino acids furnished in the amounts supplied by 20 g whole egg protein, they estimated the phenylalanine requirement with three levels of tyrosine.

With no tyrosine in the diet, the women required 600 to 700 mg and the men required 900 to 1000 mg phenylalanine/day. Both the criteria of Rose and of Leverton (positive N balance and zone of equilibrium) were applied in estimating these requirements. When 200 mg tyrosine were added, all of the men and women were maintained within the equilibrium zone with intakes of 400 to 500 mg phenylalanine/day but all were not in positive nitrogen balance. When 400 mg tyrosine were fed, the women could store nitrogen with phenylalanine intakes of 300 to 400 mg but the men required 500 to 600 mg. Burrill and Schuck calculated that tyrosine had a replacement value of 50% for men when fed at the level of either 200 or 400 mg/day. For women, tyrosine had a replacement value of 35 to 40% when fed at the 200 mg level and of 50% when fed at the 400 mg level.

Threonine was reported by Rose et al. (20, 22) to be essential for humans. Without it in the diet, two young men were in negative nitrogen balance. The addition of threonine to the diet promptly restored positive balance. Later, in studies with three young men, Rose et al. (57) determined that a) D-threonine was totally ineffective in maintaining nitrogen equilibrium and b) 0.6 to 1.0 g of DL-threonine or 0.3 to 0.5 g L-threonine were needed to permit nitrogen retention. The minimum requirement was tentatively set at 0.5 g L-threonine/day with 1.0 g/day regarded as a safe allowance. Double these amounts (1.0 and 2.0 g) would be needed if the racemic form were used.

Leverton et al. (8) studied the threonine requirements of three groups of young women, 19 to 26 years old (a total of 21 women). The minimum L-threonine intake required to maintain the women in the equilibrium zone varied from 103 to 305 mg/day. Because 305 mg were adequate or more than adequate for all the women studied, Leverton selected this level, rounding it off to 310 mg, as the tentative minimum daily requirement for young women. Some evidence suggesting that threonine requirement might be related to nitrogen intake was noted.

Later, in studies on the availability of threonine from corn, Linkswiler et al. (70)

determined nitrogen retention of ten young women with two levels of nitrogen intake and three levels of L-threonine intake (620, 280 and 195 mg/day). When the total nitrogen intake was 10 g/day the mean nitrogen balance was positive with 620 mg threonine but it was negative with 280 and 195 mg threonine. When the total nitrogen intake was 6 g/day, the mean nitrogen balance was negative at all levels of threonine intake. Reducing the threonine intake from 620 to 280 mg/day did not affect the mean balance significantly. At the higher nitrogen intake, the subjects frequently experienced nausea and vomiting when the threonine intake was lowered to 195 mg/day. When the lower level of total nitrogen was provided, no such symptoms were observed with 195 mg threonine/day. The investigators suggested that these observations indicated a possibly greater need for threonine at the higher than at the lower nitrogen intake. The threonine from corn appeared to be fully utilized. There was some evidence, in fact, for higher nitrogen balances when threonine was supplied by corn than by the purified amino acid.

Another possible index of requirement investigated by Wertz et al. (71) was urinary excretion of amino acids. In their study the urinary excretion of women during early and late pregnancy was compared with that of the same women in the fourth or fifth month postpartum. All the essential amino acids were excreted in larger amounts during pregnancy than during the postpartum period. The excretion of threonine, which showed the greatest relative increase, was two to four times higher in pregnancy than during the nonpregnant state (postpartum). Lack of quantitative data on protein and amino acid intakes, however, prevents one from concluding that the increased excretions were related to changes in requirements.

Tryptophan was first reported to be essential for nitrogen equilibrium by Holt et al. (72). In their study, four men ate a diet of fats, starch and sugar, and selected fruits and vegetables of low nitrogen content. Nitrogen was provided by an acid hydrolysate of casein supplemented with cystine. With this diet the men were in negative nitrogen balance. The addition of tryptophan to the diet restored them to positive balance. The following year, a report by Cox et al. (73) on nitrogen balance in a patient whose protein was provided either by enzymatically hydrolyzed casein or by acid-hydrolyzed casein (in which tryptophan was destroyed) supported Holt's conclusion that tryptophan is an essential amino acid. A similar conclusion was reported by Rose (18, 42). Using a diet and source of protein similar to those used in their previous study (72), Holt et al. (74) next attempted to determine the tryptophan requirement of man. With two adult male subjects they measured urinary tryptophan excretion and nitrogen retention when various levels of tryptophan were fed. Urinary tryptophan excretion decreased sharply when tryptophan was omitted from the diet. A supplement of 3.0 to 6.0 mg tryptophan/kilogram body weight restored the excretion to normal levels. Supplements of 6.3 and 9.4 mg tryptophan/kilogram body weight were necessary to restore the subjects to nitrogen balance. Holt et al. questioned which level of intake should be regarded as the requirement. They suggested that the lower level needed to restore tryptophan excretion to its normal level might have been the result of reduced tolerance developed during the 30 days when no tryptophan was fed. On the other hand, they suggested that with longer periods of supplementation (they used 3-day periods) nitrogen balance might have been attained at a lower level than 6.0 to 9.0 mg tryptophan/kilogram (approximately 0.4 to 0.6 g/day for a 70 kg man).

Denko and Grundy (75) reported a study in which seven young men maintained nitrogen balance with tryptophan intakes as low as 0.24 g/day. At this level of intake, five of the seven men excreted more tryptophan than when they received 813 mg tryptophan. When the tryptophan intake was reduced the protein content of the diet was also changed in quantity and quality. This change from 70 g presumably mixed protein in the "normal diet" to 40 g protein mainly of plant origin (corn etc.) in the restricted diet may have influenced the tryptophan excretion. Denko and Grundy reported that they found no correlation between body weight, minimum tryptophan requirement, and excretion of free L-tryptophan.

In the quantitative studies of Rose et al. (7), two young men were maintained in positive nitrogen balance with a purified diet furnishing 0.15 g L-tryptophan/day. A third subject required 0.25 g L-tryptophan/day. Rose, therefore, suggested a tentative minimum requirement of 0.25 g L-tryptophan/day with 0.50 g as a safe allowance. Rose et al. (7) reported also that no correlation was found between tryptophan requirements and body size.

Relationships between plasma tryptophan levels and dietary tryptophan intakes of young men were studied recently by Young et al. (16). Their diet contained an L-amino acid mixture simulating egg protein which supplied nitrogen equivalent to 0.5 g protein/kilogram/day. Energy was provided by cornstarch, sucrose, dextrimaltose, corn oil, butter and shortening. The tryptophan intake was varied from approximately 1 to 9 mg/kg body weight. At levels below 3 and above 5 mg/kg, plasma tryptophan levels did not respond to dietary changes. As the dietary intake increased from 3 to 5 mg/kg, however, plasma tryptophan increased linearly. Young et al. interpreted these data as suggesting a tryptophan requirement of 3 mg/kg body weight. Nitrogen balance data obtained in the same study indicated a mean minimum requirement of 2.0 to 2.6 mg tryptophan/kilogram body weight. Because integumental and sweat losses were not included in the nitrogen balance data, however, Young pointed out that the balance results probably underestimate tryptophan needs, and suggested that the values for the requirement based on nitrogen balance and plasma tryptophan values are essentially identical.

Leverton et al. (76) studied the tryptophan requirements of a group of eight college women, eating the semipurified diet customarily used in their studies. Nitrogen retention decreased with lowered tryptophan intakes. An intake of 157 mg L-tryptophan/day permitted retention within the equilibrium zone for all subjects. With an intake of 120 mg/day three subjects failed to maintain nitrogen equilibrium. One subject remained in equilibrium with an intake of 82 mg/day. A second group of eight subjects was then maintained in equilibrium with an intake of 157 mg

tryptophan/day. Leverton, on the basis of these data, suggested 160 mg tryptophan/day as a tentative minimum requirement for young women.

Subsequently, Fisher et al. (47) found that five young women could be maintained in positive nitrogen balance when their diet provided 50 mg tryptophan and 4.8 g total nitrogen/day. As noted previously, these researchers suggested that the lower requirement for both lysine and tryptophan observed in their studies might be explained by the lower level of total essential amino acids provided in their diets as compared to the level supplied in earlier work (76).

As described previously, Wertz et al. (71) studied urinary amino acid excretion in women during pregnancy and 4 to 5 months postpartum. Tryptophan excretions during pregnancy were observed to be about double the levels found during the non-pregnant state. Whether this difference in excretion was related to a difference in requirement could not be ascertained from the data.

In the studies by Rose et al. (7), D-tryptophan was apparently not utilized. Earlier, Albanese et al. (77) had reported evidence indicating that D-tryptophan was metabolized differently than the L-isomer in the human. The feeding of D-tryptophan resulted in the excretion of an "aberrant" metabolite in the urine. Later Albanese et al. (78) reported that when D-tryptophan was ingested, it was entirely excreted in the urine as judged by the appearance of the unusual metabolite, but when DL-tryptophan was acetylated, it was wholly utilized. This, they suggested, indicated that the acetylation of D-tryptophan improved its availability.

Baldwin and Berg (79) published data in essential agreement with Rose's data (7). They were able to maintain five men in positive balance with approximately 225 mg L-tryptophan/day or less. About twice as much DL-tryptophan as L-tryptophan was needed to maintain positive nitrogen balance. There was a slight indication that D-tryptophan, if fed in sufficiently large amounts, might support nitrogen balance but no attempt was made to determine the amount required. Acetylation of

D-tryptophan did not enhance its usefulness.

Rose et al. (80) with their customary nitrogen balance technique studied the utilization by five young men of acetyl-D-, acetyl-L- and acetyl-DL-tryptophan. Their data indicated that acetyl-D-tryptophan was not utilized to any significant extent and that the acetylation of L- and DL-tryptophan did not measurably change their usefulness.

Valine was first reported to be an essential amino acid by Rose et al. (12, 20). Two young men were in negative nitrogen balance when DL-valine was removed from the mixture of essential amino acids included in their purified diet. The inclusion of valine restored them to positive balance. A drop in the urinary excretion of α-amino acids when DL-valine was removed from the diet provided indirect evidence that the D-form of valine was not utilized. Later (19), quantitative studies with five young men showed that L-valine was twice as effective as DL-valine in maintaining positive nitrogen balance and that D-valine was not available for maintaining nitrogen equilibrium. Minimum daily requirements of the five men for L-valine ranged from 0.4 to 0.8 g/day. No correlation between valine requirement and body size was observed. Rose suggested that 0.8 and 1.6 g L-valine/day be regarded as the tentative minimum requirement and a safe allowance, respectively.

Leverton et al. (81) found in a study with seven college women that all subjects could be maintained in or above the equilibrium zone with an intake of 650 mg L-valine/day. With an intake of 465 mg/day, the mean nitrogen retention was in the equilibrium zone but three of the subjects were clearly in negative balance. Intakes between 465 and 650 mg L-valine/day were not studied. Eight other women studied at the 650 mg level of intake were all maintained in the equilibrium zone. This amount, therefore, (650 mg L-valine/day) was suggested as the minimum requirement for young women.

Linkswiler et al. (82), in a study on the availability of valine from corn, measured the nitrogen retention of seven college women with valine intakes varying from 530 to 230 mg/day. With intakes of 530 and 480 mg valine/day, all subjects were maintained in the equilibrium zone. At lower levels of intake, balances below the zone of equilibrium were observed. Thus 480 mg/day was an adequate level of intake judged by this criterion (zone of equilibrium). When Rose's criterion of distinctly positive balances for all subjects was applied, none of the levels of valine intake was adequate. Valine from corn was as well utilized as was the purified amino acid.

AMINO ACID REQUIREMENTS OF THE ELDERLY

Tuttle et al. (83) concluded that elderly men may have higher essential amino acid requirements than young men do. They studied five men, 52 to 68 years old. The men, who had been maintained in positive nitrogen balance with 7 g nitrogen provided by natural foods, went into negative balance when an isonitrogenous amino acid mixture, simulating the essential amino acid content of 18.75 g egg protein, plus glycine replaced the intact protein. In the latter diet, calories were provided by selected fruits, cornstarch, sucrose and margarine. Negative nitrogen balance also resulted when 18.75 g egg protein plus glycine were fed as the nitrogen source (total 7.1 g N). The amounts of essential amino acids fed in these amino acid and egg diets were greater than or almost equal to the minimum requirements suggested by Rose et al. (19) for young men. When the quantities of essential amino acids were doubled, the men were maintained in positive nitrogen balance.

In a subsequent study, Tuttle et al. (84) maintained seven men (over 50 years of age) in positive nitrogen balance with a diet containing 7 g total nitrogen and essential amino acids in the quantities found in 300 g whole egg (36 to 39 g egg protein). In another test with eight men, five of whom had been studied with the 7 g nitrogen diet, the total dietary nitrogen was increased to 15 g by the addition of glycine or diammonium citrate. With this diet, seven of the men were in negative nitrogen balance. These results suggested to Tuttle that, aside from the possible effects of the source of nonessential nitrogen, the requirement of older men for one or more of the essential amino acids may vary with total nitrogen intake.

On the other hand, Watts et al. (85) found no evidence for a greater requirement by older men than by young men for essential amino acids. In their studies six Negro men 65 to 84 years of age ate diets containing 10 g total nitrogen. The calories were provided by selected fruits, wheatstarch, sucrose, and margarine. The essential amino acids were provided in the FAO pattern and the milk pattern at varying levels. The men were in positive nitrogen balance when the FAO pattern was fed at levels supplying 200 mg (one test), 280 mg (three tests), and 400 mg (one test) of tryptophan. When the FAO pattern was fed at a level supplying 360 mg tryptophan, positive balances occurred in three out of six tests; nitrogen retentions were in or above the equilibrium zone in five out of six tests. The retentions were higher and more frequently positive than those observed previously by Swendseid et al. (86) when 10 young men (20 to 26 years old) ate diets providing 10 g of nitrogen, in which the essential amino acids were provided in the FAO pattern at levels supplying 240, 280, 320, 360, and 440 mg tryptophan. In the studies with young men, positive nitrogen balances were found only with the 440 mg tryptophan level.

Similarly, when Watts et al. compared the response of the older men with that of young men to the diets providing essential amino acids in the milk pattern, no evidence was found to indicate that the older men had greater requirements. There is a possibility that the difference between Tuttle's and Watts' results may be due to differences in response to the amino acid patterns used.

Tuttle et al. (87), in pursuing their studies further, found, using techniques similar to those of earlier studies (83, 84), that six older men (58 to 73 years) required more than 2.1 g methionine/day. Two of the men were in positive nitrogen balance with intakes of 2.4 and 2.7 g methionine/day. Two others required 3.0 g/day to maintain positive balance. The investigators suggested that, in view of the low cystine content of the test diet, the results might have been a reflection not of an increased need for S-amino acids but

rather of a decreased ability in the aged to convert methionine to cystine. In contrast, the six elderly men studied by Watts et al. (85) were in nitrogen equilibrium or were retaining nitrogen with methionine intakes of 0.29 to 0.60 g/day.

In studies on lysine requirements, Tuttle et al. (87) found in a group of four men 53 to 64 years old that 1.4 g lysine was insufficient to maintain positive nitrogen balance in two of the subjects. When 2.8 g lysine were fed, all subjects were in positive balance. These levels, much higher than Rose's tentative minimum requirements for young men (19), are also higher than levels at which positive balances were obtained by Swendseid et al. (86) when purified amino acids were fed in the egg pattern to young men.

With the exception of a paper by Albanese et al. (88) who observed that lysine supplements apparently improved nitrogen balance in eight out of 20 elderly ladies, no reports of controlled studies on the amino acid requirements of postmenopausal women have been found.

AMINO ACID REQUIREMENTS OF CHILDREN OF SCHOOL AGE

The literature on the determination of amino acid requirements of school age children is composed principally of the reports of Japanese investigators. Fukui and his associates (89) reported that additions of lysine to the normal diet of Japanese children, 4 to 14 years old, were effective in improving height and weight gains. They concluded that a lysine/tryptophan ratio of six was best for growth in these children, and they calculated a "growing stage amino acid ratio" based on previous work on amino acid requirements of infants, adult humans and growing rats. They did not, however, attempt to determine by experimental means the quantitative requirements of the growing child for amino acids. This work has been the contribution of Nakagawa and his coworkers.

Initially, Nakagawa et al. (90) ascertained that a diet containing 10 g nitrogen and the kind and minimum quantity of amino acids estimated by Rose et al. (19) to be essential for young men was not adequate for maintaining three boys, 13 to

14 years old, in positive balance. When Nakagawa doubled the quantities of the essential amino acids and increased the total nitrogen level to 14 g, all three boys were in positive nitrogen balance. One boy, however, continued to lose weight. In a second group of five 12-year-old boys, diets containing 12 g total nitrogen and triple the amount of amino acids in Rose's tentative minimum requirements were adequate to maintain nitrogen balance. With these results as a guide, Nakagawa et al. undertook the determination of the requirement for the individual amino acids. Their purified diets contained 12 g total nitrogen. The essential L-amino acids were provided in amounts equal to three times Rose's minimal requirement levels. Histidine was also included among the essential amino acids. The nonessential nitrogen was provided by a mixture of glycine, L-glutamic acid, Na-L-glutamate and L-arginine. This mixture was modified during the studies to include also L-alanine, L-aspartic acid, L-proline, and L-serine. When the level of the essential amino acid under study was lowered or raised, isonitrogenous adjustments were made in the nonessential amino acid portion. Energy was provided by cornstarch, sucrose, butterfat, and corn oil. Each amino acid was studied with three to five boys, 11 to 12 years of age. The collection periods during which nitrogen balance was determined varied from 3 to 7 days in length. The urinary excretions of creatine, creatinine, riboflavin and N-methyl-nicotinamide were also recorded. The levels of the essential amino acids found necessary to maintain the boys in positive nitrogen balance were as follows: isoleucine 1.0 g/day or 30 mg/kg, leucine 1.5 g/day or 45 mg/kg (91); lysine 1.6 g/day or 60 mg/kg, methionine 0.8 g/day or 27 mg/kg (92); phenylalanine 0.8 g/day or 27 mg/kg, threonine 1.0 g/day or 35 mg/kg (93); tryptophan 0.12 g/day (25); valine 0.9 g/day or 33 mg/kg (93). The investigators also concluded that neither histidine nor arginine was essential to maintain positive nitrogen balance (25).

Next the Japanese team found that the amounts of essential amino acids estimated as necessary for their boys to maintain positive nitrogen balance were adequate for six girls, 8 to 13 years old (94). The minimum essential amino acid requirements of the girls were not determined. The amount of total nitrogen needed by the girls varied from 8 g/day for the youngest girl to 12 g/day for two of the oldest girls. The investigators suggested that the greater range in total nitrogen requirement of the girls as compared to that of the boys might have been because the pubertal growth spurt occurs earlier in girls than in boys. It should be noted that the Japanese studies were not designed to measure growth or the amino acid requirements for growth. To date, there are no data available on the amino acid requirements of either boys or girls during puberty or afterward while they are still in the adolescent period. In the younger age group (preadolescent) there are data on the metabolic response of 7- to 9-year-old girls to diets that differed in level of protein (95). Because not only the quantity but also the kind of protein varied from study to study, estimates on the amino acid requirements of these children are difficult.

AMINO ACID REQUIREMENTS OF INFANTS

In most of the studies on infants' requirements for amino acids, nitrogen balance, weight gain and/or blood components such as plasma proteins, hemoglobin or nonprotein nitrogen were used as the criteria by which adequacy of intake was measured. In a few studies, urinary components were estimated. A large part of the work was done by Snyderman and her associates. Other investigators have made sufficient contributions, however, to warrant the review of each essential amino acid individually.

In the work of Snyderman and her associates, mixtures of 18 L-amino acids simulating the protein composition of breast milk were used. A formula diet composed of the amino acid mixture, hydrogenated vegetable fat, dextri-maltose, minerals, and vitamins was prepared to provide 125 to 150 kcal/kilogram body weight and to meet the other nutrient needs of the subjects. After a control period in which the full complement of amino acids was fed, the amino acid under study was totally replaced by glycine and then was added back into the diet in a step-wise manner (15). Nitrogen balance, weight gains, total plasma protein, plasma albumin, and plasma globulin were usually measured. An adequate amino acid intake was considered to be one which permitted growth and nitrogen retention to proceed at the same rate as was observed with the control diet.

There has been some disagreement as to whether the results of experiments in which diets based on purified amino acids and nonessential nitrogen are used, give as accurate a measure of the needs of the subject as those obtained with diets based on intact protein. Snyderman used both procedures (96). In some of her studies she used diluted cow's milk formulas with added nonessential nitrogen. The amino acid content of the most dilute formula that would maintain normal growth and nitrogen retention was regarded as an indication of the amino acid requirement of the infant. Amino acid requirements determined with the diluted milk formula were usually similar to and sometimes a little lower than those determined with mixtures of purified amino acids.

Arginine was found to be apparently nonessential. Snyderman et al. (97) using a purified amino acid mixture found that three male infants, 1.5 weeks to 3.5 months old, maintained excellent health, gained weight, and retained nitrogen adequately when arginine was completely removed from their diets for periods ranging from 14 to 35 days. Thus arginine has not been proved to be essential for any age group so far studied.

Histidine, on the other hand, found to be apparently nonessential for young adults and school-age children, was found to be essential for infants (24). Eight normal male infants, 2 weeks to 7 months in age were studied. All ceased to make adequate weight gains when histidine was removed from the diet. Six infants showed significantly reduced nitrogen retention. Among the younger babies (under 2 months) a scaly rash appeared. The rash disappeared shortly after histidine was reincorporated into the diet. Intakes of less than 35 mg histidine/kilogram/day were found to be adequate for all babies. One child was maintained with 16.6 mg/kg per day, but two babies required more than 22 mg/kg

per day. Four other infants who were fed a diluted milk plus nonessential nitrogen diet were maintained adequately with a calculated histidine intake of 24 mg/kg per day.

Isoleucine has been studied by several investigators (98–100). Albanese et al. (98) used hydrolyzed beef hemoglobin (low in isoleucine) with added tryptophan and cystine as the nitrogen source. Additional calories were supplied by olive oil, dextrimaltose and arrowroot starch. Fomon et al. (99) used soybean flour as the nitrogen source. Energy-yielding adjuncts were olive oil, corn oil, arrowroot starch, lactose, maltose and dextrin. Synderman et al. (100) as in their previously described studies (15) used a purified amino acid mixture plus hydrogenated vegetable fat and dextri-maltose.

In Albanese's study (98) the addition of L-isoleucine to the diet (containing hydrolyzed beef hemoglobin) to provide an intake of 126, 216, or 306 mg isoleucine/kilogram per day during 7-day periods at each level, permitted three male infants, 4 to 10 months old, to retain nitrogen and to gain weight at the same rate as they did with their customary evaporated milk formula. With two other male infants, 90 mg isoleucine/kilogram per day permitted normal growth and nitrogen retention, but 60 mg did not. Albanese concluded that "the infant requires approximately 90 mg of L-isoleucine/kilogram per day."

Fomon's study (99) consisted of feeding a formula based on soy flour to five healthy male infants. Food intake and gains in weight and length were measured over 28-day periods during the first 45 days of life, during the third month, and, with one child, during the fifth month of life. Nitrogen balances were determined during 3-day periods intermittently throughout the study. The data showed adequate nitrogen retention and growth increments with daily isoleucine intakes of 82 to 91 mg/kg during the first 45 days, 67 to 85 mg/kg during the third month and 63.5 mg/kg during the fifth month (a range of 63 to 91 mg/kg per day for babies under 5 months of age). There was no evidence that the isoleucine level of the soy flour was limiting.

Snyderman's six infants (100) were all under 1 month of age when the individual studies began. Most of the studies lasted 3 to 4 months. The infants, fed purified amino acids with isoleucine intakes varying from 79 to 126 mg/kg per day, were able to maintain nitrogen retentions and growth increments comparable to those obtained with evaporated milk formulas. This range is higher than, but probably not significantly different from, that observed by Fomon in his infants studied over a similar age span but with the amino acids provided in intact protein. With other infants, fed diluted milk and nonessential nitrogen formulas, Snyderman reported that adequate nitrogen retention and growth were obtained with isoleucine intakes of 71 to 84 mg/kg per day. Snyderman et al. also observed that with isoleucine deprivation the plasma amino acid pattern was changed — the concentration of isoleucine was reduced, whereas those of tyrosine, phenylalanine, valine, serine, and lysine were increased.

Leucine requirements of infants, determined by Snyderman et al. (101), showed wide divergence reminiscent of the divergence observed in Rose's studies with young men (36). Five full-term male infants, 9 days, 15 days, 1, 2, and 5 months old, and one premature infant, 6 weeks old at the beginning of the study, were observed. Adequate leucine intakes for growth and nitrogen retention of the infants listed in the above order were found to be 150, 145, 76, 154, 229, and 113 mg/kg per day. Thus, all but one child could have been maintained adequately with approximately 150 mg leucine/kilogram per day or less. Complete deprivation of leucine resulted in lower concentrations of leucine in the plasma but in higher concentrations of some other free amino acids — most notably valine.

Lysine requirement was studied by Snyderman et al. (102). Six male infants, 1 to 5 months old, fed purified amino acid mixtures, grew and retained nitrogen normally with intakes of 90 to 105 mg lysine/kilogram. Four other infants maintained on a diluted milk plus nonessential nitrogen formula throve on an average intake of 84 mg/kg. As Snyderman et al. point out, these levels are much lower than

that of 140 to 200 mg/kg reported by Albanese (103) who used a diet in which the protein was supplied by wheat gluten. The metabolic data of Albanese's study were not included in his report.

Infant response to lysine supplementation was studied by Albanese and Lein (104) and by Dubow et al. (105). Albanese and Lein observed that supplementation with D-lysine resulted in a urinary lysine excretion that was much greater than that found when an equal level of L-lysine supplement was used. They concluded from this observation that the infant does not use D-lysine for growth. Dubow et al. (105) studied the tolerance of infants to supplementation with L-lysine. Six nonfebrile convalescent infants, 4 to 11 months in age, received a whole milk formula to which were added graded supplements of lysine monohydrochloride in seven successive 3- to 4-day periods. The highest intake of lysine studied was 5.18 g/day. No adverse clinical symptoms were noted at any level of supplementation. Plasma amino acid patterns were not markedly altered although there was an initial increase in total plasma amino acids. Urinary lysine excretion was somewhat proportional to the level of supplementation. It appears, therefore, that if there is an upper limit to the infant's tolerance for lysine, it is above the range studied by Dubow.

Sulfur-containing amino acid metabolism by infants was studied by Thurau (106) with eight healthy babies fed cow's milk formulas of various dilutions. Thurau, having noted that human milk contains a greater proportion of cystine than does cow's milk, added either cystine or methionine to the milk formulas and made daily analyses of the infants' urinary excretions. When even small amounts of methionine were added to the diet, urinary excretion of methionine or sulfur compounds rose. When small quantities (0.03%) of cystine were added to the milk the urinary cystine and sulfur excretions fell, but rose again when the cystine intake was doubled or tripled. Thurau concluded from these observations that the infant is less capable than the adult of converting methionine into cystine and that cystine might have an important role in the diet of artificially fed babies.

Albanese et al. (107), however, obtained data with five healthy infants that convinced them that methionine but not cystine was essential for the human infant. The babies were fed a diet in which the protein was provided by oxidized casein hydrolysate supplemented with tryptophan. Olive oil, dextri-maltose, and arrowroot starch provided additional calories. Methionine and cystine were added in graded amounts to this diet. The addition of methionine alone to this diet to give a total intake of 85 mg methionine/kilogram body weight restored normal weight gain and nitrogen retention whereas the addition of cystine alone failed to effect any improvement. Various combinations of cystine and methionine were tried. The intake of 50 mg cystine plus 65 mg methionine/kilogram brought about the same improvement as the intake of 15 mg cystine and 85 mg methionine. These results led the investigators to conclude that while cystine is not essential for the infant, it does spare methionine (35 mg cystine spares 20 mg methionine) and that about 22% of the methionine requirement can be met by cystine. This is considerably less than the sparing value of cystine for methionine observed in adults (58).

Fomon et al. (99), using a soy flour formula as described previously, and Snyderman et al. (108), using both a purified amino acid mixture and a diluted cow's milk formula, also studied methionine requirements. Fomon's infants grew well and retained nitrogen with methionine intakes of 25 to 28 mg/kg during the first 45 days of life, 20 to 26 mg/kg during the third month and 19.6 mg/kg during the fifth month — a range of 20 to 28 mg/kg. The cystine content of the soy flour used in this study was not determined. Analysis of three similar batches, however, indicated that it was just slightly less than the methionine content (0.95, 0.95 and 1.04 mg cystine/16 mg nitrogen as compared to 0.99, 1.08 and 1.12 mg methionine/16 mg nitrogen).

Snyderman et al. (108) fed their purified amino acid diet to seven male infants who were 2 weeks to 2 months old at the beginning of the study. The methionine re-

quirement of these babies was found to range from 32 to 49 mg/kg. The cystine in the diets was kept constant at the level found in breast milk (2.14 g cystine/100 g total amino acids). The investigators suggested that their methionine requirement values might be modified if the cystine level were changed. They noted that the infants fed the diluted cow's milk with nonessential nitrogen diet were maintained adequately with methionine levels ranging from 30 to 35 mg/kg. They also noted that, during methionine deficiency, analysis of the infants' plasma showed elevated concentrations of threonine, proline, serine, phenylalanine, and, most strikingly, of tyrosine.

In contrast to the preceding studies whose objective was to determine the least amount of methionine adequate for maintenance and growth, Goldstein (109) attempted to determine how much methionine could be safely added to the diet. One hundred and eighty-nine infants were studied for about 9 to 10 months. Of these, 109 infants served as controls receiving a proprietary formula providing about 360 mg methionine/day. The others in groups of 50, 20 and 10 infants received supplements of 90, 180 and 360 mg DL-methionine/day. The infants receiving diets supplemented with 180 mg DL-methionine/day (total intake = 540 mg/day) showed weight gains superior to those in the other groups whereas those receiving a total of about 720 mg/day exhibited impaired growth and diuresis. Goldstein concluded that methionine can be toxic at high levels of intake but that the unpleasant flavor and aroma imparted by it to the milk makes it unlikely that an infant would either accidentally or voluntarily ingest a toxic amount.

Phenylalanine and tyrosine utilization was studied by Levine et al. (110). In a study with eight premature and two full-term healthy infants the urinary and fecal excretions of phenylalanine and tyrosine after supplemental feeding of either amino acid were measured. The observation that phenylalanine and its derivatives were not excreted when tyrosine was fed, whereas tyrosine and its derivatives were excreted when phenylalanine was fed, led them to conclude that, in the human infant, L-tyrosine cannot replace DL-phenylalanine. No attempt appears to have been made to determine whether tyrosine has any sparing effect on the infant's requirement for phenylalanine as has been observed in adult subjects (66–69).

Snyderman et al. (111), using their customary purified amino acid mixture with six normal male infants 1 to 9 months old, found adequate weight gains with phenylalanine intakes ranging from 47 to 94 mg/kg per day. The investigators suggested a value of 90 mg/kg per day as the infant's phenylalanine requirement. This value fell well within the calculated range of phenylalanine intake of an infant fed pooled breast milk for the first 4.5 months of life. This range of 87 to 131 mg phenylalanine/kilogram was calculated by Snyderman from food intake data of Swanson (112) and milk composition data of Macy et al. (113).

Threonine requirements were studied in a group of eight infants, 6 days to 4.5 months old (15). These studies showed that threonine intakes ranging from 45 to 87 mg/kg per day were adequate to maintain weight gains and positive nitrogen balance in five of the babies. With the other infants, adequate intakes were not determined.

Tryptophan requirements have been estimated by Albanese et al. (114) and by Snyderman et al. (115). In the Albanese study (114), three male infants, 6 to 12 months old, were fed diets based on hydrolyzed casein supplemented with cystine to which graded amounts of tryptophan were added. Intakes of 6 mg tryptophan/ kilogram were inadequate and intakes of 59 mg/kg were apparently more than adequate. One of the infants was studied with intermediate levels of 23 and 40 mg/kg. The results indicated that this infant's requirement lay between these two levels. From these data, Albanese et al. concluded that the infant requires approximately 30 mg L-tryptophan/kilogram per day for normal growth and nitrogen retention.

Seven infants (five male, two female) studied by Snyderman et al. (115) were fed the customary purified amino acid mixture. All the babies grew well and retained nitrogen with intakes of about 22 mg tryptophan/kilogram. Four of the babies who were studied with intakes of about 16 mg/kg throve with this level of intake also. Three of the babies tested at still lower levels (about 13 mg/kg) did not grow as well and nitrogen retention declined. Snyderman et al. concluded, therefore, that the tryptophan requirement of a normally growing baby probably lies between 13 and 16 mg/kg per day. They pointed out, however, that their diets contained "adequate amounts of nicotinic acid" and that, with deficient intakes of nicotinic acid, the tryptophan requirement might increase.

Valine, the last of the amino acids to be discussed here, was studied by Snyderman et al. (116) and by Fomon et al. (99). Snyderman's five infants were 3 weeks to 3.5 months old when the study began. They were fed formulas containing purified amino acid mixtures as previously described. Normal weight gains and nitrogen retentions were observed in two infants with valine intakes of 105 mg/kg per day. For the other three infants, 85 to 87 mg valine/kilogram per day sufficed. Another group of four infants was reported to have gained weight and retained nitrogen adequately with a diluted milk diet supplemented with nonessential nitrogen that supplied 80 mg valine/kilogram.

In the Fomon study, in which isoleucine and methionine requirements were also studied, five infants maintained adequate weight gains and nitrogen retention when eating sufficient amounts of the diet to provide 65 to 115 mg valine/kilogram body weight. This is a wider range than that observed by Snyderman but as in the study of isoleucine and methionine, the values observed in the two laboratories fall within the same area.

COMMENTS ON AMINO ACID REQUIREMENTS

The studies that have provided data indicating minimum quantitative requirements for essential amino acids have been tabulated in table 1. Several observations may be made on the contents of this table. One observation is that there are no data on the amino acid needs of children from 1 to 10 years of age or of adolescents. Thus, information on two critical stages — post weaning and during puberty — is

TABLE 1

Quantitative amino acid requirements

Amino acid	Infant[1]	School child[1]	Young adult[1]	Elderly[1]	Criteria	References
1. Arginine	Nonessential (3)[2]	Nonessential (3 M)[2]	Possibly essential (3 M)		N retention, growth	97
					N retention	25
					Spermatogenesis	13
			Nonessential (6 M)		N retention, spermatogenesis	18, 19
2. Histidine	16 to 34 mg/kg (6)	Nonessential (4 M)	Possibly essential (3 M)		N retention	24
					N retention	25
					Aberrant metabolite in urine	21
			Nonessential (4 M)		N retention	19, 20, 22, 23
3. Isoleucine	90 mg/kg(2)	1.0 g/day (2 M)	0.65 to 0.70 g/day (4 M)		N retention, growth	98
	17 to 126 mg/kg (6)				N retention, growth	100
	71 to 84 mg/kg (4)				N retention, growth	100
	63 to 115 mg/kg (5)				N retention, growth	99
			250 to 450 mg/day (7 F)[2]		N retention	91
					N retention	36
			>422 mg/day (3 M, 8 F)		N equilibrium	11
					N retention and equilibrium	37
4. Leucine	76 to 226 mg/kg (6)	1.0 to 1.5 g/day (3 M)	0.5 to 1.1 g/day (5 M)		N retention, growth	101
			170 to 710 mg/day (13 F)		N retention	91
					N retention	36
					N equilibrium	39
5. Lysine	140 to 200 mg/kg (?)	1.2 to 1.6 g/day (5 M)	0.4 to 0.8 g/day (6 M)		N retention, growth	103
	90 to 105 mg/kg (6)		0.4 to 0.5 g/day (14 F)		N retention	102
			500 to 900 mg/day (5 M, 5 F)		N retention	92
			400 to 1200 mg/day (5 M)		N retention	44
					N equilibrium	9
			300 to 700 mg/day (5 F)		N retention	45
			50 mg/day (5 F)		N retention	46
					N retention	46
					N retention	47
				1.4 to 2.8 g/day (4 M)	N retention	87

	Requirement	Intake	Criterion	Ref.
6. Methionine and cystine	15 mg cystine+85 mg methionine/kg or 50 mg cystine+65 mg methionine/kg (5)		N retention, growth	107
	32 to 49 mg methionine/kg with adequate cystine (7)		N retention, growth	108
	30 to 35 mg methionine/kg (4)		N retention, growth	108
	20 to 36 mg methionine/kg (5)		N retention, growth	99
		0.8 to 1.1 g/day (6 M) (no cystine)	N retention	92
		150 to 350 mg/day plus 200 mg cystine (8 F)	N retention	57
		75 mg methionine plus 100 mg cystine/day	N equilibrium	63
		300 to 550 mg total sulfur amino acids/day (20 F)	N equilibrium	10
	0.4 to 0.8 g/day (4 M)	2.4 to 3.0 g/day (6 M)	N retention	87
		0.29 to 0.60 g/day (6 M)	N retention	85
7. Phenylalanine	47 to 94 mg/kg (6)	0.8 to 1.1 g/day (6 M) (no tyrosine)	N retention, growth	111
		834 to 1184 mg/day (6 F) (no tyrosine)	N retention	93
		600 to 700 mg/day (13 F)	N retention	65
		900 to 1000 mg/day (9 M) (no tyrosine)	N retention	68
		120 to 220 mg/day (with 900 mg tyrosine) (10 F)	N retention and equilibrium	69
		400 to 500 mg/day (with 200 mg tyrosine) (9 F, 6 M)	N equilibrium	67
	0.4 to 0.8 g/day (4 M)	300 to 400 mg/day (with 400 mg tyrosine) (6 F)	N equilibrium	69
		500 to 600 mg/day (with 400 mg tyrosine) (9 M)	N retention	69
			N retention	69

TABLE 1 (continued)

Quantitative amino acid requirements

Amino acid	Infant[1]	School child[1]	Young adult[1]	Elderly[1]	Criteria	References
8. Threonine	45 to 87 mg/kg (8)	0.8 to 1.0 g/day (4 M)			N retention, growth	15
					N retention	93
			0.3 to 1.5 g/day (3 M)		N retention	57
			103 to 305 mg/day (15 F)		N equilibrium	8
9. Tryptophan	23 to 40 mg/kg (3)				N retention, growth	114
	13 to 16 mg/kg (7)				N retention, growth	115
		0.06 to 0.12 g/day (4 M)			N retention	25
			6 to 9 mg/kg (2 M)		N retention	74
			3 to 6 mg/kg (2 M)		Urinary excretion	74
			0.24 g/day (7 M)		N retention	75
			0.15 to 0.25 g/day (3 M)		N retention	7
			225 mg/day (5 M)		N retention	79
			3 mg/kg (5 M)		Plasma levels	16
			2.0 to 2.6 mg/kg (5 M)		N retention	16
			82 to 157 mg/day (8 F)		N equilibrium	76
			50 mg/day (5 F)		N retention	47
10. Valine	85 to 105 mg/kg (5)				N retention, growth	116
	80 mg/kg (4)				N retention, growth	116
	65 to 115 mg/kg (5)				N retention, growth	99
		0.6 to 0.9 g/day (4 M)			N retention	93
			0.4 to 0.8 g/day (5 M)		N retention	19
			465 to 650 mg/day (7 F)		N equilibrium	81
			230 to 480 mg/day (7 F)		N equilibrium	82

[1] The infants studied ranged in age from 6 days to 11 months. The school children were Japanese boys, 11 to 12 years old. The young adults were mainly men and women of college age. The elderly were men 52 to 84 years old.
[2] Figures in parentheses indicate number of subjects; M = male; F = female.

missing. Information on another period of great nutritional demand — pregnancy and lactation — is also unavailable. In addition, the needs of old age have not been studied fully. As yet, it is not clear whether the elderly really have requirements that are significantly different from those of young adults. In a population where the number of people surviving to old age is increasing, this should be an important subject for research.

Another observation is that, even in the population groups that have been studied (infants under 1 year of age, children 11 to 12 years of age, young men and women) the number of subjects studied has been small. The problem is a difficult one and the studies are expensive and arduous. This accounts at least in part for the relatively few subjects.

None of the authors of the publications on amino acid requirements has provided statistical estimates of the accuracy of the requirement figures. Hegsted (117) attempted to estimate the requirements from the nitrogen balance data on young men and women by calculating the regression of nitrogen balance upon amino acid intake and the estimated error in the intake at which nitrogen balance was achieved. These calculations indicated that the data obtained with young men and the data obtained with young women generally fall in the same region. Thus, for most of the amino acids, the requirement of young men does not appear to be substantially different from that of young women. The relatively higher estimates of Rose (48) are largely the result of the criteria used and do indeed appear to be high as Rose suggested they were. The data on young women, therefore, appear to provide better estimates of the minimal requirements for young adults. The error in these estimated requirements, however, at least for several of the amino acids, is very large indeed. For most of the amino acids the estimated requirement may be no more accurate than ± 50%. It is particularly distressing that the estimated requirements of lysine, methionine and isoleucine — amino acids which are thought to be limiting in many food proteins (118) — are those for which we appear to have the least satisfactory estimates. The practical significance of additional data on these amino acids, as well as others, is obvious.

Part of the disagreement between studies may be the result of differences in methodology (e.g., feeding purified amino acids versus intact protein or protein hydrolysates). Differences in criteria for judging the adequacy of amino acid intake are also sources of disagreement (e.g., urinary amino acid excretion versus nitrogen retention). In the majority of the studies, nitrogen balance has been determined. Whether the criterion for adequate intake was positive retention or retention in the equilibrium zone, the sources of error inherent in the nitrogen balance determination could cause considerable variations in apparent response to the dietary treatment. Clark et al. (49–51) have demonstrated that, even in well-controlled experiments, nitrogen balance can be manipulated by factors other than the treatment under study.

The reliability of the estimates of the requirements of young children published by Snyderman and her co-workers also cannot be determined. This is not stated as a criticism of only this excellent and painstaking series of papers. It is a general criticism of nearly all data upon nutritional requirements of man. It indicates not only the need for more data, but for continual thought toward the development of new experimental designs, more sensitive and easier criteria, and for critical statistical evaluation.

The cause of the wide variations observed in the requirements of individuals or the scatter of the data obtained is also unexplained. Inspection of the data from specific individuals strongly suggests that there are large inherent differences in individual requirements. The data, however, are insufficient to provide an estimate of the error in the apparent requirement of an individual subject and thus to prove that his requirement is truly different from that of another. In any event, an average requirement is an inadequate base from which to establish safe "allowances" or dietary recommendations. These must be established enough above average needs to provide for most subjects and thus an estimate of the range of requirements (apart from errors in the determinations of such requirements) is important.

In the final analysis, these data will not be of practical importance unless the data on amino acid requirements, protein requirements, and the nutritional quality of proteins provide a consistent understandable pattern. At present they do not do so. The sum of the essential amino acids apparently required by young women is approximately 4 grams of amino acids. These amounts may be supplied by 8 to 10 grams of high quality protein, amounts substantially less than estimated protein requirements. Indeed, this amount of nitrogen approaches the very lowest estimates of endogenous nitrogen excretion such as those achieved by Smith (119) after long periods on a nitrogen-free diet. Estimated protein requirements of either high or low quality proteins (120) appear to provide all of the essential amino acids in excess of minimal needs. It does not appear that the studies conducted so far using different levels of total nitrogen, different kinds of nonessential nitrogen, etc., reasonably explain why more protein is apparently required than is necessary to meet the essential amino acid needs. There are data indicating that some of the high quality proteins may be diluted with nonessential nitrogen without a measurable impairment in nutritional quality (96, 60). It is not clear, however, whether this dilution is sufficient to account for the discrepancy between the estimated protein requirements and the estimated essential amino acid requirements of man. Until such information is available, the data on amino acid requirements will remain of doubtful value in the development of practical nutrition standards.

ACKNOWLEDGMENTS

The authors wish to thank the staff of the Francis A. Countway Library of Medicine, Boston, Massachusetts, for their assistance and for putting the excellent facilities of the library at our disposal.

We also thank Miss Carol Fritz for her assistance in collecting documents in the early stage of the project.

LITERATURE CITED

1. Wollaston, W. H. 1810 Phil. Trans. Roy. Soc. p. 223. Cited by: Sahyun, M. 1944 Outline of the Amino Acids and Protein. Reinhold Publishing Corp., p. 13.
2. Kühne, W. 1867 Arch. Pathol. Anat. Physiol. Virchow's Arch. 39: 130. Cited by: Greenstein, J. P., and M. Winitz 1961 Chemistry of Amino Acids, vol. 1. John Wiley & Sons, Inc., New York, p. 250.
3. Blum, L. 1900 Z. Physiol. Chem. 30: 15. Cited by: Greenstein, J. P., and M. Winitz 1961 Chemistry of Amino Acids, vol. 1. John Wiley & Sons, Inc., New York, p. 253.
4. Kauffmann, M. 1905 Über den Ersatz von Eiweiss durch Leim im Stoffwechsel. Pflüger's Arch. 109: 440. Cited by: Greenstein, J. P., and M. Winitz 1961 Chemistry of Amino Acids, vol. 1. John Wiley & Sons, Inc., New York, p. 259.
5. Willcock, E. G., and F. G. Hopkins 1906 The importance of individual amino acids in metabolism. Observations on the effect of adding tryptophane to a dietary in which zein is the sole nitrogenous constituent. J. Physiol. 35: 88.
6. Osborne, T. B., and L. B. Mendel 1914 Amino acids in nutrition and growth. J. Biol. Chem. 17: 325.
7. Rose, W. C., G. F. Lambert and M. J. Coon 1954 The amino acid requirements of man. VII. General procedures; the tryptophan requirement. J. Biol. Chem. 211: 815.
8. Leverton, R. M., M. R. Gram, M. Chaloupka, E. Brodovsky and A. Mitchell 1956 The quantitative amino acid requirements of young women. 1. Threonine. J. Nutr. 58: 59.
9. Jones, E. M., C. A. Baumann and M. S. Reynolds 1956 Nitrogen balances of women maintained on various levels of lysine. J. Nutr. 60: 549.
10. Reynolds, M. S., D. L. Steel, E. M. Jones and C. A. Baumann 1958 Nitrogen balances of women maintained on various levels of methionine and cystine. J. Nutr. 64: 99.
11. Swendseid, M. E., and M. S. Dunn 1956 Amino acid requirements of young women based on nitrogen balance data. II. Studies on isoleucine and on minimum amounts of the eight essential amino acids fed simultaneously. J. Nutr. 58: 507.
12. Rose, W. C., J. E. Johnson and W. J. Haines 1950 The amino acid requirements of man. I. The role of valine and methionine. J. Biol. Chem. 182: 541.
13. Holt, L. E., Jr., and A. A. Albanese 1944 Observations on amino acid deficiencies in man. Trans. Ass. Amer. Physicians 58: 143.
14. Albanese, A. A., V. Irby and J. E. Frankston 1945 The utilization of d-amino acids by man. 3. Arginine. J. Biol. Chem. 160: 25.
15. Pratt, E. L., S. E. Snyderman, M. W. Cheung, P. Norton, L. E. Holt, Jr., A. E. Hansen and T. C. Panos 1955 The threonine requirement of the normal infant. J. Nutr. 56: 231.
16. Young, V. R., M. A. Hussein, E. Murray and N. S. Scrimshaw 1971 Plasma tryptophan response curve and its relation to

tryptophan requirements in young adult men. J. Nutr. *101:* 45.

17. Harte, R. A., and J. J. Travers 1947 Human amino acid requirements. Science *105:* 15.

18. Rose, W. C., W. J. Haines and D. T. Warner 1954 The amino acid requirements of man. V. The role of lysine, arginine, and tryptophan. J. Biol. Chem. *206:* 421.

19. Rose, W. C., R. L. Wixom, H. B. Lockhart and G. F. Lambert 1955 The amino acid requirements of man. XV. The valine requirement; summary and final observations. J. Biol. Chem. *217:* 987.

20. Rose, W. C., W. J. Haines, J. E. Johnson and D. T. Warner 1943 Further experiments on the role of the amino acids in human nutrition. J. Biol. Chem. *148:* 457.

21. Albanese, A. A., L. E. Holt, Jr., J. E. Frankston and V. Irby 1944 Observations on a histidine deficient diet in man. Bull. Johns Hopkins Hosp. *74:* 251.

22. Rose, W. C., W. J. Haines, D. T. Warner and J. E. Johnson 1951 The amino acid requirements of man. II. The role of threonine and histidine. J. Biol. Chem. *188:* 49.

23. Rose, W. C., W. J. Haines and D. T. Warner 1951 The amino acid requirements of man. III. The role of isoleucine; additional evidence concerning histidine. J. Biol. Chem. *193:* 605.

24. Snyderman, S. E., A. Boyer, E. Roitman, L. E. Holt, Jr. and P. H. Prose 1963 The histidine requirement of the infant. Pediatrics *31:* 786.

25. Nakagawa, I., T. Takahashi, T. Suzuki and K. Kobayashi 1963 Amino acid requirements of children: minimal needs of tryptophan, arginine and histidine based on nitrogen balance method. J. Nutr. *80:* 305.

26. Greenstein, J. P., and M. Winitz 1961 Chemistry of Amino Acids, vol. 1. John Wiley & Sons, Inc., New York, p. 293.

27. Cox, G. J., and W. C. Rose 1926 The availability of synthetic imidazoles in supplementing diets deficient in histidine. J. Biol. Chem. *68:* 781.

28. Harrow, B., and C. P. Sherwin 1926 Synthesis of amino acids in the animal body. IV. Synthesis of histidine. J. Biol. Chem. *70:* 683.

29. Lehniger, A. L. 1950 Role of metal ions in enzyme systems. Physiol. Rev. *30:* 393.

30. Clifford, W. M. 1921 The distribution of carnosine in the animal kingdom. Biochem. J. *15:* 725.

31. Baumann, L., and T. Ingvaldsen 1918 Concerning histidine and carnosine. The synthesis of carnosine. J. Biol. Chem. *35:* 263.

32. Barger, G., and F. Tutin 1918 Carnosine, constitution and synthesis. Biochem. J. *12:* 402.

32a. Nasset, E. S., and V. H. Gatewood 1954 Nitrogen balance and hemoglobin of adult rats fed amino acid diets low in L- and D-histidine. J. Nutr. *53:* 163.

32b. Josephson, B., J. Bergstrom, H. Bucht, D. Dahlinder, P. Fürst, E. Hultman, L. D. Norée and E. Vinnars 1969 Intravenös aminosyranutrition vid kronisk uremi. Nord. Med. *81:* 770.

32c. Anonymous 1969 How "nonessential" is histidine? Medical World News, p. 35: November 7, 1969.

33. Kofrányi, E., F. Jekat, K. Brand, K. Hackenberg and B. Hess 1969 Zur Bestimmung der biologischen Wertigkeit von Nahrungsproteinen. XIII. Die Frage der Essentialität von Arginin und Histidin. Hoppe-Seyler's Z. Physiol. Chem. *350:* 1401.

34. Munro, H. N. 1969 Evolution of protein metabolism in mammals. In: Mammalian Protein Metabolism, ed., H. N. Munro. vol. *3:* Academic Press, Inc., New York, p. 133.

35. Kapeller-Adler, R. 1941 Histidine metabolism in normal and toxaemic pregnancy. The excretion of histidine in normal pregnancy urine and in the urine of patients with toxaemia of pregnancy. J. Obstet. Gynecol. Brit. Empire *48:* 141.

36. Rose, W. C., C. H. Eades, Jr. and M. J. Coon 1955 The amino acid requirements of man. XII. The leucine and isoleucine requirements. J. Biol. Chem. *216:* 225.

37. Linkswiler, H., H. M. Fox and P. C. Fry 1960 Availability to man of amino acids from foods. 4. Isoleucine from corn. J. Nutr. *72:* 397.

38. Rose, W. C., D. T. Warner and W. J. Haines 1951 The amino acid requirements of man. IV. The role of leucine and phenylalanine. J. Biol. Chem. *193:* 613.

39. Leverton, R. M., J. Ellison, N. Johnson, J. Pazur, F. Schmidt and D. Geschwender 1956 The quantitative amino acid requirements of young women. V. Leucine. J. Nutr. *58:* 355.

40. Albanese, A. A., L. E. Holt, Jr., M. Hayes, C. Kajdi and D. M. Wangerin 1941 Nitrogen balance in experimental lysine deficiency in man. Proc. Soc. Exp. Biol. Med. *48:* 728.

41. Albanese, A. A., L. E. Holt, Jr., J. E. Frankston, C. N. Kajdi, J. E. Brumback, Jr. and D. M. Wangerin 1943 A biochemical lesion of lysine deficiency in man. Proc. Soc. Exp. Biol. Med. *52:* 209.

42. Rose, W. C. 1944 The role of protein in the diet. Proc. Inst. Med. Chicago *15:* 24.

43. Bricker, M., H. H. Mitchell and G. M. Kinsman 1945 The protein requirement of adult human subjects in terms of the protein contained in individual foods and food combinations. J. Nutr. *30:* 269.

44. Rose, W. C., A. Borman, M. J. Coon and G. F. Lambert 1955 The amino acid requirements of man. X. The lysine requirement. J. Biol. Chem. *214:* 579.

45. Clark, H. E., E. T. Mertz, E. H. Kwong, J. M. Howe and D. C. DeLong 1957 Amino acid requirements of men and women. I. Lysine. J. Nutr. *62:* 71.

46. Clark, H. E., S. P. Yang, W. Walton and E. T. Mertz 1960 Amino acid requirements of men and women. II. Relation of lysine requirement to sex, body size, basal caloric expenditure and creatinine excretion. J. Nutr. 71: 229.

47. Fisher, H., M. K. Brush and P. Griminger 1969 Reassessment of amino acid requirements of young women on low nitrogen diets. 1. Lysine and tryptophan. Amer. J. Clin. Nutr. 22: 1190.

48. Rose, W. C. 1957 The amino acid requirements of adult man. Nutr. Abst. Rev. 27: 631.

49. Clark, H. E., S. P. Yang, L. L. Reitz and E. T. Mertz 1960 The effect of certain factors on nitrogen retention and lysine requirements of adult human subjects. I. Total caloric intake. J. Nutr. 72: 87.

50. Clark, H. E., L. L. Reitz, T. S. Vacharotayan and E. T. Mertz 1962 Effect of certain factors on nitrogen retention and lysine requirements of adult human subjects. II. Interval within experiment when dietary lysine and nitrogen were constant. J. Nutr. 78: 173.

51. Clark, H. E., N. J. Yess, E. J. Vermillion, A. F. Goodwin and E. T. Mertz 1963 Effect of certain factors on nitrogen retention and lysine requirements of adult human subjects. III. Source of supplementary nitrogen. J. Nutr. 79: 131.

52. Clark, H. E., M. A. Kenney, A. F. Goodwin, K. Goyal and E. T. Mertz 1963 Effect of certain factors on nitrogen retention and lysine requirements of adult human subjects. IV. Total nitrogen intake. J. Nutr. 81: 223.

53. Daggs, R. G. 1940 The effect of cystine on human milk production. Amer. J. Obstet. Gynecol. 40: 457.

54. Rose, W. C., W. J. Haines and J. E. Johnson 1942 The role of the amino acids in human nutrition. J. Biol. Chem. 146: 683.

55. Albanese, A. A., L. E. Holt, Jr., J. E. Brumback, Jr., C. N. Kajdi, J. E. Frankston and D. M. Wangerin 1943 Nitrogen balance in experimental human deficiencies of methionine and cystine. Proc. Soc. Exp. Biol. Med. 52: 18.

56. Albanese, A. A., L. E. Holt, Jr., J. E. Brumback, Jr., J. E. Frankston and V. Irby 1944 Observations on a diet deficient in both methionine and cystine in man. Bull. Johns Hopkins Hosp. 74: 308.

57. Rose, W. C., M. J. Coon, H. B. Lockhart and G. F. Lambert 1955 The amino acid requirements of man. XI. The threonine and methionine requirements. J. Biol. Chem. 215: 101.

58. Rose, W. C., and R. L. Wixom 1955 The amino acid requirements of man. XIII. The sparing effect of cystine on the methionine requirement. J. Biol. Chem. 216: 763.

59. Food and Agriculture Organization 1957 Protein Requirements. FAO Nutritional Studies, No. 16. Food and Agriculture Organization of the United Nations, Rome, Italy.

60. Scrimshaw, N. S., V. R. Young, R. Schwartz, M. L. Piché and J. B. Das 1966 Minimum dietary essential amino acid-to-total nitrogen ratio for whole egg protein fed to young men. J. Nutr. 89: 9.

61. Albanese, A. A. 1947 The utilization of d-amino acids by man. 1. Tryptophane, methionine, and phenylalanine. Bull. Johns Hopkins Hosp. 80: 175.

62. Camien, M. N., R. B. Malin and M. S. Dunn 1951 Urinary excretion of ingested L- and DL-methionines measured microbiologically. Arch. Biochem. 30: 62.

63. Swendseid, M. E., I. Williams and M. S. Dunn 1956 Amino acid requirements of young women based on nitrogen balance data. I. The sulfur-containing amino acids. J. Nutr. 58: 495.

64. Clark, H. E., and L. Woodward 1966 Influence of variable quantities of methionine on nitrogen retention of adult human subjects. Amer. J. Clin. Nutr. 18: 100.

65. Rose, W. C., B. E. Leach, M. J. Coon and G. F. Lambert 1955 The amino acid requirements of man. IX. The phenylalanine requirement. J. Biol. Chem. 213: 913.

66. Rose, W. C., and R. L. Wixom 1955 The amino acid requirements of man. XIV. The sparing effect of tyrosine on the phenylalanine requirement. J. Biol. Chem. 217: 95.

67. Leverton, R. M., N. Johnson, J. Ellison, D. Geschwender and F. Schmidt 1956 The quantitative amino acid requirements of young women. IV. Phenylalanine, with and without tyrosine. J. Nutr. 58: 341.

68. Tolbert, B., and J. H. Watts 1963 Phenylalanine requirement of women consuming a minimal tyrosine diet and the sparing effect of tyrosine on the phenylalanine requirement. J. Nutr. 80: 111.

69. Burrill, L. M., and C. Schuck 1964 Phenylalanine requirements with different levels of tyrosine. J. Nutr. 83: 202.

70. Linkswiler, H., H. M. Fox and P. C. Fry 1960 Availability to man of amino acids from foods. III. Threonine from corn. J. Nutr. 72: 389.

71. Wertz, A. W., M. B. Derby, P. K. Ruttenberg and G. P. French 1959 Urinary excretion of amino acids by the same women during and after pregnancy. J. Nutr. 68: 583.

72. Holt, L. E., Jr., A. A. Albanese, J. E. Brumback, Jr., C. Kajdi and D. M. Wangerin 1941 Nitrogen balance in experimental tryptophane deficiency in man. Proc. Soc. Exp. Biol. Med. 48: 726.

73. Cox, W. M., A. J. Mueller and D. Fickas 1942 Nitrogen balance in human tryptophane deficiency. Proc. Soc. Exp. Biol. Med. 51: 303.

74. Holt, L. E., Jr., A. A. Albanese, J. E. Frankston and V. Irby 1944 The tryptophane requirement of man as determined by nitrogen balance and by excretion of tryptophane in urine. Bull. Johns Hopkins Hosp. 75: 353.

75. Denko, C. W., and W. E. Grundy 1949 Minimum tryptophane requirement and urinary excretion of tryptophane by normal adults. J. Lab. Clin. Med. 34: 839.
76. Leverton, R. M., N. Johnson, J. Pazur and J. Ellison 1956 The quantitative amino acid requirements of young women. III. Tryptophan. J. Nutr. 58: 219.
77. Albanese, A. A., and J. E. Frankston 1944 A difference in the metabolism of L- and DL-tryptophane in the human. J. Biol. Chem. 155: 101.
78. Albanese, A. A., J. E. Frankston and V. Irby 1945 The utilization of d-amino acids by man. 4. Acetyltryptophane. J. Biol. Chem. 160: 31.
79. Baldwin, H. R., and C. P. Berg 1949 The influence of optical isomerism and acetylation upon the availability of tryptophan for maintenance in man. J. Nutr. 39: 203.
80. Rose, W. C., M. J. Coon, G. F. Lambert and E. E. Howe 1955 The amino acid requirements of man. VIII. The metabolic availability of the optical isomers of acetyltryptophan. J. Biol. Chem. 212: 201.
81. Leverton, R. M., M. R. Gram, E. Brodovsky, M. Chaloupka, A. Mitchell and N. Johnson 1956 The quantitative amino acid requirements of young women. II. Valine. J. Nutr. 58: 83.
82. Linkswiler, H., H. M. Fox, D. Geschwender and P. C. Fry 1958 Availability to man of amino acids from foods. II. Valine from corn. J. Nutr. 65: 455.
83. Tuttle, S. G., M. E. Swendseid, D. Mulcare, W. H. Griffith and S. H. Bassett 1957 Study of the essential amino acid requirements of men over fifty. Metabolism 6: 564.
84. Tuttle, S. G., M. E. Swendseid, D. Mulcare, W. H. Griffith and S. H. Bassett 1959 Essential amino acid requirements of older men in relation to total nitrogen intake. Metabolism 8: 61.
85. Watts, J. H., A. N. Mann, L. Bradley and D. J. Thompson 1964 Nitrogen balance of men over 65 fed the FAO and milk patterns of essential amino acids. J. Gerontol. 19: 370.
86. Swendseid, M. E., J. H. Watts, C. L. Harris and S. G. Tuttle 1961 An evaluation of the FAO amino acid reference pattern in human nutrition. I. Studies with young men. J. Nutr. 75: 295.
87. Tuttle, S. G., S. H. Bassett, W. H. Griffith, D. B. Mulcare and M. E. Swendseid 1965 Further observations on the amino acid requirements of older men. II. Methionine and lysine. Amer. J. Clin. Nutr. 16: 229.
88. Albanese, A. A., R. A. Higgons, L. A. Orto and D. N. Zavattaro 1957 Protein and amino acid needs of the aged in health and convalescence. Geriatrics 12: 465.
89. Fukui, T., H. Fukui, T. Sasaki and T. Murakami 1961 Lysine supply to children of growing age. Tokushima J. Exp. Med. 8: 1.
90. Nakagawa, I., T. Takahashi and T. Suzuki 1960 Amino acid requirements of children. J. Nutr. 71: 176.
91. Nakagawa, I., T. Takahashi and T. Suzuki 1961 Amino acid requirements of children: Isoleucine and leucine. J. Nutr. 73: 186.
92. Nakagawa, I., T. Takahashi and T. Suzuki 1961 Amino acid requirements of children: Minimal needs of lysine and methionine based on nitrogen balance method. J. Nutr. 74: 401.
93. Nakagawa, I., T. Takahashi, T. Suzuki and K. Kobayashi 1962 Amino acid requirements of children: Minimal needs of threonine, valine, and phenylalanine based on nitrogen balance method. J. Nutr. 77: 61.
94. Nakagawa, I., T. Takahashi, T. Suzuki and K. Kobayashi 1965 Amino acid requirements of children: Quantitative amino acid requirements of girls based on nitrogen balance method. J. Nutr. 86: 333.
95. Moyer, E. Z., and M. I. Irwin 1967 Basic data on metabolic patterns in 7- to 10-year-old girls in selected southern states. Home Economics Research Report no. 33. Agricultural Research Service, U. S. Department of Agriculture, Washington, D. C.
96. Snyderman, S. E., L. E. Holt, Jr., J. Dancis, E. Roitman, A. Boyer and M. E. Balis 1962 Unessential nitrogen: A limiting factor for human growth. J. Nutr. 78: 57.
97. Snyderman, S. E., A. Boyer and L. E. Holt, Jr. 1959 The arginine requirement of the infant. A.M.A. J. Dis. Child. 97: 192.
98. Albanese, A. A., L. E. Holt, Jr., V. I. Davis, S. E. Snyderman, M. Lein and E. M. Smetak 1948 The isoleucine requirement of the infant. J. Nutr. 35: 177.
99. Fomon, S. J., G. M. Owen and L. N. Thomas 1964 Methionine, valine, and isoleucine requirements during infancy. Amer. J. Dis. Child. 108: 487.
100. Snyderman, S. E., A. Boyer, P. M. Norton, E. Roitman and L. E. Holt, Jr. 1964 The essential amino acid requirements of infants. IX. Isoleucine. Amer. J. Clin. Nutr. 15: 313.
101. Snyderman, S. E., E. L. Roitman, A. Boyer and L. E. Holt, Jr. 1961 Essential amino acid requirements of infants. Leucine. Amer. J. Dis. Child. 102: 157.
102. Snyderman, S. E., P. M. Norton, D. I. Fowler and L. E. Holt, Jr. (with the assistance of E. Hasselmeyer and A. Boyer) 1959 The essential amino acid requirements of infants: Lysine. A.M.A. J. Dis. Child. 97: 175.
103. Albanese, A. A. 1950 The protein and amino acid requirements of man. In: Protein and Amino Acid Requirements of Mammals, ed., A. A. Albanese. Academic Press Inc., New York, p. 115.
104. Albanese, A. A., and M. Lein 1949 The chromatographic estimation of lysine and some applications of the method. Science 110: 163.

105. Dubow, E., A. Maher, D. Gish and V. Erk 1958 Lysine tolerance in infants. J. Pediat. 52: 30.

106. Thurau, R. 1952 Beitrag zum Stoffwechsel der schwefelhaltigen Aminosäuren im Säuglingsalter. Klin. Wochenschr. 30: 978.

107. Albanese, A. A., L. E. Holt, Jr., V. I. Davis, S. E. Snyderman, M. Lein and E. M. Smetak 1949 The sulfur amino acid requirement of the infant. J. Nutr. 37: 511.

108. Snyderman, S. E., A. Boyer, P. M. Norton, E. Roitman and L. E. Holt, Jr. 1965 The essential amino acid requirements of infants. X. Methionine. Amer. J. Clin. Nutr. 15: 322.

109. Goldstein, L. S. 1953 The effect of supplementary dl-methionine on the growth of full term infants. Arch. Pediat. 70: 285.

110. Levine, S. Z., M. Dann and E. Marples 1943 A defect in the metabolism of tyrosine and phenylalanine in premature infants. 3. Demonstration of the irreversible conversion of phenylalanine to tyrosine in the human organism. J. Clin. Invest. 22: 551.

111. Snyderman, S. E., E. L. Pratt, M. W. Cheung, P. Norton, L. E. Holt, Jr., A. E. Hansen and T. C. Panos 1955 The phenylalanine requirement of the normal infant. J. Nutr. 56: 253.

112. Swanson, W. W. 1932 The composition of growth. II. The full-term infant. Amer. J. Dis. Child. 43: 10.

113. Macy, I. G., H. J. Kelly and R. E. Sloan 1953 The composition of milks. Bull. National Research Council no. 254, Washington, D. C.

114. Albanese, A. A., L. E. Holt, Jr., V. Irby, S. E. Snyderman and M. Lein 1947 Studies on the protein metabolism of infants. II. Tryptophane requirement of the infant. Bull. Johns Hopkins Hosp. 80: 158.

115. Snyderman, S. E., A. Boyer, S. V. Phansalkar and L. E. Holt, Jr. 1961 Essential amino acid requirements of infants. Tryptophan. Amer. J. Dis. Child. 102: 163.

116. Snyderman, S. E., L. E. Holt, Jr., F. Smellie, A. Boyer and R. G. Westall 1959 The essential amino acid requirements of infants: Valine. A.M.A. J. Dis. Child. 97: 186.

117. Hegsted, D. M. 1963 Variation in requirements of nutrients — amino acids. Federation Proc. 22: 1424.

118. Autret, M., J. Périssé, F. Sizaret and M. Cresta 1968 Protein value of different types of diets in the world: Their appropriate supplementation. Nutrition Newsletter 6: 1. Food and Agriculture Organization of the United Nations, Rome, Italy.

119. Smith, M. 1926 The minimum endogenous nitrogen metabolism. J. Biol. Chem. 68: 15.

120. Food and Agriculture Organization 1965 Protein Requirements. Report of a joint FAO/WHO Expert Group. FAO Nutrition Meetings Report Series, no. 37. Food and Agriculture Organization of the United Nations, Rome, Italy.

A CONSPECTUS OF RESEARCH

ON

VITAMIN A REQUIREMENTS OF MAN

by

MILDRED S. RODRIGUEZ AND M. ISABEL IRWIN

Human Nutrition Research Division
Agricultural Research Service
United States Department of Agriculture
Beltsville, Maryland 20705

THE JOURNAL OF NUTRITION

VOLUME 102, NUMBER 7, JULY 1972

(Pages 909-968)

TABLE OF CONTENTS

INTRODUCTION

Although vitamin A and its precursors were not identified chemically until the twentieth century, foods rich in this nutrient have been used for treating night blindness, the most commonly recognized symptom of vitamin A deficiency, for several thousand years. As Aykroyd (1) pointed out, Eber's Papyrus, an ancient Egyptian medical treatise of about 1500 B.C., recommended that people unable to see properly at night should eat roast ox liver or the liver of a black cock. As early as 1825, people in India recognized that night blindness was caused by bad and insufficient food (1). About the same time Magendie (2) of France observed that animals restricted to diets containing sugar, starch, olive oil and wheat gluten developed ulcers of the cornea. Similar accounts by other early investigators have been reviewed by Bicknell and Prescott (3), McCollum (4) and Moore (5).

At the turn of the century workers began to recognize the beneficial effects of certain vitamin A-containing fats. In 1904 Mori (6) reported treating conjunctivitis among Japanese children with cod-liver oil and shortly thereafter Hopkins (7) recognized that whole milk contained "minimal qualitative factors" which were necessary supplements to a diet of purified foodstuffs if life and growth were to be maintained.

During the second decade two groups of American scientists, Osborne and Mendel of Yale (8, 9) and McCollum and his associates of Wisconsin (10, 11) found that some animal fats, such as butterfat, egg yolk or cod-liver oil, contained a substance that was essential to rats for growth and it also cured eye disorders. McCollum and Davis (12) called this biologically active ether extract "fat soluble A."

Numerous cases of keratomalacia, xerophthalmia and night blindness in young children were reported from Denmark between 1909 and 1920 (13). In 1921,

Bloch (14) reported that a diet rich in fat (full milk and cod-liver oil) cured xerophthalmia in Danish infants who had been unsuccessfully treated in the Ophthalmology Department of the State Hospital. Since an intake of 250 g of butter per week per subject prevented xerophthalmia, Bloch concluded that the eye affliction was due to the absence of the "fat soluble A bodies" in the diet.

In the meantime McCollum et al. (15) and Osborne and Mendel (16) had found that green vegetables, such as cabbage, spinach, lucerne and clover, also possessed fat-soluble A activity. Observing that the substances containing fat-soluble A were yellow, Steenbock (17) of Wisconsin tested various carotenoids and found that carotene induced growth in rats but xanthophylls did not.

Using the rat growth method which Zilva and Miura (18) devised for assaying the vitamin A activity of food, von Euler et al. (19) and Moore (20) demonstrated that carotene cured vitamin A-deficient rats. However, they maintained that the active substances in cod-liver oil and carotene were quite different. Von Euler et al. (19) observed that carotene and cod-liver oil gave different colors when reacting with antimony trichloride. In 1929 and 1930 Moore fed carotene to vitamin A-depleted rats and isolated vitamin A from the livers, providing evidence that carotene was converted to vitamin A (21, 22).

Meanwhile Karrer was studying the chemical nature of the carotenoids and in 1930 he established the structural formula of β-carotene (23). About the same time it became evident that carotene was not a single substance but rather that it existed in several different isomeric forms (24–26) later designated as α-, β- and γ-carotene.

Received for publication August 30, 1971.

The existence of more than one form of β-carotene was first suggested by Gillam and El Ridi (27, 28) in 1935–1936 when they observed that after repeated chromatographic adsorption, β-carotene divided into two different zones. *Cis-trans* isomerization and its effects on the biopotency of vitamin A and the provitamins A have been reviewed by Zechmeister (29, 30).

In experimental animals at least ten different carotenoids exhibit varying amounts of vitamin A activity (5). However, a number of dietary factors, such as food source, total intake, particle size, fat, vitamin E and protein, reportedly affect the utilization of these naturally occurring compounds. Although not all of the provitamins A are carotenes, they are commonly referred to as such. In addition to preformed vitamin A and the provitamin A compounds from plants, vitamin A_2 from fresh water fish is also biologically potent in experimental animals (31).

Reports in the literature suggest that total vitamin A requirements may possibly be increased by fever, infection, reduced environmental temperature, hyperthyroidism, chemical substances and excessive exposure to ultraviolet rays.

In discussing dietary vitamin A requirements it should be kept in mind that although circulating vitamin A is normally maintained at a relatively constant level by the liver, it is possible to raise the concentration above homeostatic levels. Since 1944, when chronic vitamin A intoxication was first reported by Josephs (32), numerous accounts of both chronic and acute hypervitaminosis A have appeared in the literature from the United States and Western Europe.

Our present knowledge of human vitamin A requirements has been obtained from field surveys and controlled dietary studies. The former provide a general idea of the total vitamin A intake of populations with and without overt clinical and biochemical vitamin A deficiency symptoms but they are of limited value in quantitating human vitamin A requirements. The criteria commonly used in field surveys include: the condition of the epithelial tissues (especially of the eyes and the skin), dark-adaptation tests, plasma vitamin A concentration, and frequency of infection.

The vitamin A content of human milk and of livers from people who have died accidentally is also frequently compared with the estimated vitamin A intake of a given population. In this paper data from field surveys have been cited only when the results of controlled dietary studies were not available. No attempt has been made to cover all of the nutritional status surveys reported.

Most of the controlled studies of human vitamin A requirements have been based on dark-adaptation tests. Its role in the visual cycle is the only metabolic function for which the mechanism has been elucidated (33–35). Serum vitamin A concentration, the second most commonly used criterion, has been included in most studies since Kimble adapted the sensitive photoelectric method for measuring vitamin A in the plasma (36). Some investigators have also measured growth, susceptibility to infections and changes in the epithelial tissue. The latter is a common symptom of vitamin A deficiency in animals (37). Human vitamin A requirements have also been estimated on the basis of data obtained from controlled animal experiments. Whether these can be translated without question into recommendations for humans is not clear.

The purpose of this conspectus is to show what research has been done with human subjects on dietary vitamin A requirements, how it was done and what has been learned. This information will, in turn, point to where further research is needed in order to complete our knowledge of human needs for vitamin A. It is not intended to be another estimate of vitamin A requirements nor a critical evaluation of the individual studies although some evaluative comments have been included. For the reader's convenience, references to basic background information and critical discussions on methodology are cited.

UNITS AND STANDARDS OF MEASURE

The necessity of establishing an internationally recognized standard for use in quantitating vitamin A was recognized before the discovery of the various isomeric forms of carotene and before vitamin A had been purified and crystallized. Therefore, in 1931, the Permanent Commission of Biological Standardisation of the League of Nations (38) adopted a stock of supposedly pure crystalline β-carotene as the International Standard for vitamin A. One International Unit (IU) of vitamin A was defined as that amount which had the same vitamin A activity in rats as 1 μg of the International Standard Preparation of β-carotene (38).

It was soon discovered that the Standard of Reference contained α-carotene as well as β-carotene. Therefore, in 1934, the Second League of Nations Conference on Vitamin Standardisation (39) replaced the old standard with a stock of pure crystalline β-carotene. One IU of vitamin A was now defined as the amount of activity contained in 0.6 μg of the Standard Preparation of β-carotene. The experimental evidence which led to the conclusion has been reviewed by Hume and Chick (40). The 1934 Conference also adopted a sample of cod-liver oil from the United States as a Reference Standard. One USP unit of the oil supposedly had the same activity as 1 IU (0.6 μg) of β-carotene (39). Furthermore, the Conference recommended that a conversion factor of 1,600 (the number of biological units/gram divided by $E^{1\%}_{1\ cm}$ at 328 mμ) be adopted for relating the spectrophotometric measurement of vitamin A to the biologically determined vitamin A potency of the same sample.

In 1949, shortly after pure crystalline vitamin A became commercially available (41, 42), the Expert Committee on Biological Standardization of the World Health Organization (43) recommended that crystalline vitamin A acetate be accepted as the International Standard for vitamin A. One IU is now equivalent to 0.344 μg all-*trans* retinyl acetate or 0.3 μg all-*trans* retinol and the conversion factor for vitamin A acetate is 1900.

Vitamin A-active compounds have been quantitated by biological, chemical, spectrophotometric and fluorimetric methods. Use of the International Unit (IU) as the Standard unit of measure for vitamin A activity has led to a great deal of misunderstanding (44). This is due to differences in the provitamin A content of natural foodstuffs. The provitamins differ from one another in biological activity and in availability. Also, our knowledge of the quantity of the provitamins A and their stereoisomers in foods "as eaten" is incomplete.

After considering these variables, the FAO/WHO Group (45) proposed, in 1965, that the vitamin A activity of all compounds be expressed in terms of μg retinol. According to this recommendation 1 μg all-*trans* β-carotene would be equivalent to 0.167 μg all-*trans* retinol and 1 μg of the other mixed carotenoids with vitamin A activity would be equivalent to 0.0835 μg all-*trans* retinol.

In this paper human dietary vitamin A requirements will be discussed according to population groups who are believed to have specific needs. Whenever possible, requirements for preformed vitamin A (retinol) and provitamin A (carotene) will be discussed separately because of incomplete information on the vitamin A activity of the provitamins A. A number of qualifying terms such as minimum, average and optimum have been used in stating vitamin A requirements. They vary, in part, according to the criteria employed. The terminology and the units of measure used in describing the results of various studies will usually be the same as those used by the original authors. However, for the convenience of the reader, values for preformed vitamin A and β-carotene in oil, expressed in IU, have been converted to μg retinol on the basis that 1 IU is equivalent to 0.3 μg retinol. These converted values appear in parentheses following the IU. Due to insufficient information on the provitamin A content of the natural foods, it is not feasible to express their vitamin A activity in terms of μg retinol.

REQUIREMENTS OF ADULTS
(TABLE 1)

Adults' requirements for retinol, β-carotene in oil and provitamins A from natural food sources have been estimated by dark adaptation (visual studies), a combination of dark adaptation and blood values, and by extrapolation from animal studies. The period of time required to deplete the vitamin A liver stores of the various subjects, enough to bring about a significant change

TABLE 1

Daily vitamin A requirements of adults, controlled studies

Source	Number of studies	Number of subjects	Principal criteria	Minimal		Adequate [1]		References
				Vitamin A value IU	Retinol μg [2]	Vitamin A value IU	Retinol μg [2]	
Retinol								
	5	22	Dark adaptation	1,750–4,000	525–1,200	2,500–5,500	750–1,650	55, 63–66
	2	12	Dark adaptation and plasma	1,300–2,500	390– 750	2,500	750	67, 69
β-Carotene in oil								
	4	14	Dark adaptation	2,210–7,180	663–2,154	5,000–9,800	1,500–2,940	55, 67, 116, 117
	1	7	Dark adaptation and plasma	2,000 [3]	600	4,000 [3]	1,200	69
Plant sources								
	2	8	Dark adaptation	1,590–8,110				59, 116
	1	5	Dark adaptation and plasma			5,000–12,000		69

[1] Also includes optimal requirements.
[2] Original values converted to µg retinol on the basis that 1 IU is equivalent to 0.3 µg retinol.
[3] Computed on the basis that 75% of β-carotene is absorbed.

in dark adaptation, has ranged from 20 to 600 days or more.

In seven studies, using dark adaptation as the criterion, estimates of minimum retinol requirements varied from 1,300 to 4,000 IU daily. Both dark adaptation and plasma values were measured in two of these studies but the minimum intake to maintain normal plasma values was not established. In addition, acute and chronic hypervitaminosis A have been reported in adults.

In five studies, using β-carotene in oil as the source of vitamin A, at least 2,000 to 7,180 IU daily were required. When different vegetables were the source of provitamins A, the average minimum requirement ranged from 1,590 to 8,110 IU daily, depending on the food source and method of assaying vitamin A activity. Absorption studies by one group of investigators indicated that three times as many IU were required when vegetables, rather than preformed vitamin A, were the source of vitamin A activity.

Early Studies

After the establishment of vitamin A as a factor in the visual cycle, researchers began to investigate the possibility of testing retinal function as a method of detecting early stages of vitamin A deprivation. The most comprehensive coverage of scotopic vision and tests of its function and abnormalities was prepared by two Frenchmen, Jayle and Ourgaud (46). This work was later translated into English by Baisinger and Holmes and extended to include more recent data (47). Numerous types of apparatus and experimental procedures have been developed to measure either the rate of adaptation to darkness or the final rod threshold, i.e., the minimum light threshold after complete dark adaptation (48–51). It is generally agreed that the latter measurement is a more reliable test of vitamin A adequacy than the former (49). Results reported in the early literature concerning the effects of a vitamin A-deficient diet on the dark-adaptation curve, duration of depletion and repletion periods, and effective corrective doses of vitamin A are as varied as the methods employed for measuring dark adaptation.

For instance, Edmund and Clemmesen (52) of Denmark reported that although the visual adaptation of 52 young healthy hospital nurses, consuming 700 to 900 IU vitamin A daily, was "normal," it was poorer in the winter months — January, February and March. Giving 25,200 IU daily improved their night vision, thus suggesting a dietary deficiency of vitamin A. Later (53), these investigators examined the ability of healthy young men to discern differences in the brightness of illumination. An average intake of 1,225 IU of vitamin A daily (about 17 to 19 IU/kg body weight) did not prevent seasonal oscillations in the night vision of 14 young men. When 0.5 liter of whole fluid milk was added to the basic prison diet, however, the visual distinction of 14 other men was normal during all seasons (over a period of 6 months). Edmund and Clemmesen estimated that the latter group received about 1,400 IU (20 to 22 IU/kg body weight) daily.

In another study Jeghers (54) tested the dark adaptation of 162 medical students. The average daily intake of the 50 subjects with the best adaptation was 5,560 IU. The 50 students with the poorest adaptation averaged 2,445 IU daily. All students who consumed more than 4,000 IU daily had normal dark adaptation. Jeghers therefore concluded that 4,000 IU probably represented the minimal intake. Allowing a safety factor of 50% he recommended a daily intake of 6,000 IU. No mention was made of the source of vitamin A, i.e., retinol or provitamin A.

Preformed Vitamin A (Retinol)

Visual studies

The first quantitative work on adult vitamin A requirements was reported in 1939 by Booher et al. (55). Five healthy adult subjects (two males and three females) were fed a vitamin A-deficient diet until they showed constant and unmistakable signs of impaired dark adaptation, according to final rod threshold measurements. When their average light threshold values attained one or more log units in excess of their normal threshold values (after 26, 27, 29, 39 and 124 days), measured amounts of vitamin A as cod-liver oil were administered. Dark adaptation improved in 2 to 3 hours but this was temporary. The investigators concluded that the amount of vitamin A necessary for maintenance of normal dark adaptation varied between 25 and 55 USP units (equivalent to 7.5 and 16.5 μg retinol) per kilogram body weight. A 70-kg man would thus require 1,750 to 3,850 USP units (525 to 1,155 μg retinol) of vitamin A daily. This was considered to be a physiological minimum requirement which did not provide for an accumulation of reserves.

USP reference cod-liver oil no. 1, which had been standardized by biological assay with rats against crystalline β-carotene, was used in these experiments. Initially, this oil was assigned a biological potency of 3,000 USP units/gram. It was later found that, due to deterioration, the vitamin A activity of USP reference cod-liver oil no. 1 (56, 57) and no. 2 (58) had been overestimated by as much as 12 and 30 to 44%, respectively. In 1947, Callison and Orent-Keiles (59) stated that, in view of the reported instability of the reference oil, the human requirements for preformed vitamin A estimated by Booher et al. in 1939, were probably somewhat high. The difficulties encountered in quantitating vitamin A by biological assay should also be kept in mind (60–62). In his review of the possible sources of error in the method, Gridgeman (61) stated that when 20 rats were used, the limits of error for a 4-week assay lay between 57 and 176% of the true value.

In four other studies (63–66), which were reported at about the same time, 20 to 120 days were required for depletion. Estimates of minimum adult requirements ranged from 2,000 to 4,000 IU daily. Blanchard and Harper (63) found that depletion time was related to the weight of the subject. Two college students, who weighed more than 73 kg, were depleted of vitamin A in 29.2 days; four students weighing less than 73 kg each required 20.2 days. Vitamin A was administered in different amounts to each of the six depleted subjects, so it is difficult to draw any conclusions for the group. Five hundred USP units of vitamin A (150 μg retinol) daily produced rapid improvement in the dark adaptation of two subjects.

The authors concluded that 2,000 USP units of vitamin A (600 μg retinol) was fairly close to the minimum requirement because the dark-adaptation time of the subjects increased promptly when the supplement was suspended. Massive doses (up to 250,000 USP units) of vitamin A were not proportionately more effective in improving night vision than the smaller amounts, 1,500 to 3,600 USP units (450 to 1,080 μg retinol) daily.

Since three of the adults tested by Basu and De (64) maintained normal final rod threshold values for 30 to 37 days when they received 5,000 IU of vitamin A concentrate (1,500 μg retinol) daily, they considered this the optimum requirement of adults. Dark adaptation values remained normal in one subject fed 3,000 IU vitamin A (900 μg retinol) daily for 20 days but decreased rapidly when the supplement was withdrawn. Thus they concluded that 3,000 IU of vitamin A concentrate daily was the minimum requirement.

Batchelder and Ebbs (65) observed that, after three women had eaten a vitamin A-deficient diet for 11 weeks, their dark adaptation time had increased 1 log unit over the final threshold values observed at the beginning of the study. Massive doses (300,000 and 500,000 IU) of vitamin A from haliver oil (equivalent to 90,000 to 150,000 μg retinol) then were administered to two subjects. Following this, they received 5,500 IU daily for 11 to 12 days. In both cases their visual thresholds improved slightly. The investigators thus concluded that 5,500 IU (1,650 μg retinol) daily was more than enough to maintain a level of dark adaptation similar to or characteristic of subjects on freely chosen diets. Later, they (66) fed four healthy young subjects a vitamin A-deficient diet for 80 to 120 days. Throughout the period, one subject showed steady improvement in her ability to adapt to the dark. Individual differences were noted among the other three in their response to large doses of vitamin A and in their return to normal visual sensitivity. Thus, Batchelder and Ebbs concluded that at least 4,000 to 5,000 IU of vitamin A concentrate (1,200 to 1,500 μg retinol) were required daily.

Visual and blood studies

Wagner (67) found that the visual sensitivity of five male prisoners who had been on a vitamin A-free diet for 6 months was 1/28 of normal. These subjects required 2,500 IU (750 μg retinol) of preformed vitamin A daily to produce complete visual normality and no vitamin A was found in the plasma until this dosage was administered. Wagner therefore concluded that adult men require 2,000 to 2,500 IU of vitamin A (600 to 750 μg retinol) daily. The vitamin A concentrate which Wagner used in his experiments was the German commercial preparation, "Vogan." Reports in the literature concerning its true vitamin A value are controversial. The Germans claimed that the conversion factor between ultraviolet readings and biological activity was 3,500 (68) instead of the usual 1,600. Thus, Moore (5) calculated that "On this basis results for vitamin A would have been given more than twice their true value." On the other hand, Hume and Krebs (69) state that according to personal communications from Wagner and Scheunert, "the 'Vogan' used in Wagner's experiment was retested in Scheunert's laboratory and that the correct figure was used in this experiment."

In 1942, the British Medical Research Council at the Sorby Research Institute (69) in Sheffield, England began a carefully controlled study of adult human vitamin A requirements. Twenty-three subjects, twenty males and three females, participated in this study which lasted for more than 2 years. Sixteen subjects received a vitamin A-deficient diet containing 62 to 65 IU vitamin A activity daily as α- and β-carotene until they were dosed therapeutically with vitamin A or carotene. Seven controls received vitamin A or carotene prophylactically. The dark-adaptation time of all subjects was measured weekly with a Wald's portable adaptometer (70). Plasma carotenoid and vitamin A values were determined at 2- to 4-week intervals, using the antimony trichloride method and a conversion factor of 1,600.

The plasma carotenoids of the 16 subjects on the deficient diet rapidly declined. After about 8 months, the plasma vitamin A values of 10 of the 16 subjects "showed a definite downward trend" (69). In four of these subjects, the fall was "especially marked." Other investigators have reported a rapid decline in the serum carotenoids of subjects on a vitamin A-deficient diet but found no change in serum vitamin A concentration after 6 and 7.5 months, respectively (71, 72).

Although the dark adaptation capacity of each of the deprived subjects in the Sheffield study deteriorated somewhat during the first winter, it returned to the initial level in the spring. The investigators reported that only three subjects showed a permanent marked rise in visual threshold values after about 10, 12 and 20 months from the start of the experiment. Both the cone–rod transition time and the final rod threshold values were affected. Previous investigators had reported much shorter depletion periods, often only a matter of days (55, 73–80). The Sheffield researchers were unable to explain this pronounced difference. Follicular hyperkeratosis and infection were observed from time to time in various subjects but did not appear to be related to vitamin A intake. However, three of the five subjects deprived of vitamin A showed significant worsening of hearing which improved significantly when they were given vitamin A. Also, four of the deprived subjects contracted major illnesses (impetigo contagiosa, migraine, tuberculosis pleurisy and tuberculous disease of the spine) during or after the period of deprivation.

Of the three subjects showing permanently impaired dark adaptation, one was treated with varying amounts of retinol in order to determine the minimum requirement for preformed vitamin A. The initial plasma value of this one subject was 96 IU/100 ml. By the end of the depletion period (425 days), when his capacity to adapt to the dark decreased, his plasma vitamin A had dropped to 22 IU/100 ml. After 2 months with a diet providing 1,300 IU vitamin A (390 μg retinol) daily as distilled natural esters in oil, his plasma value rose to 88 IU/100 ml; but at the end of 199 days it had dropped to about 50 IU/100 ml. By this time, his capacity to adapt to the dark had gradually returned to normal. Treatment with 2,600 IU of vitamin A (780 μg retinol) daily for 45 days had little effect on plasma vitamin A concentration. However, when he was given 24,000 IU (7,200 μg retinol) daily and an "unrestricted" diet, his plasma vitamin A quickly returned to the initial value.

Another subject became partially depleted after eating a vitamin A-deficient diet for 325 days. During that time his plasma vitamin A dropped slightly (from 73 to 52 IU/100 ml) but his dark adaptation capacity was unaffected. When he was treated with 2,600 IU vitamin A (780 μg retinol) daily for 25 days, no changes were noted. Similarly, three other partially depleted subjects with "somewhat" depressed plasma values (53 to 63 IU/100 ml) were given 1,250 IU of vitamin A (375 μg retinol) daily for 2 to 2.5 months. No effect was noted. Large doses (24,000 IU daily) of vitamin A (7,200 μg retinol) and an "unrestricted" diet, however, raised the plasma vitamin A value of all three to 100 IU/100 ml or more. The capacity for dark adaptation did not improve beyond the range attained with the smaller dose (1,250 IU daily). No changes by either criterion were noted in two subjects maintained for 14 and 17 months on diets containing 2,500 IU of vitamin A (750 μg retinol). There was no significant change when the dose was increased to 5,800 IU (1,740 μg retinol); but, with an ad libitum diet without supplements, the average plasma values of both subjects rose.

On the basis of these data obtained with seven subjects, the research group (69) concluded that 1,300 IU of preformed vitamin A (390 μg retinol) daily represented the minimum protective dose. They recommended that 2,500 IU (750 μg retinol) daily be accepted as the requirement of a normal adult, explaining that the blood level of vitamin A necessary for optimal health was not known. The amount of vitamin A administered in these experiments was measured spectrophotometrically, using the earlier 1934 conversion factor, 1,600 (39). In discussing the measurement of vitamin A, Leitner et al. (81) have pointed out that increasing the conversion factor from 1,600 to 1,900 (43) "presumably implies that many early results must now be increased by nearly 20% to make them comparable with modern findings."

In summarizing the results of their study the Sheffield group (69) stated that "in the absence of adequate experimental evidence, which could be obtained only by intricate experiment on very large numbers of volunteers, it is difficult to decide whether doubling the dose would confer the maximum improvement in health or whether the dose should be increased fourfold, eightfold, or even more."

There is experimental evidence that an intake of vitamin A above the minimum requirements increases longevity in rats (82–84). Sherman et al. (83) reported that 12 IU/gram air-dried food, which is four times the minimum requirement, expedited development and deferred senility of rats. However, doubling this intake resulted in decreased growth and lifespan (85). No research in humans on vitamin A intake and longevity has been reported.

Due, in part, to the difficulty of sampling human liver vitamin A concentration, the intake required to attain a prescribed reserve of vitamin A and the advantages of large stores of vitamin A in the liver are both unknown. Because of the poor correlation between plasma and liver vitamin A concentrations (86–89) the British Medical Research Group (69) was not able to determine whether the recommended intake (2,500 IU of preformed vitamin A daily) would definitely allow for an accumulation of liver reserves or not. But they thought that the daily intake of the subjects before the experiment, all of whom apparently had considerable liver reserves, had not greatly exceeded 2,500 IU preformed vitamin A (750 μg retinol) or an equivalent mixture of carotene and vitamin A (69). Also, at autopsy, the average amount of vitamin A in the livers of 71 healthy adult British subjects between 1941 and 1944 was 324 IU/gram liver (97.2 μg retinol/g) (90).

Guilbert et al. (91), Callison and Knowles (92) and High (93) found that 20 IU (6 μg) retinol/kilogram body weight/day provided for normal growth and freedom from clinical symptoms in experimental animals, but three to four times this amount was required for significant vitamin A storage in the liver. Callison and Knowles (92) therefore concluded that some considerable need of the body must be met in an apparently normal animal before liver storage occurred. After considering the vitamin A requirements of five different nonprimate species, Guilbert et al. (91) estimated that a 70-kg man required 1,500 IU (450 μg) retinol daily for freedom from clinical symptoms and 4,200 IU (1,260 μg) for optimal dark adaptation, reproduction and significant storage.

Hypervitaminosis A

Although liver vitamin A reserves may be desirable, excess preformed vitamin A has adverse effects. The amount that can be tolerated by adult humans has not been established. Fifteen cases (94–107) of chronic adult hypervitaminosis A, 12 of which occurred in the United States, have been reported to date. The daily intake and the length of the latent period before the first symptoms were observed varied from 33,333 IU (9,999 μg retinol) for 8 to 12 months (103) to 600,000 IU (180,000 μg retinol) for 1 year (94). One subject took 100,000 IU (30,000 μg retinol) daily for 3.5 years before symptoms of hypervitaminosis A were observed (101). Hillman (108) experimentally induced vitamin A poisoning in a 40-year-old physician on two different occasions, using approximately 1,000,000 units (300,000 μg retinol) daily for 14 and 25 days, respectively. Others took excess vitamin A for as long as 8 years. It appears that the duration of the latent period before the onset of symptoms of hypervitaminosis A is "somewhat inversely related to the size of the daily dose" (101).

Acute hypervitaminosis A may also occur in adults but the maximum tolerance level has not been established. Although it was commonly known in the Arctic regions that eating the liver of polar bears and bearded seals caused acute illness, it was not formally recorded in the scientific literature until 1943 (109). After determining that polar bear liver contained 13,000 to 18,000 IU vitamin A (3,900 to 5,400 μg retinol) per gram, Rodahl and Moore (109) suggested that the poisonous effect of the liver was due to the high vitamin A content. Cleland and Southcott (110) have recently reviewed the history of vitamin A poisoning in the Arctic and South Aus-

tralia and reported three previously unpublished case histories of acute hypervitaminosis A.

According to Stimson (101) the principal symptoms of hypervitaminosis A, "bone or joint pain that tended to be intermittent, fatigue and insomnia, loss of hair, dryness and fissuring of the lips and other epithelial involvement, anorexia and weight loss and hepatomegaly," are all relieved promptly and almost completely when vitamin A dosing is discontinued. In 1968, Lane concluded from microscopic examination of a liver biopsy sample from a 24-year-old man who had ingested 50,000 to 5,000,000 IU vitamin A (15,000 to 1,500,000 μg retinol) daily for the last 5 years that "there are no significant abnormalities of liver structure associated with massive hepatic storage of vitamin A" (107). On the other hand, after examining two liver biopsy samples, one of which was taken from an 18-year-old girl who had taken 300,000 IU (90,000 μg retinol) daily for 1 month and 100,000 to 200,000 IU (30,000 to 60,000 μg retinol) for 1.5 years, Muenter et al. concluded that: "Hepatocellular damage, portal fibrosis and eventual cirrhosis may result from chronic vitamin A intoxication in man" (111).

Electron microscopic studies of a liver biopsy sample from a 6-year-old girl suffering from chronic hypervitaminosis A revealed increased lysosomes, focal cytoplasmic degradation and numerous light and dark cells (112). All are indicative of hepatic injury. In rats, a small excess of vitamin A caused liver mitochondria to swell; with a large excess, the liver was "extensively autolysed" (113).

Tanksale (114) of India recently found that the dark adaptation time of 10 healthy students, who were given 24,000 IU vitamin A (7,200 μg retinol) daily for 10 days, became much slower after the first day. Their adaptation time recovered to a steady value, which was less prompt than before the experiment, after 6 and after 12 days. These data suggest that excess vitamin A may affect certain stages in the photoreceptor mechanism of the eye. Recent animal experiments support this hypothesis. Dobronravova et al. (115) found that maximum tactile sensitivity of the cornea, normal electroretinograms and optimal platelet counts were obtained when rats were fed 23 μg vitamin A daily. However, when the intake was doubled (43 μg daily) there was some loss of corneal sensitivity and the platelet count fell steeply.

Provitamin A

In the developing areas of the world, the principal dietary sources of vitamin A are fruits and green leafy and yellow vegetables (45). Provitamins A often contribute 80 to 100% of the total vitamin A intake. The following studies show that dietary provitamin A requirements vary, depending on the food source and that estimates of the total IU in a given food vary with the method of assaying the vitamin A activity.

Visual studies

Estimates of human provitamin A requirements were first reported by Booher et al. (55). The dark-adaptation time of five young adult subjects, eating a vitamin A-deficient diet, increased significantly after 16 to 124 days; 43 to 103 USP units of carotene in cottonseed oil (equivalent to 13 to 31 μg retinol) per kilogram body weight/day were required to restore and maintain normal vision. This is almost twice as many units as they required when cod-liver oil was the source of vitamin A (25 to 55 IU/kg body weight).

In the same year, Booher and Callison also reported that the amount of provitamin A required to maintain normal dark adaptation in four young adults varied according to the dietary source (116). The range of daily provitamin A requirements from various food sources was as follows: β-carotene in oil, 76 to 106 (23 to 35 μg retinol); cooked peas, 47 to 57; and cooked spinach, which was chopped prior to cooking, 77 to 101 IU/kilogram body weight (116). Although these values may be somewhat high, because the cod-liver oil used as the standard in this study had probably lost potency (58), the relationship between retinol in cod-liver oil and carotene in oil or vegetables remains unchanged (59). In this study, the vitamin A activity of the various food sources was determined by the rat-growth method. Therefore, only the provitamins utilized by the rat were taken into consideration.

Experiments by Callison and Orent-Keiles (59) illustrate the difference in the IU of vitamin A activity in a given food, depending on the method of assay. Using dark adaptation as the criterion and crystalline β-carotene in cottonseed oil as the standard, they found that four young subjects required an average of 97.8 IU/kilogram body weight when vitamin A activity of carrots was determined spectrophotometrically, and 34.2 IU when vitamin A activity was determined by bioassay. The vitamin A activity of cooked and uncooked carrots was the same.

In summarizing the results of these three experiments Callison and Orent-Keiles (59) concluded that these studies emphasize the need for caution when using food composition tables for planning and evaluating diets. They also pointed to the need for further investigation of vitamin A and carotene utilization by man.

Two other estimates of provitamin A requirements, using dark adaptation as the criterion, were reported from Germany around 1940. Von Drigalski (117) restricted his vitamin A intake until his dark adaptation became abnormal (72 days). He then took a mixture of equal parts of carotene and vitamin A until his adaptation time returned to normal. After deducting for fecal losses, he concluded that the optimal vitamin A requirement of man was about 5.9 mg or 9,800 IU of β-carotene. Wagner (67) gave β-carotene in increasing doses, over various periods of time to five vitamin A-depleted subjects, who had eaten a vitamin A-deficient diet for 188 days. Five thousand IU daily restored all subjects to normal in 61 days. He concluded, from fecal analysis, that the difference in retinol and β-carotene requirements was due to poor absorption of the latter.

Visual and blood studies

The British Vitamin A Sub-committee of the Accessory Food Factors Committee (69) also studied carotene requirements. After 22 and 17.5 months with a vitamin A-deficient diet, the plasma vitamin A values of two subjects, Proctor and Watson, had decreased to 28 and 19 IU/100 ml, respectively. Their dark-adaptation time, which remained normal until their plasma values fell below 50 IU/100 ml, had also increased significantly. When Proctor was given 1,250 IU β-carotene (equivalent to 375 μg retinol) for a month, his plasma vitamin A rose to 63 IU/100 ml but his dark-adaptation time increased. Although he slowly improved by both criteria when he was given 2,500 IU (equivalent to 750 μg retinol) daily for 6 months, still the final rod threshold values had not returned to normal. It was quickly corrected after resuming an unrestricted diet. Watson, who was less depleted, responded quickly to 2,500 IU daily by all criteria. Absorption studies indicated that control subjects absorbed three-fourths of the ingested β-carotene in oil.

On the basis of these data, the Vitamin A Sub-committee proposed that 1,500 IU β-carotene (450 μg retinol) daily was the minimum protective dose, provided all the carotene was absorbed. Allowing a safety factor of 100%, 3,000 IU (900 μg retinol) was suggested as the daily requirement of β-carotene for a normal adult. They therefore reasoned that 4,000 IU of β-carotene would have to be ingested daily.

This group also estimated the required dietary provitamin A intake when vegetables were the source of vitamin A activity. Five subjects, serving as controls for varying periods of time (6.5 to 22 months) received about 5,000 IU carotene daily from various vegetable sources for varying periods of time. Capacity for dark adaptation, plasma vitamin A and carotenoid values, and fecal excretion of carotene were measured. The carotene content of the vegetables was assayed chemically.

From these data the group estimated that, in order to assure the absorption of 3,000 IU, adults would have to ingest 12,000 IU from cooked carrots; 7,500 IU from cabbage or spinach; or 5,000 IU from homogenized carrots daily. The researchers noted that there were considerable variations among the values for different persons receiving the same supplement under apparently the same conditions as well as for the same subjects receiving the same supplement in different test weeks. They also point out that it is unknown how much of the maximum effective dose was absorbed and how much was destroyed in the gut. This is a common criticism of absorption studies (118). Ishii and Iwagaki (119) reported that in the simultaneous presence of artificial gastric juice and lipoxidase in foods, 24, 18 and 27% of the carotene in spinach, carrots and dried seaweed, respectively, was decomposed.

The Committee stressed the need for more data from human subjects on the availability of the carotenes from various sources and stated that it was undesirable to fix any single figure for carotene requirements. In a preliminary report (120), the group estimated that 5,000 IU of carotene might be regarded as providing enough vitamin A for maintenance of human adults with a fair margin of safety.

The British Medical Research Council's War Memorandum on the Nutritive Values of Wartime Foods (121) recommended that, for a mixed diet, the total carotene value expressed in IU (0.6 μg β-carotene), should be divided by three, in order to equate it with the biological value of preformed vitamin A. Taking this into consideration, along with their findings that three times as many IU were required when the source was carrots vs. β-carotene in fat, Hume and Krebs (69) recommended an intake of 7,500 IU daily from vegetable sources. This is three times their recommended intake when the dietary source is preformed vitamin A (see page 918). The practice of dividing the number of IU from provitamins by three in order to determine vitamin A potency is currently used in the United Kingdom (44, 122).

In the food tables currently used in the United States (123) "no allowance has been made for the differences in physiological equivalence of vitamin A to the various precursors or for differences in availability of the precursors as sources of vitamin A values from different types of food." In the first edition of *Agriculture Handbook No. 8* (124) many of the vitamin A values were determined by biological methods, whereas in the recent edition (123) most of the values "are based on physiochemical determinations of total carotenoids or of individual carotenes and cryptoxanthin." When the individual carotenes were determined, 0.6 μg β-carotene and 1.2 μg of other carotenes or cryptoxanthin were considered equivalent to 1 IU vitamin A value.

Guilbert et al. (91) estimated from studies on the carotene requirements of nonprimate mammalia in general, that the minimum provitamin A requirement for a healthy 70-kg man was 2,800 IU daily. The minimum daily intake for significant storage, optimal dark adaptation and reproduction was estimated at 14,000 IU. Reports of research concerning the amount of dietary provitamins A required by humans for liver storage are practically nonexistent. Leitner et al. (125, 126) demonstrated that feeding extra carotenoids in the form of vegetables increased the serum levels of both carotenoids and vitamin A. However, as Roels et al. (127) pointed out, it is not known whether the "normal" level of serum vitamin A affects the transformation of β-carotene into vitamin A or not.

Reports from West Africa where carotene-rich foods are extensively consumed, suggest that ingestion of "adequate" carotenoids leads to increased storage of vitamin A in the liver. The mean serum vitamin A values of Nigerian (128) and Ghanaian (129) soldiers, consuming 60 to 120 mg carotenoids daily, were 58 and 56 $\mu g/100$ ml, respectively. Dagadu and Gillman (129) also found that one-half of the livers, obtained at necropsy in Accra, contained more than 300 μg vitamin A/gram of liver. On the other hand, Carter and Cook (128) did not find a correlation between total serum carotenoid and vitamin A levels of Nigerians. This might be explained by the fact that humans absorb many carotenoids that have no biological activity (126, 130–132). Leitner et al. (126) estimated that an average of 25 to 61% of the total serum carotenoids was carotene, depending on the total carotenoid intake. Bayfield et al. (130) found that one-third of the total plasma carotenoids was β-carotene. Serum carotenoid concentration apparently reflects the recent intake (125).

There are no reports in the literature on human requirements for carotenoids and their stereoisomers, other than β-carotene. The biological potency of these other carotenoids has been studied extensively in rats and the literature has been reviewed by several authors (30, 133, 134). John-

son and Baumann (135) reported that the amount of vitamin A stored by rats fed the stereoisomers of β-carotene was proportional to the ability of these provitamins to promote growth. On the other hand, the vitamin A potency of cryptoxanthin estimated by liver and kidney storage criteria, was twice its potency estimated by growth criterion (134). Moreover, according to the data assembled by Beeson (136), species differences in the conversion of β-carotene to vitamin A may vary fourfold.

Mixed Diet

From time to time investigators have attempted to estimate human vitamin A requirements on the basis of survey data. During the second world war Nylund and With (137) tested the dark adaptation of persons maintained on known diets containing various sources of preformed vitamin A and carotene. Although the composition could be calculated, the exact vitamin A potency of the butter which some of the subjects consumed was not known. Only one case of night blindness was found when the 30 adults consumed 600 IU (180 μg) as retinol in addition to 670 to 10,000 IU from carrots. From these and the data of other previous investigators they concluded that the optimum daily retinol requirement of humans was 25 to 40 IU (7.5 to 12 μg) per kilogram body weight. The carotene requirement was estimated to be one and one-half to twice this amount except when derived from carrots for which data were regarded as inadequate for an estimate. The minimum requirement was considered to be possibly much less.

In reviewing the vitamin A status of Czechoslovakians, Mašek reported that, in 1959, the average estimated consumption of vitamin A was 3,000 IU/person/day and the average liver vitamin A level of adults who died accidentally during this same period was relatively low, 95.5 $\mu g/gram$ fresh liver (138). Prolonged dark-adaptation time was observed among Czechoslovakians consuming approximately 2,000 IU/person/day, one-half of which was derived from retinol. Considering these data Mašek (138) concluded that the appropriate intake for adults was in the range of 5,000 to 8,000 IU daily.

In 1968, Hoppner et al. (139) reported that, at death, the average liver vitamin A concentration of 25 Canadian subjects, 20 to 50 years old, was 79 µg/gram liver. A more extensive survey showed that specimens from 95 subjects in the same age bracket contained an average of 98 µg/gram liver (140). These values are lower than the "normal" values quoted by Pearson (141), 100 to 300 µg/gram liver. The investigators concluded that, in view of the "apparent" daily vitamin A intake of Canadians (6,800 IU), "it must be assumed that disease conditions, poor nutritional habits and other unknown environmental factors were the main contributing cause of the low vitamin A status in the high percentage of subjects" (139).

REQUIREMENTS OF CHILDREN
(TABLE 2)

Infants (0 to 24 Months)

Human vitamin A requirements during the growth period have received little attention. Studies with infants show that vitamin A requirements vary with the criteria used. According to three controlled studies (142–144), 350 to 1,100 IU daily was adequate for maintaining normal growth and resistance to infection, and infants fed 150 and 335 IU vitamin A daily maintain normal dark adaptation (145, 146). But the plasma values of depleted infants did not return to "normal" until 1,200 IU was given (146–148). Vitamin A in the liver of newborn infants is negligible and survey data suggest that an intake of 300 to 600 IU daily provides for little or no storage (149–157). On the other hand, acute vitamin A intoxication during infancy is not uncommon. Among children, 2 to 8 months old, 76 cases have been reported (158). Research on the required intake of provitamin A by infants has not been reported.

Retinol

Shortly after Bloch discovered that fat-soluble "A" bodies cured xerophthalmia in Danish infants (14), he observed that there was also a higher incidence and greater severity of infections among vitamin A-deficient children. Bloch suggested

TABLE 2

Daily vitamin A requirements of children, controlled studies

Age	Source	Number of studies	Number of subjects	Principal criteria	Inadequate Vitamin A value (IU)	Inadequate Retinol (µg²)	Adequate¹ Vitamin A value (IU)	Adequate¹ Retinol (µg²)	References
yr									
0–2	Retinol	3	468	Infection and growth			350–1,100³	105–330	142–144
		2	64	Dark adaptation			150–335	45–100	145, 146
		3	16	Plasma	150–600	45–180	1,200	360	146–148
3–5	Provitamin A	1	29	Plasma			2,500–3,700		198
6–12	Mixed diet	1	2	Dark adaptation			3,000		199
		1	20	Dark adaptation and plasma	2,000		2,700–4,000		127
13–18		0	0						

¹ Also includes optimal requirements.
² Original values converted to µg retinol on the basis that 1 IU is equivalent to 0.3 µg retinol.
³ Includes calculations on the basis that 1 Sherman unit equals 0.5 to 1.5 IU (Moore, T. 1957 Vitamin A. Elsevier Publishing Co. London, p. 564).

that vitamin A was of specific importance in the resistance to and the overcoming of infections (159). In 1932, Barenberg and Lewis (142) designed experiments to test this hypothesis. After feeding diets containing varying amounts of vitamin A to four groups of infants, they concluded that those receiving the least amount of vitamin A, 750 Sherman units daily,[1] were no more susceptible to infection than those receiving the largest amount, 16,500 Sherman units.

Seven years later, Lewis and Haig reported a similar experiment (145). Fifty-one infants, 3 to 12 months old, fed diets containing 500 to 1,050 IU vitamin A (150 to 315 μg retinol) daily, one-fourth the normal average intake, were compared with 53 infants fed approximately 17,000 IU (5,100 μg retinol) daily, four to eight times the normal daily intake. After almost 7 months, the investigators did not observe any differences in the growth, in vaginal smears, in scrapings from the conjunctiva, mouth or nose, or in resistance to infections between the two groups. Thus they stated that "it would seem therefore that the average diet of infants contains at least four times as many units as the minimum requirement," as judged by the above-mentioned criteria (145).

During a 5-month experimental period, Hess et al. (143) observed no differences in growth, nutrition or immunity to infection between 80 children under 3 years of age receiving a control diet which contained 750 ml of milk daily and those fed diets supplemented with 20,000 "rat" units of vitamin A from haliver oil or carotene. Therefore, they concluded that the amount of vitamin A contained in 750 ml of cow's milk was adequate for children less than 3 years old. Reports in the literature, however, indicate wide variations (up to 15-fold) in the vitamin A content of cow's milk (160, 161).

During this same period, Mackay (162) of England reported that 60 infants fed roller dried milk, who received additional vitamin A, were less susceptible to minor skin infections than 58 infants in the control group. However, when she repeated the experiment in 1939 (163) she observed no difference between the two groups. Mackay was unable to explain the reason for this difference in the two experiments. She estimated that in the first experiment, a 9-pound baby received at least 1,000 IU of vitamin A (300 μg retinol) daily. However, she explained that several difficulties were encountered in estimating the vitamin A content of the milk. In the second experiment, the amount was not measured. Thus "it cannot be affirmed that the vitamin A content of the milk was the same over the two different periods" (163). In view of the variability in the vitamin A content of fluid cow's milk, Mackay concluded that "pending other investigations on the subject, it is desirable to give artificially-fed babies a supplement providing extra vitamin A" (163).

According to studies conducted at the University of Iowa, 750 IU vitamin A daily permitted normal growth of infants 3 to 15 weeks old (164). Although Indian infants consuming 450 to 600 ml of human milk (149, 150) containing an average of 70 IU vitamin A (21 μg retinol)/100 ml (151, 152) are somewhat smaller than normal babies in the United States, they maintain a normal rate of growth during the first 6 months of life (150). The minimal amount to maintain growth in infants for prolonged periods has not been established. Assuming that the vitamin A expenditure of an infant is similar to that of the rat, Ellison and Moore estimated that an 11-pound baby requires roughly 500 IU (150 μg retinol) daily (165).

In 1939, Lewis and Haig (145) fed 53 infants, 1.5 to 13 months old, diets containing 135 to 200 IU of vitamin A (40.5 to 60 μg retinol) daily for 3 months, i.e., approximately 25 IU (7.5 μg retinol) per kilogram body weight, which is one-twelfth the normal intake. Since the dark adaptation remained normal and the weight gain was average, Lewis and Haig concluded that the minimum daily requirement of infants was 25 to 35 IU (7.5 to 10.5 μg retinol) per kilogram body weight. This is close to the 20 to 27 IU/kilogram which Guilbert et al. (166) estimated to be the minimum daily requirement for the mammalian species, cattle, sheep and swine. On the basis of these dark-adaptation tests, Lewis and Haig (145) concluded that the vitamin A requirements of infants

---

[1] One Sherman unit equals 0.5 to 1.5 IU (5).

and children could be met with a normal diet.

In 1941, however, after studying the effects of vitamin A supplements on the plasma vitamin A values of infants less than 6 months old, Lewis and his associates (147) advised giving vitamin A concentrate routinely to infants during the early months of life. Similarly, Kübler (167) concluded from blood values and vaginal smears that the amount of vitamin A obtained by German infants from a diet of cow's milk and carbohydrates was not enough and recommended that supplements be given. As mentioned previously, the amount of vitamin A in cow's milk is variable, depending on the provitamin A intake (5, 160, 161, 166).

When Bodansky et al. (146) fed six infants, 3 weeks to 2.5 months old, diets containing 335 units of vitamin A (100 μg retinol) daily for 2 to 4 months, they observed that although dark-adaptation time remained normal, the average plasma values dropped from the initial 74 to 61 units/100 ml. Similar results were noted in a second group of 12 infants, 1.5 to 4 months of age, who were placed on a diet devoid of vitamin A for 2 weeks to 4.5 months. When five of the depleted infants were given 150 units of vitamin A (45 μg retinol) daily for 1 month, dark adaptation became normal in every instance but plasma vitamin A remained low. Thus they concluded that plasma vitamin A concentration was a more sensitive indicator of vitamin A deficiency than dark-adaptation tests. These investigators reported similar results for 144 infants fed diets containing varying amounts of vitamin A (147). The plasma vitamin A values (93 USP units/100 ml) of 62 infants less than 6 months old, receiving 17,000 additional USP units of vitamin A (5,100 μg retinol) daily were higher than those (74 USP units/100 ml) of infants who received the average diet containing about 1,340 USP units (402 μg retinol). This difference in plasma values was not observed when the diets of infants 7 to 18 months old were supplemented with the additional vitamin A. Lewis and Bodansky (148) observed that 600 USP units (180 μg retinol) given daily for 4 weeks had no appreciable effect on the plasma values of five vitamin A-depleted infants. But 1,200 USP units (360 μg retinol) brought the blood concentration into the normal range (40 to 114 USP units/100 ml) (147) in the five infants receiving this dosage. They therefore estimated that the daily minimum vitamin A requirement for infants under 7 months of age lay somewhere between 600 and 1200 USP units, or 100 to 200 USP units per kilogram body weight/day (148). Since the latter amount brought the plasma values just within the "normal" range, they reasoned that the requirement was probably closer to 200 USP units (60 μg retinol) per kilogram body weight/day. Stearns (164) reported that the mean plasma vitamin A values of 3- to 15-week-old infants receiving 750 and 1,500 IU vitamin A (225 and 450 μg retinol) daily, were 22 and 40 μg/100 ml, respectively. The minimum plasma vitamin A level of infants over 6 months of age, receiving between 2,000 and 3,000 IU (600 and 900 μg retinol) daily, was about 40 μg/100 ml.

Lewis et al. (168) and Guilbert et al. (166) have shown that the vitamin A requirement of growing rats varies according to the criterion used. Very little vitamin A (2 USP units daily) is required to maintain an optimal concentration in the retina. However, for optimal growth, blood concentration and liver stores, respectively, 12.5, 25 and 50 times this amount are required (168). Results of studies with human infants also show that estimated requirements vary with the criterion used.

None of the human studies mentioned thus far has considered the intake necessary to provide for liver storage in infants. In view of the generally low concentration of vitamin A in the livers of premature and newborn infants (139, 165, 169–178), this may be an important factor. In summarizing the reports in the literature on the vitamin A content of livers from stillborn infants, Moore (5) pointed out that with the exception of the work of Neuweiler (170), the mean values reported from various parts of the world during the 1930's (10 to 44 IU/g liver) (165, 171–174) were much lower than those reported in the more recent literature. Since 1940, mean values reported from the United States (147, 176, 177), Canada (139), New Zealand (169) and Great

Britain (178) ranged from 115 to 142 IU/gram liver. The average value for Finnish newborns was 286 IU/g (175). The reason for the difference in the values for the two periods is unexplained. Moore (5) suggested that it may be related to the recent practice of including vitamin concentrates in the diet during pregnancy. Although the more recent figures are higher than the earlier ones, the average liver vitamin A content of newborn infants is still low compared with the "normal" values for adult livers (100 to 300 μg/g liver) (141).

Survey data on the vitamin A content of livers obtained at autopsy from infants suggest that it is possible to increase infant liver reserves at a relatively rapid rate (165, 173). But the daily intake required to allow for storage, the desirability of vitamin A liver storage per se, and the optimum level of vitamin A per gram of liver are all unknown. The mature milk of Indian (149–152, 153) and Jordanian (154) mothers provides approximately 300 to 570 IU vitamin A (90 and 171 μg retinol) daily. The high incidence of vitamin A deficiency in early childhood among children from these countries (155, 156) suggests that liver storage is negligible in human infants consuming this amount of vitamin A (157). Chandra et al. (156) found that among Indian children, 2 to 5 years old, consuming diets low in vitamin A, keratomalacia was four times more prevalent in the group whose diets had not been supplemented with vitamin A-containing foods during the first year of life than it was in the group that began eating such foods by 6 months of age.

Individual investigators and advisory groups have employed various methods of calculating the vitamin A requirements of infants. On the basis of the average vitamin A content of human milk from lactating mothers in England (179) and the assumption that the average milk production of a healthy lactating woman is 850 ml/day, the Joint FAO/WHO Expert Group on vitamin A requirements recommended 420 μg retinol daily for infants during the first 6 months of life (45). This is equivalent to 50 and 65 μg per kilogram body weight/day for infants 5 and 3 months old, respectively. On the basis of

body weight increment, the Group recommended intakes of 300 and 250 μg retinol/day for infants 6 to 12 months and 1 to 2 years old, respectively.

Rønni (180) of Copenhagen calculated that the infant required 20 to 40 IU (6 and 12 μg retinol) per kilogram body weight daily. He used a formula which involved the infant's liver weight expressed as percentage of total body weight, the IU of vitamin A/kilogram liver and duration in days of a vitamin A-free dietary regimen. On the basis of the literature review of Rubin and deRitter (181), Fomon (182) estimated that infants 1, 6 and 12 months old require 70, 170 and 200 IU (21, 51 and 60 μg retinol) per day, respectively. However, "because we do not know whether the vitamin A requirement of the adult is applicable to the infant on a body weight basis, the advisable intake during the first year of life is . . . 600 IU/day or three times the estimated requirement of an infant weighing 10 kg" (182).

Hypervitaminosis A

As mentioned in the introduction, excess vitamin A may result in acute or chronic intoxication. The acute form is more commonly observed in children less than 1 year old. Ninety-seven of the 98 acute cases reviewed by Bartolozzi et al. (158) occurred in children 3 years old or less; 76 of them were infants, 2 to 8 months old. In most cases symptoms appeared in the infants 1.5 to 36 hours after receiving 300,000 to 400,000 IU vitamin A (90,000 to 120,000 μg retinol). However, in one case, symptoms were noted 8 hours after receiving 60,000 IU (18,000 μg retinol).

Bartolozzi et al. (158) cited 24 cases of chronic toxicity among children 2 years old or less from the United States and Western Europe. The daily doses of infants, 2 to 9 months old, ranged from 18,500 to 200,000 IU (5,550 to 60,000 μg retinol) for a period of 2 to 2.5 months (158, 183–188). Children 1 to 2 years old received 100,000 to 600,000 IU (30,000 to 180,000 μg retinol) for 1 to 21 months. Pease (189) reported seven additional cases of chronic hypervitaminosis A in children about 1 to 3 years old. Growth retardation was observed in three of them when they were reexamined 4 to 16 years later.

In 1965, Persson et al. (183) reported five cases of chronic intoxication in Swedish infants, 1 to 3 months old, who manifested symptoms after taking 4,000 to 15,000 IU (1,200 to 4,500 μg retinol) per kilogram for 6 to 12 weeks (18,000 to 60,000 IU daily). These data suggest that toxicity becomes manifest more rapidly in the young infant. In Sweden, infants were routinely given 7,500 to 10,000 IU of vitamin A (2,250 to 3,000 μg retinol) daily (190). After observing that daily doses as low as 18,500 IU could cause toxicity, Tunell et al. (190) compared the effects of giving 2,500 IU vs. 7,500 IU (750 vs. 2,250 μg retinol) daily from birth. The fasting blood levels of the two groups were 68 and 95 IU, respectively. Postabsorptive blood levels were 140 IU (range, 100 to 600) and 334 IU, respectively. Since the postabsorptive levels of those receiving 7,500 IU daily were in the range known to be associated with clinical toxicity, the investigators recommended that the routine daily prophylactic dose should be reduced to 2,500 IU (750 μg retinol) (190).

Children (2 to 18 Years)

Initially, we had intended to discuss the vitamin A requirements of children according to the following age-groups: 2 to 5, 6 to 12 and 13 to 18 years old. However, in view of the limited information, we have included all the studies for children 2 to 18 years of age under each of the following topics: requirements for vitamin A from retinol, provitamin A and mixed diets.

In 1934, Mackay (191) reviewed the early literature on vitamin A deficiency and concluded that "nearly all observers agree that young children develop symptoms of vitamin A deficiency more readily and suffer more severely than older persons." The nutritional status surveys which have been conducted since then in Africa (155, 192, 193), Indonesia (194), India (156, 195), Asia (155) and Latin America (155, 196) support this early statement. The peak incidence of xerophthalmia

occurs among children 3 to 4 years of age (197).

In spite of the voluminous literature documenting the common occurrence of vitamin A deficiency among preschool age children and repeatedly deploring the widespread occurrence of irreparable eye damage, we found no reports in the literature of controlled experiments on the retinol requirements of children 2 through 18 years of age. Reports were found of one controlled study with preschool children fed provitamin A as the source of vitamin A activity (198), and of two studies with children 6 through 12 years of age who ate a mixed diet (127, 199). Incidences of hypervitaminosis A have been reported for all age groups.

A few of the nutritional status surveys conducted in various parts of the world provide information on the average intake of groups of children 2 to 18 years old. However, since the vitamin A activity of the diet is usually reported in International Units, they provide little specific data regarding the original source. In the surveys which we have included in this review, vitamin A intake has been compared with growth, prevalence of skin and eye lesions, night blindness, dark adaptation and plasma vitamin A values.

When using data from nutritional status surveys, it should be kept in mind that cases of pure vitamin A deficiency are seldom encountered (197). Almost invariably, the diets of children with clinical vitamin A deficiency symptoms also lack other essential nutrients (197, 200). Protein–calorie malnutrition (155, 156, 193) and infections (155, 197) are commonly associated with xerophthalmia. In a recent review article (201) Patwardhan concluded: "It is reasonable to expect, therefore, that the conditions in infancy and early childhood that in developing countries lead to the prevalence of protein–calorie malnutrition could also be responsible largely, if not wholly, for the occurrence of vitamin A deficiency in these same groups." As discussed in a later section of this paper, the absorption, transport and metabolism of vitamin A compounds are interrelated with several other nutrients.

Retinol

In view of the widespread deficiency signs among preschool-age children, investigators have been experimenting with the administration of massive infrequent doses of vitamin A, in lieu of daily dietary intake. In 1969, Pereira and Begum (202) reported from India that a single massive oral dose of vitamin A palmitate in oil (100,000 μg) maintained "adequate" (20 μg/100 ml) serum levels in vitamin A-depleted children 2 to 5 years old, for about 15 weeks. In that same year Susheela (203) found that the serum vitamin A values of Indian children given a single dose of 100,000 μg vitamin A were significantly higher than those children who received no vitamin A. The average serum vitamin A values 4 months, 1 year and 2 years after receiving the vitamin were 37.4, 27.4 and 24.0 μg/ml, respectively. The average value for the control group was 20.4 μg/100 ml. Similarly, Srikantia and Reddy (204) found that a single dose of 300,000 IU (90,000 μg retinol) sustained the serum levels of 15 undernourished children at almost normal levels (90 IU/100 ml) for at least 6 months. Once each year for 2 years, Swaminathan et al. (205) administered 300,000 IU of vitamin A in oil orally to 1,785 children 1 to 5 years old. This dosage prevented eye lesions in 98% of the younger children; however, only 78% of the subjects 4 to 5 years old were free of lesions. Also, toxic manifestations were observed in 4% of the children. Therefore, they suggested that 200,000 IU (60,000 μg retinol) be administered once each 6 months.

Hypervitaminosis A. Both acute and chronic hypervitaminosis A have been reported in children 2 to 18 years of age. Bartolozzi et al. (158) reviewed the data on two acute and 17 chronic cases, in children 2 to 5 years old. One of the two acute cases had taken 400,000 IU (120,000 μg retinol) in a single dose. Intake in the second case was not indicated. In the chronic cases, the daily dosage ranged from 60,000 IU (18,000 μg retinol) for 9 months to 400,000 to 500,000 IU (120,000 to 150,000 μg retinol) for 2 years, taken by a 5-year-old and a 3-year-old girl, respectively.

In 1955, Gonzalez Outon (206) reported two cases of acute hypervitaminosis A in 9- and 11-year-old Spanish children who received a water-soluble preparation providing 400,000 IU vitamin A (120,000 μg retinol) and 600,000 IU vitamin D. In the four chronic cases reported for children 6 to 8 years old (112, 158, 207, 208), the daily dose ranged from 50,000 to 100,000 IU (15,000 to 30,000 μg retinol) for 1 year (208) to 200,000 to 463,000 IU (600,000 to 138,900 μg retinol) for 5.5 years (207).

In addition, ten cases, one acute and nine chronic, have been reported in children 13 to 18 years old. According to Laplane et al. (209), a dose of 500,000 IU (150,000 μg retinol) caused acute poisoning of a 16-year-old French boy. Seven of the eight chronic cases reviewed by Bartolozzi et al. occurred in the United States (158). The daily dosage ranged from 50,000 to 300,000 IU (15,000 to 90,000 μg retinol) for 6 months to 3.5 years. A similar case of an 18-year-old girl was recently reported from the Mayo Clinic (111, 210).

Provitamin A

In 1936, Aykroyd and Krishnan (211) found eye symptoms, indicative of vitamin A deficiency (dryness, smokiness and wrinkling of the conjunctiva or Bitôt's spots), in 27% of the 436 Indian children, 1 to 12 years old, that they examined. It was assumed that the diet of these children was entirely devoid of preformed vitamin A. Although several different vegetables were included in the diet, chalam (*Andropagan sorghum*) was the principal source of provitamin A. The carotene content of the various vegetables was measured spectrophotometrically but the types of. carotene were not indicated. The diets of the 1- to 5-, 5- to 8- and 8- to 12-year-old groups contained an average of 455, 710 and 785 μg carotene daily, respectively. On the basis of this information, the investigators hypothesized that "700 μg of carotene represents an inadequate intake for children" and suggested that "optimum human requirements of vitamin A activity should perhaps be set very considerably above the 'sub-minimal' figure recorded in this paper, i.e., in the neighborhood of 3,000–5,000 IU."

The following year Aykroyd and Wright (212) reported that they could cure kerato-malacia with daily doses of approximately 1.1 g of red palm oil which contained approximately 500 μg carotene/gram of oil. A "suitable allowance" was made in the dosage for younger and older individuals. The carotene was dissolved in oil, thus making it readily available. Similarly, Awdry et al. (192) have found that in Northern Rhodesia, blindness among young children is almost unknown in those villages where red palm oil is used. And Oey Khoen Lian et al. (213) recently reported that supplementing the diets of Indonesian children, 1 to 5 years old, with 4 ml red palm oil daily ("approximately 3,000 units of provitamin A") significantly increased their serum vitamin A levels. The red palm oil contained approximately 600 to 800 μg β-carotene/gram (214).

A nutritional status survey of 156 Indonesian children less than 8 years of age (71 were 2 to 5 years old), suggested that 1,600 IU from dark leafy vegetables is sufficient to prevent night blindness in preschool-age children (194). In the survey, 19 of the 20 malnourished children with night blindness were 2 to 5 years old and Bitôt's spots were observed in 11 of them. Of the remaining 52 children, 2 to 5 years old, 28 were healthy and 24 were malnourished but clinical signs of vitamin deficiency were not observed. Individual dietary surveys of 62 children, 2 to 5 years old, revealed the following average daily total vitamin A intakes: 26 healthy children, 1,624 IU; 22 malnourished children without night blindness, 884 IU; and 14 malnourished with night blindness, 973 IU. In all cases dark leafy vegetables were the primary source of vitamin A. Vitamin A values were computed on the assumption that 1 IU was equivalent to 0.3 μg retinol, 0.6 μg β-carotene or 1.2 μg other carotenoids. Blankhart (194) pointed out that the average daily vitamin A intake of the mothers of malnourished children with night blindness was 2,084 IU carotene. The average intakes of the mothers of healthy and malnourished children without night blindness were 3,583 and 3,039 IU, respectively. "This finding suggests protection by building up vitamin A liver stores during intra-uterine life and

lactation by the children without night blindness" (194). Blankhart recommended that 2- to 5-year-old children consume 50 g of dark-green leafy vegetables, which contain 2,000 to 4,000 IU of carotene daily.

Six years later when Pek Hien Liang et al. (215) examined 64 of the original 156 children, they found that 12 of those who had previously shown vitamin A deficiency symptoms now appeared to be the smallest, the most mentally retarded and in the poorest general physical condition. Lauw Tjin Giok et al. (200) reported that at this time the mean serum vitamin A values for 90 of the original 156 subjects in these three groups were 15.5, 18.2 and 20.6 μg/100 ml, respectively. In reviewing these reports, Lauw Tjin Giok et al. (200) stated that these data, though not conclusive, are indicative of a late effect of early damage caused by malnutrition especially combined with vitamin A deficiency.

In the only controlled study on the vitamin A requirements of preschool children, Pereira and Begum (198) showed that including 30 g of cooked green leafy vegetables, which provided 2,500 to 3,750 IU β-carotene, in the diets of 29 preschool-age children for 12 weeks raised the average serum vitamin A value from 21.6 to 30.6 μg/100 ml. When seven of these children were subsequently given a vitamin A-deficient diet for 24 weeks, they maintained "adequate" vitamin A levels (above 15 μg/100 ml) for 24 weeks thus indicating that at this level of intake vitamin A was stored in the liver. Pereira and Begum (198) concluded that "inclusion of greens in the diet for 3 months will afford protection to children for 4 to 5 months afterward, even when they are given a severely vitamin A-deficient diet." Lala and Reddy (216) also observed that supplementing the diet of preschool children in India with amaranth significantly increased serum vitamin A levels.

Mixed diet

Chandra et al. (156) compared the vitamin A status of children living in two different areas of India — Hyderabad and Coonoor. The diets of the vitamin A-deficient children, 2 to 5 years old, from the two areas were similar. They contained an average of 213 to 425 IU from carotenes and 90 to 106 IU from preformed vitamin A. Yet the deficiency symptoms were much more severe in Hyderabad; 28% of the 551 deficient children in Hyderabad had keratomalacia compared with 7% of the 319 children in Coonoor. The nutritional status of the mothers from these two regions was similar and their milk provided similar amounts of vitamin A, approximately 400 IU daily. However, children from Coonoor began receiving supplementary feedings by the sixth month of life. On the other hand, in the majority of cases in Hyderabad, supplemental feeding was not instituted until well after the end of the first year. Thus the vitamin A intake of the children from Hyderabad may have been more limited for a longer period of time, providing less opportunity for hepatic storage. Data collected in this study suggest that 300 to 500 IU vitamin A daily is inadequate for the 2- to 5-year-old child. In Chile, nutritional status surveys indicated that 49.2% of 138 preschool children consuming an average of 1,899 IU vitamin A daily had hyperkeratosis and 7.9% had cutaneous xerosis (217). The source of vitamin A was not indicated for this age group. In other Chilean groups, however, 62 to 82% of vitamin A intake is derived from the provitamins.

The recent Puerto Rican surveys of Fernández et al. (218–221) demonstrate the difference in the vitamin A activity of retinol versus provitamin A. These investigators surveyed the nutritional status of 184 children, 2 to 5 years old, dwelling in four different isolated villages and estimated the intake of one-fourth of the participants from 24-hour food composition records. Vitamin A deficiency symptoms (follicular hyperkeratosis and xerosis) and plasma values were reported.

In their first survey, Fernández et al. (218) found that among the 38 children from Vega Alta who consumed an average of 1,241 IU of vitamin A daily, primarily in the provitamin form, 18.4% had follicular hyperkeratosis. According to serum plasma values, 60% were deficient (less than 20 µg/100 ml). In San German (220) the children consumed only slightly more vitamin A, 1,450 IU daily. However, according to plasma values, only 12% of

them were deficient. On the other hand, the estimated intake of children in Moca (219) was 2,826 IU daily and 51% of them had plasma values in the deficient range. The average daily intake of milk was similar in the three villages. Children in San German, however, consumed whole milk (185 g daily) while those in Vega Alta and Moca consumed more skimmed milk (63 and 69% of the total intake, respectively). Mangos, a tropical fruit, were apparently the primary source of vitamin A activity in the diet of children residing in Moca. From these data, it appears that 2,800 IU of vitamin A activity primarily from mangos does not meet the daily requirement of 2- to 5-year-old children. Although the children in the fourth village (221) consumed less total vitamin A activity (854 IU daily) and 21% of them had follicular hyperkeratosis, the mean serum vitamin A value was normal (71 µg/100 ml). The investigators were unable to explain these unexpectedly high serum values.

The results of two controlled studies with 22 subjects suggest that 3,000 to 4,000 IU vitamin A from a mixed diet are adequate for maintaining normal dark adaptation and plasma vitamin A concentration in children 6 to 12 years old.

Jeans and Zentmire (222) found that 62% of the 404 Iowa school children, 6 to 15 years old, whom they examined in 1936, had abnormal dark-adaptation rates. When 78 of them were treated with halibut-liver oil or carotene in oil, equal to approximately 3 teaspoons of cod-liver oil daily, the majority of them attained normal adaptation time within 1 month. The vitamin A activity of the oil was not indicated. The next year, Jeans et al. (199) reported that the dark-adaptation time of several children promptly returned to normal when they were fed mixed diets containing 5,000 to 6,000 IU vitamin A activity daily. They also concluded that an intake of 3,000 IU daily was adequate for 11-year-old boys. At this level of intake, one subject maintained his ability to adapt to the dark for 3 months; a second subject, with an initial subnormal adaptation time, reached normality after 2 months.

Roels et al. (127) found that 39% of the 52 Indonesian boys, 3 to 13 years old, whom they examined, had marked eye symptoms of vitamin A deficiency. Their daily intake was approximately 2,000 IU, 90% of which came from carotenoids. When the diets of 10 of these boys were supplemented with palm oil containing 410 μg carotene/gram (1 g palm oil/kg body wt), all cases of night blindness were cured within 3 weeks. By the end of the first week the average plasma vitamin A value had risen from 18.9 to 33.0 μg/100 ml. Since it remained at this level during the final 2 weeks of the experiment, the investigators concluded that the supplement was more than adequate and assumed that the excess was being stored in the liver.

Roels et al. (127) supplemented the diet of 10 other boys with 2,000 IU vitamin A acetate (600 μg retinol) daily, bringing their total intake to approximately 4,000 IU daily. Initially, six of these boys showed marked clinical symptoms of vitamin A deficiency. After 3 weeks all cases of night blindness were cured and normal plasma values were maintained. Average plasma vitamin A values at the beginning of the experiment and after 1 and 3 weeks of supplementation were 20.1, 34.4 and 35.4 μg/100 ml, respectively. However, there were no detectable changes in the anatomic lesions generally ascribed to vitamin A deficiency. The researchers point out that such lesions require a much longer period of treatment to heal.

According to the final rod threshold test all but one of 144 New York City school children, 6 to 12 years of age, whom Lewis and Haig (223) examined in 1940 had normal dark-adaptation time. The daily diets of these children contained approximately 5,000 IU total vitamin A activity, thus providing 125 to 250 IU/kilogram body weight/day. Lewis and Haig (223) therefore reasoned that, compared with the adult retinol requirements estimated by Booher et al. (55) (25 to 55 units/kg body wt) and Guilbert et al. (166) (20 to 27 units/kg body wt) an allowance of 5,000 IU daily for 6- to 12-year-old children provided a large margin of safety.

In 1941, Basu and De (64) reported that, according to dark-adaptation efficiency tests, the bodies of 77% of 391 school boys from Calcutta, India contained

adequate vitamin A. By comparing data from food consumption records kept for some of the boys (the number was not indicated) and their dark-adaptation test scores, the investigators concluded that 6- to 15-year-old boys require at least 4,000 IU while the optimal intake is 5,000 IU vitamin A daily.

After finding that supplemental vitamin A (13,000 to 38,000 USP units daily) cured follicular conjunctivitis in elementary school children 6 to 12 years old, Sandels et al. (224) recorded the daily food intake of 58 children for 1 week. Thirty-one of the 34 children who received less than 100 USP units of vitamin A/kilogram body weight per day had follicular conjunctivitis. Ten of the 15 children who received 100 to 158 USP units/kilogram daily also had the deficiency symptom. The investigators concluded that, provided the ingested vitamin A was utilizable, 160 USP units/kilogram body weight per day was sufficient to prevent follicular conjunctivitis in children 6 to 12 years old. They suggested, however, that "in diets in which carotene furnishes a large proportion of the vitamin A value 200 to 250 USP units of vitamin A per kilogram of body weight per day will provide a none too generous allowance for children between the ages of 6 and 12 years" (224).

During the 1950's investigators in the United States reported the following survey data: The mean vitamin A intake of 66, 5- to 12-year-old subjects from Utah was > 6,500 IU (225). Forty-five percent of the total intake derived from vegetable sources. The plasma values of 6% of these children were < 20 μg and 42% had values < 30 μg/100 ml (226). More than 10% of the girls 10 to 12 years old had values < 20 μg/100 ml. The mean vitamin A intakes of 1,700 children from Iowa, Kansas and Ohio, 9 to 11 years old, were 8,100 for males and 7,200 IU for females (227). Twenty-five percent had relatively low intakes, 2,950 to 3,850 IU. Individual serum values among the 830 children ranged from 2 to 87 μg/100 ml; the range of the group means was 28 to 47 μg/100 ml (228). More than 25% had values less than 30 μg. Information on intake versus plasma vitamin A for individuals was not indicated.

Dietary surveys are the only source of information on the vitamin A requirements of adolescents. During the 1950's seven states reported the results of nutritional status studies involving 1,836 subjects 13 to 19 years of age (225, 226, 229–238). The mean daily vitamin A activity of the mixed diets of 531 students from Washington (229), Montana (230) and Utah (225) ranged from 5,170 to 8,000 IU. Mean serum values ranged from 32 to 52 μg/100 ml (226, 229, 231). Except for the results of the biomicroscopic examinations of the bulbar conjunctiva of the eye and epithelium of the arm of Washington children (229), the vitamin A status of the subjects from these three states appeared to be good. More than one-half of 115 students in Arizona had plasma vitamin A values lower than 20 μg/100 ml (232). The total daily intake was not indicated but the serum values of those subjects receiving the school lunch which contained approximately 2,400 IU were significantly higher than values for those not consuming this meal (232). The home diets of all Arizona students were similar and contained limited amounts of retinol.

Less than 10% of the 729 Oregon students consumed < 3,300 IU of vitamin A daily (233) and 11% of them had plasma values below 20 μg/100 ml (234). These data suggest that 3,300 IU was insufficient. The dietary source of vitamin A for these children was not indicated.

The mean intake of 170 New Mexican children, 14 to 16 years of age, was > 5,600 IU daily (3,667 to 6,927 IU) (235). The mean plasma vitamin A values for Spanish-American and Anglo children were 29 and 32 μg/100 ml, respectively, and no deficiency symptoms were noted in any of the subjects (236).

In Idaho, the mean plasma vitamin A concentration of 150 girls, 15 to 16 years old, consuming 5,500 IU daily (237) was 31.5 μg/100 ml (238); for 123 boys consuming 7,000 IU daily, 34.5 μg/1000 ml.

Calculated Vitamin A Requirements of Children 1 to 18 Years Old

Using night blindness as the criterion, Guilbert et al. (166) concluded that, regardless of age, mammals require approximately the same amount of vitamin A/kilogram body weight. On the other hand, Johnson and Baumann reported that in rats, the degree of depletion of vitamin A liver stores depended on the rate of growth and the basal metabolic rate (239). Rechcigl et al. (240) found that when growing rats were fed a vitamin A-free diet, the amount of vitamin A in the livers decreased as the amount of protein in the diet increased. A linear relationship was observed between weight gain and vitamin A utilization. These data suggest that during growth, vitamin A requirements may be related to protein intake. Although this has not been demonstrated experimentally in humans, the National Research Council in 1945 (241) based the recommended allowances for children on a combination of age, weight and dietary protein allowance. Since then, the Council has reduced the recommended protein intake for children in each of the different age groups (241a). But the recommended vitamin A intake for children has not been changed, except for boys 16 to 20 years old. Therefore, the ratio of vitamin A to protein, at each age level, is now greater and the recommended vitamin A intake is related to weight, plus additional amounts to cover growth needs.

REQUIREMENTS OF PREGNANT AND LACTATING WOMEN

Pregnant Women

Retinol

Despite the fact that investigators have demonstrated congenital malformations in animals due to both hypovitaminosis and hypervitaminosis A during gestation (5), no reports of controlled studies on the retinol requirements of pregnant women have been found. Animal studies are our only source of information. According to Guilbert et al. (166), gravid cows need three to four times the minimum required amount of retinol (6 to 8 μg/kg body wt/day) to produce and maintain normal healthy offspring.

Botella Llusiá and Hernández Araña (242) of Spain surveyed the nutritional status of 140 pregnant women. Ten percent of those who consumed 4,000 IU preformed vitamin A (1,200 μg retinol), 50 g fat and varying amounts of provitamin A had abnormal dark adaptation. Therefore, they recommended that pregnant women take in at least 4,000 IU retinol daily. Since those who consumed 12,000 IU as provitamin A and 20 g fat had poor dark adaptation, they assumed that pregnant women do not utilize carotene.

One case of human hypervitaminosis A during pregnancy was reported by Pilotti and Scorta (243). An Italian mother who had ingested excessive amounts of vitamins A and D (40,000 and 600,000 IU daily for about a month, respectively) beginning 40 days after her menses ceased, gave birth to a malformed child. Since then Gal et al. (244) have compared the vitamin A status of malformed and normally formed offspring and their respective mothers. They were unable to show any relationship between malformed fetuses and the amount of vitamin A in the fetal liver or the mother's plasma. In a recent review Della Cella (245) pointed out that in rats, doses only slightly above therapeutic levels caused malformed fetuses. The type of deformation appears to depend on when, during gestation, the excessive dose is administered. The observations of Cohlan suggest that there may be an optimal range of vitamin A intake (246).

Provitamin A

Except for one report by von Drigalski and Kunz of Germany (247), animal studies are also our only source of information on provitamin A requirements during pregnancy. On the basis of the dark-adaptation response of three women, they estimated that in late pregnancy women require 7 to 20 mg β-carotene daily. Since fetal venous blood contained significantly more carotene than fetal arterial blood, Clausen and McCoord (248) concluded that the fetus utilized carotene. They estimated that "about 1 mg of carotene per kilogram of fetus per day might be furnished to it." According to Guilbert et al. (166), during reproduction cows require at least five times the minimum maintenance level of carotene. Although gravid cows fed 75 to 100 μg carotene/kilogram body weight/day (three to four times the minimum daily maintenance requirement) gave birth to normal calves, the calves de-

veloped deficiency symptoms 3 to 4 weeks later.

Mixed diet

No xerophthalmia was observed in the 950 pregnant Chilian women ingesting a mixed diet containing an average of 4,793 IU vitamin A daily but 22% had perifollicular hyperkeratosis (217).

Physiological changes relating to vitamin A requirements

During pregnancy, additional vitamin A is apparently necessary for a number of special metabolic processes such as fetal development and liver storage, maternal formation of colostrum and storage for lactation, and possibly hormone synthesis. Although studies of human vitamin A metabolism during pregnancy offer no quantitative data on requirements, they do provide information that has a direct bearing on the subject. Therefore, some of the observed physiological changes relating to vitamin A requirements will be discussed in this section.

Increased dark-adaptation time and reduced plasma vitamin A values are commonly observed among pregnant women in various parts of the world. Supplementing the diet with retinol relieves these symptoms. In 1930, Aykroyd (249) observed that night blindness among women in Newfoundland and Labrador was usually associated with pregnancy and tended to clear spontaneously after parturition. "Three large tablespoon doses of cod oil" relieved the symptom in one pregnant woman in 3 days. Thirty-six years later, Dixit (250) reported from India that, of 203 women whom he examined, 77 stated emphatically that night blindness, which developed in the third trimester of pregnancy, disappeared spontaneously immediately after parturition. Intramuscular injections of vitamin A temporarily relieved night blindness in pregnant women. He concluded that 2,061 IU of vitamin A, the average daily intake of women from this area, was insufficient, especially in cases of repeated pregnancies.

Edmund and Clemmesen (251) found that one-half of the 50 pregnant Danish women whom they examined had dark dysadaptation which temporarily improved when they were given an intramuscular injection of 40,000 IU (12,000 μg) retinol. Since dysadaptation recurred after the injections, they concluded that vitamin A absorption from the intestinal tract is frequently reduced during pregnancy. The diet of 62% of the 123 pregnant women whom Williams et al. examined contained less than the recommended vitamin A allowance for pregnant women (6,000–10,000 Sherman units daily) (252) and 37.5% of the women had abnormal dark-adaptation time. However, there was no significant correlation between vitamin A intake and subnormal dark adaptation. Nevertheless, when 28 women were given 20,820 IU of vitamin A daily, the dark-adaptation time of 21 subjects decreased.

In 1940, after testing the dark-adaptation time of 200 pregnant Pennsylvanian women, Hirst and Shoemaker concluded that during pregnancy there was a general tendency toward improvement of vitamin A status (253). The following year they reported that of 328 pregnant women only two had dark dysadaptation (254). When, however, a single determination of serum vitamin A for each of 34 of these women was made, 14 women were found to be vitamin A deficient (< 28 USP units/100 ml). There was no correlation between dark-adaptation readings and serum vitamin A values. On the basis of these measurement, Hirst and Shoemaker concluded that dietary insufficiency in pregnancy should be assumed. They recommended routine vitamin A supplementation. No mention was made of quantitative intake. They further declared that the dark-adaptation test was "relatively worthless." Some difficulty with interfering substances in the spectrophotometric readings in the blood analysis was also mentioned.

Decreased plasma vitamin A concentration has been observed at the onset of pregnancy (255), during the last trimester (256–262), at parturition (255, 263), as well as continuously throughout pregnancy (264). Significant increases in the ratio of plasma carotene to vitamin A have also been reported (261, 263). Ozorotsii (265) found that the coefficient of correlation of vitamin A and carotene was reduced in the first and third trimester. Except for Dawson et al. (263), who found

that expressing individual vitamin A and carotene values as a ratio to the hematocrit value did not alter the observed changes, these reports did not mention a possible change in total blood volume.

Lewis et al. (266) found that the decline in blood values during the last trimester could be compensated for with daily supplements of 10,000 IU (3,000 μg) as retinol or carotene. Similarly, Hoch and Marrack (267) reported that pregnant women who took vitamin A supplements had higher plasma values than those who did not.

Several explanations for the temporary declines in plasma vitamin A concentration have been suggested. According to Bodansky et al. (258), the terminal decrease may be due to increased requirements of the fetal tissues and storage in the fetal liver. As mentioned in the section on infant requirements, the liver reserves of newborn babies generally are low. A portion of it may also be used in forming colostrum which is rich in vitamin A (255, 268).

In 1934, Debré and Busson reported that the liver of a woman who had died in shock after a cesarean section contained 544.4 IU/gram liver (269). Williams et al. (252) presented this as evidence to support the argument that excess storage takes place during pregnancy in order to prepare for the increased requirement of lactation. Moore of England (270) proposed 220 IU/g, the median value for 40 liver samples taken at autopsy during the 1930's, as a "typical" value for the healthy adult.

Neumann (271) suggested that vitamin A acts as a catalyst for transforming cholesterol into progesterone. This sharply increased demand for vitamin A might help to account for the initial temporary drop in circulating vitamin A (272). Hays and Kendall (273) found that progesterone markedly improved reproduction in vitamin A-deficient female rabbits and hypothesized that either progesterone helps to mobilize nutrients from storage or, vitamin A may be associated with the formation of progesterone. After reviewing the recent literature on the effects of vitamin A deficiency on the adrenals of experimental animals, Granguad et al. (274)

concluded that the transformation of pregnenolone into progesterone and the elaboration of androstenedione from its physiological precursor are inhibited. They presented several hypotheses for the mode of action, but the mechanism(s) and active form(s) of vitamin A are still not known. The relationship of adrenal hormone synthesis and vitamin A may have a direct effect on vitamin A requirements during pregnancy.

A report of the Indian Council of Medical Research (275) suggests that pregnant and nonpregnant women metabolize vitamin A differently. They found that oral vitamin A supplements (5,000 IU daily) brought about increases in the vitamin A concentration of the milk of mothers who had become pregnant during the course of lactation but there was no significant effect on the vitamin A values of milk from nonpregnant mothers. Furthermore, Lübke and Finkbeiner (255) observed unusual substances, possibly breakdown products of carotenoids, in the serum of some pregnant women. Morton (272) suggested that these compounds deserve further study. It is possible that such substances might be used in investigating the vitamin A requirements of pregnant women.

Little is known about fetal vitamin A metabolism or requirements. It appears that the vitamin A concentration of fetal cord blood is constant over a wide range of maternal plasma values (276, 277) but the mechanism controlling it is not understood. One-half of the 20 African mothers studied by McLaren and Ward (277) had plasma values less than 20 μg/100 ml and fetal cord blood values exceeded those of the mother. Thomson et al. (278) reported similar findings from Malayan women. Likewise, the administration of 10,000 to 200,000 IU vitamin A (3,000 to 60,000 μg retinol) daily to mothers did not change the cord blood values (259, 266, 279). These studies suggest that the vitamin A supply to the fetus is carefully controlled.

Although cord blood vitamin A values may remain constant, there is evidence from experiments with cattle (5) that increased maternal intake may lead to modest increases in fetal liver storage. Lewis et al. (266) did not observe any change

in the vitamin A concentration of cord blood from guinea pigs which had been fed excess vitamin A (5,000 IU daily) but increased amounts were stored in the fetal livers. They point out that constant cord blood values may be controlled by a fetal regulatory mechanism. Two of the 27 human placentas which Gaehtgens (280) examined were rich in vitamin A. Since these two subjects had received vitamin A therapy during pregnancy he concluded that the placenta is capable of storing considerable amounts of vitamin A. Barnes (281) concluded that fetal plasma vitamin A level is a function of fetal metabolism and is independent of the placenta.

Toverud and Ender (172) found that the amount of vitamin A in the human fetal liver corresponded with the daily intake of the mother. As indicated in the section on infant requirements, recent values for vitamin A in fetal livers are higher than those reported earlier. Some investigators (5, 169) attribute this to improved maternal diet and vitamin supplementation. It might also reflect better methods of extracting vitamin A from the liver and more sensitive methods of detection. The maternal intake necessary to bring about changes in fetal liver stores is not known. The importance or desirability of increased fetal liver stores is also an open question. It is possible that high levels of fetal vitamin A stores are the result of excessive maternal intake.

Lactating Women

Most of our knowledge about the vitamin A requirements of lactating women has been obtained indirectly from the sum of the approximate amount of vitamin A secreted in the milk and the estimated maintenance requirement of the mother. Two research groups, Macy and her associates of the United States, and Kon and Mawson of England, have supplied most of the data. Other workers have attempted to arrive at an estimated optimal intake by studying the effects of supplementing the mother's diet with varying amounts of vitamin A. The results of these experiments indicate that the problem is complex and emphasize that more information is needed on the maternal metabolism of vitamin A.

Vitamin A in human milk

During the 1920's two groups of workers in the United States investigated the vitamin A content of human milk by rat assay (282, 283). They reported differences in the vitamin A content of human milk and cow's milk (282–284), observed wide variation in the vitamin A concentration among individual subjects (285), and suggested that the maternal diet apparently affected the vitamin A content of the milk (282). Macy and her associates later calculated that the milk in these early studies (283) contained 100 to 200 USP units of vitamin A/100 ml (268).

In 1936 Dann (286) reported that the average total vitamin A activity for 104 samples of mature human milk was 346 IU/100 ml. The value may be overestimated because all of the carotenoids were computed as β-carotene. Lesher et al. (268) estimated from the results of their own work and others (287–290) that about one-fourth of the total carotenoids in human milk is β-carotene. Taking 25 μg/100 ml as an average concentration, they calculated that the vitamin A activity of the carotenoids in human milk is about 10 USP units/100 ml, assuming that 4.3 USP units are equal to 1 μg retinol (268).

Lesher et al. (268) reviewed 13 other reports by European investigators on the vitamin A and total carotenoid content of human colostrum (291–301) and mature milk (292–299, 302, 303). However, in most cases, the methods of obtaining the samples and of expressing the vitamin A values in these studies were so diverse that it is not possible to compare the results (268).

In 1945, Hrubetz et al. (304) determined the vitamin A activity of 85 samples of milk taken during various states of lactation from normal American women receiving an "adequate" diet. Analyses of 45 samples of mature milk yielded average values of 270 IU/100 ml for total vitamin A values, 206 IU/100 ml for retinol and 39 μg/100 ml for carotene. Twenty-four samples obtained more than 61 days after parturition contained an average of 216 IU (64.8 μg) retinol and 39 μg caro-

tene/100 ml. The average total vitamin A activity was 281 IU/100 ml. The number of subjects and the total amount of milk produced by the lactating women were not indicated.

In the same year Macy and her associates (268) reported the results of an extensive study on the vitamin A content of milk from 76 well-nourished lactating women. They made 91 twenty-four-hour collections of mature milk from seven women "ingesting diets of equal quality and of known compositions" (268) which contained 1,455 μg retinol and 6,248 μg carotene (305). Milk was collected for 5 consecutive days at various intervals during the experimental period (2 to 10 months). It is not clear whether the lactating women were fed the controlled diet throughout the 10-month period or whether the diet was controlled only during the 5-day collecting periods. These seven subjects secreted an average of 675 ml milk daily (305). The mean vitamin A and carotenoid content of 76 collections was 62 and 24 μg/100 ml, respectively (268).

In addition, Macy et al. reported that 188 four- to eight-hour collections of mature milk (within 1 year after parturition) from 69 women on self-chosen diets (306) contained an average of 60 μg retinol and 24 μg carotenoids/100 ml (268). Retinol and carotenoids tended to maintain the same concentration throughout the period of lactation from days 30 to 300 after parturition. Thus, the milk of women in these two groups contained approximately 1,400 and 1,350 IU vitamin A per person per day, respectively.

Perhaps the most comprehensive attempt to date to assemble average values for the constituents of human milk was carried out in England during this same period, 1941 to 1945 (179). Samples of milk were taken between 10 AM and noon from 1,032 women residing in Reading, a prosperous country town, and 358 women from Shoreditch, a town of working-class people. The milk of women from these two areas contained an average of 4.78 and 3.91 g fat/100 ml; 31.9 and 32.5 IU vitamin A/g fat or 152.5 and 126.8 IU vitamin A/100 ml of milk, respectively. The amount of milk produced by one woman for 32 weeks ranged from 215 to 870 ml daily. During weeks 13 to 21, daily secretion exceeded 800 ml. The average daily vitamin A intake of 97 women from Shoreditch was approximately 3,000 IU but there was little correlation between the vitamin A content of the mother's diet and the milk she secreted. It is possible that liver storage of vitamin A masked the effect of the current diet. As mentioned previously, data reported by Hume and Krebs (69) suggest that the average vitamin A liver store of British subjects is approximately 500,000 IU (150,000 μg retinol) per person.

Kon and Mawson (179) concluded from these data that a lactating woman would require "something in excess of 4,000 IU (1,200 μg) of retinol daily in order to have 2,500 IU (750 μg) left for herself." They pointed out that since the utilization of β-carotene is uncertain, the position is more complicated when provitamins provide a considerable portion of the vitamin A activity.

The average vitamin A concentration (39.7 IU/g fat) of 47 samples of milk which Gunther and Stanier (307) obtained from undernourished German women in 1946 to 1947, was higher than Kon and Mawson (179) reported for British women but the fat content was lower (3.15 g/100 ml milk).

Meulemans and de Haas (296) reported that the total vitamin A activity of mature milk secreted by poorly nourished Batavian women was 50 to 60 IU/100 ml. The frequent occurrences of xerophthalmia among young Batavian children, especially after weaning, suggested to them that the maternal diet influenced the vitamin A concentration in the milk (295, 308). Similar findings were obtained 20 years later in India (151, 152). The vitamin A content of milk from Indian women subsisting mainly on rice was 51 to 70 IU/100 ml. Gopalan (149, 150, 153) reports that such women secrete less milk (400 to 600 g/day) than healthy women. Dietary surveys (262) of poor Indian women in Hyderabad and Coonoor indicated that their average daily vitamin A intake was approximately 800 IU. The prevalence of xerophthalmia among young Indian children (309) suggests that the milk of

mothers subsisting on this limited intake does not provide an adequate amount of vitamin A for the infant. It appears that the offspring of poor Indian women have little or no vitamin A reserves.

These studies from various parts of the world suggest that there is a general relationship between the customary vitamin A intake of lactating mothers and the vitamin A content of their milk. However, with the exception of Kon and Mawson's work, little has been learned about the intake required to supply "adequate" vitamin A in the milk and to maintain optimal conditions in the mother. The results of the two major studies (179, 268) suggest that at least 1,400 to 1,500 additional IU (420 to 450 μg) of vitamin A are required daily during lactation. Any additional "costs" of lactation have not been investigated.

Effect of dietary supplementation

Several workers have studied the effect of supplementing the maternal diet with vitamin A during pregnancy and lactation on the vitamin A content of human milk. They have administered both physiologic and therapeutic doses.

Supplementation during pregnancy. Dann reported from Duke University, in 1936, that adding cod-liver oil to the poor diets of pregnant women did not cause any increase in the vitamin A content of colostrum or mature milk (286). The previous diet of these women was not mentioned. Earlier, he had found that the vitamin A reserve of female rats did not effect any change in the vitamin A content of the milk (310), and concluded that "some factor" limited the amount of vitamin A that passes to the milk. However, in 1934, he found that the amount of vitamin A amassed by young rats up to the time of weaning was roughly related to the vitamin A reserves of the mother (311). McCosh et al. (312) also found that supplementing the "abundant and well-chosen" diets of pregnant women with 15 g cod-liver oil had no effect on the vitamin A content of their milk.

Kon and Mawson (179) conducted several supplementation experiments in their study. They found no significant difference between the vitamin A value of milk secreted by 91 women from Shoreditch who took Multivite, a vitamin A supplement containing approximately 3,000 to 12,000 IU (900 to 3,600 μg), daily for 1 week to 3 months during pregnancy (32.8 IU/g fat) and the vitamin A value of milk from 91 control subjects who were receiving no supplement (33.0 IU/g fat). Similar results were reported for 67 women from Reading (179) who took cod-liver oil supplying 4,000 IU daily during the last 6 months of pregnancy versus 53 unsupplemented control subjects (32.5 vs. 33.0 IU/g milk fat, respectively). The investigators thus concluded that vitamin A supplements of this magnitude, given during pregnancy, had no influence on the vitamin A content of the milk fat. The writers pointed out that "we do not know whether supplements increased the stores of vitamin A in the liver; if so, it would appear that an increase of this degree in the liver reserves is without effect on the vitamin A content of full lactation milk" (179). It is possible that the vitamin A reserves of the subjects were already of such a magnitude that they were able to maintain homeostasis.

Kon and Mawson (179) and Ajans et al. (313) both found that excessive amounts of vitamin A (240,000 to 600,000 IU) administered just before or at parturition increased the amount of vitamin A in the milk but the increment was not sustained. Indian mothers given 30,000 IU (9,000 μg) responded similarly (262).

Supplementation during lactation. Most of the studies indicate that supplementing the diet of lactating women with moderate amounts of vitamin A does not increase the concentration of vitamin A in the milk. McCosh et al. in the United States reported in 1934 (312) that supplementing the diets of three lactating women with 15 g cod-liver oil daily for 3 months did not increase the vitamin A content of their milk. Likewise, Kon and Mawson (179) found no difference in the vitamin A content of milk secreted by 20 women from Shoreditch who had taken Multivite since parturition and that of the milk of the remaining 338 women, 32.1 and 32.5 IU/gram fat, respectively. In Reading, however, supplementation during lactation significantly increased the

amount of vitamin A in the milk. The mean values for 22 subjects taking various vitamin A preparations (39.6 IU/g fat) and for 19 subjects taking cod-liver oil (41.1 IU/g fat) were significantly higher than the mean value (31.9 IU/g fat) for the entire 1,032 subjects. The vitamin A dosage and the length of time the mother had been lactating when the samples were taken were not indicated.

Bhavani Belavady and Gopalan (152) supplemented the diets of nine poorly nourished lactating women in India with 2,000 to 10,000 IU vitamin A acetate (600 to 3,000 μg retinol) daily during various stages of lactation. After 3 weeks of supplementation, they concluded that, compared with the values for ten control subjects receiving no supplements (57 ± 11 IU initially vs. 51 ± 10 IU/100 ml at the end of the experimental period), the difference in the vitamin A content of milk from supplemented women at the beginning and end of the experiment (69 ± 8 vs. 78 ± 13 IU/100 ml, respectively) was not significant.

Several investigators have reported that administering massive doses of vitamin A to lactating women causes a concomitant rise in the vitamin A concentration of milk. But the threshold for homeostasis in humans, i.e., the dosage required to bring about a change in vitamin A values of milk, has not been established. Neuweiler (294) gave one woman 80,000 "units" of vitamin A and increased the milk content. Friderichsen and With (314) reported similar results with vitamin A but carotene supplementation was ineffective. During their 4-year study on the composition of human milk, Kon and Mawson (179) found that the vitamin A concentration of milk from 22 mothers who had eaten liver 20 to 22 hours before the samples were taken, was significantly higher than the mean value for milk from the 1,400 subjects who participated in the study (51.6 vs. 31.9 and 32.5 IU/g fat, respectively). The vitamin A content of a portion of liver may vary from 10,000 to 150,000 IU (3,000 to 45,000 μg) vitamin A (179).

When Hrubetz et al. (304) supplemented the diets of 42 lactating women with 50,000 or 200,000 IU (15,000 or 60,000 μg) vitamin A daily over a period of months, vitamin A content of the milk increased proportionately. Since the milk from those subjects receiving 50,000 IU (15,000 μg) did not continue to contain significantly more vitamin A for prolonged periods of time, they concluded that the threshold for humans was 50,000 IU. On the other hand, Kon and Mawson (179) contended that the threshold value may be closer to 25,000 IU (7,500 μg) daily. When they administered this quantity to one subject for 2 weeks, the amount of vitamin A in the milk almost doubled (from 25 to 44 IU/g fat). The administration of 15 mg β-carotene had no effect on the vitamin A values of the milk. They also found that supplementing the diets of ten subjects with 25,000 IU of vitamin A for the first 9 days after parturition raised the vitamin A in postpartum milk above the values for the ten controls (179). Values decreased immediately following withdrawal of the supplement.

Sobel et al. (315) observed that after administering massive doses (1,000 USP units/0.456 kg body wt) of aqueously dispersed vitamin A to well-nourished lactating women, the increases in the vitamin A concentrations of their plasma and milk were almost the same.

These reports indicate that the quantity of vitamin A in milk may be altered by prolonged maternal deprivation or excessive intakes. The mechanisms controlling the vitamin A concentration of milk have not been elucidated. It appears that the relationship between the intake and the amount secreted is complex. The results of supplementing the diet of lactating women with moderate amounts of vitamin A suggest that certain maternal requirements must be satisfied before the amount of vitamin A in the milk is increased. The metabolism of vitamin A during lactation is not understood. It is possible that the mammary gland may play an intermediary role in regulating the vitamin A in the milk. Vogt (316) found that the mammary gland of lactating women was rich in vitamin A. Members of the Expert Committee of the World Health Organization (317) recommended that the efficiency of the mammary gland as a synthesizing and secretory organism be further investigated.

Gopalan and Bhavani Belavady (318) concluded in their review of nutrition and lactation that the long-term status of the mother appears to be important, and animal work supports this hypothesis (311). They also suggested that the possible role of hormonal factors governing lactation in conditioning nutritional requirements should "receive adequate attention" (318). It will be recalled from the discussion on the requirements of pregnant women that pregnant and nonpregnant lactating women appear to metabolize vitamin A differently (275).

Carotene requirements

Very little work has been reported in this area. Friderichsen and With (314) and Kon and Mawson (179) both reported that supplementing the diets of lactating women with excessive amounts of β-carotene had no effect on the vitamin A content of the milk fat. According to von Drigalski and Kunz (247) three German lactating women required 5 to 10 mg of carotene to correct prolonged dark adaptation. As pointed out by the WHO Expert Committee (317), it is not known whether lactation has any effect on the conversion of the carotenes to vitamin A or not. Oomen (319) also emphasizes the need for studying the relationships between carotene intake, and the blood and milk vitamin A values of lactating mothers.

Mixed diet

According to nutritional status data from Chile, of the 226 nursing mothers ingesting an average of 2,958 IU vitamin A daily, 32.2% had hyperkeratosis (217).

REQUIREMENTS OF THE ELDERLY

Information on the vitamin A requirements of elderly people is limited. The results of three nutritional status surveys (320–322) suggest that a mixed diet supplying 5,000 IU of vitamin A activity daily is sufficient to maintain normal plasma values in healthy elderly people. Gillum et al. (320) found that for 514 healthy Californians more than 50 years old, the average daily total vitamin A intakes of men and women living at home and men living in a county home were 10,640, 8,450 and 5,450 IU, respectively. All groups derived more than one-half of their daily intake from carotene. Assuming that

3 IU from carotene and 1 IU from pre-formed vitamin A were equivalent to 0.344 μg vitamin A ester, these investigators calculated that men living in their own homes consumed 2,387; women 1,833; and men in the county home, 1,354 μg/day. This amounted to 33, 27 and 21 μg/kilogram body weight, respectively. The mean plasma vitamin A values of these three groups were 57, 54 and 47 μg/100 ml, respectively.

Dibble et al. (321) recently reported similar plasma vitamin A values (57 and 54 μg/100 ml) for elderly men and women consuming an average of 5,348 and 5,719 IU vitamin A daily. The average plasma vitamin A values of forty 70-year-old Yugoslavian subjects (11 men and 29 women) who were consuming approximately 3,100 IU vitamin A daily were 34.6 and 36.2 μg/100 ml, respectively (322). When the total daily vitamin A intake was increased to approximately 5,600 IU by feeding a daily supplement containing 2,500 IU (750 μg) vitamin A, 10 mg tocopherol and 50 mg vitamin C for 5 months, the average plasma vitamin A values of both sexes increased to 60 μg/100 ml.

On the other hand Rafsky et al. (323) reported that apparently healthy men and women over 65 years of age, who were consuming an average of 2,400 IU (720 μg) retinol and 6,900 IU carotene daily, had low plasma values (27 and 80 μg/100 ml, respectively).

Gillum et al. (320) and Kahan (324) observed that serum vitamin A declined in elderly people but others (321, 325) found no statistical difference in the plasma values of different age groups. The lower plasma values which some investigators have observed in elderly people may be due to reduced utilization of fat-soluble substances (323, 326). Patients with peripheral arterial circulatory disturbances of the lower extremities have significantly lower plasma vitamin A values than normal people of the same age (327). On the other hand, Rafsky et al. (323) suggested that "normal" plasma values for healthy elderly people may possibly be different from accepted values for younger adults.

Absorption tests by Yiengst and Shock (325) indicate that subjects 40 to 49 years old absorbed large doses of vitamin A (100,000 IU) at a faster rate than older subjects but there did not appear to be any difference in net absorption. On the other hand, Rafsky and Newman (328) suggested that, since 50,000 IU (15,000 μg) were required to raise the plasma values of all elderly subjects, the vitamin A requirement of elderly people may be greater than that of younger adults.

Workers in both the United States (329) and Russia (330) have found that supplemental vitamin A raised the low plasma values of elderly people living in institutions. The plasma vitamin A values of 23 infirmary inmates, approximately 70 years of age, ranged from zero to 15 μg/100 ml (329). When 30,000 IU (9,000 μg) vitamin A acetate was administered daily, in addition to the infirmary diet which contained about 10,000 IU, the mean plasma value for the group increased from 5.1 to 44.5 μg/100 ml in 4 months. It remained at this level during the next 8 months. The investigators also noted a gradual improvement in existing localized conjunctival thickening, blepharo-conjunctivitis, toad skin and dark-adaptation time of some patients. When the supplement was discontinued, the mean plasma vitamin A dropped to 18.7 μg/100 ml in 4 weeks and remained at 16 μg for the remaining 7 months of the experiment (329).

In general, the liver vitamin A stores of elderly people do not appear to differ from those of adults 40 to 60 years of age (89, 140, 169).

Chronic hypervitaminosis A was reported in two elderly people, 67 and 75 years old. Their daily vitamin A intakes were 100,000 to 200,000 IU (30,000 to 60,000 μg) for 6 years (100) and 600,000 IU (180,000 μg retinol) for about 1 year, respectively (331).

FACTORS AFFECTING DIETARY VITAMIN A REQUIREMENTS

Existing data suggest that a number of factors may affect the amount of vitamin A-active compounds an individual needs to ingest to meet his daily requirement. Utilization (absorption, transport and storage) of vitamin A-active substances (especially the vitamin A precursors) from natural foods is probably the most important factor. Other compounds and conditions (physical and environmental) that appear to affect the human vitamin A requirement include: dietary protein, exercise, exposure to sun, environmental temperature, thyroid activity, infection and fever, toxic substances and genetic aberrations.

It is not easy to determine whether an increase in dietary requirement is due to decreased utilization of compounds with vitamin A activity or increased metabolic requirement. The same criteria, such as plasma vitamin A and carotene concentration, dark-adaptation time and condition of epithelial tissue, are often used for evaluating either of them.

Because most information derives from experimental animals where data from human studies are lacking, mention will be made of animal experiments, referring whenever possible to review articles.

Utilization (Absorption, Transport and Storage) of Vitamin A

A number of factors may affect the utilization of compounds having vitamin A activity (5, 136, 332–335). These include state of dispersion; chemical form; availability from natural foods; intake of other nutrients (for example fat, vitamin E and protein); age, sex and physical condition of the subjects; and pathological conditions.

Methods which have been used to estimate the utilization of dietary vitamin A include "apparent absorption" tests, i.e., intake minus the amount excreted in the feces; vitamin A and carotene concentration in the lymph and serum; liver storage; and improvement in dark-adaptation time and epithelial tissue lesions.

Physical and chemical properties of the vitamin

State of dispersion. About the time that vitamin A became commercially available, a number of investigators compared the absorption of aqueous dispersions of vitamin A versus vitamin A in oil, as measured by vitamin A tolerance curves. Studies with premature infants (336), full-term infants (337) and humans at all ages (338) indicate that vitamin A is more readily absorbed from an aqueous dispersion than from oil. Corroboration has been found in animal studies (5, 337, 339, 340). Thus Sobel et al. concluded that "it is likely that the standard requirements for vitamin A when the vitamin is given in aqueous dispersion will ultimately be revised to a lower level than is advised at present" (338).

Adlersberg and Sobotka (341) and Kern et al. (342) both reported that lecithin increased the absorption of vitamin A in humans. On the other hand Ames (343) recently concluded from animal work that emulsified vitamin A and vitamin A in oil were biologically equivalent. Emulsification may increase the speed of absorption but it does not increase the biological utilization.

In experimental animals, a number of substances such as conjugated bile acids (344), Tween (345) and lecithin (334) enhance carotene utilization suggesting that utilization is directly related to the state of dispersion. In fact, aqueous carotene dispersions in Tween 40 are better absorbed and more efficiently converted into vitamin A than carotene in oil (345). However, cholate or conjugated bile acids are still required for the metabolism of solubilized β-carotene (344).

Alcohol vs. ester. Reports on human utilization of the alcohol, acetate or natural ester forms of vitamin A are conflicting. Kagan et al. (346) found no difference in the plasma vitamin A concentration after oral test doses of the alcohol or palmitate form in aqueous dispersion; Week and Sevigne (347) found superior absorption of vitamin A alcohol; and Popper et al. (348) reported higher plasma levels after feeding vitamin A esters than after equal doses of vitamin A alcohol. The results were the same in oily or aqueous medium.

Ascarelli (349) has reviewed the recent animal experiments on vitamin A absorption and transport. In the intestines of chickens and in rat liver, the enzymes for hydrolyzing vitamin A acetate and vitamin A palmitate are different. It also appears that sodium taurocholate, one of the bile salts, may activate the enzyme which hydrolyzes natural esters of vitamin A. On the other hand rats apparently do not require bile acids for the absorption and esterification of retinol (344). In chickens, the alcohol form is more readily absorbed but there is more storage in the liver when the palmitate form is fed (349).

Availability of the provitamins. One of the first factors to consider in the utilization of the provitamins A is their availability from the natural foodstuff.

From 1936 to 1958, 16 studies on the "apparent absorption" of vitamin A precursors from natural foods prepared in various ways were reported (69, 118, 174, 350–362). A total of 143 determinations were made, using subjects of all ages. The average amount of carotene absorbed ranged from 1 to 88% for carrots (cooked or raw) and cooked spinach, respectively. After reviewing 15 of these reports (69, 118, 174, 350–354, 356–362) the Expert Group of the FAO/WHO (45) concluded that the data were too few and variable to make any accurate predictions about the availability of the carotenes from natural foods.

In most of the studies only total carotenes were measured. Few of the investigators subtracted basal carotenoid excretion which, according to Kawaguchi and Fujita (118), is a common source of error. Further, in some cases carotenoid extraction from the feces may have been incomplete (118). It is also possible that all of the biologically active carotenoids were not initially extracted from the food by the procedures commonly used (363). The detailed carotenoid composition of many common foodstuffs is still unknown (364).

No information was reported on the microbiological destruction of the carotenes in the gastrointestinal tract. In 1970, Rao and Rao (365) separated the fecal pigments on a chromatographic column and found bands that were not in the carotene sources fed. They suggested that these compounds may have been formed by bacteria.

Two additional balance studies were reported from India in 1970. In both, basal carotenoid excretion was determined initially. Four young adult males eating diets low in fat absorbed 33, 36, 46 and 58% of the total carotenes from mixed vegetables, carrot, papaya, and amaranth (a leafy vegetable), respectively (365). The differences appeared to be related to the

amount of β-carotene and possibly the fiber content of the foodstuff. They calculated that 20% of the total carotenes in carrots were β-carotene. Earlier, cooked carrots grown in the United States were reported to contain 57.6% β-carotene (366). In the second study, four undernourished preschool children absorbed 75% of the total carotenes and 70% of the β-carotene from 50 g of amaranth (216).

A number of investigators have reported that provitamin A absorption, especially from carrots, is directly proportional to particle size (69, 352, 354–356). Leonhardi (357) suggested that absorption of the carotenes from vegetables is possible only after the destruction of the vegetable cell membranes. In 1937, Wilson et al. (350) concluded from experiments with one subject that carotene from raw carrots or cooked spinach was absorbed equally well. Similarly, Callison and Orent-Keiles found that there was no difference in the biological value of frozen carrots, cooked or raw (59). On the other hand, Eriksen and Höygaard (353) reported that cooking increased carotene absorption from both carrots and spinach. Also, the percentage of carotene absorbed is inversely proportional to the amount ingested (356, 358).

The Joint FAO/WHO Group (45) also reviewed the results of ten studies on the "apparent absorption" of carotene in oil (67, 69, 118, 174, 351, 354, 361, 367–369). The 77 subjects absorbed 25 to 98% of the trial doses. Regardless of the age of the subject, carotene in oil appears to be more readily absorbed than carotene from vegetable sources (69, 118, 351, 354, 361). Rao and Rao recently reported that crystalline β-carotene was completely absorbed by four adult subjects (365).

In 1966, Goodman and his associates (370) compared the absorption of labeled β-carotene and retinol by measuring the amount of radioactivity recovered in the thoracic duct lymph. Vitamin A precursors may be converted to retinol in the intestinal wall or absorbed "intact." Two subjects absorbed 8.74 and 16.7% of the β-carotene within 22 hours after it was administered. Twenty-two to 30% of the radioactivity was in the form of β-carotene. After feeding retinol-^{14}C, a total of 21.5%

of the radioactivity was recovered in the lymph during the next 20 hours. The following year, Blomstrand and Werner (371) administered labeled carotene to four subjects and recovered 8.7 to 52.3% of the radioactivity. Unchanged labeled β-carotene comprised 1.7 to 46.9% of the radioactivity absorbed. When preformed vitamin A was administered, they recovered 6.7 to 66.9% of the radioactivity.

Presence of other dietary components

Fat. Dietary lipids do not appear to be as important for utilizing preformed vitamin A as they are for the provitamins (350). Recently, Oey Khoen Lian et al. (213) and Figueira et al. (372) both concluded that dietary fat is not essential for vitamin A absorption since young children on low fat diets, supplemented with vitamin A and dried skimmed milk, had normal plasma values. The form of vitamin A was not indicated.

In premature infants the amount of vitamin A absorbed appeared to parallel the amount of fat absorbed (177), thus the type of dietary fat may influence vitamin A absorption. Daniels (373) and Rowntree (374) both found that bottle-fed babies excreted more vitamin A than those that were breastfed.

Animal experiments suggest that unsaturated fatty acids affect vitamin A utilization (181). In rats, it appears that they are essential for the assimilation of vitamin A in the body but excessive amounts may cause vitamin A deficiency (375).

Several investigators have reported that dietary fat enhanced carotene absorption in humans (350, 357, 118). Roels et al. (361) found that African boys receiving 200 g of carrots and their normal diet absorbed only 5% of the carotene, but a supplement of 18 g olive oil daily raised the absorption to 25% and serum levels of both carotene and vitamin A increased rapidly.

Animal experiments indicate that both the amount (376) and type of fat have a decided effect on carotene utilization (334). Carotenes are poorly utilized when indigestible fats are included in the diet (5, 332, 334).

Vitamin E. Vitamin E reportedly affects the utilization of preformed vitamin A. After reviewing numerous animal experiments Green and Bunyan (377) concluded that the effect of vitamin E is observed mainly when the diet contains highly unsaturated fat such as cod-liver oil or when the two vitamins are given together as a single dose. Many reports suggest that the effect of vitamin E is predominantly in the gastrointestinal tract. On the other hand, Ames (343) has concluded that it is also "essential for the normal in vivo utilization of vitamin A." In 1965, Hanna (378) reported from Egypt that giving vitamin E to adults suffering from night blindness shortened the period of treatment and helped in decreasing the dose of vitamin A.

Kasper and Ernst (379) gave two doses of 50 mg β-carotene in 5 ml olive, groundnut or corn oil or in olive oil with α-tocopherol to men between 24 and 60 years of age. Serum carotene values increased significantly more with corn oil than with the other oils. Adding tocopherol to the olive oil had no effect.

Animal studies also indicate that α-tocopherol under some circumstances may enhance the utilization of carotene (334, 380–383). Apparently the effectiveness of the α-tocopherol depends on the total amount of unsaturated fatty acids (380, 381) and carotene (5, 382, 383) in the diet.

Protein. The experimental evidence that vitamin A utilization (absorption, transport and storage) is closely related to the quantity and quality of dietary protein has recently been reviewed by Moore (384), Gershoff (385), Mahadevan et al. (386) and Arroyave (387). Although most of the work has been done with animals, some research involving humans has also been reported. In his review, Moore (384) suggested that a very low intake of protein can result in poor utilization of vitamin A because of fatty infiltration of the liver and deterioration of digestion and absorption processes. As Arroyave (387) has suggested, the metabolic processes that are affected probably depend on the dietary protein level and the duration of the diet. Kuming reported a significantly higher incidence of xerophthalmia among malnourished children with low protein serum values than those with normal protein concentration (388).

In 1959, Arroyave et al. (389) reported that the oral administration of 75,000 µg vitamin A palmitate to children with kwashiorkor had no effect on their plasma vitamin A values. However, when the test load was readministered, after supplementing their diets with skimmed milk for 3 to 5 days, serum vitamin A values increased. The investigators were not sure if the initial response was due to malabsorption, abnormal transport or both. They later (390) observed that even without vitamin A in the diet, protein supplements caused an increase in the plasma values of those children with vitamin A reserves in the liver but that the plasma values of those children with scant vitamin A stores did not change. Gopalan et al. (309) and Konno et al. (391) reported similar experiences from India and Africa, respectively.

Arroyave and his associates (390) observed that, as the concentrations of lipids and vitamin A decreased in the liver of children being treated for kwashiorkor, these components increased in the serum. This suggested an impairment of vitamin A transport, possibly associated with a decrease in some of the plasma protein fractions. They observed that increments in the serum vitamin A values of kwashiorkor patients receiving skimmed milk, free of vitamin A, paralleled increments in serum protein and albumin (392). Woodruff and Stewart (393) and Bagchi et al. (394) reported a similar correlation between human serum albumin and vitamin A levels.

In malnourished children, Leonard (395) and High (132) found that serum α_1-globulin and vitamin A levels were related while El-Din and Hammad (396) observed a direct relationship between total serum protein and vitamin A concentrations. On the other hand, McLaren et al. (157) found no correlation between serum vitamin A levels and total serum protein or any paper electrophoretic fractions in 31 cases of xerophthalmia unless total protein values were markedly depressed. Similarly, Garciá et al. (397) found no relationship between plasma vitamin A and any of the protein fractions. Plasma vitamin A and total protein values correlated only in those subjects with plasma vitamin A values above the mean (14.9 µg/100 ml). Kothari et al. (398) have recently found that the plasma vitamin A values of healthy children, 5 to 10 years old, correlate significantly with plasma total protein and albumin concentrations. The serum retinol-binding protein (RBP) which has α_1-globulin electrophoretic mobility has now been isolated from human plasma, purified and characterized (399). Plasma RBP complexes with another protein which has prealbumin electrophoretic mobility (399).

In 1964, Deshmukh et al. (400) reported that in rats, protein malnutrition caused a pronounced reduction in both the hydrolyzing and synthesizing enzymes of rat intestinal mucosa. Ascarelli (349) has recently reported similar effects in chicks and pointed out that, in cases of protein malnutrition, administering the alcohol form of vitamin A may be advantageous.

Reports on the effects of protein intake on the utilization of the provitamins A are conflicting. Gronowska-Senger and Wolf (401) found that feeding young men a protein-free diet for 8 or 9 days had no effect on the specific activity of intestinal carotene dioxygenase. Ehrlich et al. (402) fed 37 healthy girls, 7 to 10 years of age, varying levels of protein from plant and animal sources and a constant amount of vitamin A activity but the proportion of "plant vitamin A" varied. In two of the three experiments, plasma carotene values were higher when the girls were given the high protein diet. Multiple regression analysis of the data showed that the serum carotene levels tended to be influenced by protein from animal sources and serum vitamin A by protein from plant sources.

Other investigators have failed to observe any effect of dietary protein on the "apparent absorption" and utilization of the provitamins by humans. Roels et al. (127) reported that administering carotene-rich palm oil (13,500 IU daily) cured night blindness in Indonesian boys, 3 to 13 years old. After treatment, their serum vitamin A levels were the same as those of boys receiving 2,000 IU vitamin A acetate (600 µg retinol) and did not increase when they added 2 g skimmed milk/kilogram body weight to their experimental diets. Similarly, Moschette (360) found that, according to fecal carotene excretion and serum carotene and vitamin A values, adding protein in the form of fat-free milk to the diets of six normal preadolescent girls, 8 to 11 years old, had no effect on their utilization of 3,600 μg carotene from sweet potatoes. The recent data of Lala and Reddy (216) also suggest that a mild degree of protein–calorie malnutrition does not impair carotene absorption. When six preschool children were fed a diet containing 20% fat, they absorbed about 70% of the β-carotene from amaranth (green vegetables), a value similar to that reported for normal adults. However, severe protein deficiency did not exist in any of these cases. In 1954, Oomen (403) observed that, in spite of adequate dietary carotenes, xerophthalmia in children suffering from kwashiorkor was not cured.

Recent animal experiments suggest that there may be an optimal level of dietary protein for maximum provitamin A utilization (404, 405). Protein intake has a direct effect on intestinal protein biosynthesis and the intestinal enzyme, carotene dioxygenase (401).

Other nutrients. Animal studies have indicated that vitamin C (406), vitamin B₁₂ (407) and possibly other micronutrients (406) affect the utilization of provitamin A. The type of carbohydrate fed to rats has also been found to be effective (376). No reports were found of similar data obtained in studies with human subjects.

Sex, age and physical condition of the consumer

Age and sex. The experimental evidence reviewed by Moore suggests that males metabolize vitamin A compounds differently than females and that their vitamin A requirement may be higher (5). Since the early report of Kimble (36), most investigators have found that males have higher plasma vitamin A and lower carotene values than females (5, 81, 125, 126, 408–414). However, some have reported no sex difference in plasma values (395, 412–414). On the other hand, Leitner et al. (126) found that in mental patients females consistently had higher plasma vitamin A values than males. The plasma vitamin A concentration of women varies during the menstrual cycle (415). According to Eppright et al. (416), plasma values in children vary with age and sex. However, Hoppner et al. (140) and Abels et al. (417) found no difference in the vitamin A liver stores of males and females.

In reviewing data collected in Indonesia for the past 20 years, Oomen (197, 418) reported that a preponderance of the vitamin A-deficient children were males. The disparity between the two sexes was greatest after the age of 10 years (418). He also cites similar reports from Japan, Rumania, India and El Salvador (197). Birnbacher (419) had reported the same observations in Vienna 30 years earlier. McLaren (420) suggested that the increased susceptibility of the male may be related to the difference in the rate of growth of males and females. On the other hand, Patwardhan and Kamel found that in Jordan, the number of cases were equally divided between the two sexes (154).

Although it is generally accepted that infants utilize vitamin A precursors poorly, data from human studies are limited. Rowntree (374) fed carrots, cod-liver oil or egg to three infants, 4 to 6 months old. According to rat assays of the feces, the youngest lost much of the vitamin contained in carrots but, in the other two, excretion was similar, regardless of the dietary source. She concluded that "it was not conclusively shown whether the vitamin A of carrots was completely utilized, as the small amount the infants could take was too limited to make the results definitive." With (174) and van Zeben (354) did not find any difference between infants and adults in their apparent absorption of β-carotene in oil. Sinios (369) concluded that infants utilized β-carotene in oily suspension better than adults. When infants who had been receiving no vegetables were fed 6 to 14 mg carotene daily, plasma carotene concentration increased fourfold and "apparent absorption" increased from 59 to 81% as the dose was increased from 6 to 14 mg.

In 1933, Hess et al. (143) fed 40 infants, 0 to 3 years old, an oily solution of carotene containing "20,000 rat units, which represents the extract of about 60 Gm. of dry carrots or 500 Gm. of the fresh vegetable" for 5 months. All subjects developed varying degrees of carotenemia and no "blue units," i.e., vitamin A, were found in their blood. However, the investigators did not mention any difference in growth or in resistance to infection between children receiving carotene and those receiving various amounts of vitamin A concentrate. Two-month-old infants may absorb carotene but their ability to convert it to vitamin A may be limited (421).

In 1958–1959, Kübler (362) of Germany reported that according to apparent absorption studies, 3- to 8-month-old infants utilized carotene as well as adults. Later, however, after comparing infant and adult plasma vitamin A and carotene levels in response to large doses of β-carotene, Kübler expressed doubt that infants can absorb as much carotene unaltered, or form the same amount of vitamin A from it as adults (422).

Friderichsen and Edmund (423) reported that in infants, 2 to 11 months old, dried spinach was ten times as effective as fish-liver oils for improving poor dark adaptation but the carotene from carrots was ineffective. All subjects used in this study had been admitted to the hospital with other problems. Nicholls and Nimalasuria (424) concluded that infants and children do not absorb or at least do not convert carotene into vitamin A efficiently since 30 g red palm oil (calculated to contain 26,000 IU β-carotene) daily was not as effective for curing phyrodermia as 30 g unstandardized cod-liver oil daily.

Apparent absorption tests and plasma vitamin A values indicate that children, 2 to 5 years old, utilize β-carotene from red palm oil (213) and cooked green leafy vegetables (198, 216) quite efficiently.

Experiments with rats suggest that females may utilize carotene more efficiently than males (425, 426). Murray and Erdody recently concluded that "there can be no doubt that male rats, rather early in life, suffer a loss in ability to utilize carotene." And they point out that "If carotene utilization by human males is affected by age as it is for male rats, it would be a matter of concern" (425). At present, age and sex are not considered in calculating the vitamin A potency of provitamins.

Pregnancy. a) *Mother.* There are a few reports in the literature concerning the metabolism of the carotenes during pregnancy. Botella Llusía and Hernández Araña (242) concluded that, since 20 Spanish women who were consuming approximately 12,000 IU of vitamin A as carotene and 20 g of fat daily showed defects in night vision, carotene was not utilized during pregnancy.

Some investigators have found that plasma carotene concentration increases during pregnancy (258, 261, 263, 264). Others have reported that, except for an initial decline during the early months of pregnancy, there was little variation in plasma carotene concentration (427, 255, 267). When carotene supplements are added to the diets of pregnant women, plasma carotene and vitamin A values increase (259, 266), thus suggesting that provitamin A compounds are utilized.

b) *Fetus.* Byrn and Eastman (259) found no change in carotene cord blood values after maternal carotene supplementation but Lund and Kimble (276) and Barnes (281) both reported that fetal blood carotene concentration varied regularly with the level of maternal blood carotene concentration. Lund and Kimble stated that the fetal value could be estimated mathematically. According to Lübke and Finkbeiner (255) and Gaehtgens (428) the concentration of carotene in cord blood is usually about one-fourth that of maternal blood. Since the placenta contained more carotene than vitamin A and fetal cord blood reflected the maternal plasma concentration of carotene but not vitamin A, Barnes (281) concluded that vitamin A was transferred to the fetus primarily in the form of carotene. Hoch (429) hypothesized that, since the proportion of β-carotene in the total carotenoids of fetal serum was markedly lower than it was in maternal serum, the fetal organism takes up β-carotene from the cord blood and converts it into vitamin A leaving the xanthophylls which are more slowly returned to the maternal blood.

These data suggest that the carotenes are utilized by pregnant women and the fetus.

Pathological conditions. The utilization of vitamin A compounds may be altered in a number of pathological conditions such as acute infections and fever (147, 248, 367, 421, 430–437), tuberculosis [2] (438–440), diabetes (171, 270, 411, 434, 437, 441–443), heart conditions (165, 169, 270, 444), kidney disorders (171, 270, 411, 434) or thyroid abnormalities (248, 411, 430, 443, 445–450). Any disorder which affects fat utilization such as celiac disease (433, 451, 452), sprue (341), intestinal obstruction (452), bile duct abnormalities (411, 414, 433) or pancreatic disorders (414, 433) also reduces the utilization of vitamin A compounds. Vitamin A storage is decreased when liver abnormalities are present (139, 171, 173, 270, 453–455).

Protein

Moore (384) has suggested that the level of dietary protein, in addition to affecting utilization of vitamin A, may be directly related to the requirement for vitamin A. A good allowance of protein promotes rapid growth and thus requires a high rate of expenditure of vitamin A. Reports from various parts of the world suggest that adding protein to diets of children increases the vitamin A requirement, thus precipitating vitamin A deficiency symptoms when intake is marginal. Gopalan et al. (309) observed that protein-malnourished Indian children, who initially had no signs of vitamin A deficiency, developed conjunctival signs of deficiency after a few weeks of treatment with a high protein diet containing no additional vitamin A. The preceding year, McLaren (420) had demonstrated that the onset of vitamin A deficiency in rats could be delayed by reducing the protein intake.

According to the results of the Central American Nutrition Survey in 1965, although the protein and vitamin A intakes and serum vitamin A values of Salvadorian children were low, no cases of xerophthalmia or keratomalacia were encountered among the 3,200 individuals studied (387). Arroyave states that "this indirect evidence strongly suggests that the subsistence on a diet limited primarily in proteins, but

also in vitamin A, hinders the development of gross clinical lesions of the vitamin deficiency by decreasing protein metabolism, growth, and thereby, the requirement for vitamin A" (387).

Data reported by Roels et al. (127) also suggest that dietary protein may affect vitamin A requirement. When these workers supplemented the diet of ten Indonesian boys, 3 to 13 years of age, with 2 g protein/kilogram body weight daily, the average plasma vitamin A value for the group rose from 29.8 to 50 μg/100 ml. However, at the end of 3 weeks, the values were back to normal, 30.8 μg/100 ml. The investigators speculate that the increased protein intake may have caused a greater mobilization of vitamin A from the liver into the bloodstream, because the higher protein intake increased the vitamin A requirement. Then, when the liver stores were reduced, the serum level started to fall again (127). Thus "protein supplements alone conceivably might precipitate vitamin A deficiency in areas in which the vitamin A status of growing children is marginal" (127).

Several researchers have shown that, as the amount of protein in the diet of experimental animals is increased, the amount of vitamin A stored in the liver decreases (240, 404, 456, 457). Experiments with chickens suggest that an excessively high protein diet may put a special stress on vitamin A requirements (458). Gershoff (385) reviewed a number of papers which indicated that the severity of vitamin A deficiency symptoms increases when very high levels of protein are fed.

Exercise

Campbell and Tonks (410) found that subjects performing heavy normal labor had lower plasma vitamin A and carotenoid values than those engaged in light or sedentary occupations. Others (459, 460) have suggested that vitamin A intake should be increased during strenuous work, especially in a hot environment.

---

[2] Hekking, A. M. W. Clinische beschouwingen over het vitamin A-gebrek, en speciaal zijn beteekenis bij de tuberculose. M.D. Thesis, Univ. Utrecht. Kemink en Zoon, N. V., Utrecht, pp. 112. Cited in: Nutr. Abst. Rev. 16: (abstr. no. 968), 1946.

Stress Conditions

Exposure to sun

Recently, investigators have suggested, on the basis of changes in plasma vitamin A concentration, that exposure to the sun may increase vitamin A requirements. The data are conflicting. In 1964, for instance, Cluver (461) reported from South Africa that vitamin A–calcium tablets protected people, highly susceptible to sunburn, from such trauma. Cluver and Politzer (462) observed that in sun-sensitive white persons, exposure to the autumn sun caused an immediate drop in the serum vitamin A level. However, when 20 predominantly fair-complexioned girls were exposed to the mid-summer sun, 13 of them showed a significant immediate rise in serum vitamin A (463). They hypothesized that the difference in response might possibly be explained by the fact that the mild ultraviolet irradiation in the autumn was not enough to cause immediate liberation of vitamin A from the liver stores which was noted in the summer. On the other hand, the vitamin A plasma values of Bantus exposed to the hot summer sun dropped immediately after exposure but, 19 hours later, most plasma values had returned to normal (464).

Neither Findlay and Van Der Merwe (465) from South Africa nor Anderson (466) from Australia observed any change in the plasma vitamin A values of subjects immediately after they were exposed to ultraviolet radiation. Findlay and Van Der Merwe (465) reported that the values rose 7 hours later and then dropped 24 to 48 hours after exposure but they found that the epidermis did not take up any extra vitamin A from the plasma. Anderson (466, 467) did not find that giving 25,000 to 75,000 IU of vitamin A provided any protection from the burning of the sun's rays. Thus it appears that exposure to ultraviolet radiation affects plasma vitamin A values but the effect on vitamin A requirements remains unresolved.

Environmental temperature

Animal studies indicate that decreased environmental temperature increases vitamin A requirement (468–474). In human studies, the observed seasonal changes in dark adaptation and plasma vitamin A values may possibly be related to changes in environmental temperature. Hume and Krebs (69) found that the dark-adaptation time of their subjects increased during January and then spontaneously returned to the original values. Others (81, 265, 321, 410) reported that the average plasma vitamin A and total carotenoid concentrations of adults were lowest during March and April and highest in the summer and autumn. Roderuck et al. (475) observed similar results for girls 8 to 14 years old. When supplementary foods, rich in vitamin A compounds were given, carotene values increased but serum vitamin A continued to fluctuate seasonally. On the other hand, Železovskaja (411) found no seasonal plasma vitamin A variation in Russian adults. Phillips (472) suggested that the apparent increased vitamin A requirement of animals kept at low temperatures might possibly be related to increased thyroid activity.

Thyroid activity

It is beyond the scope of this paper to discuss in depth the possible relationship between thyroxine and the metabolism of vitamin A compounds. Low plasma vitamin A levels have been found in both hypothyroid (445–447) and hyperthyroid conditions (248, 411, 430, 446, 448, 449). Poor dark adaptation has been found in hypothyroidism (446, 476) and thyrotoxicosis (446, 476). Liver vitamin A concentration may be above average in thyrotoxicosis (171, 270). Administration of vitamin A supplements reportedy results in a decreased incidence of endemic goiter among children (477). Supplemental vitamin A has also been reported to significantly decrease plasma iodine concentration and basal metabolic rate of hyperthyroid subjects (478). It is not known whether the association of circulating thyroxin and retinol-binding protein with the prealbumin plays a role (479). In rats, supplemental vitamin A decreased the amount of circulating protein-bound iodine (474).

Hypercarotenemia has been observed in hypothyroidism (248, 430, 443, 445, 446, 450, 480) and the plasma carotene concentration of subjects with hyperthyroidism was slightly lower than average values for normal subjects (248, 443). Popper and Steigmann (434) found normal plasma carotene concentrations in hyperthyroid subjects.

Animal experiments provide evidence for and against a relationship between carotene and thyroid function (481–483). After reviewing the experimental results with animals, Thompson (334) concluded that: "There are probably no studies more controversial than those about the interrelationship between thyroid function and carotene metabolism."

Infection and fever

The relationship between infectious diseases and vitamin A is not clear. In a recent review Oomen (197) pointed out that vitamin A deficiency symptoms, such as xerophthalmia, often appear after acute contagious diseases such as a measles. It is possible that vitamin A requirements may be increased by infections or that mobilization and utilization may be altered (431).

In 1933, Clausen (421) showed that after the administration of carotene, serum carotene levels rose more slowly in children with infection than in healthy children. Others have demonstrated that carotene absorption is reduced in children with infection (367, 431). However, in those children with fever due to smallpox vaccination, absorption was normal (367). Since then, several investigators have reported that serum vitamin A (146, 248, 430–436) and carotene (248, 431, 433–436) concentrations are markedly lower in acute febrile diseases, especially pneumonia. Plasma vitamin A usually increases during recovery (431, 436) and may exceed the upper limits of the normal range, depending partially on the age of the subject (431). On the other hand, Thiele and Scherff (432) found that carotene values remained unchanged. No papers indicating that increased vitamin A intake prevented the observed decrease in plasma vitamin A during acute infections were found.

Aron et al. (484) artificially induced hyperthermia in 92 patients. The extent of plasma vitamin A and carotene depression was directly related to the duration of the fever. Carotene depression was generally not as great and occurred more slowly. Restoration of plasma vitamin A level usually occurred spontaneously by the second day after treatment. Méndez et al. (485) reported from Guatemala the results of a similar experiment. Elevation of body temperature by 2 to 3° for 2 hours caused a highly significant decrease in plasma vitamin A levels and an increase in white blood cells but not in carotene concentration.

Although the plasma vitamin A levels may drop abruptly in acute infections, liver values are often normal (165, 171, 430, 453). Others have found reduced liver stores in respiratory (165, 173, 270), renal (270) and septic infections (165, 270). The degree of liver damage appears to be an important factor (453). Reduced adrenal content (454) and increased urinary excretion (486, 487) of vitamin A have also been reported.

Little is known about vitamin A metabolism in the various pathological conditions. Recent animal experiments suggest that vitamin A may play a hormonal-like role in controlling the biosynthesis of protein (488–490), polysaccharides[3] and mucus-producing cells in the parotid duct (491).

Chemical substances

It has been suggested that the ingestion of various chemical substances may possibly increase vitamin A requirements. Despite a high per capita disappearance of vitamin A-containing foods from the Canadian consumer market, recent surveys (139, 140) have demonstrated a surprisingly high incidence of low human liver vitamin A stores. Phillips and Brien (492) have suggested that in view of the effect of cholestyramine on vitamin A absorption, further studies on factors affecting the utilization of vitamin A (e.g., food additives, therapeutic agents and environmental contaminants) are warranted.

Ignatova and Prokop'ev (440) reported that vitamin A deficiency was pronounced in patients with pulmonary tuberculosis who had been treated with antibacterial therapy. Administering vitamin A along with the chemicals increased the effec-

---

[3] Blough, H. A., and C. H. Tudor 1967 Potentiation of interferon by vitamin A and polysaccharides. Federation Proc. 26: 363 (abstr.).

tiveness of the chemotherapy. Gal et al. (415) have found that the mean plasma vitamin A level (83 μg/100 ml) of women receiving oral contraceptive pills is double the value for healthy women not receiving the pill (45 μg/100 ml). It is not known whether this significant increase affects maternal vitamin A requirements or fetal development in women who become pregnant shortly after discontinuing the oral contraceptive.

Liver vitamin A stores are reduced in animals that have ingested a number of chemicals including nitrate or nitrite (136, 493), DDT (494–496), bromobenzole (497) and ethyl alcohol (498, 499) but the mode of action is not clear (493, 495, 500–502).

Genetic Defects

After studying three generations of a family with an usually high incidence of Darier's disease, follicular keratosis, Getzler and Flint (503) suggested that genetic defects may increase the amount of vitamin A required to maintain normal epithelial tissues. When the subjects were given 100,000 to 150,000 IU of water-soluble vitamin A (30,000 to 45,000 μg retinol) daily for 3 to 5 months, the symptoms cleared. All affected family members showed the same symptoms, thus suggesting that the excessively high vitamin A requirements were due to genetic factors. Although skin abnormalities were among the first vitamin A deficiency symptoms to be recognized in experimental animals (37), in humans the relationship between vitamin A intake and various skin conditions is controversial (504, 505). We still have little information about the metabolism of vitamin A and carotene in epithelial tissue (505).

COMMENTS

Although vitamin A has been recognized as an essential nutrient for about 50 years, there are relatively few data on human dietary requirements for it. Controlled studies on retinol requirements of adults and infants have been reported. Data on requirements of adults and of children 2 to 5 years old, when the vitamin is supplied as provitamin A, are also available. But no reports of controlled studies with adolescents, pregnant women or elderly people were found. On the other hand, gross clinical symptoms of excessive intakes (hypervitaminosis A) have been observed in people of all ages. Seventy-five percent of the acute cases occurred in infants 2 to 8 months old.

One of the primary reasons for this dearth of information on human vitamin A requirements has been the lack of sensitive criteria for evaluating vitamin A status. Dark adaptation was the criterion most commonly used in the controlled studies, most of which were conducted in the late 1930's and in the 1940's. However, this vitamin A deficiency symptom is among the last to appear (69). Similarly, dark adaptation may be corrected with relatively small amounts of vitamin A but increasing amounts are required to replete the other tissues (69, 168). Lesions of the epithelial tissues also are observed but they are an imprecise index with currently used methodology.

Vitamin A storage in the liver and our inability to estimate it conveniently have added to the complexity of the problem. Plasma vitamin A levels are commonly measured in nutritional status surveys. Animal studies (148, 506) however, show that this parameter is relatively insensitive to vitamin A status until liver stores have been virtually depleted. Some investigators have thus concluded that plasma vitamin A and carotenoid values are of little value in studying vitamin A requirements. On the other hand, Patwardhan (201) has shown that potentially useful information may be obtained from a critical evaluation of blood values as related to intake. The relation of the kind and quantity of vitamin A-active compounds consumed to plasma retinol and carotenoid values, as well as the relationship between the latter two are yet to be resolved. Comparisons of these values within the various age groups might also be useful. The answers to some of these questions might be obtained from a careful analysis and correlation of data from selected individual subjects. The mass of information that the ICNND [4] has collected in 34 nutrition surveys of various population groups throughout the world

---

[4] Interdepartmental Committee on Nutrition for National Defense.

(507–540) might be considered as a source of data for such analysis.

The use of β-carotene as the International Standard, until pure crystalline vitamin A became available in 1947, has led to a great deal of confusion. The relative vitamin A value of provitamins and their stereoisomers to retinol is based primarily on the rat's ability to utilize these compounds. Beeson (136), however, has compiled data that showed greater than fourfold differences among species in their ability to utilize the provitamins. Beta-carotene is the only purified provitamin that has been fed experimentally to man.

In addition, there are differences in the provitamin A availability in natural foodstuffs. We have few data on this subject and it is a question that will have to be answered in order to arrive at the dietary vitamin A requirement.

What we need to know is first, how much retinol is required by the various population groups under the different conditions and second, how much of the various provitamins in the different foods must be consumed in order to meet this requirement. In order to determine the latter we need to know: first, how much of the different provitamin A compounds and their stereoisomers are in the foods "as eaten"; second, what is their vitamin A value in humans (i.e., in relation to retinol); and third, what percentage of these compounds is available from the foods that we eat. Only then can we arrive at the human dietary vitamin A requirement.

During the last decade, our knowledge of vitamin A metabolism and our technological capabilities have both progressed. We can now separate and quantitate the stereoisomers of different provitamins (541). Relatively rapid and reliable methods have also been developed for isolating and quantitating plasma retinol (542) and β-carotene (543). Sensitive methods such as electron microscopy and histochemistry also offer hope that we may soon be able to detect subcellular response of the epithelial cells to various levels of vitamin A intake.

Recently, methods for isolating and quantitating retinol-binding protein (RBP) from human plasma have been developed

(399, 544). After finding species differences in vitamin A binding by plasma protein, Frank et al. (545) suggested that these differences may correlate with the vitamin A requirements of the species.

Rask et al. (546) have just reported that human RBP exists in two main physiological forms, each of which displays electrophoretic heterogeneity, but only one form (RBP-1) contains vitamin A. Since the electrophoretic mobility of RBP-1 varies with its vitamin A content, this may be helpful in evaluating vitamin A status. The other form (RBP-2), which is the main RBP component of the urine, lacks vitamin A. Rask et al. suggest that it may be a catabolite of RBP-1. If this is true, it might possibly be used for determining vitamin A turnover.

Information has also become available on the urinary excretion of retinoic acid metabolites (547). Pearson (141) has suggested that "really new advances will be offshoots of basic studies of vitamin A metabolism." As we learn more about the active metabolites of vitamin A, therefore, excretory products may also become useful indices of vitamin A status.

Hopefully, through the practical application of some of these newly developed methods, we will be able to complete our knowledge of human needs for vitamin A.

ACKNOWLEDGMENTS

The authors wish to thank Mr. D. C. Borton and the National Library of Medicine, Bethesda, Maryland, for their invaluable assistance and for the use of the excellent library collection during our literature search.

We also thank Mrs. June A. Jessop and Mrs. Linda A. Watkins for their excellent secretarial and editorial work.

LITERATURE CITED

1. Aykroyd, W. R. 1944 An early reference to night-blindness in India, and its relation to diet deficiency. Curr. Sci. *13:* 149.
2. Magendie, M. F. 1816 Sur les propriétés nutritives des substances qui ne contiennent pas d'azote. Ann. Chim. Phys. *3:* 66.
3. Bicknell, F., and F. Prescott 1953 The Vitamins in Medicine, ed. 3. W. Heinemann, London, 784 pp.
4. McCollum, E. V. 1957 A History of Nutrition. Houghton Mifflin Co., Boston, 451 pp.
5. Moore, T. 1957 Vitamin A. Elsevier Publishing Co., Amsterdam, 645 pp.

6. Mori, M. 1904 Über den sog. Hikan (Xerosis conjunctivae infantum ev. Keratomalacie). Jahrbuch Kinderheilk. 59: 175. Cited by: Bicknell, F., and F. Prescott 1953 The Vitamins in Medicine, ed. 3. W. Heinemann, London.

7. Hopkins, F. G. 1912 Feeding experiments illustrating the importance of accessory factors in normal dietaries. J. Physiol. 44: 425.

8. Osborne, T. B., and L. B. Mendel 1913 The influence of butter-fat on growth. J. Biol. Chem. 16: 423.

9. Osborne, T. B., and L. B. Mendel 1914 The influence of cod liver oil and some other fats on growth. J. Biol. Chem. 17: 401.

10. McCollum, E. V., and M. Davis 1913 The necessity of certain lipins in the diet during growth. J. Biol. Chem. 15: 167.

11. McCollum, E. V., and N. Simmonds 1917 A biological analysis of pellagra-producing diets. II. The minimum requirements of the two unidentified dietary factors for maintenance as contrasted with growth. J. Biol. Chem. 32: 181.

12. McCollum, E. V., and M. Davis 1915 The nature of the dietary deficiencies of rice. J. Biol. Chem. 23: 181.

13. Blegvad, O. M. D. 1924 Xerophthalmia, keratomalacia and xerosis conjunctivae. Amer. J. Ophthalmol. 7: 89.

14. Bloch, C. E. 1921 Clinical investigation of xerophthalmia and dystrophy in infants and young children. (Xerophthalmia et Dystrophia Alipogenetica.) J. Hyg. 19: 283.

15. McCollum, E. V., N. Simmonds and W. Pitz 1917 The supplementary dietary relationship between leaf and seed as contrasted with combinations of seed with seed. J. Biol. Chem. 30: 13.

16. Osborne, T. B., and L. B. Mendel 1919 The vitamines in green foods. J. Biol. Chem. 37: 187.

17. Steenbock, H. 1919 White corn vs yellow corn and a probable relation between the fat-soluble vitamine and yellow plant pigments. Science 50: 352.

18. Zilva, S. S., and M. Miura 1921 LXXIX. The quantitative estimation of the fat-soluble factor. Biochem. J. 15: 654.

19. Euler, B. von, H. von Euler and H. Hellström 1928 A-Vitaminwirkungen der Lipochrome. Biochem. Z. 203: 370.

20. Moore, T. 1929 A note on carotin and vitamin A. Lancet 216: 499.

21. Moore, T. 1929 The relation of carotin to vitamin A. Lancet 217: 380.

22. Moore, T. 1930 LXXIX. Vitamin A and carotene. VI. The conversion of carotene to vitamin A in vivo. Biochem. J. 24: 696.

23. Karrer, P. 1932 Carotenoids and vitamin-A. In: Chemistry at the Centenary (1931) Meeting of the British Association for Advancement of Science. Heffer, Cambridge, England, p. 82.

24. Kuhn, R., and E. Lederer 1931 Fraktionierung und Isomerisierung des Carotins. Naturwissenschaften 19: 306.

25. Rosenheim, O., and W. W. Starling 1931 The purification and optical activity of carotene. Chem. Ind. 50: 443.

26. Karrer, P., A. Helfenstein, H. Wehrli, B. Pieper and R. Morf 1931 Pflanzenfarbstoffe. XXX. Beiträge zur Kenntnis des Carotins, der Xanthophylle, des Fucoxanthins und Capsanthins. Helv. Chim. Acta 14: 614.

27. Gillam, A. E., and M. S. El Ridi 1935 Adsorption of grass and butter carotenes on alumina. Nature 136: 914.

28. Gillam, A. E., and M. S. El Ridi 1936 CCXLIII. The isomerization of carotenes by chromatographic adsorption. I. Pseudo-α-carotene. Biochem. J. 30: 1735.

29. Zechmeister, L. 1962 Cis-trans Isomeric Carotenoids, Vitamins A and Arylpolyenes. Academic Press, New York, 251 pp.

30. Zechmeister, L. 1949 Stereoisomeric provitamins A. In: Vitamins and Hormones, vol. 7, eds., R. S. Harris and K. V. Thimann. Academic Press, New York, p. 57.

31. Shantz, E. M., and J. H. Brinkman 1950 Biological activity of pure vitamin A$_2$. J. Biol. Chem. 183: 467.

32. Josephs, H. W. 1944 Hypervitaminosis A and carotenemia. Amer. J. Dis. Child. 67: 33.

33. Fridericia, L. S., and E. Holm 1925 Experimental contribution to the study of the relation between night blindness and malnutrition. Amer. J. Physiol. 73: 63.

34. Yudkin, A. M. 1931 The presence of vitamin A in the retina. Arch. Ophthalmol. 6: 510.

35. Wald, G. 1935 Carotenoids and the visual cycle. J. Gen. Physiol. 19: 351.

36. Kimble, M. S. 1939 The photocolorimetric determination of vitamin A and carotene in human plasma. J. Lab. Clin. Med. 24: 1055.

37. Wolbach, S. B., and P. R. Howe 1925 Tissue changes following deprivation of fat-soluble A vitamin. J. Exp. Med. 42: 753.

38. Permanent Commission on Biological Standardisation: League of Nations Health Organisation. June 23, 1931 Report of the Permanent Commission on Biological Standardisation. Geneva.

39. Permanent Commission on Biological Standardisation: League of Nations Health Organisation. 1934 Report of the Second International Conference on Vitamin Standardisation. Quart. Bull. Health Organ. 3: 428.

40. Hume, E. M., and H. Chick, eds. 1935 IV. The Standardisation and Estimation of Vitamin A. Medical Research Council Special Report Series no. 202, H. M. Stationery Office, London.

41. Van Dorp, D. A., and J. F. Arens 1947 Synthesis of vitamin A aldehyde. Nature 160: 189.

42. Isler, O., W. Huber, A. Ronco and M. Kofler 1947 238. Synthèse des Vitamin A. Helv. Chim. Acta. 30: 1911.

43. World Health Organization, Expert Committee on Biological Standardization 1950

Report of the subcommittee on fat-soluble vitamins. Tech. Report Series no. 3, Geneva.

44. Greaves, J. P., and J. Tan 1966 Vitamin A and carotene in British and American diets. Brit. J. Nutr. 20: 819.

45. FAO/WHO 1967 Requirements of vitamin A, thiamine, riboflavin, and niacin. FAO Nutr. Meet. Report Series no. 41, WHO Tech. Report Series no. 362, Rome.

46. Jayle, G. E., and A. G. Ourgaud 1950 La Vision Nocturne et ses Troubles. Masson & Cie., Paris.

47. Jayle, G. E., A. G. Ourgaud, L. F. Baisinger and W. J. Holmes 1959 Night Vision. English ed., Chas. C Thomas, Springfield, Ill. 408 pp.

48. Jeghers, H. 1937 Night blindness as a criterion of vitamin A deficiency: Review of the literature with preliminary observations of the degree and prevalence of vitamin A deficiency among adults in both health and disease. Ann. Intern. Med. 10: 1304.

49. Yudkin, J., G. W. Robertson and S. Yudkin 1943 Vitamin A and dark adaptation. Lancet 2: 10.

50. Schmidtke, R. L. 1947 Hypovitaminosis A in ophthalmology. Arch. Ophthalmol. 37: 653.

51. McLaren, D. S. 1963 Malnutrition and the Eye. Academic Press, New York.

52. Edmund, C., and Sv. Clemmeson 1936 On Deficiency of A Vitamin and Visual Dysaptation. Levin and Munksgaard, Copenhagen; Humphrey Milford, Oxford University Press, London. Translated by C. Packness, Copenhagen, 77 pp.

53. Edmund, C., and Sv. Clemmesen 1937 On Deficiency of A Vitamin and Visual Dysaptation, vol. 2. Oxford University Press, London. Translated by C. Packness, Copenhagen, 52 pp.

54. Jeghers, H. 1937 The degree and prevalence of vitamin A deficiency in adults. J. Amer. Med. Ass. 109: 756.

55. Booher, L. E., E. C. Callison and E. M. Hewston 1939 An experimental determination of the minimum vitamin A requirements of normal adults. J. Nutr. 17: 317.

56. Hume, E. M. 1939 Estimation of vitamin A. Nature 143: 22.

57. Hume, E. M. 1943 Estimation of vitamin A. Nature 151: 535.

58. Callison, E. C., and E. Orent-Keiles 1945 Standards in vitamin A assays. U.S.P. reference cod liver oil vs. beta-carotene. Ind. Eng. Chem., Anal. Ed. 17: 378.

59. Callison, E. C., and E. Orent-Keiles 1947 Availability of carotene from carrots and further observations on human requirements for vitamin A and carotene. J. Nutr. 34: 153.

60. Coward, K. H. 1938 The Biological Standardisation of the Vitamins. Baillière, Tindall and Cox, London, 227 pp.

61. Gridgeman, N. T. 1944 The Estimation of Vitamin A. Lever Brothers and Unilever Limited, Port Sunlight, Cheshire, England, 74 pp.

62. Nelson, E. M., and J. B. DeWitt 1947 Biological assay for vitamin A. In: The Estimation of the Vitamins, vol. 12, eds., W. J. Dann and G. H. Satterfield. Biological Symposia Series, ed., J. Cattell. Jaques Cattell Press, Lancaster, Pa., p. 1.

63. Blanchard, E. L., and H. A. Harper 1940 Measurement of vitamin A status of young adults by the dark adaptation technic. Arch. Intern. Med. 66: 661.

64. Basu, N. M., and N. K. De 1941 Assessment of vitamin A deficiency amongst Bengalees and determination of the minimal and optimal requirements of vitamin A by a simplified method for measuring visual adaptation in the dark. Indian J. Med. Res. 29: 591.

65. Batchelder, E. L., and J. C. Ebbs 1942 Vitamin A metabolism and requirements as determined by the rhodometer. R. I. Agricultural Experiment Station of the Rhode Island State College, Kingston, Rhode Island, Bull no. 286, 24 pp.

66. Batchelder, E. L., and J. C. Ebbs 1944 Some observations of dark adaptation in man and their bearing on the problem of human requirement for vitamin A. J. Nutr. 27: 295.

67. Wagner, K. H. 1940 Die experimentelle Avitaminose A beim Menschen. Hoppe-Seyler's Z. Physiol. Chem. 264: 153.

68. Grab, W., and Th. Moll 1939 Über die verschiedene Wirksamkeit von Vitamin A-Konzentraten aus Fischleberolen. Wertbestimmung des Vitamin A-Konzentrates "Vogan." Klin. Wochenschr. 18: 563.

69. Hume, E. M., and H. A. Krebs 1949 Vitamin A Requirement of Human Adults. An Experimental Study of Vitamin A Deprivation in Man. Medical Research Council Special Report Series no. 264, H. M. Stationery Office, London, 145 pp.

70. Wald, G. 1941 A portable visual adaptometer. J. Ophthalmol. Soc. Amer. 31: 235.

71. Wald, G., L. Brouha and R. E. Johnson 1942 Experimental human vitamin A deficiency and the ability to perform muscular exercise. Amer. J. Physiol. 137: 551.

72. Brenner, S., and L. J. Roberts 1943 Effects of vitamin A depletion in young adults. Arch. Intern. Med. 71: 474.

73. Hecht, S., and J. Mandelbaum 1939 The relation between vitamin A and dark adaptation. J. Amer. Med. Ass. 112: 1910.

74. Hecht, S., and J. Mandelbaum 1940 Dark adaptation and experimental human vitaman A deficiency. Amer. J. Physiol. 130: 651.

75. Wald, G., H. Jeghers and J. Arminio 1938 An experiment in human dietary nightblindness. Amer. J. Physiol. 123: 732.

76. Steven, D. M. 1942 Human vitamin A deficiency. 5. Experimental human vitamin A deficiency. The relation between dark adaptation and blood vitamin A. Ophthalmol. Soc. United Kingdom Transactions 62: 259.

77. Jeans, P. C., E. L. Blanchard and F. E. Satterthwaite 1941 Dark adaptation and vitamin A. J. Pediat. 18: 170.

78. Pett, L. B., and G. A. LePage 1940 Vitamin A deficiency. III. Blood analysis correlated with a visual test. J. Biol. Chem. 132: 585.

79. Pett, L. B. 1939 Vitamin A deficiency: Its prevalence and importance as shown by a new test. J. Lab. Clin. Med. 25: 149.

80. Wald, G., and D. Steven 1939 An experiment in human vitamin A-deficiency. Proc. Nat. Acad. Sci. U. S. 25: 344.

81. Leitner, Z. A., T. Moore and I. M. Sharman 1960 Vitamin A and vitamin E in human blood. 1. Levels of vitamin A and carotenoids in British men and women 1948–57. Brit. J. Nutr. 14: 157.

82. Batchelder, E. L. 1934 Nutritional significance of vitamin A throughout the life cycle. Amer. J. Physiol. 109: 430.

83. Sherman, H. C., H. L. Campbell, M. Udiljak and H. Yarmolinsky 1945 Vitamin A in relation to aging and to length of life. Proc. Nat. Acad. Sci. 31: 107.

84. Paul, H. E., and M. F. Paul 1946 The relation of vitamin A intake to length of life, growth, tooth structure and eye condition. J. Nutr. 31: 67.

85. Sherman, H. C., and H. Y. Trupp 1949 Long-term experiments at or near the optimum level of intake of vitamin A. J. Nutr. 37: 467.

86. Popper, H., F. Steigmann, K. A. Meyer and S. S. Zevin 1943 Relation between hepatic and plasma concentrations of vitamin A in human beings. Arch. Intern. Med. 72: 439.

87. Meyer, K. A., H. Popper, F. Steigmann, W. H. Walters and S. Zevin 1942 Comparison of vitamin A of liver biopsy specimens with plasma vitamin A in man. Proc. Soc. Exp. Biol. Med. 49: 589.

88. McLaren, D. S., W. W. C. Read and M. Tchalian 1966 Extent of human vitamin A deficiency. Proc. Nutr. Soc. 25: xxviii.

89. Underwood, B. A., H. Siegel, R. C. Weisell and M. Dolinski 1970 Liver stores of vitamin A in a normal population dying suddenly or rapidly from unnatural causes in New York City. Amer. J. Clin. Nutr. 23: 1037.

90. Moore, T., and A. C. Cooper; cited by: E. M. Hume and H. A. Krebs 1949 Vitamin A Requirement of Human Adults. An Experimental Study of Vitamin A Deprivation in Man. Medical Research Council Special Report Series no. 264. H. M. Stationery Office, London.

91. Guilbert, H. R., C. E. Howell and G. H. Hart 1940 Minimum vitamin A and carotene requirements of mammalian species. J. Nutr. 19: 91.

92. Callison, E. C., and V. H. Knowles 1945 Liver reserves of vitamin A and their relation to the signs of vitamin A deficiency in the albino rat. Amer. J. Physiol. 143: 444.

93. High, E. G. 1954 Studies on the absorption, deposition and depletion of vitamin A in the rat. Arch. Biochem. 49: 19.

94. Sulzberger, M. B., and M. P. Lazar 1951 Hypervitaminosis A. Report of a case in an adult. J. Amer. Med. Ass. 146: 788.

95. Bifulco, E. 1953 Vitamin A intoxication: Report of a case in an adult. N. Engl. J. Med. 248: 690.

96. Shaw, E. W., and J. Z. Niccoli 1953 Hypervitaminosis A: Report of a case in an adult male. Ann. Intern. Med. 39: 131.

97. Gerber, A., A. P. Raab and A. E. Sobel 1954 Vitamin A poisoning in adults. With description of a case. Amer. J. Med. 16: 729.

98. Block, H. S. 1955 Chronic hypervitaminosis A; report of a probable case in man. Minn. Med. 38: 627.

99. Elliott, R. A., Jr., and R. L. Dryer 1956 Hypervitaminosis A: Report of a case in an adult. J. Amer. Med. Ass. 161: 1157.

100. Creek, D. W., K. J. McNiece and L. M. Nelson 1958 Hypervitaminosis A — toxic reaction. Amer. J. Gastroenterol. 29: 169.

101. Stimson, W. H. 1961 Vitamin A intoxication in adults: Report of a case with a summary of the literature. N. Engl. J. Med. 265: 369.

102. Soler-Bechara, J., and J. L. Soscia 1963 Chronic hypervitaminosis A. Report of a case in an adult. Arch. Intern. Med. 112: 462.

103. Bergen, S. S., Jr., and O. A. Roels 1965 Hypervitaminosis A. Report of a case. Amer. J. Clin. Nutr. 16: 265.

104. Jennekens, F. G. I., and C. W. M. van Veelen 1966 Hypervitaminose A. Presse Med. 74: 2925.

105. Wisse Smit, J., and D. Pott Hofstede 1966 Vitamine-A-intoxicatie bij volwassenen. Nederl. Tijdschr. Geneesk. 110: 10.

106. Di Benedetto, R. J. 1967 Chronic hypervitaminosis A in an adult. J. Amer. Med. Ass. 201: 700.

107. Lane, B. P. 1968 Hepatic microanatomy in hypervitaminosis A in man and rat. Amer. J. Pathol. 53: 591.

108. Hillman, R. W. (with M. E. Leogrande) 1956 Hypervitaminosis A. Experimental induction in the human subject. Amer. J. Clin. Nutr. 4: 603.

109. Rodahl, K., and T. Moore 1943 The vitamin A content and toxicity of bear and seal liver. Biochem. J. 37: 166.

110. Cleland, J. B., and R. V. Southcott 1969 Illnesses following the eating of seal liver in Australian waters. Med. J. Australia 1: 760.

111. Muenter, M. D., H. O. Perry and J. Ludwig 1971 Chronic vitamin A intoxication in adults. Hepatic, neurologic and dermatologic complications. Amer. J. Med. 50: 129.

112. Rubin, E., A. L. Florman, T. Degnan and J. Diaz 1970 Hepatic injury in chronic hypervitaminosis A. Amer. J. Dis. Child. 119: 132.

113. Baba, H., and M. Hirayama 1969 Electron microscopic observation of liver of rat fed

various levels of vitamin A. Jap. J. Nutr. 27: 42.

114. Tanksale, K. G. 1970 Paradoxical increase in dark-adaptation time after vitamin A intake. J. Postgrad. Med. Bombay 16: 65. Cited in: Nutr. Abst. Rev. 41: (abstr. no. 1069), 1971.

115. Dobronravova, N. P., N. N. Prostajakova and A. A. Tupikova 1969 Ob optimal'noj potrebnosti organizma v vitamine A. Vop. Pitan. 28: (6) 51. Cited in: Nutr. Abst. Rev. 40: (abstr. no. 7178), 1970.

116. Booher, L. E., and E. C. Callison 1939 The minimum vitamin-A requirements of normal adults. II. The utilization of carotene as affected by certain dietary factors and variations in light exposure. J. Nutr. 18: 459.

117. Drigalski, W. von 1939 Über den Vitamin A-Bedarf des Menschen. 1. Der gesunde Erwachsene. Klin. Wochenschr. 18: 1269.

118. Kawaguchi, T., and A. Fujita 1956 Studies on the absorption of carotene in man. J. Vitaminol. 2: 115.

119. Ishii, R., and C. Iwagaki 1955 Factors affecting the biological activity of carotene. I. Lipoxidase in foods and its destructive power on carotene in the synthetic gastric juice. Vitamins 9: 213.

120. Anonymous 1945 Vitamin A deficiency and the requirements of human adults. Nature 156: 11.

121. Medical Research Council (Accessory Food Factors Committee) 1945 Nutritive Values of Wartime Foods. Med. Res. Coun. War Memo. no. 14, London, 59 pp.

122. Barrett, I. M., and E. M. Widdowson 1960 Part II. Vitamins. In: The Composition of Foods, eds., R. A. McCance and E. M. Widdowson. Medical Research Council Special Report Series no. 297, H. M. Stationery Office, London, p. 161.

123. Watt, B. K., and A. L. Merrill 1963 Composition of Foods — Raw, Processed, Prepared. Agr. Handbook no. 8, Agr. Research Serv., U. S. D. A. U. S. Govt. Printing Office, Washington, D. C., 189 pp.

124. Watt, B. K., and A. L. Merrill 1950 Composition of Foods — Raw, Processed, Prepared. Agr. Handbook No. 8, Agr. Research Serv., U. S. D. A. U. S. Govt. Printing Office, Washington, D. C., 147 pp.

125. Leitner, Z. A., T. Moore and I. M. Sharman 1954 The effect of the vegetable ration on carotene and vitamin A in the blood of chronic hospital patients. Proc. Nutr. Soc. 13: xi.

126. Leitner, Z. A., T. Moore and I. M. Sharman 1964 Vitamin A and vitamin E in human blood. 3. Levels in patients in psychiatric hospitals. Brit. J. Nutr. 18: 115.

127. Roels, O. A., S. Djaeni, M. E. Trout, T. G. Lauw, A. Heath, S. H. Poey, M. S. Tarwotjo and B. Suhadi 1963 The effect of protein and fat supplements on vitamin A-deficient Indonesian children. Amer. J. Clin. Nutr. 12: 380.

128. Carter, R. A., and G. C. Cook 1963 Studies on the serum total carotenoids, vitamin A and serum colour in Nigerian soldiers. Brit. J. Nutr. 17: 515.

129. Dagadu, M., and J. Gillman 1963 Hypercarotenaemia in Ghanaians. Lancet 1: 531.

130. Bayfield, R. F., R. H. Falk and J. D. Barrett 1968 The separation and determination of a-tocopherol and carotenoids in serum or plasma by paper chromatography. J. Chromatogr. 36: 54.

131. Blankenhorn, D. H. 1957 Carotenoids in man. II. Fractions obtained from atherosclerotic and normal aortas, serum, and depot fat by separation on alumina. J. Biol. Chem. 227: 963.

132. High, E. G. 1969 Some aspects of nutritional vitamin A levels in preschool children of Beaufort County, South Carolina. Amer. J. Clin. Nutr. 22: 1129.

133. Goodwin, T. W. 1951 Vitamin A-active substances. Brit. J. Nutr. 5: 94.

134. Johnson, R. M., and C. A. Baumann 1948 Storage of vitamin A in rats fed cryptoxanthine and certain other carotenoids with parallel data on adsorbability. Arch. Biochem. 19: 493.

135. Johnson, R. M., and C. A. Baumann 1947 Storage and distribution of vitamin A in rats fed certain isomers of carotene. Arch. Biochem. 14: 361.

136. Beeson, W. M. 1965 Relative potencies of vitamin A and carotene for animals. Federation Proc. 24: 924.

137. Nylund, C. E., and T. K. With 1942 Über den Vitamin-A-Bedarf der warmblütigen Tiere und des Menschen. Eine kritische Übersicht, erweitert durch eigene Untersuchungen. Vitamine Hormone 2: 7.

138. Mašek, J. 1962 Recommended nutrient allowances. In: World Review of Nutrition and Diet, vol. 3, ed., G. H. Bourne. Hafner Publishing Co., New York, p. 149.

139. Hoppner, K., W. E. J. Phillips, T. K. Murray and J. S. Campbell 1968 Survey of liver vitamin A stores of Canadians. Can. Med. Ass. J. 99: 983.

140. Hoppner, K., W. E. J. Phillips, P. Erdody, T. K. Murray and D. E. Perrin 1969 Vitamin A reserves of Canadians. Can. Med. Ass. J. 101: 84.

141. Pearson, W. N. 1967 Blood and urinary vitamin levels as potential indices of body stores. Amer. J. Clin. Nutr. 20: 514.

142. Barenberg, L. H., and J. M. Lewis 1932 Relationship of vitamin A to respiratory infections in infants. J. Amer. Med. Ass. 98: 199.

143. Hess, A. F., J. M. Lewis and L. H. Barenberg 1933 Does our dietary require vitamin A supplement? J. Amer. Med. Ass. 101: 657.

144. Lewis, J. M., and L. H. Barenberg 1938 The relationship of vitamin A to the health of infants. Further observations. J. Amer. Med. Ass. 110: 1338.

145. Lewis, J. M., and C. Haig 1939 Vitamin A requirements in infancy as determined by dark adaptation. J. Pediat. 15: 812.

146. Bodansky, O., J. M. Lewis and C. Haig 1941 The comparative value of the blood plasma vitamin A concentration and the dark adaptation as a criterion of vitamin A deficiency. Science 94: 370.

147. Lewis, J. M., O. Bodansky and C. Haig 1941 Level of vitamin A in the blood as an index of vitamin A deficiency in infants and in children. Amer. J. Dis. Child. 62: 1129.

148. Lewis, J. M., and O. Bodansky 1943 Minimum vitamin A requirements in infants as determined by vitamin A concentration in blood. Proc. Soc. Exp. Biol. Med. 52: 265.

149. Gopalan, C. 1956 Protein intake of breastfed poor Indian infants. J. Trop. Pediat. 2: 89.

150. Gopalan, C. 1958 Studies on lactation in poor Indian communities. J. Trop. Pediat. 4: 87.

151. Bhavani Belavady, and C. Gopalan 1959 Chemical composition of human milk in poor Indian women. Indian J. Med. Res. 47: 234.

152. Bhavani Belavady, and C. Gopalan 1960 Effect of dietary supplementation on the composition of breast milk. Indian J. Med. Res. 48: 518.

153. Gopalan, C. 1958 Effect of protein supplementation and some so-called "Galactogogues" on lactation of poor Indian women. Indian J. Med. Res. 46: 317.

154. Patwardhan, V. N., and W. W. Kamel 1967 Studies on vitamin A deficiency in infants and young children in Jordan. Report to World Health Organization, Geneva. Cited by: Patwardhan, V. N. 1969 Hypovitaminosis A and epidemiology of xerophthalmia. Amer. J. Clin. Nutr. 22: 1106.

155. Oomen, H. A. P. C., D. S. McLaren and H. Escapini 1964 A global survey on xerophthalmia. Trop. Geograph. Med. 16: 271.

156. Chandra, H., P. S. Venkatachalam, Bhavani Belavady, V. Reddy and C. Gopalan 1960 Some observations on vitamin A deficiency in Indian children. Indian J. Child. Health 9: 589.

157. McLaren, D. S., E. Shirajian, M. Tchalian and G. Khoury 1965 Xerophthalmia in Jordan. Amer. J. Clin. Nutr. 17: 117.

158. Bartolozzi, G., G. Bernini, L. Marianelli and E. Corvaglia 1967 Ipervitaminosi a cronica nel lattante e nel bambino. Descrizione di due casi e rassegna critica della litteratura. Riv. Clin. Pediat. 80: 231.

159. Bloch, C. E. 1928 Decline in immunity as a symptom due to deficiency in A-vitamine and in C-vitamine. Acta Paediat. 7: (suppl. 2) 61.

160. Meulemans, O., and J. H. De Haas 1938 Vitamin A, carotene and vitamin C content of canned milk. Amer. J. Dis. Child. 56: 14.

161. Hartman, A. M., and L. P. Dryden 1965 Vitamins in Milk and Milk Products. Amer. Dairy Sci. Assoc., Champaign, Ill., 123 pp.

162. Mackay, H. M. M. 1934 Vitamin A deficiency in children. Part 2. Vitamin A requirements of babies: Skin lesions and vitamin A deficiency. Arch. Dis. Child. 9: 133.

163. Mackay, H. M. M. 1939 Vitamin A requirements of infants: The health of infants fed on roller-process dried milk, with and without a supplement of vitamin A. Arch. Dis. Child. 14: 245.

164. Stearns, G. 1950 Carotene and vitamin-A requirements in infants. In: Infant Metabolism. Proc. World Health Organization Seminars, Leyden and Stockholm. MacMillan Co., New York, p. 168.

165. Ellison, J. B., and T. Moore 1937 XIX. Vitamin A and carotene. XIV. The vitamin A reserves of the human infant and child in health and disease. Biochem. J. 31: 165.

166. Guilbert, H. R., R. F. Miller and E. H. Hughes 1937 The minimum vitamin A and carotene requirement of cattle, sheep and swine. J. Nutr. 13: 543.

167. Kübler, W. 1958 Latente A-Hypovitaminose bei künstlich genährten Säuglingen. Monatsschr. Kinderheilk. 106: 281.

168. Lewis, J. M., O. Bodansky, K. G. Falk and G. McGuire 1942 Vitamin A requirements in the rat. The relation of vitamin A intake to growth and to concentration of vitamin A in the blood plasma, liver and retina. J. Nutr. 23: 351.

169. Smith, B. M., and E. M. Malthus 1962 Vitamin A content of human liver from autopsies in New Zealand. Brit. J. Nutr. 16: 213.

170. Neuweiler, W. 1936 Der Gehalt der foetalen und Neugeborenen-Leber an Vitamin A. Z. Vitaminforsch. 5: 104.

171. Wolff, L. K. 1932 On the quantity of vitamin A present in the human liver. Lancet 223: 617.

172. Toverud, K. U., and F. Ender 1938 The vitamin A and D content of the liver of newborn infants. Acta Paediat. 18: 174.

173. Woo, T. T., and F. Chu 1940 The vitamin A content of the livers of Chinese infants, children and adults. Chinese J. Physiol. 15: 83.

174. With, T. K. 1940 Absorption, Metabolism and Storage of Vitamin A and Carotene. Oxford University Press, London, 263 pp.

175. Skurnik, L. von, H. von Heikel and T. U. Westerberg 1944 Ueber den A-Vitamin-, Carotin- und Riboflavingehalt der Leber. Z. Vitaminforsch. 15: 68.

176. Lewis, J. M., O. Bodansky and L. M. Shapiro 1943 Regulation of level of vitamin A in blood of newborn infants. Amer. J. Dis. Child. 66: 503.

177. Henley, T. H., M. Dann and W. R. C. Golden 1944 Reserves, absorption and plasma levels of vitamin A in premature infants. Amer. J. Dis. Child. 68: 257.

178. Marrack, J. R. 1948 Results of recent investigations of nutritional status in Great Britain. Laboratory investigations into the state of nutrition. Brit. J. Nutr. 2: 147.

179. Kon, S. K., and E. H. Mawson 1950 Human Milk. Wartime Studies of Certain Vitamins and Other Constituents. Medical

Research Council Special Report Series no. 269, H. M. Stationery Office, London, 188 pp.

180. Rønne, G. 1941 A-Vitaminbehov hos nyfødte og spaede. Ugeskr. Laeger. 103: 1432. Cited in: Nutr. Abst. Rev. 12: (abstr. no. 2631), 1943.

181. Rubin, S. H., and E. deRitter 1954 Vitamin A requirements of animal species. Vitamins Hormones 12: 101.

182. Fomon, S. J. 1967 Infant Nutrition. 8. Vitamins. W. B. Saunders Co., Philadelphia, p. 115.

183. Persson, B., R. Tunell and K. Ekengren 1965 Chronic vitamin A intoxication during the first half year of life. Description of 5 cases. Acta Paediat. Scand. 54: 49.

184. Arena J. M., P. Sarazen, Jr., and G. J. Baylin 1951 Hypervitaminosis A. Report of an unusual case with marked craniotabes. Pediatrics 8: 788.

185. Naz, J. F., and W. M. Edwards 1952 Hypervitaminosis A: A case report. New Engl. J. Med. 246: 87.

186. Woodard, W. K., L. J. Miller and O. Legant 1961 Acute and chronic hypervitaminosis in a 4-month-old infant. J. Pediat. 59: 260.

187. Drablös, A., and J. Slördahl 1959 Chronic vitamin A poisoning. Acta Paediat. 48: 507.

188. Varveri, A. 1967 Un caso di intossicazione cronica da vitamina. Infanzia 64: 27. Cited by: Bartolozzi, G., G. Bernini, L. Marianelli and E. Corvaglia 1967 Ipervitaminosi A cronica nel lattante e nel bambino. Rev. Clin. Pediat. 80: 231.

189. Pease, C. N. 1962 Focal retardation and arrestment of growth of bones due to vitamin A intoxication. J. Amer. Med. Ass. 182: 980.

190. Tunell, R., L. G. Allgén, B. Jalling and B. Persson 1965 Prophylactic vitamin A dose in Sweden. An investigation in connection with cases of intoxication. Acta Paediat. Scand. 54: 61.

191. Mackay, H. M. M. 1934 Vitamin A deficiency in children. 1. Present knowledge of the clinical effects of vitamin A deficiency, with special reference to children. Arch. Dis. Child. 9: 65.

192. Awdry, P. N., B. Cobb and P. C. G. Adams 1967 Blindness in the Luapula Valley. Cent. Afr. J. Med. 13: 197.

193. Kuming, B. S., and W. M. Politzer 1967 Xerophthalmia and protein malnutrition in Bantu children. Brit. J. Ophthalmol. 51: 649.

194. Blankhart, D. M. 1967 Individual intake of food in young children in relation to malnutrition and night blindness. Trop. Geogr. Med. 19: 144.

195. Venkataswamy, G. 1967 Ocular manifestations of vitamin A deficiency. Brit. J. Ophthalmol. 51: 854.

196. Pan American Health Organization, WHO 1970 Hypovitaminosis A in the Americas. Report of a Pan American Health Organization Technical Group Meeting, Scientific Publication no. 198, Washington, D. C., 28 pp.

197. Oomen, H. A. P. C. 1969 Clinical epidemiology of xerophthalmia in man. Amer. J. Clin. Nutr. 22: 1098.

198. Pereira, S. M., and A. Begum 1968 Studies in the prevention of vitamin A deficiency. Indian J. Med. Res. 56: 362.

199. Jeans, P. C., E. Blanchard and Z. Zentmire 1937 Dark adaptation and vitamin A. J. Amer. Med. Ass. 108: 451.

200. Lauw Tjin Giok, C. S. Rose and P. György 1967 Influence of early malnutrition on some aspects of the health of school-age children. Amer. J. Clin. Nutr. 20: 1280.

201. Patwardhan, V. N. 1969 Hypovitaminosis A and epidemiology of xerophthalmia. Amer. J. Clin. Nutr. 22: 1106.

202. Pereira, S. M., and A. Begum 1969 Prevention of vitamin A deficiency. Amer. J. Clin. Nutr. 22: 858.

203. Susheela, T. P. 1969 Studies on serum vitamin A levels after a single massive oral dose. Indian J. Med. Res. 57: 2147.

204. Srikantia, S. G., and V. Reddy 1970 Effect of a single massive dose of vitamin A on serum and liver levels of the vitamin. Amer. J. Clin. Nutr. 23: 114.

205. Swaminathan, M. C., T. P. Susheela and B. V. S. Thimmayamma 1970 Field prophylactic trial with a single annual oral massive dose of vitamin A. Amer. J. Clin. Nutr. 23: 119.

206. Gonzalez Outon, P. M. 1955 Hipervitaminosis A aguda en niños de edad prepuberal. (San Fernando, Cadiz) Medicamenta 24: 70.

207. Pickup, J. D. 1956 Hypervitaminosis A. Arch. Dis. Child. 31: 229.

208. Kane, A. L. 1952 Hypervitaminosis A: Study of an unusual case. Arizona Med. 9: 29.

209. Laplane, R., D. Duché, H. Jallut and M. Séligmann 1953 Oedème aigu cérébro-méningé résolutif chez un garçon de 16 ans après absorption de vitamine A à dose massive. Arch. Franc. Pédiat. 10: 979.

210. Jowsey, J., and B. L. Riggs 1968 Bone changes in a patient with hypervitaminosis A. J. Clin. Endocrinol. 28: 1833.

211. Aykroyd, W. R., and B. G. Krishnan 1936 The carotene and vitamin A requirements of children. Indian J. Med. Res. 23: 741.

212. Aykroyd, W. R., and R. E. Wright 1937 Red-palm oil in the treatment of human keratomalacia. Indian J. Med. Res. 25: 7.

213. Oey Khoen Lian, Liam Tjay Tie, C. S. Rose, D. D. Prawiranegara and P. György 1967 Red palm oil in the prevention of vitamin A deficiency. A trial on preschool children in Indonesia. Amer. J. Clin. Nutr. 20: 1267.

214. György, P. 1968 Protein–calorie and vitamin A malnutrition in Southeast Asia. Federation Proc. 27: 949.

215. Pek Hien Liang, Tjiook Tiauw Hie, Oey Henk Jan and Lauw Tjin Giok 1967 Evaluation of mental development in relation to early malnutrition. Amer. J. Clin. Nutr. 20: 1290.

216. Lala, V. R., and V. Reddy 1970 Absorption of β-carotene from green leafy vegetables in undernourished children. Amer. J. Clin. Nutr. 23: 110.

217. Arteaga, A., S. Valiente, E. Rosales and C. Urteaga 1969 La hipovitaminosis A: un problema nutricional colectivo en Chile. Bol. Of. Sanit. Pan-am. 66: 200.

218. Fernández, N. A., J. C. Burgos, I. C. Plough, L. J. Roberts and C. F. Asenjo 1965 Nutritional status of people in isolated areas of Puerto Rico. Survey of Barrio Mavilla, Vega Alta, Puerto Rico. Amer. J. Clin. Nutr. 17: 305.

219. Fernández, N. A., J. C. Burgos, I. C. Plough, L. J. Roberts and C. F. Asenjo 1966 Nutritional status of people in isolated areas of Puerto Rico. Survey of Barrio Naranjo, Moca, Puerto Rico. Amer. J. Clin. Nutr. 19: 269.

220. Fernández, N. A., J. C. Burgos, L. J. Roberts and C. F. Asenjo 1967 Nutritional status of people in isolated areas of Puerto Rico. Survey of Barrio Duey Alto, San German, Puerto Rico. Arch. Latinoamer. Nutr. 17: 215.

221. Fernández, N. A., J. C. Burgos, L. J. Roberts and C. F. Asenjo 1967 Nutritional status of people in isolated areas of Puerto Rico. Survey of Barrio Masas 2, Gurabo, Puerto Rico. Bol. Ass. Med. Puerto Rico 59: 503.

222. Jeans, P. C., and Z. Zentmire 1936 The prevalence of vitamin A deficiency among Iowa children. J. Amer. Med. Ass. 106: 996.

223. Lewis, J. M., and C. Haig 1940 Vitamin A status of children as determined by dark adaptation. J. Pediat. 16: 285.

224. Sandels, M. R., H. D. Cate, K. P. Wilkinson and L. J. Graves 1941 Follicular conjunctivitis in school children as an expression of vitamin A deficiency. Amer. J. Dis. Child. 62: 101.

225. Wilcox, E. B., and L. S. Galloway 1954 Children with and without rheumatic fever. I. Nutrient intake, physique, and growth. J. Amer. Diet. Ass. 30: 345.

226. Wilcox, E. B., L. S. Galloway, P. Wood and F. L. Mangelson 1954 Children with and without rheumatic fever. III. Blood serum vitamins and phosphatase data. J. Amer. Diet. Ass. 30: 1231.

227. Eppright, E. S., A. L. Marlatt and M. B. Patton 1955 Nutrition of 9-, 10-, and 11-year-old public school children in Iowa, Kansas and Ohio. I. Dietary findings. Iowa Agr. Exp. Sta. Res. Bull. no. 434, Ames, Iowa, p. 614.

228. Patton, M. B., E. S. Eppright and A. L. Marlatt 1957 Nutritional status of 9-, 10-, and 11-year-old public school children in Iowa, Kansas, and Ohio. II. Blood findings. North Central Res. Pub. 72, Ohio Exp. Sta. Res. Bull. no. 794, Wooster, Ohio, 63 pp.

229. Donald, E. A., N. C. Esselbaugh and M. M. Hard 1958 Nutritional status of selected adolescent children. II. Vitamin A nutrition assessed by dietary intake and serum levels. Biomicroscopic and gross observations. Amer. J. Clin. Nutr. 6: 126.

230. Odland, L. M., L. Page and L. P. Guild 1955 Nutrient intakes and food habits of Montana students. J. Amer. Diet. Ass. 31: 1134.

231. Odland, L. M., and R. J. Ostle 1956 Clinical and biochemical studies of Montana adolescents. J. Amer. Diet. Ass. 32: 823.

232. Vavich, M. G., A. R. Kemmerer and J. S. Hirsch 1954 The nutritional status of Papago Indian children. J. Nutr. 54: 121.

233. Storvick, C. A., B. Schaad, R. E. Coffey and M. B. Deardorff 1951 Nutritional status of selected population groups in Oregon. I. Food habits of native born and reared school children in two regions. The Milbank Memorial Fund Quarterly, vol. 29, no. 2. Published by Milbank Memorial Fund, New York.

234. Storvick, C. A., M. L. Hathaway and R. M. Nitchals 1951 Nutritional status of selected population groups in Oregon. II. Biochemical tests on the blood of native born and reared school children in two regions. The Milbank Memorial Fund Quarterly, vol 29, no. 3. Published by Milbank Memorial Fund, New York.

235. Lantz, E. M., and P. Wood 1958 Nutrition of New Mexican Spanish-American and "Anglo" adolescents. I. Food habits and nutrient intakes. J. Amer. Diet. Ass. 34: 138.

236. Lantz, E. L., and P. Wood 1958 Nutrition of New Mexican Spanish-American and "Anglo" adolescents. II. Blood findings, height and weight data and physical condition. J. Amer. Diet Ass. 34: 145.

237. Bring, S. V., K. P. Warnick and E. Woods 1955 Nutritional status of school children 15 and 16 years of age in three Idaho communities: Blood biochemical tests. J. Nutr. 57: 29.

238. Warnick, K. P., S. V. Bring and E. Woods 1955 Nutritional status of adolescent Idaho children. I. Evaluation of seven-day dietary records. J. Amer. Diet. Ass. 31: 486.

239. Johnson, R. M., and C. A. Baumann 1948 Relative significance of growth and metabolic rate upon the utilization of vitamin A by the rat. J. Nutr. 35: 703.

240. Rechcigl, M., Jr., S. Berger, J. K. Looski and H. H. Williams 1962 Dietary protein and utilization of vitamin A. J. Nutr. 76: 435.

241. National Research Council Food and Nutrition Board 1945 Recommended Dietary Allowances. Reprint and Circular Series no. 122, Washington, D. C.

241a. National Research Council Food and Nutrition Board 1968 Recommended Dietary Allowances. Seventh revised edition, publication 1694. National Academy of Sciences, Washington, D. C.

242. Botella Llusiá, J., and J. M. Hernández Araña 1942 El problema de la vitamina A en la alimentación de la embarazada. Rev. Clin. Espan. 7: 203.

243. Pilotti, G., and A. Scorta 1965 Ipervitaminosi A gravidica e malformazioni neonatali dell'apparato urinario. Minerva Ginec. 17: 1103.

244. Gal, I., I. M. Sharman, J. Pryse-Davies and T. Moore 1969 Vitamin A as a possible factor in human teratology. Proc. Nutr. Soc. 28: 9A.

245. Della Cella, G. 1967 Vitamine e gravidanza. Acta Vitaminol. (Milano) 21: 179.

246. Cohlan, S. Q. 1954 Congenital anomalies in the rat produced by excessive intake of vitamin A during pregnancy. Pediatrics 13: 556.

247. Drigalski, W. von, and H. Kunz 1939 Über den Vitamin A-Bedarf des Menschen. 2. Schwangere, Stillende und Kranke. Klin. Wochenschr. 18: 1318.

248. Clausen, S. W., and A. B. McCoord 1938 The carotinoids and vitamin A of the blood. J. Pediat. 13: 635.

249. Aykroyd, W. R. 1930 Beriberi and other food-deficiency diseases in Newfoundland and Labrador. J. Hyg. 30: 357.

250. Dixit, D. T. 1966 Night-blindness in third trimester of pregnancy. Indian. J. Med. Res. 54: 791.

251. Edmund, C., and Sv. Clemmesen 1936 On parenteral A vitamin treatment of dysaptatio (nyctalo-hemeralopia) in some pregnant women. Acta Med. Scand. 89: 69.

252. Williams, P. F., B. Hark and F. G. Fralin 1940 Nutrition study in pregnancy. Correlation between dietary survey of vitamin A content and dark adaptation time. Amer. J. Obstet. Gynecol. 40: 1.

253. Hirst, J. C., and R. E. Shoemaker 1940 Vitamin A in pregnancy. 1. Average capacity according to the Feldman adaptometer. Amer. J. Obstet. Gynecol. 40: 12.

254. Hirst, J. C., and R. E. Shoemaker 1941 Vitamin A in pregnancy. II. Comparison of dark adaptation and serum tests. Amer. J. Obstet. Gynec. 42: 404.

255. Lübke, F., and H. Finkbeiner 1958 Beitrag zum Verhalten des Vitamin-A- und β-Carotin-Spiegels in der Gravidität, unter der Geburt und im Wochenbett. Z. Vitaminforsch. 29: 45.

256. Wendt, H. 1936 Ueber den Carotin-Vitamin A Stoffwechsel des menschlichen Fetus, Carotin und Vitamin A Bestimmungen im Schwangerenblut, in Placenten, in Nabelschnurblut und in fetalen Lebern. Klin. Wochenschr. 15: 222. Cited by: Popper, H., and F. Steigmann 1943 The clinical significance of the plasma vitamin A level. J. Amer. Med. Ass. 123: 1108.

257. Abt, A. F., H. C. S. Aron, H. N. Bundesen, M. A. Delaney, C. J. Farmer, R. S. Greenebaum, O. C. Wenger and J. L. White 1942 Studies on plasma vitamin A. Part II. Relationship of the plasma vitamin A to pregnancy and anemia in syphilitic patients. Quart. Bull. Northwestern Medical School, Chicago 16: 245.

258. Bodansky, O., J. M. Lewis and C. C. Lillienfeld 1943 The concentration of vitamin A in the blood plasma during pregnancy. J. Clin. Invest. 22: 643.

259. Byrn, J. N., and N. J. Eastman 1943 Vitamin A levels in maternal and fetal blood plasma. Bull. Johns Hopkins Hospital 73: (No. 2) 132.

260. Cayer, D., V. Crescenzo and S. Cody 1947 Plasma vitamin A levels in pregnancy. Amer. J. Obstet. Gynecol. 54: 259.

261. Pulliam, R. P., W. N. Dannenburg, R. L. Burt and N. H. Leake 1962 Carotene and vitamin A in pregnancy and the early puerperium. Proc. Soc. Exp. Biol. Med. 109: 913.

262. Venkatachalam, P. S., Bhavani Belavady and C. Gopalan 1962 Studies on vitamin A nutritional status of mothers and infants in poor communities of India. J. Pediat. 61: 262.

263. Dawson, E. B., R. R. Clark and W. J. McGanity 1969 Plasma vitamins and trace metal changes during teen-age pregnancy. Amer. J. Obstet. Gynecol. 104: 953.

264. McGanity, W. J., R. O. Cannon, E. B. Bridgforth, M. P. Martin, P. M. Densen, J. A. Newbill, G. S. McClellan, A. Christie, J. C. Peterson and W. J. Darby 1954 The Vanderbilt cooperative study of maternal and infant nutrition. VI. Relationship of obstetric performance to nutrition. Amer. J. Obst. Gynecol. 67: 501.

265. Ozorotsii, F. F. 1965 Zalezhnist' fizychnoho rozvytku novonarodzhenykh vid mistu vitamin A i karotynu v. syvorottsi krovi vahitnykh zhinok u zv'yazkuz profilaktychnoyu vitaminizatsiyeyu. Pediat. Akush. Ginekol. (Ukr) 27: 44. Cited in: Biol. Abstr. 47: (abstr. no. 71145), 1966.

266. Lewis, J. M., O. Bodansky, M. C. C. Lillienfeld and H. Schneider 1947 Supplements of vitamin A and of carotene during pregnancy. Their effect on the levels of vitamin A and carotene in the blood of mother and of newborn infant. Amer. J. Dis. Child. 73: 143.

267. Hoch, H., and J. R. Marrack 1948 The composition of the blood of women during pregnancy and after delivery. J. Obstet. Gynecol. Brit. Emp. 55: 1.

268. Lesher, M., J. K. Brody, H. H. Williams and I. G. Macy 1945 Human milk studies. XXVI. Vitamin A and carotenoid contents of colostrum and mature human milk. Amer. J. Dis. Child. 70: 182.

269. Debré, R., and A. Busson 1934 La vitamine A, son métabolisme, son rôle dans certains états pathologiques chez l'homme. Rev. Fr. Pediat. 10: 413.

270. Moore, T. 1937 XVIII. Vitamin A and carotene. XIII. The vitamin A reserve of the adult human being in health and disease. Biochem. J. 31: 155.

271. Neumann, O. 1950 Ueber das Corpus luteum-Hormon. Wien. Klin. Wochenschr. 62: 909.

272. Morton, R. A. 1960 Summary discussion. Part of symposium on vitamin A and metabolism. In: Vitamins and Hormones, vol. 18, eds., R. S. Harris and D. J. Ingle, Academic Press, New York, p. 543.

273. Hays, R. L., and K. A. Kendall 1956 The beneficial effect of progesterone on preg-

nancy in the vitamin A-deficient rabbit. J. Nutr. 59: 337.

274. Grangaud, R., M. Nicol and D. Desplanques 1969 Effect of vitamin A on enzymic conversion of the Δ^5-3-β-hydroxy- into Δ^4-3-oxosteroids by adrenals of the rat. Amer. J. Clin. Nutr. 22: 991.

275. Indian Council of Medical Research 1961 Annual Report of 1st July, 1960 to 30th Sept., 1961. The Nutrition Research Laboratories, Hyderabad. Cited by: Dixit, D. T. 1966 Night-blindness in third trimester of pregnancy. Indian J. Med. Res. 54: 791.

276. Lund, C. J., and M. S. Kimble 1943 Plasma vitamin A and carotene of the newborn infant. Amer. J. Obstet. Gynecol. 46: 207.

277. McLaren, D. S., and P. G. Ward 1962 Malarial infection of the placenta and foetal nutrition. E. Afr. Med. J. 39: 182.

278. Thomson, D. L., E. Ruiz and M. Bakar 1964 Vitamin A and protein deficiency in Malayan children. Trans. Roy. Soc. Trop. Med. Hyg. 58: 425.

279. Neuweiler, W. 1943 Karotin- und Vitamin A-Resorption aus der Plazenta. Z. Vitaminforsch. 13: 275.

280. Gaehtgens, G. 1937 Der Gehalt der Placenta an Carotin und Vitamin A. Arch. Gynäkol. 164: 588.

281. Barnes, A. C. 1951 The placental metabolism of vitamin A. Amer. J. Obstet. Gynecol. 61: 368.

282. Kennedy, C., L. S. Palmer and F. W. Schultz 1923 The vitamin content of breast milk. milk. Trans. Amer. Pediat. Soc. 35: 26.

283. Macy, I. G., J. Outhouse, A. Graham and M. L. Long 1927 Human milk studies. II. The quantitative estimation of vitamin A. J. Biol. Chem. 73: 175.

284. Outhouse, J., I. G. Macy, V. Brekke and A. Graham 1927 Human milk studies. IV. A note on the vitamin A and B content of cow's milk. J. Biol. Chem. 73: 203.

285. Macy, I. G., J. Outhouse and H. Hunscher 1928 The variability in vitamin content of human milks. J. Home Econ. 20: 897.

286. Dann, W. J. 1936 The transmission of vitamin A from parents to young in mammals. V. The vitamin A and carotenoid contents of human colostrum and milk. Biochem. J. 30: 1644.

287. Willstaedt, H., and T. K. With 1938 Über die chromatographische Adsorptionsanalyse kleiner Carotinoidmengen (Mikrochromatographie) mit besonderer Berücksichtigung der Carotinoide der Milch und des Serums. Z. Physiol. Chem. 253: 40.

288. Truka-Tuzson, J. 1939 Über das Lipochrom des menschlichen Kolostrum, mit besonderer Berücksichtigung des Karotins. Z. Geburtsh. Gynäkol. 120: 86. Cited by: Lesher, M., J. K. Brody, H. A. Williams and I. G. Macy 1945 Human milk studies. XXVI. Vitamin A and carotenoid contents of colostrum and mature human milk. Amer. J. Dis. Child. 70: 182.

289. Truka-Tuzson, J. 1940 As Emberi Colostrum Lipochromjáröl Különös Tekintettel A Carotinra. Magyar. Orvosi. Arch. 41: 145. Cited by: Lesher, M., J. K. Brody, H. A. Williams and I. G. Macy 1945 Human milk studies. XXVI. Vitamin A and carotenoid contents of colostrum and mature human milk. Amer. J. Dis. Child. 70: 182.

290. Thompson, S. Y., S. K. Kon and E. H. Mawson 1942 The application of chromatography to the study of the carotenoids of human and cow's milk. Biochem. J. 36: xvii.

291. Menken, J. G. 1934 Over het gehalte aan vitamine-A en carotenoïden in het bloedserum van den mensch en in moedermelk. Maandschr. Kindergeneesk. 4: 22.

292. Van Eekelen, M., and J. H. de Haas 1934 Over carotine en vitamine A in moedermelk in het bijzonder in colostrum. Geneesk. Tijdschr. Nederland-Indië 74: 1201.

293. Waltner, K. 1934 Ueber den A-Vitamingehalt einiger Nahrungsstoffe. Z. Vitaminforsch. 3: 245.

294. Neuweiler, W. 1935 Der Vitamin A- und Carotingehalt der Frauenmilch. Z. Vitaminforsch. 4: 259.

295. Meulemans, O., and J. H. de Haas 1936 The carotene and vitamin A contents of mother's milk at Batavia. Indian J. Pediat. 3: 57.

296. Meulemans, O., and J. H. de Haas 1936 The carotene and vitamin A contents of mother's milk at Batavia. Indian J. Pediat. 3: 133.

297. Svensson, E. 1936 Biologische Bestimmungen des Gehaltes an A-Vitamin plus seinem Provitamin in Milch von Frauen nordischen Rasse, samt in Hagebutten und schwarzen Johannisbeeren. Skand. Arch. Physiol. 73: 237.

298. Nylund, C. E. 1937 Vitamin-A och karotin i modersmjölken. Finska Läk.-Sällsk. Handl. 80: 733.

299. Chevallier, A., P. Giraud and C. Dinard 1939 Sur les teneurs comparées du sang et du lait en vitamin A. C. R. Soc. Biol. 131: 396.

300. Portes, L., and J. Varangot 1942 Sur la richesse actuelle du lait de femme en caroténoïdes en vitamine A au début de la lactation. C. R. Soc. Biol. 136: 168.

301. Escudero, P. 1943 La función biológica del calostro en la alimentación del recién nacido. Resenha Clin. Cient. 12: 409.

302. Skurnik, L., and M. Stenberg 1937 Untersuchungen über den Vitamin A- und Karotingehalt der Milch und des Blutes. Skand. Arch. Physiol. 77: 77.

303. Chevallier, A., P. Giraud, and C. Dinard 1939 Sur la teneur du lait de femme en vitamine A. C. R. Soc. Biol. 131: 373.

304. Hrubetz, M. C., H. J. Deuel, Jr. and B. J. Hanley 1945 Studies on carotenoid metabolism. V. The effect of a high vitamin A intake on the composition of human milk. J. Nutr. 29: 245.

305. Kaucher, M., E. Z. Moyer, A. J. Richards, H. H. Williams, A. L. Wertz and I. G. Macy 1945 Human milk studies. XX. The diet of

lactating women and the collection and preparation of food and human milk for analysis. Amer. J. Dis. Child. 70: 142.

306. Macy, I. G., H. H. Williams, J. P. Pratt and B. M. Hamil 1945 Human milk studies. XIX. Implications of breast feeding and their investigation. Amer. J. Dis. Child. 70: 135.

307. Gunther, M., and J. E. Stanier 1951 The volume and composition of human milk. In: Medical Research Council Special Report Series no. 275, H. M. Stationery Office, London, p. 379.

308. De Haas, J. H., and O. Meulemans 1938 Vitamin A and carotinoids in blood: Deficiencies in children suffering from xerophthalmia. Lancet 1: 1110.

309. Gopalan, C., P. S. Venkatachalam and Belavady Bhavani 1960 Studies of vitamin A deficiency in children. Amer. J. Clin. Nutr. 8: 833.

310. Dann, W. J. 1932 CXXV. The transmission of vitamin A from parents to young in mammals. Biochem. J. 26: 1072.

311. Dann, W. J. 1934 The transmission of vitamin A from parents to young in mammals. IV. Effect of the liver reserves of the mother on the transmission of vitamin A to the foetal and suckling rat. Biochem. J. 28: 2141.

312. McCosh, S. S., I. G. Macy, H. A. Hunscher, B. N. Erickson and E. Donelson 1934 Human milk studies. XIII. Vitamin potency as influenced by supplementing the maternal diet with vitamin A. J. Nutr. 7: 331.

313. Ajans, Z. A., A. Sarrif and M. Husbands 1965 Influence of vitamin A on human colostrum and early milk. Amer. J. Clin. Nutr. 17: 139.

314. Friderichsen, C., and T. K. With 1939 Ueber den Gehalt der Frauenmilch an Karotinoiden und A-Vitamin, besonders in Bezug auf seine Abhängigkeit von der Kost. Ann. Paediat. 153: 113.

315. Sobel, A. E., A. Rosenberg and B. Kramer 1950 Enrichment of milk vitamin A in normal lactating women. A comparison following administration of vitamin A in aqueous and oily mediums. Amer. J. Dis. Child. 80: 932.

316. Vogt, E. 1932 Ueber die Vitaminbestände des weiblichen Organismus. Münch. Med. Wochenschr. 79: 1570. Cited in: Chem. Abstr. 27: (abstr. no. 1383), 1933.

317. Expert Committee on Pregnancy and Lactation 1965 Nutrition in Pregnancy and Lactation. World Health Organization Tech. Report Series no. 302, Geneva, 54 pp.

318. Gopalan, C., and Bhavani Belavady 1961 Nutrition and lactation. Federation Proc. 20: (suppl. 7) 177.

319. Oomen, H. A. P. C. 1958 In: Hypovitaminosis A. Federation Proc. 17: (suppl. 2) 103. Proceedings of a conference on beriberi, endemic goiter and hypovitaminosis A, eds., T. D. Kinney and R. H. Follis, Jr.

320. Gillum, H. L., A. F. Morgan and F. Sailer 1955 Nutritional status of the aging. V. Vitamin A and carotene. J. Nutr. 55: 655.

321. Dibble, M. V., M. Brin, V. F. Thiele, A. Peel, N. Chen and E. McMullen 1967 Evaluation of the nutritional status of elderly subjects, with a comparison between fall and spring. J. Amer. Geriat. Soc. 15: 1031.

322. Simić, B. S., S. Šibalić, M. Naumović, A. Simić, R. Marković, V. Raković 1963 Relation between vitamin A, tocopherol and cholesterol serum levels in the elderly. Int. J. Vitamin Res. 33: 48.

323. Rafsky, H. A., B. Newman and N. Jolliffe 1947 A study of the carotene and vitamin A levels in the aged. Gastroenterology 8: 612.

324. Kahan, J. 1969 The vitamin A absorption test. Studies on children and adults without disorders in the alimentary tract. Scand. J. Gastroenterol. 4: 313.

325. Yiengst, M. J., and N. W. Shock 1949 Effect of oral administration of vitamin A on plasma levels of vitamin A and carotene in aged males. J. Gerontol. 4: 205.

326. Pelz, K. S., S. P. Gottfried and E. Soos 1968 Intestinal absorption studies in the aged. Geriatrics 23: 149.

327. Kalbe, I., and I. Lübeck 1966 Vitamin-A- und E-Untersuchungen bei peripheren Durchblutungsstörungen. Deut. Gesundheitsw. 21: 1654.

328. Rafsky, H. A., and B. Newman 1948 A study of the vitamin A and carotene tolerance tests in the aged. Gastroenterology 10: 1001.

329. Kirk, J. E., and M. Chieffi 1952 Hypovitaminemia A. Effect of vitamin A administration on plasma vitamin A concentration, conjunctival changes, dark adaptation and toad skin. Amer. J. Clin. Nutr. 1: 37.

330. Efremow, V. V., E. M. Maslenikowa, E. A. Krajko, L. G. Gwozdowa, B. K. Skirko, J. M. Nemenowa, L. J. Solowjewa, A. N. Smirnowa and A. Sch. Wainerman 1967 Vitamine und Alternsprozess. Z. Alternsforsch. 20: 213. Cited in: Nutr. Abstr. Rev. 8: (abstr. no. 7686), 1968.

331. Bolgert, M., J. P. Noble, J. P. Lichtenberg and A. M. Gehanno 1968 Epithéliomatose multiple. Lésions kératosiques et pigmentées diffuses des avant-bras avec hypervitaminémie. A. Bull. Soc. Franc. Dermatol.. Syphiligr. 75: 285.

332. Deuel, H. J., Jr. 1955 The Lipids, vol. 2: Biochemistry. Interscience Publishers, New York and London, 919 pp.

333. Goodwin, T. W. 1952 The Comparative Biochemistry of the Carotenoids. Chapman and Hall, Ltd., London, 356 pp. Goodwin, T. W. 1954 Carotenoids: Their Comparative Biochemistry (1st Amer. ed.), New York Chemical Publishing Company, New York, 356 pp.

334. Thompson, S. Y. 1964 Factors affecting the absorption of carotene and its conversion into vitamin A. Exp. Eye Res. 3: 392.

335. Thompson, S. Y. 1965 Occurrence, distribution and absorption of provitamins A. Proc. Nutr. Soc. 24: 136.

336. Clifford, S. H. 1946 Vitamin A absorption in premature infants. Pediat. Res. Soc., Skytop, Pa. Cited by: Lewis, J. M., O. Bodansky, J. Birmingham and S. Q. Cohlan 1947 Comparative absorption, excretion, and storage of oily and aqueous preparations of vitamin A. J. Pediat. 31: 496.

337. Lewis, J. M., O. Bodansky, J. Birmingham and S. Q. Cohlan 1947 Comparative absorption, excretion, and storage of oily and aqueous preparations of vitamin A. J. Pediat. 31: 496.

338. Sobel, A. E., L. Besman and B. Kramer 1949 Vitamin A absorption in the newborn. Amer. J. Dis. Child. 77: 576.

339. Sobel, A. E., M. Sherman, J. Lichtblau, S. Snow and B. Kramer 1948 Comparison of vitamin A liver storage following administration of vitamin A in oily and aqueous media. J. Nutr. 35: 225.

340. Sobel, A. E. 1952 The problem of the absorption and transportation of fat-soluble vitamins. Vitamins Hormones 10: 47.

341. Adlersberg, D., and H. Sobotka 1943 Influence of lecithin feeding on fat and vitamin A absorption in man. J. Nutr. 25: 255.

342. Kern, C. J., T. Anthoshkiw and M. R. Maiese 1949 Vitamin A alcohol stability and absorption. Influence of antioxidants. Ind. Eng. Chem. 41: 2849.

343. Ames, S. R. 1969 Factors affecting absorption, transport, and storage of vitamin A. Amer. J. Clin. Nutr. 22: 934.

344. Olson, J. A. 1964 The effect of bile and bile salts on the uptake and cleavage of β-carotene into retinol ester (vitamin A ester) by intestinal slices. J. Lipid Res. 5: 402.

345. Kon, S. K., W. A. McGillivray and S. Y. Thompson 1955 Metabolism of carotene and vitamin A given by mouth or vein in oily solution or aqueous dispersion to calves, rabbits and rats. Brit. J. Nutr. 9: 244.

346. Kagan, B. M., D. A. Jordan and P. S. Gerald 1950 Absorption of aqueous dispersions of vitamin A alcohol and vitamin A ester in normal children. J. Nutr. 40: 275.

347. Week, E. F., and F. J. Sevigne 1950 Vitamin A utilization studies. III. The utilization of vitamin A alcohol, vitamin A acetate and vitamin A natural esters by humans. J. Nutr. 40: 563.

348. Popper, H., F. Steigmann and H. A. Dyniewicz 1950 Difference in intestinal absorption between vitamin A alcohol and ester. Proc. Soc. Exp. Biol. Med. 73: 188.

349. Ascarelli, I. 1969 Absorption and transport of vitamin A in chicks. Amer. J. Clin. Nutr. 22: 913.

350. Wilson, H. E. C., S. M. Das Gupta and B. Ahmad 1937 Studies on the absorption of carotene and vitamin A in the human subject. Indian J. Med. Res. 24: 807.

351. Van Eekelen, M., and W. Pannevis 1938 Absorption of carotinoids from the human intestine. Nature 141: 203.

352. Kreula, M., and A. I. Virtanen 1939 Absorption of carotene from carrots in humans. Upsala Läkarefören. Förh. 45: 357.

353. Eriksen, B., and A. Höygaard 1941 The absorption of carotene in man. Klin. Wochenschr. 20: 200. Cited in: Chem. Abstr. 36: (abstr. no. 7075), 1942.

354. Van Zeben, W. 1946 The absorption of carotene by man. Z. Vitaminforsch. 17: 74.

355. Van Zeben, W., and T. F. Hendriks 1948 The absorption of carotene from cooked carrots. Int. Z. Vitaminforsch. 19: 265.

356. Kreula, M. S. 1947 Absorption of carotene from carrots in man and the use of the quantitative chromic oxide indicator method in the absorption experiments. Biochem. J. 41: 269.

357. Leonhardi, G. 1947 Über die Resorption von Karotin aus Gemüsen beim Menschen. 1. Mitteilung. Z. Gesamte Inn. Med. 2: 376. Cited in: Chem. Abstr. 42: (abstr. no. 3473ᶠ), 1948.

358. Wilbrand, U. 1950 Untersuchungen über die Karotinresorption unter besonderer Berücksichtigung der Resorption bei Unterernährten. Med. Monatsschr. 4: 923.

359. James, W. H., and M. E. Hollinger 1954 The utilization of carotene. II. From sweet potatoes by young human adults. J. Nutr. 54: 65.

360. Moschette, D. S. 1955 Metabolic studies with pre-adolescent girls. I. Utilization of carotene. J. Amer. Diet. Ass. 31: 37.

361. Roels, O. A., M. Trout and R. Dujacquier 1958 Carotene balances on boys in Ruanda where vitamin A deficiency is prevalent. J. Nutr. 65: 115.

362. Kübler, W. 1958–1959 Studien am Säugling zur Resorption von Carotin aus Möhren. Int. Z. Vitaminforsch. 29: 339.

363. Almendinger, R., and F. C. Hinds 1969 Apparent carotenoid increases in the digestive tract of beef cattle. J. Nutr. 97: 13.

364. McLaren, D. S. 1966 Present knowledge of the role of vitamin A in health and disease. Trans. Roy. Soc. Trop. Med. Hyg. 60: 436.

365. Nageswara Rao, C., and B. S. Narasinga Rao 1970 Absorption of dietary carotenes in human subjects. Amer. J. Clin. Nutr. 23: 105.

366. Weckel, K. G., B. Santos, E. Hernan, L. Laferriere and W. H. Gabelman 1962 Carotene components of frozen and processed carrots. Food Technol. 16: 91.

367. Heymann, W. 1936 Absorption of carotene. Amer. J. Dis. Child. 51: 273.

368. Wald, G., W. R. Carroll and D. Sciarra 1941 The human excretion of carotenoids and vitamin A. Science 94: 95.

369. Sinios, A. 1949 Vitamin A und β-Carotin beim gesunden Säugling. Ein Beitrag zur Frage der Bilanz. Int. Z. Vitaminforsch. 21: 151.

370. Goodman, D. S., R. Blomstrand, B. Werner, H. S. Huang and T. Shiratori 1966 The intestinal absorption and metabolism of vitamin A and β-carotene in man. J. Clin. Invest. 45: 1615.

371. Blomstrand, R., and B. Werner 1967 Studies on the intestinal absorption of radioactive β-carotene and vitamin A in man.

Conversion of β-carotene into vitamin A. Scand. J. Clin. Lab. Invest. 19: 339.

372. Figueira, F., S. Mendonça, J. Rocha, M. Azevedo, G. E. Bunce and J. W. Reynolds 1969 Absorption of vitamin A by infants receiving fat-free or fat-containing dried skim milk formulas. Amer. J. Clin. Nutr. 22: 588.

373. Daniels, A. L. 1925–1926 Vitamin A content of fecal excretion of a breast fed and artificially fed infant. Preliminary report. Proc. Soc. Exp. Biol. Med. 23: 824.

374. Rowntree, J. I. 1930 A study of the absorption and retention of vitamin A in young children. J. Nutr. 3: 265.

375. Iwanowska, J., and K. Paczek 1967 Wpływ podstawowych nienasyconych kwasow tłuszczowych na witamine. A. Acta Physiol. Pol. 18: 963.

376. Berger, S., M. Korycka, M. Miler, T. Białek and K. Chabrowski 1969 Studies on availability and mechanism of carotene and vitamin A utilization from different dietary sources and under different experimental conditions. Final Report from Warsaw Agricultural University (July 1964–June 1969), Warsaw, Poland.

377. Green, J., and J. Bunyan 1969 Vitamin E and the biological antioxidant theory. Nutr. Abstr. Rev. 39: 321.

378. Hanna, M. B. 1965 Management of nightblindness with vitamins A and E. Bull. Ophthal. Soc. Egypt 58: 219.

379. Kasper, H., and B. Ernst 1969 Der Einfluss des Nahrungsfettes auf die Vitamin-A-und Carotinresorption. Int. Z. Vitaminforsch. 39: 23. Cited in: Nutr. Abstr. Rev. 39: (abstr. no 6761), 1969.

380. Sherman, W. C. 1941 Activity of alpha tocopherol in preventing antagonism between linoleic and linolenic esters and carotene. Proc. Soc. Exp. Biol. Med. 47: 199.

381. Guggenheim, K. 1944 The biological value of carotene from various sources and the effect of vitamin E on the utilization of carotene and of vitamin A. Biochem. J. 38: 260.

382. Koehn, C. J. 1948 Relative biological activity of beta-carotene and vitamin A. Arch. Biochem. 17: 337.

383. Burns, M. J., S. M. Hauge and F. W. Quackenbush 1951 Utilization of vitamin A and carotene by the rat. I. Effects of tocopherol, Tween, and dietary fat. Arch. Biochem. 30: 341.

384. Moore, T. 1960 Vitamin A and proteins. Vitamins Hormones 18: 431.

385. Gershoff, S. N. 1964 Effects of dietary levels of macronutrients on vitamin requirements. Federation Proc. 23: 1077.

386. Mahadevan, S., P. Malathi and J. Ganguly 1965 Influence of proteins on absorption and metabolism of vitamin A. World Rev. Nutr. Dietet. 5: 209.

387. Arroyave, G. 1969 Interrelations between protein and vitamin A and metabolism. Amer. J. Clin. Nutr. 22: 1119.

388. Kuming, B. S. 1967 The evolution of keratomalacia. Trans. Ophthal. Soc. UK. 87: 305.

389. Arroyave, G., F. Viteri, M. Béhar and N. S. Scrimshaw 1959 Impairment of intestinal absorption of vitamin A palmitate in severe protein malnutrition (kwashiorkor). Amer. J. Clin. Nutr. 7: 185.

390. Arroyave, G., D. Wilson, J. Méndez, M. Béhar and N. S. Scrimshaw 1961 Serum and liver vitamin A and lipids in children with severe protein malnutrition. Amer. J. Clin. Nutr. 9: 180.

391. Konno, T., J. D. L. Hansen, A. S. Truswell, R. Woodd-Walker and D. Becker 1968 Vitamin-A deficiency and protein–calorie malnutrition in Cape Town. S. Afr. Med. J. 42: 950.

392. Arroyave, G., D. Wilson, C. Contreras and and M. Béhar 1963 Alterations in serum concentration of vitamin A associated with hypoproteinemia of severe protein malnutrition. J. Pediat. 62: 920.

393. Woodruff, A. W., and R. J. C. Stewart 1962 Correlation of albumin and vitamin A in human serum. Proc. Nutr. Soc. 21: iv.

394. Bagchi, K., K. Halder and S. R. Chowdhury 1959 Study of Bitôt's spot with special reference to protein malnutrition. J. Indian Med. Ass. 33: 401.

395. Leonard, P. J. 1964 Serum and liver levels of vitamin A in Ugandans. E. Afr. Med. J. 41: 133.

396. El-Din, M. K. B., and S. Hammad 1966 Serum vitamin A in infancy and childhood. II. In the malnourished. J. Trop. Pediat. 12: 63.

397. Garciá, H., M. A. Tangle, D. Ballesier and G. Donoso 1963 Caracteristicas del sindrome pluricarencial infantil. IV. Vitamina A y caroteno en suero. Nutr. Bromat. Toxicol. 2: 40.

398. Kothari, L. K., K. B. Lal, D. K. Srivastava and Rameshwar Sharma 1971 Correlation between plasma levels of vitamin A and proteins in children. Amer. J. Clin. Nutr. 24: 510.

399. Kanai, M., A. Raz and DeW. S. Goodman 1968 Retinol-binding protein: the transport protein for vitamin A in human plasma. J. Clin. Invest. 47: 2025.

400. Deshmukh, D. S., P. Malathi and J. Ganguly 1964 Studies on metabolism of vitamin A. 5. Dietary protein content and metabolism of vitamin A. Biochem. J. 90: 98.

401. Gronowska-Senger, A., and G. Wolf 1970 Effect of dietary protein on the enzyme from rat and human intestine which converts β-carotene to retinal. J. Nutr. 100: 300.

402. Ehrlich, S. T., B. R. Farthing and D. S. Moschette 1964 Metabolic patterns in preadolescent children. 11. Response of vitamin A and carotene serum levels to dietary protein and vitamin A. J. Nutr. 84: 389.

403. Oomen, H. A. P. C. 1954 Xerophthalmia in the presence of kwashiorkor. Brit. J. Nutr. 8: 307.

404. Jagannathan, S. N., and V. N. Patwardhan 1960 Dietary protein in vitamin A metabolism. Part 1. Influence of level of dietary protein on the utilization of orally fed pre-

formed vitamin A and β-carotene in the rat. Indian J. Med. Res. 48: 775.

405. Deshmukh, D. S., and J. Ganguly 1964 Effect of dietary protein contents on the intestinal conversion of β-carotene to vitamin A in rats. Indian J. Biochem. 1: 204.

406. Mayfield, H. L., and R. R. Roehm 1956 The influence of ascorbic acid and the source of the B vitamins on the utilization of carotene. J. Nutr. 58: 203.

407. High, E. G., and S. S. Wilson 1953 Effects of vitamin B₁₂ on the utilization of carotene and vitamin A by the rat. J. Nutr. 50: 203.

408. Leitner, Z. A., T. Moore and I. M. Sharman 1952 Vitamin A, carotenoids and tocopherol levels in the blood of two different classes of patient. Brit. J. Nutr. 6: x.

409. Gravesen, K. J. 1967 Vitamin A and carotene in serum from healthy Danish subjects. Scand. J. Clin. Lab. Invest. 20: 57.

410. Campbell, D. A., and E. L. Tonks 1949 Vitamin A, total carotenoids, and thymol turbity levels in plasma. Test in normal subjects residing in the Midlands during 1947. Brit. Med. J. 2: 1499.

411. Železovskaja, I. B. 1969 Koncentracija vitamina A v krovi i svjaz' ce s soderžaniem belkov, holesterina i β-lipoproteidov v krovi bol'nyh aterosklerozom. Vop. Med. Him. 15: 506. Cited in: Nutr. Abstr. Rev. 40: (abstr. no. 8215), 1970.

412. Kirk, E., and M. Chieffi 1948 Vitamin studies in middle-aged and old individuals. 1. The vitamin A, total carotene and α + β carotene concentrations in plasma. J. Nutr. 36: 315.

413. Morse, E. H., S. B. Merrow and R. F. Clarke 1965 Some biochemical findings in Burlington (Vt.) junior high school children. Amer. J. Clin. Nutr. 17: 211.

414. Kahan, J. 1970 The vitamin A absorption test. II. Studies on children and adults with disorders in the alimentary tract. Scand. J. Gastroenterol. 5: 5.

415. Gal, I., C. Parkinson and I. Craft 1971 Effects of oral contraceptives on human vitamin-A levels. Brit. Med. J. 2: 436.

416. Eppright, E. S., C. Roderuck, V. D. Sidwell and P. P. Swanson 1954 Relationship of estimated nutrient intakes of Iowa school children to physical and biochemical measurements. J. Nutr. 54: 557.

417. Abels, J. C., A. T. Gorham, G. T. Pack and C. P. Rhoads 1941 Metabolic studies in patients with gastrointestinal cancer. III. The hepatic concentrations of vitamin A. Proc. Soc. Exp. Biol. Med. 48: 488.

418. Oomen, H. A. P. C. 1958 The incidence of xerophthalmia in relation to age and sex in Java. Proc. Nutr. Soc. 17: viii.

419. Birnbacher, T. 1928 Zur Physiologie des Fettlöslichen Vitamins A. Münch. Med. Wochenschr. 75: 1114.

420. McLaren, D. S. 1959 Influence of protein deficiency and sex on the development of ocular lesions and survival time of the vitamin A-deficient rat. Brit. J. Ophthalmol. 43: 234.

421. Clausen, S. W. 1933 Limits of the anti-infective value of provitamin A (carotene). J. Amer. Med. Ass. 101: 1384.

422. Kübler, W. 1963 Carotin als Provitamin A beim Menschen. Deut. Med. Wochenschr. 88: 1319.

423. Friderichsen, C., and C. Edmund 1937 Studies of hypovitaminosis A. 3. Clinical experiments in the vitamin A balance in children after various diets. Amer. J. Dis. Child. 53: 1179.

424. Nicholls, L., and A. Nimalasuria 1941 Carotene preparations as substitutes for vitamin A preparations. Brit. Med. J. 2: 406.

425. Murray, T. K., and P. Erdody 1971 The utilization of vitamin A and of β-carotene by rats of increasing age. Nutr. Rept. Int. 3: (2) 129.

426. Booth, V. H. 1952 Liver storage of vitamin A by male and female rats. J. Nutr. 48: 13.

427. Gaehtgens, G. 1937 Bestimmungen von Carotin und Vitamin A im Schwangerenblut. Klin. Wochenschr. 16: 893. Cited in: Nutr. Abstr. Rev. 7: (abstr. no. 2413), 1937–1938.

428. Gaehtgens, G. 1937 Bestimmungen von Carotin und Vitamin A im Nabelschnurblut. Klin. Wochenschr. 16: 894. Cited in: Nutr. Abstr. Rev. 7: (abstr. no. 2413), 1937–1938.

429. Hoch, H. 1944 Chromatographic investigation of the β-carotene content of serum of the newborn infant. Biochem. J. 38: 304.

430. Lindqvist, T. 1938 Studien über das Vitamin A beim Menschen. Acta Med. Scand. Suppl. no. 97, Appelberg Boktryckeriaktiebolag, Uppsala, 314 pp. Cited by: Leitner, Z. A. 1951 The clinical significance of vitamin-A deficiency. Brit. Med. J. 1: 1110.

431. Josephs, H. W. 1943 Studies on vitamin A. Vitamin A and total lipid of the serum in pneumonia. Amer. J. Dis. Child. 65: 712.

432. Thiele, W., and I. Scherff 1939 Der Serum-Vitamin A-Spiegel im Fieber. Klin. Wochenschr. 18: 1275.

433. May, C. D., K. D. Blackfan, J. F. McCreary and F. H. Allen 1940 Clinical studies of vitamin A in infants and in children. Amer. J. Dis. Child. 59: 1167.

434. Popper, H., and F. Steigmann 1943 The clinical significance of the plasma vitamin A level. J. Amer. Med. Ass. 123: 1108.

435. Panchenko, V. I. 1968 Pro vmist vitamin A karotynu v syvorottsi krovi u ditei rann'oho viku pry pnevmoniyi. (Ukr). Pediat. Akush. Ginekol. Issue no. 3, p. 13. Cited in: Biol. Abstr. 50: (abstr. no. 46680), 1969.

436. Gracheva, A. G. 1969 Vitamin A and carotene level in the blood of children in pneumonia. Pediatriia 48: 9.

437. Kimble, M. S., O. A. Germek and E. L. Sevringhaus 1946 Vitamin A and carotene metabolism in the diabetic as reflected by blood levels. Amer. J. Med. Sci. 212: 574.

438. Breese, B. B., Jr., E. Watkins and A. B. McCoord 1942 The absorption of vitamin A in tuberculosis. J. Amer. Med. Ass. 119: 3.

439. Smurova, T. F., and D. I. Prokop'ev 1969 Soderžanie vitamina A i karotina v krovi bol'nyh tuberkulezom legkih i saharnym diabetom. Probl. Tuberkul. 47: 50. Cited in: Nutr. Abstr. Rev. 40: (abstr. no. 7970), 1970.

440. Ignatova, A. V., and D. I. Prokop'ev 1966 Vitamin A i karotin u bol'nykh tuberkulezom legkikh s pobochnymi Yavleniy ami pri antibakterialnoi terapii. Probl. Tuberkul. 44: 36. Cited in: Biol. Abstr. 48: (abstr. no. 122280), 1967.

441. Ralli, E. P., A. C. Pariente, H. Brandaleone and S. Davidson 1936 Effect of carotene and vitamin A on patients with diabetes mellitus. III. The effect of the daily administration of carotene on the blood carotene of normal and diabetic individuals. J. Amer. Med. Ass. 106: 1975.

442. Brazer, J. G., and A. C. Curtis 1940 Vitamin A deficiency in diabetes mellitus. Arch. Intern. Med. 65: 90.

443. Cadman, E. F. B. 1954 The interrelationships of the thyroid hormone and carotene and vitamin A. M. D. thesis, University of Liverpool. Cited by: Cohen, H. 1958 Observations on carotenemia. Ann. Intern. Med. 48: 219.

444. Wang, P., H. L. Glass, L. Goldenberg, G. Stearns, H. G. Kelly and R. L. Jackson 1954 Serum vitamin A and carotene levels in children with rheumatic fever. Amer. J. Dis. Child. 87: 659.

445. Wendt, H. 1935 Ueber Veränderungen im Karotin-Vitamin-A-Haushalt beim Myxödem und bei Kretins. München. Med. Wochenschr. 82: 1679. Cited in: Chem. Abstr. 30: (abstr. no. 3470), 1936.

446. Walton, K. W., D. A. Campbell and E. L. Tonks 1965 The significance of alterations in serum lipids in thyroid dysfunction. I. The relation between serum lipoproteins, carotenoids and vitamin A in hypothyroidism and thyrotoxicosis. Clin. Sci. 29: 199.

447. del Pozo, E. 1968 Hypothyreose, Hypovitaminose A, und Hyperkeratosis cutis (Vilanova-Canadell-Syndrom). Endokrinologie 53: 249. Cited in: Biol. Abstr. 51: (abstr. no. 19270), 1970.

448. Wendt, H. 1935 Beiträge zur Kenntnis des Carotin und Vitamin A Stoffwechsels. Klin. Wochenschr. 14: 9.

449. Thiele, W., and I. Scherff 1939 Über die pathogenetische und diagnostiche Bedeutung des Carotin- und Vitamin A-Spiegels im Serum. Klin. Wochenschr. 18: 1208. Cited by: Popper, H., and F. Steigmann 1943 The clinical significance of the plasma vitamin A level. J. Amer. Med. Ass. 123: 1108.

450. Josephs, H. W. 1952 The carotenemia of hypothyroidism. J. Pediat. 41: 784.

451. May, C. D., and J. F. McCreary 1941 The absorption of vitamin A in celiac disease. Interpretation of the vitamin A absorption test. J. Pediat. 18: 200.

452. Breese, B. B., Jr., and A. B. McCoord 1939 Vitamin A absorption in celiac disease. J. Pediat. 15: 183.

453. Ralli, E. P., E. Papper, K. Paley and E. Bauman 1941 Vitamin A and carotene content of human liver in normal and in diseased subjects: An analysis of one hundred and sixteen human livers. Arch. Intern. Med. 68: 102.

454. Popper, H. 1941 Histologic distribution of vitamin A in human organs under normal and under pathologic conditions. Arch. Pathol. 31: 766.

455. Haig, C., and A. J. Patek, Jr. 1942 Vitamin A deficiency in Laennec's cirrhosis. The relative significance of the plasma vitamin A and carotenoid levels and the dark adaptation time. J. Clin. Invest. 21: 309.

456. Rechcigl, M., Jr., S. Berger, J. K. Loosli and H. H. Williams 1959 Effect of protein-free diet on the vitamin A storage in the rat liver. Nature 183: 1597.

457. Esh, G. C., S. Bhattacharya and J. M. Som 1960 Studies on the utilization of vitamin A. Part IV: Influence of the level of protein on the storage and utilization of vitamin A. Ann. Biochem. Exp. Med. 20: 15.

458. Stoewsand, G. S., and M. L. Scott 1964 Effect of stress from high protein diets on vitamin A metabolism in chicks. J. Nutr. 82: 188.

459. Prokop, L. 1961 Vitamine and Sportleistung. Med. Ernährung 2: 174; 199. Cited in: Nutr. Abstr. Rev. 33: (abstr. no. 1064), 1963.

460. Efremov, V. V. 1958 Gipovitaminozy i perspektivy bor'by s nimi v SSSR. (Hypovitaminosis. Aspects of their control in the USSR). Vop. Pitan. 17: (no. 6) 21. Cited by: Mašek, J. 1962 Recommended nutrient allowances. World Rev. Nutr. Diet. 3: 167.

461. Cluver, E. H. 1964 Sun-trauma prevention. S. Afr. Med. J. 38: 801.

462. Cluver, E. H., and W. M. Politzer 1965 Sunburn and vitamin A deficiency. S. Afr. J. Sci. 61: 306.

463. Cluver, E. H., and W. M. Politzer 1965 The pathology of sun trauma. S. Afr. Med. J. 39: 1051.

464. Politzer, W. M., and E. H. Cluver 1967 Serum vitamin-A concentration in healthy white and Bantu adults living under normal conditions on the Witwatersrand. S. Afr. Med. J. 41: 1012.

465. Findlay, G. H., and L. W. Van Der Merwe 1965 Epidermal vitamin A and sunburn in man. Brit. J. Dermatol. 77: 622.

466. Anderson, F. E. 1969 Studies in the relationship between serum vitamin A and sun exposure. Aust. J. Dermatol. 10: 26.

467. Anderson, F. E. 1968 "Sylvasun" and sunburn protection. Med. J. Aust. 1: 802.

468. Keener, H. A., S. I. Bechdel, N. B. Guerrant and W. T. S. Thorp 1942 Carotene in calf nutrition. J. Dairy Sci. 25: 571.

469. Ershoff, B. H. 1950 Effect of prolonged exposure to cold on the vitamin A require-

ment of the rat. Proc. Soc. Exp. Biol. Med. 74: 586.

470. Ershoff, B. H. 1952 Effects of vitamin A malnutriture on resistance to stress. Proc. Soc. Exp. Biol. Med. 79: 580.

471. Porter, E., and E. J. Masoro 1961 Effect of cold acclimation on vitamin A metabolism. Proc. Soc. Exp. Biol. Med. 108: 609.

472. Phillips, W. E. J. 1962 Low-temperature environmental stress and the metabolism of vitamin A in the rat. Can. J. Biochem. Physiol. 40: 491.

473. Sundaresan, P. R., V. G. Winters and D. G. Therriault 1967 Effect of low environmental temperature on the metabolism of vitamin A (retinol) in the rat. J. Nutr. 92: 474.

474. Anderson, T. A., F. Hubbert, Jr. and C. B. Roubicek 1964 Effect of thyroxine, thiouracil and ambient temperature on the utilization of vitamin A by vitamin A-deficient rats. J. Nutr. 82: 457.

475. Roderuck, C. E., V. D. Sidwell, E. H. Jebe and E. S. Eppright 1963 Studies of serum carotenoids and vitamin A in Iowa school children. Amer. J. Clin. Nutr. 13: 186.

476. Wohl, M. G., and J. B. Feldman 1939 Vitamin A deficiency in disease of the thyroid gland: its detection by dark adaptation. Endocrinology 24: 389.

477. Horvat, A., and H. Maver 1958 The role of vitamin A in the occurrence of goitre on the island of Krk, Yugoslavia. J. Nutr. 66: 189.

478. Hirsch, W., and G. Woschée 1967 Hyperthyreose-therapie mit Vitamin A. Ther. Gegenw. 106: 251.

479. Raz, A., and D. S. Goodman 1969 The interaction of thyroxine with human plasma prealbumin and with the prealbumin–retinol-binding protein complex. J. Biol. Chem. 244: 3230.

480. Anderson, H. H., and M. H. Soley 1938 The effects of carotenemia on the function of thyroid and the liver. Amer. J. Med. Sci. 195: 313.

481. Euler, H. von, and E. Klussmann 1932 Carotin (Vitamin A) und Thyroxin. Z. Physiol. Chem. 213: 21. Cited in: Chem. Abstr. 1933, p. 754.

482. Johnson, R. M., and C. A. Baumann 1947 The effect of thyroid on the conversion of carotene into vitamin A. J. Biol. Chem. 171: 513.

483. Cama, H. R., N. C. Pillai, P. R. Sundaresan and C. Venkateshan 1957 The effect of thyroid activity on the conversion of carotene and retinene to vitamin A and on serum proteins. J. Nutr. 63: 571.

484. Aron, H. C. S., R. M. Craig, C. J. Farmer, H. W. Kendell and G. X. Schwemlein 1946 Effect of elevated body temperature on plasma vitamin A and carotene. Proc. Soc. Exp. Biol. Med. 61: 271.

485. Méndez, J., N. S. Scrimshaw, C. Salvadó and M. López Selva 1959 Effects of artificially induced fever on serum proteins, vitamin levels and hematological values in human subjects. J. Appl. Physiol. 14: 768.

486. Moore, T., and I. M. Sharman 1951 Vitamin A levels in health and disease. Brit. J. Nutr. 5: 119.

487. Lawrie, N. R., T. Moore and K. R. Rajagopal 1941 The excretion of vitamin A in urine. Biochem. J. 35: 825.

488. Wolf, G. 1970 Recent progress in research on the metabolic function of vitamin A. In: Nutrition: Proceeding of the Eighth International Congress, Sept. 1969, Prague, p. 111. eds. J. Mašek, K. Osancová and D. P. Cuthbertsón. Pub. Excerpta Medica, Amsterdam.

489. Johnson, B. C., M. Kennedy and N. Chiba 1969 Vitamin A and nuclear RNA synthesis. Amer. J. Clin. Nutr. 22: 1048.

490. Tryfiates, G. P., and R. F. Krause 1971 Effect of vitamin A deficiency on the protein synthetic activity of rat liver ribosomes. Proc. Soc. Exp. Biol. Med. 136: 946.

491. Hayes, K. C., H. L. McCombs and T. B. Faherty 1970 The fine structure of vitamin A deficiency. I. Parotid duct metaplasia. Lab. Invest. 22: 81.

492. Phillips, W. E. J., and R. L. Brien 1970 Effect of pectin, a hypocholesterolemic polysaccharide, on vitamin utilization in the rat. J. Nutr. 100: 289.

493. Phillips, W. E. J. 1966 Effect of dietary nitrite on the liver storage of vitamin A in the rat. Can. J. Biochem. Physiol. 44: 1.

494. Tinsley, I. J. 1969 DDT effect on rats raised on alpha-protein rations: growth and storage of liver vitamin A. J. Nutr. 98: 319.

495. Phillips, W. E. J., G. Hatina, D. C. Villeneuve and D. L. Grant 1971 Multigeneration studies on the effect of dietary DDT on the vitamin A status of the weanling rat. Can. J. Physiol. Pharmacol. 49: 382.

496. Read, S. I., T. K. Murray and W. P. McKinley 1965 The effect of DDT on the liver carboxylesterase and vitamin A utilization of mother rats and their young. Can. J. Biochem. 43: 317.

497. Bohdal, M., and F. Hrubá 1962 Der Vitamin-A-Haushalt des Organismus im Verlauf der Brombenzolvergiftung. Acta Biol. Med. Germ. 8: 66.

498. Baumann, C. A., E. G. Foster and P. R. Moore 1942 The effect of dibenzanthracene, of alcohol, and of other agents on vitamin A in the rat. J. Biol. Chem. 142: 597.

499. Miller, R. W., R. W. Hemken, D. R. Waldo and L. A. Moore 1969 Effect of ethyl alcohol on the vitamin A status of holstein heifers. J. Dairy Sci. 52: 1998.

500. Meunier, P., R. Ferrando, J. Jouanneteau and G. Thomas 1949 Vitamine A et phénomènes de détoxication. I. Influence de la vitamine a sur les conditions de la détoxication du benzoate de sodium par l'organisme du rat en voie de croissance. Bull. Soc. Chim. Biol., Paris 31: 1413.

501. Meunier, P., R. Ferrando and G. Perrot-Thomas 1950 Vitamine A et phénomènes de détoxication. 2. Influence de la vitamine A sur la détoxication du bromobenzène

par l'organisme du rat en voie de croissance. Bull. Soc. Chim. Biol., Paris 32: 50.

502. Mameesh, M. S., F. Utne and O. R. Braekkan 1965 Studies on glucuronide detoxication mechanisms in vitamin A deficient rats. Acta Pharmacol. Toxicol. 22: 235.

503. Getzler, N. A., and A. Flint 1966 Keratosis follicularis. A study of one family. Arch. Dermatol. 93: 545.

504. Leitner, Z. A. 1951 Pathology of vitamin A deficiency and its clinical significance. Brit. J. Nutr. 5: 130.

505. Youmans, J. B. 1960 Vitamin A nutrition and the skin. Amer. J. Clin. Nutr. 8: 789.

506. Dowling, J. E., and G. Wald 1958 Vitamin A deficiency and night blindness. Proc. Nat. Acad. Sci. 44: 648.

507. Interdepartmental Committee on Nutrition for National Defense 1956 Iran: Nutrition Survey of the Armed Forces. National Institutes of Health, DHEW.

508. Interdepartmental Committee on Nutrition for National Defense 1957 Korea: Nutrition Survey of the Armed Forces. National Institutes of Health, DHEW.

509. Interdepartmental Committee on Nutrition for National Defense 1957 Philippines: Nutrition Survey of the Armed Forces. National Institutes of Health, DHEW.

510. Interdepartmental Committee on Nutrition for National Defense 1957 Libya: Nutrition Survey of the Armed Forces and Civilians, 1957. National Institutes of Health, DHEW.

511. Interdepartmental Committee on Nutrition for National Defense 1958 Turkey: Nutrition Survey of the Armed Forces. National Institutes of Health, DHEW.

512. Interdepartmental Committee on Nutrition for National Defense 1958 Spain: Nutrition Survey of the Armed Forces. National Institutes of Health, DHEW.

513. Interdepartmental Committee on Nutrition for National Defense 1959 Ethiopia: Nutrition Survey. National Institutes of Health, DHEW.

514. Interdepartmental Committee on Nutrition for National Defense 1959 Peru: Nutrition Survey of the Armed Forces. National Institutes of Health, DHEW.

515. Interdepartmental Committee on Nutrition for National Defense 1959 Alaska: An Appraisal of the Health and Nutritional Status of the Eskimo, 1958. National Institute of Arthritis and Metabolic Diseases, DHEW.

516. Interdepartmental Committee on Nutrition for National Defense 1960 Ecuador: Nutrition Survey. National Institutes of Health, DHEW.

517. Interdepartmental Committee on Nutrition for National Defense 1960 Republic of Vietnam: Nutrition Survey, October -- December 1959. National Institutes of Health, DHEW.

518. Interdepartmental Committee on Nutrition for National Defense 1961 Colombia: Nutrition Survey, May — August 1960. National Institutes of Health, DHEW.

519. Interdepartmental Committee on Nutrition for National Defense 1961 Republic of China: Nutrition Survey of the Armed Forces, September — October 1960. National Institutes of Health, DHEW.

520. Interdepartmental Committee on Nutrition for National Defense 1961 Chile: Nutrition Survey, March — June 1960. National Institutes of Health, DHEW.

521. Interdepartmental Committee on Nutrition for National Defense 1962 The Kingdom of Thailand: Nutrition Survey, October — December 1960. National Institutes of Health, DHEW.

522. Interdepartmental Committee on Nutrition for National Defense 1962 The West Indies: Nutrition Survey, August — September 1961. National Institutes of Health, DHEW.

523. Interdepartmental Committee on Nutrition for National Defense 1962 Republic of Lebanon: Nutrition Survey, February — April 1961. National Institutes of Health, DHEW.

524. Interdepartmental Committee on Nutrition for National Defense 1963 Union of Burma: Nutrition Survey, October — December 1961. National Institute of Arthritis and Metabolic Diseases, DHEW.

525. Interdepartmental Committee on Nutrition for National Defense 1963 Republic of Uruguay: Nutrition Survey, March — April 1962. National Institute of Arthritis and Metabolic Diseases, DHEW.

526. Interdepartmental Committee on Nutrition for National Defense 1964 Federation of Malaya: Nutrition Survey, September — October 1962. National Institutes of Health, DHEW.

527. Interdepartmental Committee on Nutrition for National Defense 1964 Bolivia: Nutrition Survey. National Institute of Arthritis and Metabolic Diseases, DHEW.

528. Interdepartmental Committee on Nutrition for National Defense and the Interdepartmental Committee on Nutrition for Jordan 1964 The Hashemite Kingdom of Jordan: Nutrition Survey on Infants and Preschool Children in Jordan, November 1962 — October 1963. National Institutes of Health, DHEW.

529. Interdepartmental Committee on Nutrition for National Defense 1964 Venezuela: Nutrition Survey, May — June 1963. National Institute of Arthritis and Metabolic Diseases, DHEW.

530. Interdepartmental Committee on Nutrition Defense 1964 Blackfeet Indian Reservation: Nutrition Survey, August — September 1961. U.S. Public Health Service, DHEW.

531. Interdepartmental Committee on Nutrition for National Defense and the Division of Indian Health 1964 Fort Belknap Indian Reservation: Nutrition Survey, August — October 1961. U.S. Public Health Service, DHEW.

532. Interdepartmental Committee on Nutrition for National Development 1965 Northeast

Brazil: Nutrition Survey, March — May 1963. National Institutes of Health, DHEW.

533. Ministry of Health, Government of Pakistan, and the Nutrition Section, Office of International Research, National Institutes of Health 1966 Pakistan: Nutrition Survey of East Pakistan, March 1962 — January 1964. U.S. Public Health Service, DHEW.

534. Nutrition Section, Office of International Research, National Institutes of Health 1967 Republic of Nigeria: Nutrition Survey, February — April 1965. U.S. Public Health Service, DHEW.

535. Instituto de Nutritión de Centro América y Panamá (INCAP), Oficina de Investigaciones Internacionales de los Institutos Nacionales de Salud (EEUU) y Ministerio de Salud Pública y Asistencia Social 1969 Guatemala: Evaluación Nutricional de la Población de Centro América y Panamá, febrero a abril de 1965. INCAP, Guatemala, C.A.

536. Instituto de Nutrición de Centro América y Panamá (INCAP), Oficina de Investigaciones Internacionales de los Institutos Nacionales de Salud (EEUU) y Ministerio de Salud Pública y Asistencia Social 1969 El Salvador: Evaluación Nutricional de la Población de Centro América y Panamá, septiembre a noviembre de 1965 y mayo de 1967. INCAP, Guatemala, C.A.

537. Instituto de Nutrición de Centro América y Panamá (INCAP), Oficina de Investigaciones Internacionales de los Institutos Nacionales de Salud (EEUU) y Ministerio de Salubridad Pública 1969 Nicaragua: Evaluación Nacional de la Población de Centro América y Panamá, enero a marzo de 1966. INCAP, Guatemala, C.A.

538. Instituto de Nutrición de Centro América y Panamá (INCAP), Oficina de Investigaciones Internacionales de los Institutos Nacionales de Salud (EEUU) y Ministerio de Salubridad Pública 1969 Costa Rica: Evaluación Nacional de la Población de Centro América y Panamá, abril a junio de 1966. INCAP, Guatemala, C. A.

539. Instituto de Nutrición de Centro América y Panamá (INCAP), Oficina de Investigaciones Internacionales de los Institutos Nacionales de Salud (EEUU) y Ministerio de Salud Pública y Asistencia Social 1969 Honduras: Evaluación Nutricional de la Población de Centro América y Panamá, septiembre a noviembre de 1966. INCAP, Guatemala, C.A.

540. Instituto de Nutrición de Centro América y Panamá (INCAP), Oficina de Investigaciones Internacionales de los Institutos Nacionales de Salud (EEUU) y Ministerio de Salud Pública 1969 Panamá: Evaluación Nacional de la Población de Centro América y Panamá, enero a marzo de 1967. INCAP, Guatemala, C.A.

541. Sweeney, J. P., and A. C. Marsh 1970 Separation of carotene stereoisomers in vegetables. J. Ass. Off. Anal. Chem. 53: 937.

542. Awdeh, Z. L. 1965 Separation of vitamin A from carotenoids in micro samples of serum. Anal. Biochem. 10: 156.

543. Targan, S. R., S. Merrill and A. D. Schwabe 1969 Fractionation and quantification of β-carotene and vitamin A derivatives in human serum. Clin. Sci. 15: 479.

544. Smith, F. R., A. Raz and DeW. S. Goodman 1970 Radioimmunoassay of human plasma retinol-binding protein. J. Clin. Invest. 49: 1754.

545. Frank, O., A. V. Luisada-Opper, S. Feingold and H. Baker 1970 Vitamin binding by human and some animal plasma proteins. Nutr. Rept. Int. 1: 161.

546. Rask, L., A. Vahlquist and P. A. Peterson 1971 Studies on two physiological forms of the human retinol-binding protein differing in vitamin A and arginine content. J. Biol. Chem. 246: 6638.

547. Sundaresan, P. R., and H. N. Bhagavan 1971 Metabolic studies on retinoic acid in the rat. Biochem. J. 122: 1.

A CONSPECTUS OF RESEARCH

ON

CALCIUM REQUIREMENTS OF MAN[1]

by

M. ISABEL IRWIN

Nutrition Institute
Agricultural Research Service
United States Department of Agriculture
Beltsville, Maryland 20705

and

ELDON W. KIENHOLZ

Department of Avian Science
Colorado State University
Fort Collins, Colorado 80521

THE JOURNAL OF NUTRITION

VOLUME 103, NUMBER 7, JULY 1973

(Pages 1019-1095)

TABLE OF CONTENTS

INTRODUCTION

The problem of calcium requirements of man has been under investigation for at least a century. In spite of the obvious need for calcium in bone formation, indisputable symptoms of calcium deficiency are lacking. Calcium, it is true, is involved in two major bone disorders, osteomalacia or rickets and osteoporosis. In osteomalacia or rickets, the primary defect seems to be vitamin D deficiency or a hormonal imbalance that prevents the efficient use of calcium supplies (363). It is not inconceivable that a deficient calcium intake would cause rickets. To date, however, only one report (323) has been found of a clearly identified case of calcium deficiency rickets. The etiology of osteoporosis is still in doubt. Some hold it to be a defect of the bone matrix (9). Others hold it to be the result of prolonged negative calcium balance (363). Negative calcium balance may be caused by a number of factors. Among them are inadequate calcium intake, malabsorption and high urinary output. Although osteoporosis has been produced in animals fed low calcium diets (28, 165, 348, 405), there is little agreement in the literature on whether there is a similar relationship between calcium intake and osteoporosis in human subjects (141). Krook and Lutwak (276), for instance, in reviewing Nordin's study on international patterns of osteoporosis (366) called attention to an inverse relationship between radiological evidence of bone density and the amount of calcium provided in the diet. Walker (499), on the other hand, concluded from a review of the literature that "there is no unequivocal evidence that osteoporosis or its pathological sequelae are promoted by an habitually low intake of calcium."

Poor growth and low serum calcium levels have been suggested as possible indicators of inadequate calcium intake. There is little clear evidence in human subjects, however, of response in either growth or serum calcium levels that can be attributed solely to changes in calcium intake.

The balance method (intake minus fecal and urinary output) has been the principal tool used in assessing calcium requirements. The data obtained have been subjected to a variety of statistical treatments. The resulting estimates of requirements have been noteworthy for their great range.

Equally noteworthy is the wide range of intakes with which people in various parts of the world maintain themselves without apparent signs of either calcium deficiency or calcium excess. Such an observation led Brull (78) to suggest in 1936 that people may be able to adapt to various intakes. This suggestion was made again by other investigators (25, 358, 467), and many seemingly conflicting results have thus been explained.

Clear evidence of adaptation was obtained by Malm (322) in his long-term study with male prison inmates. In his work, 23 of a squad of 26 men immediately, or over a period of time, achieved calcium equilibrium when their calcium intake was reduced from about 930 or 650 mg/day to about 450 mg/day. Three men, however, did not adapt but remained in negative calcium balance as long as they were receiving the lower calcium intake (266 to 532 days). These data have been interpre-

Received for publication June 19, 1972.

[1] In accordance with the general policy of *The Journal of Nutrition*, metric units have been used throughout, using appropriate conversions when the original source of data used different units, except when the metric equivalent was not clearly indicated or when the conversion to the metric system seemed to give an illusion of greater precision than the actual data conveyed. In some cases, an estimate of the approximate measure in the metric system is included.

ted by Nordin (364) as indicating that the majority of the population probably can adjust to intakes much lower than they normally consume but that a significant proportion cannot.

This ability of many people to adapt to different calcium intakes hinders the determination of either minimal or optimal requirements (if they are different) by the balance method and suggests the need for long-term studies. These are difficult to carry out with human subjects, particularly in populations not confined to institutions. In addition, the results of studies may not be comparable from one laboratory to another because of differences in experimental diets and methods.

At the present time the majority of the available data on calcium requirements of man have been obtained in short-term studies. In many studies, observations have been made on a small number of subjects eating a controlled diet. In a few studies, large numbers of subjects (70 to 136 persons) ate weighed portions of self-selected diets. The reports of these latter studies provide information on the range of intakes over which health seems to be maintained. Usually, estimates of requirements were made by extrapolation from the observed data.

The purpose of this conspectus is not to produce another estimate of calcium requirements. Nor is it intended to be a critical review, although some evaluative comment is inevitable. Rather, the purpose is to show what work has been done on determining human requirements for calcium, how it has been done, and where the greatest need for research lies. The body of literature on calcium metabolism is very large. For this review, the reports covered have been restricted as much as possible to those on human studies and principally to those on studies dealing specifically with human requirements for calcium and with factors affecting those requirements.

EARLY STUDIES

Early attempts to define calcium requirements were based on food intake records and on observations of fecal and urinary calcium excretion. The food intake records showed wide variation in the calcium in-

take of apparently healthy people. For instance, Tigerstedt (484) obtained 72 dietary records of 3 to 5 days' duration from 64 Finns including 23 children, 2 to 12 years old, 4 girls and 5 boys, 12 to 16 years old, 21 women and 11 men. Daily calcium intakes varied from 2.21 g CaO for the 2- to 3-year-old children to 5.31 g CaO for the men. Hornemann (218), on the other hand, collected 18 two- or three-day records from four men, two women and one 6-year-old boy in Berlin. The average daily calcium intake was calculated to be 1.716, 0.862, and 0.667 g CaO per person for the men, women, and boy, respectively. Hornemann considered on the basis of earlier studies that the adults had adequate intakes. The boy, who was apparently healthy, was judged to be eating enough to provide for a retention of at least 0.13 g CaO per day which Hornemann calculated was needed for normal growth.

Data resembling those of the Berlin study were obtained by Sherman et al. (439) in a dietary study in the eastern United States. Food intake records of 7 to 31 days' duration were obtained from families of various economic levels and from work camps and college dining halls. A total of 167 men, 165 women and 53 children were included in the 20 families and groups studied. Taking into account the number, age, and sex of the participants in each family or dining group, the calcium intakes per man per day were calculated. These ranged from 0.08 to 1.48 g CaO per man per day. Sherman expressed doubts as to the adequacy of the intakes of many of the families.

One of the earliest recommended allowances for calcium based on calcium excretion was proposed by Smith in 1865 (450). This allowance (2.3 to 6.3 grains of "lime"/day, equivalent to 145 to 400 mg/day) was based on determination of urinary and fecal calcium excretion of people who were eating a presumably adequate diet. The subjects' calcium intakes were not estimated. Smith's proposed allowance was lower than those suggested by the work of German scientists who studied excretion of adult individuals during relatively short experimental periods (2 to 11 days) with various controlled levels of calcium intake (10, 13, 47, 174,

177, 201, 256, 374, 406). The number of subjects observed in these investigations varied from one to five per study. The intakes at which slightly positive calcium balance or equilibrium could be maintained varied from 0.4 g to 1.8 g of CaO (0.3 to 1.5 g calcium). Hornemann (218), from the results of these previous studies, calculated an average requirement of 0.74 to 1.2 g CaO/day (0.6 to 1.0 g calcium). Sherman et al. (439) similarly concluded from the results of previous workers and from their own observations in six 3-day metabolism studies with one subject that a calcium requirement of about 0.7 g CaO/day (0.6 g calcium) was indicated. They suggested, however, that much more experimentation must be done before such an estimate could be accepted as satisfactory.

STUDIES ON CALCIUM REQUIREMENTS BY THE BALANCE METHOD (APPENDIX TABLE 1)

Following the early work of Sherman et al. (439), Sherman (435) collected data on calcium intake and output of young men and women eating relatively low calcium diets (437, 440–442). A compilation of these data together with some from early German work and from contemporary studies by Rose (417) was made. Of the 97 experiments listed, 69 were by Sherman and his co-workers, 22 by Rose and 6 were by German workers (47, 212, 406, 510). Each experiment consisted of one 3- to 8-day dietary study with one subject. Minimum calcium requirement was estimated from the sum of the mean daily fecal and urinary excretion when the calcium intake was "somewhat insufficient." In order to be comparable, the values were adjusted to represent those of a 70-kg individual. The average minimal daily calcium requirement so calculated was 0.45 g Ca (0.63 g CaO). The standard deviation was 0.12 g and the coefficient of variation was 27%. The individual values ranged from 0.27 to 0.82 g calcium per day. After comparing these data with a similar compilation on protein requirements, Sherman recommended that the diet should provide 1.0 g Ca or 1.4 g CaO for every 100 g of protein. On reexamining his previously collected food intake data (439), he concluded that one

of every six dietaries failed to meet this recommended allowance.

Some years later calcium balance studies with adult and adolescent Africans, reported from Nairobi (195, 196, 259), yielded requirement values which when recalculated to the basis of 70 kg body weight fell within the range of Sherman's values. In this study, male prisoners received a prison diet supplying approximately 300 mg Ca/day. Balance studies with 12 adults and five 15- to 17-year-old boys showed that most of the subjects were in negative balance with this intake.

Subsequent to Sherman's report of 1920, many balance studies were carried out. The primary objective of many of the studies was to study the usefulness of various foods as sources of calcium, for instance, vegetables (51, 252, 319, 336), cereals (25, 82, 104, 398) and other plant foods (25, 394, 398). Another objective was to study the effect of food processing on the retention of calcium from a food such as milk (271, 272, 318, 467, 469, 520) or vegetables (92). A third objective was to study the effect of other dietary components on the availability of calcium from various foods. Among the dietary components or adjuncts studied were fat (61, 157, 320, 470), yeast (61, 227), cod-liver oil (185, 227) and cocoa (66).

The collection periods used in the early studies varied from 3 to 7 days in length. Frequently they were preceded by adjustment periods of 1 to 3 days. In many studies, data from several consecutive collection periods were used. The number of subjects observed in any one of the early studies varied from one to ten. In some of the later studies (469, 470) more subjects were used. In most of the studies the subjects were women. In addition to information on utilization, these studies frequently yielded data from which estimates of calcium requirements were derived. Usually the experimental diet was planned to provide just enough or slightly less than enough calcium to meet the subject's calculated minimum requirement (approximately 6.4 mg/kg body weight) (435). At low levels of intake, absorption was expected to be most efficient and the amount of unabsorbed calcium to be inversely related to the availability of calcium from the dietary source. By comparing the balance data obtained for one source with those obtained for a source of reputedly highly available calcium, such as milk, the relative usefulness of a food as a source of calcium could be estimated. Calcium requirements were calculated by estimating the amount of calcium required to balance the urinary and fecal losses. The requirements thus estimated varied, of course, with the dietary source of calcium. Requirement estimates were expressed either in terms of total daily intake or in terms of body weight. Among the estimates of calcium requirement resulting from these studies were 5 to 6 mg/kg (nine women) reported by Rose and MacLeod (418), 9.2 mg/kg (one man) reported by Steggerda and Mitchell (466), 0.56 g/day obtained with four women studied by Kramer et al. (271), and 0.45 g/day found with two male and one female Chinese subjects studied by Adolph and Chen (6). In all of these studies, the principal source of calcium was milk.

In 1937, Leitch (289) assembled data from the literature on calcium intake and excretion of women. These data included those reported by Sherman and his associates (437, 440–442), as well as those reported in subsequent years (approximately 397 balance studies on 60 women) (6, 51, 82, 271, 272, 318–320, 336, 394, 417, 418, 520). The data were grouped according to intake and were analyzed by two methods. By one method, the number of negative and positive balances reported for each intake level were noted. The level at which the number of negative balances equalled the number of positive balances was assumed to be the average maintenance requirement. This value was 0.55 g calcium/day. By the second method, the average positive and negative balances at each intake were plotted about the equilibrium line. Straight lines were fitted by the method of least squares to the negative balance data and to the positive balance data. The point on the equilibrium line that was equidistant from both plotted lines indicated an intake of 0.55 g/day. Leitch therefore estimated the "true maintenance requirement" for healthy women to be 0.55 g calcium/day. She suggested that, because the few data available for

men did not indicate otherwise, this standard might be used for both sexes. In her summary, Leitch remarked that "there is no evidence to show what additional allowance is required 'for health,' but it is probable that such an allowance should be made." In the available data, Leitch could find no statistical support for expressing the requirement in terms of body weight. Later Mitchell and Curzon (345), agreeing that it was difficult with the available data to prove that a correlation existed between calcium output and body size, nevertheless declared that "it is hardly conceivable that the endogenous output of calcium in urine and feces would be independent of body size." Calculating the average weight of the subjects in Leitch's compilation to be 55.6 kg, they restated her "true maintenance requirement" as 10.0 mg calcium per kilogram body weight per day.

Another compilation of balance data from the literature was made by Mitchell and Curzon (345). It contained the data used by Sherman (435) and by Leitch (289) and data from additional studies (27, 30, 31, 59–61, 143, 158, 185, 195, 273). In some of these studies calcium output under fasting conditions or with very low calcium intakes was studied (27, 158); in others, calcium output with various diets and dietary adjuncts was measured (30, 59, 61). There was a total of 139 average observations on 107 subjects (89 women and 18 men). The data were expressed as milligrams of calcium per kilogram body weight per day. When the regression of output (y) on intake (x) was calculated and plotted, Mitchell and Curzon found that the regression line crossed a) the equilibrium line $(x = y)$ at 9.75 mg/kg and b) the y axis at 3.09 mg/kg. These data, therefore, indicated a daily maintenance requirement of 9.75 mg calcium per kilogram body weight and a daily endogenous loss of 3.09 mg per kilogram. From these values, an average utilization of about 30% of the dietary calcium was deduced.

The estimates of requirement derived from the compilations of Sherman (435), Leitch (289), and Mitchell and Curzon (345) were based on the equation:

Intake − Balance = Requirement.

This same calculation refined by an allowance for incomplete utilization of dietary calcium was used by Steggerda and Mitchell (467) and Outhouse et al. (380). Requirement estimates of 9.55 mg/kg (9 men) (467) and of 8.3 to 13.3 mg/kg (4 women, 3 men) (380) were made when the subjects ate low calcium diets supplemented with milk or calcium gluconate.

Some years later, Steggerda and Mitchell (469) reported observations on 19 men, 17 to 39 years old, eating a low calcium basal diet for 20 to 192 days and the same diet supplemented with milk or calcium gluconate for 20 to 256 days. Calcium requirements calculated from the individual balance data ranged from 222 to 1,018 mg/day. The mean requirement for the group was 644 ± 181 mg/day. When the requirement was expressed in terms of body weight (9.21 ± 2.71 mg/kg), body surface (343 ± 93.8 mg/m²), or basal energy needs (0.366 ± 0.101 mg/basal kilocalorie), the coefficients of variation were not reduced appreciably. Maintaining that calcium requirements logically must be related to body size, Steggerda and Mitchell interpreted these observations as indicating "that other factors are so much more potent in causing variation in calcium metabolism as to completely obscure the effect of variable body size." They also pointed out that the variability from one subject to another in utilization of calcium and in calcium requirement makes observations on food consumption alone inadequate for assessing calcium nutriture.

Calcium requirements have been calculated also by means of other treatments of balance data. One such treatment was the regression calculation. Steggerda and Mitchell (470) obtained data in a controlled study on the effect of high and low levels of dietary fat on calcium metabolism. After ascertaining that the data were homogeneous they calculated and plotted the regression of calcium retention on calcium intake. Sixty-five observations were made on 13 men eating controlled diets for 8 to 20 days. Reported calcium intakes ranged from 2.59 to 10.10 mg/kg body weight. Calcium balances ranged from −2.70 to 1.99 mg/kg. Positive balances occurred with intakes as low as 2 to 3 mg/kg, and negative balances were observed with intakes as high as 9 to 10 mg/kg. The regression calculation indicated that, for this group of subjects, the mean calcium intake necessary for equilibrium was 7.40 mg/kg, the mean endogenous calcium excretion was 3.72 mg/kg, and that 50.2% of the dietary calcium was utilized. The estimate of endogenous calcium excretion is reasonably close to that calculated by Mitchell and Curzon (345). The reason for the lower estimate of maintenance requirement and higher estimate of utilization than those obtained previously in the same laboratory (466, 467, 469) was not clear. The difference in method of calculation may have contributed to the discrepancies.

Much lower values for calcium requirement and endogenous calcium excretion were obtained by Hegsted et al. (194) when they studied the calcium intake and excretion of 10 inmates in a Peruvian prison. The subjects received a basal diet to which was added one, two, or three cups of milk in successive 10-day dietary periods. In another dietary period, meat was substituted for some of the food in the basal diet. The data were submitted to several mathematical treatments. In one, the regression of output on intake was calculated and plotted for each individual subject. Calcium requirements for equilibrium calculated in this way varied from 0 to 596 mg/day. The mean requirement was 216 mg calcium/day. The investigators noted that in almost every case the estimated urinary excretion accounted for the total estimated excretion at zero intake (endogenous calcium excretion).

In a second mathematical treatment, all of the data were subjected to one regression calculation of output on intake. The mean calcium requirement for equilibrium was estimated to be 126 mg/day (1.8 mg/kg/day). The mean endogenous calcium excretion was 20 mg/day. When the data were expressed in terms of body weight and the regression of output on intake was calculated, the mean calcium requirement for equilibrium was 3.25 mg/kg. The mean endogenous calcium excretion was 0.91 mg/kg. Besides showing that the estimated requirement depends, in part, on how it is calculated, these values indicated that some people apparently could maintain themselves with calcium intakes much lower than those commonly believed to be necessary.

More recently, a study has been reported from Russia (130) in which calcium intake and output of 36 men were measured. Regression equations indicated that a calcium intake of 600 to 700 mg/day was necessary for equilibrium. The English abstract of this report did not indicate which parameters were correlated in the regression calculation.

In earlier work, McKay et al. (334) studied the calcium intake and excretion of 109 young women eating their customary self-selected diets. Observations were made during one or more 7- or 10-day periods. A total of 124 balances was calculated. Calcium intakes ranged from 322 to 2,323 mg/day. Positive balances were observed with intakes as low as 400 to 500 mg, but negative balances were also observed with intakes as high as 1,500 to 1,600 mg/day. The mean intake and mean retention were 941 mg and 30 mg/day, respectively. When the regression of retention on intake was plotted, the point of intersection of the regression line and the equilibrium line (retention = 0) indicated that a mean calcium intake of 816 mg was required for equilibrium in this group.

A treatment somewhat similar to the regression calculation was used by Leverton and Marsh (295) in their examination of the data resulting from 100 seven-day balance studies with 70 young women eating self-selected diets. Calcium intake varied from 421 to 1,679 mg/day, and retention varied from −463 to 377 mg/day. The mean intake and retention were 857 and 13 mg/day, respectively. The data were grouped according to level of intake and the mean intake and retention at each level were calculated. The mean retention increased as the mean intake increased, but the percentage of intake retained (mean percentage retention) did not. When the mean percentage retentions were plotted against the mean intakes and the points were joined by straight lines, the resultant graph showed a percentage retention line that rose steeply crossing the line of equilibrium at an intake of about 830 mg. When it reached an intake of about 1,083 mg it began to level off. Leverton and Marsh suggested that this treatment of the data indicated a mean minimum calcium requirement of 830 mg and an optimum

intake of about 1,083 mg/day. By this method of calculation the optimal intake was about 30% higher than the minimum requirement. In another treatment of the data, Leverton and Marsh grouped the balances as negative (27 balances), positive (40 balances), and equilibrium (31 balances). The mean intake of the equilibrium balances was 875 ± 34 mg. The close agreement between the "minimum daily requirement" (830 mg), the mean daily intake of the balances in equilibrium (875 mg) and the mean daily intake of the entire group of subjects (857 mg) suggested to the investigators that a total daily intake of 0.83 to 0.88 g of calcium was required for maintenance of young women similar to the group studied. Other calculations of the data revealed no significant correlation between body size and calcium requirement.

STUDIES ON CALCIUM REQUIREMENTS BY THE FACTORIAL METHOD (APPENDIX TABLES 1 AND 2)

Another approach to estimating calcium requirements is the factorial method. By this method, the sum of the individual minimum calcium losses through various routes is regarded as the "net calcium requirement." The amount of dietary calcium needed to satisfy the net requirement depends on the availability or absorbability of the calcium in the diet. In recent years, isotopic calcium (^{45}Ca or ^{47}Ca) has been used in estimating some of the losses. Drawing on data from the literature on endogenous fecal, urinary, and skin losses, and on intestinal absorption rates of calcium, Whedon (513) proposed an allowance of 1,086 mg calcium per day. This intake would allow for obligatory losses of 380 mg/day and an absorption rate of 35%. Lower values were derived from a study by Blau et al. (53) in which two subjects, eating a low calcium diet, were given a single dose of ^{45}Ca orally. The results revealed rather wide differences between individuals in their endogenous fecal excretion, intestinal absorption, and urinary losses of calcium. From the data of this study and those accumulated in additional work with the same subjects Blau et al. (52) calculated minimum daily calcium requirements of 431 mg/day or 8.1 mg/kg body weight for one subject and 240 mg/day or 3.5 mg/kg body weight for the other. These estimates did not make any allowances for skin losses.

Endogenous fecal calcium
(Appendix table 2)

Prior to the use of isotope studies, there were a few attempts to determine endogenous fecal calcium excretion. In the late nineteenth century and early part of the twentieth century when observations on fasting subjects were being made, some data were collected.

Lehmann et al. (286) studied the metabolic response of two "professional fasters," Cetti and Breithaupt. They reported that Cetti excreted 690 mg of fecal calcium during a 10-day fast (69 mg/day) and Breithaupt excreted 189 mg fecal calcium during a 6-day fast (32 mg/day). Benedict (42), who studied one man during a fast of 31 days, reported that no defecation occurred during the entire fasting period and that it was difficult to determine what proportion of the feces passed after the fast should be ascribed to the fasting period. He expressed some reservations on the validity of the data reported earlier. Bauer et al. (27) approached the problem by feeding a diet containing very low levels of calcium. They studied the calcium excretion of 13 "normal" subjects during 3-day periods (one to eight periods per subject). With an average daily intake of 109 mg calcium the average fecal calcium output was 200 mg/day.

Observations such as these of fecal excretion greater than the intake had suggested that calcium is excreted from the body through the gastrointestinal tract. They also suggested that variations in the rate of excretion might be a means of controlling the calcium levels in the body. McCance and Widdowson (326) explored this possibility in a study with six subjects. In two 4-day periods, the subjects ate diets containing two levels of calcium, approximately 582 mg and 734 mg calcium/day. Then in a third 14-day period, when their dietary calcium intake was about 628 mg/day, the subjects received an additional 186 mg of calcium intravenously each day. Comparisons of the urinary/fecal Ca and fecal/food Ca ratios during the three periods convinced McCance and Widdowson that all or almost all of the intravenously administered calcium was excreted in the urine, and that the gastrointestinal tract excretion of calcium does not vary with plasma levels or the needs of the body. It should be noted that this conclusion was not that calcium excretion does not take place through the gastrointestinal tract but rather that excretion through the gut is not a regulatory pathway. Nicolaysen et al. (361) reached a similar conclusion saying "all the carefully conducted experiments in this group . . . have led to the conclusion that no regulated secretion takes place." Nicolaysen et al. (361) postulated further that "endogenous" calcium is actually calcium secreted into the gut in the digestive juices, and that the amount of endogenous calcium lost in the feces depends on the efficiency of absorption. In other words, endogenous fecal calcium is unreabsorbed digestive juice calcium.

Brine and Johnston (67) assembled data on calcium intake and fecal excretion of normal subjects from 51 reports in the literature. The studies included were those in which the collection period had been at least 6 days in length and in which the dietary calcium intake did not differ by more than 200 mg from that eaten prior to the study. Experiments involving factors suspected of affecting calcium absorption were excluded. Fecal calcium excretion was plotted against calcium intake. A best fitting curve extrapolated to zero intake indicated an endogenous fecal excretion of 75 mg/day. This value, Brine and Johnston suggested, might vary considerably from person to person. If Nicolaysen's (361) assumption is correct, it might also vary with factors affecting the absorption of calcium from the gastrointestinal tract. Barnes et al. (23) have suggested also that such apparent obligatory losses may occur only in people conditioned to high calcium intakes.

Isotope studies have been used to determine how much of the total fecal calcium is unreabsorbed digestive juice calcium. Blau et al. (53) estimated endogenous excretions of 91 mg/day and 117 mg/day by two subjects given ^{45}Ca orally. In this study the radioactive calcium was detected in the blood and urine within 1 hour after a 50 μCi dose had been ingested. Within

2 hours the specific activities of the plasma and urine became equal. In the feces, the specific activity was high for several days and then fell to a level below that in the urine and plasma. Blau et al. based their calculations of endogenous fecal calcium on the assumption that the digestive juice calcium enters the gut with the same specific activity as that of the plasma or urine, becomes diluted with food calcium, and is reabsorbed at the same rate as the food calcium is absorbed. The fraction of the fecal calcium that is endogenous calcium, then, is the ratio of the specific activity of the feces to that of the urine or plasma.

In additional work with the same two subjects, Blau et al. (52) fed calcium gluconate with the basal low calcium diet. Endogenous fecal calcium excretions were estimated with three levels of intake (107 and 135 mg, 529 and 638 mg, 1,446 and 1,740 mg). The excretions calculated from the ratio of the specific activity of the feces to that of the urine were 91, 91, and 73 mg/day for one subject and 118, 87, and 93 mg/day for the other. Blau concluded that the endogenous fecal calcium was similar in amount to the urinary calcium (about 100 mg/day) and was independent of level of calcium intake.

Bronner and Harris (72) injected [45]Ca intravenously in a study of calcium absorption by human subjects. From determinations of the mean specific activity of the serum and the total [45]Ca excretion in the feces during a given length of time, they calculated the endogenous fecal calcium excretion. When these values were recalculated on the basis of 24-hour excretion, they ranged for seven subjects from 46 to 116 mg/day with a mean of 85 mg/day. In this study, from 5 to 15% of the total fecal calcium output was endogenous.

Heaney and Skillman (191) also used intravenous injections of [45]Ca. From measures of fecal radioactivity during 14 days after the injection, they calculated the mean endogenous fecal calcium excretion of 33 subjects to be 130 ± 47 mg/day. They reported, in contrast to Blau et al. (52), that the endogenous fecal excretion was correlated directly with both calcium intake and fecal output and was correlated inversely with rate of absorption.

Nordin et al. (369) estimated fecal ex-

cretion of endogenous calcium by means of intravenously administered [47]Ca and [85]Sr. Estimates ranged from 1.3 to 4.5 mg/kg daily when [47]Ca was used (7 normal and 7 osteoporotic patients) and from 0.5 to 5.0 mg/kg when [85]Sr was used (12 patients with various degenerative disorders). Their estimates were based as were those of Blau et al. (52, 53), Bronner and Harris (72), and Heaney and Skillman (191) on the assumption that dietary calcium and secreted digestive juice calcium are absorbed to the same extent. There is some evidence that this may not be true. Briscoe and Ragan (69), for instance, studying patients with fistulated bile ducts, concluded that biliary calcium was completely reabsorbed. Rose et al. (416), on the other hand, concluded from estimates of "net" and "true" absorption that very little of the secreted digestive juice calcium was reabsorbed. By their method, combining oral administration of [47]Ca and the conventional balance measurement, net secreted calcium (digestive juice calcium) was estimated from the difference between the true absorption and the net absorption of calcium. They suggested that, if their conclusion is true, estimates of endogenous fecal calcium based on the assumption that secreted calcium and food calcium are absorbed at the same rate may need reappraisal.

Urinary calcium excretion
(Appendix table 2)

Urinary calcium excretion seems to be a highly individual matter. Knapp (267) assembled data from 1494 studies with 533 subjects ranging in age from less than 1 year to 80 years. The objective of this study was to delineate the normal range of calcium excretion as an aid to diagnostics. In this collection of data, urinary calcium excretion increased with age during the growing period and it was greater in males than in females. Both the differences apparently due to age and to sex could be explained as due largely to differences in body size. Knapp suggested that skeletal size probably influenced the urinary calcium excretion during the growth period. In a more recent study with 59 young adults, a highly significant correlation was observed between urinary calcium and creatinine excretion (105, 411). Evidence of great variability in the relationship between urinary calcium and creatinine has been reported, however, by Garrido and Orozco (161). In their study of calcium–creatinine relationships in 665 persons, 1 to 90 years old, the mean calcium excretion was 256 mg per gram of creatinine with a coefficient of variation of 89.5%.

Knapp's collection of data showed also that urinary calcium excretion increased with increasing calcium intake. For instance, with intakes of 0 to 5 mg calcium per kilogram body weight the urinary calcium excretion ranged from 0.4 to 4.7 mg/kg, whereas with intakes above 75 mg/kg urinary calcium excretions between 0.9 and 11.4 mg/kg were recorded. When, however, the urinary calcium excretion was expressed as a percentage of the calcium intake, the proportion of ingested calcium that was excreted in the urine declined as intake increased. Wide variation in urinary calcium excretion was found among individuals of the same age, size, and with similar intakes. Knapp suggested that this variation indicated that, in addition to size and calcium intake, other factors "presumably endocrine" must govern urinary calcium output.

Nicolaysen et al. (361) have also reported wide variation in urinary calcium among subjects at any one level of calcium intake. Nicolaysen et al. (361) and Malm (322), however, reported only insignificant decreases in urinary output when the calcium intake of male prison inmates was reduced from about 900 to 450 mg/day. These intakes, as Malm pointed out, were approximately 13.4 mg and 6.5 mg/kg body weight. The intakes on which Knapp based her conclusions ranged from 0 to more than 75 mg/kg body weight. The differences in urinary excretion at the lower segment of the intake range were not great. It is likely, therefore, that the two collections of data are in closer agreement on this point than the investigators' conclusions indicate. Recently, however, Paunier et al. (388) studied urinary calcium excretion of 38 children (1 month to 14 years old) with a wide range of calcium intakes, 21.0 to 162.0 mg/kg. Urinary excretions also varied greatly from 1.1 to 7.4 mg/kg but were not significantly related to intake. Nicolaysen et al. (361) found that there

was variation in urinary excretion within the individual which "occurred mostly in the form of waves developing over some months." Day to day urinary calcium variations in an individual did coincide with variations in intake. Nicolaysen concluded from the results of 4 years of study that the "urinary calcium level, considered over some time, is an individual constant which presumably is conditioned by endogenous factors (hormonal status). Day to day variations occur frequently and are considerable. They closely reflect variations in the daily calcium intake."

If urinary calcium excretion does increase with increasing calcium intake, one would expect that urinary levels during fasting would be minimal levels. Studies with fasting men (42, 87, 286) did show declining excretion values during the course of the fast. With the resumption of food intake there was an increase in urinary calcium with some subjects (87), whereas in other studies (42, 286) there was a further decrease.

Bauer et al. (27), in reporting their study of calcium excretion of 13 subjects with low calcium diets containing 109 mg/day, summarized the data from the literature and found, as Knapp did, that calcium excretion was lower with their low calcium diets than it was with high calcium diets. They also found that the urinary excretion with their low calcium diets (about 63 mg Ca/day) was lower than that observed during fasting (about 256 mg Ca/day) (42, 87, 286). Bauer et al. explained this by suggesting that the fasting men were consuming their own flesh and therefore were subsisting on a "very acid" diet. Similar low levels of calcium excretion with low calcium intakes have been reported by Blau et al. (52, 53) (51 and 90 mg/day for two subjects) and Bassir (24) (84 mg/day for 99 men and women).

The effect of "acid-forming" and "base-forming" diets upon calcium metabolism has been the subject of numerous studies and reviews (59, 144, 285, 292, 303, 350, 355, 422, 443, 445). Lavan (285) has summarized the hypotheses that have been proposed to explain the increase in urinary calcium that is observed in acidotic subjects as follows: . . . "Albright et al. (1964) (8) maintained that in tubular acidosis 'calcium being a base, will appear in increased amounts in the urine,' whereas Epstein (1960) (139) considered that the urinary calcium excretion of metabolic acidosis was the result of a primary dissolution of bone rather than the requirement for calcium as a urinary buffer. Walser and Robinson (1963) (502) suggested that the augmented urinary calcium excretion in acute acidosis was directly related to, and dependent on a concomitant increase in urinary sodium excretion. On the basis of an increased urine calcium in spite of a reduction in the calculated filtered load of this substance, Lemann et al. (1967) (293) considered the calcium excretion in cases of metabolic acidosis to be the result of a direct effect of such acidosis on the metabolic processes within the renal tubular cells. Finally, it is possible that the increased urine calcium in acidosis results from the increased ultrafilterable fraction of calcium that is found with reduction of blood pH (Myers, 1962) (354)." [2]

Among other factors that may affect urinary calcium excretion are protein intake, phosphorus intake (in particular, the calcium to phosphorus ratio in the diet), other minerals, and dietary factors that affect absorption.

Protein intake. Numerous investigators have noted an increase in urinary calcium excretion when the level of dietary protein was raised (178, 194, 239, 321, 330, 331, 429, 435). In most of the studies the increase in urinary calcium was offset by an increase in absorbed calcium so that calcium balance was unchanged. In a study by Johnson et al. (239), however, when the protein intake of six youths was raised from 48 to 141 g/day, urinary calcium excretion almost doubled while calcium absorption increased only slightly. Johnson et al. (239) suggested that the increased level of urinary calcium with higher protein intake was due to changes in acid–base balance. Knapp (267), however, concluded from reviewing her own work as well as that of others that there is a small but consistent protein effect even when acid–base balance is not changed.

Phosphorus intake. The "protein effect" has been confounded at times by changes in Ca/P ratio. An increase in calcium intake without a proportional increase in

phosphorus intake is reflected in greater urinary calcium excretion (267, 288, 299, 300). Conversely, an increase in phosphorus without a proportional increase in calcium intake is accompanied by a decrease in urinary calcium (119, 170, 267, 321). The effect of the Ca/P ratio is not as great on calcium balance as it is on urinary calcium. Patton et al. (387), for instance, in a study with 18 women on the effect of the Ca/P ratio on calcium balance found that, when calcium intake was held constant, additions of phosphorus to the diet did not affect calcium retention. On the other hand, when phosphorus intake was held constant, calcium retention rose with increasing levels of calcium in the diet. Malm (321) also found that the addition of phosphates to the diet did not affect calcium balance. Patton et al. (387) concluded that calcium retention is much more closely related to calcium intake than to the Ca/P ratio.

Other minerals. Among the other minerals that have been reported to affect calcium excretion in the urine are sodium, fluorine and magnesium. Kleeman et al. (266) have reported that, in a study with six healthy adults, urinary calcium was directly related to urinary sodium which, in turn, varied with sodium chloride intake. Sodium fluoride ingestion, on the other hand, has been reported to be accompanied by decreases in urinary calcium excretion (45). Previously, however, Wagner and Muhler (495) had reported finding no relationship between urinary calcium excretion and fluoride intake. Increased magnesium intakes with an otherwise constant diet have been reported to result in increased urinary calcium output and decreased fecal output. The overall effect was an improvement in calcium balance (193).

Other factors. Numerous other factors have been reported to influence urinary calcium excretion. For instance, Phang et al. (392) reported that feeding milk in six equal doses during the day resulted in a greater urinary calcium excretion than feeding the same amount of milk in a single dose. Lactose when substituted for sucrose in the diets of five children reduced urinary calcium excretion signifi-

---

[2] Quoted with permission of the Editor, Irish J. Med. Sci.

cantly and thereby improved calcium retention (344). Vitamin D administration was reported by Chu et al. (90) to result in increased urinary calcium and decreased fecal calcium output. McKay et al. (335), on the other hand, could detect no marked change in either urinary or fecal output when vitamin D was added to the diet. Chu's subjects included three patients with osteomalacia whereas McKay's study was carried out with healthy women.

Decreased fecal excretion indicates increased apparent absorption. McCance and Widdowson (330) observed a close correlation between urinary calcium excretion and apparent calcium absorption. They suggested that changes in urinary calcium output could be used as an indicator of changes in absorption. Their studies were with adult subjects. Knapp (267) could fiind no evidence in her compilation of data for a similar relationship during the growth period.

The facts that a) there has not been a clear determination of minimum urinary calcium excretion and b) urinary calcium is influenced by factors as yet not clearly defined, introduce an unavoidable element of speculation into the estimation of calcium requirements by the factorial method. Nicolaysen et al. (361) using Knapp's (267) collection of data estimated an average urinary calcium excretion of 175 mg/day (minimum 35 mg, maximum 420 mg) for a 70-kg man eating 10 mg calcium/kg body weight. He pointed out that the data indicated little reduction in urinary excretion if the calcium intake were reduced from 10 to 2 mg/kg. Whedon (513) using the same data (267) as the basis of his estimations suggested 200 mg/day as a "reasonable upper limit" for urinary calcium excretion of healthy adults.

Dermal calcium losses (Appendix table 2)

Calcium losses through the skin, principally in sweat, were reported in 1931 (64, 324). Concentrations ranging from 0 to 20 mg/100 cc of sweat were found (64, 147, 475). In these studies with adult subjects the total quantity of sweat excreted was not recorded. Swanson and Iob (474) studied five normal infants, 2 to 24 weeks old. Data were obtained from 14 observations. Each observation consisted of a 6-

day period during which an infant was kept on a metabolism frame that allowed the separate collection of urine and feces. Skin losses of minerals were estimated by analyzing the distilled water in which the baby and his clothing were washed every 24 hours. Calcium losses varied from 0.07 to 0.23 mmoles per day (2.8 to 9.2 mg/day). The data did not show any trend toward increasing or decreasing excretion of calcium with age. Much later Paupe (389) studying a group of subjects that ranged in age from infants to adults (47 infants, 41 children and 10 adults) found no significant differences in calcium concentration in sweat due to age. The mean concentrations were estimated as 102, 99, and 105 mg Ca/liter of sweat for the infants, children, and adults, respectively. The total daily calcium loss through the skin was not measured.

Swanson and Iob (474) considered that the dermal calcium losses observed in their study were negligible. Later Hawawini and Schreier (187) came to a different conclusion. In their study of dermal losses of nitrogen and minerals by 17 infants 2 to 13 weeks of age, they observed calcium losses of 10 to 30 mg/day. They concluded that "in balance studies of any kind, the skin as a metabolic and excreting organ should not be disregarded."

Quantitative studies of calcium losses through the skin of adults also have yielded variable data. Freyberg and Grant (155), for instance, found no trace of calcium losses through the skin of two healthy subjects when precautions were taken to avoid sweating. During the experimental period the subjects wore special underclothing. They continued to carry out their routine laboratory work. Later Mitchell and Hamilton (346) studied dermal losses of 6 men in a controlled environment chamber under "comfortable" conditions (27 to 28°, relative humidity 43 to 45%). Total sweat loss was estimated by weight changes. Sweat for analysis was obtained by mopping the body with towels which, together with the subjects' clothing, were washed with distilled water. The average dermal calcium loss under comfortable conditions was found to be 6.2 mg/hour, accounting for 14.4% of the total calcium excretion. The calcium loss under comfortable or minimal sweating conditions when calculated on a 24-hour basis was 149 mg. This loss, Mitchell and Hamilton suggested, represented a potential source of considerable error in balance experiments.

A similar conclusion was reached by Isaksson et al. (231, 232). By a combination of the conventional balance technique and an isotope dilution technique, they estimated the dermal loss of potassium. Then, after determining the Ca/K ratio in sweat, they estimated the cutaneous excretion of calcium. In one study (231) the dermal losses ranged from 19 to 300 mg calcium/day. In another report, dermal calcium losses estimated for 13 patients suffering from a variety of disorders ranged from 20 to 365 mg/day (232). The mean loss was about 120 mg calcium/day.

Consolazio et al. (97) and Gitelman and Lutwak,[3] on the other hand, reported losses of much smaller magnitude. In Consolazio's study, three young men were observed in an environmental chamber at 24° and 30% relative humidity for four 4-day periods. They exercised moderately for 30 minutes each day. The calcium excretion in the sweat under these conditions was found to approximate 70 mg/day or 3 mg/hour. Gitelman and Lutwak as reported by Whedon (513) studied total body skin losses for two consecutive 3-day periods in seven women, some of whom were ambulatory patients and others normal subjects. The mean dermal loss of calcium determined in two consecutive 3-day periods with each subject was 15.4 ± 10.8 mg/day.

Whedon (513) suggested on the basis of these data that in balance studies conducted at "minimal activity and in comfortable environmental temperatures" skin losses of calcium could be ignored. In a more recent study by Lutwak et al. (307) the sweat losses of two astronauts undergoing orbital space flight were estimated. During the preflight control phase, 24-hour sweat collections yielded 26 and 23 mg of calcium. During the 14-day orbital flight the mean dermal calcium excretions were 14 and 16 mg/day. Another 24-hour sweat collection by each man during the postflight period contained 43 and 45 mg calcium. These losses were considered to be insignificant in the overall balance estimate.

Mitchell and Hamilton (346) observed higher dermal losses in a hot humid environment than under comfortable conditions. When their subjects were studied at 37 to 39° with relative humidity 65 to 73%, the average dermal calcium loss was 20.2 mg/hour, accounting for 29.9% of the total calcium excretion. When total sweat loss was estimated from weight loss during the observation period, the calcium concentration was calculated to be 26.0 mg/kg sweat.

A similar mean concentration of 29.1 mg calcium/kg sweat was found with four women by Johnston et al. (241). The women, however, who were observed during periods of about 1 hour at 36° with relative humidity 74 to 90%, excreted much less sweat as estimated by weight changes than did the men. Their average dermal loss was about 8.54 mg calcium/hour. In this study, sweat losses from the scalp were not collected.

Consolazio et al. (99) observed high calcium excretion (0.79 to 1.95 g/day) by eight men undergoing energy requirement tests in a hot environment. The men had high calcium intakes (about 3.5 g/day). Subsequently, Consolazio et al. (97) reported a series of studies which were undertaken to determine the extent of dermal calcium losses under varying atmospheric conditions and with varying amounts of exercise. In these studies the total sweat loss was estimated from weight changes, and the concentration of calcium in sweat was determined on samples collected in arm bags. The data indicated that calcium excretion in sweat increased as atmospheric temperature increased. When the amount of controlled exercise was kept constant (100 minutes per day with a bicycle), mean sweat calcium excretion rates increased from 8.1 to 11.6 to 20.2 mg/hour as the environmental temperature rose from 21.1° to 29.4° to 37.8°. These values were obtained when four men spent 7.5 hours daily in a controlled environment chamber. Assuming an excretion of 3 mg calcium/hour for the 16.5 hours spent outside the environmental chamber, daily dermal calcium excretions of 111, 137 and 201 mg were calculated.

When exercise was restricted to 30 min-

---

[3] Gitelman, H. J. & Lutwak, L. (1963) Dermal losses of minerals in elderly women under nonsweating conditions. Clin. Res. 11, 42, (abstr.).

utes daily and the temperature in the environmental chamber was held at 37.8°, the calcium concentration in sweat of three men decreased during the 7.5-hour period spent each day in the chamber. The concentration dropped from day to day during the 16 days of observation. The amount of calcium excreted decreased also throughout the study from a mean of 36 mg/hour during the first 4-day period to 17 mg/hour during the fourth period. Evidence of acclimatization has been reported by others (136, 217, 346). No reports have indicated, however, that dermal losses, even in prolonged exposure to heat, drop to levels observed in temperate environments.

Consolazio et al. (97) noted that sweat calcium accounted for 22.7% of the total calcium excretion during exposure to hot temperatures. They suggested sweat losses might be in part responsible for retarded growth of children from semitropical or tropical regions where calcium intakes are relatively low. Walker and Richardson (501), however, measured height and weight in Zulu and Bantu children and reported no evidence of differences that could be attributed to environmental temperatures or sweat losses.

Lower sweat calcium losses than those shown in Consolazio's studies with high environmental temperatures were reported by Vellar and Askevold (489). In their study, total body sweat was collected from 27 men exposed for 60 minutes to temperatures of 40 to 45° with 80 to 90% relative humidity. The mean calcium concentration in sweat was 6.7 mg/liter and the mean calcium loss was 8.4 mg/hour. Vellar and Askevold attributed these lower values to the difference between total body sweat and arm bag sweat. Earlier, van Heyningen and Weiner (488) had found that sweat collected in an arm bag contained higher concentrations of chloride, lactate and urea than total body sweat. Consolazio et al. (98) compared the calcium content of arm bag sweat with that of total body sweat in a study with 12 men. The mean calcium excretion in total body sweat during 24 hours of observation at high atmospheric temperatures (38.5° in the day and 33.1° at night) was 7.7 mg/hour. Calcium excretion estimated from total body sweat analysis was 71 to 76% of that estimated by extrapolation from arm bag sweat analysis. The agreement was improved when more than 15 g of arm bag sweat was collected in any one exposure. Consolazio suggested that, though the mean loss of 7.7 mg calcium/hour was much lower than values reported earlier by his group, it represented a loss that should be considered in estimating calcium requirements.

No precise data have been found showing the effect of exercise on calcium excretion through the skin. In Consolazio's studies, comparisons from one level of exercise to another at any one temperature are difficult because of changes in subjects and in level of dietary calcium. Gontzea et al. (171) reported studies on calcium balance of men doing work. They measured sweat losses only during the work periods, however, so that valid comparisons cannot be made.

Consolazio et al. (97) intimated that the high dermal calcium excretions observed during their earlier studies in a hot environment might have been influenced by the high calcium intakes (3.6 and 3.5 g/day). In their subsequent studies the diets contained lower levels of calcium (1.5 to 1.7 g, 441 mg, and 581 mg/day). Again, however, because of differences in other experimental conditions from one experiment to another, it is difficult to draw conclusions on the effect of level of dietary calcium on dermal excretion.

While dermal calcium losses have usually been measured as sweat losses, one study has been reported in which the loss of calcium in hair was measured. In this study Johnston (240) estimated the average hair calcium loss of 12 young women to be 90 ± 63 mg per year. The color of the hair did not affect its calcium content.

Calcium absorption

Besides the obligatory fecal, urinary, and skin losses, the estimation of calcium requirements by the factorial method must take into account the losses due to incomplete absorption of dietary calcium. The absorption of some nutrients can be estimated by assuming that what is not excreted in the feces must have been absorbed into the body. The evidence of a secretion of calcium into the gut from the body makes this assumption untenable in calcium studies.

Before the development of radioactive isotope techniques, some methods were developed whereby indirect estimates of calcium absorption were attempted. The earliest of these (152), for obvious reasons, could not be used with human subjects. It consisted of feeding a food with or without added calcium to an experimental animal. Then, after an interval of several hours, the animal was killed and the contents of various parts of the gastrointestinal tract were analyzed for calcium. Similar information can be obtained now with reasonable safety in human subjects by collecting gastrointestinal contents with multilumen tubes (140, 511). The method, however, does not distinguish between food calcium and digestive juice calcium.

Kinsman et al. (264) noted that previous studies on availability of calcium in foods had provided comparative rather than quantitative values. Usually fluid whole milk was the reference standard. They proposed a method whereby a quantitative value might be obtained. It consisted of determining calcium balances at two levels of intake, both of which were "above the maintenance requirement but neither of which was in excess of the minimum requirement for maximum retention of calcium by the subjects." The proportion of dietary calcium utilized was determined by relating the increment in retention to the increment in intake. This, then, was a measure of utilized or retained calcium rather than a measure of available or absorbed calcium. It was based on the premise that the proportion of calcium retained was not influenced by changes in intake.

Reports in the literature indicated that with Kinsman's method or some variation of it, the utilization of milk calcium was observed to range from 19 to 32% (65, 264, 466, 467, 469). In one report (467) data on fecal excretion as well as on calcium retention were included. For nine men, absorption values, calculated by relating differences in absorption to differences in intake, ranged from 24 to 61% with a mean of 36% for calcium provided mainly by milk.

Malm (322) from a review of the literature, estimated that 400 to 1100 mg of

digestive juice calcium is secreted daily into the gut. The estimated average secretion, 760 mg/day, was used in a formula previously proposed by Nicolaysen et al. (361),

$$\% \text{ absorbed} = \frac{(1 - Ca_{feces}) \times 100}{Ca_{food} + Ca_{secretion}}$$

Malm pointed out that this average secretion value might be quite unrealistic when applied to an individual.

When radioactive tracers became available, more informative methods for determining calcium absorption and for distinguishing quantitatively between secreted digestive juice calcium and ingested dietary calcium were developed. Both ^{45}Ca (53) and ^{47}Ca (235) have been used. The former is usually employed only in patients with limited life expectancy. The isotopes are administered either orally or intravenously.

Relative absorption measurements with isotopic calcium. With oral administration of the isotope, relative absorption has been estimated by measuring the specific activity of the plasma drawn at selected intervals after ingestion of the isotope (16, 48). Kinney et al. (263), however, reported that they found no significant correlation between peak plasma ^{47}Ca levels and absorption of ^{47}Ca. They reported that they did find a relationship between urinary excretion of the isotope and absorption, but that the variability was too high for this relationship to have practical application. Lutwak and Shapiro (306) have reported also the estimation of relative absorption by means of the specific activity of the forearm as measured in a liquid scintillation counter after isotopic calcium has been ingested. The whole body counter has been used by Deller et al. (118) and by Agnew et al. (7).

Quantitative absorption measurements with one isotope. The conventional balance method has been used to obtain absolute or "net" absorption values of isotopic calcium. The absorption data thus calculated are applied to the total dietary calcium, but they are potentially no more precise than those calculated from measurements of stable calcium. The use of isotopic calcium, however, does permit the estimation of calcium absorption without a precise determination of total dietary calcium intake or fecal calcium output.

Unabsorbed food calcium may be estimated more precisely by determining how much of the fecal calcium is digestive juice calcium. To do this, both oral and intravenous administration of isotopic calcium have been used. The assumption is made that after administration, the isotope will eventually become uniformly distributed throughout the body in relation to stable calcium. Thus, the ratio of isotopic calcium to stable calcium will be the same in plasma, urine, and digestive juices.

When the isotope is administered orally, sufficient time must be allowed for all the unabsorbed tracer to be excreted. Then when it is reasonably certain that all tracer in the feces must be calcium that has been absorbed and then secreted back into the gut in the digestive juices, the specific activity of the feces is compared with that of the urine or the plasma. The total amount of unabsorbed digestive juice calcium is thus estimated, and the rest of the fecal calcium is assumed to be unabsorbed food calcium (52, 53).

Similarly when the isotope is administered intravenously, some of it eventually is secreted into the gut with the digestive juices. By comparing specific activities of feces and urine an estimate of the total unabsorbed digestive juice calcium can be made (72).

Another approach is to compare the specific activity of plasma (421) or of urine (75), after intravenous administration of tracer calcium, with that observed after the same amount of isotope is administered orally at a different time but under similar experimental conditions. The validity of this approach depends on the maintenance, as far as is possible, of identical experimental and metabolic conditions when the two doses are given. Samachson (421) compared the absorption coefficients calculated from plasma specific activity with those calculated from fecal values corrected for estimated secretion of digestive juice calcium. He reported that when absorption was low, plasma activity levels yielded more accurate (less variable) absorption data than fecal values did.

Quantitative absorption measurements with two isotopes. Some investigators have used two isotopes, ^{45}Ca and ^{47}Ca, simultaneously, one administered orally and the other intravenously (114, 304, 325). Unabsorbed ingested calcium thus can be distinguished from secreted calcium (digestive juice calcium) in the feces more quickly than when only one isotope is used. DeGrazia and Rich (114) calculated intestinal absorption from the ratio of specific activities of the two isotopes in the urine 24 hours after the oral and intravenous doses were administered. Mautalen et al. (325) compared absorption values obtained by measuring a) fecal excretion corrected for endogenous calcium, b) the ratio of orally to intravenously administered calcium appearing in the urine, and c) the ratio of orally to intravenously administered calcium in the plasma in 14 subjects. They found that the three methods gave similar mean values and were equally reliable as indicated by similar standard errors of the means.

In all of these methods the assumptions are made that the body does not distinguish between ^{40}Ca and ^{45}Ca or ^{47}Ca and that secreted digestive juice calcium and dietary calcium are absorbed to the same extent. Lutwak (304) in reviewing the available methods, decided that the most reliable information could be obtained by using two tracers and prolonged fecal collections. Isaksson and Sjögren (233) agreed that, in addition to isotope methods, the balance technique is necessary. In a critical evaluation of the balance method, however, they pointed out that variation in measured fecal output is a serious limitation. They advocated that cumulative calcium balances be recorded and that the fecal collection be continued until the cumulative balance has reached a plateau for at least three periods. In their studies, 4-day collection periods apparently were used.

The results of studies using radioactive calcium indicate that calcium is not well absorbed. Furthermore, there is much variation from one study to another and from one individual to another in the same study. For example, Blau et al. (52, 53) used orally administered ^{45}Ca with two patients believed to have normal calcium metabolism. They found absorption rates of 44 and 67% when the subjects were eating low calcium diets. In five subjects studied with varying calcium intakes and experimental treatments, Samachson (421) found absorption rates that varied from 18 to 69% when estimated from specific activity of the feces and from 20 to 81% when measured by plasma activity. In studying gastrointestinal absorption after oral administration of ^{47}Ca plus intravenous administration of ^{45}Ca, Mautalen et al. (325) found "true absorption" values ranging from 30.7 to 60.6% in 20 subjects.

Many factors are believed to influence calcium absorption. Among them are vitamin D, the level of calcium intake, other dietary components, the age of the subject, and hormonal activity.

Vitamin D. Bauer and Marble (29) with two adult subjects eating carefully controlled diets, found evidence that the administration of 30 mg irradiated ergosterol resulted in a decrease in fecal calcium excretion. In additional studies (30) with two other subjects, increases in the level of serum calcium following the administration of irradiated ergosterol convinced Bauer et al. that vitamin D increases the absorption of calcium from the gastrointestinal tract. They noted in some subjects, however, that urinary calcium also rose indicating that the extra absorbed calcium was "not necessarily retained." Other studies reviewed and reported by Chu et al. (91) showed improved calcium absorption with irradiation of the body or with administration of vitamin D. Studies with rats reviewed by Harrison (183) and by Nicolaysen (360) indicated that vitamin D is most effective in increasing absorption when the concentration of calcium in the gut is low. Nicolaysen (360) was of the opinion that vitamin D is "the primary regulating factor of importance throughout life." He postulated further that there is another regulating factor, "'the endogenous factor,' hypothetically a hormonal factor, which will strongly regulate absorption in the presence of vitamin D in the body but not in the vitamin D-free body." Heaney (189) suggested that this "endogenous factor" is probably the parathyroid hormone. Nordin (367), in reviewing animal studies on calcium absorption, observed that both vitamin D and parathyroid hormone are of primary importance in calcium transport.

Whether the hormone is fully dependent upon the vitamin is not clear (12).

Level of intake. The "endogenous factor" is responsible in Nicolaysen's opinion for the adjustment of absorption to the level of calcium intake. Clark (92) in studying nitrogen and mineral retention of five prison inmates noted that increases in calcium intake of from 28 to 53% resulted in no significant changes in retention. An examination of the balance data shows that when the calcium intake was increased, fecal excretion (and, to a much lesser extent, urinary excretion) increased also. The result of increased intake was a decreased rate of absorption but not necessarily decreased quantity of calcium absorbed. Similar evidence was provided later by Kraut and Wecker (274).

Clark also suggested that the calcium retention of the men was influenced by their previous diet. This hypothesis was based on the observation that prisoners whose previous calcium intake could be assumed to be low retained much more calcium than those who were known to have had an adequate diet. An examination of the data indicates that differences among the subjects in level of retention were largely due to differences in fecal output and, therefore, presumably due to differences in rate of absorption.

Thorangkul et al. (483) using a diet providing 200 to 300 mg calcium per day, studied absorption and retention of calcium by subjects accustomed to low (350 to 700 mg) and high (1,250 to 2,000 mg) calcium intakes. The subjects accustomed to low calcium intakes had slightly higher mean absorption rates than those accustomed to high intakes. When, however, the means of two subjects who were believed to be still growing were excluded, there was little diference between the two groups. During 95 days of study, five of seven subjects appeared to be adapting to reduced calcium intake by reducing their fecal excretion. One of these subjects, however, had an increase in urinary excretion resulting in a reduced retention. Leitch and Aitken (291) pointed out, in reviewing this work, that the balance studies included only one level of intake and that this intake was "well below probable endogenous loss."

In Malm's study with Norwegian prisoners (322), adaptation to reduced calcium intake depended largely on reduction in fecal excretion. Assuming a calcium secretion into the gut of 750 mg/day, Malm calculated the mean absorption of 20 men who adapted in 28 to 252 days to reduced intakes as follows. With intakes of about 940 mg, absorption was 62%; with intakes of about 450 mg, absorption before adaptation was 72%; and after adaptation 78%. The differences in mean absorption rates were statistically significant ($P = <0.001$). When no allowance was made for secretion of calcium in digestive juice, the "net absorption" was calculated to be 31% with the high intake and 27 and 43% before and after adaptation to the low intake. Three men adapted immediately when their calcium intake was reduced from 940 to 450 mg/day. When allowance was made for calcium secretion into the gut, their mean rate of absorption was 65% with the higher intake and 83% with the lower intake. When no allowance was made for secreted calcium, their mean "net absorption" was 37 and 54% with the higher and lower intakes.

Nordin (367) reported on the basis of 56 balance studies that fecal calcium (y) was related to dietary calcium (x) according to the following equation:

$$y = 0.742\,x + 0.45\ \text{mg/kg.}$$

When net absorption (ingested calcium minus fecal calcium) was calculated from this formula, he found that as intake increased from very low levels, net absorption increased from zero until it reached a maximum level of 12.5 mg/kg with an intake of 45 mg/kg. He suggested that 10 to 15 mg/kg body weight should be regarded as the "maximum absorptive capacity for calcium of normal subjects."

Other dietary components. Malm (322) was confident that the differences in rate of absorption in his study were due principally to adaptation to different levels of intake. In other studies, changes in absorption have been effected by changes in dietary components accompanying the calcium. One such dietary component is protein. Early Chinese work (6) indicated that calcium absorption was higher with a high protein diet (13 to 15 g N/day equivalent

to 81 to 94 g protein/day) than with a low protein diet (6 to 7 g N/day equivalent to 37 to 44 g protein/day). Similarly, Kunerth and Pittman (279) and Pittman and Kunerth (395) found increased absorption of calcium (dietary calcium minus fecal calcium) when dietary protein was almost tripled (from 4 to 11 g N/day or from 25 to 69 g protein/day). In their studies and in the Chinese study, urinary calcium was not appreciably affected. The net result therefore was an improvement in calcium balance. McCance et al. (330) also found increased calcium absorption when diets containing 45 to 70 g of protein were supplemented with 100 to 130 g of purified protein. Urinary calcium excretion, however, increased with increasing protein intake but not to the same extent as absorption was improved. In an extension of this work, Hall and Lehmann (178) developed a "peptone powder" that was found in studies with normal subjects and mentally disturbed patients to enhance calcium absorption. Hall and Lehmann measured urinary calcium rather than fecal calcium excretion. They assumed that urinary calcium reflects the amount of calcium entering the body from the gastrointestinal tract. Their observed increases in urinary calcium when the "peptone powder" was eaten were interpreted as indicating greater calcium absorption. Hegsted et al. (194) also observed improved calcium absorption by Peruvian prison inmates when meat was added to the diet. Urinary calcium excretion also increased so that calcium retention was not improved. Hegsted interpreted these observations as indicating that the subjects "were not in great need of additional calcium."

Schofield and Morrell (429), on the other hand, found no significant difference in mean calcium absorption by preadolescent girls when the protein intake varied from approximately 1 g/kg per day to 2 to 3 g/kg per day. Urinary calcium excretion was greater with the two higher protein intakes but not enough greater to change the calcium balance.

More recently Johnson et al. (239) studied calcium absorption of 18- to 20-year-old youths. The diets provided 1.4 g calcium and 48 or 141 g protein per day. With the high protein diet, calcium absorption was greater by a mean of 69 mg/day than with the low protein diet. This increase was not statistically significant. Mean urinary calcium excretion (175 mg and 338 mg/day with the low protein and high protein diets respectively) was significantly increased with the result that mean calcium balance was lowered from +10 mg to −84 mg/day.

In Johnson's study the change in quantity of protein was effected without a change in quality of protein. Studies with animals indicate that quality of protein may affect calcium absorption (121) and that the addition of certain amino acids (e.g., lysine, arginine) to the diet promotes absorption (507).

Evidence of an effect of phosphorus, in particular of the calcium to phosphorus ratio on calcium absorption, is conflicting. Leichsenring et al. (288) studied calcium and phosphorus retention by young women eating a basal diet providing approximately 300 mg calcium and 800 mg phosphorus (Ca/P = 0.38). About 24% of the calcium was absorbed (ingested calcium minus fecal calcium). When the diet was supplemented with about 1200 mg of calcium as calcium carbonate (Ca/P = 1.85), about 27% of the calcium was absorbed and retention increased. When, however, in addition to the supplemental calcium, about 600 g of phosphorus (dibasic calcium phosphate and dibasic sodium phosphate) was added (Ca/P = 1.06), calcium absorption declined to about 12%. Calcium retention decreased also. Leichsenring concluded that the amount of phosphorus was a factor of importance in influencing calcium utilization. Widdowson et al. (517) also concluded that phosphorus intake influenced calcium retention. In their study, however, when breast-fed infants were given 120 mg of phosphorus as the neutral sodium and potassium salt, changing the Ca/P ratio from 1.96 to 0.77, calcium absorption and retention *increased*. Widdowson suggested that their results supported an earlier hypothesis that calcification of bone and growth of soft tissue were limited in early infancy by the amount of phosphorus in breast milk.

Unlike Leichsenring et al. (288) and Widdowson et al. (517), Spencer et al.

(458) found no clear evidence of an effect of phosphorus intake on calcium absorption. They studied the absorption of calcium by adult patients at two levels of calcium intake with and without supplemental glycerophosphate. With both the low calcium diet (140 to 272 mg Ca/day) and the high calcium diet (1180 to 2080 mg Ca/day), the addition of phosphorus (972 and 893 mg) did not result in consistent changes in fecal calcium excretion.

When dietary phosphorus occurs as phytin there is evidence that calcium absorption is impaired. McCance and Widdowson (327) observed in a study with 10 men and women that calcium was more highly absorbed from 69% extraction flour than from 92% extraction flour. Similarly, Krebs and Mellanby (275) observed that six men absorbed less calcium from diets containing "National wheatmeal" (85% extraction) than from those containing white flour (75% extraction). To confirm their hypothesis that it was the phytin component of the high extraction flour that was responsible for the difference in absorption, McCance and Widdowson (327) compared the response of eight men and women to diets containing white bread with and without sodium phytate. The results of this experiment showed that a marked decrease in calcium absorption accompanied the addition of sodium phytate to the diet. A second study (328) in which the subjects ate diets containing bread made with dephytinized flour provided further confirmation.

Cullumbine et al. (104) studied the response of 12 men to diets containing polished or unpolished rice. With the unpolished rice, containing 225 mg phytic phosphorus/100 g, fecal calcium output was higher and balances were lower than with the polished rice diet containing 81 mg phytic phosphorus/100 g. When a second polished rice containing more calcium but also somewhat more phytin than the first one was used, the proportion of dietary calcium excreted in the feces remained the same but the calcium retention increased. Cruickshank et al. (103), on the other hand, found that the rate of calcium absorption improved when calcium was added to a diet based on oatmeal (containing approximately 574 mg phytic phosphorus), but the effect on calcium retention was not consistent.

In most of these studies (275, 327, 328) the periods of observation varied from 12 days to 4 weeks in length. Hoff-Jørgensen et al. (206) observed that two 10-year-old boys tended to "adapt" after the first 5 days of a 15-day period with a high phytin diet. Calcium balances that had been negative in the first 5 days became positive but were much lower than those observed before phytin was added to the diet. They suggested that if the boys had continued to eat the high phytin diet for a longer time their absorption might have continued to improve. When Cullumbine et al. (104) maintained their subjects on the unpolished rice diet for 18 weeks, there was improved retention of calcium indicating possible adaptation to the high phytin diet. Walker et al. (500) studied the effect of high phytin diets on the calcium metabolism of three men in periods ranging from 3 to 19 consecutive weeks. They observed that, over the course of the study, fecal calcium excretion gradually declined. On the basis of their observations in this study and on the calculated calcium and phytin contents of cereal diets "commonly consumed in various parts of the world," they suggested that adaptation to low calcium, high phytin intakes probably occurs.

In later studies using [45]Ca, Bronner et al. (73) observed that calcium uptake from "low-calcium breakfasts" (83 to 91 mg calcium) was reduced when the breakfast contained oatmeal with naturally occurring phytate (116 to 118 mg phytic phosphorus) or farina plus sodium phytate (78 mg phytic phosphorus) as compared to farina with no phytate. The absolute amount of calcium rendered unavailable, however, was very small (15 mg). When a "moderate-calcium breakfast" (234 to 244 mg Ca) was used (74), no significant difference in calcium absorption was observed between oatmeal (80 mg phytic phosphorus) and farina (no phytate). Bronner et al. concluded that the effect of phytate on calcium was of no nutritional concern in the United States.

Other minerals that have been suggested as influencing calcium absorption are magnesium and fluorine. An increase in dietary magnesium has been accompanied by a decrease in fecal calcium excretion (70, 133, 193). As noted previously (page 1031) in some studies (70, 193), urinary calcium excretion increased when fecal excretion decreased. Fluoride has been reported to improve calcium balance in osteoporotic patients (408). Spencer et al. (454, 455) found, however, in studies with [47]Ca that fluoride had little effect on calcium absorption. In one study (454) the addition of 20.6 mg sodium fluoride per day to the diet resulted in a small but statistically significant decrease in absorption. In another study (455) calcium absorption remained unchanged. In both studies urinary calcium excretion decreased.

The excretion of large amounts of calcium in the feces in steatorrhea had sugguested that diets high in fat might affect calcium absorption (14). Early studies with young children (214, 215, 355) and adults (14, 320) indicated that the quantity of fat in the diet had little effect on fecal calcium excretion. Studies with animals, however (153, 154, 359), produced conflicting data. In later work with three men, Steggerda and Mitchell (470) found that raising the dietary levels of milk fat from 1 to 32% of the dry matter did not significantly affect the proportion of calcium excreted in the feces. Similarly in studies with six young women, Meyer et al. (340) found that lowering the fat intake from 76 to 24 g/day did not significantly change fecal excretion of calcium. Fuqua and Patton (157) also found no relationship between level of fat intake and calcium balance. Their report did not give detailed information on fecal calcium excretion.

Annual studies reviewed by Speckmann and Brink (453) suggest that the effect of fat on calcium absorption may depend on the kind of fat in the diet. There is some evidence that this may be true also in human subjects. Basu and Nath (26) studied the mineral metabolism of four young men eating diets which provided 187 to 512 mg calcium per day and in which the fat was supplied principally by mustard oil, coconut oil, groundnut oil, sesame oil or butterfat. Response to an almost fat-free diet was also studied. The addition of each of the fats except coconut oil resulted in a slightly decreased excretion of fecal calcium. With coconut oil there was a distinct increase in fecal calcium and also in urinary calcium. Basu and Nath concluded that coconut oil should not be recommended for use as the main dietary fat.

Other dietary components that have been suggested as influencing calcium absorption are orange juice, citric acid and ascorbic acid. Studies with both children (88, 108, 508) and adults (287, 468), however, provide conflicting data.

The food source of the calcium that is incorporated into the diet may also affect its absorbability. Schroeder et al. (430), for instance, found that the calcium in whole cooked soybeans was less well utilized than the calcium in "soybean milk." They attributed most of the difference to differences in fecal excretion. They suggested that the bulk of the whole soybeans interfered with calcium absorption. Bricker et al. (66) found that the inclusion of cocoa in a diet in which a large part of the calcium was provided by milk resulted in increased fecal calcium excretion. Urinary calcium decreased, however, so that calcium balances were·not significantly affected. Brine and Johnston (67) suggested that the effect of cocoa was probably due to its oxalic acid content. Johnston et al. (242) added spinach to a diet providing about 820 mg calcium/day. The resultant increase in fecal calcium excretion was just slightly greater than the amount of calcium provided by the spinach (160 mg). Johnston et al. concluded that the spinach (containing 0.6 g oxalic acid) prevented the absorption of "an amount of calcium equivalent to that in the spinach." They suggested that there was a possibility that more calcium might have been excreted in the feces if the spinach had been served in a meal containing milk and cheese, the main sources of calcium in the diet. In their study, the spinach was served in the morning or evening meal whereas the milk and cheese were served in the noon meal. Bonner et al. (63), however, had previously been unable to show that the daily addition of 100 g of spinach containing 0.7 g oxalic acid to the diet of preadolescent children had any deleterious effect on calcium absorption.

The usefulness of different calcium salts as dietary supplements has been studied (128, 261, 385, 386, 430, 465, 466, 469). These studies indicated that the calcium in bone meal, dicalcium phosphate, and calcium gluconate, sulfate, lactate or carbonate were as well utilized as the calcium of milk. Radiocalcium studies on absorption per se, however (459), indicated that calcium from the lactate salt was absorbed significantly better than calcium from gluconate. The inclusion of lactose itself in the diet has been found to improve calcium absorption in elderly patients whose absorption was poor (175).

Data summarized by Harrison (183) indicate that calcium absorption decreases as the subject ages from infancy to adulthood. Whether elderly people absorb calcium less well than young adults is not as clear (68). Avioli et al. (15) compared absorption of 59 normal women 12 to 85 years of age by measuring plasma activity 1 hour after an oral test dose of ^{47}Ca. The mean plasma ^{47}Ca concentrations of premenopausal women 16 to 32 years old, postmenopausal women 36 to 54 years old, and postmenopausal women 55 to 85 years old (2.67%, 2.14%, 1.92% of the administered dose per liter plasma, respectively) indicated that changes in hormonal activity may be responsible for some changes in absorptive ability with age. An earlier study by Cofer et al. (94), in which increased fecal calcium excretion was observed in two of three women after the withdrawal of diethylstilbestrol therapy or of natural estrogens, provided corroborating evidence.

Bullamore et al. (79) studied calcium absorption in 75 men and 115 women, 20 to 95 years old. Absorption was estimated by plasma radioactivity after oral administration of ^{45}Ca or ^{47}Ca. Their data indicated that absorption fell with age, starting at age 55 to 60 years in women and at 65 to 70 years in men. Observations on the effect of vitamin D supplementation indicated that vitamin D deficiency in older people may be a contributing factor to the decline in calcium absorption.

Seasonal changes also, with greater absorption in July and August than in February and March, have been reported by McCance and Widdowson (329). These changes were observed in three out of six people studied at intervals throughout the years from 1940 to 1942. Evidence of cyclical changes in absorption from year to year as well as from season to season within the year was noted. Urinary calcium excretion rose and fell parallel to absorption. Malm (322) reported calcium balance data obtained with 43 men during 8 to 22 months of continuous observation. Balances were better in June through December than in January through May. The largest number of better retentions was found in August and September. Malm considered these data to be strong corroboration of the English work (329).

STUDIES ON ADDITIONAL FACTORS
THAT MAY AFFECT CALCIUM
REQUIREMENTS

Immobilization

Increased urinary and fecal excretion of calcium during immobilization has been reported frequently (115–117, 124, 170, 222, 234, 307, 309, 310, 404). Reifenstein's early observations (404) were obtained with patients undergoing surgery and subsequent bed rest. He reported that with immobilization after surgery there was a twofold increase in urinary calcium and a 30% increase in fecal calcium but no change in serum calcium levels. Similar observations were reported by Howard et al. (22) in a study with 17 patients immobilized with bone fractures. Studies by Deitrick et al. (115–117) with four healthy young men confined in plaster casts, or ambulatory with controlled exercise, for periods as long as 6 to 8 weeks, provided similar data and clearly indicated that the calcium losses observed by Reifenstein and Howard were not due principally to the stress of injury. Deitrick (115) pointed out that urinary calcium excretion was most significantly affected and because there was no change in other factors influencing calcium solubility such as urinary pH and citric acid excretion, there was an increased danger of urinary calculi formation during immobilization.

Since those early studies, investigations on the effect of immobilization have focused principally on two aspects, inactivity and recumbency. With the rapidly developing technology in space flight, a third feature, high altitude and weightlessness has become of interest also.

Radiocalcium (^{45}Ca) studies by Heaney (189) showed that in paralyzed adults with acutely developing osteoporosis, bone formation rates were normal or as high as twice normal. Bone resorption rates were increased to two to three times normal. Negative calcium balances were more than accounted for by the increased bone resorption rates. Studies with rats (282) however, indicated that depressed bone formation as well as increased bone destruction occurred. In these studies, bone formation was estimated by the uptake of tetracycline. When a rat's hind limb was immobilized by nerve section, there was first diminished bone formation, then increased bone formation and increased bone destruction, then finally, decreased bone formation. The overall effect was a diminished rate of bone formation and an increased rate of bone destruction.

Further evidence of a decreased amount of bone with decreased activity has been reported by Vose and Keele (494). They estimated bone density by radiological densitometry in 553 mentally retarded patients 5 to 30 years old. Of these, 254 were ambulatory. The others were bedfast but were classified as active, moderately active, or inactive. Bone density decreased with diminished activity. All classes of bedfast patients had lower bone density than the ambulatory patients. In the active and moderately active bedfast patients there was an increase in bone density with age as is characteristic in ambulatory patients in this age range. In the completely inactive bedfast group, however, there was an 18% decrease in bone density as age progressed from 5 to 30 years.

Donaldson et al. (124) studied calcium excretion and bone mass changes in three healthy young men who were restricted to complete bed rest for 30 to 36 weeks. Urinary calcium excretion rose during the first 7 weeks, then gradually fell but did not return to baseline levels during the bed rest period. Fecal calcium excretion also rose during the bed rest period. Calcium balance was, of course, depressed. During a 3-week reambulation period, calcium excretions fell and calcium balances returned to normal. Gamma ray transmission scanning indicated large mineral losses (25 to 45%) from the *os calcis* during bed rest.

The bone mineral was reaccumulated during reambulation at a rate similar to the rate at which it was lost during bed rest. Calcium balance data indicated that about 4.2% of the total body calcium was lost during the bed rest period. The disproportionately large loss from the *os calcis* suggested to the investigators that the major mineral loss is from the weight-bearing bones during immobilization.

Whether the increased calcium loss during immobilization was due to inactivity or recumbency or both cannot be ascertained from Donaldson's data. Earlier, Issekutz et al. (234) concluded from a study with 14 men that the supine position itself with the absence of longitudinal pressure on the long bones was responsible for their observed increased excretion of calcium. In this study, the subjects underwent complete bed rest for 18 days. Then they were subjected to combinations of either bed rest (23 hours) and exercise (bicycle ergometer) in the supine or sitting position (1 hour), bed rest (16 hours) and quiet sitting (8 hours), or bed rest (21 hours) and quiet standing (3 hours). Neither exercise nor quiet sitting decreased calcium excretion. When, however, the quiet standing program was instituted, calcium excretion declined slowly in four out of five subjects.

In an additional experiment, two men underwent complete bed rest for 21 days followed by another similar period when each man was subjected for 3 hours each day to pressure equal to his weight along the longitudinal axis of the body. In one subject this treatment was accompanied by decreased calcium excretion. In the other man there was no change in excretion.

The observation by radiographic densitometry of small losses in bone mass from the *os calcis* by astronauts in space flight (310, 311) had suggested that weightlessness may impose a demineralizing stress (186). Lynch et al. (309) however, found that men subjected to bed rest at ground level had higher urinary calcium excretions than men subjected to bed rest at simulated altitudes of 10,000 and 12,000 feet. Lutwak et al. (307) suggested, in view of the Lynch study, that the increased calcium excretion during space flight might have been due to hyperoxic conditions in the spacecraft.

Whether the increased excretion can be balanced by increased intake has not been shown. Indeed, the danger of urinary calculi has suggested that calcium intake of paralyzed patients should be restricted. Heaney (189), however, pointed out that because of depressed absorption with immobilization, this type of therapy is probably not needed.

Mack et al. (311) have reported that in a study with healthy men subjected to 14-day periods of bed rest, the proportion of bone lost from the *os calcis* decreased as calcium intake increased from 300 to 2,000 mg/day. Urinary and fecal calcium excretion increased quantitatively but decreased proportionately as intake increased. In the Gemini IV and V missions the mean proportion of bone loss was greater than that of earthbound men undergoing bed rest with similar calcium intakes. In the Gemini VII flight the mean proportion of bone loss of the crew was less than that of the crews of Gemini IV and V. Mack and LaChance (310) pointed out that the Gemini VII crew consumed a larger portion of their diet than did the crews of Gemini IV and V. They thus had calcium intakes of approximately 900 mg/day as compared to intakes of approximately 700 to 350 mg/day in the earlier flights. Another difference was that an isometric exercise program was included in the Gemini VII mission. In the study of Lynch et al. (309), however, the inclusion of isometric exercises at each simulated altitude level did not significantly affect calcium excretion.

Goldsmith et al. (170) reported that with subjects immobilized in body casts for 40 days, those who received a phosphate supplement had lowered urinary calcium excretion and no crystalluria. Hypercalciuria and crystalluria which occurred in subjects not receiving phosphate supplements were reversed when supplementation began. Keele and Vose (257), on the other hand, observed no significant change in bone density when phosphate supplements were administered to bedfast patients in an 18-month study. Supplements of sodium fluoride or an anabolic steroid (oxymetholone) resulted in faster increases in bone density than in a control group receiving no supplements. In a 15-month follow-up study, however, following discontinuation of the supplements (258), the investigators found that the gains in bone mass had been lost as rapidly as they had been made. Keele and Vose suggested that the results indicated that the bone mineral deposits added as a result of the supplementation were in a less stable state than those naturally occurring. They suggested further that continuous treatment with low doses of fluorides might be indicated to prevent the development of osteoporosis with prolonged bed rest.

Activity

In controlled studies reported by Konishi (269) and Shore and Consolazio (446), young men excreted less urinary calcium during periods of controlled exercise than in periods of sedentary activity. Calcium absorption and serum calcium levels were not significantly affected, but calcium retention was significantly increased during the exercise periods (269). Shore and Consolazio (446) studied immediate effects of exercise on serum levels and the urinary excretion of calcium, phosphorus and various metabolites involved in energy exchange. They found that neither serum calcium levels nor urinary calcium excretion was immediately affected by exercise. When exercise was sustained at a high level over a period of several hours, calcium excretion eventually decreased. Immediate changes in serum levels of phosphorus and citrate, both involved in energy metabolism, suggested to Shore and Consolazio that there is probably a relationship between calcium and some of the metabolites produced during exercise. Whether this relationship would significantly affect calcium requirements during physical activity was not indicated.

Contradictory to these results (269, 446), Gontzea et al. (171) found that young men eating controlled diets providing approximately 800 mg calcium daily were in positive calcium balance when they were engaged in sedentary activity but were in negative balance when subjected to controlled exercise programs. During the exercise periods, absorption decreased and urinary calcium excretion increased. When the intake was reduced to 700 mg/day calcium balances were positive during "rest periods" but were negative during "work periods." During five successive 4-day periods the negative balances fluctuated but gave some indication of an adaptation toward equilibrium. When the intake was raised to 1.2 or 2.0 g calcium all balances were positive.

Radioactive calcium (^{47}Ca) levels in blood, feces and urine were measured by Ragan and Briscoe (401) after intravenous administration of the isotope to three patients. Calculations based on these measurements indicated that when the patients were subjected to exercise there was an increase in the "total exchangeable calcium pool" with a postulated increase in bone formation rate. Ragan and Briscoe (401) suggested on examining their data that calcium retention during exercise as compared with during rest can be roughly assessed by comparing fecal excretions of the isotopic calcium. "In three pairs of studies . . . the percentage of the injected dose in the feces and the specific activity of fecal calcium decreased during exercise" (401).

Recently Fiorica et al. (146) reported what appeared to be a circadian rhythm in urinary calcium excretion. Eight boys 16 to 17 years old ate a controlled diet at four-hour intervals for 144 hours. Calcium was excreted in a circadian periodicity with maximum excretion occurring from 2200 to 0600 hours (sleeping hours) and minimum excretion occurring at 1000 to 1400 hours. In a second study two groups of 10 men (20 to 29 years old) were observed. One group (control) was recumbent throughout the study. The test group underwent an alternating rest and exercise program. Calcium excretion decreased during and after exercise. Fiorica et al. concluded that the apparent circadian excretion pattern observed in their first study was actually reflective of the circadian activity pattern of the boys. The investigators pointed out, however, that this study did not indicate whether their calcium excretion may also follow an endogenous circadian cycle.

Stress

There is evidence that calcium excretion is increased by stress of various kinds. Malm (322) for example, reported on the effect of what was believed to be emotional stress in two subjects, both of whom had increased urinary and fecal calcium excretions during periods when they were uncooperative, tense and depressed. In studies with young women (76, 294, 523, 524), reduced caloric intake for the purpose of weight reduction was accompanied by reduced calcium retention and in some cases by negative calcium balance. Both decreased calcium absorption (76) and increased urinary calcium excretion (523) were observed during the periods of low caloric intake. Whether this effect was due simply to reduced caloric intake or possibly to increased proportion of protein in the diet is not clear. Exposure to carbon monoxide was reported to result in increased urinary calcium excretions in eight subjects studied by Kjeldsen and Damgaard (265). Beisel et al. (40) reported that when hyperthermia was induced during a 24-hour period in eight men eating a controlled diet, urinary calcium increased but fecal calcium excretion was unchanged. Calcium balance became negative. Serum calcium levels dropped but slowly recovered. Calcium losses were rapidly regained during the posthyperthermic days. Beisel et al. concluded that many metabolic alterations attributed to the activity of an infecting agent are in fact due to fever. Whether increased calcium intake during the time of stress will prevent the losses has not been clearly shown.

STUDIES ON REQUIREMENTS FOR SPECIFIC POPULATION GROUPS

In addition to the requirements for maintenance, calcium is needed to provide for body increments during growth. From analysis of aborted or stillborn bodies, information has been obtained on the rate of calcification *in utero*. The full-term newborn infant's body contains approximately 0.8% calcium, about 24 g (179, 289). The adult body contains approximately 1.6% calcium, about 1,100 g (347). Thus between birth and physical maturation, 1,000 g or more of calcium is incorporated into the bones and soft tissues of the body. Reliable data on body composition and rates of calcification between infancy and maturity, however, are lacking. Some information has been obtained indirectly through observations on calcium retention by healthy children in various stages of growth. The conclusions drawn from these observations must be regarded as of limited applicability in view of the diversity of factors that affect calcium absorption and urinary calcium excretion.

Premature infants (Appendix table 3)

The infant born 8 to 10 weeks before term contains only about 30% as much calcium as is contained in a full-term infant (168, 230, 260, 315, 342, 519). Leitch and Aitken (291) calculated that about 200 mg of calcium is laid down daily in the fetus during the last 2 months of intrauterine life. Whether it is desirable for the premature newborn infant to accumulate calcium at this rate is not clear. Only one report (221) of daily retentions of 200 mg or greater by premature infants has been found in the literature.

The early literature (50, 426) reviewed by Hamilton (179) reported intakes of 352 and 210 mg CaO per day (251 and 150 mg calcium) for two infants. The respective retentions were 168 and 71 mg CaO (120 and 51 mg calcium). Hamilton reported data on calcium intake and retention in four premature breast-fed infants (two to four 10-day periods with each infant). The babies were 3 weeks to 1 month old at the beginning of the studies. Mean daily intakes ranged from 134 to 310 mg CaO (96 to 221 mg calcium, mean 162 mg) and retentions ranged from 1 to 98 mg CaO (1 to 70 mg calcium, mean 32 mg, 20% of the intake). Data from the literature reviewed by Hamilton showed that 10 full-term infants, 2 to 4 months old, had calcium intakes ranging from 170 to 260 mg/day (mean 220 mg) and retentions of 30 to 129 mg/day (mean 79 mg, 36%). Hamilton concluded that "premature infants would not, as a rule, until the age of about two months receive with the milk an amount of calcium comparable with the calcium intake of infants born at full-term." After 2 months of age, the data indicated that the intakes and retentions of the premature infants were comparable with those of the full-term infants. Supplemental calcium ($CaCl_2$) given to one premature infant resulted in an increase in retention from a very low level to one within the range found for the full-term infants. All of

Hamilton's premature infants developed rickets.

Benjamin et al. (43) observed that Hamilton's study and others like it had been carried out without administration of vitamin D (351, 384). In their study (43) with five healthy premature infants, approximately 4,000 USP units of vitamin D was provided for each child daily. The infants, whose birth weights ranged from 1,200 to 2,170 g, were studied for periods lasting 3 to 28 days. They were 13 to 41 days old at the beginning of the studies. Two subjects received breast milk, two were given a cow's milk–olive oil mixture, and one infant was studied with both diets. The mean daily calcium intakes were 56.4 and 164.6 mg/kg body weight with the breast milk and cow's milk diets, respectively. The calcium retention both in amount and proportion was less with human milk (27 mg/kg, 45%) than with cow's milk (114 mg/kg, 71%). Benjamin suggested that the poorer calcium retention with human milk as compared to cow's milk was probably due to "the limited total dietary supply of phosphorus, part of which is preferentially used for building up of protoplasm rather than for skeletal calcification." The Ca/P ratio of the human milk was 2.1:1 whereas that of the cow's milk was 1.5:1. Support for this hypothesis was provided later by Widdowson et al. (517) in a study with neonatal full-term infants (see page 1038). On the other hand, Baum et al. (32) suggested that the higher phosphorus content of cow's milk as compared to human milk might have contributed to the increased incidence of hypocalcemic tetany in neonates that they had observed among formula-fed babies.

In comparing their observed retentions with standards calculated to allow theoretically desired growth performance, Benjamin et al. (43) concluded that the human milk diet supplemented with vitamin D was inadequate to meet even the lowest degree of calcification that had been reported to be compatible with health. The cow's milk diet was adequate to enable the premature infant to reach, within 1 year, the degree of calcification of a full-term one-year-old infant's body (0.8% calcium). Higher daily calcium intakes (about 340 mg intake with 130 mg retained) have

been achieved by Hoffman et al. (207) by using evaporated milk diets. These diets, however, also had high levels of electrolytes which Hoffman suggested might be objectionable.

In contrast to Benjamin's findings, Gohshi (169) has reported calcium balance studies with four premature Japanese infants. Their intakes varied from 20 to 142 mg calcium/day. All but the smallest infant (body weight 1670 g, calcium intake 45 mg/day) were in negative balance.

Also in contrast to Benjamin's findings, Hövels et al. (221) observed mean daily calcium intakes varying from 114 mg with breast milk (retention 63 mg, 54%) to 589 mg with acidified cow's milk plus calcium phosphate (retention 265 mg, 45%). The subjects were 17 premature infants (birth weight 1,300 to 2,260 g) who were 12 to 59 days old at the beginning of the study. They each received at least 800 IU vitamin D/day. The calcium retention appeared to depend more on level of intake than on kind of diet or on calcium to phosphorus ratio. In a later report Hövels and Stephan (220) suggested on the basis of their previous work that the premature infant needs about 90 to 120 mg calcium per kilogram body weight and 60 to 90 mg phosphorus per kilogram daily. These amounts, they suggested, can be provided by an allowance of 100 g whole cow's milk per kilogram of body weight.

Besides the level of intake and the calcium/phosphorus ratio the effect of dietary components or adjuncts on calcium retention has been studied. Reports from Hövels' group (255, 270, 471) indicated that, in studies with a total of 40 premature infants, the inclusion of vitamin D in the diet increased the urinary excretion of calcium but not of phosphorus. With mineral intakes considered to be adequate (90 to 120 mg calcium and 60 to 90 mg phosphorus/kg), calcium retention increased slightly when vitamin D intake was increased from 400 to 800 IU/day. Further increases in the supply of vitamin D were of no value in increasing calcium retention. When the lactose content of the diet was altered, little change in calcium retention was noted. The investigators concluded that lactose has no effect on calcium retention.

In a study with six premature infants Sereni et al. (432) reported that the proportion of calcium retained did not change, but the total amount retained was greater with a diet containing a mixture of sugars and starch as compared to one in which lactose was the sole source of carbohydrate. The diets, however, were not alike in their other ingredients. The "mixed carbohydrate" diet provided more calcium and phosphorus, less fat of a different composition, and more protein of a different composition than the lactose diet did.

Benjamin et al. (43) suggested that poor absorption of fat might diminish retention of calcium. Their data, however, did not support this hypothesis. Later Gassmann et al. (164) observed in a study with premature infants 7 to 14 weeks old that neither the quantity nor the degree of emulsification or homogenization of dietary fat affected calcium retention.

Low serum calcium levels are commonly found in premature infants (77). Cohen (95) reported that administration of calcium lactate and viosterol resulted in increased levels of serum calcium. No conclusive evidence has been found of other dietary effects on serum calcium levels in premature infants.

Full-term infants (Appendix table 3)

Neonatal and young infants, 0–12 months old. Early attempts to assess the calcium requirements of infants were based on calcium intakes from breast milk (216, 379, 478). Hoobler (216) noted that the calcium content of breast milk was lower than that of cow's milk, but that a greater proportion of calcium was retained from the former than from the latter. Furthermore, he suggested that "since a healthy nursing infant shows no signs of a deficiency of calcium" the amount of calcium he gets from breast milk might be regarded as his true calcium need. From information available in the literature, Hoobler calculated that during the first 12 months of life approximately 157.6 g CaO (112.6 g calcium) is provided in a diet of breast milk (308 mg calcium per day). With a cow's milk diet, an infant would ingest 344.0 g CaO (245.7 g calcium) in the first year of life (673 mg calcium/day). Because of great differences among individuals in absorption of calcium,

Hoobler suggested that unless a child is sustained with human milk he should receive 1 to 1.5 g CaO daily (0.714 to 1.071 g calcium/day).

Also using information from the literature, Orgler (379) tabulated intakes of breast-fed neonatal infants (under 1 month of age) ranging from 62 to 296 mg CaO/day (44 to 211 mg calcium). The retentions ranged from 42 to 193 mg CaO (30 to 138 mg calcium). Breast-fed infants, 1 to 5 months old, ingested 272 to 423 mg CaO (194 to 302 mg calcium) and retained 54 to 183 mg CaO (39 to 131 mg calcium). In the same tabulation, the intakes of artificially fed infants, 2.5 to 10.5 months old, ranged from 611 mg CaO from a malt gruel diet to 2,084 mg CaO from a whole milk diet (436 to 1,488 mg calcium). Orgler estimated that the daily calcium intake of breast-fed infants should provide for a retention of 0.13 to 0.17 g CaO (86 to 120 mg calcium). The data tabulated by Orgler showed an average retention equivalent to about 53% of the mean intake. From these data, a minimum required intake of about 160 to 225 mg calcium/day may be calculated. Telfer (478), some 20 years later, also using data on the infant's consumption of human milk, estimated the calcium requirement of a baby weighing 3 kg to be 260 mg CaO (186 mg calcium) per day.

Another approach to the infant's calcium requirement was through body composition data. Leitch (289) estimated from growth rates and from data on body composition at birth (179) that an infant in the first 4 months of life would have to retain 130 to 310 mg calcium/day in order to maintain the proportion of calcium found in the full-term newborn infant's body. Hoobler (216), on the other hand, by comparing the calcium content of a newborn infant with that of a 4-month-old child, calculated that during the first 4 months of life a child must add 11.75 g CaO (8.39 g calcium) to his body weight. This would require a retention of approximately 70 mg calcium/day. Studies on calcium intake and output (412, 413, 473) indicate that the full-term infant in the first few weeks of life does not retain enough calcium to maintain the calcium content of his body at the level with which he was born. Stearns (461, 464) concluded from information available in the literature that, during the first 6 to 8 weeks of life, there is a rapid decrease in calcium content. With a cow's milk diet, the decrease is not as great with a human milk diet, and after the first 3 months the calcium content of the body begins to increase at a rate parallel to that observed in fetal life. With a diet of human milk only, an infant is not able to regain the proportion of calcium (0.8%) with which he was born. Wake (497) studied 22 breast-fed infants during the first 6 months of life. No difference in retention of calcium and phosphorus was found between those children (10 infants) whose calcification was found by radiologic examination to be defective and those (12 infants) with normal calcification. The defective calcification was presumed to be of prenatal origin. Whether it could have been corrected by calcium intakes higher than are possible with breast feeding is not clear.

Recently Kahn et al. (251) reported a long-term study with 30 infants receiving modified cow's milk and evaporated milk diets with daily calcium intakes ranging from 472 mg at 31 to 60 days of age to 522 mg at 271 to 300 days of age. From the calcium retention data, Kahn calculated calcium deposition values that indicated that the infants would have body calcium contents of approximately 0.8 to 0.9% at 300 days of age. Fomon and Owen (149) suggested, however, that metabolic balance data are not suitable bases for estimating body composition. They pointed out that errors inherent in the balance calculation usually result in an overestimation of retention.

Most of the calcium studies with infants have been balance studies. Estimates of calcium requirements, however, are not easily derived from these studies because of the wide range of intakes and retentions reported for presumably healthy infants. Early balance studies with breast milk (49, 296, 343, 390, 424, 485) summarized by Hamilton (179) showed daily intakes increasing from 62 mg CaO (44 mg calcium) for a newborn infant to 377 and 364 mg CaO (269 and 260 mg calcium) for a 3- and 4-month-old child, respectively. Daily retention (intake minus output) increased in amount from 14 mg CaO (10

mg calcium) for the newborn to 181 mg CaO (129 mg calcium) for a 4-month-old infant. The rate of retention was 68% for the newborn infant and varied from 17 to 50% for infants ranging in age from 2 to 4 months.

More recent studies with neonates (less than 1 month old) showed considerable variation in the calcium intake and retention when breast milk was the source. In seven reports (150, 181, 449, 452, 516–518) the mean daily calcium intake of groups of infants 6 to 18 days of age varied from 31 to 73 mg calcium/kg body weight. Mean retention varied from 15 to 24 mg calcium/kg body weight (32 to 66% of the intake). In these studies, the infants were either fed at the breast or were given weighed amounts of pooled pasteurized breast milk. The infants fed at the breast were weighed before and after suckling. The difference in body weight was assumed to be due to the weight of the milk consumed.

When babies of similar age (4 to 30 days) were fed various cow's milk preparations (150, 181, 449, 452, 516, 518), intakes were usually higher and retentions were more varied than those observed with human milk. In Slater's study (449), for instance, nine infants fed a formula based on dried whole milk had a mean intake four times as great as 13 breast-fed babies (135 vs. 36 mg calcium/kg). The mean calcium retention of the formula-fed babies (80 mg/kg, 59% of the intake) was also higher than that of the breast-fed babies (15 mg/kg, 43% of the intake). In a later study, coordinated in the same research institution, Southgate et al. (452) again observed a higher mean intake with the dried whole milk formula (576 mg calcium/day) than with breast milk (102 mg calcium/day). These intakes are approximately equivalent to 166 and 31 mg/kg body weight. The mean retention with the whole milk formula, however, was only slightly greater than that with human milk (88 ± 66 vs. 60 ± 21 mg/day; equivalent to approximately 25 vs. 18 mg/kg). When related to intake the retention of the formula-fed infants was much less (16% vs. 66%) than that of the infants fed human milk.

There was another unexpected observation in the Southgate study. Two groups of infants, one in Birmingham and the other in Dundee, were fed a formula based on partially demineralized whey and dried skim milk designed to resemble human milk more closely than cow's milk does. Due to differences in management of the infants, the Dundee babies had higher intakes than the Birmingham babies (238 vs. 191 mg Ca/day). The mean calcium retention of the Dundee babies, however, was much lower than that of the Birmingham babies both in amount (16 vs. 74 mg/day) and in relation to intake (7 vs. 38%). The reason for the difference in performance between the two groups was not apparent. The calcium retention of the Dundee babies was similar to that observed by Widdowson (516) when babies were fed a similar formula. Widdowson suggested that the poor calcium retention was due to failure to absorb calcium. She suggested, further, that the calcium absorption was hindered by unabsorbed fatty acids which combined with the calcium and were excreted as soaps. The fat content of the formula given to the Dundee infants, however, had been modified to improve the fat absorption. Widdowson (516) commented that this failure to absorb calcium satisfactorily from such "filled" milks "is most certainly peculiar to the baby during the first weeks after birth." Mean calcium retentions observed by Fomon (150) and Hanna (181) resembled more closely that of Southgate's (452) Birmingham infants than those of the Dundee infants and the Widdowson (516) babies.

With infants beyond the neonatal period, human milk has been used in only a few calcium balance studies. In most of these studies, calcium retention from human milk was compared with that from cow's milk or from formulas compounded to resemble human milk. In early studies (54, 296, 341, 343, 390, 424, 485) summarized by Wang et al. (506), infants, 1.5 to 3.75 months of age, fed breast milk had daily intakes of 209 to 364 mg CaO (149 to 260 mg calcium). They retained from 3.6 to 60.6% of the calcium. Other infants, 1.5 to 15.0 months old, fed cow's milk ingested daily 728 to 1,413 mg CaO (520 to 1,009 mg calcium). Retention varied from 1.2 to 30.9% of the intake (102, 390, 477). Wang et al. (506) and Boldt et al. (62) compared the intake and retention of calcium from human milk and cow's milk by a total of seven infants during alternating periods. Calcium intakes were higher with cow's milk than with breast milk (627 to 1,629 mg/day from cow's milk vs. 218 to 637 mg/day from breast milk). The infants usually retained more calcium from cow's milk, but the proportion of intake retained was usually higher from breast milk. In Wang's study with five infants, for instance, the retention varied from 453 to 1,815 mg CaO/day (324 to 1,296 mg calcium/day) from cow's milk and from 363 to 566 mg CaO/day (259 to 404 mg calcium/day) from breast milk. The mean proportion of calcium retained was 46% from cow's milk and 61% from human milk. In Boldt's study with two infants, the cow's milk period was preceded and followed by human milk periods. Each period was 25 to 36 days long. The infants retained 20 and 23% of the calcium from cow's milk. In the first human milk period they retained 26 and 42% of the calcium. In the second human milk period, intakes were slightly greater than in the first (227 mg/day in the first and 296 mg/day in the second period) but the retentions were much less (12 and 8%). The reason for this reduction in retention is not clear from the data.

Fomon et al. (150) studied calcium and phosphorus intake and retention in 25 normal infants during the first 6 months of life. One group of infants received pooled human milk for all or nearly all of the time. Two other groups were fed one or another of two formulas, based on dried nonfat cow's milk and whey for the first 3 to 5 months of life. A fourth group received a formula based on dried nonfat cow's milk (Similac) for the first 6 months. The mean intake of calcium from human milk, when expressed in terms of body weight (mg calcium/kg), decreased during the study from 72.9 mg/kg in month 1 to 45.5 mg/kg in month 6. Retention also decreased but the proportion of intake that was retained was higher in month 6 (47%) than it was in months 1 and 2 (33 and 40%). When the formula based on dried nonfat milk was fed, the calcium intakes, much larger than when human milk was fed, also decreased during the course of the study from 140.7 mg/kg in month 1 to 105.9

mg/kg in month 6. Retention, however, increased and the proportion retained was considerably higher during month 6 (39%) than during months 1 and 2 (25 and 23%). The calcium intakes from the formulas based on nonfat milk and whey in month 1 and 2 resembled in amount those from human milk but tended to be a little higher. They did not decline in proportion to body weight as the study progressed, however, and retentions increased both in amount and in proportion to intake. Fomon et al. (150) compared their data with those of Nelson (356) who had fed infants, 1 to 10 months old, formulas based on undiluted whole milk. In Nelson's study, intakes increased quantitatively from 887 mg/day at 1 month to 1,301 mg/day at 10 months, but decreased in proportion to the weight of the infant. Retention paralleled intake until the infants were 7 months old and then declined somewhat. Retention in terms of body weight remained fairly constant until month 7 after which it declined. Intakes and retentions were both greater in Nelson's study than in comparable months in Fomon's study.

The significance of higher apparent retentions that are not reflected in greater growth rates is difficult to assess. Slater (449) having observed higher retentions in week-old infants fed formulas based on dried whole cow's milk than in breast-fed infants, suggested that chemical maturation of the soft tissues and skeleton might proceed faster in infants fed cow's milk than in those fed human milk. Fomon et al. (150), recalling their previous conclusion (149) that balance data are not sound bases for calculations of body composition, suggested that such speculations would not likely prove fruitful. Kahn et al. (251) agreed that the use of data from metabolic studies is likely to lead to high errors in estimating deposition in the body. They suggested that the error could be as high as 30% for phosphorus and 10% for calcium. They suggested, however, that the probable error could be reduced by including inert tracers in the diet, by collecting saliva lost between meals, and by measuring skin losses.

Calcium retention from other milk preparations has been studied also. Harrison (182) measured calcium retention of five infants, 4 to 7 months old, when they were fed a formula based on sweetened condensed milk and again when they had an evaporated milk formula. The mean calcium intake and retention with the condensed milk formula (0.604 g and 0.206 g/day) were lower than with the evaporated milk diet (1.048 g and 0.244 g/day). Harrison suggested, however, that the lower intake and retention were sufficient for normal growth and that there was no evidence that higher retention was necessary.

When whole cow's milk is acted on by rennin, a large tough curd is formed. This curd is difficult for the young infant to digest (238). Hess et al. (202, 203), in a study first with one infant (203) and later with six infants, 16 to 48 weeks old (202) found that a greater proportion of calcium was absorbed and retained from cow's milk modified by base exchange treatment than from untreated cow's milk. There was, however, a reduction of about 20% in the calcium content of the milk due to the base exchange treatment. The absolute retention of calcium, therefore, from base exchange milk was not as great as from boiled whole milk.

Jeans et al. (238) studied calcium retention from whole cow's milk whose curd had been modified either by the evaporation process or by the addition of organic acid (citric or lactic) or a pepsin–rennin solution. Calcium retention and growth were satisfactory with each diet studied. Jeans et al. concluded that each type of milk (unacidified evaporated milk or whole milk curded by organic acid or by a pepsin–rennin mixture) was a good food for infants. The modified milks were not compared with unacidified, untreated whole milk.

Calcium retentions observed in early studies with infants had been highly variable and not obviously related to intake (464). Daniels et al. (112) showed that the addition of a source of vitamin D to the diet improved calcium and phosphorus absorption and retention. The sources of vitamin D included cod-liver oil, irradiated evaporated milk, and irradiated olive oil. Jeans and Stearns (236, 237) studied the effect of various sources and different amounts of vitamin D. This work was summarized by Stearns (464) who reported that not only was calcium retention improved but it was related positively to intake when vitamin D was given. Calcium losses were prevented when 135 IU of vitamin D was given, and calcium retention was further improved when 340 to 400 IU of vitamin D was provided. Increasing the vitamin D daily intake to 800 IU did not result in any additional improvement in calcium retention. With vitamin D intakes of 1,800 IU, the rate of calcium retention was similar to that observed when 400 to 800 IU of vitamin D was provided. The food intake, however, decreased so that the actual amount of calcium retained was decreased.

The effect of other dietary components on calcium absorption and retention by infants has been studied. Holt et al. (213) with healthy infants and Hickmans (204) with atrophic children concluded that the proportion of calcium to fat in the diet was important. Holt et al. suggested that the diet should contain 45 to 60 mg CaO (32 to 43 mg calcium) for every gram of fat and that the fat intake should be not less than 4.0 g/kg body weight. Similar levels of intake, 40 to 78 mg CaO (29 to 56 mg calcium) per gram of fat and 2 to 6 g fat/kg body weight, were suggested by Hickmans. These studies were contemporary with or just subsequent to the work of Mellanby (339) and McCollum et al. (332) in which the existence of vitamin D and its requirement by dogs and rats was demonstrated. It is not surprising therefore that neither investigator intentionally included a source of vitamin D in the infants' diets. Holt noted that one child, who had previously been receiving cod-liver oil, had a higher rate of calcium absorption than the other infants. Hickmans suggested that lower calcium retentions from skim milk diets than from whole milk diets might be due to the absence of the "antirachitic" or "calcium-depositing" vitamin in the former.

Stearns (460) declared that the ratio between the amounts of calcium and phosphorus retained was of equal importance to the absolute retentions. From data available on bone and soft tissue composition, she calculated that a calcium to phosphorus retention ratio of 1.5:1 or 1.6:1 would indicate that bone and soft tissues were growing at the same rate. The data available on calcium and phosphorus retention in infants indicated that a retention ratio between 1.5:1 and 2:1 was normal for infants under 1 year of age. Daniels et al. (112) had previously decided that a retention ratio of 2:1 was optimal. Stearns suggested that such a high ratio might indicate previous depletion of calcium. She concluded from a review of her own data and those of others that an artificially fed infant, given sufficient vitamin D, should retain daily at least 40 mg calcium and 20 to 25 mg phosphorus per kilogram body weight. This estimate was similar to one made previously by Daniels (40 to 50 mg calcium and 20 to 25 mg phosphorus/kg).

While it seems logical to assume that the calcium to phosphorus ratio of human milk would be most advantageous for the human infant, Fomon (148) pointed out that metabolic balance data do not support this assumption. He cited the study of Widdowson et al. (517) (see page 1038) in which the administration of phosphate to breast-fed week-old infants increased the absorption of calcium. Paradoxically, the higher phosphorus content of cow's milk as compared to human milk has been suggested as a factor contributing to neonatal hypocalcemia (32, 159, 378). Graham et al. (173), however, found higher serum phosphorus levels but no difference in serum calcium levels in infants fed evaporated milk formulas as compared to breastfed infants. A transient hypoparathyroidism has been suggested as a cause of neonatal hypocalcemic tetany (19). Gittleman et al. (167) found corroborating evidence in a metabolic study of an infant with tetany. Gardner et al. (159) suggested that in the neonate fed a cow's milk formula, the resultant elevated serum phosphorus level superimposed on limited parathyroid and renal function (due to immaturity) may predispose the infant toward tetany. While at present there is no agreement on the basic cause of the disorder (172, 176, 349, 431, 509), inadequate calcium intake has not been implicated. Nevertheless, the addition of calcium to cow's milk formulas has proved beneficial in preventing the condition (22). Dilution of cow's milk and formulation of feeds more closely resembling human milk particularly in its phosphorus content have been advocated as preventive measures (32, 378).

Older infants, 12 to 24 months old. Few data are available on the calcium needs of the older infant. Leitch (289) cited three studies (412, 414, 477) in which intakes of 0.470 to 2.222 g and retentions of 0.336 to 0.623 g calcium/day had been observed. Estimates of calcium needs for skeletal growth include 290 mg/day (289), 86 to 116 mg/day (345), 105 mg/day (347) and 172 mg/day at 12 months of age decreasing to 107 mg/day at 24 months (211). The amount of dietary calcium needed to provide for these varied retentions depends on the efficiency of utilization. No data have been found on the ability of the older infant to utilize dietary calcium. For younger infants, retention values ranging from 27 to 41% have been summarized from the literature by Holmes (211). Leitch (289) assumed a retention of 50% and suggested a requirement of approximately 0.7 g calcium/day for infants between 1 and 2 years of age. Holmes (211) suggested that for the weaned infant the amount of cow's milk necessary to meet other nutrient needs will insure an adequate supply of calcium.

Food consumption surveys (36, 145) indicate that deficient calcium intake is not likely to be a problem with the milk-fed infant. Filer and Martinez' questionnaires giving information on the food intake of 4,146 6-month-old infants in the United States showed an average intake of 1,134 mg of calcium/day. Ninety percent of the calcium was provided by milk (145). Beal (36) reported similar intakes for this age group. She compiled data on food and nutrient intake during the first 2 years of life of 94 children living in the Denver area. The calcium intake rose from birth until about 7 months of age and then gradually declined. Boys had slightly higher intakes than girls. The median calcium intake for boys rose from 0.58 g/day during the first month of life to 1.06 g/day during months 6 to 9 and then slowly declined to 0.75 g/day at 2 years of age. For girls the values were 0.54 g/day during month 1, 0.99 g/day during months 5 and 6, and 0.79 g/day at 2 years. Milk contributed 100% of the calcium at birth, 81% at 1 year, and 77% at 2 years of age. Beal also

noted that the increased use of feeds formulated to resemble breast milk has been accompanied by decreasing calcium intakes.

Preschool children, 2 to 5 years old (Appendix table 3)

Calcium requirements of children, 2 to 5 years of age, have been estimated by means of balance studies, observations on growth rate, dietary surveys, and from estimates of bone accretion.

Early balance studies carried out before the need for vitamin D had been established were concerned principally with the effect of acidosis (422) and dietary fat (214, 215, 476) on calcium absorption and retention. Holt et al. (214), having previously studied calcium metabolism of infants taking cow's milk formulas, next reported on calcium intake and absorption of children, 1 to 5 years old, eating mixed diets. In 79 observations, the intakes ranged from 0.043 to 0.178 g CaO/kg body weight (0.031 to 0.127 g Ca/kg). The children had lower calcium intakes and much lower calcium absorption than the milk-fed infants had. Calcium absorption ranged from 0 to 0.147 g CaO/kg (0 to 0.105 g Ca/kg) with a mean of 0.055 g CaO/kg (0.039 g Ca/kg). The highest calcium absorption was observed when the fat intake exceeded 3.0 g/kg body weight and when there was 0.03 to 0.05 g CaO (0.021 to 0.036 g Ca) per gram of dietary fat. Holt et al. also observed that when the daily calcium oxide intake was 0.09 g/kg (0.064 g Ca/kg) or less, the amount of calcium absorbed barely covered the normal urinary calcium excretion. They concluded that "an intake of less than 0.09 gm. of calcium oxide per kilo is insufficient to supply the calcium need of young children taking a mixed diet." In a later controlled study with seven children, 2 to 6 years old, Holt and Fales (215) again found evidence of impaired calcium absorption with low fat intakes. They concluded, therefore, that "conditions for proper calcium absorption are much better when the fat intake is generous." How much of the apparent effect of fat was due to vitamin D cannot be ascertained.

In 1922, Sherman and Hawley (438) reported a series of experiments with children to study "the rate of storage of calcium in normal children of different ages and the nature and amount of the intake required to support optimum calcium storage in the growing child." In the first series of experiments an intake of approximately 1 g calcium/day, supplied largely by milk, resulted in retentions that increased with age and size. The intakes of the three preschool children studied ranged from 46 to 58 mg/kg (mean 53 mg/kg). Their retentions ranged from 9 to 11 mg/kg (mean 10 mg/kg). These retentions were similar to the mean of data (198, 423, 425) summarized from the literature by Sherman and Hawley. In succeeding series of experiments, Sherman and Hawley observed calcium retention when calcium intake was increased by raising the level of milk intake and when vegetables were substituted for milk as sources of calcium. With three children, 4, 5, and 12 years old, calcium retention increased as calcium intake supplied by milk increased from approximately 400 mg to 1,000 mg. Further increases in intake resulted in either decreases or in only slight increases in retention. When vegetables (carrots and spinach) were added to the diet instead of milk, lower calcium retentions were observed than when milk was added. Sherman and Hawley concluded that children, 3 to 13 years old, need about 1 g of calcium/day to induce optimum storage, and that this can best be assured by providing one quart of milk/day for each child.

Several years later Willard and Blunt (520) studied calcium retention in two adults, two school children 8 and 12 years old, and two preschool children 3 and 4 years old when pasteurized or evaporated milk supplied most of the calcium. The calcium intakes of the younger children (1.01 to 1.12 g/day) were similar to those observed by Sherman and Hawley. The retentions, 7 to 14 mg/kg body weight (mean 10 mg/kg), were also similar. Similar data were obtained by Wang et al. (503) in a study with 60 underweight children. The six preschool children (4 and 5 years old) included in the study had a mean daily intake of 1.365 g CaO (0.975 g Ca) and a mean retention of 17 mg CaO/kg body weight (12 mg Ca/kg). The data indicated wide variation among the children

both in intake (0.932 to 2.033 g CaO/day) and in retention (8 to 28 mg CaO/kg). In none of these reports (438, 503, 520) was there an indication that the children had been provided with a specific source of vitamin D.

In subsequent reports found in the literature, provisions for some form of vitamin D supplementation were indicated. The methods for doing so included irradiation of the children, irradiation of the foods and/or provision of cod-liver oil or other vitamin D-rich dietary adjuncts. In these later studies, data were obtained that indicated that adequate retentions could be achieved with intakes lower than that recommended by Sherman and Hawley (438). Daniels et al. (109, 110), for instance, studied calcium metabolism of eight healthy children, 3 to 5 years old. The children ate a controlled mixed diet with either 475 ml (1 pint) or 950 ml (1 quart) of milk. The calcium intakes were approximately 800 mg (51 mg/kg) and 1350 mg (82 mg/kg) with the lower and higher milk diets, respectively. The mean daily retentions of the children ranged from 2 to 18 mg calcium/kg body weight. The mean retention with the higher calcium intake (8.9 mg/kg) did not differ significantly from that with the lower calcium intake (8.8 mg/kg). Because "these findings were so out of harmony with the generally accepted hypothesis that one quart of milk is necessary to supply the calcium for children of the ages considered," Daniels et al. (111) continued the work with 10 children, 3 to 6 years old. The experimental procedures were modified by lengthening the preliminary adjustment periods and the collection periods to allow more time for metabolic adjustment. Calcium intakes ranged from 35 to 100 mg/kg body weight. The balance data indicated that the highest mean retention (12 mg/kg body weight) was obtained with intakes between 60 and 64 mg/kg. There was no apparent relationship between retention and intake. The observed wide variation in retention suggested to Daniels et al. that calcium retentions were more likely related to the physical condition of the children and to their growth pattern than to their intakes. The data also suggested that the calcium requirements of healthy preschool children receiving adequate amounts of vitamin D could be met by diets supplying 45 to 50 mg of calcium/kg body weight or 7 to 9 mg/cm height.

Outhouse et al. (381) observed evidence in the literature of great variation in calcium retention within and among individuals (228, 397, 503). They recalled also that data obtained with rats by Fairbanks and Mitchell (142) indicated that calcium retention was inversely related to the calcium intake immediately preceding the period of observation. This suggested to Outhouse et al. that the observed variation in studies with young growing children might be related to differences in the degree of calcium saturation of the bones. Furthermore, Porter-Levin (397) had observed with three children, 2 to 6 years old, ingesting 1 g of calcium/day, that retentions varied in a "wave-like" fashion. She found that 15 to 21 days of continuous observation were required to cover the complete range of retention in an individual. With these considerations in mind, Outhouse et al. planned a study to estimate the calcium needs of preschool children. The study involved feeding liberal amounts of calcium for an initial period judged to be long enough to assure saturation of body tissues with calcium. In subsequent periods, varying levels of calcium were fed in order to determine the maximum retention (assumed to represent the requirement for growth) and the minimum intake that would support this retention. The periods were planned to be long enough to show the characteristic fluctuation in retention within the individual. Two studies were carried out, one with five girls, 3 to 6 years old (381) and one with seven boys, 2 to 6 years of age (337). During the saturation period the basal diet was supplemented with dicalcium phosphate (presumably CaHPO$_4$) to provide 1,800 mg calcium for the girls and 1600 mg for the boys. During the subsequent periods the calcium intake was altered by adding varying amounts of milk.

The data obtained in the two studies were used by Kinsman et al. (264) to estimate the utilization of calcium from milk. By their calculations the mean utilization, estimated as the proportion of the increase in intake that was retained, was 19.3% for the girls and boys. The value agreed well with utilization estimates similarly calculated for calcium from milk from data available in the literature (63, 109, 110, 397, 503). Kinsman et al. observed that the percentage retention and percentage utilization of calcium were very similar in these studies. They reasoned that if there is an appreciable maintenance requirement for calcium, the percentage retention should be less than the percentage utilization. Because the two values were similar, they concluded that the children did not have an appreciable maintenance requirement. Leitch and Aitken (291) disagreed with this conclusion. They said that, when intakes are in a range that gives almost maximum retention, regression calculations are not sufficiently sensitive to estimate maintenance requirements. By their own calculations based on Kinsman's data, using ascending retention slopes only, they calculated a maintenance requirement of 40 to 60 mg calcium/day.

Assuming, on the basis of Kinsman's calculations, that "the child's only requirement is for growth," McLean et al. (337) calculated calcium requirements for the five girls (381) and the seven boys (337) using observed or assumed maximum retention values and the utilization values calculated for milk calcium. The calcium requirements for the girls ranged from 535 to 855 mg/day (mean 699 mg/day), 30 to 61 mg/kg body weight (mean 43 mg/kg), or 4.8 to 8.7 mg/cm height (mean 7.0 mg/cm). Corresponding values for the boys were 685 to 1165 mg/day (mean 839 mg/day), 35 to 53 mg/kg body weight (mean 45 mg/kg), or 6.6 to 10.3 mg/cm height (mean 7.8 mg/cm). Assuming that the nonmilk portion of the diet supplied 300 mg calcium, McLean et al. concluded that the requirements of all the children but one boy could have been met by a milk supplement of one pint (about 475 ml). The one boy would have needed about 0.75 quart (about 700 ml).

Because milk was not a practical source of calcium in the diets of Chinese children, Yeh and Adolph (522) investigated the calcium requirements of 11 girls, 30 to 54 months old, when their diet was supplemented with bone meal or bone ash. The basal diet was representative of the North

China diet. With it, the children had a mean intake of 208 mg calcium/day (16 mg/kg) and they retained 5 mg/kg. When the calcium intake was varied during successive 6-day periods (3 days preliminary and 3 days collection), a maximum mean retention of 13 mg/kg was observed with a mean daily intake of 460 mg calcium. Additional increases in intake up to 1400 mg/day did not result in higher retentions. This mean intake (460 mg) required for maximum retention is lower than any calculated by Outhouse et al. (381) or McLean et al. (337). Most of the Chinese children, however, were smaller than any of the United States children. When the Chinese intake is expressed in terms of body weight (37.4 mg/kg), it falls within the range observed in the United States studies. It should be pointed out, however, that no attempt was made to "saturate" the Chinese children with calcium before measuring retention.

Higher requirements for maximum retention were estimated by Pierce et al. (393) in a study with 10 children 3 to 6 years old. The children were first "saturated" with intakes of approximately 1.3 g calcium/day over a 6-week period. During a subsequent 5-week period the children's intake was approximately 1.1 g calcium/day. The retention with this level was the same as with the saturation intake. When approximately 0.7 g calcium was fed for 2 weeks, retention decreased. Pierce et al. concluded that an intake of 700 mg calcium/day was not sufficient to promote maximum retention. They also concluded that an intake of 1.0 g calcium/day would "more nearly fulfill the needs of the preschool child than smaller amounts." There was no indication that the response to intakes between 0.7 and 1.1 g calcium/day had been studied. Pierce et al., in noting the difference between their results and those of Outhouse et al. (381) and McLean et al. (337) suggested that children living in a rigorous climate may have greater calcium requirements than those living in more moderate regions.

Attempts to estimate calcium requirements by means of measurements of growth or skeletal maturation have not been successful. Aykroyd and Krishnan (17) in 1938 observed significantly greater increases in height and weight in young South Indian children, 2 to 7 years old, receiving a daily supplement of 0.5 g calcium lactate for approximately 4 months than in similar children receiving no supplement. Many years later Bansal et al. (21) reported that they were unable to observe similar results in a study with South Indian infants and young children 6 months to 2.5 years of age. Bansal pointed out that in addition to differences in the subjects' age between the two studies, there were probably differences in nutritional status. Aykroyd's children came from middle and lower middle class families whereas Bansal's children were from poor rural families. Dietary surveys had indicated that the diets of the latter children were deficient in a number of nutrients. Bansal suggested that "in order to obtain the beneficial effects of calcium supplementation in children consuming low calcium diets, the dietary intake with respect to other nutrients must be adequate."

Daniels (107) pointed out that differences in response may be due to differences in growth pattern. The infant, according to Stearns (463), retains calcium much more avidly than does the preschool child. In addition, the degree of saturation of the tissues at the time of the study and the availability of the mineral as fed may affect retention (107). Daniels (107) studied three boys, 3 to 5 years of age, over a period of 280 days. All three children at the beginning of the study were below the average in height for age and in skeletal development. The diet provided 53 to 76 mg calcium/kg body weight. During the last 2 months of the study the protein intake, previously 3.0 to 3.4 g/kg, was reduced to 2.6 g/kg. During the study, growth in height and weight proceeded at faster than the normal rate. By the end of the study the children were normal by all growth standards used. It had been anticipated that calcium retention would decrease as the children achieved normal size, and that an estimate could then be made of the calcium retention necessary for healthy children. This, however, did not occur. At the end of the study, calcium retention was as great or greater than it had been at the beginning. Daniels concluded that, at the end of the study, the tissues were not yet saturated.

Dietary surveys combined with measurements of growth and skeletal maturation of children 1 to 6 years old in Canada (11) (166 children) and 2 to 7 years old in Australia (83) (120 children) showed no correlation between calcium intake and growth. In the Canadian study roentgenological studies showed adequate calcification with calcium intakes ranging from 0.2 to 0.7 g/day in some children but not in others (11). In the Australian study skeletal maturation was not correlated significantly with either calcium intake or with frequency and kind of illness (83).

Intakes of healthy children apparently vary widely. Beal (34, 35) reported on mineral intakes of 58 healthy children in the Denver area during their first 5 years of life. At 2 years of age, the calcium intake varied from 0.36 to 1.33 g/day. The intake at the fiftieth percentile was 0.76 g/day. At 5 years of age the range of intake was similar, 0.38 to 1.44 g/day, but the fiftieth percentile value had risen to 1.01 g/day. The recorded intakes included only calcium taken in food. The intake of calcium from mineral concentrates was not reported. Milk was the major source of dietary calcium. After about 3 years of age boys had a higher median intake than girls.

Burke et al. (80) also reported great variation in intake at any one age level. They studied the food intake pattern of 125 children (64 boys, 61 girls) from 1 to 18 years of age. The range of intakes of boys, 2 to 3 years old, was 0.40 to 1.30 g calcium/day. The mean intake was 0.88 g/day. The intakes of girls in the same age group ranged from 0.50 to 1.40 g/day with a mean of 0.90 g/day. Between 5 and 6 years of age, the range of boys' intakes was 0.55 to 1.80 g/day with a mean of 1.03 g/day. At the same age, the range of intakes of girls was 0.50 to 1.55 g/day with a mean of 1.03 g/day. Similar ranges of intakes were also reported by Widdowson (515) in her report on food intake of British boys and girls 1 to 18 years of age. The mean intakes of the 2-year-old children (0.76 and 0.73 g/day for boys and girls) were similar to Beal's median value.

At 5 years of age, the mean intakes of Widdowson's boys and girls (0.80 and 0.82 g/day) were just slightly lower than Beal's median or Burke's mean intakes. In Widdowson's study as in Beal's, milk provided most of the dietary calcium.

Calcium requirements have also been calculated from estimates of increases in the calcium content of the body during growth. Leitch (289) for instance, assumed that the fresh weight of the skeleton bears a constant relationship to body weight through the growth period. Calcium increments during growth were calculated from weight increments indicated in the growth standards of Baldwin (20) and Bayley and Davis (33). Assuming also that the body is able to utilize (retain) 50% of the dietary calcium, the dietary requirement for growth was estimated by doubling the calculated calcium increment during growth. On the basis of a private communication from Stearns, Leitch calculated the maintenance calcium requirement as 10 mg/kg body weight. The total calcium requirement, therefore, was estimated as calcium required for skeletal growth × 2 plus 10 mg/kg mean body weight. The requirement thus calculated for preschool children varied from 650 to 849 mg/day. She suggested that in round figures the daily requirement might be stated as 0.8 g from 0.5 to 2 years and 0.9 g from 2 to 10 years. The data used for estimating calcium increments with growth were found later to be in error (291). Shohl (444) using data collected from the literature on mineral content of the whole body, calculated calcium increments that were less than half of those calculated by Leitch.

Mitchell and Curzon (345) also calculated the increments in body weight to be expected at different ages from data of Bayley and Davis (33) and Brody (71). Their calculations of the calcium content of the weight increments were based on the assumptions that a) the newborn infant's body contains 0.8% and the adult body contains 1.5% calcium, b) the calcium content of the weight gains increases from 0.8% at birth to 2.3% with an average content of 1.55%, and c) the calcium content of girls' weight gains is 10% higher than that of boys' gains. The estimates based on these calculations were for the amount of retained calcium needed for growth. To this was added a maintenance requirement of 3.1 mg/kg. The dietary calcium requirement was based on the observations of Kinsman (264) that approximately 20% of the food calcium is utilized (retained). Requirements thus estimated for children over 3 years of age were 30 to 45 mg calcium/kg body weight. Suggested total daily requirements increased from 600 mg at 3 years to 1 g at 9 years of age.

Holmes (211) compared calcium accretion data calculated by Shohl (444) and Mitchell and Curzon (345) with that based on data obtained by Venar and Todd (490) from weights of fresh skeletons of children. The latter data, Holmes suggested, were indicative of children with poor skeletal development. She therefore included, for further comparison, estimates of calcium accretion based on the application of the calcification pattern of the rat to data on percentage increments in body size obtained primarily by Simmons (448) from children of families of high economic status. The calcium accretions thus calculated suggested a retention of approximately 100 mg calcium/day for the healthy preschool child. Assuming that 20% of the dietary calcium is utilized (264), Holmes suggested that 500 mg calcium/day should be enough for the preschool child who has been well nourished from birth. This estimate was based also on the assumptions that a) there is no maintenance calcium requirement for the growing child, and b) that there is no consistent difference between the needs of boys and girls under 10 years of age.

Many of the calcium balance studies with preschool children have been designed to compare the usefulness of various sources of calcium or to examine interactions of calcium with other nutrients. Calcium retention from evaporated milk was found to be as great or slightly better than the retention from pasteurized whole milk (520) or from raw fluid milk (451). When the evaporated milk was irradiated, Souders et al. (451) observed greater increases in recumbent length of children 5 to 6 years old than when they were fed fluid whole milk or nonirradiated evaporated milk. Evidence of improved retention of calcium

has been reported by Porter-Levin (396) with diets containing irradiated oatmeal and by Vorob'eva (493) when the subjects themselves were irradiated. On the other hand, Rakowska et al. (402) observed no significant difference in calcium retention between children receiving 400 to 800 IU cholecalciferol/day and those who received none.

Rakowska's children (40 children initially 4 years old) retained 167 mg calcium of a mean intake of 577 mg/day (approximately 29% retention). During the 3 years of the study, skeletal age, judged to be retarded, did not improve. The investigators suggested that the study indicated that the FAO recommendation (151) of 400 to 500 mg calcium/day for this age group is not enough. Begum and Pereira (39) in India, however, found that 28 children 3 to 5 years old were in positive balance with a mean intake of about 200 mg calcium/day. When the calcium intake was raised to about 280 mg/day by the addition of green vegetables to the diet, calcium retention increased from 38.5 to 54.0%. Growth, however, was maintained at the same rate as with the lower intake. Begum and Pereira concluded that children in the tropics, if adequately provided with calories and protein, can maintain positive calcium balance. The Indian children's diet provided about 2 g protein/kg. This was considered to be adequate. Hawks et al. (188) in a study with U. S. children observed no significant increase in calcium retention when the dietary intake of 2 g protein/kg was raised to 3 g/kg.

Whether the Ca/P intake ratio significantly influences calcium retention is open to question (39). Nevertheless when calcium is supplied as calcium phosphate salts, Stearns and Jeans (465) suggested that calcium retention is enhanced if the intakes of calcium and phosphorus are approximately equal. They found that calcium retentions from calcium phosphate salts were similar to retention of calcium from milk. Kempster et al. (261) reported similar results when the retention of calcium from dicalcium phosphate was studied with six preschool boys.

School children, 6 to 12 years old
(Appendix table 3)

Stearns (462) reviewing information on nutrient requirements during childhood said that steady growth occurs during the period from 4 to 11 years of age. Calcium retention during this time depends both on the rate of growth and the calcium intake. A child who has an ample intake tends "to store calcium most heavily during the year or so which precedes the period of rapid growth in height."

One of the earliest suggestions of calcium requirements of the school age child was that of Herter (200). He estimated that there must be an average annual storage of about 37 g calcium (approximately 0.1 g/day) to support normal growth in children from 2 to 15 years old. This required retention for growth was in addition to any requirement there might be for maintenance. A few years later Herbst (198) studied the mineral metabolism of five normally developed boys 6 to 13 years old. He reported a mean daily intake of 1.188 g CaO (0.849 g calcium) and a mean retention of 0.459 g CaO (0.328 g calcium). In terms of body weight the intake and retention were, respectively, 30 and 12 mg calcium/kg.

In subsequent attempts to assess calcium requirements, data have been examined on calcium retention (balance trials), on intakes during growth, and on estimated bone accretion. Sherman and Hawley (438) included nine children 6 to 13 years old in their first study designed to investigate the relation of calcium retention to age. The data showed that total calcium intake increased with age from 0.741 g (one 6-year-old child) to 1.017 g/day (the 13-year old child). In terms of body weight, the intakes tended to decrease from 43 mg/kg for one of the 6-year-old children to 18 mg/kg for the 13-year-old. There was considerable variation among the children, however, with an 8-year-old child having the lowest intake both in total quantity and in terms of body weight (0.654 g/day, 17 mg/kg). Total retention increased with age from 0.207 to 0.622 g/day. In terms of body weight, retention ranged between 7 mg/kg

(the 8-year-old child) and 14 mg/kg (an 11-year-old child).

Observing Sherman's recommendation that children should be provided with at least 1 g of calcium/day (see page 1052), Willard and Blunt (520) provided their two school age subjects with 1.2 and 1.3 g calcium/day. The subjects, 8 and 12 years old, retained from 0.37 to 0.64 g calcium/day—retentions similar to those observed by Sherman and Hawley (438).

In neither of these studies (438, 520) was there an attempt to estimate the minimum calcium requirement of the school age child. Wang et al. (505), in studying the metabolism of undernourished children, often observed negative calcium balances. In order to estimate the minimum calcium requirement, Wang et al. compiled the data from 38 studies (each at least 1 week long) on 18 children, 8 to 12 years old. The children's daily intakes ranged from 13 to 145 mg CaO/kg body weight (9 to 104 mg calcium/kg). The tabulated data showed negative balances with all intakes below 32 mg CaO/kg (23 mg Ca/kg). With intakes greater than 23 mg calcium/kg the retentions varied from 2.8 to 17.8 mg/kg body weight. Based on these observations, Wang et al. suggested that the minimum requirement of an 8-year-old child weighing 20 kg would be 0.64 g CaO (0.457 g calcium) per day supplied by a mixed diet.

Similar data were obtained by Petrunkina (391) when she studied the mineral metabolism of 14 healthy children, 7 to 8 years old, eating a mixed diet. With intakes less than 20 mg calcium/kg the mean balance and most of the individual balances were negative. With intakes between 20 and 30 mg/kg, 8 of the 11 balances were positive with a mean balance of only 2.06 mg/kg. With intakes between 30 and 40 mg/kg, all balances were positive ranging from 6.13 to 16.26 mg calcium/kg body weight. The diets, providing 30 to 40 mg calcium/kg body weight, contained about 500 ml of milk/day.

Indications of lower minimum requirements were observed by Holemans and Lambrechts (209). In their study with 17 healthy African boys 6 to 12 years old, calcium intake and output were measured in 39 three- to five-day periods. The basal diet, which was the customary village diet, was supplemented with varying amounts of milk powder. Calcium intakes ranged from 6.9 to 77.4 mg/kg body weight. The data were grouped according to intake as follows: a) 6.9 to 15 mg/kg, b) 15 to 20 mg/kg, c) 20 to 30 mg/kg, and d) intakes higher than 50 mg/kg. The mean retention was plotted against the mean intake of each group and the points were joined by straight lines. The line thus drawn indicated that the mean maintenance requirement of calcium (intake when retention is zero) was 12 mg/kg body weight (range 7 to 22 mg/kg). Holemans and Lambrechts also calculated that with calcium intakes below 24 mg/kg the boys retained 100% of the fraction of calcium above the maintenance requirement. These high retentions were explained as being the result, not of adaptation to low intakes, but rather of previous depletion "and this in spite of the absence of clinical evidence of shortages."

Response to high calcium intakes has been studied by Lutwak et al. (305). In their study, two groups of ten and eight American Indian girls, 8 to 11 years old, ate diets providing either 2.286 g or 1.295 g calcium/day. The diets were similar in composition except that one was supplemented with dibasic calcium phosphate. The girls had had calcium intakes similar to these for 1 or 2 years before the study. Intake and output of calcium was measured in four consecutive 6-day periods. The data indicated that the ten girls with the higher calcium intake (2.286 g) had balances ranging from 0.129 to −0.119 g calcium/day (mean −0.003 g/day). Five of the ten girls were in negative balance. Of the eight girls with the lower calcium intake (1.295 g), all were in positive balance with retentions ranging from 0.085 to 0.426 g/day (mean 0.272 g/day). Evidence of high fecal fat excretions among the girls eating the high calcium diet suggested to Lutwak et al. that "negative balances of calcium and the development of steatorrhea may result when high dietary calcium is given."

Earlier Macy (312) had observed in her metabolic studies with children that less than 2 g of fecal fat was excreted when 400 g of milk was included in the diet. When, however, the milk intake was increased to 800 g, the fecal fat increased to over 3 g/day. She reported that "the greater part of the increased fecal fat excretion seemed to be due to the excess soap and this in turn to the augmented calcium intake."

The information gained from balance studies is limited in applicability because of the apparent ability of children to adapt to low calcium intakes. Nicholls and Nimalasuriya (358) and Murthy et al. (353) reported positive balances with low intakes of about 200 mg/day. The children in both studies were small by European and United States standards. Whether higher levels of calcium intake would have resulted in greater stature was not studied. In studies in which growth was measured, both Aykroyd and Krishnan (18) and Doraiswamy et al. (126) found greater height increments in Indian children receiving calcium supplements than in those eating unsupplemented diets. Neither study, however, provided an estimate of the amount of calcium needed to promote normal growth. Walker (498) has suggested furthermore that, because of the numerous factors that influence growth, such an estimation is probably impossible. Evidence of the difficulties involved has been furnished by Luyken et al. (308) who studied the nutritional contribution of the food supply in four boarding schools in Surinam. The calcium provided in the diets of the four schools varied in quantity from 340 to 915 mg/day; protein varied from 45 to 71 g/day; and riboflavin varied from 524 to 1,390 µg/day. The children, 6 to 12 years of age, did not differ from school to school in mean height, weight or skeletal age. One group of children in each of the three schools with the lower calcium supply (340 to 634 mg/day) was given a daily supplement of 400 mg calcium/child for 15 months. After this time there still were no significant differences in height or weight increments between the supplemented and unsupplemented groups in each school or among the four schools. Luyken et al. suggested that, in order to draw conclusions on requirements of calcium from studies such as these, much longer periods of observation on large numbers of individuals would be needed. They suggested, further, that the studies should, if possible, cover a whole generation.

Longitudinal or cross-sectional food consumption studies (35, 81, 515) indicate that there is great variation in calcium intakes among healthy children. Beal (35) observed substantial differences in intake not only among children of the same socioeconomic class but also between children within the same family. Ohlson and Stearns (377) also pointed out that there are great differences among children in their ability to utilize calcium. These differences presumably would be reflected in their calcium requirements and possibly in their intakes. Macy (312) suggested that the observed differences among children in utilization of calcium may be due to the need for longer periods of adjustment to the experimental conditions. She provided evidence, obtained with children, 4 to 8 years old, that, as the study progressed, the children became more alike in their response. Macy concluded that "since the study was carried out for only eight months it is not known whether the subjects would have become even more nearly alike in the selective retention of food constituents, and therefore in their daily retentions of this element, irrespective of body size, nor is it possible to determine whether season was an influencing factor."

Because of reported seasonal variation in growth (515) and because growth had been suggested to be related to calcium intake (312), Widdowson (515) examined mean calcium intakes for boys and girls during 11 months of the year. No evidence was found of seasonal trends in intake. Similarly, Young et al. (525) examined calcium intake data of grade school children in the state of New York and found no significant differences between the mean intakes in fall and those in spring. Vorob'-eva (492) on the other hand, in a series of balance trials with boarding school children, 5 to 7 years old, found that calcium intakes tended to increase from January to July and then to decrease. Retention was better in summer and fall than in winter and spring. The children got more milk and milk products and had greater exposure to sunlight in summer.

Calcium requirements based on calculated increases in body calcium have been estimated for children 6 to 12 years old as follows: 0.850 increasing to 1.000 g/day

(289); 0.690 increasing to 1.450 g/day for boys and 0.710 increasing to 1.530 g/day for girls (345); 0.500 increasing to 0.800 g/day (211). The methods used in arriving at these estimates have been described previously (pages 1055–1056). Holmes' estimates (211), it should be remembered, were based only on growth requirements, whereas those of Leitch (289) and Mitchell and Curzon (345) included a maintenance allowance.

Nicholls and Nimalasuriya (358) noted that Ceylonese children were able to retain calcium with much lower intakes than the requirements suggested by Leitch (289). They found, for instance, that four children, 4 and 7 years old, retained 34 to 89% of calcium intakes that ranged from 70 to 245 mg/day. In order to arrive at more realistic estimates of requirements, they derived data on calcium increments in the body based on measurements of Ceylonese skeletons and on tables of heights and weights developed for Ceylonese boys and girls. Then applying Leitch's formula (skeletal increment × 2 plus 10 mg/kg) they calculated calcium requirements ranging from 350 to 700 mg/day for boys and 285 to 570 mg/day for girls 6 to 12 years old.

Leitch and Aitken (291) in 1959 reassessed calcium requirements on the basis of skeletal increment and endogenous loss. In the 20 years since Leitch (289) had first published her estimate of requirements, more data had been obtained on the calcium content of the infant and adult body, on growth rates, and on endogenous calcium loss. Calcium increments to the body between infancy and adulthood were assumed to be in proportion to increments of body weight. From data available in the literature, Leitch and Aitken estimated the daily endogenous calcium loss to be approximately 100 mg in infants, 50 or 60 mg in children, 150 mg in adolescents and 200 to 260 mg in adults. The total daily calcium requirements based on these data were approximately 250 mg in infancy, decreasing to 120 to 140 mg in preschool years, then increasing through childhood to reach a peak of about 550 mg in adolescence. These values did not include an allowance for availability or incomplete utilization of the dietary calcium. To translate these values into dietary requirements, Leitch and Aitken recommended further metabolic research aimed at determining "what levels of calcium in different diets will supply a given skeletal increment."

Ohlson and Stearns (377) compared the calcium retention of Iowa children from infancy to 12 years of age with a "theoretical requirement" calculated from growth rates, calcium content of the bone and the proportion of body weight due to skeleton. The theoretical requirement and the mean retentions at different ages and different calcium and vitamin D intakes were plotted on a graph. The resultant retention curves showed that vitamin D was essential for adequate calcium retention. The retention curve of children consuming 1.5 pints (about 710 ml) of milk and 300 to 400 units of vitamin D almost duplicated the theoretical requirement curve. The curve of those receiving one quart (about 950 ml) of milk plus vitamin D fell above, and the curves of those receiving 1 or 1.5 pints (about 475 or 710 ml) of milk without vitamin D fell below the theoretical requirement curve. No information was given on the calcium content of the total diet or on other possible combinations of milk and vitamin D.

No reports were found in which serum calcium levels were used in estimating calcium requirements of children. There is conflicting evidence in the literature on the response of serum calcium to dietary intakes. Houet (219) reported that serum levels of five patients with hypocalcemia, presumed to be due to low calcium intakes, returned to normal when tricalcium phosphate and vitamin D were administered. Karnani et al. (254) found that the serum calcium levels of six children, 7 to 9 years old, who had been subsisting on a low calcium diet (244 mg calcium/day), rose when the dietary calcium level was raised to about 360 mg/day by the addition of soya milk or cow's milk. Schoenthal and Lurie (428) on the other hand, reported that administration of viosterol or one quart (about 950 ml) of milk did not have a consistent effect in raising serum calcium levels of children 5 to 16 years of age regardless of whether their diets were "poor" or "well balanced."

Various nutrients and food components have been reported to influence calcium absorption and retention. The beneficial effect of vitamin D in promoting calcium retention and in preventing rickets has been reaffirmed recently in Russian and Scottish studies (134, 491). Calcium retention was improved when orange juice was added to the diet (88, 434). Shepherd's data (434) indicated that oranges or orange juice contained other effective components than vitamin C. Chaney and Blunt (88) suggested that the "basic residue" might be responsible. Davis (113), however, observed no difference in the mean calcium retention of 12 children, 7 to 12 years old, when they were eating "acid-forming" and "base-forming" diets.

In cultures where milk is not habitually consumed, low calcium intake has been recognized as having a possibly limiting effect on growth. Various studies in India (247, 248, 254, 472) have shown that improvement in calcium intake and retention can be effected by a dietary supplement of indigenously produced plant foods such as ragi, groundnut curd, fortified soya milk, or macaroni made of tapioca, groundnuts and wheat.

Adolescents (Appendix table 3)

Adolescence has been defined as "the period of life beginning with the appearance of secondary sex characters and terminating with the cessation of somatic growth" (127). Because of differences among individuals in rate of biological maturation, it is difficult to restrict a review of adolescents to a relatively narrow age range. Reports on adolescents have been found that included girls 10 years old while others have included boys up to 21 years old. Research on requirements of adolescents has included balance studies, food intake measurements and estimates of calcium increments in the body during growth.

The reports available on balance studies show much variability in calcium intake and retention from one study to another and from one subject to another. In 1936 Wang et al. (504) summarized data from preceding studies on calcium balance of children 12 to 16 years old. The summary included six studies with five girls and nine boys, a total of 14 children (198, 199,

419, 438, 503, 520). The daily calcium intakes varied from 666 mg (17 mg/kg) (199) to 1520 mg (55 mg/kg) (503). The latter value was included in a report on calcium metabolism of undernourished children. The daily calcium retention varied from 141 to 523 mg (4 to 13 mg/kg). Retention was not obviously related to intake. In their own study, Wang et al. (504) studied mineral intake and excretion of 23 girls, 12 to 15 years of age, for 11 days (5 days' adjustment and 6 days' collection). The calcium intakes ranged from 1,186 to 1,806 mg/day (mean 1,604 mg). The intake per kilogram of body weight (30 to 53 mg/kg) decreased as body weight increased. The range of retentions (1 to 19 mg/kg) was similar to that observed in the summary of preceding studies. There was, as before, no close relationship between retention and intake or between retention and body weight.

Previously, Henderson and Kelly (195) had been able to show that increased intake was accompanied by increased retention. In their study with five 15- to 17-year-old African boys in a Nairobi prison, much lower calcium intakes were observed than were reported by Wang et al. (504). Three of the boys were in negative calcium balance when subsisting on the customary prison diet supplying approximately 300 mg calcium/day. All were in negative balance with the prison hospital diet providing about 346 mg calcium/day. When calcium was added to the hospital diet either in a pint of milk (770 mg calcium) or in a mineral mixture resembling the mineral content of one pint of milk (680 mg calcium), the boys began to retain calcium. On the basis of Sherman's (435) estimated maintenance requirement of 0.45 g calcium/day for a 70-kg adult, Henderson and Kelly assumed a maintenance requirement of about 0.5 g/day for their rapidly growing boys who weighed only about 50 kg. Based on weight changes observed during the study and on calcium retentions of growing children reported by previous investigators (198, 438), Henderson and Kelly estimated that the boys required a retention of approximately 500 mg calcium/day for growth. The balance data indicated that only about half of the calcium ingested in excess of the estimated maintenance requirement was retained. Henderson and Kelly therefore suggested that the growth allowance be doubled to allow for incomplete absorption. The proposed total calcium requirement of these African boys, therefore, was 1.5 g/day.

Some of the great differences in retention observed by Wang et al. (504) may have been due to differences in the subjects' physical maturity. Johnston (244) observed in studies with six girls at puberty that sexual maturation was accompanied by reduced calcium and nitrogen retention. The menarche did not necessarily coincide with the time of reduced retention but might precede it or follow it by several months. Three of the girls were convalescing from "a childhood type of tuberculosis" and three girls "had been hospitalized with minimal adult type lesions." Johnston suggested that the reduced calcium and nitrogen retention coinciding with puberty might have an unfavorable effect on the course of tuberculosis. Additional work with adolescent girls indicated that the administration of estrogen was accompanied by a reduction in calcium retention (245). In a later review of his work and that of others with adolescents Johnston (246) recommended an intake of 1.4 g calcium/day as optimal during adolescence.

Suspecting that part of the variation in retention observed in past studies might be due to differences from one individual to another in calcium stores, Johnston, Schlaphoff and McMillan (243) chose subjects whose diet history showed that they habitually drank at least "three glasses of milk a day." Six girls 13 and 14 years old were fed a diet providing 1,050 to 1,131 mg calcium/day for 8 weeks. The mean intake was 1,079 mg/day. Mean calcium retentions varied from 174 to 444 mg/day. Johnston et al. then estimated the daily calcium accretion to be expected in 11-, 12-, 13- and 14-year-old girls with early, medium and late menarches. When the mean daily retentions of the six girls were compared to the appropriate estimated accretions, Johnston observed that all of the subjects when ingesting about 1 g of calcium/day had retained more than the amount estimated to be required.

Food intake studies indicate that during

adolescence, boys' intakes tend to be higher and to approach the suggested requirements more closely than girls' intakes do (81, 138, 180, 377, 515). Boys' daily intakes tend to increase from 12 to 17 years of age whereas girls' intakes tend to decline. Widdowson (515) found that the intakes in terms of body weight for boys and girls paralleled each other, indicating that part of the observed difference in daily intakes was due to difference in size. Intakes/kg body weight for both boys and girls declined as age increased from 13 to 18 years. Wait and Roberts (496) on the basis of food intake studies with 38 girls, 10 to 17 years old, suggested "that smoothed curves of the intakes per kilogram per age" might be used as tentative minimum standards for requirements. Their data, however, were obtained with a small fairly homogeneous population in one institution which provided daily approximately 3.5 cups of milk/individual. The daily intakes of the subjects, therefore, were less variable than those observed in other studies (81, 180, 515).

Estimated requirements based on calculated calcium accretion rates (211, 289, 291, 345, 358) indicate greatest need during the pubertal growth spurt with gradually decreasing need as the individual achieves physical maturity. Leitch and Aitken's (291) estimates allowed for an endogenous loss of 150 mg/day and a calcium accretion of 280 to 375 mg/day for 13- to 15-year-old boys. The total requirement for maintenance and growth (430 to 525 mg/day) did not make any allowance for incomplete absorption of dietary calcium. Holmes' (211) estimates were based on calcium accretion data and utilization rates of 20 to 25% but made no allowance for maintenance requirements. She suggested a daily intake of about 1.1 g calcium at the peak of the pubertal growth spurt. Mitchell and Curzon (345) added estimated calcium accretion to a maintenance allowance of 3.1 mg/kg body weight and assumed a utilization rate of about 20%. They calculated that the dietary calcium requirement should increase from about 1 g/day at 9 years of age to 2.6 g/day at 13 years for girls and 2.4 g at 15 years for boys. The requirement would then decrease gradually to about 1 g/day at 20 years. Nicholls and

Nimalasuriya (358) calculated a similar peak in requirements at the height of the growth spurt. Their proposed requirements based on Ceylonese growth data and skeletal composition estimates were, as noted previously, much lower than the English and the United States estimates. As a practical standard, they suggested 1 g calcium/day for adolescents from 12 to 20 years of age.

Because milk in many areas is the principal dietary source of calcium, nutritionists have frequently translated calcium requirements into milk requirements. Studies by Kung and Yeh (280) and Hsu and Adolph (223) indicated, however, that the calcium needs of adolescent Chinese boys could be met satisfactorily with mixtures of wheat, soybeans and vegetables or by supplementation of the diet with bone ash.

Pregnant women (Appendix table 4)

The calcium intake during pregnancy should cover the needs of the mother and, in addition, those of the developing fetus. In developing estimates of requirements two main approaches have been used—the factorial approach and the balance study. In the former the requirement estimate is derived by adding the calculated calcium content of the fetus at various stages of development to the maintenance requirement of the mother. Usually an allowance is made for incomplete utilization of dietary calcium. In the second approach, the calcium intake and output of the pregnant woman is measured. The adequacy of the intake is evaluated by comparing the apparent retention with the estimated calcium content of the fetus and the other products of pregnancy.

Serum calcium levels, dental health and obstetrical performance have been considered at times to reflect adequacy of calcium intake during pregnancy. The evidence supporting such relationships is unclear and of limited value in estimating calcium requirements.

The calcium needs of the fetus. Information on the calcium needs of the developing fetus have been obtained from body composition studies of human fetuses of various sizes. Data are available on over 100 fetuses. These data have been summarized a number of times (101, 168, 229, 260,

315). Estimates of the calcium content of the full-term fetus vary from 13 to 33 g. Most estimates fall between 21 and 28 g. About half of the accumulation of calcium occurs in the last lunar month of pregnancy (168, 230, 260, 315). Coons et al. (101) calculated from data obtained from 85 analyses that approximately 0.306 g calcium/day are deposited in the fetal body during the last lunar month. Hytten and Leitch (229) in a later estimate arrived at a value of 0.250 g calcium/day. The placenta accumulates about 0.65 g calcium during the gestation period. Most of this accumulation occurs in the last stages of pregnancy (229).

Macy and Hunscher (315) in 1934 summarized the then available data from the literature on calcium intake and output of gravid women during the last 8 lunar months of pregnancy (118 balance studies). They compared the retention values with data similarly summarized from the literature on fetal calcium content during the same stage of pregnancy (69 fetuses). The assembled data indicated that the mother's retention was greater than the estimated fetal requirements except in the tenth month when the fetus deposited about 200 mg/day more than the mother retained. Concluding that calcium obviously "must be withdrawn from the maternal reserve to satisfy the fetal demands," Macy and Hunscher asked what effect this would have on the bones and teeth of the mother and child. Hytten and Leitch (229) concluded that, since the total calcium requirement of the fetus is only about 2.5% of the calcium content of the mother's body, fetal needs in excess of the mother's retention can be satisfied from the mother's stores. They pointed out, however, that in a succession of pregnancies, such imbalance between maternal retention and fetal needs may result in maternal osteomalacia and fetal rickets. They suggested, further, that since the calcium requirement during lactation is much greater than during pregnancy, adding calcium to the mother's body (rather than withdrawing from it) in pregnancy would probably be desirable.

Various estimates of calcium requirements based on the needs for maintenance and for fetal development have been made. Garry and Stiven (162), for instance, used Sherman's (435) estimate of 0.46 g/day for maintenance with an estimated fetal requirement of 0.3 g/day during the last 2 months based on data of Coons et al. (101). Allowing for incomplete utilization they proposed a requirement of "not less than 1.3 g and probably 1.8 g or more daily."

Mitchell and Curzon (345) estimated a maintenance requirement of 3.1 mg calcium/kg body weight. Their estimate of fetal needs, based on Coons' data (101), varied from about 9 mg/day in lunar month 3 to 300 mg/day in lunar month 10. Assuming that about 30% of the dietary calcium is retained, they estimated a requirement of 1.56 g/day in the last month and an average requirement of about 1.2 g/day during the last 5 months of pregnancy.

Beaton (38) questioned the applicability of such estimates based on information obtained with nonpregnant subjects. He pointed out that calcium absorption is increased in late pregnancy and that women have been observed to bear children successfully over a wide range of intakes. Leitch (290) earlier had made similar observations that the pregnant woman is physiologically much different from the nonpregnant woman and that "there is an almost incredible range in the extent of the changes that occur."

Balance studies. Most of the balance studies with gravid women have taken place during the last half of pregnancy. The early ones were conducted with women who were accustomed to relatively high calcium intakes (208, 283). In more recent studies somewhat lower intakes were studied. There have been few studies of calcium intake and output of pregnant women who habitually eat low levels of calcium. The data obtained show much variability both within the individual subject and from one subject to another. In one of the early studies, Hoffström (208) measured calcium intake and output of one woman from week 17 through week 40 of pregnancy. The woman's daily calcium intake ranged from 1.013 to 2.385 g (mean 1.712 g). Retention varied from −0.330 to 0.951 g/day. The calculated accumulated retention of calcium between week 17 and parturition was 34.3 g. This accumulated retention was somewhat larger than could be accounted for by the estimates of fetal calcium content.

The only other long continuous study reported in the literature on calcium intake and output during pregnancy was that of Hummel et al. (225). They measured nutrient intake and output by one healthy multipara from day 135 of pregnancy to day 53 of lactation with only one interruption (the first 10 days postpartum). The observation time was divided into 5-day collection periods. Calcium intake fluctuated between 2.78 and 3.35 g/day (mean 3.09 g/day). Retention was positive varying from 0.09 to 0.66 g/day (mean 0.37 g/day). There was no apparent relationship between the amount of calcium retained and the calcium intake or the estimated needs of gestation.

The total amount of calcium apparently accumulated during the last 145 days of pregnancy was 52.90 g. Assuming, as did Hummel et al., that about 24 g of calcium was laid down in the fetus, the woman completed her pregnancy with a "maternal reserve" of a least 29 g of calcium. Negative balances observed during the first 2 months of lactation depleted her of about 21 g of this "rest material." Hummel et al. suggested that the accumulation of a generous reserve beyond that needed for fetal growth may be helpful in preventing serious consequences of losses that occur during lactation.

A second woman, a poorly nourished primapara, was studied continuously during the last 65 days of pregnancy (224). During this time the woman's mean calcium intake ranged from 1.91 to 1.98 g/day (mean 1.95 g/day). She retained from 0.35 to 1.18 g/day (mean 0.71 g/day). The total calcium gain during the 65 days was 46.3 g. This accumulation, when compared to that observed in the corresponding period by the previously studied healthy multipara (225) (24.7 g) and the woman studied by Hoffström (208) (20.0 g), suggested to Hummel et al. (224) that the physiological state of the gravid mother may greatly influence her utilization of the nutrients in her diet. They concluded that "maternal nutritive state and physiological constitution . . . should be considered when interpreting dietary requirements for preg-

nancy." A similar opinion was expressed by Thomson (479) when he stated that the "nutritional status of a pregnant woman depends more upon her life-experience of diet than upon the nature of the diet she happens to take during pregnancy."

Landsberg (283) also noted calcium retentions in excess of the estimated needs of the developing fetus ranging from a mean of 0.024 g/day in lunar month 2 to a mean of 0.422 g/day in lunar month 10. Because no woman among the 13 subjects in his studies was followed throughout the entire pregnancy period, the total accumulated calcium could not be calculated.

In all of these studies the calcium intakes were high, ranging from 1.013 to 2.385 g/day in Hoffström's work and from 2.78 to 3.35 g/day in Hummel's study of the multipara. With similar intakes (1.5 to 2.7 g/day), Macy et al. (317) observed what they called "excessive excretions" of calcium by three women studied at intervals from week 14 to week 38. One subject was in negative balance both times she was studied (weeks 30 and 34). The other two, each studied five times, had calcium balances ranging from −1.276 to 0.166 and from −0.220 to 0.278 g/day. These balances were adjusted for the fetal calcium uptake. Larger retentions were reported later by Macy et al. (314). In this second study one woman was observed in months 7 and 8 of gestation. With intakes of 1.93 (month 7) and 1.55 g/day (month 8) she retained 0.62 and 0.64 g calcium/day—much larger amounts than those observed with the first three women in similar stages of pregnancy. According to calculations of Coons et al. (101), the retention of the woman in the second study would be ample and in excess of the needs of the fetus.

Coons et al. studied nutrient intake and output during pregnancy in nine women in Chicago (100) and in six women in Oklahoma (101). The women ate self-selected diets which were sampled and analyzed for their nutrient content. In Chicago, data were obtained from 23 4- to 6-day balance studies from week 11 to week 39 of pregnancy. Calcium intakes in Chicago ranged from 0.603 to 1.705 g/day (mean 1.096 g/day) and retention varied from −0.138 to 0.306 g. Most of the women were not retaining enough to meet the calculated needs of the fetus (101). In Oklahoma, calcium intakes ranged from 0.697 to 2.375 g/day (mean 1.418 g/day) and retentions ranged from 0.059 to 0.488 g/day. There were no negative balances and all but one woman retained enough calcium to meet the estimated needs of the fetus. The higher intakes of the Oklahoma women were thought to be partly responsible for their superior performance. When retentions of women with similar intakes were compared, however, the Oklahoma women retained more than the Chicago women. The mean retention of the Oklahoma women was 21% while that of the Chicago women was 9% of the intake. With the Chicago group, mean retention increased as the mean intake increased, but with the Oklahoma women no improvement in retention was shown with intakes over 1.6 g calcium/day. Coons et al. (101), after examining various possible factors, concluded that the superior performance of the Oklahoma women was most probably due to their greater exposure to sunshine. Two women in Chicago and one in Oklahoma took cod-liver oil intermittently during their pregnancy. Their calcium retentions, however, were not demonstrably superior to those of other women in their group.

Toverud and Toverud (487) found that the beneficial effect of vitamin D supplements depended on the level of calcium and phosphorus in the diet. They observed calcium intake and output in 44 four-day balance studies in 17 women. There were no positive calcium balances in the last 2 months of pregnancy with intakes lower than 1.6 g/day. Toverud and Toverud found that vitamin D did not help to make the balance positive when the calcium intake was below 1.6 g/day. With calcium intakes higher than 1.6 g/day the addition of vitamin D helped to raise negative balances to positive. The addition of fresh vegetables and an egg to the daily diet also helped to promote calcium retention.

Unlike Toverud and Toverud (487), Adair et al. (5) observed positive balances with calcium intakes ranging from 0.702 g to 1.653 g/day. Their 14 subjects were divided into four groups. One group received the basal diet (1.3 g calcium/day). The other three groups received either a supplement of cereal as a source of added calcium, a supplement of 39,900 IU vitamin A and 5,550 IU vitamin D, or both cereal and vitamin A and D. Adair et al. reported that they could see "no change in the metabolism of calcium or phosphorus in those patients who received added calcium or vitamins A and D." Most of the individual retentions appeared to be adequate to cover the estimated needs of a developing fetus.

Obermer (371) studied calcium intake and retention of pregnant women in wartime Britain. Unlike Adair et al. (5), he found that calcium retention was strikingly related to calcium intake. He reported that in his study 12 pregnant women served as controls. They ate the typical wartime diet which included calcium additives in the bread and a pint of milk/day. Another group of 10 women received supplements of calcium phosphate supplying 0.64 g of calcium from month 3 to month 5, 0.95 g from month 6 to month 7 and 1.26 g from month 8 to term. Calcium balances during 2-day collection periods were calculated at various times from week 9 to week 38 of pregnancy. The proportion of negative balances was much higher in the control group than in the experimental group. When the balances were related to intake Obermer found that 93% of the balances were negative when intakes were less than 1 g calcium/day. As the intake increased, the proportion of negative balances decreased. When calciferol as well as calcium was added, balances were further improved (370). Additional analysis of the data suggested that calcium and phosphorus intake might be related to successful implantation of the ovum (372) and to length of labor (373). Obermer concluded from the findings "that an intake of not less than 2 g of calcium element from the beginning of pregnancy to the end of the seventh month and 2.5 g from the eighth month to term should be considered as the minimum 'safety' levels" (371).

Liu et al. (297) suggested that the calcium requirement during pregnancy depended in part on the customary intake prior to pregnancy. In their study with three pregnant Chinese women, adequate retentions (0.253 to 0.284 g/day) were observed when the diet provided 1.00 g or 1.25 g of calcium/day. When the vitamin D supply was inadequate, more than 1.3 g of calcium was needed. Liu et al. suggested that with optimum vitamin D intake the calcium requirement might be even lower than 1.00 g/day. On the basis of additional studies with pregnant women with moderate to severe osteomalacia they suggested further "that the so-called calcium requirement . . . must be regarded as a variable quantity conditioned by such factors as the prior skeletal store, the previous dietary custom, and the state of vitamin D nutrition."

More recently Shenolikar (433) reported balance data obtained with 6 to 12 pregnant Indian women during each of the three trimesters of pregnancy. The mean calcium intake was 0.423, 0.414 and 0.381 g/day in the first, second and third trimester, respectively. Absorption rose from 41.9% in the first trimester to 52.7% in the second, and 53.4% in the third. Retention also rose from 0.037 g/day in trimester 1 to 0.124 g/day in trimester 2 and 0.132 g/day in trimester 3. Shenolikar calculated that approximately 27.0 g of calcium was retained during pregnancy. Calculations based on the average size of the babies born to women of the class studied (2,600 g) indicated that this accumulated retention was sufficient to meet the calcium needs of the fetus. Whether larger babies might be born if the mothers had higher nutrient intakes was not indicated.

Shenolikar (433) reported that the increase in retention from trimester 1 to trimester 2 was due to improved absorption, and the additional increase from trimester 2 to trimester 3 was due to decreased urinary excretion. Knapp and Stearns (268) had previously concluded from data assembled from their own studies and those of others that urinary calcium excretion rises until after week 20 when it may level off and then fall abruptly just before term. Their data were so variable that it is difficult to perceive the trend their calculations indicated.

In a recent study, however, Heaney and Skillman (192) reported similar trends in urinary calcium excretion. In this study 15 pregnant women, 15 to 28 years old, were studied in balance periods lasting 3 to 6 weeks (24 balances in all). Nine nonpregnant women, 20 to 26 years old, were also studied. Midway through each balance period each pregnant subject was given an intravenous dose of $CaCl_2$, enriched to provide 30 mg of the stable isotope [48]Ca. The nonpregnant women received [45]Ca. The results of the study indicated that significant adjustments take place in a woman's metabolism during pregnancy.

These adjustments were reflected in changes in calcium balance. The mean calcium balance of the nonpregnant woman was −0.087 g/day with a mean intake of 0.757 g/day. Calcium balance was significantly more positive in the pregnant women at weeks 20 to 24 (0.039 g/day) than the mean balance of the nonpregnant women. During pregnancy, calcium balance improved progressively to 0.134 g/day in weeks 35 to 40. Then, during postpartum and lactation, it dropped until it was not significantly different from the mean balance of the nonpregnant controls. The mean calcium intake of the pregnant women which varied from 0.660 to 0.931 g/day did not differ significantly from that of the nonpregnant controls (0.757 g/day). Taking the nonpregnant balance as a baseline, Heaney and Skillman (192) calculated that the relative accumulative balance in the pregnant women was approximately equal to fetal needs (20 to 24 g calcium).

As compared with the nonpregnant women, calcium absorption in the pregnant women was significantly greater by weeks 20 to 24, calcium accretion was significantly increased by weeks 25 to 29, calcium resorption rose slowly but was significantly increased by weeks 30 to 34, endogenous fecal calcium did not change significantly, and total digestive juice calcium was significantly increased in weeks 35 to 40. During pregnancy, calcium turnover and pool size increased. Most of the increase in pool size could be attributed to the fetus.

In exploring the governing mechanism for these changes in maternal metabolism, Heaney and Skillman attempted to induce pseudopregnancy in one nonpregnant volunteer by administering large doses of estrogen and progesterone for 7 weeks. The metabolic changes that had been observed in the pregnant women did not occur. The investigators speculated that the changes observed in pregnancy were based on an interaction between placental lactogen (which exhibits some of the properties of growth hormone), estrogens and parathyroid hormone.

Serum calcium levels. In studies of pregnancy, serum calcium levels have been measured frequently but as yet have not been found to be an efficient parameter of calcium requirements. Serum calcium levels fall gradually during pregnancy (55, 166, 352, 357, 362, 403, 420, 514) usually reaching the nadir in lunar month 9 and then rising slightly during lunar month 10. There is usually a sharp rise immediately following delivery. Mull and Bill (352) suggested that the decrease coincides with the greatest fetal demand for calcium made on the maternal system and that recovery follows immediately. after the demand ceases. Roth (420), however, calculated that the fetal requirement, assumed to be 100 mg/day during the last 2 months of pregnancy, was not enough to cause the observed drop in maternal serum calcium levels.

Mull and Bill (352) with 900 patients and Nishihara (362) with 115 patients found evidence of a seasonal effect with lower maternal serum calcium levels in winter and spring than in summer and fall. Dieckmann et al. (123), however, could find no evidence of a significant seasonal effect in their data obtained with 553 patients. Mull and Bill (352) also reported some evidence of decreased serum calcium levels with successive pregnancies. Ghosh (160), however, could find no significant effect of parity in data obtained with 187 Indian women.

Hormones have also been implicated. Bodansky and Duff (56) suggested that low serum calcium levels might reflect either parathyroid deficiency or dietary deficiency. Roth (420) on the other hand, in studies involving 85 pregnant women, could find no evidence that their subjects' parathyroid activity differed from normal. Administration of estrogen and testosterone were also ineffective in altering the serum calcium level (407, 420).

The possibility that serum calcium levels can be affected by dietary intake or intravenous administration of calcium has been explored. Pyle et al. (400), in five subjects, could find no significant relationship between serum calcium and ingested calcium. Serum calcium was "somewhat related" to absorbed calcium (ingested calcium minus fecal calcium). Dieckmann et al. (123) found that the addition of 0.76 g calcium/day in cereal with or without 39,900 IU vitamin A and 5,550 IU vitamin D to the diet had no significant effect on serum calcium levels. Similarly, Lapan and Friedman (284) and Roth (420) found that the administration of calcium orally or intravenously had no lasting effect. Kerr et al. (262), however, in studies with 24 women in month 6 through month 8 of pregnancy found that hypercalcemia could be produced when 2 g of calcium/day was administered orally in the form of calcium lactate. Similar amounts of calcium administered in nonfat milk, calcium sulfate or dicalcium phosphate had no effect on serum calcium levels. Ghosh (166) reported that, with 185 pregnant Indian women, there was a trend toward higher serum calcium levels in those whose diets included milk. The actual calcium intakes of the women were not reported.

Dental studies. There is evidence that during pregnancy gingival inflammation is prevalent (302). This has been suspected by some of being induced by hormones (84). Löe (302) and Camilleri (84) suggested that it can be controlled by good dental hygiene. On the other hand, Krook et al. (276, 278) have concluded that the primary lesion in periodontal disease is alveolar bone loss due to insufficient calcium intake. Teeth become loose and mobile when the bone supporting them is resorbed. Gingivitis and hemorrhage are the consequences of this pathological movement of the teeth. Evidence to support this hypothesis was found when Krook et al. (276, 278) studied 10 men and women, all of whom had severe periodontal disease. When the patients were given a supplement of 1 g calcium/day for 6 months, radiological evidence of new bone formation was obtained. At the same time, gingival inflammation and bleeding, calculus formation, and tooth mobility were reduced. Whether increased calcium intake would be similarly beneficial in reducing gingivitis in pregnancy has not yet been reported.

Clinical and dietary surveys. The findings of some early dietary and clinical surveys (80, 135) were interpreted as indicating that the quality of the mother's diet was related to the events of pregnancy and to the condition of the infant. In others (521) no correlation could be found between the occurrence of complications in pregnancy and the mother's diet. Nor was the infant's birthweight significantly related to the mother's dietary intake. Similar data have been accumulated in more recent studies (37, 333, 480–482). Thomson (482) has concluded that "diets of pregnant women can vary widely, in quantity as well as in quality, without clinically obvious impairment of the reproductive process." In these studies the average calcium intakes ranged from 0.7 g (521) to 1.19 g calcium/day (481).

Lactating women (Appendix table 4)

In assessing calcium requirements of lactating women, the calcium intake of the nursing infant has been estimated. Balance studies have been used with a few subjects. In addition, requirements have been calculated from the sum of the estimated maintenance requirement and the amount of calcium actually secreted in the milk. There have been also a few dietary surveys from which the intakes of presumably healthy lactating women with healthy infants were estimated.

Stearns (461) estimated that a young baby receives about 200 mg calcium/day when he ingests 650 ml of breast milk. By the time he is 8 months old, his daily intake has increased to 350 mg of calcium. Macy and Hunscher (315) measured the voluntary intake of breast milk of known composition by a healthy infant during the first 5 months of postnatal life. The calcium intake rose from 252 mg/day (54.6 mg/kg body weight) in month 1 to 418 mg/day (57.2 mg/kg) in month 5.

Most of the balance studies were carried out by Macy and Hunscher and their associates (125, 225, 226, 316, 447). Three healthy women who were copious milk producers were studied at intervals through successive reproductive cycles. Two, who were first studied late (week 60 and week 50) in lactation, were in positive calcium balance. Pregnancy immediately followed the cessation of lactation. In the next lactation period calcium balances were determined in week 7 and week 27. The third woman was also studied in weeks 7 and 27 of lactation. All three women, with calcium intakes ranging from 2.82 to 3.62 g/day were in negative balance in week 7. The amount of calcium secreted in the milk ranged from 0.47 to 1.24 g/day. Twenty weeks later (week 27), with higher calcium intakes (3.39 to 4.42 g/day) their balances had become more negative. Milk calcium secretion had risen to range from 0.53 to 1.30 g/day. Fecal calcium excretion had also increased. This increase in fecal excretion was greater than the increase in intake, suggesting that factors inhibiting assimilation were operating (226). During the next 2 months the women received daily supplements of cod-liver oil and yeast. The fecal calcium excretion decreased, improving balance to the extent that one woman began to retain calcium. The other two women were losing less calcium but remained in negative balance (316). At the end of this lactation period (weeks 62 and 63) and in the post-lactation rest period that followed, all three women were in negative balance even though the secretion of calcium in milk had ceased (125). These observations suggested to Donelson et al. (125) that in frequent pregnancies with long copious lactation there is danger of depleting the mother's body of calcium. Hummel et al. (225), however, concluded from observations with one of the women who was studied in a subsequent reproductive cycle (see page 1064), that sufficient reserves may be built up during pregnancy so that losses during lactation are not deleterious. When Shukers et al. (447) related the calcium secretion to the calcium intake of the three women during 3- to 10-day periods, they found an inverse relationship. The woman with the highest mean intake (3.08 g calcium/day) had the lowest milk calcium output (0.45 g calcium/day) whereas the woman with the lowest intake (2.71 g calcium/day) had the highest milk calcium output (1.17 g calcium/day). These women were exceptionally high milk producers (1.4 to 3.1 liters/day). The calcium intakes required by them would probably not be needed by women with less copious flows.

Toverud and Toverud (487) for instance, observed six women at various times during lactation from months 1 to 5 (a total of 12 balance studies). With intakes varying from 0.8 to 2.4 g/day, milk calcium secretion varied from 0.09 to 0.26 g/day. Negative balances were observed in 4 of the 12 studies. These became positive when the calcium intake was raised by adding milk or a calcium salt to the diet. The addition of cod-liver oil to the lactating women's diets did not have any significant effect on calcium balance. Toverud and Toverud also found that the calcium content of the breast milk of 14 women was raised from a range of 0.0177 to 0.0314% to a range of 0.0213 to 0.0417% when the women received a supplement of about 0.5 g calcium/day as calcium lactate. They pointed out that their subjects were all primaparae whereas those of Macy and her associates (125, 225, 226, 316, 447) were multiparae. They suggested that it might be more difficult to establish a positive balance in multiparae. Oberst and Plass (375) also found that three young primaparae, 17 to 18 years old, were able to maintain themselves in positive balance with intakes ranging from 1.92 to 2.18 g calcium/day when studied during the first 2 months of lactation. Their milk calcium secretion ranged from 0.04 to 0.38 g/day. The amount of calcium secreted in the milk, however, did not appear to be related to the calcium intake.

Karmarkar and Ramakrishnan (253) and Devadas and Prema (122) in studies with 59 and 30 lactating Indian women, respectively, found no significant difference in the calcium concentration in breast milk that could be related to the mothers' calcium intakes. In the Karmarkar study the mothers' intakes ranged from 0.08 to 1.90 g calcium/day. In the Devadas study the unsupplemented diets of five women contained about 1040 mg calcium/day. No information was given in these Indian reports on the volume of milk produced. The calcium concentration in the milk in Karmarkar's study (253) was reported to be about 0.02 g/100 ml. This is lower than the estimates of Stearns (461) (30.0 mg/

100 ml), Macy (313) (34.4 mg/100 cc) or Drummond et al. (129) (25 to 41 mg/100 ml). It is in reasonable agreement, however, with the values (17.6 to 38.4 mg/100 ml) reported by Holemans and Martin (210) for African mothers during the first 6 months of lactation.

Other investigators have reported that the calcium concentration of breast milk can be raised by increasing calcium intake (298, 301, 409). Garry and Wood (163) have suggested in reviewing these reports that the vitamin D content of the milk may be more important than the calcium content in preventing rickets in breast-fed infants.

Garry and Stiven (162) concluded from the data reported by Hunscher (226) that "with good mixed diets not less than four times the milk calcium is required for positive balance." Therefore, they calculated that, to cover maintenance requirements of 0.46 g with a 50% margin of safety plus a milk yield of 500 to 1,000 ml containing 20 to 30 mg calcium/100 ml, the lactating woman needs 1 to 2 g calcium/day.

Mitchell and Curzon (345) based their calculations on an estimated maintenance requirement of 3.1 mg/kg body weight and an efficiency of utilization of 30% (0.57 g/day for a 56-kg woman). Assuming a milk production of 500 ml/day at 1 month after parturition rising to 1,000 ml/day at peak of production and a calcium concentration of 36 mg/100 ml of milk, they calculated a calcium requirement of 1.16 to 1.75 g/day for the lactating woman.

These calculated estimates are in reasonable agreement with the intakes of 41 lactating Australian women as reported by Hitchcock and English (205). According to their data the suckling infants were healthy and gaining weight adequately when their mothers had a mean intake of 1.28 g calcium/day when studied during weeks 6 to 20 after parturition. Trinidad lactating women, however, were reported by Chopra et al. (89) to have intakes of about 0.55 g/day which suggested to Chopra that chronic low dietary intakes may lead to adjustments in efficiency of utilization. The Joint FAO/WHO Expert Group on Calcium Requirements (151) agreed that an allowance of 1.0 to 1.2 g calcium/day is probably sufficient during the third trimester of pregnancy and throughout lactation. The committee noted, however, that women in many parts of the world maintained themselves and lactated adequately with lower intakes, and suggested that more observations were needed.

The elderly (Appendix table 5)

In recommending dietary allowances, the elderly are not usually classed separately from other adults (526). There is, however, some question as to whether the nutrient requirements of the elderly, specifically the calcium requirement, is the same as that of younger adults. The small amount of work done with older people has consisted mainly of balance studies that have yielded conflicting results. The problem is complicated by the evidence of bone loss with aging and by the prevalence of senile osteoporosis.

Rose (415) described osteoporosis as "the condition resulting from a diffuse lack of bone with no detectable chemical abnormality in the bone that remains." This definition, Rose suggested, has the advantage of being acceptable to researchers (9, 120, 281, 365) who are in disagreement on many aspects of the disorder. Its principal disadvantage is that it does not distinguish between causes or conditions which result in osteoporosis but which have nothing else in common. Rose pointed out that "this is analogous to considering anemia as a single entity because all causes lead to low hemoglobin levels" (415).

Heaney (190) classified osteoporosis into homeostatic and nonhomeostatic categories. The homeostatic varieties develop "whenever bone is forced to provide calcium which the organism fails to obtain from its environment." Conceivably this could occur because of a dietary deficiency or malabsorption although Heaney suggests that it is more commonly due to imbalance between the responses of bone and those of intestine and kidney to hormonal stimulation. Studies with pre- and postmenopausal women by Young and Nordin (527) tend to support Heaney's opinion.

In attempting to develop a "unified concept of osteoporosis" Heaney (190) cited earlier work with animals in which deprivation of dietary calcium resulted in osteoporosis (28, 348, 405). More recently Gershon-Cohen and Jowsey (165) have reported the development of osteoporosis in rats fed a calcium-deficient diet for 10 months or more. When the rats were then fed a high calcium diet for more than a year, the bones appeared to have been reconstructed normally. In the 40 to 50 years in which osteoporosis has been studied extensively, a deficient calcium intake has not been shown conclusively to be one of its causes in man (368), although in some cases dietary calcium deficiency has been found to accompany the condition (86). Some of the symptoms, moreover, may be relieved by high calcium intakes (132, 184, 250). There is a possibility that because some kinds of osteoporosis (e.g., senile osteoporosis) are insidious, whatever the underlying cause, the condition may be beyond correction before it becomes apparent (106, 165). Bernstein et al. (44) have pointed out that roentgenographic evidence of decreased bone density is not apparent until 30% or more of the bone tissue has been lost.

Garn et al. (160) in examining the relationship of calcium intake to bone size and bone loss in about 400 adults, found no evidence that high calcium intakes prevented or low calcium intakes accelerated bone loss. They reported, however, that the taller individuals lost "less" bone than the shorter individuals. They concluded that all people lose bone but that those developing greater bone mass by decade 4 show less evidence of bone loss in later life. Similarly Rose (415), in a critique on methods of diagnosis and treatment of osteoporosis, suggested that bone loss begins to occur in most people between 20 and 30 years of age. Whether or not the condition of osteoporosis eventually becomes detectable may depend on whether an adequate amount of bone was amassed before the gradual loss began.

In contrast, Pratt (399) cited observations with rats by Henry and Kon (197). In this study (197), senescent rats, raised on a low calcium intake, remained in equilibrium under conditions which led to calcium loss in rats raised on a more liberal diet. Pratt suggested that "if humans could be shown to behave in a similar manner, calcium intakes lower than those generally advocated might be desirable for children."

Whedon (512) has reviewed reports of animal experiments (28, 41, 85, 137, 436) in which increases in bone mass have resulted from high calcium intakes. Few similar data with human subjects, however, have been found in the literature. Schmid (427) reported in 1963 that the administration of large amounts of calcium gluconate (4 g daily) was accompanied by improvement in bone density in 60 osteoporotic patients. Bone density was estimated radiographically. Anabolic steroid administration had a similar result and was somewhat more effective than calcium dosage as the age of the patient increased. Recently Cohn et al. (96) reported a combination of calcium balance studies and ^{47}Ca tracer studies with seven elderly osteoporotic patients whose intake was increased from about 0.5 to 2.5 g/day. The data were interpreted as showing that with the high calcium diet there was a slight increase in bone accretion but a much more substantial decrease in bone resorption.

Rose (415) suggested that efforts to prevent the manifestation of osteoporosis should be made in the first 20 years of life. He suggested further that Bernstein's work (46), showing that formation of harder bone and lower incidence of osteoporosis accompanied high–normal fluoride intake, might indicate a productive approach to the problem.

Recently Jowsey et al. (249) reported a study with 11 osteoporotic patients, 54 to 72 years old, who were treated with a combination of sodium fluoride, calcium and vitamin D for 12 to 17 months. Mean bone formation increased and mean bone resorption decreased during the study. Increases in bone formation were directly related to the fluoride dosage and total fluoride intake ($P < 0.01$) but not to the calcium intake. The bone was morphologically normal with daily sodium fluoride intakes of 45 mg or less. With daily intakes of 60 or more mg sodium fluoride, the new bone was abnormal. Changes in bone resorption were inversely related to the calcium intake ($P < 0.05$) but were not related to fluoride intake. On the basis of their observations, Jowsey et al. suggested that daily doses of 50 mg sodium fluoride supplemented by 600 mg calcium/day and 50,000 IU vitamin D/week would result in modest increases in bone mass without undesirable effects on the skeleton. Jowsey et al. also noted that before treatment began, bone resorption was positively related ($P < 0.05$) to the estimated phosphorus intake but was not related to the calcium intake. This observation suggested to them that "dietary phosphorus may be an important factor in the etiology of osteoporosis."

Calcium balance studies with elderly people have indicated much variation in requirement from one study to another as well as from one individual to another. In some studies the subjects were confined to bed and were served a controlled diet. In others, the subjects lived at home and ate a self-selected diet. The estimated requirements have been expressed as grams or milligrams per day or per kilogram of body weight. Comparison among some of the studies is difficult because in some reports the weight of the subjects is not recorded. There is some indication that the subject's response to the experimental diet was influenced by his customary calcium intake. In a number of studies, subjects, well below the age conventionally thought of as elderly, were included.

Owen (382) for instance, studied 10 men, 32 to 69 years of age, only four of whom were 65 years or older. Diet histories for the previous 6 months were known and the experimental diet was planned to resemble the previous diet. During the experiment the men were confined to bed. Two levels of calcium, approximately 0.520 and 0.880 g/day, were provided. All subjects were in positive balance with the higher intake. The mean balance with the lower intake was −0.004 g/day. Five men, 53 to 69 years old, were in positive balance or in equilibrium. One 66-year-old man and the four younger men 32 to 45 years old were in negative balance. Owen concluded that the mean daily minimum requirement for maintenance was probably about 0.520 g/day for older men. In a subsequent study, Owen et al. (383) found that seven men,

69 to 76 years old, could be maintained in positive balance with calcium intakes of 0.556 to 0.593 g/day or less. Some were in equilibrium with intakes as low as 0.241 to 0.266 g/day. Further increases in intake led to increased retention in some subjects. In one man, increased intake was balanced by increased fecal calcium excretion. The men's customary intake was low and all but one subject showed evidence of being osteoporotic. Owen et al. suggested that equilibrium at low intakes indicated adaptation to low intake and that increased retention indicated replenishment of body stores.

Roberts et al. (410) found evidence of much higher requirements in nine women 52 to 74 years old than those observed by Owen et al. (382, 383). With self-selected diets, the women's calcium intakes ranged from 0.515 to 1.303 g/day (mean 0.850 g/day). The women, who were active, lived at home and weighed all food eaten. Calcium intake was adjusted by adding various amounts of milk or calcium gluconate. Roberts et al. found that there were great variations in retention among the women with similar intakes. Losses were more frequent than retention with intakes below 1.100 g/day. The intakes with which equilibrium was achieved ranged from 0.448 to 1.301 g/day (9.4 to 23.7 mg/kg). When balance was plotted against intake the mean intake necessary for equilibrium was found to be 1.067 g calcium/day. Roberts et al. concluded that at least 1 g calcium/day is desirable for older women.

A requirement fairly close to this was estimated by Bogdonoff et al. (57) in a study with seven ambulatory men 66 to 83 years old in a metabolic ward. Calcium intakes ranging from 107 to 1600 mg were observed. Balances were consistently negative with the lowest intakes (107 and 131 mg). All subjects could be maintained approximately in equilibrium with 850 mg calcium/day.

A similar mean requirement was calculated by Ackermann and Toro (1) from data obtained in a study with eight men 69 to 88 years old. The men were ambulatory inmates of an infirmary. The basal diet was one to which they were accustomed. Calcium intakes ranged from 13.65 to 33.15

mg/kg or from 0.560 to 2.100 g/day. When retention was plotted against intake, the mean intake necessary for equilibrium was found to be 18.5 mg/kg. Applying this value to the mean weight of the men during the study as reported for each level of calcium intake, a mean intake of about 992 mg calcium/day may be calculated.

In a study with eight women, of whom one was 48 years old and the other seven ranged from 68 to 83 years, Ackermann and Toro (3) estimated a mean calcium requirement of 16.7 mg/kg which when applied to the mean weight of the subjects yields a requirement of approximately 900 mg/day. They reported, in addition, that in their studies the estimated requirements of the women were consistently lower than those of the men even when balances were being determined with men and women at the same time. They concluded, from a review of the studies that had been carried out with young men and women, that the calcium requirements of elderly people are greater than those of young adults.

The data of Ohlson et al. (376), however, are not in agreement with the conclusions of Ackermann and Toro (3). Ohlson et al. studied the calcium intake and output of 136 women, 30 to 85 years old, 37 of whom were over 60 years old. The women ate their customary self-selected diets which were weighed, sampled and analyzed. Calcium intake tended to decrease from a mean of 0.95 g/day for the 30- to 39-year-old group to 0.82 g/day for the 60- to 69-year-old group. The decrease was not significant. The mean intake of the 70- to 79-year old group, 0.65 g/day, was, however, significantly lower than those of the younger age groups. No negative balances in any age group were observed with intakes greater than 1.10 g calcium/day. When retention was plotted against intake in each age group the intakes calculated to be necessary for equilibrium were similar in the groups between 30 and 69 years old (0.88 to 0.92 g/day). The requirement predicted for the 70- to 79-year-old group was lower (0.73 g/day) than that calculated in the younger groups. The data suggested to Ohlson et al. that when diets are self-selected the calcium requirement remains fairly constant for the average vigorous woman between the age of 30 and 70 years but after 70 years, the requirement appears to decrease.

Much lower requirements were calculated by Fujitani (156) for elderly Japanese men and women. In his study, seven men and women 63 to 81 years old were studied during the winter with calcium intakes ranging from 0.090 to 0.300 g/day, and eight men and women 63 to 78 years old were studied during the summer with intakes ranging from 0.185 to 0.450 g/day. Each subject was studied at three levels of calcium intake. In the winter study, only three of the 21 balances were positive. In the summer study, 14 of the 24 balances were positive. When balance and intake, expressed as milligrams calcium per kilogram body weight, were plotted against each other, the mean intake calculated to be required for equilibrium was found to be 7.0 mg/kg in winter and 8.0 mg/kg in summer. When these values are applied to the mean weights of the subjects, mean calcium requirements of approximately 0.290 g/day in winter and 0.330 g/day in summer may be calculated. There was no indication of differences between men and women. Nor was it clear whether the somewhat higher intakes during the summer study might have influenced the estimated requirement.

Ackermann and Toro (2) in examining their data and those of others suggested that the vitamin D intake might have influenced calcium retention. With six of the elderly men studied previously they observed calcium intake and output with intakes ranging from 0.555 to 2.065 g/day with or without vitamin D. When 25,000 IU of vitamin D was provided, all subjects were in positive calcium balance regardless of their calcium intake. The addition of 600 or 1,800 IU of vitamin D improved calcium retention but positive balances were not always achieved. When vitamin D was fed, fecal calcium excretion was decreased. Ackermann and Toro concluded that the relatively high calcium requirements calculated from their data were due to the elderly subjects' decreased ability to absorb food calcium or to an increased fecal excretion of previously absorbed calcium. According to their data, 25,000 IU vitamin D increased daily calcium retention by approximately 5 mg/kg body weight. In

radioisotope and balance studies with elderly osteoporotic patients, Spencer et al. (456, 457) found that osteoporotic patients retained less calcium than normal subjects. Furthermore, the poor retention was due to poor absorption of food calcium rather than to increased excretion of endogenous fecal calcium.

The possibility that hormones might influence the calcium requirements of the elderly was examined by Ackermann et al. (4). In a study with seven elderly women whose calcium requirements had been previously estimated (3) they found estradiol benzoate injected intramuscularly (2 mg/week) had little effect on calcium balance. Testosterone administered in large doses (30 mg/day) increased calcium retention principally by reducing fecal excretion in the two subjects to whom it was given. Progesterone had a similar but much smaller effect. From the results of a later study, Toro et al. (486) reported that the administration of thyroid, insulin, cortisone or ACTH did not increase or depress calcium retention in five patients, 69 to 88 years old. In other studies with elderly patients, estrogen has been found to reduce urinary calcium excretion (281) but with little effect on calcium retention except in osteoporotic patients (58). Lafferty et al. (281) also found that androgen reduced both fecal and urinary calcium excretion and temporarily reduced bone resorption. With continued administration, the androgen ceased to affect bone resorption so that the skeleton apparently failed to utilize the additionally absorbed calcium.

CONCLUSIONS

The observed ability of populations in different geographic areas to live in apparent health with widely varying calcium intakes has made food intake studies of little use in assessing calcium requirements or calcium nutriture. Such studies do, however, indicate the diversity in human subjects and thereby indicate some of the difficulties involved in attempting to make calcium requirement estimates of general applicability.

The lack of a clear-cut calcium deficiency syndrome is a major impediment in the determination of calcium requirements for maintenance in man. It is possible that with more information on calcium metabolism, on how calcium functions in maintaining tonicity of the muscles, clotting of the blood and neural irritability as well as on how it is laid down structurally, we might be able to devise clinical tests that could indicate calcium nutritional status.

The recent reports of Krook et al. (276–278), Lutwak et al.,[4] and Coulston and Lutwak[5] indicate a promising approach. Their studies suggest that spontaneous periodontal disease in human subjects is similar to that developed experimentally in dogs and may be the forerunner of more serious disorders of the spinal column and the long bones[6] (276–278). Furthermore, these investigators found evidence of the regression of signs and symptoms of periodontal disease, and of increased bone density of the mandible when human subjects were fed daily calcium supplements in studies lasting 6 and 12 months[7, 8] (276). The findings suggest, therefore, a possible approach toward estimating calcium requirements.

In obtaining the necessary information on calcium nutriture and calcium requirements and in developing the research methods, isotopic studies with animals would be a logical approach. As safe precise methods are developed, their application to human subjects should be tested. Ideally, methods for measuring calcium nutriture should be applicable under field study conditions. It is not realistic to expect that such methods will be developed in the near future. In lieu of them, the currently available balance method may be used to obtain more needed information on calcium retention and excretion under varying experimental conditions. While the meaning of positive calcium balances is debatable (131, 149), observations on changes in excretion patterns might yield useful data. Isotope studies combined with balance studies as suggested by Lutwak (304) might yield information that would help to explain the changes observed in excretion patterns. There is understandable reluctance to use radioactive isotopes freely with human subjects. Some progress has been made, however, in developing the use of stable calcium isotopes (338). Heaney and Skillman's study with pregnant women

(192) has demonstrated the feasibility of this approach.

In order to assess accurately the calcium requirements for growth much more information is needed on rates and patterns of calcification during childhood. These data cannot be obtained adequately by the balance method. Other methods, possibly involving anthropometry, bone density and body composition estimates need to be devised. Again, studies with animals may provide useful guidelines.

The physiological changes that take place during puberty, pregnancy, lactation and menopause are believed to affect calcium metabolism and possibly calcium requirement (244, 290, 527). As yet, little is known on how calcium is involved in these changes and few data are available on which to base recommendations for calcium intake during these periods of physiological change. Also of concern is the effect on calcium nutriture of successive pregnancies with and without intervening periods of lactation, and of pregnancy occurring during adolescence.

Whether or not the elderly have calcium needs that differ from those of young adults is not clear. Much of the research with the elderly has involved osteoporotics. Until more information is obtained on causative factors and on the metabolic and physiological changes involved in osteoporosis, the potential for preventing or curing the disorder by means of dietary calcium will remain speculative.

If it is determined that osteoporosis can be relieved or prevented in the elderly by increased dietary calcium, the effect of high calcium intakes on other physiological aspects such as renal function must be ascertained (93). This is a problem that may have to be solved also in dealing with stress conditions that are accompanied by hypercalciuria. The upper limit of calcium intake in all age groups has had little research.

[4] Lutwak, L., Krook, L., Henrikson, P. A., Uris, R., Whalen, J., Coulston, A. & Lesser, G. (1971) Calcium deficiency and human periodontal disease. Israel J. Med. Sci. 7, 504 (abstr.).
[5] Coulston, A. & Lutwak, L. (1972) Dietary calcium deficiency and human periodontal disease. Federation Proc. 31, 721 (abstr.).
[6] See footnote 4.
[7] See footnote 4.
[8] See footnote 5.

The evidence of negative calcium balances with protein intakes that are high but not unusually high for rapidly growing boys and youths (239) indicates the need for much more information on the interaction of calcium with other nutrients. Not only the effect of other nutrients on calcium metabolism but also the effect of calcium on the metabolism and utilization of other nutrients needs clarification. It may be that a practical approach will be to recommend calcium intakes in relation to the intake of one or another nutrient, as for instance, Sherman (435) and Holt et al. (214) did.

Finally, much of our current information has been obtained in cultures where milk is a major source of dietary calcium. More information is needed on the availability and utilization of calcium from diets eaten in areas where milk is not customarily consumed. Until this information is available, data obtained with groups who habitually consume milk and who, presumably, have generous calcium intakes may have little applicability to the majority of the world's population.

ACKNOWLEDGMENTS

The authors wish to thank Miss Catherine E. Walsh for her assistance in collecting citations, abstracting papers and procuring documents. Her efforts in acquiring copies of the early literature were especially helpful.

LITERATURE CITED

1. Ackermann, P. G. & Toro, G. (1953) Calcium and phosphorus balance in elderly men. J. Gerontol. 8, 289–300.

2. Ackermann, P. G. & Toro, G. (1953) Effect of added vitamin D on the calcium balance in elderly males. J. Gerontol. 8, 451–457.

3. Ackermann, P. G. & Toro, G. (1954) Calcium balance in elderly women. J. Gerontol. 9, 446–449.

4. Ackermann, P. G., Toro, G., Kountz, W. B. & Kheim, T. (1954) The effect of sex hormone administration on the calcium and nitrogen balance in elderly women. J. Gerontol. 9, 450–455.

5. Adair, F. L., Dieckmann, W. J., Michel, H., Dunkle, F., Kramer, S. & Lorang, E. (1943) The effect of complementing the diet in pregnancy with calcium, phosphorus, iron, and vitamins A and D. Amer. J. Obstet. Gynecol. 46, 116–121.

6. Adolph, W. H. & Chen, S-C. (1932) The utilization of calcium in soy bean diets. J. Nutr. 5, 379–385.

7. Agnew, J. E., Kehayoglou, A. K. & Holdsworth, C. D. (1969) Comparison of three isotopic methods for the study of calcium absorption. Gut 10, 590–597.

8. Albright, F., Burnett, C. H., Parsons, W., Reifenstein, E. C. & Roos, A. (1946) Osteomalacia and late rickets. The various etiologies met in the United States with emphasis on that resulting from a specific form of renal acidosis, the therapeutic indications for each etiological sub-group, and the relationship between osteomalacia and Milkman's syndrome. Medicine 25, 399–479.

9. Albright, F. & Reifenstein, E. C. (1948) The Parathyroid Glands and Metabolic Bone Disease, Selected Studies, p. 135–150, Williams and Wilkins Co., Baltimore.

10. Albu, A. & Neuberg, K. (1906) Physiologie und Pathologie des Mineralstoffwechsels. Berlin. Cited by: Hornemann (1913) Zur Kenntnis des Salzgehaltes der täglichen Nahrung des Menschen. Z. Hyg. Infektionskrankh. 75, 553–568.

11. Allen, T., MacLeod, A. V. & Young, E. G. (1953) On the nutritional requirements of young children with particular reference to calcification. Can. J. Med. Sci. 31, 447–461.

12. Arnaud, C., Rasmussen, H. & Anast, C. (1966) Further studies on the interrelationship between parathyroid hormone and vitamin D. J. Clin. Invest. 45, 1955–1964.

13. Aron, H. (1907) Über die physiologische Bedeutung der Kalksalze und ihre therapeutische Verwendung. Therapeut. Monatshefte 21, 194–198.

14. Aub, J. C., Tibbetts, D. M. & McLean, R. (1937) The influence of parathyroid hormone, urea, sodium chloride, fat and of intestinal activity upon calcium balance. J. Nutr. 13, 635–655.

15. Avioli, L. V., McDonald, J. E. & Sook Won Lee (1965) The influence of age on the intestinal absorption of ^{47}Ca in women and its relation to ^{47}Ca absorption in postmenopausal osteoporosis. J. Clin. Invest. 44, 1960–1967.

16. Avioli, L. V., McDonald, J. E., Singer, R. A. & Henneman, P. H. (1965) A new oral isotopic test of calcium absorption. J. Clin. Invest. 44, 128–139.

17. Aykroyd, W. R. & Krishnan, B. G. (1938) Effect of calcium lactate on children in a nursery school. Lancet 2, 153–155.

18. Aykroyd, W. R. & Krishnan, B. G. (1939) A further experiment on the value of calcium lactate for Indian children. Indian J. Med. Res. 27, 409–412.

19. Bakwin, H. (1939) Tetany in newborn infants. Relation to physiologic hypoparathyroidism. J. Pediat. 14, 1–10.

20. Baldwin, B. T. (1921) The physical growth of children from birth to maturity. Univ. Iowa Studies in Child Welfare 1, 1–411. Cited by: Leitch, I. (1937) The determination of the calcium requirement of man. Nutr. Abstr. Rev. 6, 553–578.

21. Bansal, P., Rau, P., Venkatachalam, P. S. & Gopalan, C. (1964) Effect of calcium supplementation on children in a rural community. Indian J. Med. Res. 52, 219–223.

22. Barltrop, D. & Oppé, T. E. (1970) Dietary factors in neonatal calcium homoeostasis. Lancet 2, 1333–1335.

23. Barnes, B. A., Cope, O. & Harrison, T. (1958) Magnesium conservation in the human being on a low magnesium diet. J. Clin. Invest. 37, 430–440.

24. Bassir, O. (1959) Urinary excretion of electrolytes by healthy Nigerians fed on an unrestricted salt diet. W. Afr. J. Biol. Chem. 3, 32–34.

25. Basu, K. P., Basak, M. N. & Rai Sircar, B. C. (1939) Studies in human metabolism. Part II. Calcium and phosphorus metabolism in Indians on rice and on wheat diets. Indian J. Med. Res. 27, 471–499.

26. Basu, K. P. & Nath, H. P. (1946) The effect of different fats on calcium utilization in human beings. Indian J. Med. Res. 34, 27–31.

27. Bauer, W., Albright, F. & Aub, J. C. (1929) Studies of calcium and phosphorus metabolism. II. The calcium excretion of normal individuals on a low calcium diet, also data on a case of pregnancy. J. Clin. Invest. 7, 75–96.

28. Bauer, W., Aub, J. C. & Albright, F. (1929) Studies of calcium and phosphorus metabolism. V. A study of the bone trabeculae as a readily available reserve supply of calcium. J. Exp. Med. 49, 145–161.

29. Bauer, W. & Marble, A. (1932) Studies on the mode of action of irradiated ergosterol. II. Its effect on the calcium and phosphorus metabolism of individuals with calcium deficiency diseases. J. Clin. Invest. 11, 21–35.

30. Bauer, W., Marble, A. & Claflin, D. (1932) Studies on the mode of action of irradiated ergosterol. I. Its effect on the calcium, phosphorus and nitrogen metabolism of normal individuals. J. Clin. Invest. 11, 1–18.

31. Bauer, W., Marble, A. & Claflin, D. (1932) Studies on the mode of action of irradiated ergosterol. IV. In hypoparathyroidism. J. Clin. Invest. 11, 47–62.

32. Baum, D., Cooper, L. & Davies, P. A. (1968) Hypocalcaemic fits in neonates. Lancet 1, 598–599.

33. Bayley, N. & Davis, F. C. (1935) Growth changes in bodily size and proportions during the first three years: a developmental study of sixty-one children by repeated measurements. Biometrika 27, 26–87. Cited by: Leitch, I. (1937) The determination of the calcium requirement of man. Nutr. Abstr. Rev. 6, 553–578.

34. Beal, V. A. (1954) Nutritional intake of children. 2. Calcium, phosphorus and iron. J. Nutr. 53, 499–510.

35. Beal, V. A. (1961) Dietary intake of individuals followed through infancy and childhood. Amer. J. Pub. Health 51, 1107–1117.

36. Beal, V. A. (1968) Calcium and phosphorus in infancy. J. Amer. Diet. Ass. 53, 450–459.

37. Beal, V. A. (1971) Nutritional studies during pregnancy: (1) Changes in intakes of calories, carbohydrate, fat, protein, and calcium. J. Amer. Diet. Ass. 58, 312–326.

38. Beaton, G. H. (1961) Nutritional and physiological adaptations in pregnancy. Federation Proc. 20, 196–201.

39. Begum, A. & Pereira, S. M. (1969) Calcium balance studies on children accustomed to low calcium intakes. Brit. J. Nutr. 23, 905–911.

40. Beisel, W. R., Goldman, R. F. & Joy, R. J. (1968) Metabolic balance studies during induced hyperthermia in man. J. Appl. Physiol. 24, 1–10.

41. Bell, G. H., Cuthbertson, D. P. & Orr, J. (1941) Strength and size of bone in relation to calcium intake. J. Physiol. 100, 299–317.

42. Benedict, F. G. (1915) A study of prolonged fasting. Carnegie Institution of Washington, Publ. no. 203, pp. 1–416.

43. Benjamin, H. R., Gordon, H. H. & Marples, E. (1943) Calcium and phosphorus requirements of premature infants. Amer. J. Dis. Child. 65, 412–425.

44. Bernstein, D. S., Baylink, D. J. & Guri, C. D. (1969) The therapy of osteoporosis. J. Amer. Med. Women's Ass. 24, 36–41.

45. Bernstein, D. S. & Cohen, P. (1967) Use of sodium fluoride in the treatment of osteoporosis. J. Clin. Endocrinol. 27, 197–210.

46. Bernstein, D. S., Sadowsky, N., Hegsted, D. M., Guri, C. D. & Stare, F. J. (1966) Prevalence of osteoporosis in high- and low-fluoride areas in North Dakota. J. Amer. Med. Ass. 198, 499–504.

47. Bertram, J. (1878) Ueber die Ausscheidung der Phosphorsäure bei den Pflanzenfressern. Z. Biol. 14, 335–382.

48. Bhandarkar, S. D., Bluhm, M. M., MacGregor, J. & Nordin, B. E. C. (1961) An isotope test of calcium absorption. Brit. Med. J. 2, 1539–1541.

49. Birk, W. (1911) Beiträge zur Physiologie des neugeborenen Kindes. III. Die Bedeutung des Kolostrums. Analysen und Stoffwechselversuche. Monatsschr. Kinderheilk. 9, 595–612. Cited by Hamilton, B. (1922) The calcium and phosphorus metabolism of prematurely born infants. Acta Paediat. 2, 1–84.

50. Birk, W. & Orgler, A. (1911) Der Kalkstoffwechsel bei Rachitis. Monatsschr. Kinderheilk. 9, 544–548.

51. Blatherwick, N. R. & Long, M. L. (1922) The utilization of calcium and phosphorus of vegetables by man. J. Biol. Chem. 52, 125–131.

52. Blau, M., Spencer, H., Swernov, J., Greenberg, J. & Laszlo, D. (1957) Effect of intake level on the utilization and intestinal excretion of calcium in man. J. Nutr. 61, 507–521.

53. Blau, M., Spencer, H., Swernov, J. & Laszlo, D. (1954) Utilization and intestinal excretion of calcium in man. Science 120, 1029–1031.

54. Blauberg, M. (1900) Experimentelle Beiträge zur Frage über den Mineralstoffwechsel

beim künstlich en rährten Säugling. Z. Biol. *40*, 1. Cited by: Wang, C. C. et al. (1924) A comparison of the metabolism of some mineral constituents of cow's milk and of breast milk in the same infant. Amer. J. Dis. Child. *27*, 352–368.

55. Bodansky, M. (1938) Nutritional vs. endocrine factors in bone metabolism during pregnancy. Texas State J. Med. *34*, 339–343.

56. Bodansky, M. & Duff, V. B. (1939) Regulation of the level of calcium in the serum during pregnancy. J. Amer. Med. Ass. *112*, 223–229.

57. Bogdonoff, M. D., Shock, N. W. & Nichols, M. P. (1953) Calcium, phosphorus, nitrogen, and potassium balance studies in the aged male. J. Gerontol. 8, 272–288.

58. Bogdonoff, M. D., Shock, N. W. & Parsons, J. (1954) The effects of stilbestrol on the retention of nitrogen, calcium, phosphorus, and potassium in aged males with and without osteoporosis. J. Gerontol. 9, 262-275.

59. Bogert, L. J. & Kirkpatrick, E. E. (1922) Studies in inorganic metabolism. II. The effects of acid-forming and base-forming diets upon calcium metabolism. J. Biol. Chem. *56*, 375–386.

60. Bogert, L. J. & McKittrick, E. J. (1922) Studies in inorganic metabolism. I. Interrelations between calcium and magnesium metabolism. J. Biol. Chem. 56, 363–374.

61. Bogert, L. J. & Trail, R. K. (1922) Studies in inorganic metabolism. III. The influence of yeast and butterfat upon calcium assimilation. J. Biol. Chem. 56, 387–397.

62. Boldt, F., Brahm, C. & Andresen, G. (1929) Langfristige Mineralstoffuntersuchungen an zwei gesunden Säuglingen bei mineralstoffarmer und -reicher Kost. Arch. Kinderheilk. *87*, 277–296.

63. Bonner, P., Hummel, F. C., Bates, M. F., Horton, J., Hunscher, H. A. & Macy, I. G. (1938) The influence of a daily serving of spinach or its equivalent in oxalic acid upon the mineral utilization of children. J. Pediat. *12*, 188–199.

64. Borchardt, W. (1931) Aufgaben der Tropenphysiologie. Ergeb. Physiol. *31*, 96–131.

65. Breiter, H., Mills, R., Dwight, J., McKey, B., Armstrong, W. & Outhouse, J. (1941) The utilization of the calcium of milk by adults. J. Nutr. *21*, 351–362.

66. Bricker, M. L., Smith, J. M., Hamilton, T. S. & Mitchell, H. H. (1949) The effect of cocoa upon calcium utilization and requirements, nitrogen retention and fecal composition of women. J. Nutr. *39*, 445–461.

67. Brine, C. L. & Johnston, F. A. (1955) Endogenous calcium in the feces of adult man and the amount of calcium absorbed from food. Amer. J. Clin. Nutr. *3*, 418–420.

68. Brine, C. L. & Johnston, F. A. (1955) Factors affecting calcium absorption by adults. J. Amer. Diet. Ass. *31*, 883–888.

69. Briscoe, A. M. & Ragan, C. (1965) Bile and endogenous fecal calcium in man. Amer. J. Clin. Nutr. *16*, 281–286.

70. Briscoe, A. M. & Ragan, C. (1966) Effect

of magnesium on calcium metabolism in man. Amer. J. Clin. Nutr. *19*, 296–306.

71. Brody, S. (1927) Growth and development with special reference to domestic animals. IX. A comparison of growth curves of man and other animals. Missouri Agr. Exp. Sta. Res. Bull. *104*, 31. Cited by: Mitchell, H. H. & Curzon, E. G. (1939) The dietary requirement of calcium and its significance. Actualitées Scientifiques et Industrielles no. 771, pp. 36–101, Hermann & Co., Paris.

72. Bronner, F. & Harris, R. S. (1956) Absorption and metabolism of calcium in human beings, studied with [45]calcium. Ann. N. Y. Acad. Sci. *64*, 314–325.

73. Bronner, F., Harris, R. S., Maletskos, C. J. & Benda, C. E. (1954) Studies in calcium metabolism. Effect of food phytates on calcium[45] uptake in children on low-calcium breakfasts. J. Nutr. *54*, 523–542.

74. Bronner, F., Harris, R. S., Maletskos, C. J. & Benda, C. E. (1956) Studies of calcium metabolism. Effect of food phytates on calcium[45] uptake in boys on a moderate calcium breakfast. J. Nutr. *59*, 393–406.

75. Bronner, F., Saville, P. D., Nicholas, J. A., Cobb, J. R., Wilson, P. D., Jr. & Wilson, P. D. (1962) Calcium metabolism in man. Quantitation of calcium absorption and the excretion index. In: Radioisotopes and Bone (McLean, F. C., LaCroix, P. & Budy, A. M., eds.), pp. 17–33, Blackwell Scientific Publications, Oxford.

76. Brown, E. G., Herman, C. & Ohlson, M. (1946) Weight reduction of obese women of college age. 2. Nitrogen, calcium and phosphorus retentions of young women during weight reduction. J. Amer. Diet. Ass. *22*, 858–863.

77. Bruck, E. & Weintraub, D. H. (1955) Serum calcium and phosphorus in premature and full-term infants. A longitudinal study in the first three weeks of life. Amer. J. Dis. Child. *90*, 653–668.

78. Brull, L. (1936) Recherches sur le métabolisme minéral. La grandeur des besoins d'entretien en calcium, phosphore et magnésium. Bull. Acad. Roy. Med. Belg. *1*, 444–456.

79. Bullamore, J. R., Gallagher, J. C., Wilkinson, R., Nordin, B. E. C. & Marshall, D. H. (1970) Effect of age on calcium absorption. Lancet 2, 535–537.

80. Burke, B. S., Beal, V. A., Kirkwood, S. B. & Stuart, H. C. (1943) Nutrition studies during pregnancy. 1. Problems, methods of study, and group studied. Amer. J. Obstet. Gynecol. *46*, 38–52.

81. Burke, B. S., Reed, R. B., Van den Berg, A. S. & Stuart, H. C. (1962) A longitudinal study of the calcium intake of children from one to eighteen years of age. Amer. J. Clin. Nutr. *10*, 79–88.

82. Burton, H. B. (1930) The influence of cereals upon the retention of calcium and phosphorus in children and adults. J. Biol. Chem. *85*, 405–419.

83. Cahn, A. & Roche, A. F. (1961) The influence of illness and calcium intake on

rate of skeletal maturation in children. Brit. J. Nutr. 15, 411–417.

84. Camilleri, A. P. (1968) Dental obstetrics. Brit. Dent. J. 124, 219–222.

85. Campbell, H. L., Bessey, O. A. & Sherman, H. C. (1935) Adult rats of low calcium content. J. Biol. Chem. 110, 703–706.

86. Caniggia, A. (1965) Medical problems in senile osteoporosis. Geriatrics 20, 300–311.

87. Cathcart, E. P. (1907) Über die Zusammensetzung des Hungerharns. Biochem. Z. 6, 109–148.

88. Chaney, M. S. & Blunt, K. (1925) The effect of orange juice on the calcium, phosphorus, magnesium and nitrogen retention and urinary organic acids of growing children. J. Biol. Chem. 66, 829–845.

89. Chopra, J., Perelta, F., Villegas, N. & Everette, L. (1964) Anaemia in lactation. W. Indian Med. J. 13, 252–265. Cited in: Nutr. Abstr. Rev. 35, 801, (1965).

90. Chu, H. I., Liu, S. H., Yu, T. F., Hsu, H. C., Cheng, T. Y. & Chao, H. C. (1940) Calcium and phosphorus metabolism in osteomalacia. X. Further studies on vitamin D action: early signs of depletion and effect of minimal doses. J. Clin. Invest. 19, 349–363.

91. Chu, H. I., Yu, T. F., Chang, K. P. & Liu, W. T. (1939) Calcium and phosphorus metabolism in osteomalacia. VII. The effect of ultraviolet irradiation from mercury vapor quartz lamp and sunlight. Chin. Med. J. 55, 93–124.

92. Clark, G. W. (1926) Studies in the mineral metabolism of adult man. Univ. Calif. Publ. Physiol. 5, 195–269.

93. Clarkson, E. M., McDonald, S. J. & DeWardener, H. E. (1966) The effect of a high intake of calcium carbonate in normal subjects and patients with chronic renal failure. Clin. Sci. 30, 425–438.

94. Cofer, E. S., Porter, T. & Davis, M. E. (1957) The effect of withdrawal of estrogens on the nitrogen, calcium and phosphorus balances of women. J. Nutr. 61, 357–371.

95. Cohen, P. (1933) Tetany in very young infants with special reference to etiology. Amer. J. Dis. Child. 45, 331–342.

96. Cohn, S. H., Dombrowski, C. S., Hauser, W. & Atkins, H. L. (1968) High calcium diet and the parameters of calcium metabolism in osteoporosis. Amer. J. Clin. Nutr. 21, 1246–1253.

97. Consolazio, C. F., Matoush, L. O., Nelson, R. A., Hackler, L. R. & Preston, E. E. (1962) Relationship between calcium in sweat, calcium balance, and calcium requirement. J. Nutr. 78, 78–88.

98. Consolazio, C. F., Matoush, L. O., Nelson, R. A., Isaac, G. J. & Canham, J. E. (1966) Comparisons of nitrogen, calcium and iodine excretion in arm and total body sweat. Amer. J. Clin. Nutr. 18, 443–448.

99. Consolazio, C. F., Shapiro, R., Masterson, J. E. & McKinzie, P. S. L. (1961) Energy requirements of men in extreme heat. J. Nutr. 73, 126–134.

100. Coons, C. M. & Blunt, K. (1930) The retention of nitrogen, calcium, phosphorus and magnesium by pregnant women. J. Biol. Chem. 86, 1–16.

101. Coons, C. M., Schiefelbusch, A. T., Marshall, G. B. & Coons, R. R. (1935) Studies in metabolism during pregnancy. Oklahoma Agr. Exp. Sta. Res. Bull no. 223, pp. 1–113.

102. Cronheim, W. & Müller, E. (1908) Stoffwechselversuche an gesunden und rachitischen Kindern mit besonderer Berücksichtung des Mineralstoffwechsels. Biochem. Z. 9, 76. Cited by: Wang, C. C. et al. (1924) A comparison of the metabolism of some mineral constituents of cow's milk and of breast milk in the same infant. Amer. J. Dis. Child. 27, 352–368.

103. Cruickshank, E. W. H., Duckworth, J., Kosterlitz, H. W. & Warnock, G. M. (1945) The digestibility of the phytate-P of oatmeal in adult man. J. Physiol. 104, 41–46.

104. Cullumbine, H., Basnayake, V., Lemottee, J. & Wickramanayake, T. W. (1950) Mineral metabolism on rice diets. Brit. J. Nutr. 4, 101–111.

105. Dale, N. E. (1968) A study of the urinary calcium, phosphorus, creatinine and sodium excretion of young adults in Sydney. Med. J. Aust. 1, 791–793.

106. Dallas, I. & Nordin, B. E. C. (1962) The relation between calcium intake and roentgenologic osteoporosis. Amer. J. Clin. Nutr. 11, 263–269.

107. Daniels, A. L. (1941) Relation of calcium, phosphorus and nitrogen retention to growth and osseous development. A long time study of three preschool boys. Amer. J. Dis. Child. 62, 279–294.

108. Daniels, A. L. & Everson, G. J. (1937) The relation of ascorbic acid ingestion to mineral metabolism in children. J. Nutr. 14, 317–328.

109. Daniels, A. L., Hutton, M. K., Knott, E., Everson, G. & Wright, O. (1933) Relation of milk ingestion to calcium metabolism in children. Proc. Soc. Exp. Biol. Med. 30, 1062–1063.

110. Daniels, A. L., Hutton, M. K., Knott, E., Everson, G. & Wright, O. (1934) Relation of ingestion of milk to calcium metabolism in children. Amer. J. Dis. Child. 47, 499–512.

111. Daniels, A. L., Hutton, M. K., Knott, E. M., Wright, O. E. & Forman, O. (1935) Calcium and phosphorus needs of preschool children. J. Nutr. 10, 373–388.

112. Daniels, A. L., Stearns, G. & Hutton, M. K. (1929) Calcium and phosphorus metabolism in artificially fed infants. 1. Influence of cod liver oil and irradiated milk. Amer. J. Dis. Child. 37, 296–310.

113. Davis, N. J. (1935) Calcium, phosphorus and nitrogen retention of children. Effects of acid-forming and base-forming diets. Amer. J. Dis. Child. 49, 611–624.

114. DeGrazia, J. A. & Rich, C. (1965) Studies of intestinal absorption of calcium[45] in man. Metabolism 13, 650–660.

115. Deitrick, J. E. (1948) The effect of immobilization on metabolic and physiological

functions of normal men. Bull. N. Y. Acad. Med. *24*, 364–375.

116. Deitrick, J. E., Whedon, G. D. & Shorr, E. (1948) Effects of immobilization upon various metabolic and physiologic functions of normal men. Amer. J. Med. *4*, 3–36.

117. Deitrick, J. E., Whedon, G. D., Shorr, E. & Barr, D. P. (1945) Effects of bed rest and immobilization upon various physiological and chemical functions of normal men. In: Conference on Metabolic Aspects of Convalescence including Bone and Wound Healing, Ninth Meeting, Feb. 2–3, 1945, (Reifenstein, E. C., Jr., ed.), pp. 62–81, Josiah Macy Jr. Foundation, New York.

118. Deller, D. J., Worthley, B. W. & Martin, H. (1965) Measurement of calcium-47 absorption by whole-body gamma spectrometry. Australasian Ann. Med. *14*, 223–231.

119. Dent, C. E., Harper, C. M. & Parfitt, A. M. (1964) The effect of cellulose phosphate on calcium metabolism in patients with hypercalciuria. Clin. Sci. *27*, 417–425.

120. Dent, C. E. & Watson, L. (1966) Osteoporosis. Postgraduate Med. J. *42*, 583–608. Cited by: Rose, G. A. (1967) A critique of modern methods of diagnosis and treatment of osteoporosis. Clin. Orthop. *55*, 17–41.

121. Desikachar, H. S. R. & Subrahmanyan, V. (1956) The level of protein intake and the quality of protein on calcium and phosphorus absorption. Indian J. Med. Res. *37*, 85–90.

122. Devadas, R. P. & Prema, L. (1965) The nutritional status of nursing mothers and infants in an applied nutrition area in Madras State. J. Nutr. Diet., India *2*, 149–153.

123. Dieckmann, W. J., Adair, F. L., Michel, H., Kramer, S., Dunkle, F., Arthur, B., Costin, M., Campbell, A., Wensley, A. C. & Lorang, E. (1944) The effect of complementing the diet in pregnancy with calcium, phosphorus, iron and vitamins A and D. Amer. J. Obstet. Gynecol. *47*, 357–368.

124. Donaldson, C. L., Hulley, S. B., Vogel, J. M., Hattner, R. S., Bayers, J. H. & McMillan, D. E. (1970) Effect of prolonged bed rest on bone mineral. Metabolism *19*, 1071–1084.

125. Donelson, E., Nims, B., Hunscher, H. A. & Macy, I. G. (1931) Metabolism of women during the reproductive cycle. IV. Calcium and phosphorus utilization in late lactation and during subsequent reproductive rest. J. Biol. Chem. *91*, 675–686.

126. Doraiswamy, T. R., Daniel, V. A., Rajalakshmi, D., Swaminathan, M. & Parpia, H. A. B. (1971) Effect of supplementing a poor diet based on rice and wheat consumed by school children with vitamins, minerals, lysine and protein-rich foods, on their growth and nutritional status. Nutr. Rep. Int. *3*, 67–78.

127. Dorland's Illustrated Medical Dictionary (1965) 24th Ed., p. 39, W. B. Saunders Co., Philadelphia.

128. Drake, T. G. H., Jackson, S. H., Tisdall, F. F., Johnstone, W. M. & Hurst, L. M. (1949) The biological availability of the calcium in bone. J. Nutr. *37*, 369–376.

129. Drummond, J. C., Gray, C. H. & Richardson, N. E. G. (1939) The antirachitic value of human milk. Brit. Med. J. *2*, 757–760. Cited by: Garry, R. C. & Wood, H. O. (1946) Dietary requirements in human pregnancy and lactation. A review of recent work. Nutr. Abstr. Rev. *15*, 591–621.

130. Dubrovina, Z. V., Sarapul'cev, I. A. & Fadeev, A. P. (1967) K voprosu ob obmene stroncija i kal'cija u celoveka. Gigiena Sanit. no. 4, 43–46. Cited in: Nutr. Abstr. Rev. *38*, 138, 1968.

131. Duncan, D. L. (1958) The interpretation of studies of calcium and phosphorus balance in ruminants. Nutr. Abstr. Rev. *28*,. 695–715.

132. Dunn, A. W. (1967) Senile osteoporosis. Geriatrics *22*, 175–180.

133. Dunn, M. J. & Walser, M. (1966) Magnesium depletion in normal man. Metabolism *15*, 884–895.

134. Dunnigan, M. G. & Smith, C. M. (1965) The aetiology of late rickets in Pakistani children in Glasgow. Report of a diet survey. Scot. Med. J. *10*, 1–9.

135. Ebbs, J. H., Tisdall, F. F. & Scott, W. A. (1941) The influence of prenatal diet on the mother and child. J. Nutr. *22*, 515–526.

136. Ejsmont, W., Bartnicki, C. & Dubrawski, R. (1966) The problem of acclimatization in the tropical zone. VI. Changes in the calcium and phosphate levels in serum urine and sweat. Bull. Inst. Mar. Med. Gdansk. *17*, 521–528.

137. Ellinger, G. M., Duckworth, J. & Dalgarno, A. C. (1952) Skeletal changes during pregnancy and lactation in the rat: effect of different levels of dietary calcium. Brit. J. Nutr. *6*, 235–257.

138. Eppright, E. S., Sidwell, V. D. & Swanson, P. P. (1954) Nutritive value of the diets of Iowa school children. J. Nutr. *54*, 371–388.

139. Epstein, F. H. (1960) Calcium and the kidney. J. Chron. Dis. *11*, 255–277.

140. Ewe, K. (1968) Resorption und Sekretion von Calcium im menschlichen Jejunum. Klin. Wochenschr. *46*, 661–666.

141. Exton-Smith, A. N. (1972) Physiological aspects of aging: relationship to nutrition. Amer. J. Clin. Nutr. *25*, 853–859.

142. Fairbanks, B. W. & Mitchell, H. H. (1936) The relation between calcium retention and the store of calcium in the body, with particular reference to the determination of calcium requirements. J. Nutr. *11*, 551–572. Cited by: Outhouse et al. (1939) The calcium requirements of five pre-school girls. J. Nutr. *17*, 199–211.

143. Farquharson, R. F., Salter, W. T. & Aub, J. C. (1931) Studies of calcium and phosphorus metabolism. XIII. The effect of ingestion of phosphates on the excretion of calcium. J. Clin. Invest. *10*, 251–269. Cited by: Mitchell, H. H., & Curzon, E. G. (1939) The dietary requirement of calcium and its significance. Actualités Scientifiques et Industrielles no. 771, pp. 36–101, Hermann & Co., Paris.

144. Farquharson, R. F., Salter, W. T., Tibbetts

D. M. & Aub, J. C. (1931) Studies of calcium and phosphorus metabolism. XII. The effect of the ingestion of acid-producing substances. J. Clin. Invest. 10, 221–249.

145. Filer, L. J., Jr. & Martinez, G. A. (1964) Intake of selected nutrients by infants in the United States: an evaluation of 4,000 representative six-month-olds. Clin. Pediat. 3, 633–645.

146. Fiorica, F., Burr, M. J. & Moses, R. (1968) Contribution of activity to the circadian rhythm in excretion of magnesium and calcium. Aerosp. Med. 39, 714–717.

147. Fishberg, E. H. & Bierman, W. (1932) Acid-base balance in sweat. J. Biol. Chem. 97, 433–441.

148. Fomon, S. J. (1967) Infant Nutrition, pp. 142–146, W. B. Saunders Co., Philadelphia.

149. Fomon, S. J. & Owen, G. M. (1962) Comment on metabolic balance studies as a method of estimating body composition of infants. (With special consideration of nitrogen balance studies). Pediatrics 29, 495–498.

150. Fomon, S. J., Owen, G. M., Jensen, R. L. & Thomas, L. N. (1963) Calcium and phosphorus balance studies with normal full term infants fed pooled human milk or various formulas. Amer. J. Clin. Nutr. 12, 346–357.

151. Food and Agriculture Organization (1962) Calcium Requirements. Report of an FAO/WHO Expert Group. FAO Nutrition Meetings Report Series no. 30, Rome.

152. Forster, J. (1884) Beiträge zur Kenntnis der Kalkresorption im Thierkörper. Arch. Hyg. 2, 385–411.

153. French, C. E. (1942) The interrelation of calcium and fat utilization in the growing albino rat. J. Nutr. 23, 375–384.

154. French, C. E. & Elliot, R. F. (1943) The interrelation of calcium and fat utilization. J. Nutr. 25, 17–21.

155. Freyberg, R. H. & Grant, R. L. (1937) Loss of minerals through the skin of normal humans when sweating is avoided. J. Clin. Invest. 16, 729–731.

156. Fujitani, M. (1960) Studies on calcium, phosphorus, sodium and chlorine balances in the aged. J. Osaka City Med. Center 9, 2063–2082.

157. Fuqua, M. E. & Patton, M. B. (1953) Effect of three levels of fat intake on calcium metabolism. J. Amer. Diet. Ass. 29, 1010–1013.

158. Gamble, J. L., Ross, G. S. & Tisdall, F. F. (1923) The metabolism of fixed base during fasting. J. Biol. Chem. 57, 633–695. Cited by: Mitchell, H. H. & Curzon, E. G. (1939) The dietary requirement of calcium and its significance. Actualités Scientifique et Industrielles no. 771, pp. 36–101, Hermann & Co., Paris.

159. Gardner, L. I., MacLachlen, E. A., Pick, W., Terry, M. L. & Butler, A. M. (1950) Etiologic factors in tetany of newly born infants. Pediatrics 5, 228–240.

160. Garn, S. M., Rohmann, C. S. & Wagner, B.

(1967) Bone loss as a general phenomenon in man. Federation Proc. 26, 1729–1736.

161. Garrido, M. & Orozco, F. (1968) Excreción urinaria de calcio. Una constante biologica? Rev. Clin. Española 109, 411–416.

162. Garry, R. C. & Stiven, D. (1936) A review of recent work on dietary requirements in pregnancy and lactation, with an attempt to assess human requirements. Nutr. Abstr. Rev. 5, 855–887.

163. Garry, R. C. & Wood, H. O. (1946) Dietary requirements in human pregnancy and lactation. A review of recent work. Nutr. Abstr. Rev. 15, 591–621.

164. Gassmann, B., Plenert, W. & Heine, W. (1965) Zur Frage der Notwendigkeit einer Fetthomogenisierung bei Säuglingsfertignahrungen mit Pflanzenölzusatz. Deutsch. Gesundheitswesen 20, 1097–1100.

165. Gershon-Cohen, J. & Jowsey, J. (1964) The relationship of dietary calcium to osteoporosis. Metabolism 13, 221–226.

166. Ghosh, C. (1951) Studies on some aspects of mineral and lipid metabolism in relation to normal pregnancy. Part 1. Calcium metabolism. Calcutta Med. J. 48, 287–301.

167. Gittleman, I. F., Pinkus, J. B. & Schmertzler, E. (1964) Interrelationship of calcium and magnesium in the mature neonate. Amer. J. Dis. Child. 107, 119–124.

168. Givens, M. H. & Macy, I. G. (1933) The chemical composition of the human fetus. J. Biol. Chem. 102, 7–17.

169. Gohshi, N. (1960) Studies on the calcium and phosphorus metabolism in infancy and childhood. J. Osaka City Med. Center 9, 2301–2315.

170. Goldsmith, R. S., Killian, P., Ingbar, S. H. & Bass, D. E. (1969) Effect of phosphate supplementation during immobilization of normal men. Metabolism 18, 349–368.

171. Gontzea, I., Dumitrache, S., Rujinski, A. & Schutzesku, P. (1966) Die Calciumbilanz des körperlich arbeitenden Menschen. Int. Z. angew. Physiol. Arbeitsphysiol. 22, 103–114.

172. Goodman, D. B. P. (1968) Neonatal hypocalcemia. N. Engl. J. Med. 279, 326.

173. Graham, G. G., Barness, L. A. & György, P. (1953) Serum calcium and inorganic phosphate in the newborn infant, and their relation to different feedings. J. Pediat. 42, 401–408.

174. Gramatchikov (1890) Inaug. Diss. St. Petersburg. Cited by: Sherman, H. C., Mettler, A. J. & Sinclair, J. E. (1910) Calcium, magnesium and phosphorus in food and nutrition. U. S. Dept. Agr. Off. Exp. Sta. Bull. no. 227.

175. Greenwald, E., Samachson, J. & Spencer, H. (1963) Effect of lactose on calcium metabolism in man. J. Nutr. 79, 531–538.

176. Gribetz, D., Mizrachi, A. & London, R. B. (1968) Neonatal hypocalcemia. N. Engl. J. Med. 279, 327.

177. Gumpert, E. (1905) Beitrag zur Kenntnis des Stickstoff-, Phosphor-, Kalk- und Mag-

nesia-Umsatzes beim Menschen. Med. Klinik I(41), 1037–1041.

178. Hall, T. C. & Lehmann, H. (1944) Experiments on the practicability of increasing calcium absorption with protein derivatives. Biochem. J. 38, 117–119.

179. Hamilton, B. (1922) The calcium and phosphorus metabolism of prematurely born infants. Acta Paediat. 2, 1–84.

180. Hampton, M. C., Huenemann, R. L., Shapiro, L. R. & Mitchell, B. W. (1967) Caloric and nutrient intakes of teen-agers. J. Amer. Diet. Ass. 50, 385–396.

181. Hanna, F. M., Navarrete, D. A. & Hsu, F. A. (1970) Calcium–fatty acid absorption in term infants fed human milk and prepared formulas simulating human milk. Pediatrics 45, 216–224.

182. Harrison, H. E. (1936) The retentions of nitrogen, calcium, and phosphorus of infants fed sweetened condensed milk. J. Pediat. 8, 415–419.

183. Harrison, H. E. (1959) Factors influencing calcium absorption. Federation Proc. 18, 1085–1092.

184. Harrison, M., Fraser, R. & Mullan, B. (1961) Calcium metabolism in osteoporosis. Acute and long-term responses to increased calcium intake. Lancet 1, 1015–1019.

185. Hart, M. C., Tourtellotte, D. & Heyl, F. W. (1928) The effect of irradiation and cod liver oil on the calcium balance in the adult human. J. Biol. Chem. 76, 143–148.

186. Hattner, R. S. & McMillan, D. E. (1968) Influence of weightlessness upon the skeleton: a review. Aerosp. Med. 39, 849–855.

187. Hawawini, E. & Schreier, K. (1965) Die ernährungsphysiologische Bedeutung der Stickstoff- und Ionenverluste durch die Haut. Z. Kinderheilk. 92, 333–342.

188. Hawks, J. E., Bray, M. M., Wilde, M. O. & Dye, M. (1942) The interrelationship of calcium, phosphorus and nitrogen in the metabolism of pre-school children. J. Nutr. 24, 283–294.

189. Heaney, R. P. (1962) Radiocalcium metabolism in disuse osteoporosis in man. Amer. J. Med. 33, 188–200.

190. Heaney, R. P. (1965) A unified concept of, osteoporosis. Amer. J. Med. 39, 877–880.

191. Heaney, R. P. & Skillman, T. G. (1964) Secretion and excretion of calcium by the human gastrointestinal tract. J. Lab. Clin. Med. 64, 29–41.

192. Heaney, R. P. & Skillman, T. G. (1971) Calcium metabolism in normal human pregnancy. J. Clin. Endocrinol. Metab. 33, 661–670.

193. Heaton, F. W. & Parsons, F. M. (1961) The metabolic effect of high magnesium intake. Clin. Sci. 21, 273–284.

194. Hegsted, D. M., Moscoso, I. & Collazos Ch., C. (1952) A study of the minimum calcium requirements of adult men. J. Nutr. 46, 181–201.

195. Henderson, J. McA. & Kelly, F. C. (1929–1930) The influence of certain dietary supplements in relation to the calcium require-

196. Henderson, J. McA. & Kelly, F. C. (1929–1930) A note of the influence of the addition of certain supplements to the diets of African natives. III. J. Hyg. 29, 439–442.

197. Henry, K. M. & Kon, S. K. (1953) The relationship between calcium retention and body stores of calcium in the rat: effect of age and of vitamin D. Brit. J. Nutr. 7, 147–159.

198. Herbst, O. (1912) Beiträge zur Physiologie des Stoffwechsels im Knabenalter mit besonderer Berücksichtigung einiger Mineralstoffe. Jahrb. Kinderheilk. 76, 40. Cited by: Sherman, H. C. & Hawley, E.(1922) Calcium and phosphorus metabolism in childhood. J. Biol. Chem. 53, 375–399.

199. Herbst, O. (1913) Calcium und Phosphor beim Wachstum am Ende der Kindheit. Z. Kinderheilk. 7, 161. Cited by: Wang, C. C. et. al. (1936) Metabolism of adolescent girls. Amer. J. Dis. Child. 52, 41–53.

200. Herter, C. A. (1908) On Infantilism from Chronic Intestinal Infection, pp. 52–53, MacMillan Co., New York.

201. Herxheimer (1897) Berlin klin. Wochenschr. 34 423. Cited by: Sherman, H. C., Mettler, A. J. & Sinclair, J. E. (1910) Calcium, magnesium and phosphorus in food and nutrition. U. S. Dept. Agr. Off. Exp. Sta. Bull. No. 227.

202. Hess, J. H., Poncher, H. G., Wade, H. W. & Ricewasser, J. C. (1940) Cow's milk treated by base exchange for infant feeding. Metabolism of calcium, phosphorus and nitrogen. Amer. J. Dis. Child. 60, 535–547.

203. Hess, J. H., Poncher, H. G. & Woodward, H. (1934) Factors influencing the utilization of calcium and phosphorus of cow's milk. Amer. J. Dis. Child. 48, 1058–1071.

204. Hickmans, E. M. (1924) The calcium metabolism of atrophic infants and its relationship to their fat metabolism. Biochem. J. 18, 925–936.

205. Hitchcock, N. E. & English, R. M. (1966) Nutrient intake during lactation in Australian women. Brit. J. Nutr. 20, 599–607.

206. Hoff-Jørgensen, E., Andersen, O. & Nielsen, G. (1946) The effect of phytic acid on the absorption of calcium and phosphorus. 3. In children. Biochem. J. 40, 555–557.

207. Hoffman, W. S., Parmelee, A. H. & Grossman, A. (1949) Electrolyte balance studies on premature infants on a diet of evaporated milk. Amer. J. Dis. Child. 77, 49–60.

208. Hoffström, K. A. (1910) Eine Stoffwechseluntersuchung während der Schwangerschaft. Skand. Arch. Physiol. 23, 326–409.

209. Holemans, K. & Lambrechts, A. (1958) Calcium and phosphorus balances in African children. (Retention and minimum requirements). J. Trop. Pediat. 4, 43–49.

210. Holemans, K. & Martin, H. (1954) Étude de l'allaitement maternal et des habitudes alimentaires du sevrage chez les indigènes du Kwango. Ann. Soc. Belg. Med. Trop. 34, 915–923.

ments of growing African natives. II. J. Hyg. 29, 429–438.

211. Holmes, J. O. (1945) The requirement for calcium during growth. Nutr. Abstr. Rev. 14, 597–612.

212. Holsti, O. (1910) Zur Kenntnis des Phosphorumsatzes beim Menschen. Skand. Arch. Physiol. 23, 143–153.

213. Holt, L. E., Courtney, A. M. & Fales, H. L. (1920) Calcium metabolism of infants and young children, and the relation of calcium to fat excretion in the stools. 1. Infants taking modifications of cow's milk. Amer. J. Dis. Child. 19, 97–113.

214. Holt, L. E., Courtney, A. M. & Fales, H. L. (1920) Calcium metabolism of infants and young children and the relation of calcium to fat excretion in the stools. Part 2. Children taking a mixed diet. Amer. J. Dis. Child. 19, 201–222.

215. Holt, L. E. & Fales, H. L. (1923) Calcium absorption in children on a diet low in fat. Amer. J. Dis. Child. 25, 247–256.

216. Hoobler, B. R. (1911) The role of mineral salts in the metabolism of infants. Amer. J. Dis. Child. 2, 107–140.

217. Hopf, G. (1935) Chemisch-physikalische Untersuchungen über den menschlichen Schweiss. Arch. Dermatol. Syphilis 171, 301–312.

218. Hornemann (1913) Zur Kenntnis des Salzgehaltes der täglichen Nahrung des Menschen. Z. Hyg. Infektionskrankh. 75, 553–568.

219. Houet, R. (1945) Recherches sur le métabolisme du calcium et du phosphore dans l'enfance. 1. L'hypocalcémie de carence chez l'enfant. Rev. Belge Sci. Méd. 16, 301–312. Cited in: Nutr. Abstr. Rev. 16, 150, (1946).

220. Hövels, O. & Stephan, U. (1961) Der Calcium- und Phosphorstoffwechsel Frühgeborener und seine Bedeutung für die Rachitisprophylaxe. Med. Ernährung 2, 178–181.

221. Hövels, O., Thilenius, O. G. & Krafczyk, S. (1960) Untersuchungen zum Calcium- und Phosphatstoffwechsel Frühgeborener. 1. Der Einfluss des Angebotes, der Grundnahrung und des Calciumphosphorquotienten der Zufuhr auf die Calciumretention. Z. Kinderheilk. 83, 508–518.

222. Howard, J. E., Parson, W. & Bigham, R. S. Jr. (1945) Studies on patients convalescent from fracture. 3. The urinary excretion of calcium and phosphorus. Bull. Johns Hopkins Hosp. 77, 291–313.

223. Hsu, P. C. & Adolph, W. H. (1940) Nitrogen, calcium and phosphorus balances of adolescent boys. Chin. J. Physiol. 15, 317–325.

224. Hummel, F. C., Hunscher, H. A., Bates, M. F., Bonner, P., Macy, I.G. & Johnston, J. A. (1937) A consideration of the nutritive state in the metabolism of women during pregnancy. J. Nutr. 13, 263–278.

225. Hummel, F. C., Sternberger, H. R., Hunscher, H. A. & Macy, I. G. (1936) Metabolism of women during the reproductive cycle. 7. Utilization of inorganic elements (a con-

tinuous case study of a multipara). J. Nutr. 11, 235–255.

226. Hunscher, H. A. (1930) Metabolism of women during the reproductive cycle. II. Calcium and phosphorus utilization in two successive lactation periods. J. Biol. Chem. 86, 37–57.

227. Hunscher, H. A., Donelson, E., Erickson, B. N. & Macy, I. G. (1934) Results of the ingestion of cod liver oil and yeast on calcium and phosphorus metabolism of women. J. Nutr. 8, 341–346.

228. Hunscher, H. A., Hummel, F. C. & Macy, I. G. (1936) Variability of metabolic response of different children to a given intake of calcium. Proc. Soc. Exp. Biol. Med. 35, 189–192.

229. Hytten, F. C. & Leitch, I. (1964) The Physiology of Human Pregnancy, pp. 319–353, Blackwell Scientific Publications, Oxford.

230. Iob, V. & Swanson, W. W. (1934) Mineral growth of the human fetus. Amer. J. Dis. Child. 47, 302–306.

231. Isaksson, B., Lindholm, B. & Sjögren, B. (1966) Dermal losses of nutrients and their significance for human metabolic balance studies. Acta Med. Scand. 179 (suppl. 445), 416–420.

232. Isaksson, B., Lindholm, B. & Sjögren, B. (1967) A critical evaluation of the calcium balance technic. II. Dermal calcium losses. Metabolism 16, 303–313.

233. Isaksson, B. & Sjögren, B. (1967) A critical evaluation of the calcium balance technic. I. Variation in fecal output. Metabolism 16, 295–302.

234. Issekutz, B., Jr., Blizzard, J. J., Birkhead, N. C. & Rodahl, K. (1966) Effect of prolonged bed rest on urinary calcium output. J. Appl. Physiol. 21, 1013–1020.

235. Jaworski, Z. F., Brown, E. M., Fedoruk, S. & Seitz, H. (1963) A method for the study of calcium absorption by the human gut using a standard dose of calcium labelled with calcium[47]. N. Engl. J. Med. 269, 1103–1111.

236. Jeans, P. C. & Stearns, G. (1934) Effectiveness of vitamin D in infancy in relation to the vitamin source. Proc. Soc. Exp. Biol. Med. 31, 1159–1161.

237. Jeans, P. C. & Stearns, G. (1935) Retention of calcium by infants fed evaporated milk containing cod liver oil concentrate. Proc. Soc. Exp. Biol. Med. 32, 1464–1466.

238. Jeans, P. C., Stearns, G., McKinley, J. B., Goff, E. A. & Stinger, D. (1936) Factors possibly influencing the retention of calcium, phosphorus and nitrogen by infants given whole milk feedings. 1. The curding agent. J. Pediat. 8, 403–414.

239. Johnson, N. E., Alcantara, E. N. & Linkswiler, H. (1970) Effect of level of protein intake on urinary and fecal calcium and calcium retention of young adult males. J. Nutr. 100, 1425–1430.

240. Johnston, F. A. (1958) The loss of calcium, phosphorus, iron, and nitrogen in hair from the scalp of women. Amer. J. Clin. Nutr. 6, 136–141.

241. Johnston, F. A., McMillan, T. J. & Evans, E. R. (1950) Perspiration as a factor influencing the requirement for calcium and iron. J. Nutr. 42, 285–296.

242. Johnston, F. A., McMillan, T. J. & Falconer, G. D. (1952) Calcium retained by young women before and after adding spinach to the diet. J. Amer. Diet. Ass. 28, 933–938.

243. Johnston, F. A., Schlaphoff, D. & McMillan, T. (1950) Calcium retained from one level of intake by six adolescent girls. J. Nutr. 41, 137–147.

244. Johnston, J. A. (1940) Factors influencing retention of nitrogen and calcium in period of growth. III. Puberty in the normal girl and in the girl with the minimal reinfection type of tuberculosis. Amer. J. Dis. Child. 59, 287–309.

245. Johnston, J. A. (1941) Factors influencing retention of nitrogen and calcium in period of growth. IV. Effect of estrogen. Amer. J. Dis. Child. 62, 708–715.

246. Johnston, J. A. (1947) Nutritional requirement of the adolescent and its relation to the development of disease. Amer. J. Dis. Child. 74, 487–494.

247. Joseph, K., Kurien, P. P., Swaminathan, M. & Subrahmanyan, V. (1959) The metabolism of nitrogen, calcium and phosphorus in undernourished children. 5. The effect of partial or complete replacement of rice in poor vegetarian diets by ragi (Eleusine coracana) on the metabolism of nitrogen, calcium and phosphorus. Brit. J. Nutr. 13, 213–218.

248. Joseph, K., Narayanarao, M., Swaminathan, M. & Subrahmanyan, V. (1958) The metabolism of nitrogen, calcium and phosphorus in undernourished children. 4. The effect of replacing rice in the diet by tapioca macaroni on the metabolism of nitrogen, calcium and phosphorus. Brit. J. Nutr. 12, 429–432.

249. Jowsey, J., Riggs, B. L., Kelly, P. J. & Hoffman, D. L. (1972) Effect of combined therapy with sodium fluoride, vitamin D and calcium in osteoporosis. Amer. J. Med. 53, 43–49.

250. Jowsey, J., Schenk, R. K. & Reutter, F. W. (1968) Some results of the effect of fluoride on bone tissue in osteoporosis. J. Clin. Endocrinol. 28, 869–874.

251. Kahn, B., Straub, C.P., Robbins, P. J., Wellman, H. N., Seltzer, R. A. & Telles, N. C. (1969) Retention of radiostrontium, strontium, calcium and phosphorus by infants. 2. Intake and excretion of calcium and phosphorus by infants; calcium retention and model. Pediatrics 43, 668–686.

252. Kamalanathan, G., Sankari, L. & Devadas, R. P. (1965) The effect of supplementing a basal rice diet with wild green leafy vegetables on the retention of nitrogen, calcium and phosphorus in adolescent girls. J. Nutr. Diet. (India) 2, 37–41.

253. Karmarkar, M. G. & Ramakrishnan, C. V. (1960) Studies on human lactation. Relation between the dietary intake of lactating women and the chemical composition of milk with regard to principal and certain inorganic constituents. Acta Paediat. 49, 599–604.

254. Karnani, B. T., De, S. S., Subrahmanyan, V. & Cartner, D. (1948) Relative utilization of calcium from soya milk (fortified with di-calcium phosphate) and cow's milk by growing children. Indian J. Med. Res. 36, 355–360.

255. Kasper, W., Hövels, O. & Thilenius, O. G. (1963) Untersuchungen zur Calcium- und Phosphatstoffwechsel Frühgeborener. 5. Untersuchungen zum Vitamin D-Bedarf Frühgeborener. Z. Kinderheilk. 87, 472–489.

256. Kaufmann & Mohr (1903) Berlin. Klin. Wochenschr. no. 8. Cited by: Renvall, G. (1904) Zur Kenntniss des Phosphor-, Calcium-, und Magnesiumumsatzes beim erwachsenen Menschen. Skand. Arch. Physiol. 16, 94–138.

257. Keele, D. K. & Vose, G. P. (1969) A study of bone density: comparison of the effects of sodium fluoride, inorganic phosphates, and an anabolic steroid (oxymetholone) on demineralized bone. Amer. J. Dis. Child. 118, 759–764.

258. Keele, D. K. & Vose, G. P. (1971) Bone density in nonambulatory children. Follow-up after termination of treatment with sodium fluoride, inorganic phosphates, and oxymetholone. Amer. J. Dis. Child. 121, 204–206.

259. Kelly, F. C. & Henderson, J. McA. (1929–1930) The influence of certain dietary supplements on the nutrition of the African native. I. J. Hyg. 29, 418–428.

260. Kelly, H. J., Sloan, R. E., Hoffman, W. & Saunders, C. (1951) Accumulation of nitrogen and six minerals in the human fetus during gestation. Human Biol. 23, 61–74.

261. Kempster, E. R., Breiter, H., Mills, R., McKey, B., Bernds, M. & Outhouse, J. (1940) The utilization of the calcium of di-calcium phosphate by children. J. Nutr. 20, 279–287.

262. Kerr, C., Loken, H. F., Glendening, M. B., Gordan, G. S. & Page, E. W. (1962) Calcium and phosphorus dynamics in pregnancy. Amer. J. Obstet. Gynecol. 83, 2–8.

263. Kinney, V. R., Tauxe, W. N. & Dearing, W. H. (1965) Isotopic tracer studies of intestinal calcium absorption. J. Lab. Clin. Med. 66, 187–203.

264. Kinsman, G., Sheldon, D., Jensen, E., Bernds, M., Outhouse, J. & Mitchell, H. H. (1939) The utilization of the calcium of milk by pre-school children. J. Nutr. 17, 429–441.

265. Kjeldsen, K. & Damgaard, F. (1968) Influence of prolonged carbon monoxide exposure and high altitude on the composition of blood and urine in man. Scand. J. Clin. Lab. Invest. 22 (Suppl. 103), 20–25.

266. Kleeman, C. R., Bohannan, J., Bernstein, D., Ling, S. & Maxwell, M. H. (1964) Effect of variations in sodium intake on calcium excretion in normal humans. Proc. Soc. Exp. Biol. Med. 115, 29–32.

267. Knapp, E. L. (1947) Factors influencing the urinary excretion of calcium. 1. In normal persons. J. Clin. Invest. 26, 182–202.

268. Knapp, E. L. & Stearns, G. (1950) Factors influencing the urinary excretion of calcium. 2. Pregnancy and lactation. Amer. J. Obstet. Gynecol. 60, 741–751.
269. Konishi, F. (1957) The effect of exercise on calcium and phosphorus balance in young adult men. U. S. Army Med. Nutr. Lab. Rept. no. 211, pp. 1–19.
270. Kornhuber, B., Hövels, O. & Thilenius, O. G. (1962) Untersuchungen zum Calcium- und Phosphatstoffwechsel Frühgeborener. 3. Der Einfluss des Vitamin D auf die Calcium- und Phosphatclearance. Z. Kinderheilk. 86, 439–446.
271. Kramer, M. M., Latzke, E. & Shaw, M. M. (1928) A comparison of raw, pasteurized, evaporated, and dried milks as sources of calcium and phosphorus for the human subject. J. Biol. Chem. 79, 283–295.
272. Kramer, M. M., Potter, M. T. & Gillum, I. (1931) Utilization by normal adult subjects of the calcium and phosphorus in raw milk and in ice cream. J. Nutr. 4, 105–114.
273. Krane, W. (1927) Mineralstoffwechsel bei Kalkzufuhr. Arch. Ges. Physiol. (Pflügers) 217, 24–35. Cited by. Mitchell, H. H. & Curzon, E. G. (1939) The dietary requirement of calcium and its significance. Actualités Scientifique et Industrielles no. 771, pp. 36–101, Hermann & Co., Paris.
274. Kraut, H. & Wecker, H. (1943) Kalkbilanz und Kalkbedarf. Biochem. Z. 315, 329–344.
275. Krebs, H. A. & Mellanby, K. (1943) The effect of national wheatmeal on the absorption of calcium. Biochem. J. 37, 466–468.
276. Krook, L. & Lutwak, L. (1972) The Ca to P ratio: its significance to bone health. Personal Communication.
277. Krook, L., Lutwak, L., Henrikson, P.-A. & Whalen, J. (1970) Periodontal disease and calcium nutrition. Proc. 1970 Cornell Nutrition Conference for Feed Manufacturers, Nov. 3–5, Buffalo, N. Y., pp. 10–14.
278. Krook, L., Lutwak, L., Whalen, J. P., Henrikson, P.-A., Lesser, G. V. & Uris, R. (1972) Human periodontal disease. Morphology and response to calcium therapy. Cornell Vet. 62, 32–53.
279. Kunerth, B. L. & Pittman, M. S. (1939) A long-time study of nitrogen, calcium, and phosphorus metabolism on a low protein diet. J. Nutr. 17, 161–171.
280. Kung, L. C. & Yeh, H. L. (1938) Nitrogen, calcium and phosphorus balances of rural adolescent boys on low cost diets. Chin. J. Physiol. 13, 285–305.
281. Lafferty, F. W., Spencer, G. E. & Pearson, O. H. (1964) Effects of androgens, estrogens and high calcium intakes on bone formation and resorption in osteoporosis. Amer. J. Med. 36, 514–528.
282. Landry, M. & Fleisch, H. (1964) The influence of immobilisation on bone formation as evaluated by osseous incorporation of tetracyclines. J. Bone Joint Surg. 46B, 764–771.
283. Landsberg, E. (1915) Eiweiss und Mineralstoffwechseluntersuchungen bei der schwangeren Frau nebst Tierversuchen mit besonderer Beruchsichtigung der Funktion endokriner Drüsen. Z. Geburtsch. Gynäk. 76, 53–98.
284. Lapan, B. & Friedman, M. M. (1958) Blood studies in normal pregnancy and the newborn: the effects of iron and calcium administration. Amer. J. Obstet. Gynecol. 76, 96–102.
285. Lavan, J. N. (1969) The effect of oral ammonium chloride on the urinary excretion of calcium, magnesium and sodium in man. Irish J. Med. Sci. 2, 223–227.
286. Lehmann, C., Mueller, F., Munk, I:, Senator, H. & Zuntz, N. (1893) Untersuchungen an zwei hungernden Menschen. Virchows Arch. Pathol. Anat. Physiol. Klin. Med. 131 (Suppl), 1–228.
287. Leichsenring, J. M., Norris, L. M. & Halbert, M. L. (1957) Effect of ascorbic acid and of orange juice on calcium and phosphorus metabolism of women. J. Nutr. 63, 425–436.
288. Leichsenring, J. M., Norris, L. M., Lamison, S. A., Wilson, E. D. & Patton, M. B. (1951) The effect of level of intake on calcium and phosphorus metabolism in college women. J. Nutr. 45, 407–418.
289. Leitch, I. (1937) The determination of the calcium requirements of man. Nutr. Abst. Rev. 6, 553–578.
290. Leitch, I. (1957) Changing concepts in the nutritional physiology of human pregnancy. Proc. Nutr. Soc. 16, 38–45.
291. Leitch, I. & Aitken, F. C. (1959) The estimation of calcium requirement: a reexamination. Nutr. Abstr. Rev. 29, 393–411.
292. Lemann, J., Jr., Lennon, E. J., Goodman, A. D., Litzow, J. R. & Relman, A. S. (1965) The net balance of acid in subjects given large loads of acid or alkali. J. Clin. Invest. 44, 507–517.
293. Lemann, J., Jr., Litzow, J. R. & Lennon, E. J. (1967) Studies of the mechanism by which chronic metabolic acidosis augments urinary calcium excretion in man. J. Clin. Invest. 46, 1318–1328.
294. Leverton, R. M. & Gram, M. R. (1951) Further studies of obese young women during weight reduction. Calcium, phosphorus, and nitrogen metabolism. J. Amer. Diet. Ass. 27, 480–484.
295. Leverton, R. M. & Marsh, A. G. (1942) One hundred studies of the calcium, phosphorus, iron, and nitrogen metabolism and requirement of young women. Nebraska Agr. Exp. Sta. Res. Bull. no. 125, pp. 1–39.
296. Lindberg, G. (1917) Über den Stoffwechsel des gesunden, natürlich ernährten Säuglings und dessen Beeinflussung durch Frauenmilchfett. Z. Kinderheilk. 16, 90–175.
297. Liu, S. H., Chu, H. I., Hsu, H. C., Chao, H. C. & Cheu, S. H. (1941) Calcium and phosphorus metabolism in osteomalacia. XI. The pathogenetic role of pregnancy and relative importance of calcium and vitamin D supply. J. Clin. Invest. 20, 255–271.
298. Liu, S. H., Chu, H. I., Su, C. C., Yu, T. F. & Cheng, T. Y. (1940) Calcium and phosphorus metabolism in osteomalacia. IX.

Metabolic behaviour of infants fed on breast milk from mothers showing various states of vitamin D nutrition. J. Clin. Invest. *19*, 327–347. Cited by: Garry, R. C. & Wood, H. O. (1946) Dietary requirements in human pregnancy and lactation. A review of recent work. Nutr. Abst. Rev. *15*, 591–621.

299. Liu, S. H., Hannon, R. R., Chou, S. K., Chen, K. C., Chu, H. I. & Wang, S. H. (1935) Calcium and phosphorus metabolism in osteomalacia. III. The effects of varying levels and ratios of intake of calcium and phosphorus on their serum levels, paths of excretion and balances. Chin. J. Physiol. *9*, 101–118.

300. Liu, S. H., Su, C. C., Chou, S. K., Chu, H. I., Wang, C. W. & Chang, K. P. (1937) Calcium and phosphorus metabolism in osteomalacia. V. The effect of varying levels and ratios of calcium to phosphorus intake on their serum levels, paths of excretion and balances in the presence of continuous vitamin D therapy. J. Clin. Invest. *16*, 603–611.

301. Liu, S. H., Su, C. C., Wang, C. W. & Chang, K. P. (1937) Calcium and phosphorus metabolism in osteomalacia. VI. The added drain of lactation and beneficial action of vitamin D. Chin. J. Physiol. *11*, 271–294. Cited by: Garry, R. C. & Wood, H. O. (1946) Dietary requirements in human pregnancy and lactation. A review of recent work. Nutr. Abst. Rev. *15*, 591–621.

302. Löe, H. (1965) Periodontal changes in pregnancy. J. Periodontol. *36*, 209–217.

303. Loeb, R. F., Atchley, D. W., Richards, D. W., Jr., Benedict, E. M. & Driscoll, M. E. (1932) On the mechanism of nephrotic edema. J. Clin. Invest. *11*, 621–639.

304. Lutwak, L. (1969) Tracer studies of intestinal calcium absorption in man. Amer. J. Nutr. *22*, 771–785.

305. Lutwak, L., Laster, L., Gitelman, H. J., Fox, M. & Whedon, G. D. (1964) Effects of high dietary calcium and phosphorus on calcium, phosphorus, nitrogen and fat metabolism in children. Amer. J. Clin. Nutr. *14*, 76–82.

306. Lutwak, L. & Shapiro, J. R. (1964) Calcium absorption in man: based on large volume liquid scintillation counter studies. Science *144*, 1155–1157.

307. Lutwak, L., Whedon, G. D., LaChance, P. A., Reid, J. M. & Lipscomb, H. S. (1969) Mineral, electrolyte and nitrogen balance studies of the Gemini-VII fourteen-day orbital space flight. J. Clin. Endocrinol. *29*, 1140–1156.

308. Luyken, R., Luyken-Koning, F. W. M., Cambridge, T. H, Dohle, T. & Bosch, R. (1967) Studies on physiology of nutrition in Surinam. 10. Protein metabolism and influence of extra calcium on the growth of and calcium metabolism in boarding school children. Amer. J. Clin. Nutr. *20*, 34–42.

309. Lynch, T. N., Jensen, R. L., Stevens, P. M., Johnson, R. L. & Lamb, L. E. (1967) Metabolic effects of prolonged bed rest: their modification by simulated altitude. Aerosp. Med. *38*, 10–20.

310. Mack, P. B. & LaChance, P. L. (1967) Effects of recumbency and space flight on bone density. Amer. J. Clin. Nutr. *20*, 1194–1205.

311. Mack, P. B., LaChance, P. A., Vose, G. P. & Vogt, F. B. (1967) Bone demineralization of foot and hand of Gemini-Titan IV, V and VII astronauts during orbital flight. Amer. J. Roentgenol. Radium Ther. Nucl. Med. *100*, 503–511.

312. Macy, I. G. (1942) Nutrition and Chemical Growth in Childhood. Vol. 1. Evaluation, pp. 161–167, Charles C Thomas, Springfield, Ill.

313. Macy, I. G. (1949) Composition of human colostrum and milk. Amer. J. Dis. Child. *78*, 589–603.

314. Macy, I. G., Donelson, E., Long, M. L., Graham, A., Sweeney, M. E. & Shaw, M. M. (1931) Nitrogen, calcium and phosphorus balances in late gestation under a specified dietary regime, a record of one case. J. Amer. Diet. Ass. *6*, 314–320.

315. Macy, I. G. & Hunscher, H. A. (1934) An evaluation of maternal nitrogen and mineral needs during embryonic and infant development. Amer. J. Obstet. Gynecol. *27*, 878–888.

316. Macy, I. G., Hunscher, H. A., McCosh, S. S. & Nims, B. (1930) Metabolism of women during the reproductive cycle. III. Calcium, phosphorus, and nitrogen utilization in lactation before and after supplementing the usual home diets with cod liver oil and yeast. J. Biol. Chem. *86*, 59–74.

317. Macy, I. G., Hunscher, H. A., Nims, B. & McCosh, S. S. (1930) Metabolism of women during the reproductive cycle. 1. Calcium and phosphorus utilization in pregnancy. J. Biol. Chem. *86*, 17–35.

318. Mallon, M. G., Johnson, L. M. & Darby, C. R. (1932) A study of the calcium retention on a diet containing American cheddar cheese. J. Nutr. *5*, 121–126.

319. Mallon, M. G., Johnson, L. M. & Darby, C. R. (1933) The calcium retention on a diet containing leaf lettuce. J. Nutr. *6*, 303–311.

320. Mallon, M. G., Jordon, R. & Johnson, M. (1930) A note on the calcium retention on a high and low fat diet. J. Biol. Chem. *88*, 163–167.

321. Malm, O. J. (1953) On phosphates and phosphoric acid as dietary factors in the calcium balance of man. Scand. J. Clin. Lab. Invest. *5*, 75–84.

322. Malm, O. J. (1958) Calcium requirement and adaptation in adult men. Scand. J. Clin. Lab. Invest. *10* (Suppl.), 1–289.

323. Maltz, H. E., Fish, M. B. & Holliday, M. A. (1970) Calcium deficiency rickets and the renal response to calcium infusion. Pediatrics *46*, 865–870.

324. Marchionini, A. & Ottenstein, B. (1931) Stoffwechselveränderungen im Schwitzbad bei Hautgesunden und Hautkranken. 1. Einfluss auf Säurebasenhaushalt und Mineralstoffwechsel. Klin. Wochenschr. *10*, 969–971.

325. Mautalen, C. A., Cabrejas, M. L. & Soto,

R. J. (1969) Isotopic determination of intestinal calcium absorption in normal subjects. Metabolism 18, 395–405.

326. McCance, R. A. & Widdowson, E. M. (1939) The fate of calcium and magnesium after intravenous administration to normal persons. Biochem. J. 33, 523–529.

327. McCance, R. A. & Widdowson, E. M. (1942) Mineral metabolism of healthy adults on white and brown bread dietaries. J. Physiol. 101, 44–85.

328. McCance, R. A. & Widdowson, E. M. (1942) Mineral metabolism on dephytinized bread. J. Physiol. 101, 304–313.

329. McCance, R. A. & Widdowson, E. M. (1943) Seasonal and annual changes in the calcium metabolism of man. J. Physiol. 102, 42–49.

330. McCance, R. A., Widdowson, E. M. & Lehmann, H. (1942) The effect of protein intake on the absorption of calcium and magnesium. Biochem. J. 36, 686–691.

331. McClellan, W. S., Rupp, V. R. & Toscani, V. (1930) Clinical calorimetry. XLVI. Prolonged meat diets with a study of the metabolism of nitrogen, calcium, and phosphorus. J. Biol. Chem. 87, 669–681.

332. McCollum, E. V., Simmonds, N., Shipley, P. G. & Park, E. A. (1921) Studies on experimental rickets. J. Biol. Chem. 45, 333–348.

333. McGanity, W. J., Cannon, R. O., Bridgforth, E. B., Martin, M. P., Densen, P. M., Newbill, J. A., McClellan, G. S., Christie, A., Peterson, J. C. & Darby, W. J. (1954) The Vanderbilt cooperative study of maternal and infant nutrition. VI. Relationship of obstetric performance to nutrition. Amer. J. Obstet. Gynecol. 67, 501–527.

334. McKay, H., Patton, M. B., Ohlson, M. A., Pittman, M. S., Leverton, R. M., Marsh, A. G., Stearns, G. & Cox, G. (1942) Calcium, phosphorus and nitrogen metabolism of young college women. J. Nutr. 24, 367–384.

335. McKay, H., Patton, M. B., Pittman, M. S., Stearns, G. & Edelblute, N. (1943) The effect of vitamin D on calcium retentions. J. Nutr. 26, 153–159.

336. McLaughlin, L. (1927) Utilization of the calcium of spinach. J. Biol. Chem. 74, 455–462.

337. McLean, D. S., Lewis, G. K., Jensen, E., Hathaway, M., Breiter, H. & Holmes, J. O. (1946) Further studies on the calcium requirement of preschool children. J. Nutr. 31, 127–140.

338. McPherson, D. (1964) Stable Ca^{48} as a tracer in studies of mineral metabolism in man. In: Medical Uses of Ca^{47}. Second Panel Report, pp. 17–20, Int. Atomic Energy Agency Tech. Rep. Series, no. 32, Vienna.

339. Mellanby, E. (1921) Experimental rickets. Medical Research Council, Special Report Series no. 61, London.

340. Meyer, F. L., Brown, M. L., Wright, H. J. & Hathaway, M. L. (1955) A standardized diet for metabolic studies. Its development and application. USDA Technical Bull. 1126, 81 pp.

341. Michel, C. (1896) Recherches, sur la nutrition normale, du nouveau-né échanges nutritifs azotés et salins. L'Obstetrique 1, 140. Cited by: Wang, C. C. et al. (1924) A comparison of the metabolism of some mineral constituents of cow's milk and of breast milk in the same infant. Amer. J. Dis. Child. 27, 352–368.

342. Michel, C. (1899) Sur la composition chimique de l'embryon et du foetus humains aux différentes périodes de la grossesse. C. R. Soc. Biol. 51, 422–423.

343. Michel, C. & Perret, M. (1899) Étude des échanges nutritifs azotés et minéraux chez un nourrisson. Bull. Soc. d'Obstet. Paris 2, 98. Cited by: Hamilton, B. (1922) The calcium and phosphorus metabolism of prematurely born infants. Acta Paediat. 2, 1–84.

344. Mills, R., Breiter, H., Kempster, E., McKey, B., Pickens, M. & Outhouse, J. (1940) The influence of lactose on calcium retention in children. J. Nutr. 20, 467–476.

345. Mitchell, H. H. & Curzon, E. G. (1939) The dietary requirement of calcium and its significance. Actualités Scientifiques et Industrielles No. 771, pp. 36–101, Hermann & Co., Paris.

346. Mitchell, H. H. & Hamilton, T. S. (1949) The dermal excretion under controlled environmental conditions of nitrogen and minerals in human subjects, with particular reference to calcium and iron. J. Biol. Chem. 178, 345–361.

347. Mitchell, H. H., Hamilton, T. S., Steggerda, F. R. & Bean, H. W. (1945) The chemical composition of the adult human body and its bearing on the biochemistry of growth. J. Biol. Chem. 158, 625–637.

348. Miwa, S. & Stoeltzner, W. (1898) Ueber die bei jungen Hunden durch kalkarme Fütterung entstehende Knochenerkrankung. Beitr. Pathol. Anat. 24, 578–595.

349. Mizrahi, A., London, R. D. & Gribetz, D. (1968) Neonatal hypocalcemia—its causes and treatment. N. Engl. J. Med. 278, 1163–1165.

350. Morris, N. & MacRae, O. (1930) Metabolic reactions to acidosis produced by ammonium chloride. Arch. Dis. Child. 5, 207–228.

351. Muhl, G. (1926) The fat absorption and the calcium metabolism of prematurely born infants. Acta Paediat. 5, 188–222.

352. Mull, J. W. & Bill, A. H. (1934) Variations in serum calcium and phosphorus during pregnancy. 1. Normal variations. Amer. J. Obstet. Gynecol. 27, 510–517.

353. Murthy, H. B. N., Reddy, S. K., Swaminathan, M. & Subrahmanyan, V. (1955) The metabolism of nitrogen, calcium and phosphorus in undernourished children. 1. Adaptation to low intakes of calories, protein, calcium and phosphorus. Brit. J. Nutr. 9, 203–209.

354. Myers, W. P. L. (1962) Studies of serum calcium regulation. Advan. Intern. Med. 11, 163–213.

355. Nelson, M. van K. (1928) Calcium and

phosphorus metabolism of epileptic children receiving a ketogenic diet. Amer. J. Dis. Child. *36*, 716–719.

356. Nelson, M. van K. (1931) Calcium and phosphorus metabolism of infants receiving undiluted milk. Amer. J. Dis. Child. *42*, 1090–1099.

357. Newman, R. L. (1947) Blood calcium: a normal curve for pregnancy. Amer. J. Obstet. Gynecol. *53*, 817–822.

358. Nicholls, L. & Nimalasuriya, A. (1939) Adaptation to a low calcium intake in reference to the calcium requirements of a tropical population. J. Nutr. *18*, 563–577.

359. Nicolaysen, R. (1938) Fett- og Kalkstoffskiftet. Tidsskr. Kjemi *18*, 141–143. Cited in: Nutr. Abstr. Rev. *9*, 130, (1939).

360. Nicolaysen, R. (1960) The calcium requirement of man as related to diseases of the skeleton. Clin. Orthop. *17*, 226–234.

361. Nicolaysen, R., Eeg-Larsen, N. & Malm, O. J. (1953) Physiology of calcium metabolism. Physiol. Rev. *33*, 424–444.

362. Nishihara, O. (1959) Polarographic studies on the calcium metabolism. 1. Change of the calcium concentration in serum by month of pregnancy. Shikoku Acta Med. *15*, 1063–1074. Cited in: Nutr. Abstr. Rev. *30*, 980, (1960).

363. Nordin, B. E. C. (1960) Osteomalacia, osteoporosis and calcium deficiency. Clin. Orthop. *17*, 235–257.

364. Nordin, B. E. C. (1960) Osteoporosis and calcium deficiency. In: Bone as a Tissue (Rodahl, K., Nicholson, J. T. & Brown, E. M. eds.), pp. 46–66, McGraw-Hill Book Co., New York.

365. Nordin, B. E. C. (1961) The pathogenesis of osteoporosis. Lancet *1*, 1011–1015.

366. Nordin, B. E. C. (1966) International patterns of osteoporosis. Clin. Orthop. *45*, 17–30.

367. Nordin, B. E. C. (1968) Measurement and meaning of calcium absorption. Gastroenterology *54*, 294–301.

368. Nordin, B. E. C. (1971) Clinical significance and pathogenesis of osteoporosis. Brit. Med. J. *1*, 571–576.

369. Nordin, B. E. C., Bluhm, M. & MacGregor, J. (1962) In vitro and in vivo studies with bone-seeking isotopes. In: Radioisotopes and Bone (McLean, F. C., LaCroix, P. & Budy, A. M., eds.), pp. 105–125, Blackwell Scientific Publications, Oxford.

370. Obermer, E. (1946) Calcium and phosphorus metabolism in pregnancy. (A survey under war and post-war conditions.) First communication on the calciferol factor. J. Obstet. Gynaecol. Brit. Empire *53*, 362–367.

371. Obermer, E. (1946) Calcium and phosphorus metabolism in pregnancy. (A survey under war and post-war conditions.) Preliminary communication. J. Obstet. Gynaecol. Brit. Empire *53*, 269–277.

372. Obermer, E. (1947) Calcium and phosphorus metabolism in pregnancy. (A survey under war and post-war conditions.) 4. Calcium and phosphorus balances and antenatal

findings. J. Obstet. Gynaecol. Brit. Empire *54*, 817–823.

373. Obermer, E. (1948) Calcium and phosphorus metabolism in pregnancy. (A survey under war and post-war conditions.) 5. Calcium and phosphorus balances and labour findings. J. Obstet. Gynaecol. Brit. Empire *55*, 142–148.

374. Oberndörffer (1904) Berlin. Klin. Wochenschr. no 41. Cited by: Hornemann (1913) Zur Kenntnis des Salzgehaltes der täglichen Nahrung des Menschen. Z. Hyg. Infektionskrankh. *75*, 553–568.

375. Oberst, F. W. & Plass, E. D. (1940) Calcium, phosphorus, and nitrogen metabolism in women during the second half of pregnancy and in early lactation. Amer. J. Obstet. Gynecol. *40*, 399–413.

376. Ohlson, M. A., Brewer, W. D., Jackson, L., Swanson, P. P., Roberts, P. H., Mangel, M., Leverton, R. M., Chaloupka, M., Gram, M. R., Reynolds, M. S. & Lutz, R. (1952) Intakes and retentions of nitrogen, calcium and phosphorus by 136 women between 30 and 85 years of age. Federation Proc. *11*, 775–783.

377. Ohlson, M. A. & Stearns, G. (1959) Calcium intake of children and adults. Federation Proc. *18*, 1076–1085.

378. Oppé, T. E. & Redstone, D. (1968) Calcium and phosphorus levels in healthy newborn infants given various types of milk. Lancet *1*, 1045–1048.

379. Orgler, A. (1912) Der Kalkstoffwechsel des gesunden und des rachitischen Kindes. Ergebn. Inn. Med. Kinderheilk. *8*, 142–182.

380. Outhouse, J., Breiter, H., Rutherford, E., Dwight, J., Mills, R. & Armstrong, W. (1941) The calcium requirement of man: balance studies on seven adults. J. Nutr. *21*, 565–575.

381. Outhouse, J., Kinsman, G., Sheldon, D., Twomey, I., Smith, J. & Mitchell, H. H. (1939) The calcium requirements of five pre-school girls. J. Nutr. *17*, 199–211.

382. Owen, E. C. (1939) The calcium requirements of older male subjects. Biochem. J. *33*, 22–26.

383. Owen, E. C., Irving, J. T. & Lyall, A. (1940) The calcium requirements of older male subjects with special reference to the genesis of senile osteoporosis. Acta Med. Scand. *103*, 235–250.

384. Paffrath, H. & Massart, J. (1933) Langfristige Untersuchungen des Mineral- und Wasserstoffwechsels bei Frühgeborenen. Z. Kinderheilk. *54*, 343–366.

385. Patton, M. B. (1955) Further experiments on the utilization of calcium from salts by college women. J. Nutr. *55*, 519–526.

386. Patton, M. & Sutton, T. S. (1952) The utilization of calcium from lactate, gluconate, sulfate and carbonate salts by young college women. J. Nutr. *48*, 443–452.

387. Patton, M. B., Wilson, E. D., Leichsenring, J. M., Norris, L. M. & Dienhart, C. M. (1953) The relation of calcium-to-phosphorus ratio to the utilization of these min-

erals by 18 young college women. J. Nutr. 50, 373–382.

388. Paunier, L., Borgeaud, M. & Wyss, M. (1970) Urinary excretion of magnesium and calcium in normal children. Helv. Paediat. Acta 25, 577–584.

389. Paupe, J. (1958) Élimination cutanée sudorale du calcium. C. R. Soc. Biol. 152, 424–427.

390. Peiser, A. (1915) Beiträge zur Kentniss des Stoffwechsels, besonders der Mineralien im Säuglingsalter. Jahrb. Kinderheilk. 81, 437. Cited by: Hamilton, B. (1922) The calcium and phosphorus metabolism of prematurely born infants. Acta Paediat. 2, 1–84.

391. Petrunkina, A. (1934) Über die Bilanzen von Stickstoff, Kalk, Magnesium, Phosphor und Eisen bei Kindern von 7–8 Jahren. Z. Kinderheilk. 56, 219–226.

392. Phang, J. M., Kales, A. N. & Hahn, T. J. (1968) Effect of divided calcium intake on urinary calcium excretion. Lancet 2, 84–85.

393. Pierce, H. B., Daggs, R. G., Meservey, A. B. & Simcox, W. J. (1940) The retention of calcium and phosphorus by pre-school children. J. Nutr. 19, 401–414.

394. Pittman, M. S. (1932) The utilization by human subjects of the nitrogen, calcium, and phosphorus of the navy bean (*Phaseolus vulgaris*), with and without a supplement of cystine. J. Nutr. 5, 277–294.

395. Pittman, M. S. & Kunerth, B. L. (1939) A long-time study of nitrogen, calcium and phosphorus metabolism on a medium protein diet. J. Nutr. 17, 175–185.

396. Porter-Levin, T. (1933) Calcium and phosphorus metabolism of normal pre-school children. 1. On diets containing plain and irradiated cereals. J. Amer. Diet. Ass. 8, 482–488.

397. Porter-Levin, T. (1933) Calcium and phosphorus metabolism of normal pre-school children. 2. Successive balance studies showing the range of variation in calcium and phosphorus storage. J. Amer. Diet. Ass. 9, 22–25.

398. Potgieter, M. (1940) The utilization of the calcium and phosphorus of taro by young women. J. Amer. Diet. Ass. 16, 898–904.

399. Pratt, E. L. (1957) Dietary prescription of water, sodium, calcium and phosphorus for infants and children. Amer. J. Clin. Nutr. 5, 555–560.

400. Pyle, S. I., Potgieter, M. & Comstock, G. (1938) On certain relationships of calcium in the blood serum to calcium balance and basal metabolism during pregnancy. Amer. J. Obstet. Gynecol. 35, 283–289.

401. Ragan, C. & Briscoe, A. M. (1964) Effect of exercise on the metabolism of [40]calcium and [47]calcium in man. J. Clin. Endocrinol. 24, 385–392.

402. Rakowska, M., Czarnowska-Misztal, E., Brzezińska, Z. & Krupowicz, J. (1969) Wyniki badań nad retencją wapnia ze zwyczajowo spożywanej diety w wybranej grupie dzieci w wieku przedszkolnym. Rocz. Państwowego Zakl. Hig. 20, 533–542. Cited in: Nutr. Abst. Rev. 40, 962, (1970).

403. Reding, R. & Slosse, A. (1931) Des variations du pH, de la réserve alcaline et du calcium sanguin au cours de la grossesse et la parturition. Leurs rapports avec l'évolution des néoplasmes. Bruxelles-Medical 11, 503–518.

404. Reifenstein, E. C., Jr. (1942) Comments on nitrogen and calcium retention in immobilization. In: Conference on Bone and Wound Healing, Second meeting, Dec. 11–12, 1942. (Reifenstein, E. C., Jr., ed.), pp. 96–98, Josiah Macy Jr. Foundation, New York.

405. Reimers, P. & Boye (1905) Ein Beitrag zur Lehre von der Rachitis. Zentralblat. Inn. Med. 26, 953–962.

406. Renvall, G. (1904) Zur Kenntniss des Phosphor-, Calcium-, und Magnesiumumsatzes beim erwachsenen Menschen. Skand. Arch. Physiol. 16, 94–138.

407. Rice, B. F., Schneider, G. & Weed, J. (1969) Serum calcium and magnesium concentration during early labor and the postpartum period. Amer. J. Obstet. Gynecol. 104, 1159–1162.

408. Rich, C., Ensinck, J. & Ivanovich, P. (1964) The effects of sodium fluoride on calcium metabolism of subjects with metabolic bone diseases. J. Clin. Invest. 43, 545–556.

409. Ritchie, B. V. (1942) The calcium and phosphorus content of milk from Australian women. Med. J. Aust. 1, 331–336.

410. Roberts, P. H., Kerr, C. H. & Ohlson, M. A. (1948) Nutritional studies of older women. Nitrogen, calcium, phosphorus retentions of nine women. J. Amer. Diet. Ass. 24, 292–299.

411. Rogers, J. F., Brown, B. & Pang, M. (1968) A dietary assessment of a group of young adults in Sydney. Med. J. Aust. 1, 789–791. Cited by: Dale, N. E. (1968) A study of the urinary calcium, phosphorus, creatinine and sodium excretion of young adults in Sydney. Med. J. Aust. 1, 791–793.

412. Rominger, E. & Meyer, H. (1927) Mineralstoffwechseluntersuchungen beim Säugling. 1. Die Salzretention des gesunden Brust- und Flaschenkindes. Arch. Kinderheilk. 80, 195–234.

413. Rominger, E. & Meyer, H. (1928) Mineralstoffwechseluntersuchungen beim Säugling. 3. Die Mineralbilanz bei dystrophischen Zuständen. Arch. Kinderheilk. 85, 23–58.

414. Rominger, E., Meyer, H. & Bomskov, C. (1930) Rachitisstudien. 1. Langfristige Kalk- und Phosphorstoffwechseluntersuchungen bei gesunden und rachitischen Säuglingen. Zugleich ein Beitrag zur Wirkungsweise des Vigantols. Z. Ges. Exp. Med. 73, 343–381.

415. Rose, G. A. (1967) A critique of modern methods of diagnosis and treatment of osteoporosis. Clin. Orthop. 55, 17–41.

416. Rose, G. A., Reed, G. W. & Smith, A. H. (1965) Isotopic method for measurement

of calcium absorption from the gastro-intestinal tract. Brit. Med. J. *1*, 690–692.

417. Rose, M. S. (1920) Experiments on the utilization of the calcium of carrots by man. J. Biol. Chem. *41*, 349–355.

418. Rose, M. S. & MacLeod, G. (1923) Experiments on the utilization of the calcium of almonds by man. J. Biol. Chem. *57*, 305–315.

419. Rost, E., Herbst, O. & Weitzel, A. (1923) Die Ernährungsverhältnisse der Berliner Waisenhauszöglinge mit besonderer Berücksichtigung des Kalkstoffwechsels. Arch. Kinderheilk. *72*, 81. Cited by: Wang, C. C. et al. (1936) Metabolism of adolescent girls. Amer. J. Dis. Child. *52*, 41–53.

420. Roth, F. (1961) Die Hypocalcämie in letzten Drittel der Gravidität. Arch. Gynäkol. *194*, 493–509. Cited in: Nutr. Abstr. Rev. *31*, 1282, (1961).

421. Samachson, J. (1963) Plasma values after oral [45]calcium and [85]strontium as an index of absorption. Clin. Sci. *25*, 17–26.

422. Sawyer, M., Baumann, L. & Stevens, F. (1918) Studies of acid production. II. The mineral loss during acidosis. J. Biol. Chem. *33*, 103–109.

423. Schabad, J. A. (1909) Der Phosphor in der Therapie der Rachitis. Der Einfluss des Phosphors auf den Kalkstoffwechsel bei rachitischen und gesunden Kindern. Z. Klin. Med. *67*, 454–494. Cited by: Sherman, H. C. & Hawley, E. (1922) Calcium and phosphorus metabolism in childhood. J. Biol. Chem. *53*, 375–399.

424. Schabad, J. A. (1910) Zur Bedeutung des Kalkes in der Pathologie der Rachitis 1. Der Mineralgehalt gesunder und rachitischer Knochen. Arch. Kinderheilk. *52*, 47–106.

425. Schabad, J. A. (1910) Zur Bedeutung des Kalkes in der Pathologie der Rachitis. IV. Der Phosphorstoffwechsel bei Rachitis. Arch. Kinderheilk. *54*, 83–110. Cited by: Sherman, H. C. & Hawley, E. (1922) Calcium and phosphorus metabolism in childhood. J. Biol. Chem. *53*, 375–399.

426. Schlossman, A. (1905) Über Mange, Art und Bedeutung des Phosphors in der Milch und über einige Schicksale desselben im Säuglingsorganismus. Arch. Kinderheilk. *40*, 1–39.

427. Schmid, J. (1963) Kalktherapie bei Osteoporose. Bestimmung der Knochendichte als Kriterium. Schweiz. Med. Wochenschr. no. 51, 1815–1820.

428. Schoenthal, L. & Lurie, D. K. (1933) Concentration of calcium and phosphorus in the serum of children. Amer. J. Dis. Child. *46*, 1038–1044.

429. Schofield, F. A. & Morrell, E. (1960) Symposium on metabolic patterns in preadolescent children. Calcium, phosphorus and magnesium. Federation Proc. *19*, 1014–1016.

430. Schroeder, L. J., Cahill, W. M. & Smith, A. H. (1946) The utilization of calcium in soybean products and other calcium sources. J. Nutr. *32*, 413–422.

431. Segal, A. J. (1968) Neonatal hypocalcemia. N. Engl. J. Med. *279*, 327.

432. Sereni, F., Pototschnig, C. & Piceni Sereni, L. (1965) Latti vaccini a diverso contenuto proteico e salino: loro influenza su alcuni aspetti del metabolismo e dell'accrescimento dell'immaturo. 1. I bilanci metabolici dell'azoto, del calcio e del fosforo. Minerva Pediat. *17*, 1019–1024.

433. Shenolikar, I. S. (1970) Absorption of dietary calcium in pregnancy. Amer. J. Clin. Nutr. *23*, 63–67.

434. Shepherd, M. L., Macy, I. G., Hunscher, H. A. & Hummel, F. C. (1940) Synthesized, processed, and natural sources of vitamin C in the mineral metabolism of normal children. J. Pediat. *16*, 704–716.

435. Sherman, H. C. (1920) Calcium requirement of maintenance in man. J. Biol. Chem. *44*, 21–27.

436. Sherman, H. C. & Booher, L. E. (1931) The calcium content of the body in relation to that of the food. J. Biol. Chem. *93*, 93–103.

437. Sherman, H. C., Gillett, L. H. & Pope, H. M. (1918) Monthly metabolism of nitrogen, phosphorus and calcium in healthy women. J. Biol. Chem. *34*, 373–381.

438. Sherman, H. C. & Hawley, E. (1922) Calcium and phosphorus metabolism in childhood. J. Biol. Chem. *53*, 375–399.

439. Sherman, H. C., Mettler, A. J. & Sinclair, J. E. (1910) Calcium, magnesium, and phosphorus in food and nutrition. U. S. Dept. Agr. Off. Exp. Sta. Bull. no. 227, pp. 1–70.

440. Sherman, H. C., Wheeler, L. & Yates, A. B. (1918) Experiments on the nutritive value of maize protein and on the phosphorus and calcium requirements of healthy women. J. Biol. Chem. *34*, 383–393.

441. Sherman, H. C. & Winters, J. C. (1918) Efficiency of maize protein in adult human nutrition. J. Biol. Chem. *35*, 301–311.

442. Sherman, H. C., Winters, J. C. & Phillips, V. (1919) Efficiency of oat protein in adult human nutrition. J. Biol. Chem. *39*, 53–62.

443. Shohl, A. T. (1923) Mineral metabolism in relation to acid–base equilibrium. Physiol. Rev. *3*, 509–543.

444. Shohl, A. T. (1939) Mineral Metabolism. Amer. Chem. Soc. Monograph Series no. 82, Reinhold Publishing Corp., New York.

445. Shohl, A. T. & Sato, A. (1923) Acid–base metabolism. II. Mineral metabolism. J. Biol. Chem. *58*, 257–266.

446. Shore, J. D. & Consolazio, C. F. (1959) The immediate effect of exercise on calcium and phosphorus metabolism. U. S. Army Med. Res. Nutr. Lab. Rept. no. 241, pp. 1–13.

447. Shukers, C. F., Macy, I. G., Nims, B., Donelson, E. & Hunscher, H. A. (1932) A quantitative study of the dietary of the human mother with respect to the nutrients secreted into breast milk. J. Nutr. *5*, 127–139.

448. Simmons, K. (1944) The Brush Foundation study of child growth and development. II. Physical growth and development. Monograph Soc. Res. Child Development *9* (no.

1), pp. 1–87. Cited by: Holmes, J. O. (1945) The requirement for calcium during growth. Nutr. Abstr. Rev. 14, 597–612.

449. Slater, J. E. (1961) Retentions of nitrogen and minerals by babies 1 week old. Brit. J. Nutr. 15, 83–97.

450. Smith, E. (1865) Practical dietary for families, schools, and the labouring classes, pp. 22–23, Walton and Maberly, London.

451. Souders, H. J., Hunscher, H. A., Hummel, F. C. & Macy, I. G. (1939) Influence of fluid and of evaporated milk on mineral and nitrogen metabolism of growing children. Amer. J. Dis. Child. 58, 529–539.

452. Southgate, D. A. T., Widdowson, E. M., Smits, B. J., Cooke, W. T., Walker, C. H. M. & Mathers, N. P. (1969) Absorption and excretion of calcium and fat by young infants. Lancet 1, 487–489.

453. Speckmann, E. W. & Brink, M. F. (1967) Relationships between fat and mineral metabolism—A review. J. Amer. Diet. Ass. 51, 517–522.

454. Spencer, H., Lewin, I., Fowler, J. & Samachson, J. (1969) Effect of sodium fluoride on calcium absorption and balances in man. Amer. J. Clin. Nutr. 22, 381–390.

455. Spencer, H., Lewin, I., Osis, D. & Samachson, J. (1970) Studies of fluoride and calcium metabolism in patients with osteoporosis. Amer. J. Med. 49, 814–822.

456. Spencer, H., Menczel, J. & Lewin, I. (1964) Metabolic and radioisotope studies in osteoporosis. Clin. Orthop. 35, 202–219.

457. Spencer, H., Menczel, J., Lewin, I. & Samachson, J. (1964) Absorption of calcium in osteoporosis. Amer. J. Med. 37, 223–234.

458. Spencer, H., Menczel, J., Lewin, I. & Samachson, J. (1965) Effect of high phosphorus intake on calcium and phosphorus metabolism in man. J. Nutr. 86, 125–132.

459. Spencer, H., Scheck, J., Lewin, I. & Samachson, J. (1966) Comparative absorption of calcium from calcium gluconate and calcium lactate. J. Nutr. 89, 283–292.

460. Stearns, G. (1931) The significance of the retention ratio of calcium:phosphorus in infants and in children. Amer. J. Dis. Child. 42, 749–759.

461. Stearns, G. (1939) The mineral metabolism of normal infants. Physiol. Rev. 19, 415–438.

462. Stearns, G. (1952) Nutritional health of infants, children and adolescents. Proc. National Food and Nutr. Institute, U. S. Dept. Agr., Agr. Handbook no. 56, pp. 59–63.

463. Stearns, G. (1954) Comments on the intake of calcium and phosphorus required for bone growth. In: Metabolic interrelationships with special reference to calcium. Transactions of the fifth conference. Jan. 5–6, 1953. (Reifenstein, E. C. Jr., ed.), pp. 185–188, Josiah Macy Jr. Foundation, New York.

464. Stearns, G. (1956) Calcium, phosphorus, and vitamin D requirements in infants. In: Infant Metabolism. (Scheinberg, I. H., ed.), pp. 64–80. MacMillan Co., New York.

465. Stearns, G. & Jeans, P. C. (1934) Utilization of calcium salts by children. Proc. Soc. Exp. Biol. Med. 32, 428–430.

466. Steggerda, F. R. & Mitchell, H. H. (1939) The calcium requirement of adult man and the utilization of the calcium in milk and in calcium gluconate. J. Nutr. 17, 253–262.

467. Steggerda, F. R. & Mitchell, H. H. (1941) Further experiments on the calcium requirement of adult man and the utilization of the calcium in milk. J. Nutr. 21, 577–588.

468. Steggerda, F. R. & Mitchell, H. H. (1946) The effect of the citrate ion on the calcium metabolism of adult human subjects. J. Nutr. 31, 423–438.

469. Steggerda, F. R. & Mitchell, H. H. (1946) Variability in the calcium metabolism and calcium requirements of adult human subjects. J. Nutr. 31, 407–422.

470. Steggerda, F. R. & Mitchell, H. H. (1951) The calcium balance of adult human subjects on high- and low-fat (butter) diets. J. Nutr. 45, 201–211.

471. Stephan, U., Hövels, O. & Thilenius, O. G. (1962) Untersuchungen zum Calcium- und Phosphatstoffwechsel Frühgeborener. 4. Der Einfluss der Lactose auf die Calciumretention. Z. Kinderheilk. 86, 447–451.

472. Sur, G., Reddy, S. K., Swaminathan, M. & Subrahmanyan, V. (1955) The metabolism of nitrogen, calcium and phosphorus in undernourished children. 2. The effect of supplementary groundnut-milk curds on the metabolism of nitrogen, calcium and phosphorus. Brit. J. Nutr. 9, 210–215.

473. Swanson, W. W. (1932) The composition of growth. II. The full-term infant. Amer. J. Dis. Child. 43, 10–18.

474. Swanson, W. W. & Iob, L. V. (1933) Loss of minerals through the skin of infants. Amer. J. Dis. Child. 45, 1036–1039.

475. Talbert, G. A., Haugen, C., Carpenter, R. & Bryant, J. E. (1933) Simultaneous study of the constituents of the sweat, urine and blood: also gastric acidity and other manifestations resulting from sweating. 10. Basic metals. Amer. J. Physiol. 104, 441–442.

476. Telfer, S. V. (1921) The influence of free fatty acids in the intestinal contents on the excretion of calcium and phosphorus. Biochem. J. 15, 347–354.

477. Telfer, S. V. (1922) Studies on calcium and phosphorus metabolism. 1. The excretion of calcium and phosphorus. Quart. J. Med. 16, 45–62.

478. Telfer, S. V. (1930) Mineral metabolism in infancy. 1. The mineral constituents of human milk and cow's milk. Glasgow Med. J. 113, 246–256.

479. Thomson, A. M. (1957) Technique and perspective in clinical and dietary studies of human pregnancy. Proc. Nutr. Soc. 16, 45–51.

480. Thomson, A. M. (1958) Diet in pregnancy. 1. Dietary survey technique and the nutritive value of diets taken by primagravidae. Brit. J. Nutr. 12, 446–461.

481. Thomson, A. M. (1959) Diet in preg-

nancy. 2. Assessment of the nutritive value of diets, especially in relation to differences between classes. Brit. J. Nutr. *13*, 190–204.

482. Thomson, A. M. (1959) Diet in pregnancy. 3. Diet in relation to the course and outcome of pregnancy. Brit. J. Nutr. *13*, 509–525.

483. Thorangkul, D., Johnston, F. A., Kime, N. S. & Clark, S. J. (1959) Adaptation to a low-calcium intake. J. Amer. Diet. Ass. *35*, 23–30.

484. Tigerstedt, R. (1910) Zur Kenntnis der Aschenbestandteile in der frei gewahlten Kost des Menschen. Skand. Arch. Physiol. *24*, 97. Cited by: Hornemann (1913) Zur Kenntnis des Salzgehaltes der täglichen Nahrung des Menschen. Z. Hyg. Infektionskrankh. *75*, 553–568.

485. Tobler, L. & Noll, F. (1911) Zur Kentniss des Mineralstoffwechsels beim gesunden Brustkind. Monatsschr. Kinderheilk. *9*, 210. Cited by: Hamilton, B. (1922) The calcium and phosphorus metabolism of prematurely born infants. Acta Paediat. *2*, 1–84.

486. Toro, G., Ackermann, P. G. & Kountz, W. B. (1958) Effect of some hormones on calcium balance in elderly subjects. Proc. Soc. Exp. Biol. Med. *97*, 819–821.

487. Toverud, K. U. & Toverud, G. (1931) Studies on the mineral metabolism during pregnancy and lactation and its bearing on the disposition to rickets and dental caries. Acta Paediat. *12* (Suppl. 2), 1–116.

488. Van Heyningen, R. & Weiner, J. S. (1952) A comparison of arm-bag sweat and body sweat. J. Physiol. *116*, 395–403.

489. Vellar, O. D. & Askevold, R. (1968) Studies on sweat losses of nutrients. 3. Calcium, magnesium, and chloride content of whole body cell-free sweat in healthy unacclimatized men under controlled environmental conditions. Scand. J. Clin. Lab. Invest. *22*, 65–71.

490. Venar, Y. A. & Todd, T. W. (1933) White House Conference on Child Health and Protection. 2. Anatomy and Physiology. Century Co., New York, p. 93. Cited by: Holmes, J. O. (1945) The requirement for calcium during growth. Nutr. Abstr. Rev. *14*, 597–612.

491. Vorob'eva, A. M. (1961) K voprosu o profilaktike kal'cievoj i fosfornoj nedostatočnosti u detej doškol'nogo vozrasta. Vop. Pitan. *20*, (4), 23–28.

492. Vorob'eva, A. M. (1964) Sezonnye izmenenija v usvoenii kal'cija i fosfora pisci rastuscim organizmon. Vop. Pitan *23* (2), 64–67. Cited in: Nutr. Abstr. Rev. *34*, 1040, (1964).

493. Vorob'eva, A. M. (1968) Rol' ul'trafioletovogo oblucenija v usvoenii piscevogo kal'cija rastuscim organismom rebenka. Pediatrija, no. 12, 69. Cited in: Nutr. Abstr. Rev. *39*, 1259, (1969).

494. Vose, G. P. & Keele, D. K. (1970) Hypokinesia of bedfastness and its relationship to X-ray determined skeletal density. Texas Rep. Biol. Med. *28*, 123–131.

495. Wagner, M. J. & Muhler, J. C. (1959) The relationship between fluoride ingestion and urinary calcium. J. Dental Res. *38*, 1078–1081.

496. Wait, B. & Roberts, L. J. (1933) Studies in the food requirement of adolescent girls. 4. The mineral intake of 38 well-nourished girls 10 to 16 years of age. J. Amer. Diet. Ass. *9*, 124–137.

497. Wake, N. D. (1944) Calcium and phosphorus absorption in breast fed infants and its relationship to bone decalcification (rickets). Med. J. Austral. *1*, 27–30.

498. Walker, A. R. P. (1954) Does a low intake of calcium retard growth or conduce to stuntedness? Amer. J. Clin. Nutr. *2*, 265–271.

499. Walker, A. R. P. (1972) The human requirement of calcium: should low intakes be supplemented? Amer. J. Clin. Nutr. *25*, 518–530.

500. Walker, A. R. P., Fox, F. W. & Irving, J. T. (1948) Studies in human mineral metabolism. I. The effect of bread rich in phytate phosphorus on the metabolism of certain mineral salts with special reference to calcium. Biochem. J. *42*, 452–462.

501. Walker, A. R. P. & Richardson, B. D. (1964) Growth rate in relation to calcium losses through sweat. Amer. J. Clin. Nutr. *15*, 309–311.

502. Walser, M. & Robinson, B. H. B. (1963) Renal excretion and tubular reabsorption of calcium and strontium. In: The Transfer of Calcium and Strontium across Biological Membranes. (Wasserman, R. H., ed.), pp. 305–326, Academic Press, New York.

503. Wang, C. C., Kaucher, M. & Frank, M. (1928) Metabolism of undernourished children. IV. Calcium metabolism. Amer. J. Dis. Child. *35*, 856–861.

504. Wang, C. C., Kaucher, M. & Wing, M. (1936) Metabolism of adolescent girls. 4. Mineral metabolism. Amer. J. Dis. Child. *52*, 41–53.

505. Wang, C. C., Kern, R. & Kaucher, M. (1930) Minimum requirement of calcium and phosphorus in children. Amer. J. Dis. Child. *39*, 768–773.

506. Wang, C. C., Witt, D. B. & Felcher, A. R. (1924) A comparison of the metabolism of some mineral constituents of cow's milk and of breast milk in the same infant. Amer. J. Dis. Child. *27*, 352–368.

507. Wasserman, R. H., Comar, C. L. & Nold, M. M. (1956) The influence of amino acids and other organic compounds on the gastrointestinal absorption of calcium[45] and strontium[80] in the rat. J. Nutr. *59*, 371–383.

508. Watson, E. K., McGuire, E. W., Meyer, F. L. & Hathaway, M. L. (1945) Calcium metabolism of preschool children. J. Nutr. *30*, 259–268.

509. Weintraub, M. (1968) Neonatal hypocalcemia. N. Engl. J. Med. *279*, 327.

510. Wendt, G. von (1905) Untersuchungen über den Eiweiss- und Salz-Stoffwechsel beim Menschen. Skand. Arch. Physiol. *17*, 211–289.

511. Wensel, R. H., Rich, C., Brown, A. C. & Volwiler, W. (1969) Absorption of calcium measured by intubation and perfusion of the intact human small intestine. J. Clin. Invest. 48, 1768–1775.

512. Whedon, G. D. (1959) Effects of high calcium intakes on bones, blood and soft tissue; relationship of calcium intake to balance in osteoporosis. Federation Proc. 18, 1112–1118.

513. Whedon, G. D. (1964) The combined use of balance and isotopic studies in the study of calcium metabolism. In: Proceedings of the Sixth International Congress of Nutrition, Edinburgh, Aug. 9–15, 1963. (Mills, C. F. & Passmore, R., eds.), pp. 425–438, E. & S. Livingstone, Ltd. Edinburgh.

514. Widdows, S. T. (1923) Calcium content of the blood during pregnancy. Biochem. J. 17, 34–40.

515. Widdowson, E. M. (1947) A study of individual children's diets. Med. Res. Council Special Report Series no. 257, pp. 1–196, H. M. Stationery Office, London.

516. Widdowson, E. M. (1965) Absorption and excretion of fat, nitrogen, and minerals from "filled" milks by babies one week old. Lancet 2, 1099–1105.

517. Widdowson, E. M., McCance, R. A., Harrison, G. E. & Sutton, A. (1963) Effect of giving phosphate supplements to breast-fed babies on absorption and excretion of calcium, strontium, magnesium, and phosphorus. Lancet 2, 1250–1251.

518. Widdowson, E. M., Slater, J. E., Harrison, G. E. & Sutton, A. (1960) Absorption, excretion, and retention of strontium by breast-fed and bottle-fed babies. Lancet 2, 941–944.

519. Widdowson, E. M. & Spray, C. M. (1951) Chemical development in utero. Arch. Dis. Child. 26, 205–214.

520. Willard, A. C. & Blunt, K. (1927) A comparison of evaporated with pasteurized milk as a source of calcium, phosphorus, and nitrogen. J. Biol. Chem. 75, 251–262.

521. Williams, P. F. & Fralen, F. G. (1942) Nutrition study in pregnancy. Dietary analyses of seven-day food intake records of 514 pregnant women, comparison of actual food intakes with variously stated requirements, and relationship of food intake to various obstetric factors. Amer. J. Obstet. Gynecol. 43, 1–20.

522. Yeh, H. L. & Adolph, W. H. (1939) Calcium, phosphorus and nitrogen balances with pre-school children. Chin. J. Physiol. 14, 303–314.

523. Young, C. M. (1952) Weight reduction using a moderate-fat diet. 2. Biochemical responses. J. Amer. Diet. Ass. 28, 529–533.

524. Young, C. M., Ringler, I. & Greer, B. J. (1953) Reducing and post-reducing maintenance on the moderate-fat diet. Metabolic studies. J. Amer. Diet. Ass. 29, 890–896.

525. Young, C. M., Smudski, V. L. & Steele, B. F. (1951) Fall and spring diets of school children in New York State. J. Amer. Diet. Ass. 27, 289–292.

526. Young, E. G. (1964) Dietary Standards, In: Nutrition, a Comprehensive Treatise, vol. 2, Vitamins, Nutrient Requirements and Food Selection. (Beaton, G. H. & McHenry, E. W., eds.), pp. 299–350, Academic Press, New York.

527. Young, M. M. & Nordin, B. E. C. (1967) Calcium metabolism and the menopause. Proc. Roy. Soc. Med. 60, 1137–1138.

APPENDIX TABLE 1

Studies on maintenance requirements for calcium

Kind of study	Description of subjects	Number of studies	Suggested daily requirement	References
Balance method, controlled diets, intake minus output	18 women, 34 men	7	0.45, 0.56 g 5.0 to 13.3 mg/kg	6, 271 380, 418, 466, 467, 469
regression	59 men	3	126 to 700 mg 1.8 to 7.4 mg/kg	130, 194 194, 470
Self-selected diets, regression	179 women	2	816 to 880 mg	295, 334
Calculations based on data in the literature		5	0.45 to 1.00 g 9.75 mg/kg	218, 289, 435, 439 345
Factorial method isotope studies	1 woman, 1 man	1	240, 431 mg 3.5, 8.1 mg/kg	52 52
Calculation based on data in the literature		1	1,086 mg	513

APPENDIX TABLE 2

Studies on quantitative determination of obligatory calcium losses

Kind of loss	Condition of study	Description of subjects	Number of studies	Amount of daily[1] loss	References
Endogenous fecal calcium	fasting	2 men	1	32, 69 mg	286
	low calcium intake	13 men and women	1	200 mg	27
	regression—data from the literature		1	75 mg	67
	isotopic calcium	54 normal and osteoporotic	5	46 to 290 mg 1.3 to 4.5 mg/kg	52, 53, 72, 191, 369 369
	isotopic strontium	12 patients various disorders	1	0.5 to 5.0 mg/kg	369
Urinary calcium	fasting	4 men	3	102 to 326 mg	42, 87, 286
	low calcium intakes	114 men and women	3	51 to 90 mg	24, 27, 52, 53
	estimates based on the literature		2	175,[2] 200 mg[3]	267, 361, 513
Dermal calcium sweat	comfortable environment	22 infants	2	3 to 30 mg	187, 474
		22 men	3	70 to 149 mg	97, 231, 232, 346
		14 women	1	15.4 mg	513
	hot environment	57 men	5	7.7 to 20.2 mg/hr 0.79 to 1.95 g	97, 98, 346, 489 99
		4 women	1	8.5 mg/hr	241
	space flight preflight inflight postflight	2 men	1	26, 23 mg 14, 16 mg 43, 45 mg	307
hair		12 women	1	90 ± 63 mg/year	240

[1] Except where otherwise stated.   [2] Average urinary excretion (361) based on Knapp's compilation of data (267).   [3] Reasonable upper limit for healthy adults (513) based on Knapp's collection of data (267).

APPENDIX TABLE 3

Studies on calcium requirements of children since 1920

Subjects	Number of subjects	Number of studies	Principal criteria	Suggested daily requirement	References
Infants Premature	76	8	retention	90 to 120 mg/kg	43, 169, 179, 220, 221, 255, 270, 432, 471
Full-term 0–12 months		1	intake from breast milk	62 mg/kg	478
		1	estimated calcium accretion	retention of 130 to 310 mg	289
	325	15	retention	40 to 120 mg/kg	62, 150, 181, 182, 214, 238, 251, 356, 449, 452, 497, 506, 516–518
12–24 months		4	estimated calcium accretion	retention of 86 to 290 mg intake of 0.7 g	211, 289, 345, 347 289
	3	3	retention	0.470 to 2.222 g	412, 417, 477
Preschool children	166	1	roentgenology	0.2 to 0.7 g	11
2–5 years		3	calcium accretion	500 to 900 mg 30 to 45 mg/kg	211, 289 345
	69	10	retention	0.46 to 1.12 g	337, 381, 393, 438, 503, 520, 522
				43 to 64 mg/kg	109–111, 215, 337
School children 6–12 years		5	calcium accretion	285 to 1530 mg 140 to 550 mg plus allowance for incomplete utilization	211, 289, 345, 358 291
	69	7	retention	0.2 to 1.3 g 12 to 40 mg/kg	358, 438, 520 209, 391, 505
Adolescents 13–18 years		4	calcium accretion	1 to 2.6 g 430 to 525 mg plus allowance for incomplete utilization	211, 345, 358 291
	32 girls 9 boys	6	retention	0.9 to 1.6 g	195, 243, 419, 438, 504, 520

APPENDIX TABLE 4

Studies on calcium requirements of pregnant and lactating women

Subjects	Number of subjects	Number of studies	Principal criteria	Suggested daily requirement	References
Pregnant women		2	fetal growth	1.2 to 1.8 g	162, 345
	173	7	retention	0.4 to 2.5 g	5, 100, 101, 297, 314, 371, 433, 487
Lactating women		2	infant's calcium intake from breast milk	200 to 418 mg plus mother's needs	315, 461
	101	6	retention	no clear indication of requirement	122, 125, 225, 226, 253, 316, 375, 447, 487
		2	calculations based on data from the literature	1 to 2 g	162, 345

APPENDIX TABLE 5

Studies on calcium requirements of the elderly (60 to 88 years)

Subjects	Number of studies	Principal criterion	Suggested daily requirement	References
95 men and women	8	retention	290 to 1000 mg	1, 3, 57, 156, 376, 382, 383, 410
7 men and women (winter)	1	retention	7.0 mg/kg	156
8 men and women (summer)	1	retention	8.0 mg/kg	156
8 men	1	retention	18.5 mg/kg	1
8 women	1	retention	16.7 mg/kg	3

A CONSPECTUS OF RESEARCH ON ZINC REQUIREMENTS OF MAN

by

JAMES A. HALSTED

Albany Medical College
Albany, New York 12208

J. CECIL SMITH, JR.

Trace Element Research Laboratory
Veterans Administration Hospital
Washington, D. C. 20422

and

M. ISABEL IRWIN

Nutrition Institute
Agricultural Research Service
United States Department of Agriculture
Beltsville, Maryland 20705

THE JOURNAL OF NUTRITION

VOLUME 104, NUMBER 3, MARCH 1974

(Pages 345-378)

TABLE OF CONTENTS

INTRODUCTION

The 1934 report by Todd et al. (300) that zinc was necessary for life in animals suggested that it was probably an essential nutrient for man also. Nevertheless the ubiquity of zinc made it seem unlikely that alterations in zinc metabolism could lead to significant problems in human nutrition or clinical medicine. For example, in 1962 Underwood (303) stated that "an uncomplicated dietary deficiency of zinc has never been observed in man." Since then, zinc deficiency has been observed in man, and thus, in 1971 Underwood (304) included man among the species in whom a deficiency syndrome had been demonstrated. This was the result of reports of primary zinc deficiency in Egypt by Prasad et al. (224, 226, 228) and in Iran by Halsted et al. (80, 84). In addition, Caggiano et al. (27), in the United States, observed zinc deficiency secondary to intestinal malabsorption. More recently, also in the United States, Hambidge et al. (87) reported cases of low hair zinc concentration and low taste acuity that were responsive to zinc supplementation.

The literature on the metabolic aspects of zinc is extensive (223) and is growing. Much of our knowledge of zinc has stemmed however from clinical observations in plant, animal and, most recently, human pathology. It is still necessary to rely on indirect information in estimating human requirements for zinc and in delineating those factors that may accentuate requirements. This indirect information comes from all branches of available knowledge including geochemistry and the zinc content of the earth's crust. Many bits of information gleaned from widely disparate experimental approaches, including those from the few reported metabolic balance studies and from cultural eating practices, shed some light on the role of zinc in human nutrition.

The objective of this conspectus is to bring together the information that bears on human requirements for zinc, to show how the information was obtained, and to point out areas where research is needed.

ZINC IN NATURE

Zinc has been estimated to rank 25th in abundance (305) and to make up 0.004 to 0.01% of the earth's crust (216, 305). However, it is less abundant than titanium, barium, zirconium, or vanadium (264), elements not yet shown to be essential to man. Although zinc is ubiquitous it is unevenly distributed in the earth's crust, ranging from 10 to 300 ppm with a mean of 50 ppm (264). Rocks average 16 to 95 ppm (21). Shales have the highest concentration and sandstone has the lowest.

Analysis of moon samples brought back by the astronauts of Apollo 11, 12, and 14 revealed a much lower concentration of zinc in both the rocks and soils than in materials found on earth (39, 253, 254). Specifically, igneous rock samples (basalt and gabbro) contained from 0.2 to 3.0 ppm zinc (Apollo 11). Eight rocks returned by Apollo 12 contained between 0.2 and 4.3 ppm zinc with a mean of slightly less than 4.0 ppm. Lunar soil samples showed a range of 4.0 to 8.2 ppm with a mean of 6.7 ppm zinc, less than 15% the mean concentration of earth soil.

The zinc content of certain land plant species grown in the United States has been summarized (100). The contents vary widely around a mean of 23 ppm. Some land plants reportedly accumulate up to 16% of their ash weight as zinc (330). Marine animals have a wide range of zinc concentrations with oysters having the highest level (21).

As an inorganic element, zinc is not destroyed but remains in "cycle." This cycle in its simplest form is from the rock (soil) →plants→animals→soil or ocean. There is however a net loss of elemental zinc from the soil due to natural leaching and erosion

Received for publication February 7, 1972.
Requests for reprints should be addressed to M. Isabel Irwin.

and because sewage is directed toward the oceans. Thus, it is theoretically possible that zinc and other trace elements may be depleted from the soil. In a like manner, constant removal of crops without repletion results in deficiency of zinc in the soil. Mitchell (172) has calculated that the uptake of zinc by plants is relatively high compared with soil concentration. That is, when a crop containing 100 ppm zinc is removed from the soil, 1 ppm zinc is lost from the surface soil (assuming a yield of 10 tons/acre). The feasibility of zinc-enriched fertilizers as a method for soil repletion has been discussed by Viets (310).

DEVELOPMENT OF KNOWLEDGE ABOUT ZINC

Early discovery—uses in metallurgy

Zinc does not occur naturally in a free, uncombined state. It was discovered by accident in the fourth century A.D. that brass was produced when a certain earth (zinc bearing) was heated with copper. In India during the 13th century, metallic zinc was produced by reducing calamine (zinc oxide plus a small percentage of ferric oxide) with organic substances such as wool (88). Ebener of Nürnberg is reported to have recognized zinc as a discrete element in 1509 (223). In 1746 Marggraf rediscovered the metal in Europe (88). Zinc as a bipositive ion is combined with sulfide in the mineral sphalerite which contains 67% zinc. Other naturally occurring zinc-containing minerals of the earth's crust include zincite, ZnO; smithsonite $ZnCO_3$; willemite, Zn_2SiO_4; and hemimorphite, $Zn_4(OH)(Si_2O_7) \cdot H_2O$.

Chemistry

Zinc has an atomic number of 30 and an atomic weight of 65.4. It has a relatively low melting point of 419°. Fifteen isotopes of zinc have been described ranging from ^{60}Zn to ^{72}Zn. Ten of these isotopes are not stable. Their half-lives vary from 1.48 minutes (^{61}Zn) to 245 days (^{65}Zn) (98). Metallic zinc is a good reducing agent, is amphoteric and will dissolve in mineral acids and strong bases. Zinc exists in solution only in the oxidized state of Zn^{2+}. The soluble salts of zinc include chloride, bromide, iodide, formate, acetate, sulfate, and nitrate (98). The insoluble salts include carbonate, sulfide, hydroxide, ammonium phosphate, oxalate, and phytate (98).

Today elemental zinc is obtained by heating ores containing zinc to form zinc oxide, reducing the oxide with carbon and then distilling the metal. Metallic zinc is bluish white.

Biological essentiality

Over 100 years ago (1869) Raulin (236), a pupil of Pasteur, discovered that zinc was indispensable for the growth of a black bread mold, *Aspergillus niger*. This finding was confirmed in 1911, 40 years later, by Bertrand and Javillier (16). According to Bertrand and de Wolf (12–15) *Aspergillus niger* requires zinc in order to synthesize phenylalanine, tryptophan, and tyrosine as well as several enzymes. Growth of penicillin-producing fungi is greatly retarded by zinc deficiency of the culture medium (60). Evidence indicating that zinc is essential to the growth of microorganisms has been summarized recently (330).

In 1919 Birckner (18) reported that egg yolk, human milk, and cow's milk contained zinc and suggested that zinc was of nutritive value. Shortly thereafter, Sommer and Lipman (278) demonstrated that zinc was essential for plant life. Lutz (137) noted that there had been reports from time to time indicating that zinc was a common and nearly universal constituent of animal as well as plant tissues. He emphasized that zinc was not present in "traces" but in amounts not greatly different from that found for other heavy metals such as iron. Analyses of many foods at that time showed amounts somewhat greater than in present day analyses, presumably the result of contamination of samples and less precise analytical methods than those used at present. After extensive and meticulous analyses of tissues from rats, cats, and man, Lutz (137) calculated that the human body contained a total of 2.2 g of zinc, an amount about half that of iron. This value has been widely quoted. The only other similar work is that of Widdowson et al. (325), who reported human body zinc content to be between 1.4 and 2.3 g.

Some plant diseases have been traced to zinc deficiency, such as leaf rosette in apples, mottle leaf in citrus crops and probably dwarfing of trees. Agronomists have traced zinc deficiency in plants to deficient soils in parts of California and Texas and in the Ninety Mile Desert in South Australia. These lands have been reclaimed for productivity by zinc supplementation (305).

Although many attempts were made to provide a controlled zinc-deficient diet, this was not accomplished until 1934 when Todd et al. (300) were successful in demonstrating that zinc is essential for growth and development of rats. The disease of swine, porcine parakeratosis, which had been long recognized in animal husbandry, was shown to be the result of zinc deficiency by Tucker and Salmon (302) in 1955. Their findings led to the general practice of supplementing animal feeds with zinc. O'Dell and Savage (193) showed that zinc was essential for growth in birds also. At present, at least 15 animal species, man included, have been shown to require zinc.

A dwarfism syndrome in man was first described by Lemann in 1910 (129). This syndrome was reported subsequently in Turkey by Reimann (237) in 1956 and by Okçuoğlu et al. (195) in 1968, in Portugal by LeCour (128), and in Morocco by Faure (53). In 1960 and 1961 Prasad et al. (224) and Halsted and Prasad (83) published a detailed clinical description of 11 dwarfs with extreme iron deficiency anemia who were studied in a hospital at Pahlavi University, Shiraz, Iran. They suggested that the endocrinopathies (growth and sexual retardation) observed in the dwarfs might be caused by zinc deficiency. Subsequent biochemical investigations (225, 226, 257) in similar dwarfs residing in the Nile delta of Egypt demonstrated abnormalities of zinc metabolism. Daily oral supplementation with zinc sulfate resulted in significantly more rapid growth and sexual development. These findings were confirmed in Iran by Halsted et al. (80, 84) in a study on 17 nutritional dwarfs. In this study sexual function occurred in 224 ± 72 days (mean $\pm$ SD) in nine dwarfs who were fed a well-balanced hospital diet. In contrast, seven dwarfs, fed the same diet plus 100 mg of zinc sulfate daily, developed sexual function in 59 ± 40 days. In 6 months the mean growth incre-

ment in the nine dwarfs fed the hospital diet alone was 4.2 ± 1.9 cm, whereas in dwarfs who were fed the same diet plus zinc sulfate, the growth increment was 10.5 ± 3.7 cm.

The extreme degree of dwarfism and total lack of sexual development noted in the above reports probably represent one end of a spectrum, the other end being represented by outwardly healthy but short adolescents with delayed puberty and mild anemia. Two studies have been published designed to determine whether oral zinc supplementation of such mildly growth retarded individuals would cause a growth response. Carter et al. (31) in Egypt gave daily zinc supplementation for 5 months with negative results. Ronaghy et al. (251) in Iran administered a complete supplement that provided all essential trace elements and vitamins with and without added zinc to each of two groups. Those receiving zinc developed sexually more rapidly than those who did not ($P < 0.02$). It thus appears that zinc, in addition to other essential nutrients and calories, may be a limiting factor in normal growth and well-being of certain populations in underdeveloped regions of the world.

Biological functions

The biochemical functions in which zinc has been implicated as necessary include: 1) enzymes and enzymatic function, 2) protein synthesis, and 3) carbohydrate metabolism.

Keilin and Mann in 1939 (116) and 1940 (117) first showed that zinc was an integral and necessary component of carbonic anhydrase of red blood cells. Since then, at least 18 metalloenzymes have been shown to contain zinc (202). Several enzymes necessary for cellular oxidation, such as human alcohol dehydrogenase, are zinc dependent. More complete information on the importance of zinc in enzymatic function may be found in recent reviews (160, 202).

Zinc has been shown to be related to protein synthesis in microorganisms, animals, and animal tissues. The synthesis of both DNA (63, 132) and RNA (315, 321, 327) is inhibited when zinc is lacking. Protein synthesis appears to be reduced or altered in zinc-deficient rats (295, 326).

Somers and Underwood (277), in a controlled study, found that the output of urinary nitrogen and sulfur was significantly higher in zinc-deficient lambs than in control animals. This observation suggested impaired protein or amino acid utilization. The data did not show whether the defect was due to impaired tissue synthesis or to increased catabolism.

Hsu et al. (104–107) recently elaborated on the relationship of zinc to protein synthesis. They showed that, in vivo, the incorporation of ^{35}S amino acids into organ and skin protein was significantly altered in zinc-deficient rats.

The role of zinc in carbohydrate metabolism is controversial. In 1937 Hove et al. (103) and more recently Quarterman et al. (235) reported decreased glucose tolerance in rats that were zinc deficient. In contrast, Macapinlac et al. (139) could find no difference in fasting blood sugar, or in glucose and insulin tolerance curves between zinc-deficient rats and ad libitum controls. Studies by Mills et al. (169) indicated that zinc influences the membrane transport and utilization of glucose. Although Harding et al. (89) showed that the insulin molecule contains 2 zinc atoms, it has not been demonstrated that these are necessary for the biological activity of insulin. Kinetic studies by Weil et al. (322) have indicated, however, that the stability of zinc-free insulin is less than that of zinc insulin. It is evident that the exact role of zinc in carbohydrate metabolism has yet to be elucidated.

METHODS OF MEASURING ZINC

Because of the lack of precise analytical procedures for the determination of zinc by the earliest workers, zinc was assigned to the category of a "trace" element. The element could be detected but not accurately quantitated. As methods became more sensitive, the problem of contamination due to the ubiquitous nature of zinc became evident. For example, blood for zinc analysis is easily contaminated by the needles and syringes used for venepuncture. Vacutainers, now widely used to draw venous blood, have been shown to be a source of contamination (86, 91). The use of all-plastic polyethylene syringes [1] and certain stainless steel needles,[2] however, prevents contamination from these sources (81). Anticoagulants also may be a source of extraneous zinc.

Early analytical determinations of zinc relied upon gravimetric and volumetric methods that were relatively insensitive. Beamish and Westland (7) have reviewed such methods.

Among the more modern techniques are atomic absorption spectrophotometry, emission spectrochemical methods (173), and X-ray emission spectrography (1). Of these, atomic absorption spectrophotometry is at present the most popular method for analyzing zinc in biological samples (76, 249, 271). Walsh (318), an Australian physicist, developed the method in 1955 and since then several commercial instruments have become available. The general advantages of this method include: 1) simplicity and ease of operation, 2) sensitivity, precision and accuracy, and 3) cost. In its simplest form the instrumentation consists of a hollow cathode lamp (light source), a flame atomizer, grating or prism, and a photodetector. Sample preparation is a persistent problem in this method because the sample must be aspirated into the instrument. Dry ashing may result in losses of zinc, presumably due to volatilization (296). At present, the most popular method of preparing biological solid material for atomic absorption analysis of zinc is acid (wet) digestion (274).

Although many of the techniques for the analysis of zinc are extremely sensitive, each method is no better than the standards available. The same standards rarely have been used by different laboratories. Biological reference standards are now available from the U. S. National Bureau of Standards.[3] For an accurate comparison of zinc analyses between laboratories it is imperative that a universal reference standard be used.

ZINC IN FOOD

Content in classes of foods

Classes of foods cannot be rigidly categorized according to zinc concentration be-

[1] Peel-A-Way Scientific. So. El Monte, California 91733.
[2] Monoject-250, Sherwood Medical Industries, Inc., Delano, Florida 32720.
[3] U. S. National Bureau of Standards. Washington, D. C. 20204.

TABLE 1

Zinc contents of selected foods[1]

Food item	Zinc
	mg/100 g (wet wt)
Meat products	
Roast beef	6.4
Beef patty (raw)	4.7
Chicken breast	1.1
Chicken thigh	2.8
Dairy products	
Milk	0.34
Cream (half and half)	0.40
Breads	
White	0.57
Rye	1.34
Whole Wheat	1.04
Vegetables and fruits	
Peas	0.69
Potatoes	0.29
Green beans	0.21
Carrots	0.25
Tomatoes	0.20
Apricots	0.12
Peaches	0.07
Pears	0.08
Applesauce	0.08
Orange juice	0.11
Apple juice	0.07
Grapefruit juice	0.10
Beverages	
Tea	0.02
Coffee	0.03
Decaf coffee	0.04

[1] Taken from Osis et al. (197).

cause of the variability of the zinc contents of foods within each class. There is a wide range of values published in the literature for the same food because of the differences in analysis, source, and variety. In general, meat, eggs, milk products, and shellfish (oysters in particular) are the best sources of zinc. Fruits and vegetables usually are poor sources. Berfenstam (11) reported human milk to contain 3 to 5 ppm (wet weight) which is comparable to cow's milk (189). More recent analyses of infant foods showed that 22 mature human milk samples contained a mean zinc concentration of 1.34 ppm and four commercially prepared infant formulas, as consumed, contained 1.47 to 3.99 ppm (180). These concentrations are markedly lower than that of 20 ppm previously reported for human colostrum (147). The importance

of zinc in colostrum was demonstrated by Nishimura (184) who showed that zinc deficiency developed in suckling mice deprived of colostrum. Oral administration of zinc prevented the deficiency. Mutch and Hurley [4] reported that dietary zinc deficiency in lactating female rats resulted in zinc deficiency in the suckling young due to a lowered zinc content of the milk. These studies suggest that consideration be given to the adequacy of zinc in infant formulas.

Content of typical meals or diets

During the course of metabolic balance studies, Osis et al. (197) analyzed numerous diets. The average total zinc content of 138 diets used in metabolic balance studies sampled and analyzed over a 4-year period was 12.2 mg/day. The zinc contents of a standard hospital diet according to individual meals were: breakfast, 2.2 mg; lunch, 4.7 mg; and dinner, 4.4 mg. Thus the total zinc content of the daily standard hospital diet was 11.3 mg, very similar to the mean of the experimental diets. Murphy et al. (178) published analyses of trace minerals in "Type A" school lunches collected from 300 schools in 19 states. The average zinc content of these lunches, served to sixth grade children, was 3.91 mg. The zinc content of selected foods as reported by Osis et al. (197) is shown in table 1.

An estimation of the zinc content of several diets from other cultures was summarized by Eggleton in 1938 (47). The diet of native sailors in the Dutch East Indian Navy prior to 1874 was estimated to contain 7.3 mg of zinc. The diet consisted mainly of meat (beef, pork, or fish) and rice. (Its caloric content was not known.) The Steffanssen all-meat diet (lean beef, fatty tissue, liver, marrow) eaten by Arctic explorers in the 1920's contained about 24 mg/day. The zinc content of a North China diet was estimated as 9.5 mg/day. Grain products and legumes furnished most of the protein. Eggleton (47) estimated that the daily zinc intake of the poorest class of Chinese in South China at that time was

[4] Mutch, P. B. & Hurley, L. S. (1971) Zinc deficiency in suckling rats. Fed. Proc. 30, 643 (Abstr.). Complete paper to be published in The Journal of Nutrition 1974.

less than 6 mg/day. He suggested that zinc might be limiting at this level. The southern China diet consisted mainly of polished rice, sea fish, and cooked cabbage.

Factors influencing zinc content of foods

Manufacturing techniques. The refining of foods usually results in a decrease in the zinc content. For example, Czerniejewski et al. (40) found that during the milling process of wheat for flour, up to 80% of the zinc may be lost. Schroeder et al. (263, 264) reported similar data. Thus, bread made from white flour has a lower zinc content than whole wheat bread (197). Cornstarch contains much less zinc than the whole corn kernel (165). The possibly deleterious effects of refining foods have been discussed by Mertz (157) and Schroeder (263).

Preparation of foods. Food preparation methods also affect zinc concentration. For example, water added for cooking purposes will vary markedly in zinc content among different regions, thus changing the zinc level of the prepared food. Kopp (123) analyzed 380 samples of tap (finished) water and reported the average zinc concentration to be 79.2 µg/liter. The range was from 3 to 2010 µg/liter. The zinc content of foods will also be affected by the equipment and utensils used to prepare and store the food. For instance, the corrosive action of acid foods in contact with galvanized metal increases the zinc concentration. This source of contamination, however, has decreased with the increased use of stainless steel, plastic, and plastic-coated cooking utensils.

METABOLIC ASPECTS OF ZINC IN HUMAN NUTRITION

Distribution in the body

Several studies have been published on the distribution of zinc in tissues. Extensive work on trace-element concentration in the tissues of man has been carried out by Tipton et al. (298). They analyzed, by emission spectrography, 24 trace elements, including zinc, in 10 different tissues of 162 adult subjects from various countries outside the continental United States. About half of the subjects had died from accidental causes, but the remainder had died

of various diseases. The tissues were collected from primitive African cultures, Lebanon, India, the Far East and Europe (Switzerland and Scandinavia). These samples represented people of a wide geographical distribution as well as with a variety of dietary habits. Surprisingly, little variation was found in the zinc content. The results were similar to data obtained by Perry et al. (211) from 150 healthy American adults who died suddenly of accidents.

Other data have been reported by Netsky et al. (182), Tipton and Cook (297), Butt et al. (25), Eggleton (47, 49), Galin et al. (66), Schrodt et al. (262), and McBean et al. (148). The results are summarized in table 2. The distribution of stable zinc in various tissues of rats (231), calves (163), and pigs (232) is included for comparison in this table.

A highly significant correlation among dietary, plasma, and bone zinc contents has been demonstrated in rats (274). Often the zinc concentrations of the kidney and liver are not decreased when there is zinc deficiency.

The concentrations of zinc in plasma or serum, blood cells, and hair have been extensively studied and will be considered in more detail.

Plasma and serum. Although plasma and serum have usually been regarded as possessing similar zinc concentrations (305, 311), Foley et al. (55) reported that serum invariably has a higher zinc content than plasma (about 16%). They attributed the greater serum content to the liberation of zinc by disintegrated platelets, to a dilution factor and to invisible hemolysis which always occurs (268). In a sense, serum is always slightly contaminated by the zinc contained in platelets and by hemolysis of red cells.

Values for the concentrations of zinc in plasma under normal conditions obtained by different laboratories using different methods are, with a few exceptions, in reasonably good agreement (table 3). The constancy of most estimates since 1965 coincides with better methods for avoiding contamination and with more precise analytical methods.

Red blood cells. The reported zinc content of red blood cells varies from about

TABLE 2

Zinc concentrations in human and animal tissues
(mg/kg dry weight)[1]

	Human		Rat (231)[2]		Calf (163)[2]		Pig (232)[2]	
		Reference	Normal	Zinc deficient	Normal	Zinc deficient	Normal	Zinc deficient
Liver	141–245	(25, 49, 66, 182, 297)	101±13	89±12	101	84	150.8±12	96.1±8
Kidney	184–230	(25, 49, 66, 182, 297)	91± 3	80± 3	73	76	97.8± 3.0	90.8±4.0
Lung	67–86	(25, 49, 182, 297)	81± 3	77± 9	81	72		
Muscle	197–226	(49, 148)	45± 5	31± 6	86	78		
Pancreas	115–135	(49, 148)						
Heart	100	(49)	73±16	67± 9	78	63	139.5± 4.0	88.3±4.0
Bone	218	(148)	168± 8	69± 6			95 ± 1.8	47 ±1.6
Prostate								
normal	520	(262)						
hyperplasia	2330	(262)						
cancer	285	(262)						
Eye								
retina	571	(66)						
choroid	562	(66)						
ciliary body	288	(66)						
Testis			176±12	132±16	79	70	54 ± 2.0	59 ±2.0
Esophagus			108±17	88±10			88.1± 3.0	97.6±5.0

[1]Mean ±SD except human data which are expressed as distribution of published mean values. [2]Literature reference.

10 to 14 μg/ml. Ross et al. (256) using the dithizone method found that the red cells of 48 normal subjects contained 11.8 ± 1.8 μg zinc/g. Also using the dithizone method, Prasad et al. (229) found a mean red cell zinc content of 13.7 ± 1.2 μg/ml in a study with 14 normal subjects. When samples of the same blood were analyzed by atomic absorption spectrophotometry, a mean value of 14.0 ± 1.5 μg/ml was obtained. Mansouri et al. (144) also using atomic absorption spectrophotometry found a mean zinc content of 11.8 ± 1.7 μg/ml in the red blood cells of 51 normal subjects. In the same laboratory, McBean and Halsted (149) obtained a mean value of 10.1 ± 1.2 μg/ml in 10 fasting controls. After a meal, the mean value $(10.1 \pm 1.0$ μg/ml) was not significantly changed. Differences in technique, for instance in speed of centrifugation, may account for part of the difference in estimates.

Leucocytes. The zinc content of leucocytes has been determined (44, 170, 214, 306) with general agreement that these cells are rich in zinc.

Hair. Hair zinc concentration has been reported to be affected by zinc intake in rats (242), swine (130), cattle and goats (164, 168), and in man (87).

Absorption of Zinc

As with iron, apparently only a small percentage of ingested zinc is absorbed. Absorption is difficult to ascertain precisely and intake–output studies are not valid

TABLE 3

Plasma or serum zinc concentration in normal adults[1]
(μg/100 ml)

Investigator	Reference	Year	Mean ±SD	Range	Method	Notes
Wolff	(328)	1950	130 ± 14(S)[2]	—	Dithizone	
Vikbladh	(311)	1950	126 ± 18(S)	84–163	Dithizone	Same for males and females
Berfenstam	(11)	1952	109 ± 2(P)[3]		Dithizone	Newborn, 125 ± 5
Koch et al.	(122)	1956	120 ± 23(P)	70–170	Dithizone	Males, 121 ± 29
Vallee et al.	(308)	1956	121 ± 19(S)	101–139	Dithizone	
Smit	(272)	1960	139 ± 29(S)	·		55 adults
Fuwa et al.	(65)	1964	122 ± 3(S)		A.A.S.[4]	Adults
Gofman et al.	(67)	1964	98 ± 2(S)[5]			39 adults
Butt et al.	(26)	1964	140 ± 6(S)[5]			170 adults
Prasad et al.	(229)	1965	104 ± 14(P)	—	A.A.S.	
			103 ± 9(P)		Dithizone	
Kahn et al.	(115)	1965	84 ± 30(S)		A.A.S.	
Sullivan & Lankford	(292)	1965	94 ± 12(S)	72–112	A.A.S.	
Olehy et al.	(196)	1966	93 ± 5(P)		Neutron Activation	
Helwig et al.	(92)	1966	91 ± 17(S)		Dithizone	64 adults
Parker et al.	(205)	1967	90 ± 10(S)		A.A.S.	23 adults
Rosner & Gorfien	(255)	1968	138 ± 13(P)	87–234	A.A.S.	
Halsted et al.	(81)	1968	96 ± 13(P)		A.A.S.	
Mahanand et al.	(143)	1968	94(P)	86–102	Fluorometry	Children, 108 ± 15
Davies et al.	(41)	1968	95 ± 13(P)	76–125	A.A.S.	Males, 95 ± 13 Females, 16 ± 11
Halsted & Smith	(85)	1970	96 ± 12(P)	72–115	A.A.S.	Children, 89 ± 13 Males, 96 ± 13 Females, 97 ± 11
Sinha & Gabrieli	(269)	1970	120 ± 20(S)	76–160	A.A.S.	100 males 121 ± 18 100 females 118 ± 21
Meret & Hankin	(156)	1971	92 ± 3(S)[5]	63–147	A.A.S.	45 females 90 ± 3 37 males 94 ± 3
Lindeman et al.	(134)	1971	96(P)	68–138	A.A.S.	Males, 96 Females, 88
Kurz et al.	(125)	1972	119(S)		A.A.S.	11 adults 110 ± 21 37 children 128 ± 17
Pekarek et al.	(209)	1972	102 ± 17(S)	68–136	A.A.S.	99 males

[1] Zinc concentration has been found to be 16% higher in serum than in plasma in one study (298).   [2] (S); serum.   [3] (P); plasma.   [4] A.A.S.; atomic absorption spectrophotometry.   [5] SE.

indicators because excretion of zinc is nearly all via the gut. Thus data indicating an *increased* absorption may also be interpreted as indicating a *decreased* excretion and vice versa.

Data on the site or sites of absorption in man and on the mechanism(s) of absorption, whether this be by active, passive or facultative transport, are meager. Pearson et al. (207) using the everted gut sac of the rat provided evidence that zinc is actively absorbed into the intestinal mucosa against a concentration gradient. They reported that zinc was most efficiently absorbed from the distal gut segments. More recently, Methfessel and Spencer (159) using $^{65}ZnCl_2$, studied specific absorption sites in rats by means of ligated intestinal sacs. They concluded that the absorption of ^{65}Zn was significantly greater from the duodenum than from the more distal segments of the small intestine. Over a 2-hour observation period, absorption was much less from the midjejunum and ileum. Only minimal amounts were observed from the stomach, cecum and colon. These data suggest that sites of zinc absorption may be similar to those of iron.

Becker and Hoekstra (9) recently reviewed the available information on intestinal absorption of zinc. They concluded that "zinc absorption is variable in extent and is highly dependent upon a variety of factors." Among the factors that they suggested might affect zinc absorption were body size, the level of zinc in the diet, and the presence in the diet of other potentially interfering substances such as calcium, phytate, other chelating agents, and vitamin D.

Availability of zinc

Edwards (46) using chicks studied the availability of zinc from various compounds and ores. He reported that zinc was most available from zinc sulfate, zinc metal and zinc oxide, and least available from sphalerite and franklinite. Later Roberson and Schaible (247) confirmed these observations.

Other factors influence the absorption and retention of zinc and thus its availability. Phytate (inositol hexaphosphate), which is present in cereal grains, markedly impairs the availability (absorption) of zinc. This was first shown in 1960 by O'Dell and Savage (194). Later Oberleas et al. (186) showed that phytic acid added to an animal protein diet depressed growth in swine. Using rats, Oberleas and Prasad (190) demonstrated a close relationship between zinc and the utilization of soybean protein. Without zinc supplementation, rats fed a 12% soybean diet gained less than half as much as rats that were supplemented with zinc. O'Dell (192) reported that autoclaving soybeans destroyed most of the phytic acid. In contrast, Lease (127) autoclaved sesame meal and found no reduction in phytate despite the fact that there was a marked increase in zinc availability to the chick. Likuski and Forbes (133) showed that phytic acid depressed the availability of zinc whether the protein source was pure amino acids or casein.

Such studies have a close relationship to zinc in human nutrition because there is strong evidence that phytate exerts a similar effect in man. Reinhold (238, 239) found that unleavened bread, consumed in large amounts by the Iranian villagers (often providing the major source of protein), contains significantly more phytate than urban breads which are leavened and allowed to ferment ($P < 0.001$). Leavening results in destruction of phytate. The omission of the leavening process in Iranian village breadmaking is presumably responsible for the high content of phytate.

The data suggesting that phytate enhances the possibility of zinc deficiency in man were strengthened by the reports from Egypt (225, 226, 257) and Iran (83, 84) that zinc deficiency occurred under conditions where unleavened bread was consumed in great amounts. Reinhold et al. (244) tested the hypothesis that phytate ingestion may result in zinc deficiency. Three adult subjects were studied. During an initial 16-day control period a diet providing approximately 0.7 g phytic acid was fed. Following the control period, sodium phytate (4.5 g/day) was added to the diet for 28 days yielding a total intake of about 2.5 g phytic acid/day. Then during the next 32 days, no sodium phytate was fed, but tanok replaced the low phytate bread in the experimental diet. The tanok, a bread consumed by villagers of Southern Iran, provided 2.6 to 3.4 g of phytate daily. During the sodium phytate period (28 days) zinc balances became significantly less positive. Occasionally, negative balances were observed. During the tanok period (32 days), zinc balances became more negative. After these two experimental periods, a white bread low in phytate was given to two of the subjects for 32 days. During this period of low phytate ingestion, zinc balances became positive again in both subjects.

The availability of zinc from foodstuffs, with major emphasis on the effect of phytate, was reviewed by Oberleas et al. (188) in 1966. More recently Oberleas (185), studying phytate–mineral complexes, suggested that the chelating properties of phytate may induce a wide variety of mineral deficiencies depending on which element first becomes limiting. Chemical studies indicate that phytate decreases zinc availability by forming an extremely insoluble calcium–zinc–phytate salt at the pH ranges found in the upper small intestine where most minerals are absorbed (141, 187, 313). Judging from the information now available on the deleterious effect of phytate in cereals on optimum growth and protein utilization, some amino acid supplementation programs may not be fully successful without careful consideration of the possibility of abnormal zinc metabolism associated with cereal diets.

Other factors that possibly may affect the availability of zinc include the zinc status of the organism, geophagia, the presence of chelating agents (other than phytate), and vitamin D.

Zinc status. Heth et al. (96), working with rats, and Prasad (222), studying human subjects, observed that the proportion of orally administered zinc lost in the feces decreased when the animals or human subjects were zinc deficient. Prasad et al. (225) suggested, however, that this increased apparent absorption was probably due to decreased excretion of zinc rather than to the increased true absorption.

Geophagia. Minnich et al. (171) found that clay from Turkey inhibited iron absorption in human subjects. Nearly all subjects with severe nutritional dwarfism studied in Iran gave a history of eating large amounts of clay for many years. Because the evidence indicated that zinc deficiency was the basic cause of this dwarfism syndrome, it was logical to suspect that Iranian clay might hinder zinc absorption. Furthermore, when a solution of ^{65}Zn was mixed with this clay, 97% of the radioactivity was removed from the solution. When, however, Iranian clay was fed to zinc-deficient rats, it proved to be a lifesaving source of zinc (274). A plausible deduction, therefore, is that the subjects in Iran may have sought zinc through the ingestion of clay.

Chelating agents. Considerable work has been reported on the effect of chelating agents on zinc absorption. Most of these studies were carried out in animals and have been summarized by Vohra and Kratzer (314) and Maddaiah et al. (141). The ability of EDTA(ethylenediaminetetraacetic acid) to complex readily with zinc has led to its use in removing radioactive zinc from the body (279).

Vitamin D. Worker and Migicovsky (329) found that the movement of zinc into the bones of chicks was enhanced by vitamin D. They suggested that the site of the vitamin's effect on zinc metabolism might be "in the absorption mechanism." Later Becker and Hoekstra (8) observed increased absorption of dietary zinc in rats treated with vitamin D. Additional studies with ^{65}Zn convinced them that the increased absorption of zinc was not the primary response but rather was the result of an increased need for zinc secondary to increased skeletal growth.

Excretion of zinc

McCance and Widdowson (153) found that regardless of whether zinc enters the body orally or parenterally, it is excreted almost wholly via the feces. Animal experiments have shown that fecal excretion is chiefly by way of the pancreatic juice regardless of the route of zinc intake. Negligible amounts are excreted by the liver into bile (153, 267). Urinary zinc excretion in normal individuals and those with diseases was summarized by Roman (250). In normal subjects, most of published means ranged between 400 and 600 $\mu g/24$ hours.

Steele (284) recently reported data suggesting that renal handling of zinc is different from that of other divalent cations.

For instance, when saline-loaded subjects were infused with a NaCl solution, zinc excretion decreased, whereas that of calcium and magnesium increased. Furthermore, when a diuretic, either ethacrynic acid or furosemide, was administered, urinary zinc concentration decreased significantly while the concentrations of calcium and magnesium increased. The mechanism governing renal excretion of zinc is not clear.

Increased urinary zinc excretion (zincuria) has been reported to accompany nephrosis (52), diabetes (36, 154, 215), postalcoholic hepatic cirrhosis (229, 291, 307), and porphyria (213, 267). McCance and Widdowson (153) found the urinary zinc excretion in two patients with albuminuria to be 3.3 and 2.0 mg/day—about seven times the amount excreted by their healthy subjects.

Spencer and Samachson (282) noted that urinary zinc excretion rose to high levels during total starvation in extreme obesity. They found a tenfold increase in daily excretion during their ten 6-day balance periods. Despite the urinary losses, plasma zinc levels did not change.

Recently Fell et al. (54) studied urinary zinc excretion by two patients after surgery for total hip replacement. They administered ^{65}Zn to the patient in sufficient time before surgery to allow its incorporation into the muscles. They found large increases in urinary excretion of ^{65}Zn, total zinc and nitrogen after surgery. The excretions rose to a maximum about 10 days postoperation. The close correlation between the excretion of ^{65}Zn and total zinc suggested that the zinc was being withdrawn mainly from the skeletal muscles. Because urinary total zinc was also closely correlated with urinary nitrogen, Fell et al. (54) suggested that urinary zinc may provide an index by which to estimate muscle catabolism.

Binding of zinc to serum protein

Early work by Laurel on zinc binding was summarized and amplified by Vikbladh in 1951 (312). The portion of plasma zinc bound to albumin was described as "loosely bound," whereas that associated with the globulin fractions was more "tightly bound" (312). The relative amounts of loosely and tightly bound zinc are at present some-

what controversial, but it appears that most is in a tightly bound form. The loosely bound zinc complex according to Vikbladh (312) is concerned with zinc transport. These findings on zinc binding with serum proteins have been confirmed by others (22, 203, 305). The identity of the fraction to which zinc is firmly bound has been the subject of several studies. Surgenor et al. (293) reported that zinc could combine with a β_1 globulin (transferrin) in vitro. Later Boyett and Sullivan (22) from studies of the distribution of protein-bound zinc suggested that transferrin and alpha-2 macroglobulin may have "an important role in internal zinc exchange." Parisi and Vallee (203) isolated alpha-2 macroglobulin and found that it contained 30 to 40% of the total serum zinc. They suggested that alpha-2 macroglobulin is the principal zinc metalloprotein in human serum.

Prasad and Oberleas (227) using ^{65}Zn incubated serum found that from 2 to 8% of the total serum zinc was ultrafilterable. In their in vitro studies they found also that several amino acids, specifically histidine, glutamine, threonine, cystine, and lysine, when added to predialyzed serum, increased the amount of ultrafilterable ^{65}Zn several fold. They suggested that this amino acid bound fraction of zinc may play a significant role in biological transport.

Factors influencing the concentration of zinc in plasma

As noted in table 3 the mean plasma zinc concentration reported in recent years has been reasonably constant. Most of these results were derived by atomic absorption spectrophotometry, but the neutron activation, fluorometric, and dithizone methods have given similar values. The use of polyethylene materials, which became available in the 1960's, has undoubtedly aided in eliminating sources of contamination.

Little work has been done on the effects of age or sex differences on plasma zinc levels. Somewhat higher levels have been found in newborn infants and children than in adults (11, 143), but another report showed contradictory data (85). No significant differences between males and females have been reported (85).

Inconclusive data exist on the effect of

meals on plasma zinc concentration. Davies et al. (41) reported that the zinc level decreased following intravenous or oral glucose loading, but this has not been confirmed. In another study (149), the effect of a meal containing 3.92 mg of zinc on the plasma zinc level was negligible in 10 normal individuals who had fasted 12 hours prior to eating the meal. There are few data on the effect of fasting on the plasma zinc levels of man. As noted previously, Spencer and Samachson (282) reported no change in plasma level in one obese patient treated by total starvation despite a tenfold increase in urinary zinc excretion.

Many factors, including pregnancy and oral contraceptives, various diseases, and stress, induce the lowering of the plasma zinc concentration (41, 85). Whether this reflects zinc deficiency, a redistribution of zinc, or an emergency call on available circulating zinc loosely bound to albumin is not clear. Wacker et al. (316) in 1956 noted that serum zinc concentration was lowered after an acute myocardial infarct. Lindeman et al. (134) also noted that the zinc level fell rapidly after extensive surgery, myocardial infarct, and acute infections. It rose to normal during convalescence. Similarly, after injection of endotoxin in man [5] and rats (208) a sharp fall in serum zinc level was noted. As the infection subsided, the serum zinc level returned toward normal (208, 210, 319). In pulmonary tuberculosis and in various types of chronic liver diseases the plasma zinc level was usually depressed, rising toward normal as the patient recovered (85).

Observations with burned and wounded rats suggested to Strain et al. (288, 289) that zinc was essential for wound healing. Other investigators using rats (258, 126, 191), cattle (166), and hamsters (289) also observed improved healing when zinc was administered. Sandstead et al. (258) suggested that collagen formation is impaired in conditions of zinc deficiency. Recently Stephan and Hsu (285) found that in zinc-deficient rats, there was decreased DNA synthesis as indicated by reduced thymidine-methyl-^{3}H incorporation into the DNA of skin. They suggested that this observation of impaired skin DNA synthesis together with a previous observation of "de-creased incorporation of ^{14}C-labeled amino acids in skin proteins of zinc deficient rats" (105) might "indicate a molecular basis for the relationship of zinc to healing" (285).

At present there is conflicting evidence on the effect of zinc on wound healing in human subjects. Pories and Strain (219) in 1966 reported that, with oral administration of zinc sulfate heptahydrate, healing time was apparently decreased. Their observations included the measurement of wound volume during the healing of pilonidal sinus tract excision wounds in two unsupplemented patients and one zinc-supplemented patient. When the work was extended to include 20 young men (217, 218), 10 of whom received zinc supplements, healing time was significantly reduced in the supplemented group (45.8 vs. 80.1 days). Studies on healing of leg ulcers (72, 77, 78, 113, 266) also indicated significantly higher rates of healing in patients to whom zinc was administered as compared with nonsupplemented controls. Other investigators, however, failed to find that healing was accelerated after zinc supplementation. Brewer et al. (23), for instance, in a double blind study with 14 patients with decubitus ulcers did not find any difference in healing time between zinc-treated and control patients. Likewise, Myers and Cherry (181), studying 51 patients, 36 to 80 years old, with chronic leg ulcers, and Barcia (5), with 20 young men who underwent surgical treatment for chronic pilonidal disease, failed to show an improvement in healing time in those patients who were treated with zinc. Pories and Strain (220) in reviewing these studies, suggested that the patient's initial zinc status may influence his response to zinc therapy. Holböök and Lanner (78), for instance, observed significant differences in healing time between zinc treated and untreated patients in a group whose individual serum zinc levels were less than 110 μg/100 ml but not in a group whose serum zinc levels were 110 μg/100 ml or higher.

For many years there has been interest in a possible relationship of zinc to malig-

[5] Smith, J. C., Jr., McDaniel, E. G., McBean, L. D., Doft, F. S. & Halsted, J. A. (1971) Effect of microorganisms upon zinc metabolism. Proc. Western Hemisphere Nutr. Cong., Bal Harbour, Florida (Abstr.).

nant disease. Ross et al. (256), using [65]Zn in patients with neoplastic disease, found that uptake of zinc in leukemia leucocytes was about one-half that of normal subjects. The zinc content of blood constituents in Hodgkin's disease has been reported to be low (4). Davies et al. (42) and Morgan (176) reported low plasma or serum zinc levels in patients treated for bronchogenic carcinoma. Smith et al. (275), however, found no differences in serum zinc levels between patients with untreated bronchogenic carcinoma and normal controls. DeWys et al. (45) found that Walker 256 sarcoma implanted in zinc-deficient rats grew at a markedly reduced rate compared with ones implanted in control, pair-fed rats. These results suggest an increased zinc requirement for tumor growth.

The wide variety of pathological states in which plasma zinc concentration has been found to be depressed suggests that there may be several mechanisms involved whereby zinc metabolism is altered in disease. On the other hand, there also may be a fundamental mechanism common to all. It is attractive to speculate that zinc is required rapidly for enzyme formation or protein synthesis when bodily insults occur, and that the zinc that is loosely bound to albumin is immediately available for these purposes. Of interest is the fact that the zinc level rarely falls below 30 to 35% of the normal. This may correspond to that amount loosely bound to albumin.

Relationship of zinc to endocrine functions

Endocrine abnormalities in human zinc deficiency have been studied only in cases of nutritional dwarfism reported from Egypt (34, 226). Somewhat ambiguous results were obtained in assessing growth hormone, gonadotropin, adrenocortical, and testicular function. In human pregnancy, plasma zinc concentration is usually depressed to about two-thirds that of normal (114). In a study with rats, McBean et al. (151) confirmed the findings, previously observed in women (82), that depression of plasma zinc concentration occurs when contraceptive hormones are fed. McBean et al. (151) found that the estrogen component of the contraceptive compounds was responsible for the plasma zinc lowering effect. Additional work is needed to establish more precisely the interrelationships between zinc and endocrine function.

Interrelationships with other minerals

Calcium. Tucker and Salmon (302) first demonstrated that increasing the calcium content of practical diets for swine enhanced zinc-deficiency symptoms (skin lesions and growth retardation). Because the basal diets fed were relatively high in zinc, 34 to 44 ppm, this was an apparent demonstration of the antagonism of calcium to zinc. Numerous investigations with swine using diets containing plant protein have confirmed the calcium–zinc antagonism (35, 130, 131, 135, 136, 183, 286). In contrast, when swine were fed animal protein diets the deleterious effect of calcium on zinc utilization was not demonstrable (10, 324). In 1960 (57) Forbes reviewed the interrelationship of zinc and calcium. As pointed out by Forbes (58, 59) and more recently by O'Dell (192), the conflicting results regarding the antagonistic effect of calcium toward zinc can be explained by the presence of phytate. That is, excess calcium in the presence of phytate (which accompanies plant but *not* animal protein) results in decreased zinc absorption, enhancing zinc deficiency. The interrelationships of calcium, zinc, and phytic acid in promoting growth of pigs are shown in figure 1.[6]

It is doubtful whether the calcium antagonism to zinc absorption plays an important role in a well-balanced diet containing animal protein. Spencer et al. (283) could not demonstrate a calcium–zinc antagonism in human subjects fed meat as a protein source when calcium was varied in the diet tenfold. However, the antagonism may be a factor in diets high in plant protein, i.e., beans, peas, and cereal grains.

Cadmium. Cadmium and zinc have several similar chemical properties, including a usual coordination number of 4, tetrahedral configuration, and isoelectronic valence shells. In 1957 Pařízek (204) showed that the destructive effect of injected cadmium upon testicular tissue could be alleviated by zinc, and suggested that the injury was due to interference with

---

[6] By permission of the author B. L. O'Dell and the publisher American Journal of Clinical Nutrition.

zinc function. Gunn et al. (74, 75), and Mason and Young (146) confirmed the antagonistic zinc–cadmium effects on testicular function.

In human nutrition, the zinc–cadmium interrelationship has not been demonstrated. Schroeder et al. (264) have elaborated on the close association between cadmium and zinc. Cadmium, a nonessential element, is invariably associated with zinc in both geological and biological matter.

Copper. In animal studies, excessively high levels of zinc resulted in interference with copper metabolism (70, 142). Studies such as those by Hoefer et al. (101) and Wallace et al. (317) indicated that the severity of parakeratosis in swine could be alleviated by either zinc or copper, although zinc was usually more effective. Ritchie et al. (246) reported that, in addition to preventing parakeratosis in swine, zinc gave protection against copper toxicity.

The plasma zinc concentration was decreased but copper concentration was increased in pregnant women (114) and in those taking oral contraceptives (82). At present the significance of these observations is not understood.

When a diet composed entirely of meat was fed to rodents, an anemia developed that was responsive to copper (73, 174, 175). It was proposed that this "meat anemia" resulted not only from a relative excess of zinc over copper present in meat but also from the lower calcium levels found in meat. The meat anemia, however, could be reduced or prevented by cooking the meat (174). This suggests that it was not due simply to a high zinc–copper ratio but that a heat labile factor may have been involved. Hoekstra (102) has reviewed this subject briefly.

Others. In 1958 Sivarama Sasty and Sarma (270) suggested that iron metabolism was affected by toxic levels of zinc. In addition, decreased concentrations of iron in the liver were reported by Cox and Harris (37), Magee and Matrone (142), and Kinnamon (120) when rats were fed toxic levels of zinc.

An interaction of zinc and molybdenum was suggested by the investigations of Gray and Ellis (71).

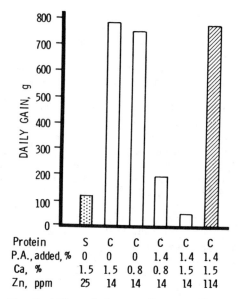

Fig. 1 Effect of phytic acid on growth rate of pigs fed diets based on soybean (S) or casein (C) with varying levels of calcium and zinc. Phytic acid (P.A.) was added to the casein diet. Reproduced from Amer. J. Clin. Nutr. (1969) 22, 1316, by permission of the author and publisher.

The interrelationships of zinc with other minerals are obviously not limited to single elements, i.e., zinc–copper or zinc–cadmium. There have been some reports involving a simultaneous interaction of several minerals (99, 136, 177, 243, 287). No information on such multiple interactions in humans was found.

Interrelationships with vitamins

Vitamin A. Early studies on dark adaptation indicated that another nutrient might be necessary for vitamin A utilization (206). Observations of reduced plasma zinc concentration in cirrhotic patients (85) suggested that this necessary nutrient might be zinc. Studies with animals tended to support this hypothesis. Stevenson and Earle (286), for instance, reported that zinc-deficient swine had depressed serum vitamin A levels. These levels did not return to normal even after massive oral doses of vitamin A. Later, Saraswat and Arora (260) reported that zinc supplementation was necessary for maximum efficiency of vitamin A therapy in lambs that were deficient in both zinc and vitamin A.

More recently, Smith et al. (276) found in rats that zinc was necessary for the mobilization of vitamin A from the liver into the plasma. In addition, retinal reductase, an alcohol dehydrogenase of the retina involved in the metabolism of vitamin A, is most probably a zinc metalloenzyme (307).

Vitamin D. In 1958 Whiting and Bezeau (324) reported that vitamin D decreased the absorption and retention of zinc when diets low in zinc were fed to pigs. Wasserman (320) observed no significant change in ^{65}Zn absorption from the ligated duodenum when rachitic chicks were fed vitamin D_3. As noted previously (page 356), however, Worker and Migicovsky (329) with chicks and Becker and Hoekstra (8) with rats observed that zinc absorption and zinc uptake in the bones were enhanced when vitamin D_3 was fed. A positive effect of vitamin D on zinc metabolism was observed by others also (33, 118, 145). Becker and Hoekstra (8) suggested that the effect of vitamin D was primarily on calcification and skeletal growth and that the increased uptake of zinc by the bone was only a secondary effect. Chang et al. (33), however, concluded from studies in which bone growth and calcification of rats were stimulated by either vitamin D or protein that vitamin D probably exerts an effect on zinc metabolism that is not related to calcification or bone growth.

Riboflavin. In 1941, Follis et al. (56) reported histological corneal lesions in zinc-deficient rats and suggested that they were apparently similar to lesions described by Bessey and Wolbach (17) in uncomplicated riboflavin deficiency in rats. This was the first suggestion of an apparent similarity in the effect of riboflavin and zinc deficiencies upon specific tissues. More recently, French investigators noted a similarity in the effects of riboflavin and zinc deficiency in rats (221). Specifically, in deficiencies of either zinc or riboflavin, similar bony malformations were observed. In addition, fetuses from riboflavin-deficient females had lower body zinc contents than fetuses from riboflavin-sufficient mothers.

ZINC DEFICIENCY

Animals

In animals, zinc deficiency has been described in rats (300), mice (43), swine (302), chickens (193), turkeys (124), cattle (162), goats (167), lambs (200), dogs (248), Japanese quail (62), rabbits (69), squirrel monkeys (138), hamsters (20), and guinea pigs (152).

The signs and symptoms of zinc deficiency are markedly similar in different animals. They include dermatitis, emaciation, alopecia, ocular lesions, testicular atrophy, retarded growth, and anorexia. All of these conditions with the possible exception of testicular lesions are reversed by zinc supplementation (6, 161).

Malformations of embryos and/or fetuses due to zinc deficiency were reported for a number of species. Blamberg et al. (19) reported gross malformations involving the brain, vertebrae, limbs, beak, and head of chick embryos produced from eggs laid by zinc-deficient hens. Kienholz et al. (119) confirmed these findings. Hurley and co-workers (108–111) demonstrated congenital malformations in rat fetuses delivered from zinc-deficient females. The malformations included a high incidence of short or missing mandibles, clubbed feet, fused or missing digits, cleft palate, and brain abnormalities. Related studies by Apgar (3) and Hurley and Swenerton (112) indicated that female rats fed a zinc-deficient diet during pregnancy cannot mobilize zinc from tissue stores in amounts sufficient to supply the needs of normal fetal development. Swenerton et al. (294) suggested that the high incidence of gross congenital malformations resulting from zinc deficiency may be caused by impaired DNA synthesis. The evidence of a relationship between zinc deficiency and congenital malformations in the rat was reviewed in 1967 (2). To our knowledge no congenital malformations due to zinc deficiency have been reported in humans. It is of interest, nevertheless, that a brother of one patient with the dwarfism syndrome originally reported in 1961 (224) had pronounced bony abnormalities as well as extreme dwarfism.

Behavioral impairment was reported in zinc-deficient adult rats (28, 29). Performance tests indicated that zinc-deficient rats were inferior to zinc-sufficient animals in both learning ability and emotional stability.

Man—clinical and metabolic features

In man, the clinical aspects of zinc deficiency are similar to those described above for animals. In summary, they consist of severe iron deficiency anemia, hepatosplenomegaly, short stature, infantile testes, open epiphyses, spoon nails, frequently a history of geophagia, and rough skin with hyperpigmentation.

An interesting feature of the syndrome is the rather prolonged rise in alkaline phosphatase (a zinc-dependent enzyme) which occurs when zinc is administered. This could be due either to a regeneration of enzyme activity or to an increase in bone growth. It was at first thought that the syndrome was limited to males because considerably higher concentrations of zinc have been found in the testes than in the ovaries. However, two well-documented cases in females were included in a recent report from Iran (84).

Ronaghy et al. (252) conducted a 6-year follow-up study on the Iranian dwarfs in whom zinc deficiency had first been suspected (224). They found that the patients remained well if they continued to eat a well-balanced diet including meat. If, however, they resumed the village diet in which unleavened bread was predominant, their symptoms of zinc deficiency reappeared.

Reinhold et al. (240) measured zinc, calcium, phosphorus, and nitrogen intake and output of 13 Iranian apparently healthy villagers in a metabolic ward (table 4). The subjects were studied over a 6- to 7-day period during which a well-balanced diet was fed. The zinc data showed a wide range of retention (−6.7 to 61.4%). More than half of the group had positive retentions greater than 25%. This observation suggested to Reinhold et al. (240) that these villagers had been depleted of zinc previously.

Sandstead et al. (259) and Smit and Pretorius (273) found very low serum zinc levels in kwashiorkor. The latter workers also found low urinary zinc excretion. Al-

TABLE 4

Zinc balance studies of adult Iranian villagers[1,2]

Subject number	Sex	Age	Weight	Weight gain	Retention	
		yr	kg	kg/day	mg	%
1	M	32	N.A.[3]	N.A.	−1.6[4]	−6.7
2	M	25	56	0.07	−2.2	−9.7
3	M	38	61	0.07	+3.5	12.4
4	F	25	48	0.18	+3.2	13.0
5	M	35	60	−0.06	+3.8	14.9
6	M	47	60	0.03	+5.1	23.1
7	F	30	N.A.	N.A.	+5.9	25.2
8	M	30	56	0.24	+6.0	26.5
9	F	24	45	0.08	+6.7	28.8
10	M	37	57	0.21	+7.0	29.3
11	F	22	40	0.25	+8.5	30.5
12	M	40	58	0.30	+15.9	58.5
13	F	17	39	0.46	+15.4	61.4

[1] From Reinhold et al. (240).   [2] All were sufficiently healthy to carry out normal activities of a villager.   [3] Not available. [4] Mean for a 6- to 7-day period during which intakes in food and losses in excreta were measured. The hospital diet provided 2,400 calories, 75 g of protein (15% from pulses, 21% from meat, 28% from bread, and 36% from milk and cheese), 80 to 120 g of fat from butter and corn oil, 24.6 mg of zinc, 1,031 mg of calcium, and 1,513 mg of phosphorus.

though kwashiorkor is an extreme example of protein–calorie malnutrition, zinc deficiency may be a secondary factor. To date, little account of this possibility has been taken.

Zinc deficiency, secondary to intestinal malabsorption, recurrent infection and hypogammaglobulinemia, has been reported by Caggiano et al. (27). One suspects that zinc deficiency might be implicated in growth retardation that may occur in cystic fibrosis, inflammatory bowel disease, and other malabsorption states, but these have not yet been adequately investigated.

Reports by Henkin et al. (93–95) and Schechter et al. (261) indicated that a decrease in acuity of taste and/or smell may occur spontaneously (idiopathic hypogeusia, hyposmia) or after the administration of d-penicillamine. These investigators reported that this disorder may be corrected by the administration of either copper or zinc.

Recently Hambidge et al. (87) reported that 10 children over 4 years old in the Denver area had hair zinc concentrations of less than 70 ppm—a level similar to that reported for Egyptian adolescents suffering from symptomatic zinc deficiency (290). Seven of the 10 children had a history of poor appetite and eight had heights that fell on or below the 10th percentile when "plotted on growth charts based on data compiled by the Harvard School of Public Health and the Iowa Child Welfare Research Station." Of six children whose taste acuity was measured, five showed evidence of lowered acuity. After 1 to 3 months with daily dietary zinc supplementation (1 to 2 mg $ZnSO_4$/kg body weight), the taste acuity returned to normal and hair zinc concentrations increased in the five children. These children were from a group of 338 subjects who were apparently healthy Caucasians in the upper and middle socioeconomic class.

Eggleton in 1938 (47) commenting on a possible role of zinc deficiency in beriberi, said: "Attention is drawn, however, to the fact that a diet producing beriberi may supply minimal quantities of zinc, and presumably also copper and manganese. To what extent shortage of minor elements may be the cause of certain symptoms usually associated with beriberi remains to be shown, but it is considered possible that this shortage may account, in part at least, for the peculiar appearance of the hair, the dry skin and the abnormal finger and toe nails . . ." The integumentary changes to which Eggleton referred also are found in zinc-deficient dwarfs as well as in animals with experimental or spontaneous zinc deficiency. It seems possible that spoon nails (koilonychia), long attributed to chronic iron deficiency, might actually be the result of associated zinc deficiency.

PARAMETERS FOR ASSESSING ZINC STATUS IN MAN

Parameters that have been used in assessing zinc status in man are as follows: 1) plasma or serum concentration, 2) hair zinc concentration, 3) metabolic balance of zinc, 4) isotope turnover studies, 5) excretion of urinary sulfate, and 6) response of growth and sexual development to zinc supplementation.

The simplest method is measurement of plasma zinc concentration. As discussed previously (pages 357–359), there are many factors that influence the plasma zinc level so that a lower than normal value cannot be said to be more than suggestive of zinc deficiency. In some instances directly after a stressful situation, such as the injection of endotoxin, a myocardial infarct, surgery, and other trauma, a very rapid drop in the plasma zinc level occurs. It appears unlikely that such a transiently low level occurring so rapidly is a sign of zinc deficiency. Nevertheless, demonstrable zinc deficiency in man is accompanied by a low plasma zinc concentration.

Measurement of a specific zinc-binding protein, alpha-2 macroglobulin, possibly may become a useful tool in assessment of zinc deficiency. Boyett and Sullivan (22) found a slight increase in this globulin fraction in patients with alcoholic cirrhosis as compared with normals. McBean et al.,[7] studying a variety of diseases, found no significant correlation, however, between serum zinc and alpha-2 macroglobulin.

Hair zinc concentration has been studied by several investigators with varying results (table 5). McBean et al. (150) could find no correlation between plasma and hair zinc concentration in growth-retarded 6- to 11-year-old children. These subjects had lower than normal plasma zinc levels, but hair zinc concentrations were normal. They concluded that the zinc content of hair was not a reliable indicator of body zinc metabolism at the time of sampling. Others (121, 212) have shown that various factors, including age, affect the zinc concentration in hair.

Reinhold's zinc balance studies on Iranian villagers (240) point to the value of the balance method (table 4). His data indicate that a zinc balance study, cumbersome though it may be, is likely to shed light on possible subclinical zinc deficiency.

Isotope turnover studies in man are scarce, probably because the half-life of ^{65}Zn is 245 days making it an unacceptable procedure except in patients with a limited life expectancy. Richmond et al. (245) reported that the biological half-life of this isotope in human subjects averaged 154 days. Zinc isotope turnover studies have been carried out by Ross et al. (256), Prasad (225), and Spencer et al. (280, 281, 283). Ross et al. (256) injected ^{65}Zn intra-

---

[7] McBean, L. D., Smith, J. C., Bernard, B. H. & Halsted, J. A. (1972) Serum zinc and alpha-macroglobulin concentration in patients with various disorders. Proc. IX Int. Congr. Nutr., Mexico City, Mexico, September 2–9, 1972 (Abstr.).

TABLE 5

Hair zinc concentration as reported by various investigators

Investigator	Reference	Year	Subjects	Hair zinc	Method
				ppm	
Eggleton	(48)	1938	11 Chinese adults	255	Dithizone
Reinhold et al.	(241)	1966	19 male adult Iranian villagers	139±16.4[1]	Zincon
			20 male control adult subjects (Shiraz, Iran)	181±36.3[1]	Zincon
Strain et al.	(290)	1966	10 zinc deficient Egyptian male dwarfs 16 to 20 years	54± 6[2]	E.S.[3]
			8 zinc-treated dwarfs 16 to 20 years	121± 5[2]	E.S.
			12 normal Egyptians 27 to 40 years	103± 4[2]	E.S.
			6 normal Rochester residents 23 to 37 years	120± 5[2]	E.S.
Eminians et al.	(50)	1967	12 healthy village children 11 years old	163±22[2]	A.A.S.[4]
Klevay	(121)	1970	31 Panamanian males 6 to 10 years	127±49[1]	A.A.S.
McBean et al.	(150)	1971	14 normal adults (Washington, D. C.)	176±37[1]	A.A.S.
			75 Iranian village children 6 to 12 years (growth retarded)	199±22[1]	A.A.S.

[1] Mean±SD.   [2] Mean±SE.   [3] E.S.; emission spectrography.   [4] A.A.S.; atomic absorption spectrophotometry.

venously into patients with malignancy, finding that it disappeared rapidly from the plasma. Prasad's studies indicated that, in zinc deficiency, plasma zinc turnover was increased, the 24-hour exchangeable zinc pool was decreased, cumulative excretion of ^{65}Zn was low, and 6-hour plasma ^{65}Zn disappearance was rapid. Spencer's reports were limited to metabolic aspects of zinc without consideration of zinc deficiency.

Hsu and Anthony (104) showed that, in zinc-deficient rats, urinary sulfate is markedly increased after an injection of cystine-^{35}S. Somers and Underwood (277) confirmed the significantly elevated sulfur excretion in zinc-deficient lambs. The mechanism suggested by Hsu and Anthony (104) was the inability of the zinc-deficient animal to utilize sulfur-containing amino acids for protein synthesis, with consequent excretion of sulfate. No reports of similar work in man were found.

At present the critical test for zinc deficiency in man or animals is a definitive response to oral supplementation with zinc under controlled conditions. The data for primary zinc deficiency in the cereal-eating populations of Iran and Egypt now appear unequivocal. No reports of similar studies in other geographic locations have been found.

ZINC TOXICITY

In comparison with the trace elements lead, cadmium, arsenic, and antimony, zinc is relatively nontoxic. Many of the toxic effects ascribed to zinc by early investigators may be due actually to other contaminating elements such as lead, cadmium, or arsenic (90). Zinc is noncumulative, and the proportion absorbed is thought to be inversely related to the amount ingested (64, 96). Vomiting, a protective mechanism, occurs after ingestion of large quantities or after extended exposure to fumes containing zinc. In fact, an oral dose of 2 g of zinc sulfate (454 mg of zinc) has been recommended as an emetic (155). In addition to severe vomiting, the symptoms of zinc toxicity in humans include dehydration, electrolyte imbalance, stomach pain, nausea, lethargy, dizziness, and muscular incoordination. Acute renal failure caused by zinc chloride poisoning was reported by Csata et al. (38). The symptoms occurred within 3 hours after large quantities of zinc were ingested.

There are reports in the literature indicating that the zinc content of acidic food in contact with zinc-coated (galvanized) containers for long periods possibly may rise to toxic levels (24, 30). Toxic symptoms were observed also after the voluntary ingestion of 12 g of elemental zinc over a 2-day period (179). Death is reported to have occurred after the ingestion of 45 g of zinc sulfate (199). Toxic symptoms, such as pulmonary distress, chills, and fever, may be caused also by inhalation of fumes or dust containing high levels of zinc (201). This so-called "metal-fume fever" usually has been seen in industrial workers such as welders of galvanized metal.

Numerous studies on the toxicity of zinc in lower animals have been summarized by Van Reen (309).

HUMAN REQUIREMENTS FOR ZINC
(TABLE 6)

The apparent enteroenteric circulation of zinc makes precise estimation of absorption and excretion impossible by a simple measurement of intake and output. Nevertheless, the balance method has been the principal technique used in estimating zinc requirements of man. Adult subjects and school children have been most studied. There have been a few observations on infants and preschool children. No reports were found on zinc requirements of healthy adolescents, pregnant or lactating women, or of the elderly. All of the balance studies with presumably healthy subjects indicated that urinary zinc excretion was low and not apparently related to intake. Fecal zinc excretion tended to fluctuate with intake.

In the studies with adults, the intakes varied from relatively low (about 5 mg/day) to relatively high (about 22 mg/day). McCance and Widdowson (153), for instance, reported data on two men and one woman eating a specially formulated diet that provided 4.9 to 6.1 mg of zinc/day. Zinc analysis was carried out by the method described by Keilin and Mann (116). During dietary periods of "about a fortnight," balances of −0.8 to 0.0 mg zinc/day were observed. When the zinc intake was raised to 9.1 or 13.8 mg/day by adding zinc salts or by providing 40 to 50% of the calories from white flour, balances rose slightly to range from −0.1 to 2.7 mg/day. For two subjects, the zinc intake was increased to 19.6 and 22.0 mg/day by replacing the white flour with 90% extraction flour. With these intakes, retentions of 1.1 and 2.6 mg/day were observed. The possible effect of phytate in the high extraction flour on zinc absorption was not discussed in this report.

In other studies in which moderate zinc intakes (about 9 to 14 mg/day) were recorded, retentions ranged from −4.0 to 8.8 mg/day. The highest retentions with this range of intake were recorded by Tribble and Scoular (301). They studied a group of 13 young women, 17 to 27 years old, eating self-selected diets that were sampled and analyzed for zinc by Hibbard's dithizone method (97). With mean intakes that ranged from 11.8 to 14.1 mg/day, the young women retained from 5.1 to 8.8 mg/day. Osis et al. (198) on the other hand, observed much smaller retentions with similar intakes. They studied one subject whose mean zinc intake during four 6-day periods ranged from 11.7 to 13.1 mg/day.

TABLE 6

Controlled studies on human requirements for zinc

Subjects	Number of subjects	Number of studies	Daily intake[1]	Daily retention[1]	Estimated daily requirement[1]	Reference
Infants 5 to 8 days old	10	1	0.20 to 1.19 mg/kg	−0.85 to 0.08 mg/kg		(32)
Preschool 3 to 6 years old	3	1	3.80 to 5.87	−2.70 to 3.39	0.300 to 0.307 mg/kg	(265)
School children 7 to 12 years old	58	3	4.6 to 9.2 13.85 to 18.35	0.5 to 3.8 4.92 ± 2.94	6.2	(51, 234) (140)
Adolescents	0	0				
Adults men and women	51	6	4.9 to 6.1 9.0 to 14.1 18.0 to 22.0	−0.8 to 0.0 −4.0 to 8.8 1.0 to 8.3		(153) (153, 198, 299, 301, 323) (68, 153, 299)

[1] In mg/day except where otherwise stated.

With these intakes, the subject's retentions ranged from 0.28 to 0.63 mg of zinc/day. In an additional 24-day study, nine subjects ate a diet providing 12.3 mg of zinc/day with either 200 or 1300 mg of calcium. Four subjects with the low calcium diet retained 0.73 mg of zinc/day whereas those with the higher calcium diet retained 0.17 mg of zinc/day. The data indicated that the difference in mean retention was due mainly to a difference in mean fecal zinc excretion. Zinc analysis was carried out by atomic absorption spectrophotometry.

White and Gynne (323) also observed low retentions in their study with nine young women, 19 to 20 years old. The women ate a controlled diet for 30 days (six 5-day collection periods). The average zinc intake was 11.5 mg/day. Urinary losses were too small to be accurately measured by emission spectroscopy. Four women absorbed 1 to 21% of the dietary zinc. Fecal losses of four other subjects were greater than the intakes. The average fecal excretion was 11.4 mg/day. White and Gynne (323) concluded that, for zinc, the subjects were "essentially in equilibrium."

A still lower mean balance was recorded by Tipton et al. (299). They reported on the mineral intake and excretion of two young men, 23 and 25 years old, who recorded their food intake and collected samples of food, urine, and feces over a 50-week period. The samples were analyzed for zinc by atomic absorption photometry. One subject whose mean zinc intake was 11 mg/day had a mean balance of −4.0 mg/day. The second subject had a mean intake of 18 mg of zinc/day. He retained 1.0 mg/day. This retention is in reasonably close agreement with those (1.1 to 2.6 mg/day) reported by McCance and Widdowson (153) in studies with similar high intakes. It is much lower, however, than those reported recently by Gormican and Catli (68). They studied mineral balances in five young men, 21 to 24 years old. The men were given a liquid diet based on milk solids, calves' liver, corn oil, and purified carbohydrates for 28 days (four 7-day periods). The zinc contents of food, feces, and urine were determined by emission spectroscopy. The average zinc intake was 19.5 mg/day with mean retention ranging from 7.3 to 8.3 mg/day. The apparent dif-

ferences in retention of zinc as indicated by these studies may be due in part to differences in dietary composition. The differences in retention may be due also to differences in nutritional status among the subjects. Fox (61) recently reviewed the status of zinc and factors that affect its requirement in human nutrition.

In studies with school children, the intakes covered a range similar to that observed in studies with adults. Low to moderate intakes were reported by Engel et al. (51). They studied a total of 36 girls, 7 to 10 years old, in groups of 12 in three separate studies of 56, 48, and 36 days duration. The controlled diets provided from 4.6 to 9.2 mg of zinc/day. All subjects were in apparent positive balance with these intakes. When retentions were plotted against intakes, the retentions during study 2 were found to be much higher than those during study 1 or 3. No explanation for this "unusual behavior" was found. Using the data from studies 1 and 3, Engel et al. (51) plotted a regression line that, when extrapolated, indicated a mean endogenous zinc loss of 0.874 mg/day and a minimum requirement of 2.75 mg of zinc/day for equilibrium. The regression calculation also indicated that the children retained 31.8% of the dietary zinc. Assuming a dermal loss of 0.874 mg/day and an allowance for growth of 0.25 mg/day, Engel et al. (51) calculated a daily dietary zinc requirement of 6.2 mg for the preadolescent child.

In a continuation of these studies Price et al. (234) reported data obtained with another group of 15 girls, 7 to 9 years old. In this study, both protein and calcium levels were adjusted in diets composed of foods representative of those eaten by low income groups in the southeastern United States. The daily calcium intake was 0.26 or 0.62 g and the daily protein intake was 25 or 46 g. After a 6-day adjustment period, the subjects were randomly assigned to the four experimental diets for 30 days (five 6-day periods). The variations in calcium intake did not affect zinc retention. With the low protein diets, the mean zinc intakes were 4.83 and 4.53 mg/day, and the mean retentions were 0.54 and 0.81 mg/day. With the high protein diets, the mean zinc intakes were 6.93 and 6.88 mg/day, and the mean retentions were 1.99 and 1.79

mg/day. Price et al. (234) pointed out that the low protein diets provided less zinc than the approximate 6 mg/day recommended by Engel et al. (51) for preadolescent girls. Assuming a sweat loss of 0.5 mg zinc/day (233), Price et al. (234) suggested that the subjects would be barely in positive zinc balance with the low protein diets.

Much higher levels of zinc intake were reported by Macy (140) who studied six boys and one girl, 8 to 12 years old. In experimental periods of about 55 consecutive days, zinc intakes ranged from 13.85 to 18.35 mg/day. The mean intake was 15.92 mg of zinc/day and the mean retention was 4.92 mg/day. Macy (140) concluded that, "on the basis of body weight, the children's intakes average 500 ± 65 micrograms, and their retentions 154 ± 88 micrograms per kilogram per day, indicating a relatively high zinc requirement for children and contradicting classification of zinc as a trace element."

Intakes to provide similar retentions were recommended for preschool children by Scoular (265). She studied zinc intake and output of three boys, 3 to 6 years old, in 12 successive 5-day periods. The zinc intakes varied from 3.80 to 5.87 mg/day (0.218 to 0.307 mg/kg body weight). Zinc retention varied from −2.70 mg to 3.39 mg/day (from −0.159 to 0.171 mg/kg). Two of the boys had highest retentions (0.171 and 0.123 mg/kg) with their highest intakes (0.300 and 0.307 mg/kg). Therefore, Scoular (265) concluded that, "an ingestion of not less than 0.300 to 0.307 mg of zinc per kilogram of body weight is necessary for the preschool age child."

The one report available on zinc balance in healthy infants suggests that neonates behave differently from older children (32). Cavell and Widdowson (32) determined the zinc content of the meconium excreted by six newborn infants during the first 24 hours of life. They found the mean zinc excretion to be 0.66 mg/kg body weight. Next, they measured zinc intake and output of 10 full-term neonates nourished only by breast milk during days 6, 7, and 8 of life. Analysis of the breast milk from the mothers of the babies indicated that the zinc content varied considerably from woman to woman (from 0.142 to 0.677

mg/100 ml). The mean zinc content of the milk was 0.408 mg/100 ml. The infants' daily zinc intake also varied widely from child to child (0.20 to 0.89 mg/kg) with a mean daily intake of 0.67 mg/kg. All but one baby were in negative balance and all but two excreted more zinc in the feces than they ingested in the milk. The balances ranged from −0.85 to 0.08 mg/kg body weight (mean = −0.23 mg/kg). Cavell and Widdowson (32) calculated that the babies were losing more than 1% of the body's total zinc each day. They pointed out that these large losses could not go on indefinitely without serious depletion. It is not known how long they continue and how extensive the losses are.

CONCLUSIONS

The concept of possible or probable zinc deficiency in man is relatively new, and the deficiency syndrome, as yet, is not clearly defined. Many of the manifestations of inadequate zinc intake observed in animals and poultry, such as reduced bone growth, skeletal abnormalities, and retarded sexual development (304) may be more difficult to detect in human subjects because of their slower growth pattern. The evidence obtained in Egypt and Iran showing that more rapid growth and sexual development could be induced in dwarfs by feeding a well-balanced diet plus zinc than by feeding a well-balanced diet alone (80, 84, 257) suggests, however, that man's qualitative zinc needs are similar to those of other species.

At present we have few data on the quantitative zinc needs of human subjects at any age level. Most of the few studies with healthy human subjects were conducted with young adults and school children. No reports were found of studies designed to determine zinc requirements of healthy adolescents, pregnant and lactating women, or elderly people.

The data that are available were obtained by the balance method. The studies differed from each other in experimental design and analytical technique. As might be expected, the results also lacked agreement. In only two of these studies (51, 234) were allowances made for skin losses.

The balance study per se tells us whether the subject was ingesting enough zinc to cover his measured losses. It does not tell us what was happening to the zinc in the body, from where zinc was being withdrawn in negative balances, and where it was being stored or used in positive balances. Nor does it tell us whether zinc equilibrium is the optimum condition or whether positive zinc balance might be beneficial or potentially toxic. In growing children, we have no information on the amount of zinc needed for growth and development. This information is especially important during puberty if, as the evidence indicates, a deficiency of zinc may delay sexual development.

Controlled studies, with graduated levels of zinc intake, in which various parameters of zinc metabolism are measured in addition to zinc output, might yield useful information for estimating requirements. Among the parameters that might be studied are, zinc concentrations in blood plasma, red blood cells, hair and bone, hormone and enzyme activities, and urinary sulfate excretion after a load dose of cystine. Parallel studies carried out with normal subjects and with patients with diagnosed nutritional dwarfism might be fruitful.

More information is needed on zinc absorption, excretion, and enteroenteric circulation in man. Such information is difficult to obtain without the use of tracers. There are, at present, a number of stable zinc isotopes available commercially and the analytical methods necessary for their use are becoming available also. With such stable isotopes as ^{67}Zn, ^{68}Zn, and ^{70}Zn, much information, currently lacking, on zinc turnover, zinc deposition in bones and hair, the roles of zinc in wound healing, in endocrine function, and in enzyme activity could be obtained safely during different periods of growth. The interaction of zinc with other nutrients such as protein, calcium, and copper could be studied more effectively also.

The study of Hambidge et al. (87) suggests that marginal zinc deficiency may be more widely spread in terms of geographic area and economic status than has been believed formerly. Whether this is due to food consumption practices or to food composition as influenced by modern agricultural practices and food processing techniques is not known.

Low plasma zinc concentrations have been observed under various temporary stress conditions (85, 134). In certain chronic diseases, also, low blood zinc levels are common. The significance of these low concentrations is not clear. They may be transient phenomena due to the redistribution of zinc in the various body compartments. On the other hand, they may be the result of inadequate dietary intake or of decreased absorption or increased excretion associated with the stress condition. If the latter is the cause, will increased zinc intake correct the apparent deficiency? Although the literature suggesting that zinc is beneficial in a variety of clinical disorders is growing, the conclusions are often based on inadequately controlled studies. More observations under carefully defined conditions are needed.

In summary, much more information on indices of marginal zinc deficiency and on factors affecting availability and utilization of dietary zinc is needed in order to make sound recommendations on the nutritional requirements and dietary allowances for different population groups.

ACKNOWLEDGMENTS

The authors want to thank Dr. Herta Spencer of the Veterans Administration Hospital, Hines, Illinois, Dr. E. J. Underwood of the University of Western Australia, and Dr. John G. Reinhold of the University of Pennsylvania for their thoughtful advice and criticism.

LITERATURE CITED

1. Adler, I. & Rose, H. J., Jr. (1965) X-ray emission spectrography. In: Trace Analysis: Physical Methods (Morrison, G. H., ed.), pp 271–324, Interscience Publishers, New York.
2. Anonymous (1967) Zinc deficiency and congenital malformations in the rat. Nutr. Rev. 25, 157–159.
3. Apgar, J. (1968) Effect of zinc deficiency on parturition in the rat. Amer. J. Physiol. 215, 160–163.
4. Auerbach, S. (1965) Zinc content of plasma, blood, and erythrocytes in normal subjects and in patients with Hodgkin's disease and various hematologic disorders. J. Lab. Clin. Med. 65, 628–637.

5. Barcia, P. J. (1970) Lack of acceleration of healing with zinc sulfate. Ann. Surg. *172,* 1048–1050.

6. Barney, G. H., Orgebin-Crist, M. C. & Macapinlac, M. P. (1968) Genesis of esophageal parakeratosis and histologic changes in the testes of the zinc-deficient rat and their reversal by zinc repletion. J. Nutr. *95,* 526–534.

7. Beamish, F. E. & Westland, A. D. (1958) Inorganic gravimetric and volumetric analysis. Anal. Chem. *30,* 805–822.

8. Becker, W. M. & Hoekstra, W. G. (1966) Effect of vitamin D on ^{65}Zn absorption, distribution and turnover in rats. J. Nutr. *90,* 301–309.

9. Becker, W. M. & Hoekstra, W. G. (1971) The intestinal absorption of zinc. In: Intestinal Absorption of Metal Ions, Trace Elements and Radionuclides (Skoryna, S. C. & Waldron-Edward, D., eds.), pp 229–256, Pergamon Press, New York.

10. Bellis, D. B. & Philp, J. McL. (1957) Effect of zinc, calcium and phosphorus on the skin and growth of pigs. J. Sci. Food Agr. *8* (Suppl.) s119–s127.

11. Berfenstam, R. (1952) Studies on blood zinc. A clinical and experimental investigation into the zinc content of plasma and blood corpuscles with special reference to infancy. Acta Paediat. *41,* (Suppl. 87) 3–97.

12. Bertrand, D. & de Wolf, A. (1959) Premières recherches sur le rôle de l'oligoélément zinc chez l'*Aspergillus niger.* Bull. Soc. Chim. Biol. *41,* 545–554.

13. Bertrand, D. & de Wolf, A. (1960) Sur la nécessité du zinc, comme oligoélément, pour la synthèse de la tyrosine par l'*Aspergillus niger.* C. R. Acad. Sci. *250,* 2951–2952.

14. Bertrand, D. & de Wolf, A. (1961) Nécessité de l'oligoélément zinc pour la synthèse des acides nucléiques chez l'*Aspergillus niger.* C. R. Acad. Sci. *252,* 2613–2615.

15. Bertrand, D. & de Wolf, A. (1961) Sur la nécessité du zinc, comme oligoélément, pour la synthése de la phénylalanine par l'*Aspergillus niger* et son remplacement partiel possible par le cadmium. C. R. Acad. Sci. *252,* 799–801.

16. Bertrand, G. & Javillier, M. (1911) Influence du zinc et du manganèse sur la composition minérale de l'*Aspergillus niger.* C. R. Acad. Sci. *152,* 1337–1340.

17. Bessey, O. A. & Wolbach, S. B. (1939) Vascularization of the cornea of the rat in riboflavin deficiency with a note on corneal vascularization in vitamin A deficiency. J. Exp. Med. *69,* 1–12.

18. Birckner, V. (1919) The zinc content of some food products. J. Biol. Chem. *38,* 191–203.

19. Blamberg, D. L., Blackwood, U. B., Supplee, W. C. & Combs, G. F. (1960) Effect of zinc deficiency in hens on hatchability and embryonic development. Proc. Soc. Exp. Biol. Med. *104,* 217–220.

20. Boquist, L. & Lernmark, A. (1969) Effects on the endocrine pancreas in Chinese hamsters fed zinc deficient diets. Acta Pathol. Microbiol. Scand. *76,* 215–228.

21. Bowen, H. J. M. (1966) Trace Elements in Biochemistry. pp 209–210, Academic Press, New York.

22. Boyett, J. D. & Sullivan, J. F. (1970) Distribution of protein-bound zinc in normal and cirrhotic serum. Metabolism *19,* 148–157.

23. Brewer, R. D., Jr., Mihaldzic, N. & Dietz, A. (1967) The effect of oral zinc sulfate on the healing of decubitus ulcers in spinal cord injured patients. Proc. 16th Annual Clin. Spinal Cord Injury Conf. *17,* 70–72. Veterans Administration Hospital, Long Beach, Calif.

24. Brown, M. A., Thom, J. V., Orth, G. L., Cova, P. & Juarez, J. (1964) Food poisoning involving zinc contamination. Arch. Environ. Health *8,* 657–660.

25. Butt, E. M., Nusbaum, R. E., Gilmour, T. C. & DiDio, S. L. (1954) Use of emission spectrograph for study of inorganic elements in human tissues. Amer. J. Clin. Pathol. *24,* 385–394.

26. Butt, E. M., Nusbaum, R. E., Gilmour, T. C., DiDio, S. L. & Sr. Mariano (1964) Trace metal levels in human serum and blood. Arch. Environ. Health *8,* 52–57.

27. Caggiano, V., Schnitzler, R., Strauss, W., Baker, R. K., Carter, A. C., Josephson, A. S. & Wallach, S. (1969) Zinc deficiency in a patient with retarded growth, hypogonadism, hypogammaglobulinemia and chronic infection. Amer. J. Med. Sci. *257,* 305–319.

28. Caldwell, D. F. & Oberleas, D. (1969) Effects of protein and zinc nutrition on behavior in the rat. Perinatal factors affecting human development. PAHO Scientific Publication no. 185, 2–8.

29. Caldwell, D. F., Oberleas, D., Clancy, J. J. & Prasad, A. S. (1970) Behavioral impairment in adult rats following acute zinc deficiency. Proc. Soc. Exp. Biol. Med. *133,* 1417–1421.

30. Callender, G. R. & Gentzkow, C. J. (1937) Acute poisoning by the zinc and antimony content of limeade prepared in a galvanized iron can. Milit. Surg. *80,* 67–71.

31. Carter, J. P., Grivetti, L. E., Davis, J. T., Nasiff, S., Mansour, A., Mousa, W. A., Atta, A., Patwardhan, V. N., Moneim, M. A., Abdou, I. A. & Darby, W. J. (1969) Growth and sexual development of adolescent Egyptian village boys. Effects of zinc, iron, and placebo supplementation. Amer. J. Clin. Nutr. *22,* 59–78.

32. Cavell, P. A. & Widdowson, E. M. (1964) Intakes and excretions of iron, copper, and zinc in the neonatal period. Arch. Dis. Child. *39,* 496–501.

33. Chang, I. H., Harrill, I. & Gifford, E. D. (1969) Influence of zinc and vitamin D on bone constituents of the rat. Metabolism *18,* 625–629.

34. Coble, Y. D., Jr., Bardin, C. W., Ross, G. T. & Darby, W. T. (1971) Studies on endocrine function in boys with retarded growth, delayed sexual maturation, and zinc de-

ficiency. J. Clin. Endocrinol. Metab. *32*, 361–367.

35. Conrad, J. H. & Beeson, W. M. (1957) Effect of calcium level and trace minerals on the response of young pigs to unidentified growth factors. J. Anim. Sci. *16*, 589–599.

36. Constam, G. R., Leemann, W., Almasy, F. & Constam, A. G. (1964) Weitere Beobachtungen über den Zinkstoffwechsel bei Diabetes mellitus. Schweiz. Med. Wochenschr. *94*, 1104–1109.

37. Cox, D. H. & Harris, D. L. (1960) Effect of excess dietary zinc on iron and copper in the rat. J. Nutr. *70*, 514–520.

38. Csata, S., Gallays, F. & Toth, M. (1968) Akute Niereninsuffizienz als Folge einer Zinkchloridvergiftung. Z. Urol. *61*, 327–330.

39. Cuttitta, F., Rose, H. J., Jr., Annell, C. S., Carron, M. K., Christian, R. P., Dwornik, E. J., Greenland, L. P., Helz, A. W. & Ligon, D. T., Jr. (1971) Elemental composition of some Apollo 12 lunar rocks and soils. Proc. Second Lunar Sci. Conf., Geochim. Cosmochim. Acta *2*, 1217–1229.

40. Czerniejewski, C. P., Shank, C. W., Bechtel, W. G. & Bradley, W. B. (1964) The minerals of wheat, flour, and bread. Cereal Chem. *41*, 65–72.

41. Davies, I. J. T., Musa, M. & Dormandy, T. L. (1968) Measurements of plasma zinc. Part I. In health and disease. J. Clin. Pathol. *21*, 359–365.

42. Davies, I. J. T., Musa, M. & Dormandy, T. L. (1968) Measurements of plasma zinc. II. In malignant disease. J. Clin. Pathol. *21*, 363–365.

43. Day, H. G. & Skidmore, B. E. (1947) Some effects of dietary zinc deficiency in the mouse. J. Nutr. *33*, 27–38.

44. Dennes, E., Tupper, R. & Wormall, A. (1961) The zinc content of erythrocytes and leucocytes of blood from normal and leukaemic subjects. Biochem. J. *78*, 578–587.

45. DeWys, W., Pories, W. J., Richter, M. C. & Strain, W. H. (1970) Inhibition of Walker 256 carcinosarcoma growth by dietary zinc deficiency. Proc. Soc. Exp. Biol. Med. *135*, 17–22.

46. Edwards, H. M., Jr. (1959) The availability to chicks of zinc in various compounds and ores. J. Nutr. *69*, 306–308.

47. Eggleton, W. G. E. (1938) The occurrence of zinc in foodstuffs and in the human body. Caduceus *17*, 103–128.

48. Eggleton, W. G. E. (1938) The zinc content of epidermal structures. Chinese J. Physiol. *13*, 399–404.

49. Eggleton, W. G. E. (1940) The zinc and copper contents of the organs and tissues of Chinese subjects. Biochem. J. *34*, 991–997.

50. Eminians, J., Reinhold, J. G., Kfoury, G. A., Amirhakimi, G. H., Sharif, H. & Ziai, M. (1967) Zinc nutrition of children in Fars province of Iran. Amer. J. Clin. Nutr. *20*, 734–742.

51. Engel, R. W., Miller, R. F. & Price, N. O. (1966) Metabolic patterns in preadolescent children: XIII. Zinc balance. In: Zinc Metabolism (Prasad, A. S., ed.), pp. 326–338, Charles C Thomas, Springfield.

52. Fairhall, L. T. & Hoyt, L. H. (1929) The excretion of zinc in health and disease. J. Clin. Invest. *7*, 537–541.

53. Faure, H. (1958) Les cirrhoses nutritionelles au Maroc. Algerie Med. *62*, 737–744.

54. Fell, G. S., Fleck, A., Cuthbertson, D. P., Queen, K., Morrison, C., Bessent, R. G. & Husain, S. L. (1973) Urinary zinc levels as an indication of muscle catabolism. Lancet *1*, 280–282.

55. Foley, B., Johnson, S. A., Hackley, B., Smith, J. C., Jr. & Halsted, J. A. (1968) Zinc content of human platelets. Proc. Soc. Exp. Biol. Med. *128*, 265–269.

56. Follis, R. H., Jr., Day, H. G. & McCollum, E. V. (1941) Histological studies of the tissues of rats fed a diet extremely low in zinc. J. Nutr. *22*, 223–233.

57. Forbes, R. M. (1960) Nutritional interactions of zinc and calcium. Fed. Proc. *19*, 643–647.

58. Forbes, R. M. (1964) Mineral utilization in the rat. III. Effects of calcium, phosphorus, lactose and source of protein in zinc-deficient and in zinc-adequate diets. J. Nutr. *83*, 225–233.

59. Forbes, R. M. (1967) Studies of zinc metabolism. In: Newer Methods of Nutritional Biochemistry, Vol. 3 (Albanese, A. A., ed.), pp 339–364, Academic Press, New York.

60. Foster, J. W. (1949) Chemical Activities of Fungi. pp 567–570, Academic Press, New York.

61. Fox, M. R. S. (1970) The status of zinc in human nutrition. World Rev. Nutr. Diet. *12*, 208–226.

62. Fox, M. R. S. & Harrison, B. N. (1964) Use of Japanese quail for the study of zinc deficiency. Proc. Soc. Exp. Biol. Med. *116*, 256–259.

63. Fujioka, M. & Lieberman, I. (1964) A Zn^{++} requirement for synthesis of deoxyribonucleic acid by rat liver. J. Biol. Chem. *239*, 1164–1167.

64. Furchner, J. E. & Richmond, C. R. (1962) Effect of dietary zinc on the absorption of orally administered Zn^{65}. Health Phys. *8*, 35–40.

65. Fuwa, K., Pulido, P., McKay, R. & Vallee, B. L. (1964) Determination of zinc in biological materials by atomic absorption spectrophotometry. Anal. Chem. *36*, 2407–2411.

66. Galin, M. A., Nano, H. D. & Hall, T. (1962) Ocular zinc concentration. Invest. Opththalmol. *1*, 142–148.

67. Gofman, J. W., deLalla, O. F., Kovich, E. L., Lowe, O., Martin, W., Piluso, D. L., Tandy, R. K. & Upham, F. (1964) Chemical elements of the blood of man. Arch. Environ. Health *8*, 105–109.

68. Gormican, A. & Catli, E. (1971) Mineral balance in young men fed a fortified milk-base formula. Nutr. Metab. *13*, 364–377.

69. Graham, E. R. & Telle, P. (1967) Zinc retention in rabbits: effect of previous diet. Science 155, 691–692.

70. Grant-Frost, D. R. & Underwood, E. J. (1958) Zinc toxicity in the rat and its interrelation with copper. Austral. J. Exp. Biol. 36, 339–345.

71. Gray, L. F. & Ellis, G. H. (1950) Some interrelationships of copper, molybdenum, zinc and lead in the nutrition of the rat. J. Nutr. 40, 441–452.

72. Greaves, M. W. & Skillen, A. W. (1970) Effects of long-continued ingestion of zinc sulphate in patients with venous leg ulceration. Lancet 2, 889–891.

73. Guggenheim, K., Ilan, J., Fostick, M. & Tal, E. (1963) Prevention of "meat anemia" in mice by copper and calcium. J. Nutr. 79, 245–250.

74. Gunn, S. A., Gould, T. C. & Anderson, W. A. (1961) Zinc protection against cadmium injury to rat testis. Arch. Pathol. 71, 274–281.

75. Gunn, S. A., Gould, T. C. & Anderson, W. A. D. (1963) The selective injurious response of testicular and epididymal blood vessels to cadmium and its prevention by zinc. Amer. J. Pathol. 42, 685–702.

76. Hackley, B. M., Smith, J. C. & Halsted, J. A. (1968) A simplified method for plasma zinc determination by atomic absorption spectrophotometry. Clin. Chem. 14, 1–5.

77. Haeger, K., Lanner, E. & Magnusson, P. O. (1972) Oral zinc sulphate in the treatment of venous leg ulcers. J. Vascular Dis. 1, 62–69.

78. Hallböök, T. & Lanner, E. (1972) Serum-zinc and healing of venous leg ulcers. Lancet 2, 780–782.

79. Halsted, J. A. (1968) Geophagia in man: its nature and nutritional effects. Amer. J. Clin. Nutr. 21, 1384–1393.

80. Halsted, J. A. (1970) Human zinc deficiency. Trans. Amer. Clin. and Climat. Ass. 82, 170–176.

81. Halsted, J. A., Hackley, B., Rudzki, C. & Smith, J. C., Jr. (1968) Plasma zinc concentration in liver diseases. Comparison with normal controls and certain other chronic diseases. Gastroenterology 54, 1098–1105.

82. Halsted, J. A., Hackley, B. M. & Smith, J. C., Jr. (1968) Plasma zinc and copper in pregnancy and after oral contraceptives. Lancet 2, 278.

83. Halsted, J. A. & Prasad, A. S. (1960) Syndrome of iron deficiency anemia, hepatosplenomegaly, hypogonadism, dwarfism and geophagia. Trans. Amer. Clin. Climat. Ass. 72, 130–149.

84. Halsted, J. A., Ronaghy, H. A., Abadi, P., Haghshenass, M., Amirhakemi, G. H., Barakat, R. M. & Reinhold, J. G. (1972) Zinc deficiency in man: The Shiraz experiment. Amer. J. Med. 53, 277–284.

85. Halsted, J. A. & Smith, J. C., Jr. (1970) Plasma-zinc in health and disease. Lancet 1, 322–324.

86. Halsted, J. A., Smith, J. C., Jr., Hackley, B. M. & McBean, L. D. (1969) Plasma zinc and copper levels. Amer. J. Obstet. Gynecol. 105, 645–646.

87. Hambidge, K. M., Hambidge, C., Jacobs, M. & Baum, J. D. (1972) Low levels of zinc in hair, anorexia, poor growth, and hypogeusia in children. Pediat. Res. 6, 868–874.

88. Handbook of Chemistry and Physics, 46th Edition (1965–1966) The Chemical Rubber Co., p B-146, Cleveland.

89. Harding, M. M., Hodgkin, D. C., Kennedy, A. F., O'Connor, A. & Weitzmann, P. D. J. (1966) The crystal structure of insulin. II. An investigation of rhombohedral zinc insulin crystals and a report of other crystalline forms. J. Molec. Biol. 16, 212–226.

90. Heller, V. G. & Burke, A. D. (1927) Toxicity of zinc. J. Biol. Chem. 74, 85–93.

91. Helman, E. Z., Wallick, D. K. & Reingold, I. M. (1971) Vacutainer contamination in trace element studies. Clin. Chem. 17, 61.

92. Helwig, H. L., Hoffer, E. M., Thielen, W. C., Alcocer, A. E., Hotelling, D. R. & Rodgers, W. H. (1966) Modified zinc analysis method and serum and urinary zinc levels in control subjects. Amer. J. Clin. Pathol. 45, 160–165.

93. Henkin, R. I. & Bradley, D. F. (1970) Hypogeusia corrected by Ni++ and Zn++. Life Sci. 9, 701–709.

94. Henkin, R. I., Graziadei, P. P. G. & Bradley, D. F. (1969) The molecular basis of taste and its disorders. Ann. Intern. Med. 71, 791–821.

95. Henkin, R. I., Schechter, P. J., Hoye, R. & Mattern, C. F. T. (1971) Idiopathic hypogeusia with dysgeusia, hyposmia, and dysosmia. A new syndrome. J. Amer. Med. Ass. 217, 434–440.

96. Heth, D. A., Becker, W. M. & Hoekstra, W. G. (1966) Effect of calcium, phosphorus and zinc on zinc-65 absorption and turnover in rats fed semipurified diets. J. Nutr. 88, 331–337.

97. Hibbard, P. L. (1937) A dithizone method for the measurement of small amounts of zinc. Ind. Eng. Chem. 9, 127–131. Cited by: Tribble, H. M. & Scoular, F. I. (1954) Zinc metabolism of young college women on self-selected diets. J. Nutr. 52, 209–216.

98. Hicks, H. G. (1960) The Radiochemistry of Zinc. National Academy of Sciences, NRC Publ. no. N3015—National Research Council, Washington, D. C.

99. Hill, C. H., Matrone, G., Payne, W. L. & Barber, C. W. (1963) In vivo interactions of cadmium with copper, zinc and iron. J. Nutr. 80, 227–235.

100. Hodgson, J. F., Allaway, W. H. & Lackman, R. B. (1971) Regional plant chemistry as a reflection of environment. In: Environmental Geochemistry in Health and Disease. (Cannon, H. L. & Hopps, H. C., eds.), pp 57–72, The Geological Society of America Memoir.

101. Hoefer, J. A., Miller, E. R., Ullrey, D. E., Ritche, H. D. & Luecke, R. W. (1960) In-

terrelationships between calcium, zinc, iron and copper in swine feeding. J. Anim. Sci. *19*, 249–259.

102. Hoekstra, W. G. (1964) Recent observations on mineral interrelationships. Fed. Proc. *23*, 1968–1076.

103. Hove, E., Elvehjem, C. A. & Hart, E. B. (1937) The physiology of zinc in the nutrition of the rat. Amer. J. Physiol. *119*, 768–775.

104. Hsu, J. M. & Anthony, W. L. (1970) Zinc deficiency and urinary excretion of taurine-³⁵S and inorganic sulfate-³⁵S following cystine-³⁵S injection in rats. J. Nutr. *100*, 1189–1196.

105. Hsu, J. M. & Anthony, W. L. (1971) Impairment of cystine-³⁵S incorporation into skin protein by zinc-deficient rats. J. Nutr. *101*, 445–452.

106. Hsu, J. M., Anthony, W. L. & Buchanan, P. J. (1969) Zinc deficiency and incorporation of ¹⁴C-labeled methionine into tissue proteins in rats. J. Nutr. *99*, 425–432.

107. Hsu, J. M., Anthony, W. L. & Buchanan, P. J. (1970) Zinc deficiency and the metabolism of labelled cystine in rats. In: The Proceedings of the First International Symposium on Trace Element Metabolism in Animals (Mills, C. F., ed.), pp 151–158, E. and S. Livingstone, Edinburgh.

108. Hurley, L. S. (1967) Studies on nutritional factors in mammalian development. J. Nutr. *91*, (Suppl. 1), 27–38.

109. Hurley, L. S. (1968) Approaches to the study of nutrition in mammalian development. Fed. Proc. 27, 193–198.

110. Hurley, L. S. (1969) Zinc deficiency in the developing rat. Amer. J. Clin. Nutr. 22, 1332–1339.

111. Hurley, L. S. & Swenerton, H. (1966) Congenital malformations resulting from zinc deficiency in rats. Proc. Soc. Exp. Biol. Med. *123*, 692–696.

112. Hurley, L. S. & Swenerton, H. (1971) Lack of mobilization of bone and liver zinc under teratogenic conditions of zinc deficiency in rats. J. Nutr. *101*, 597–603.

113. Husain, S. L. (1969) Oral zinc sulphate in leg ulcers. Lancet *1*, 1069–1071.

114. Johnson, N. C. (1961) Study of copper and zinc metabolism during pregnancy. Proc. Soc. Exp. Biol. Med. *108*, 518–519.

115. Kahn, A. M., Helwig, H. L., Redecker, A. G. & Reynolds, T. B. (1965) Urine and serum zinc abnormalities in disease of the liver. Amer. J. Clin. Pathol. *44*, 426–435.

116. Keilin, D. & Mann, T. (1939) Carbonic anhydrase. Nature *144*, 442–443.

117. Keilin, D. & Mann, T. (1940) Carbonic anhydrase. Purification and nature of the enzyme. Biochem. J. *34*, 1163–1176.

118. Kienholz, E. W., Sunde, M. L. & Hoekstra, W. G. (1964) Influence of dietary zinc calcium and vitamin D for hens on zinc content of tissues and eggs and on bone composition. Poultry Sci. *43*, 667–675.

119. Kienholz, E. W., Turk, D. E., Sunde, M. L. & Hoekstra, W. G. (1961) Effects of zinc deficiency in the diets of hens. J. Nutr. *75*, 211–221.

120. Kinnamon, K. E. (1966) The role of iron in the copper–zinc interrelationship in the rat. J. Nutr. *90*, 315–322.

121. Klevay, L. M. (1970) Hair as a biopsy material: I. Assessment of zinc nutriture. Amer. J. Clin. Nutr. *23*, 284–289.

122. Koch, H. J., Jr., Smith, E. R., Shimp, N. F. & Connor, J. (1956) Analysis of trace elements in human tissues. I. Normal tissues. Cancer *9*, 499–511.

123. Kopp, J. F. (1970) The occurrence of trace elements in water. In: Trace Substances in Environmental Health III. Proceedings of University of Missouri's 3rd Annual Conference on Trace Substances in Environmental Health (Hemphill, D. D., ed.), pp 59–73, University of Missouri, Columbia.

124. Kratzer, F. H., Allred, J. B., Davis, P. N., Marshall, B. J. & Vohra, P. (1959) The effect of autoclaving soybean protein and the addition of ethylenediaminetetracetic acid on the biological availability of dietary zinc for turkey poults. J. Nutr. *68*, 313–322.

125. Kurz, D., Roach, J. & Eyring, E. J. (1972) Direct determination of serum zinc and copper by atomic absorption spectrophotometry. Biochem. Med. *6*, 274–281.

126. Lavy, U. I. (1972) The effect of oral supplementation of zinc sulfate on primary wound healing in rats. Brit. J. Surg. *59*, 194–196.

127. Lease, J. G. (1966) The effect of autoclaving sesame meal on its phytic acid content and on the availability of its zinc to the chick. Poultry Sci. *45*, 237–241.

128. LeCour, H., Jr. (1962) Síndrome de anemia hipocrómica, hepato-esplenomegalia, hipodenvolvimento e geofagia. J. Med. (Portugal) *49*, 389–392.

129. Lemann, I. I. (1910) A study of the type of infantilism in hookworm disease. Arch. Intern. Med. *6*, 139–146.

130. Lewis, P. K., Jr., Hoekstra, W. G. & Grummer, R. H. (1957) Restricted calcium feeding versus zinc supplementation for the control of parakeratosis in swine. J. Anim. Sci. *16*, 578–588.

131. Lewis, P. K., Jr., Hoekstra, W. G., Grummer, R. H. & Phillips, P. H. (1956) The effect of certain nutritional factors including calcium, phosphorus and zinc on parakeratosis in swine. J. Anim. Sci. *15*, 741–751.

132. Lieberman, I. & Ove, P. (1962) Deoxyribonucleic acid synthesis and its inhibition in mammalian cells cultured from the animal. J. Biol. Chem. *237*, 1634–1642.

133. Likuski, H. J. A. & Forbes, R. M. (1964) Effect of phytic acid on the availability of zinc in amino acid and casein diets fed to chicks. J. Nutr. *84*, 145–148.

134. Lindeman, R. D., Bottomley, R. G., Cornelison, R. L., Jr. & Jacobs, L. A. (1972) Influence of acute tissue injury on zinc metabolism in man. J. Lab. Clin. Med. *79*, 452–460.

135. Luecke, R. W., Hoefer, J. A., Brammell, W. S. & Schmidt, D. A. (1957) Calcium and zinc in parakeratosis of swine. J. Anim. Sci. 16, 3–11.
136. Luecke, R. W., Hoefer, J. A., Brammell, W. S. & Thorp, F., Jr. (1956) Mineral interrelationships in parakeratosis of swine. J. Anim. Sci. 15, 347–351.
137. Lutz, R. E. (1926) The 'normal occurrence of zinc in biologic materials: a review of the literature, and a study of the normal distribution of zinc in the rat, cat, and man. J. Indust. Hyg. 8, 177–207.
138. Macapinlac, M. P., Barney, G. H., Pearson, W. N. & Darby, W. J. (1967) Production of zinc deficiency in the squirrel monkey (Saimiri sciureus), J. Nutr. 93, 499–510.
139. Macapinlac, M. P., Pearson, W. N. & Darby, W. J. (1966) Some characteristics of zinc deficiency in the albino rat. In: Zinc Metabolism (Prasad, A. S., ed.), pp 142–168, Charles C Thomas, Springfield.
140. Macy, I. G. (1942) Nutrition and Chemical Growth in Childhood, Vol. 1. Evaluation, pp198–202, Charles C Thomas, Springfield.
141. Maddaiah, V. T., Kurnick, A. A. & Reid, B. L. (1964) Phytic acid studies. Proc. Soc. Exp. Biol. Med. 115, 391–393.
142. Magee, A. C. & Matrone, G. (1960) Studies on growth, copper metabolism and iron metabolism of rats fed high levels of zinc. J. Nutr. 72, 233–242.
143. Mahanand, D. & Houck, J. C. (1968) Fluorometric determination of zinc in biologic fluids. Clin. Chem. 14, 6–11.
144. Mansouri, K., Halsted, J. A. & Gombos, E. A. (1970) Zinc, copper, magnesium, and calcium, in dialyzed and nondialyzed uremic patients. Arch. Intern. Med. 125, 88–93.
145. Martin, W. G. & Patrick, H. (1961) Radionuclide mineral studies. 3. The effect of breed and dietary zinc, calcium, and vitamin D₃ on the retention of zinc-65 in chicks. Poultry Sci. 40, 1004–1009.
146. Mason, K. E. & Young, J. O. (1967) Effects of cadmium upon the excurrent duct system of the rat testis. Anat. Rec. 159, 311–323.
147. Mayer, J. (1964) Zinc deficiency: a cause of growth retardation? Postgrad. Med. 35, 206–209.
148. McBean, L. D., Dove, J. T., Halsted, J. A. & Smith, J. C., Jr. (1972) Zinc concentrations in human tissues. Amer. J. Clin. Nutr. 25, 672–676.
149. McBean, L. D. & Halsted, J. A. (1969) Fasting versus postprandial plasma zinc levels. J. Clin. Pathol. 22, 623.
150. McBean, L. D., Mahloudji, M., Reinhold, J. G. & Halsted, J. A. (1971) Correlation of zinc concentrations in human plasma and hair. Amer. J. Clin. Nutr. 24, 506–509.
151. McBean, L. D., Smith, J. C., Jr. & Halsted, J. A. (1971) Effect of oral contraceptive hormones on zinc metabolism in the rat. Proc. Soc. Exp. Biol. Med. 137, 543–547.
152. McBean, L. D., Smith, J. C., Jr. & Halsted, J. A. (1972) Zinc deficiency in guinea pigs. Proc. Soc. Exp. Biol. Med. 140, 1207–1209.
153. McCance, R. A. & Widdowson, E. M. (1942) The absorption and excretion of zinc. Biochem. J. 36, 692–696.
154. Meltzer, L. E., Rutman, J., George, P., Rutman, R. & Kitchell, J. R. (1962) The urinary excretion pattern of trace metals in diabetes mellitus. Amer. J. Med. Sci. 244, 282–289.
155. The Merck Index, Seventh Edition (1960) p 1118, Merck and Company, Inc., Rahway.
156. Meret, S. & Henkin, R. I. (1971) Simultaneous direct estimation by atomic absorption spectrophotometry of copper and zinc in serum, urine, and cerebrospinal fluid. Clin. Chem. 17, 369–373.
157. Mertz, W. (1970) Some aspects of nutritional trace element research. Fed. Proc. 29, 1482–1488.
158. Mesrobian, A. Z. & Shklar, G. (1968) The effect on gingival wound healing of dietary supplements of zinc sulfate in the Syrian hamster. Periodontics 6, 224–229.
159. Methfessel, A. H. & Spencer, H. (1973) Zinc metabolism in the rat. I. Intestinal absorption of zinc. J. Appl. Physiol. 34, 58–62.
160. Mikac-Dević, D. (1970) Methodology of zinc determinations and the role of zinc in biochemical processes. Adv. Clin. Chem. 13, 271–333.
161. Millar, M. J., Fisher, M. I., Elcoate, P. V. & Mawson, C. A. (1958) The effects of dietary zinc deficiency on the reproductive system of male rats. Can. J. Biochem. Physiol. 36, 557–569.
162. Miller, J. K. & Miller, W. J. (1960) Development of zinc deficiency in Holstein calves fed a purified diet. J. Dairy Sci. 43, 1854–1856.
163. Miller, W. J. (1969) Absorption, tissue distribution, endogenous excretion, and homeostatic control of zinc in ruminants. Amer. J. Clin. Nutr. 22, 1323–1331.
164. Miller, W. J., Blackmon, D. M., Gentry, R. P., Powell, G. W. & Perkins, H. F. (1966) Influence of zinc deficiency on zinc and dry matter content of ruminant tissues and on excretion of zinc. J. Dairy Sci. 49, 1446–1453.
165. Miller, W. J. & Miller, J. K. (1963) Zinc content of certain feeds, associated materials, and water. J. Dairy Sci. 46, 581–583.
166. Miller, W. J., Morton, J. D., Pitts, W. J. & Clifton, C. M. (1965) Effect of zinc deficiency and restricted feeding on wound healing in the bovine. Proc. Soc. Exp. Biol. Med. 118, 427–430.
167. Miller, W. J., Pitts, W. J., Clifton, C. M. & Schmittle, S. C. (1964) Experimentally produced zinc deficiency in the goat. J. Dairy Sci. 47, 556–559.
168. Miller, W. J., Powell, G. W., Pitts, W. J. & Perkins, H. F. (1965) Factors affecting zinc content of bovine hair. J. Dairy Sci. 48, 1091–1095.
169. Mills, C. F., Quarterman, J., Chesters, J. K., Williams, R. B. & Dalgarno, A. C. (1969)

Metabolic role of zinc. Amer. J. Clin. Nutr. 22, 1240–1249.

170. Milunsky, A., Hackley, B. M. & Halsted, J. A. (1970) Plasma, erythrocyte and leucocyte zinc levels in Down's syndrome. J. Ment. Defic. Res. 14, 99–105.

171. Minnich, V., Okçuoğlu, A., Tarcon, Y., Arcasoy, A., Cin, S., Yörükoğlu, O., Renda, F. & Demirağ, B. (1968) Pica in Turkey. II. Effect of clay upon iron absorption. Amer. J. Clin. Nutr. 21, 78–86.

172. Mitchell, R. L. (1964) Trace elements in soils. In: Chemistry of the Soil, Ed. 2 (Bear, F. E., ed.), pp 253–285, Reinhold Publishing Corp., New York.

173. Mitteldorf, A. J. (1965) Emission spectrochemical methods. In: Trace Analysis: Physical Methods (Morrison, G. H., ed.), pp 193–244, Interscience Publishers, New York.

174. Moore, T. (1962) Copper deficiency in rats fed upon meat. Brit. Med. J. 1, 689–691.

175. Moore, T. (1964) Meat diets for rats. Proceedings 6th International Congress on Nutrition, pp 526–527, Livingstone, Edinburgh.

176. Morgan, J. M. (1970) Cadmium and zinc abnormalities in bronchogenic carcinoma. Cancer 25, 1394–1398.

177. Morris, E. R. & O'Dell, B. L. (1963) Relationship of excess calcium and phosphorus to magnesium requirement and toxicity in guinea pigs. J. Nutr. 81, 175–181.

178. Murphy, E. W., Page, L. & Watt, B. K. (1971) Trace minerals in type A school lunches. J. Amer. Diet. Ass. 58, 115–122.

179. Murphy, J. V. (1970) Intoxication following ingestion of elemental zinc. J. Amer. Med. Ass. 212, 2119–2120.

180. Murthy, G. K. & Rhea, U. S. (1971) Cadmium, copper, iron, lead, manganese, and zinc in evaporated milk, infant products, and human milk. J. Dairy Sci. 54, 1001–1005.

181. Myers, M. B. & Cherry, G. (1971) Pathophysiology and treatment of stasis ulcers of the leg. Amer. Surg 37, 167–174.

182. Netsky, M. G., Harrison, W. W. Brown, M & Benson, C. (1969) Tissue zinc and human disease. Relation of zinc content of kidney, liver and lung to atherosclerosis and hypertension. Amer. J. Clin. Pathol. 51, 358–365.

183. Newland, H. W., Ullrey, D. E., Hoefer, J. A. & Luecke, R. W. (1958) The relationship of dietary calcium to zinc metabolism in pigs. J. Anim. Sci. 17, 886–892.

184. Nishimura, H. (1953) Zinc deficiency in suckling mice deprived of colostrum. J. Nutr. 49, 79–97.

185. Oberleas, D. (1973) Phytates. In: Toxicants Occurring Naturally in Foods (Strong, F. M., ed.), chapter 17, pp 363–371, National Academy of Sciences, Washington, D. C.

186. Oberleas, D., Muhrer, M. E. & O'Dell, B. L. (1962) Effects of phytic acid on zinc availability and parakeratosis in swine. J. Anim. Sci. 21, 57–61.

187. Oberleas, D., Muhrer, M. E. & O'Dell, B. L. (1966) Dietary metal-complexing agents and zinc availability in the rat. J. Nutr. 90, 56–62.

188. Oberleas, D., Muhrer, M. E. & O'Dell, B. L. (1966) The availability of zinc from foodstuffs. In: Zinc Metabolism (Prasad, A. S., ed.), pp 225–238, Charles C Thomas, Springfield.

189. Oberleas, D. & Prasad, A. S. (1969) Adequacy of trace minerals in bovine milk for human consumption. Amer. J. Clin. Nutr. 22, 196–199.

190. Oberleas, D. & Prasad, A. S. (1969) Growth as affected by zinc and protein nutrition. Amer. J. Clin. Nutr. 22, 1304–1314.

191. Oberleas, D., Seymour, J. K., Lenaghan, R., Hovanesian, J., Wilson, R. F. & Prasad, A. S. (1971) Effect of zinc deficiency on wound-healing in rats. Amer. J. Surg. 121, 566–568.

192. O'Dell, B. L. (1969) Effect of dietary components upon zinc availability. A review with original data. Amer. J. Clin. Nutr. 22, 1315–1322.

193. O'Dell, B. L. & Savage, J. E. (1957) Potassium, zinc and distillers dried solubles as supplements to a purified diet. Poultry Sci. 36, 459–460.

194. O'Dell, B. L. & Savage, J. E. (1960) Effect of phytic acid on zinc availability. Proc. Soc. Exp. Biol. Med. 103, 304–306.

195. Okçuoğlu, A., Arcasoy, A., Minnich, V., Tarcon, Y., Cin, S., Yörükoğlu, O., Demirag, B. & Renda, F. (1966) Pica in Turkey. 1. The incidence and association with anemia. Amer. J. Clin. Nutr. 19, 125–131.

196. Olehy, D. A., Schmitt, R. A. & Bethard, W. F. (1966) Neutron activation analysis of magnesium, calcium, strontium, barium, manganese, cobalt, copper, zinc, sodium, and potassium in human erythrocytes and plasma. J. Nucl. Med. 7, 917–927.

197. Osis, D., Kramer, L., Wiatrowski, E. & Spencer, H. (1972) Dietary zinc intake in man. Amer. J. Clin. Nutr. 25, 582–588.

198. Osis, D., Royston, K., Samachson, J. & Spencer, H. (1969) Atomic-absorption spectrophotometry in mineral and trace-element studies in man. Develop. Appl. Spectrosc. 7A, 227–235.

199. Osol, A., Farrar, G. E., Jr. & Pratt, R. (1955) Dispensatory of the U. S., 25th Ed. pp 1520–1521, J. P. Lippincott, Philadelphia.

200. Ott, E. A., Smith, W. H., Stob, M. & Beeson, W. M. (1964) Zinc deficiency syndrome in the young lamb. J. Nutr. 82, 41–50.

201. Papp, J. P. (1968) Metal fume fever. Postgrad. Med. 43, 160–163.

202. Parisi, A. F. & Vallee, B. L. (1969) Zinc metalloenzymes: characteristics and significance in biology and medicine. Amer. J. Clin. Nutr. 22, 1222–1239.

203. Parisi, A. F. & Vallee, B. L. (1970) Isolation of a zinc α_2-macroglobulin from human serum. Biochemistry 9, 2421–2426.

204. Parízek, J. (1957) The destructive effect

of cadmium ion on testicular tissue and its prevention by zinc. J. Endocrinol. *15*, 56–63.

205. Parker, M. M., Humoller, F. L. & Mahler, D. J. (1967) Determination of copper and zinc in biological material. Clin. Chem. *13*, 40–48.

206. Patek, A. J., Jr. & Haig, C. (1939) The occurrence of abnormal dark adaptation and its relation to vitamin A metabolism in patients with cirrhosis of the liver. J. Clin. Invest. *18*, 609–616.

207. Pearson, W. N., Schwink, T. & Reich, M. (1966) In vitro studies of zinc absorption in the rat. In: Zinc Metabolism (Prasad, A. S., ed.), pp 239–249, Charles C Thomas, Springfield.

208. Pekarek, R. S. & Beisel, W. R. (1969) Effect of endotoxin on serum zinc concentrations in the rat. Appl. Microbiol. *18*, 482–484.

209. Pekarek, R. S., Beisel, W. R., Bartelloni, P. J. & Bostian, K. A. (1972) Determination of serum zinc concentrations in normal adult subjects by atomic absorption spectrophotometry. Amer. J. Clin. Path. *57*, 506–510.

210. Pekarek, R. S., Burghen, G. A., Bartelloni, P. J., Calia, F. M., Bostian, K. A. & Beisel, W. R. (1970) The effect of live attenuated Venezuelan equine encephalomyelitis virus vaccine on serum iron, zinc and copper concentrations in man. J. Lab. Clin. Med. *76*, 293–303.

211. Perry, H. M., Jr., Tipton, I. H., Schroeder, H. A. & Cook, M. J. (1962) Variability in the metal content of human organs. J. Lab. Clin. Med. *60*, 245–253.

212. Petering, H. G., Yeager, D. W. & Witherup, S. O. (1971) Trace metal content of hair: I. Zinc and copper content of human hair in relation to age and sex. Arch. Environ. Health *23*, 202–207.

213. Peters, H. A. (1960) Chelation therapy in acute, chronic and mixed porphyria. In: Metal Binding In Medicine. Proceedings of a symposium sponsored by Hahnemann Medical College and Hospital, Philadelphia, (Seven, M. J., ed.), pp 190–199, J. B. Lippincott, Philadelphia.

214. Pidduck, H. G., Keenan, J. P. & Price Evans, D. A. (1971) Leucocyte zinc in diabetes mellitus. Diabetes *20*, 206–213.

215. Pidduck, H. G., Wren, P. J. J. & Price Evans, D. A. (1970) Hyperzincuria of diabetes mellitus and possible genetical implications of this observation. Diabetes *19*, 240–247.

216. Pimentel, G. C. (1963) Chemistry, An Experimental Science. W. H. Freeman, San Francisco.

217. Pories, W. J., Henzel, J. H., Rob, C. G. & Strain, W. H. (1967) Acceleration of healing with zinc sulfate. Ann. Surg. *165*, 432–436.

218. Pories, W. J., Henzel, J. H., Rob, C. G. & Strain, W. H. (1967) Acceleration of wound healing in man with zinc sulphate given by mouth. Lancet *1*, 121–124.

219. Pories, W. J. & Strain, W. H. (1966) Zinc and wound healing. In: Zinc Metabolism (Prasad, A. S., ed.), pp 378–394, Charles C Thomas, Springfield.

220. Pories, W. J. & Strain, W. H. (1974) Zinc sulfate therapy in surgical patients. In: Clinical Applications of Zinc Metabolism (Pories, W. J., ed.), chapt. 13 (in press), Charles C Thomas, Springfield.

221. Potier de Courcy, G., Susbielle, H. & Terroine, T. (1970) Étude du zinc dans de l'ariboflavinose tératogène chez le rat. Arch. Sci. Physiol. *24*, 409–417.

222. Prasad, A. S. (1966) Metabolism of zinc and its deficiency in human subjects. In: Zinc Metabolism (Prasad, A. S., ed.), pp 250–303, Charles C Thomas, Springfield.

223. Prasad, A. S. (1966) Zinc Metabolism. Charles C Thomas, Springfield.

224. Prasad, A. S., Halsted, J. A. & Nadimi, M. (1961) Syndrome of iron deficiency anemia, hepatosplenomegaly, hypogonadism, dwarfism, and geophagia. Amer. J. Med. *31*, 532–546.

225. Prasad, A. S., Miale, A., Jr., Farid, Z., Sandstead, H. H. & Schulert, A. R. (1963) Zinc metabolism in patients with the syndrome of iron deficiency anemia, hepatosplenomegaly, dwarfism and hypogonadism. J. Lab. Clin. Med. *61*, 537–549.

226. Prasad, A. S., Miale, A., Jr., Farid, Z., Sandstead, H. H., Schulert, A. R. & Darby, W. J. (1963) Biochemical studies on dwarfism, hypogonadism and anemia. Arch. Intern. Med. *111*, 407–428.

227. Prasad, A. S. & Oberleas, D. (1970) Binding of zinc to amino acids and serum proteins in vitro. J. Lab. Clin. Med. *76*, 416–425.

228. Prasad, A. S. & Oberleas, D. (1970) Zinc: human nutrition and metabolic effects. Ann. Intern. Med. *73*, 631–636.

229. Prasad, A. S., Oberleas, D. & Halsted, J. A. (1965) Determination of zinc in biological fluids by atomic absorption spectrophotometry in normal and cirrhotic subjects. J. Lab. Clin. Med. *66*, 508–516.

230. Prasad, A. S., Oberleas, D. & Halsted, J. A. (1966) Determination of zinc in biological fluids by atomic absorption spectrophotometry. In: Zinc Metabolism (Prasad, A. S., ed.), pp 27–37, Charles C Thomas, Springfield.

231. Prasad, A. S., Oberleas, D., Wolf, P. & Horwitz, J. P. (1967) Studies on zinc deficiency: changes in trace elements and enzyme activities in tissues of zinc deficient rats. J. Clin. Invest. *46*, 549–557.

232. Prasad, A. S., Oberleas, D., Wolf, P., Horwitz, J. P., Miller, E. R. & Luecke, R. W. (1969) Changes in trace elements and enzyme activities in tissues of zinc-deficient pigs. Amer. J. Clin. Nutr. *22*, 628–637.

233. Prasad, A. S., Schulert, A. R., Sandstead, H. H., Miale, A. & Farid, Z. (1963) Zinc, iron, and nitrogen content of sweat in normal and deficient subjects. J. Lab. Clin. Med. *62*, 84–89.

234. Price, N. O., Bunce, G. E. & Engel, R. W. (1970) Copper, manganese, and zinc bal-

ance in preadolescent girls. Amer. J. Clin. Nutr. 23, 258–260.

235. Quarterman, J., Mills, C. F. & Humphries, W. R. (1966) The reduced secretion of, and sensitivity to insulin in zinc-deficient rats. Biochem. Biophys. Res. Commun. 25, 354–358.

236. Raulin, J. (1869) Études cliniques sur la végétation. Ann. Sci. Natur. Botan. Biol. Végétale. 11, 93–299.

237. Reimann, F. (1955) Wachstumsanomalien und Missbildungen bei Eisenmangelzuständen (Asiderosen). In: Fünfter Kongress der europäischen Gesellschaft für Hämatologie, pp 546–550, Freiburg, Germany.

238. Reinhold, J. G. (1971) High phytate content of rural Iranian bread: a possible cause of human zinc deficiency. Amer. J. Clin. Nutr. 24, 1204–1206.

239. Reinhold, J. G. (1972) Phytate concentrations of leavened and unleavened Iranian breads. Ecol. Food Nutr. 1, 187–192.

240. Reinhold, J. G., Hedayati, H., Lahimgarzadeh, A. & Nasr, K. (1973) Zinc, calcium, phosphorus, and nitrogen balances of Iranian villagers following a change from phytate-rich to phytate-poor diets. Ecol. Food Nutr. 2, 1–6.

241. Reinhold, J. G., Kfoury, G. A., Ghalambor, M. A. & Bennett, J. C. (1966) Zinc and copper concentrations in hair of Iranian villagers. Amer. J. Clin. Nutr. 18, 294–300.

242. Reinhold, J. G., Kfoury, G. A. & Arslawian, M. (1968) Relation of zinc and calcium concentrations in hair to zinc nutrition in rats. J. Nutr. 96, 519–524.

243. Reinhold, J. G., Kfoury, G. A. & Thomas, T. A. (1967) Zinc, copper and iron concentrations in hair and other tissues: effects of low zinc and low protein intakes in rats. J. Nutr. 92, 173–182.

244. Reinhold, J. G., Nasr, K., Lahimgarzadeh, A. & Hedayati, H. (1973) Effects of purified phytate and phytate-rich bread upon metabolism of zinc, calcium, phosphorus, and nitrogen in man. Lancet 1, 283–288.

245. Richmond, C. R., Furchner, J. E., Trafton, G. A. & Langham, W. H. (1962) Comparative metabolism of radionuclides in mammals. I. Uptake and retention of orally administered Zn^{65} by four mammalian species. Health Phys. 8, 481–489.

246. Ritchie, H. D., Luecke, R. W., Baltzer, B. V., Miller, E. R., Ullrey, D. E. & Hoefer, J. A. (1963) Copper and zinc interrelationships in the pig. J. Nutr. 79, 117–123.

247. Roberson, R. H. & Schaible, P. J. (1960) The availability to the chick of zinc as the sulfate, oxide or carbamate. Poultry Sci. 39, 835–837.

248. Robertson, B. T. & Burns, M. J. (1963) Zinc metabolism and the zinc-deficiency syndrome in the dog. Amer. J. Vet. Res. 24, 997–1002.

249. Robinson, J. W. (1966) Atomic Absorption Spectroscopy. Marcel Dekker, New York.

250. Roman, W. (1969) Zinc in porphyria. Amer. J. Clin. Nutr. 22, 1290–1303.

251. Ronaghy, H., Fox, M. R. S., Garn, S. M.,

Israel, H., Harp, A., Moe, P. G. & Halsted, J. A. (1969) Controlled zinc supplementation for malnourished school boys: a pilot experiment. Amer. J. Clin. Nutr. 22, 1279–1289.

252. Ronaghy, H. A., Moe, P. G. & Halsted, J. A. (1968) A six-year follow-up of Iranian patients with dwarfism, hypogonadism, and iron-deficiency anemia. Amer. J. Clin. Nutr. 21, 709–714.

253. Rose, H. J., Jr., Cuttitta, F., Annell, C. S., Carron, M. K., Christian, R. P., Dwornik, E. J., Greenland, L. P. & Ligon, D. T., Jr. (1972) Compositional data for twenty-one Fra Mauro lunar materials. Proc. Third Lunar Sci. Conf., Geochim. Cosmochim. Acta 2, 1215–1229.

254. Rose, H. J., Jr., Cuttitta, F., Dwornik, E. J., Carron, M. K., Christian, R. P., Lindsay, J. R., Ligon, D. T., Jr. & Larson, R. R. (1970) Semimicro X-ray fluorescence analysis of lunar samples. Proc. Apollo 11 Lunar Sci. Conf., Geochim. Cosmochim. Acta 2, 1493–1497.

255. Rosner, F. & Gorfien, P. C. (1968) Erythrocyte and plasma zinc and magnesium levels in health and disease. J. Lab. Clin. Med. 72, 213–219.

256. Ross, J. F., Ebaugh, F. G., Jr. & Talbot, T. R., Jr. (1958) Radioisotopic studies of zinc metabolism in human subjects. Trans. Ass. Amer. Physicians 71, 322–336.

257. Sandstead, H. H., Prasad, A. S., Schulert, A. R., Farid, Z., Miale, A., Jr., Bassilly, S. & Darby, W. J. (1967) Human zinc deficiency, endocrine manifestations and response to treatment. Amer. J. Clin. Nutr. 20, 422–442.

258. Sandstead, H. H. & Shepard, G. H. (1968) The effect of zinc deficiency on the tensile strength of healing surgical incisions in the integument of the rat. Proc. Soc. Exp. Biol. Med. 128, 687–689.

259. Sandstead, H. H., Shukry, A. S., Prasad, A. S., Gabr, M. K., El Hifney, A., Mokhtar, N. & Darby, W. J. (1965) Kwashiorkor in Egypt. I. Clinical and biochemical studies, with special reference to plasma zinc and serum lactic dehydrogenase. Amer. J. Clin. Nutr. 17, 15–26.

260. Saraswat, R. C. & Arora, S. P. (1972) Effect of dietary zinc on the vitamin A level and alkaline phosphatase activity in blood sera of lambs. Indian J. Anim. Sci. 42, 358–362.

261. Schechter, P. J., Friedewald, W. T., Bronzert, D. A., Raff, M. S. & Henkin, R. I. (1972) Idiopathic hypogeusia: a description of the syndrome and a single-blind study with zinc sulfate. Int. Rev. Neurobiol. Suppl. 1, 125–140.

262. Schrodt, G. R., Hall, T. & Whitmore, W. F., Jr. (1964) The concentration of zinc in diseased human prostate glands. Cancer 17, 1555–1566.

263. Schroeder, H. A. (1971) Losses of vitamins and trace minerals resulting from processing and preservation of foods. Amer. J. Clin. Nutr. 24, 562–573.

264. Schroeder, H. A., Nason, A. P., Tipton, I. H. & Balassa, J. J. (1967) Essential trace metals in man: zinc. Relation to environmental cadmium. J. Chronic Dis. *20*, 179–210.

265. Scoular, F. I. (1939) A quantitative study, by means of spectrographic analysis, of zinc in nutrition. J. Nutr. *17*, 103–113.

266. Serjeant, G. R., Galloway, R. E. & Gueri, M. C. (1970) Oral zinc sulphate in sickle-cell ulcers. Lancet *2*, 891–892.

267. Sheline, G. E., Chaikoff, I. L., Jones, H. B. & Montgomery, M. L. (1943) Studies on the metabolism of zinc with the aid of its radioactive isotope. I. The excretion of administered zinc in urine and feces. J. Biol. Chem. *147*, 409–414.

268. Shinowara, G. Y. (1961) The nature of the lipoprotein of human platelets and erythrocytes. In: Blood Platelets. Henry Ford Hospital Symposium (Johnson, S. A., Monto, R. W., Rebuck, J. W. & Horn, R. C., Jr., eds.), pp 347–356, Little Brown, Boston.

269. Sinha, S. N., Gabrieli, E. R. (1970) Serum copper and zinc levels in various pathologic conditions. Amer. J. Clin. Pathol. *54*, 570–577.

270. Sivarama Sastry, K. & Sarma, P. S. (1958) Effect of copper on growth and catalase levels of *Corcyra cephalonica* St. in zinc toxicity. Nature *182*, 533–544.

271. Slavin, W. (1968) Atomic Absorption Spectroscopy. Interscience Publishers, New York.

272. Smit, Z. M. (1960) Studies in metabolism of zinc. Part I. Serum zinc levels in outwardly healthy adults, white and Bantu. S. Afr. J. Lab. Clin. Med. *6*, 29–36.

273. Smit, Z. M. & Pretorius, P. J. (1964) Studies in metabolism of zinc. Part 2. Serum zinc levels and urinary zinc excretions in South African Bantu kwashiorkor patients. J. Trop. Pediat. *9*, 105–112.

274. Smith, J. C., Jr. & Halsted, J. A. (1970) Clay ingestion (geophagia) as a source of zinc for rats. J. Nutr. *100*, 973–980.

275. Smith, J. C., Jr., Hansen, H. H., Howard, M. P., McBean, L. D. & Halsted, J. A. (1971) Plasma-zinc concentration in patients with bronchogenic cancer. Lancet *2*, 1323.

276. Smith, J. C., Jr., McDaniel, E. G., Fan, F. F. & Halsted, J. A. (1973) Zinc: a trace element essential in vitamin A metabolism. Science *181*, 954–955.

277. Somers, M. & Underwood, E. J. (1969) Studies of zinc nutrition in sheep. II. The influence of zinc deficiency in ram lambs upon the digestibility of the dry matter and the utilization of the nitrogen and sulphur of the diet. Austral. J. Agric. Res. *20*, 899–903.

278. Sommer, A. L. & Lipman, C. B. (1926) Evidence on the indispensable nature of zinc and boron for higher green plants. Plant Physiol. *1*, 231–249.

279. Spencer, H. & Rosoff, B. (1966) The effect of chelating agents on the removal of zinc-65 in man. Health Physics *12*, 475–480.

280. Spencer, H., Rosoff, B., Feldstein, A., Cohn, S. H. & Gusmano, E. (1965) Metabolism of zinc-65 in man. Radiat. Res. *24*, 432–445.

281. Spencer, H., Rosoff, B., Lewin, I. & Samachson, J. (1966) Studies of zinc-65 metabolism in man. In: Zinc Metabolism (Prasad, A. S., ed.), pp 339–362, Charles C Thomas, Springfield.

282. Spencer, H. & Samachson, J. (1970) Studies of zinc metabolism in man. In: Trace Element Metabolism in Animals (Mills, C. F., ed.), pp 312–320, E. and S. Livingstone, Edinburgh.

283. Spencer, H., Vankinscott, V., Lewin, I. & Samachson, J. (1965) Zinc-65 metabolism during low and high calcium intake in man. J. Nutr. *86*, 169–177.

284. Steele, T. H. (1973) Dissociation of zinc excretion from other cations in man. J. Lab. Clin. Med. *81*, 205–213.

285. Stephan, J. K. & Hsu, J. M. (1973) Effect of zinc deficiency and wounding on DNA synthesis in rat skin. J. Nutr. *103*, 548–552.

286. Stevenson, J. W. & Earle, I. P. (1956) Studies on parakeratosis in swine. J. Anim. Sci. *15*, 1036–1045.

287. Stewart, A. K. & Magee, A. C. (1964) Effect of zinc toxicity on calcium, phosphorus and magnesium metabolism of young rats. J. Nutr. *82*, 287–295.

288. Strain, W. H., Dutton, A. M., Heyer, H. B. & Ramsey, G. H. (1953) Experimental Studies on the Acceleration of Burn and Wound Healing. University of Rochester Reports. Cited by: Pories, W. J. & Strain, W. H. (1966) Zinc and wound healing. In: Zinc Metabolism (Prasad, A. S., ed.), pp 378–394, Charles C Thomas, Springfield.

289. Strain, W. H., Pories, W. J. & Hinshaw, J. R. (1960) Zinc studies in skin repair. Surg. Forum *11*, 291–292.

290. Strain, W. H., Steadman, L. T., Lankau, C. A., Jr., Berliner, W. P. & Pories, W. J. (1966) Analysis of zinc levels in hair for the diagnosis of zinc deficiency in man. J. Lab. Clin. Med. *68*, 244–249.

291. Sullivan, J. F. & Heaney, R. P. (1970) Zinc metabolism in alcoholic liver disease. Amer. J. Clin. Nutr. *23*, 170–177.

292. Sullivan, J. F. & Lankford, H. G. (1965) Zinc metabolism and chronic alcoholism. Amer. J. Clin. Nutr. *17*, 57–63.

293. Surgenor, D. M., Koechlin, B. A. & Strong, L. E. (1949) Chemical, clinical, and immunological studies on the products of human plasma fractionation. XXXVII. The metal-combining globulin of human plasma. J. Clin. Invest. *28*, 73–78.

294. Swenerton, H., Shrader, R. & Hurley, L. S. (1969) Zinc-deficient embryos: reduced thymidine incorporation. Science *166*, 1014–1015.

295. Theuer, R. C. & Hoekstra, W. G. (1966) Oxidation of ^{14}C-labeled carbohydrate, fat and amino acid substrates by zinc-deficient rats. J. Nutr. *89*, 448–454.

296. Thiers, R. E. (1957) Contamination in trace element analysis and its control. Methods Biochem. Anal. *5*, 273–335.

297. Tipton, I. H. & Cook, M. J. (1963) Trace elements in human tissue. Part II. Adult subjects from the United States. Health Physics 9, 103–145.

298. Tipton, I. H., Schroeder, H. A., Perry, H. M., Jr. & Cook, M. J. (1965) Trace elements in human tissue. Part III. Subjects from Africa, the Near and Far East, and Europe. Health Physics 11, 403–451.

299. Tipton, I. H., Stewart, P. L. & Dickson, J. (1969) Patterns of elemental excretion in long term balance studies. Health Physics 16, 455–462.

300. Todd, W. R., Elvehjem, C. A. & Hart, E. B. (1934) Zinc in the nutrition of the rat. Amer. J. Physiol. 107, 146–156.

301. Tribble, H. M. & Scoular, F. I. (1954) Zinc metabolism of young college women on self-selected diets. J. Nutr. 52, 209–216.

302. Tucker, H. F. & Salmon, W. D. (1955) Parakeratosis or zinc deficiency disease in the pig. Proc. Soc. Exp. Biol. Med. 88, 613–616.

303. Underwood, E. J. (1962) Trace Elements in Human and Animal Nutrition. Ed. 2, pp 157–186, Academic Press, New York.

304. Underwood, E. J. (1971) Trace Elements in Human and Animal Nutrition. Ed. 3, pp 208–252, Academic Press, New York.

305. Vallee, B. L. (1959) Biochemistry, physiology and pathology of zinc. Physiol. Rev. 39, 443–490.

306. Vallee, B. L. & Gibson, J. G., 2nd (1948) The zinc content of normal human whole blood, plasma, leucocytes, and erythrocytes. J. Biol. Chem. 176, 445–457.

307. Vallee, B. L., Wacker, W. E. C., Bartholomay, A. F. & Hoch, F. L. (1957) Zinc metabolism in hepatic dysfunction. II. Correlation of metabolic patterns with biochemical findings. New Engl. J. Med. 257, 1055–1065.

308. Vallee, B. L., Wacker, W. E. C., Bartholomay, A. F. & Robin, E. D. (1956) Zinc metabolism in hepatic dysfunction. I. Serum zinc concentrations in Laënnec's cirrhosis and their validation by sequential analysis. New Engl. J. Med. 255, 403–408.

309. Van Reen, R. (1966) Zinc toxicity in man and experimental species. In: Zinc Metabolism (Prasad, A. S., ed.), pp 411–426, Charles C Thomas, Springfield.

310. Viets, F. G., Jr. (1966) Zinc deficiency in the soil–plant system. In: Zinc Metabolism (Prasad, A. S. ed.), pp 90–128, Charles C Thomas, Springfield.

311. Vikbladh, I. (1950) Studies on zinc in blood. I. Scand. J. Clin. Lab. Invest. 2, 143–148.

312. Vikbladh, I. (1951) Studies on zinc in blood. II. Scand. J. Clin. Lab. Invest. 3, (Suppl. 2) 5–73.

313. Vohra, P., Gray, G. A. & Kratzer, F. H. (1965) Phytic acid–metal complexes. Proc. Soc. Exp. Biol. Med. 120, 447–449.

314. Vohra, P. & Kratzer, F. H. (1964) Influence of various chelating agents on the availability of zinc. J. Nutr. 82, 249–256.

315. Wacker, W. E. C. (1962) Nucleic acids and metals. III. Changes in nucleic acid, protein, and metal content as a consequence of zinc deficiency in Euglena gracilis. Biochemistry 1, 859–865.

316. Wacker, W. E. C., Ulmer, D. D. & Vallee, B. L. (1956) Metalloenzymes and myocardial infarction. II. Malic and lactic dehydrogenase activities and zinc concentrations in serum. New Engl. J. Med. 255, 449–456.

317. Wallace, H. D., McCall, J. T., Bass, B. & Combs, G. E. (1960) High level copper for growing-finishing swine. J. Anim. Sci. 19, 1153–1163.

318. Walsh, A. (1955) The application of atomic absorption spectra to chemical analysis. Spectrochim. Acta 7, 108–117.

319. Wannemacher, R. W., Pekarek, R. S., Bartelloni, P. J., Vollmer, R. T. & Beisel, W. R. (1972) Changes in individual plasma amino acids following experimentally induced sand fly fever virus infection. Metabolism 21, 67–76.

320. Wasserman, R. H. (1962) Studies on vitamin D₃ and the intestinal absorption of calcium and other ions in the rachitic chick. J. Nutr. 77, 69–80.

321. Wegener, W. S. & Romano, A. H. (1963) Zinc stimulation of RNA and protein synthesis in Rhizopus nigricans. Science 142, 1669–1670.

322. Weil, L., Seibles, T. S. & Herskovits, T. T. (1965) Photooxidation of bovine insulin sensitized by methylene blue. Arch. Biochem. Biophys. 111, 308–320.

323. White, H. S. & Gynne, T. N. (1971) Utilization of inorganic elements by young women eating iron-fortified foods. J. Amer. Diet. Ass. 59, 27–33.

324. Whiting, F. & Bezeau, L. M. (1958) The calcium, phosphorus, and zinc balance in pigs as influenced by the weight of pig and the level of calcium, zinc and vitamin D in the ration. Can. J. Anim. Sci. 38, 109–117.

325. Widdowson, E. M., McCance, R. A. & Spray, C. M. (1951) The chemical composition of the human body. Clin. Sci. 10, 113–125.

326. Williams, R. B., Mills, C. F., Quarterman, J. & Dalgarno, A. C. (1965) The effect of zinc deficiency on the in vivo incorporation of ³²P into rat-liver nucleotides. Biochem. J. 95, 29P–30P.

327. Winder, F. & Denneny, J. M. (1959) Effect of iron and zinc on nucleic acid and protein synthesis in Mycobacterium smegmatis. Nature 184, 742–743.

328. Wolff, H. P. (1950) Der normale Zinkgehalt in Blut, Serum, und Erythrocyten. Deutsch. Arch. Klin. Med. 197, 263–267.

329. Worker, N. A. & Migicovsky, B. B. (1961) Effect of vitamin D on the utilization of zinc, cadmium and mercury in the chick. J. Nutr. 75, 222–224.

330. Zajic, J. E. (1969) Microbial Biogeochemistry. Microbes and Zinc, pp 142–155, Academic Press, New York.

A CONSPECTUS OF RESEARCH ON

VITAMIN C REQUIREMENTS OF MAN

by

M. ISABEL IRWIN [1]

Nutrition Institute
Agricultural Research Service
United States Department of Agriculture
Beltsville, Maryland 20705

and

BOBBIE K. HUTCHINS [2]

Department of Nutrition
Harvard School of Public Health
Boston, Massachusetts 02115

THE JOURNAL OF NUTRITION

VOLUME 106, NUMBER 6, JUNE 1976

(Pages 821-897)

TABLE OF CONTENTS

INTRODUCTION

An exploration of the literature on vitamin C leads immediately to papers on scurvy, one of man's oldest and most studied deficiency diseases. The history of this disease and the contributions of such men as Cartier, Bachstrom and Lind to its cure or prevention have been related fully (18, 73, 102, 205, 262, 281). The concept of dietary deficiency as a major cause of ill health is usually believed to be a development of the early twentieth century (196). Attempts to estimate tangible cost benefits from improved nutrition (425) are considered to be an even more recent development. In the field of scurvy research, both of these developments were anticipated by about two centuries. In 1734, for instance, Bachstrom (20) declared that the primary cause of scurvy was a lack of fresh vegetables and greens in the diet. In that same century, when Lind's recommended daily ration of lemon juice was adopted in the British Navy, the fighting force of the navy was reported to be doubled without "adding a penny to the naval estimates or a man to the total strength" (102).

The major contribution of the twentieth century in the control of scurvy has been to support these earlier observations and to concentrate, isolate and eventually identify the potent dietary factor responsible for the prevention of scurvy (223, 389, 424). The name "vitamin C" was adopted following Drummond's proposal in 1920 for simplifying "the nomenclature of the so-called accessory food factors" (101). In 1933, the name ascorbic acid was proposed for this vitamin by Szent-Gyorgyi and Haworth (391). In 1953, these studies were recounted with citations of the pertinent literature (222, 390) in a symposium observing the bicentenary of the publication of Lind's "A Treatise of the Scurvy" (257).

Research of the twentieth century has also included investigations of methods for establishing the requirements for ascorbic acid and the factors influencing these requirements. The purpose of this conspectus is to review what has been done, how it has been done and what yet needs to be done in determining the requirements of man for vitamin C. It is not intended to be a critical review although some evaluative comments are inevitable. Although some reference to animal studies was necessary, the literature reviewed has been restricted as much as possible to reports of studies with humans and specifically to reports of studies on vitamin C requirements of human subjects.

STUDIES ON THE VITAMIN C REQUIREMENT FOR MAINTENANCE (APPENDIX TABLE 1)

There is currently, and has been for some years, a difference of opinion on the amount of vitamin C to be recommended for daily ingestion (447). This difference of opinion arises in part from the criteria by which the requirements were estimated and from our lack of knowledge of the metabolic role of vitamin C. Moreover the analytical techniques available for many of the experiments fail to recognize the instability of ascorbic acid to air oxidation or to differentiate between L-ascorbic acid and other related forms of ascorbic acid.

The primary known nutritional role of ascorbic acid is in the prevention and cure of scurvy. Attempts to estimate maintenance requirments for vitamin C have been made in studies of experimental scurvy. Other estimates have been obtained from saturation studies. These are studies of the amount of vitamin C required to saturate whole blood, blood plasma, serum or white cells, body tissues or the "body pools." The saturation of body tissues has been indicated by urinary ascorbic acid excretion. The body pool of ascorbic acid has been estimated from white blood cell content and by use of radioactive isotopes. Other estimates of requirements have been based on balance studies, lingual and skin tests, morbidity studies and health surveys.

[1] Deceased.

[2] Present address, Department of Preventive and Community Medicine, Albany Medical College of Union University, New Scotland Avenue, Albany, New York, 12208.

Experimental scurvy

Among the signs and symptoms of scurvy commonly observed are weakness and fatigue, hyperkeratosis of the hair follicles, perifollicular hemorrhages, petechiae and ecchymoses, and swollen, bleeding gums (162). Additional clinical manifestations observed during the development of experimental scurvy in man include edema, ocular hemorrhages, Sjögren's syndrome, neuropathy, arthralgia, and mental and emotional changes (186, 188).

Reports have been found of five studies in which scurvy was produced experimentally in a total of 34 men and three women (23–25, 34, 85, 86, 186, 188, 241, 326). These studies differed from each other in the procedures used to deplete or saturate the subjects with ascorbic acid and in the length of time required to produce definite signs of scurvy. The results are in agreement, however, indicating that the amount of dietary vitamin C required to prevent or cure scurvy is very small (less than 10 mg/day). They are also in agreement that plasma ascorbic acid levels and urinary ascorbic acid excretion are not good predictors of scurvy. Hyperkeratosis was one of the first signs noted in each study whereas gum changes occurred much later in the development of scurvy.

In the first reported study of experimentally produced scurvy in man, Crandon et al. (86) observed the responses of one 27-year-old man to a diet containing no milk, fruit or vegetables. They found that the first clinical sign of scurvy, hyperkeratosis, occurred after the subject had been eating the vitamin C deficient diet for 132 days. The plasma vitamin C level fell rapidly during the study, reaching zero after 41 days. The white cell-platelet (buffy coat) vitamin C level fell more slowly and reached zero at 121 days, just 11 days before the first clinical sign of scurvy was observed (85).

The subject was saturated following the depletion period by providing daily 1,000 mg doses of ascorbic acid intravenously. Taking into account the total amount lost in the urine (about 1 g) Crandon et al. estimated that from 4 to 6 g ascorbic acid was necessary to saturate the subject. They concluded that, since the first sign of scurvy occurred after 132 days of ascorbic acid

deprivation, the maximal utilization of vitamin C must have been between 30 and 45 mg/day. They suggested, further, that the true requirement possibly lay "somewhat below this figure."

Pijoan and Lozner (326), a few years later, reported a study in which a lower estimate was obtained. Their procedure differed from that of Crandon et al. in that the saturation period preceded the depletion period instead of following it. In a preliminary experiment with one man (325) they had ascertained that no signs of scurvy developed over a 20 month period and that wound healing took place normally when the ascorbic acid intake varied between 12 and 25 mg/day (mean 16 mg/day). In a second study (326), four men and two women, 26 to 64 years old, were first saturated with large doses of ascorbic acid (300 to 400 mg daily for 5 days) and then were given a diet planned to be devoid of vitamin C but adequate in all other known nutrients. Plasma ascorbic acid levels dropped to traces or to zero by the end of 2 months consuming this diet. About 5 to 6 months were required before physical signs of scurvy (petechiae and perifollicular hemorrhages) were observed. Pijoan and Lozner suggested on the basis of these results, that saturation with approximately 2 g ascorbic acid every 4 months would protect from scurvy. They calculated further that about 8,000 mg/year or about 22 mg/day would approximate the minimum protective dose.

Najjar et al. (300) provided corroborating evidence in a study of thiamin requirements with seven young adults, 17 to 21 years old. The subjects ate an experimental diet providing 25 mg crystalline ascorbic acid daily for 18 months. Although chemical studies of ascorbic acid status were not made, clinical evidences of scurvy were sought at regular intervals. No evidence of follicular keratosis was noted nor were there hemorrhages in the skin, the mucous membranes or from the urinary tract.

In the studies of both Crandon et al. (85, 86) and Pijoan and Lozner (326), although scurvy was developed, no attempt was made to determine the minimum intake of vitamin C that would prevent or cure it. This has been essayed in three more recent studies (13, 34, 186, 188, 241).

In the first of these, carried out at the Sorby Research Institute, Sheffield, England (13, 34, 241), 19 men and one woman, 21 to 34 years old, ate a basal diet containing only 1 mg of ascorbic acid but adequate amounts of all other known required nutrients. The subjects were given a supplement of 70 mg of vitamin C daily for about 6 weeks. Then they were divided into three groups. Group 1; 10 subjects received no additional vitamin C. Group 2; four subjects ate the basal diet plus a daily supplement of 10 mg vitamin C for 252 to 424 days; three ate the basal diet plus 10 mg daily for 160 days followed by 71 days with no supplement. Group 3; three subjects ate the basal diet plus 70 mg vitamin C daily. The subjects "lived a normal life without strenuous physical work" (241). During the study, which lasted as long as 424 days for some of the subjects, no physical signs of scurvy were observed in the group receiving the supplement of 70 mg vitamin C daily. Nor were any physical signs of scurvy observed in the group receiving 10 mg of vitamin C/day, even though three of these subjects received no supplement at all for 71 days. In Group 1, the unsupplemented subjects, no definite signs of scurvy were observed for 17 weeks. Then follicular keratosis was recognized and, by 26 weeks, all 10 subjects showed follicular changes on their limbs and backs. These changes were followed by follicular hemorrhages between weeks 26 and 34 and, eventually, by swelling and hemorrhaging of the gums between weeks 30 and 38.

Seven of the subjects who developed scurvy were given supplemental vitamin C (10 mg/day to six subjects and 20 mg/day to one subject). In those receiving 10 mg/day, hemorrhages stopped within a week and all signs of scurvy had disappeared within 10 to 18 weeks.

Blood values followed the same pattern as was observed in earlier studies (85, 86, 326). Plasma vitamin C in the deprived subjects and in those receiving 10 mg ascorbic acid/day declined rapidly, and after 37 days the levels of the subjects in both groups fluctuated below 0.5 mg/100 ml. The white cell-platelet levels fell more slowly. In the totally deprived group, the white cell vitamin C reached its lowest

level about 3 to 6 weeks before clinical signs of scurvy were noted. After day 109, in the group receiving 10 mg ascorbic acid/day, the white cell level remained about 1 mg/100 g higher than the level of the totally deprived group. Plasma and white cell-platelet levels of vitamin C did not fall in the group receiving 70 mg ascorbic acid/day.

These observations suggested to the investigators (13) that the minimum requirement of vitamin C to prevent the appearance of scurvy was somewhat less than 10 mg/day. They questioned, however, whether this minimal dose was optimal on the basis of small differences between the groups receiving 10 and those receiving 70 mg ascorbic acid when subjected to a modified "agility test" designed to measure physical fatigue. They suggested that it would not "seem too generous to treble the minimal protective dose of 10 mg and thereby confirm the figure of 30 mg of vitamin C daily recommended by the League of Nations Technical Commission on Nutrition" (248).

Data obtained in the two most recent studies of scurvy (23–25, 186, 188) support the conclusion that scurvy can be prevented with intakes of less than 10 mg vitamin C/day. In one study (186), four men, 33 to 44 years old, consumed a liquid formula diet containing no vitamin C for 113 days and then a controlled solid diet containing 2.5 mg ascorbic acid for an additional 97 days (210 days in all). On day 100, when mild scurvy was evident, the diet was supplemented with controlled levels of L-[1-^{14}C]ascorbic acid. The levels of ascorbic acid added to the diet ranged from 4 to 64 mg/day. The clinical signs of scurvy included hyperkeratosis, follicular hemorrhage, some hemorrhagic spots in the eyes, and swollen or bleeding gums. The results indicated that the lowest level of supplement fed, 4 mg ascorbic acid added to a diet containing 2.5 mg (6.5 mg vitamin C in all) was sufficient to cure the symptoms of scurvy shown by the man who was fed at this level (24).

In the second of these two studies (188) five men, 26 to 52 years old, ate a solid diet providing 77.5 mg ascorbic acid daily for 13 days. They then consumed a liquid formula diet containing no ascorbic acid for 84 to 97 days at which time the subjects had obvious evidence of clinical scurvy. Signs and symptoms of scurvy developed somewhat sooner and with greater severity than had been observed in the preceding study. The symptoms were reversed with intakes of 6.5, 66.5 or 130.5 mg vitamin C/day. The time required varied inversely with the vitamin C intake. With 6.5 mg ascorbic acid/day, for instance, approximately 90 days were required, whereas with 66.5 mg/day, 3 to 6 days were required (25).

In this, as in the preceding scurvy studies, plasma and urinary ascorbate fell rapidly (188). By using radioactive labeled compounds, L-[1-14C]ascorbic acid and L-[4-3H]ascorbic acid, Baker et al. (25) were able to ascertain that the normal body pools of ascorbic acid in the five subjects of the second study were remarkably constant ranging from 1,486 to 1,542 mg (mean 1,500) despite substantial variation in age, height and body weight. During the vitamin C-free intake period, the body pools were depleted at the rate of 2.6% to 4.1% per day of the total available pool. No free ascorbic acid was observed in the urine after 23 days of depletion. Four unknown organic metabolites of ascorbic acid however were excreted throughout the depletion period (24). One of these was identified as ascorbate-3-sulfate (23), later shown to be ascorbate-2-sulfate (49).

These findings are comparable to those of Hellman and Burns (176) who fed L-[1-14C]ascorbic acid to three patients weighing 65.0, 59.1 and 75.4 kg. These patients were consuming the usual hospital diets, were free from acute symptoms of their disease and were normal with respect to liver and kidney function. Body ascorbic acid pools were calculated to be 26, 21 and 19 mg/kg respectively. The turnover rates were calculated to be 1.4, 1.0 and 0.66 mg/kg/day. Most of the administered 14C was found in the urine as L-ascorbic acid, diketo-1-gulonic acid and oxalic acid.

In the studies of Hodges et al. (186, 188) whole blood ascorbate levels reflected the pool size until the pools fell to 300 mg. As the pool size fell below 300 mg there was no longer an apparent relationship between blood ascorbate and pool size. Clinical signs of scurvy were clearly identified

when the pool was reduced to 300 mg. As the pool size rose above 300 mg the clinical signs began to clear away. In some of the men, they had completely disappeared before the normal pool size was reached.

Hodges and Canham (187) compared the data obtained in the two studies with the criteria for evaluating vitamin C status used by the Interdepartmental Committee on Nutrition for National Defense (ICNND) (206). They found that when the vitamin C-free diet was fed, the plasma levels dropped within a month to the low or deficient range. Then even when obvious signs of scurvy appeared, plasma levels fluctuated more frequently in the range considered low (0.10–0.19 mg/100 ml) than in the range considered deficient (< 0.10 mg/100 ml) according to ICNND standards. They concluded that whole blood ascorbic acid levels were more dependable than plasma levels in providing an estimate of pool size and vitamin C status.

Capillary fragility

Göthlin (143), drawing on observations by clinicians of a "reduction in strength of the vascular walls in fully developed scurvy," devised a method for estimating vitamin C requirements based on capillary fragility. Göthlin developed standards for normal and deficient subjects based on the number of petechiae that appeared when a rubber tourniquet was applied to the arm at standard pressure. The method was applied first to two mental patients fed a vitamin C-free diet supplemented by varying levels of fresh orange juice (143) and later to four schizophrenic patients fed graduated levels of ascorbic acid (145). On the basis of the latter study, Göthlin calculated the vitamin C requirement of a 60 kg man to be 23.9 to 28.8 mg/day (145).

In later studies by other investigators, capillary fragility was not found to be a sufficiently sensitive method for estimating vitamin C requirements or for determining vitamin C status. Levcowich and Batchelder (252), for instance, using Dalldorf's method (87) of applying "reverse pressure" (suction) rather than "overpressure," failed to perceive a differential response when ascorbic acid intake was raised from 40 to 130 mg/day. It may be that they fed the ascorbic acid at too high a range to elicit a difference in response. Crandon et al. (86), however, in their study on experimental scurvy, were not able to observe a positive response using either Göthlin's or Dalldorf's method even after an essentially vitamin C-free diet had been fed for 5 months and clinical signs of scurvy other than capillary fragility had appeared. Crandon et al. (86) remarked that their results did not indicate that capillary fragility is not part of the pathology of scurvy but rather that neither the Göthlin test (143) nor the Dalldorf test (87) is a good measure of capillary fragility in early scurvy.

Levels of ascorbic acid in blood

The estimated requirement for vitamin C as indicated by blood levels of ascorbic acid varies with the criteria used. The intake required to saturate the blood or its fractions is greater than the amount required to maintain "adequate" levels in the blood (115). When it is saturated, whole blood contains about 1.4 to 1.5 mg vitamin C/100 ml (174, 412, 414), plasma contains about 1.0 to 1.4 mg/100 ml (62, 115, 396), and white blood cells contain about 35 mg/100 g (295, 296). The amount of dietary vitamin C needed to saturate the blood or its components was estimated by several methods. By one method, the subject was first saturated with ascorbic acid. Next he was gradually depleted by feeding him a diet deficient in vitamin C. Then, large doses were fed until he was resaturated as judged by the restoration of blood ascorbic acid levels to their predepletion levels or by a significant increase in urinary excretion of vitamin C. (Because urinary excretion fluctuated considerably, van Eekelen (407) preferred to use blood ascorbic acid levels in ascertaining that saturation had been achieved.) The amount of vitamin C required for saturation was considered to be the total intake during resaturation minus the amount excreted in the urine in excess of the excretion during depletion. By another method, the subject was saturated and the minimum amount of vitamin C needed to maintain the blood ascorbic acid at the saturation level was determined. By a third method, varying levels of vitamin C were fed over extended periods and the level with which saturation was achieved was recorded.

By the first method, van Eekelen (407) found that the amount of ascorbic acid required to resaturate himself depended on the length of the experiment and particularly on the length of time during which he ate the depletion diet. When he depleted himself for 84 days in a 94-day experiment, 3,220 mg of ascorbic acid was needed to resaturate his blood. From this, he calculated a daily requirement of 34 mg vitamin C. When, in another 27-day study, with a 20-day depletion period, he required 1,712 mg ascorbic acid for saturation, he calculated a requirement of 63 mg/day. In both cases, the amounts needed to resaturate the blood have been corrected by subtracting the surplus ascorbic acid excreted above the normal average during the last few days of intake. On the basis of his weight (90 kg), van Eekelen calculated that a 70 kg man would require about 50 mg of vitamin C/day. When data from studies by van Wersch (414) with one man and one woman and by Heinemann (170) with one man were added to those of van Eekelen (407, 408), requirements varying from 44 to 63 mg/day or from 0.83 to 0.84 mg/kg body weight were observed (413). Heinemann (171) suggested that this amount, approximating 60 mg/day for a 70 kg man, was the "actual requirement" for vitamin C as compared to the "indispensable minimum" (19 to 27 mg/day) deduced by Göthlin (144) from observations on capillary fragility in man and prevention of scurvy in guinea pigs.

More recently, Tani (392) reported from Japan that 1.2 to 1.6 mg vitamin C/kg body weight was required to saturate the blood with vitamin C. From the results of his study, Tani recommended a daily intake of 77 mg of vitamin C for Japanese adults. Tani's English summary of his work did not indicate how many subjects were studied or how blood saturation was ascertained.

Camcam (66, 67), in a study with 13 young women in the Philippines, found that "normal" levels of blood ascorbic acid (0.6 mg/100 ml) could be achieved with an intake of 55 to 70 mg vitamin C/day. This intake however was not sufficient to saturate all the subjects. Camcam concluded therefore that the currently recommended allowance of 70 mg/day for adults "may not be enough to cover requirements and allowance for individual differences."

Todhunter and Robbins (396) observed the plasma ascorbic acid levels of three women (51.3 to 66.7 kg in weight) after their diets had been supplemented with 200 mg of ascorbic acid daily for 4 days. When the plasma ascorbic acid levels did not rise after the administration of 400 mg vitamin C, saturation was assumed. Next, varying amounts of vitamin C were added to the diets of the saturated subjects for 6-day periods. The supplements ranged from 40 to 100 mg, providing a total intake of 60 to 120 mg vitamin C/day. No level of intake was sufficient to maintain the women in their saturated state (plasma levels of 1.36 to 1.68 mg/100 ml). Todhunter and Robbins suggested that plasma saturation with vitamin C may not be necessary for optimum health. They noted that Wright (444) had reported that "normal" plasma levels of vitamin C ranged from 0.7 to 1.3 mg/100 ml. In their study, intakes of 60 mg vitamin C were more than enough to maintain plasma levels above 0.7 mg/ml. Indeed, the data indicated that no plasma vitamin C levels below 1.0 mg/100 ml were observed during the 6-day period in which 60 mg of vitamin C was fed.

Bryan et al. (62) reported a study in which the plasma ascorbic acid levels of 56 men and women were correlated with their dietary vitamin C intake. They found that plasma ascorbic acid rose with increasing dietary intake until the intake reached 1.7 to 1.9 mg/kg body weight at which time the plasma level was about 1.0 mg/100 ml. With higher levels of intake there was little increase in plasma ascorbic acid concentration. The plasma therefore was assumed to be saturated when it contained about 1.0 mg ascorbic acid/100 ml. The intakes required for saturation in Bryan's study (1.7 to 1.9 mg/kg) are not very different from those indicated to be necessary by Todhunter and Robbins (in excess of 1.8 to 2.3 mg/kg). The plasma levels regarded as saturation levels in the latter study, however, were much higher than that suggested by Bryan's data. The difference may be due, at least in part, to differences in analytical methods. Todhunter and Robbins reported that they used a micro method of Farmer and Abt (109) whereas Bryan et al.

used a method similar to the macro method of Farmer and Abt (109).

Using a procedure similar to that of Todhunter and Robbins (396), Fincke and Landquist (115) determined the vitamin C intakes needed to maintain plasma ascorbic acid at saturation levels (1.1 to 1.2 mg/100 ml) in three women. The data indicated that intakes of 131, 111 and 111 mg/day equivalent to 2.0, 1.8 and 1.7 mg/kg body weight were necessary for plasma saturation. On comparing their findings with those of others reported in the literature, Fincke and Landquist suggested that there is probably no relation "between body weight and ascorbic acid required to maintain saturation levels in the blood."

Goldsmith et al. (141), on the other hand, found that blood plasma ascorbic acid levels could be maintained at or near saturation with much smaller intakes. After their 12 ambulatory patients had been saturated with vitamin C, they were given daily supplements of 50 mg ascorbic acid which brought their total intakes to 70 mg/day. After 7 weeks with this intake, all of the patients had plasma ascorbic acid levels of more than 1.0 mg/100 ml. Intakes lower than 70 mg/day were not studied. Wirths (439), however, found that intakes of about 50 mg/day were insufficient to maintain the mean plasma ascorbic acid level at 0.93 mg/100 ml in a group of eight apprentices during a period of about 1 month. During the observation period, the plasma level fell to 0.77 mg ascorbic acid/100 ml. Two other groups of apprentices eating similar diets but supplemented with 1,000 mg vitamin C every second or every fourth day (500 or 250 mg/day) showed mean increases in their plasma ascorbic acid from initial levels of 0.87 and 0.86 mg/100 ml to 1.75 and 1.10 mg/100 ml, respectively.

Noting that various investigators had estimated that plasma concentrations of 0.7 to 0.9 mg ascorbic acid/100 ml were indications of good or adequate vitamin C nutriture (110, 148, 306), Fincke and Landquist (115) attempted to determine the ascorbic acid intake needed to maintain plasma levels of 0.8 mg/100 ml in three women and two men. They found that with a diet containing 8 to 11 mg of ascorbic acid, supplements of 30 mg vitamin C/day were insufficient to maintain the women. A supplement of 60 mg/day was sufficient for one man but insufficient for the other. From observations with higher intakes, Fincke and Landquist estimated that total daily intakes of 38, 49 and 61 mg ascorbic acid or 0.8, 1.1 and 1.0 mg/kg were sufficient for the women and total daily intakes of 59 to 69 and at least 89 mg ascorbic acid or 1.1 and 1.2 mg/kg were sufficient for the two men.

Horwitt (197) and Kyhos et al. (243) studied groups of men in institutions. In both studies, the men eating the regular institution diet had low plasma ascorbic acid levels (<0.2 mg/100 ml). In Horwitt's study (197), the plasma ascorbic acid levels of 20 schizophrenic men were gradually raised to over 0.7 mg/100 ml when 25 mg of crystalline ascorbic acid was added to their diet which already contained 25 mg of vitamin C (a total intake of 50 mg/day). Kyhos et al. (243), on the other hand, with 45 prison inmates, found that supplements of 50 mg of ascorbic acid added to the prison diet increased the plasma ascorbic acid levels but were not sufficient to maintain plasma levels of 0.8 mg/100 ml during the winter and spring months when fresh fruit and vegetables were not available. For most of the men, supplements of 75 mg/day were adequate. Three men who had chronic nose and throat infections required 100 mg/day.

Davey et al. (92), in a study with five women found that neither plasma nor serum ascorbic acid could be maintained at acceptable levels (0.6 to 0.8 mg/100 ml) with an intake of 25 mg vitamin C/day. Furthermore with this intake (25 mg/day), white blood cell levels of ascorbic acid were reduced to about 50% (10.8 to 14.8 mg/100 g) of their original values (about 25 mg/100 g). One woman studied with a daily intake of 75 mg of ascorbic acid did maintain her white blood cell level at its original value (about 21 mg/100 g). These observations are similar to those of Lowry et al. (263) who found in a study with 100 men of the Royal Canadian Air Force that a daily intake of 78 mg vitamin C would maintain white blood cell ascorbic acid levels at about 24.2 mg/100 g, whereas intakes of 8 or 23 mg vitamin C/ day resulted in mean white blood cell

values of 11.9 and 12.9 mg/100 g respectively.

Steele et al. (380, 381) noted decreases in white blood cell and serum levels of ascorbic acid when men and women were fed diets providing 7 or 10 mg vitamin C/day. When the diets were supplemented to provide 20, 30 or 40 mg vitamin C/day, significant increases in white cell ascorbic acid levels were noted only when the highest supplemental level (40 mg/day) was fed (381). With this level of intake over a 14-day period, white blood cell ascorbic acid levels did not reach saturation levels previously observed when 800 mg vitamin C was fed daily for 4 days (380).

Morse et al. (295) in a study with 19 women, 27 to 64 years old, found that white blood cell ascorbic acid levels rose from 19.6 to 26.7 and then to 34.6 mg/100 g as vitamin C intake was raised from 33 to 58 and then to 83 mg/day. A further increase in vitamin C intake to 133 mg/day did not elicit any higher level of ascorbic acid in the white blood cells. In an additional study, Morse et al. (296) studied 15 women, 28 to 34 years old, and 13 women, 56 to 77 years old when they were fed 32, 47, 57, 72, 82 and 107 mg of vitamin C in successive 14-day periods. The white blood cell ascorbic acid levels in the younger women increased from 25.6 mg/100 g with the 32 mg intake to 35.2 mg/100 g with the 57 mg intake. There was no further increase at higher intake levels. In the older women, white blood cell levels increased from 22.2 mg to 34.9 mg ascorbic acid/100 g as intakes increased from 32 to 72 mg/ day. In both older and younger women, serum ascorbic acid levels continued to increase with increasing intakes even after white blood cells apparently had been saturated. Serum ascorbic acid levels were significantly correlated with white blood cell levels only in the younger women, and only with the lower intakes (32 and 47 mg ascorbic acid/day).

Mašek (275) examined the results of previous work (277) showing that, with concentrations above 1 mg ascorbic acid/ 100 ml in the serum, the concentration of ascorbic acid in the leukocytes did not change significantly. He noted that, with serum concentrations ranging from 0.9 to 1.8 mg ascorbic acid/100 ml, the leukocyte concentration fluctuated between 24.9 and 27.2 mg/100 g. He concluded that the "doses of vitamin C needed in the population to achieve this saturation" were about 60 to 100 mg/day.

A more recent report from India indicated that saturation of blood leukocytes was possible with much lower levels of vitamin C intake (379). In this study, 19 men, 16 to 45 years old were observed for 30 to 90 days. Four men ate a basal diet providing 10 to 12 mg vitamin C/day. To this was added a supplement of 10 mg/day (a total daily intake of 20 to 22 mg). The vitamin C content of their leukocytes increased steadily throughout the period of observation (30 to 50 days). Fifteen men received large doses of vitamin C until their leukocytes were saturated. The supplementation then stopped and the men ate the basal diet providing 10 to 12 mg vitamin C/day. In eight men, this intake was sufficient to maintain the leukocyte ascorbic acid at saturation levels (10 to 18 $\mu g/10^8$ cells) for 45 to 80 days. In the other seven men, the leukocyte ascorbic acid levels began to fall after 10 to 15 days consuming the basal diet. When supplements of 10 mg/day were given (total intake 20 to 22 mg vitamin C), the leukocyte ascorbic acid levels stopped falling and, in some men, began to rise again. Srikantia et al. (379) concluded from these observations that leukocyte ascorbic acid saturation could be maintained with "as little as 10 mg a day in some and by intakes of less than 22 mg a day in all subjects investigated."

Davey et al. (92) noted that there was a great deal of variation in blood levels of ascorbic acid as reported in the literature. Suggesting that some of the variation might be due to the analytical methods used and also to the fraction of blood that was analyzed, Davey et al. (92) compared plasma and serum levels of four women receiving 25 mg and of one woman receiving 75 mg ascorbic acid/day. They found that regardless of the ascorbic acid intake, there was a significant difference between the amount of total ascorbic acid and the amount of reduced ascorbic acid in both plasma and serum. In addition the levels of total and reduced ascorbic acid were higher in plasma than in serum. Davey et al. (92)

concluded that "when comparison of results from various laboratories is made, account must be taken of the method used and of the fraction of the blood analyzed."

Another source of variation was investigated by Dodds and MacLeod (100). They studied daily plasma ascorbic acid levels of 12 subjects who were fed four levels of vitamin C varying from 32 to 110 mg/day in successive 2-week periods. During the course of the study there was an apparent adjustment to the level of intake during each 2-week period. There was also a marked rhythmical fluctuation from day to day in the plasma ascorbic acid levels of the individual subjects. A similar phenomenon had also been noted earlier by Storvick and Hauck (387). Because of this fluctuation, Dodds and MacLeod (100) concluded that weekly averages of daily plasma values gave better estimates of the vitamin C status of the individual subject than single determinations did. Whitacre et al. (427) also observed a seasonal fluctuation with plasma ascorbic acid levels higher in winter than in summer when intakes were held constant.

In addition, Dodds (99), upon examining data on blood ascorbic acid levels related to vitamin C intakes as reported in the literature for boys and girls 4 to 12 years old, adolescents 13 to 20 years old and adults 20 years and over (2,130 females, 2,865 males), found that there was little difference in blood response to vitamin C intake between male and female subjects under 12 years of age. In the adolescent groups, boys began to show lower blood ascorbic acid levels than girls with equivalent intakes. This difference was also found in the adult groups. Dodds suggested that there may be a sexual difference in metabolism stemming from hormonal interrelationships, and consequently the blood levels of ascorbic acid indicative of metabolic adequacy may differ between the sexes. Recently, Loh and Wilson (260) reported that the process by which ascorbic acid is taken up and stored in the white cells is the same for both men and women. They concluded that "the higher concentration of ascorbic acid reported in leucocytes and plasma of females is therefore a metabolic phenomenon characteristic of this sex and is not attributable to any differences between the sexes in their ability to store the vitamin."

Levels of ascorbic acid in urine

The main excretion of vitamin C is in the urine (25, 74, 176, 408). Interpretation of the results of investigations based on urinary excretion of vitamin C, however, are complicated by many factors. The accuracy of the procedures used to measure ascorbic acid differed and the techniques available for many of the studies failed to differentiate between L-ascorbic acid and other urinary metabolites. Moreover, the nutritional status of the subjects varied as well as the criteria for measuring the amounts of vitamin C needed for saturation. Early attempts to determine the "normal" baseline level of excretion provided values ranging from zero (181) to 33 mg/day (166). Harris et al. (166), for instance, in a study with four men eating "normal" diets found that about 33 mg of reducing substance was excreted daily in the urine by each subject. They called this reducing substance vitamin C, but pointed out that the indicator used (2:6-dichloroindophenol) was not of proven specificity. Using a similar analytical method, Youmans et al. (446) studied the urinary excretion of 15 patients whose diets were suspected of being deficient and of 16 people believed to have adequate diets. Their results indicated to them that the lower limit of urinary "vitamin C" excretion was about 20 mg/day. Van Eekelen (407) refined the analytical method by removing interfering reducing substances with mercuric acetate. With this refined technique, he found that the daily output of urinary ascorbic acid was 10 to 15 mg.

In contrast to these estimates by refined or unrefined methodology Hess and Benjamin (181) on the basis of a study with seven children concluded that vitamin C "is not excreted in appreciable amounts in human urine." They suggested, further, that when urinary excretion of ascorbic acid does occur, it is only after the ingestion of "excessively large" amounts of vitamin C and the complete saturation of the body tissues. Harris and Ray (165), however, reported that urinary vitamin C excretion of children was on the same order as that of adults when the excretion was expressed in terms of body weight. Furthermore, Abbasy et al. (4), in attempting to develop a method for estimating vitamin C nutritional status based on urinary vitamin C excretion, concluded that, with subjects weighing 63.5 kg, excretions below 10 to 15 mg ascorbic acid/day indicated inadequate vitamin C intake. An adequate intake was assumed to be about 25 mg/day. In additional corroborating work, Harris et al. (164) found that the mean urinary excretion of vitamin C by six subjects was 13.8 mg/day when the vitamin C intake was 25 mg/day. Their determinations were not corrected for interfering reducing substances. Youmans et al. (446), in view of these findings, suggested that the children studied by Hess and Benjamin (181) probably had deficient stores and low intakes of vitamin C.

Johnson and Zilva (212) deduced from the results of studies with four men that ascorbic acid excretion in the urine was variable depending not only on the dietary intake but also on the degree of saturation of the body tissues. Faulkner and Taylor (114) plotted urinary excretion values against blood serum ascorbic acid values using data obtained in over 100 observations on one normal subject, three patients with scurvy, and four cases of chronic infection. From the plotted data a smooth curve was drawn. A projection of the linear portion of the curve indicated that urinary output began to rise after a blood serum level of about 1.37 mg/100 ml had been reached. Further observations showed that the renal threshold of vitamin C was about 1.4 mg/100 ml serum and that serum values at or above the threshold level indicated a state of saturation. Similar threshold values were reported by van Eekelen (408), Goldsmith and Ellinger (139) and Friedman et al. (118). Crandon et al. (86), however, found in their one subject a renal threshold of 0.85 mg/100 ml plasma.

When Lewis et al. (255) determined renal thresholds in 12 healthy adults, they found that the thresholds varied from 1.1 to 1.8 mg/100 ml plasma. For 10 of the 12 subjects, they varied from 1.1 to 1.3 mg/100 ml. Data on mean fasting plasma ascorbic acid levels were available for nine subjects. For five of the nine subjects for whom data were available, the renal thresholds were the same as the fasting plasma values when the tissues were saturated. For three subjects, the renal threshold was slightly higher and for one it was slightly lower than the mean fasting plasma level at saturation.

Ralli et al. (341) concluded from studies on concentration of vitamin C and insulin in plasma and urine that the excretion of vitamin C depended on the plasma ascorbic acid level, the rate of glomerular filtration and the rate of tubular reabsorption. Furthermore, the reabsorption process was such that some excretion took place even when plasma values were below threshold levels.

Hawley et al. (169) had suggested on the basis of studies with four women and eight men that factors other than the state of saturation might influence urinary vitamin C excretion. They reached this conclusion after observing "wide fluctuations . . . in the urinary response to repeated daily test doses" after the subjects apparently had been saturated. Protein intake was suggested by Ahmad (5) to be a source of variation. He found that the urinary excretion of reducing compounds was higher with a high meat diet than with a low meat intake. Heinemann (172), however, found that, though the total amount of reducing substances in the urine increased when protein intake increased, the excretion of vitamin C per se was not significantly affected.

Although early work (166, 410) had indicated that vitamin C excretion in the urine was influenced by the intake of vitamin C or vitamin C rich foods, Ralli et al. (342) reported that, in a study with three men, 35 to 57 years old, urinary excretion was not sensitive to changes in vitamin C intake between 50 and 100 mg/day. In their study, the average daily ascorbic acid excretion determined by photoelectric colorimetry (107) varied from 6 to 13 mg when 50 mg of vitamin C was fed and from 6 to 20 mg when 100 mg was fed. Mean plasma ascorbic acid levels were 0.4 mg/100 ml with an intake of 50 mg vitamin C and 1.0 mg/100 ml with an intake of 100 mg. With intakes higher than 100 mg/day, urinary ascorbic acid reflected the intake. With intakes below 100 mg/day, plasma ascorbic acid levels were a better indicator

of intake. Tissue saturation as indicated by plasma ascorbic acid levels of 1.0 mg/100 ml could not be maintained with intakes lower than 100 mg/day. Ralli et al. (342), therefore, recommended that 100 mg be considered the optimum daily intake. At this level of intake the average urinary excretion of ascorbic acid did not exceed 13 mg/day. No relationship was observed between vitamin C requirement and body size.

Other investigators (66, 251, 353) also found that urinary ascorbic acid excretion was very variable when intakes were low or normal. Consequently, attempts to determine vitamin C requirements by means of urinary ascorbic acid excretion have usually involved saturation of the tissues by feeding large intakes over a period of time or by administering a test dose. The assumption is made that, once the tissues are saturated, the urinary excretion will vary mainly with the intake. The requirements thus estimated have varied from the amount necessary to balance the "baseline" excretion previously determined with low intakes (430) to the amount necessary to restore or maintain the saturated state (43, 218, 308, 407, 408). The estimates of the amount necessary to restore or maintain saturation have varied according to the criteria for saturation.

The lowest estimate (the amount necessary to balance the baseline excretion after saturation) was made by Widenbauer (430). By his method, the "baseline" excretion was determined with a diet containing very little vitamin C. The subject was then saturated with load doses of 200 to 500 mg vitamin C/day. Next, by trial and error, the intake which would result in an excretion just slightly higher than the baseline level was found. Once determined, this amount of vitamin C was fed daily for 7 consecutive days and the mean daily urinary excretion was estimated. The daily requirement (R) was calculated by subtracting the difference between the mean daily excretion (A) and the baseline value (B) from the mean daily intake (I) as follows:

$$R = I - (A - B)$$

Studies in which this method was used yielded values of 26 to 28 mg/day for a man and 21 to 22 mg/day for a two- to three-year-old boy. Inasmuch as the basal diet contained a small but unknown amount of vitamin C, these values probably underestimated the actual requirements.

Larger requirements were estimated by Chen et al. (68) in a study with two men, 37 and 54 years old, both of whom had scurvy. The method used was that of van Eekelen (407) which estimates the amount of vitamin C necessary to restore saturation (p. 827). Chen et al. assumed that saturation had been achieved when, after administering large doses of vitamin C, they observed a "sudden and rapid rise" in urinary ascorbic acid excretion. The daily vitamin C requirements of the two men were calculated to be 73.5 and 70.2 mg/day or 1.60 and 1.46 mg/kg.

O'Hara and Hauck (308) reported a study in which they estimated "the vitamin C intake necessary to reestablish saturation after prolonged administration of a low C diet." Four young women were saturated during a 4- to 5-day period in which liberal amounts of orange juice were fed. When the women were assumed to be saturated, urinary vitamin C excretion varied from 42 to 62 mg/day. The women were then depleted for a period of 29 or 30 days during which the basal diet, containing about 5 mg vitamin C, was fed. At the end of this period, the mean daily urinary excretion of vitamin C had fallen to 9 to 11 mg. In a subsequent period, the basal diet was supplemented with orange juice providing 200 mg vitamin C/day. The subjects continued on this regimen (15 to 17 days) until urinary vitamin C levels ceased to increase, indicating that saturation had been achieved. From 2,200 to 2,800 mg vitamin C was required to restore the women to a state of saturation. O'Hara and Hauck (308) did not calculate a daily requirement. If, however, the amount required for resaturation is divided by the number of days of the experiment as van Eekelen (407) did, daily requirements of 44 to 54 mg vitamin C may be estimated.

Kellie and Zilva (218) used a criterion similar to that of O'Hara and Hauck (308) when judging the state of saturation. They considered an individual to be saturated "when the amount of ascorbic acid voided in the urine after a continued consumption of a certain dose becomes more or less constant." In their studies with one man, they attempted to find the minimum intake that would maintain "saturation." They found that urinary ascorbic acid output became constant with intakes of 30, 50, and 100 mg vitamin C/day. The urinary excretion with an intake of 30 mg/day was very low. Kellie and Zilva concluded that the minimum requirement to assure "saturation" was probably close to 30 mg/day. Drawing on information obtained with guinea pigs that showed that the vitamin C requirement for "saturation" was much higher than that required to prevent scurvy, Kellie and Zilva suggested that a daily intake of 15 mg/day should be enough to maintain a man in health. They suggested further, however, that to ensure a margin of safety, the minimum "saturation" dose of 30 to 40 mg vitamin C/day should be recommended.

Belser et al. (43) also estimated the minimum intake of vitamin C that would maintain saturation. Their criterion for saturation was different from that of Kellie and Zilva (218). By their method, an experimental diet containing 10 mg vitamin C and supplemented with 200 mg of vitamin C was given for 4 or 5 days (the saturation period). Then, the subject was given a test dose of 400 mg vitamin C and his urinary ascorbic acid excretion was recorded for 24 hours. This urinary excretion by the presumably saturated subject after a test dose was used to estimate the state of saturation in subsequent periods when experimental levels of the vitamin were fed. After each experimental 6-day period, a test dose of 400 mg vitamin C was given. If the subject excreted an amount of ascorbic acid equal to or greater than that excreted after the test dose following the saturation period, he was assumed to be fully saturated. They found that, in a study with five women and two men, the minimum requirement for saturation varied from a range of 70 to 80 mg to a range of 110 to 125 mg/day or from 1.0 to 1.6 mg/kg body weight. In other studies using the same method, requirements for saturation were estimated to be 75 to 160 mg/day (two men and four women) (387), 90 to 110 mg/day or 1.6 to 1.7 mg/kg (three women) (396) and 75 to 115 mg/day or 1.17 to 2.17 mg/kg (two men, two women) (199).

When the method was modified to accept an excretion of 50% of the test dose as the criterion of saturation, requirements varying from 0.6 to 2.2 mg/kg were estimated by Kline and Eheart (236) in a study with 14 young women. With a similar modification in methodology, De and Chakravorty (95) estimated vitamin C requirements ranging from 75 to 100 mg/day or from 1.6 to 2.0 mg/kg in a study with five adult subjects.

Basu and Ray (36) accepted an excess urinary excretion of 30% of the administered dose of vitamin C as indicative of saturation. By their method, six subjects whose customary ascorbic acid intake and excretion had been ascertained, were saturated with high daily doses of vitamin C. The dose was then reduced until the excess urinary excretion (excretion with the test dose minus customary excretion) became relatively constant at about 30% of the dose. This was referred to as the "lower state of saturation." The mean vitamin C requirement calculated as the total intake minus the total urinary excretion was 44.2 mg/day and the mean total daily intake needed to provide for this requirement was 66.2 mg.

Belser et al. (43) commented that there was not, at that time, any clear evidence that it was desirable to maintain the body in a state of saturation with vitamin C. The amount required for such saturation would indicate, however, the "upper limit to the amount of ascorbic acid which the adult can use under normal conditions of health and activity." (43).

Later, Haines et al. (154), in the same laboratory, studied the effect of different levels of vitamin C intake (33 to 70 mg/day) on tissue reserves of ascorbic acid. They found that, with five men and one woman, 23 to 31 years old, an intake of 70 mg vitamin C/day was insufficient to maintain saturation as indicated by urinary excretion. The blood plasma and daily urinary ascorbic acid levels indicated, however, that the subjects were probably being maintained at a level just slightly below saturation.

Another method involving saturation by either oral or intravenous administration of a test dose was reported by Purinton and Schuck (334). They provided their subjects, 52 women and 11 men, with a controlled diet supplying 14 or 15 mg vitamin C/day for two consecutive 24-hour periods (periods 1 and 2, respectively). The vitamin C content of the urine excreted in each 24-hour period was estimated. At the beginning of period 2 a test dose of 500 mg vitamin C was administered. "Retained" vitamin C was estimated by subtracting the urinary output from the total intake (diet plus test dose) during period 2. "Metabolized" vitamin C was calculated by subtracting the urinary vitamin C output of period 1 from the "retained" vitamin C value. Purinton and Schuck suggested that this "metabolized" vitamin C value probably was the requirement. Vitamin C requirements estimated by this method decreased with age from 112.5 mg/day (1.95 mg/kg) for women 15 to 20 years old to 80.9 mg/day (1.5 mg/kg) for women 25 to 50 years old. The requirement for men, 20 to 25 years old, was estimated to be 124.7 mg/day (1.71 mg/kg). Purinton and Schuck commented that, with orally administered test doses, the estimated "retained" vitamin C was much higher than with intravenously administered test doses. Hawley et al. (169) had previously reported that vitamin C was excreted much faster and in higher amounts in the urine after intravenous test doses than after oral administration.

Other studies

Besides studies on experimental scurvy, capillary fragility, blood ascorbic acid levels and urinary excretion, other criteria have been proposed by which estimates of vitamin C requirement might be attempted. These criteria include balance studies in which exhaled end products of vitamin C were considered, skin tests for vitamin C status, morbidity studies and health surveys.

Exhalation of end products of vitamin C. Studies in which ^{14}C-labeled ascorbic acid was fed to human subjects (24, 25, 176) indicated that the respiratory route is not a significant excretory route for ascorbic acid catabolism. Only 2% or less of the ingested ^{14}C was excreted by exhalation as long as a freshly prepared solution of labeled ascorbic acid was fed, thus preventing air oxidation in the sample before ingestion (26).

Skin tests. A test for vitamin C status depending on the length of time required to decolorize the dye 2:6-dichloroindophenol injected intradermally was proposed by Rotter (356). Portnoy and Wilkinson (332) found an inverse relationship between the decolorization time and the level of vitamin C in the blood. Other investigators (330, 210), however, did not find evidence of a reliable relationship between blood ascorbic acid levels and decolorization times. Goldsmith et al. (140), in fact, were unable to demonstrate any such correlation whatsoever in a carefully controlled study comprised of 100 observations on 45 patients.

A variant of this test was reported more recently by Giza et al. (134) and Cheraskin and Ringsdorf (69). It was a lingual test in which a drop of the dye 2:6-dichloroindophenol was placed on the tongue. The time required for decolorization of the dye, designated as the lingual time, was found to be inversely related to the plasma ascorbic acid level. Cheraskin and Ringsdorf reported that the test was highly reproducible (69). The relationship between lingual time and dietary vitamin C intake was not as obvious as the relationship between plasma vitamin C and dietary intake levels (70). Giza et al. (134) found that the lingual time was inversely correlated with the vitamin C content of the liver. No reports of controlled studies to determine vitamin C requirements by this method were found.

Morbidity studies. Scheunert (364) estimated the vitamin C requirements of German adults working in an industrial complex in Leipzig. The workers were divided into 10 groups of 241 to 447 persons. One group, which was untreated, was the control group. Nine groups received supplements of vitamin C (20 to 300 mg), of vitamin C plus quinine, of quinine alone or of vitamin C plus thiamin. During the 242 days of the study, records of absence due to illness were kept and the illnesses were classified into 20 types. The only groups having a lower number of illnesses per 100 workers than the control group (78/100)

were those receiving 100 (32/100) or 300 mg vitamin C (34/100) and those receiving 50 mg vitamin C plus 500 μg thiamin (62/100). Scheunert concluded that an intake of 125 mg vitamin C/day was desirable for "optimal nutritional conditions."

Health surveys. Information on vitamin C requirements obtained from health surveys varies with the criteria used in judging health or vitamin status. Sigurjonsson (371), for instance, observed that the vitamin C intake of the population of Iceland varied from a range of 40 to 50 mg/day in autumn to 20 mg or less/day in spring, with an overall average intake of about 34 mg/day. The health of the people was generally good, infant mortality was relatively low and the physical development of the children was adequate. Sigurjonsson concluded therefore that the allowance of 30 mg vitamin C/day recommended by the League of Nations Technical Committee on Nutrition (248) was probably adequate. Mašek (276), on the other hand, on the basis of dietary surveys and his own work (72, 311) concluded that an intake of 50 to 70 mg vitamin C/day (1 mg/kg body weight) was needed to maintain saturation of the leukocytes in healthy adults engaged in light work.

In some nutrition surveys vitamin C intake has been related to condition of the gums. Plough and Bridgforth (328), for instance, summarized the results of eight nutrition surveys conducted by the Interdepartmental Committee on Nutrition for National Defense (ICNND). These surveys included 58 military kitchen surveys in eight countries as well as clinical and biochemical examinations of men eating in the military messes. Plough and Bridgforth reported that there was a good correlation between the measured dietary vitamin C intake and the clinical findings of "scorbutic type" gums. The survey data of the individual military messes showed "a rather definite cutoff point at about 30 mg vitamin C/day." Below this point there was an increased incidence of scorbutic type gum lesions.

In a study with Royal Canadian Air Force (RCAF) personnel, Linghorne et al. (258) found very little difference in levels of ascorbic acid in blood plasma and white blood cells between subjects receiving 7.9

mg vitamin C/day and those receiving 22.3 mg/day during an 8-month period. Two groups of RCAF personnel, receiving approximately 78 mg/day (77.9 and 78.3 mg), had distinctly higher plasma and white cell ascorbic acid levels than the first two groups (intake 7.9 and 22.3 mg/ day). All four groups had comparable amounts of gingival disorders suggestive of vitamin C deficiency when the study began. Furthermore the final examinations at the end of the study showed that the incidence of gingival bleeding, tenderness, redness and swelling increased in each of the four groups. The increase, however, was much less in the two groups ingesting about 78 mg vitamin C/day than in those receiving 7.9 or 22.3 mg/day. Linghorne et al. pointed out that the histological appearance of the gingival tissues did not resemble that seen in scurvy. Pierce et al. (324) also found that gingival changes (pitting, color, thickening, recession, blunting, swelling) occurred in two groups of subjects over a 2-year period regardless of whether the subjects were eating 47 to 60 mg vitamin C/day or 340 to 412 mg/day. There was no difference in the severity of the signs.

Goldsmith (138) in reviewing these studies concluded that they suggested that no benefit to the gums would result from vitamin C intakes greater than 50 mg/day but that a daily intake of 30 mg ascorbic acid is necessary to maintain healthy gums.

STUDIES ON FACTORS THAT MAY AFFECT VITAMIN C REQUIREMENTS

Environmental temperature and pressure

Studies with monkeys (103, 104) indicated that ascorbic acid fed in large daily doses increased resistance to cold. The animals fed 325 mg ascorbic acid/day showed a significantly smaller mean decrease in rectal temperature and intramuscular temperature when transferred from room temperature to an environment at −20° than did other monkeys who had received 25 mg ascorbic acid/day. A similar study conducted more recently with human subjects in Japan provided somewhat similar evidence (301). In this study, 20 healthy medical students, eating apparently adequate diets, were observed. Ten of the subjects were given 200 mg vitamin C/day

orally for 17 days. The other 10 subjects were the control group. Basal metabolic rates, blood ascorbic acid levels and skin temperatures were measured before supplementation began and at intervals during the experimental period. The skin temperatures were measured at 13 areas on the head, trunk and limbs, 40 minutes after exposure to 20° and then 40 minutes after exposure to 5°. During the 17-day experimental period the basal metabolic rate (BMR) rose slightly in both the test group and the control group. There was no significant difference between the two groups in BMR. Blood ascorbic acid levels remained at about 0.6 to 0.7 mg/100 ml in the control group but rose significantly in the supplemented group to about 1.2 mg/ 100 ml. There appeared to be no significant relationship between BMR and blood ascorbic acid concentration. The investigators noted however that, when blood values were below 1.1 mg/100 ml, there was a positive correlation ($r = +0.228$; $P < 0.07$) between BMR and blood ascorbic acid level. The changes in mean skin temperature observed when the subjects were transferred from the warm to the cold environment were not correlated significantly with blood ascorbic acid levels. There was, however, a negative correlation between skin temperature changes in the trunk and arms and blood ascorbic acid levels when the latter were less than 1.0 mg/100 ml ($r = -0.46$; $P < 0.05$). The investigators concluded from these observations that the blood ascorbic acid level is related to changes in skin temperature and BMR when the subject is exposed to cold. They suggested further that acclimatization to cold becomes greater as the blood ascorbic acid level rises until the latter reaches approximately 1.0 mg/100 ml. This level, which is close to saturation, they regarded as "the critical level for maintaining sufficient resistance to cold."

Studies in the Arctic (331) and the Antarctic (406) both indicated higher requirements for vitamin C in cold climates. Popov and Osetrov (331) measured the blood ascorbic acid levels of 130 healthy people who had lived in the Arctic for 6 to 30 months. They found levels varying from 0.2 to 0.9 mg/100 ml with the majority within a range of 0.2 to 0.4 mg/100 ml (96 persons). Assuming that these observations indicated a deficient vitamin C intake, Popov and Osetrov recommended that the customary allowance of 100 to 150 mg vitamin C/day be raised to 250 or 300 mg/day for men doing physical work in the Arctic.

In the Antarctic, van der Merwe (406) reported that hemoglobin and red blood cell levels fell significantly during the first 5 months of the first South African Antarctic Expedition to Queen Maud Land. Administration of 25 mg vitamin C/day to each member of the expedition reversed the trend. Van der Merwe reported, further, that, in order to maintain normal hemoglobin and red blood cell levels, total intakes of 96 mg vitamin C in winter and 171 mg/day in summer were needed. He recommended that the daily allowance of vitamin C for adults in the Antarctic be 2.0 to 3.3 mg/kg body weight or 150 to 250 mg/day.

In contrast to these studies, United States and Canadian investigators reported little evidence for an increased vitamin C requirement in cold environments. Glickman et al. (136), for instance, with 12 young men, found that the addition of ascorbic acid (200 mg) and vitamins of the B complex to a basal diet did not enhance mental or physical performance when men were exposed to cold or cool environments. No differences attributable to the vitamin supplement were observed in changes in rectal or skin temperatures when the men were exposed for 8 hours to cool (15.5°) or intensely cold (−28.9°) temperatures. During the last 5 months of the study, the basal diet provided only 33 to 34 mg ascorbic acid/3,000 kcal.

Similarly, Ryer et al. (357, 358) reported a study in which soldiers were engaged in heavy activity in a cold climate (−3° with wind at 13 mph) for 9 weeks. One group of 42 men ate the basal diet plus a supplement of 24 mg vitamin C/day. Their total ascorbic acid intake was 56 to 68 mg/day. Another group of 44 men received supplements providing them with a total intake of 1,231 to 1,244 mg ascorbic acid/day plus additional B complex vitamins. During the first 6 weeks, the men consumed about 3,500 kcal/day, and during the last 3 weeks, their intake was reduced to about 2,250 kcal/day. Various standardized tests of physical fitness revealed no differences in performance between the test and control group (357).

The urinary ascorbic acid excretion of the control group (intake 57 to 65 mg vitamin C) varied from 12.2 to 13.0 mg/day (approximately 21% of the intake). In the supplemented group (intake 1,231 to 1,244 mg vitamin C/day) the urinary ascorbic acid excretion varied from 988 to 1,044 mg/day (about 83% of the intake). Neither activity nor cold appeared to affect total ascorbic acid excretion. The excretion of the oxidized forms of ascorbic acid, however, increased with exposure to cold (358).

The whole blood ascorbic acid level varied from 0.53 to 0.77 mg/100 ml in the control group. In the supplemented group, the mean level rose to 1.7 mg/100 ml by the third week. During caloric restriction, the blood ascorbic acid level rose temporarily to 2.0 and then fell back again to 1.7 mg/100 ml. Exposure to cold did not significantly affect blood ascorbic acid levels. The investigators observed however that, after a 4-hour exposure to cold there was a slight rise in the mean level of the control group and a slight decrease in that of the supplemented group (358).

In other studies with military personnel during a 78-day trek across the Arctic (213, 215) and with soldiers flown in to bivouac for 12 days in a very cold environment (−37°) after acclimatization to warm temperatures (47), no remarkable changes in vitamin C metabolism were noted. Ascorbic acid intakes of 30 to 50 mg/day were adequate to meet the needs of the men.

In studying the response to stress of short duration, Kuhl et al. (242) submerged 21 healthy men for 8 minutes in water cooled to 9.5°. Blood samples were drawn before, immediately after, and 1, 2 and 4 hours after the stress was applied. Blood ascorbic acid levels did not show any significant changes. Urinary ascorbic acid excretion, measured in 12 men, rose significantly during 1 and 2 hours after the stress. At the end of 4 hours, however, the excretion was normal. Kuhl et al. suggested that this change in urinary ascorbic acid excretion might be indicative of increased adrenal cortical activity or it might be due to an increased rate of glomerular filtration.

There is conflicting evidence also on whether vitamin C requirements are affected by hot environments. Boiko (48) reported that symptoms of vitamin C deficiency were observed in the crew of a ship sailing in the northern hemisphere between latitudes 20° and 65° (from the tropics to close to the Arctic circle). The addition of 50 mg vitamin C to the customary intake of 100 mg/day cleared up the symptoms when the ship was in the northern latitudes. An additional 100 to 150 mg/day was needed to clear up the symptoms in the tropics. Boiko, therefore, recommended allowances of 150 to 175 mg/day in the northern regions and 200 to 225 mg/day for tropical conditions. Vitamin C deficiency was apparently judged by urinary ascorbic acid excretion.

Olivová (310) and Hindson (183) both reported reductions in blood ascorbic acid levels with exposure to heat. In Olivová's study, the mean blood ascorbic acid level of seven persons unacclimatized to heat fell from 0.55 mg/100 ml to 0.45 mg/100 ml when they were exposed for 2 hours to a temperature of 50°. Hindson (183) measured white blood cell ascorbic acid levels in healthy European men and women in Singapore. He found that the mean levels in people who had resided in the tropics for more than 4 months was lower than that of those who had lived there for less than 4 months. For the men, but not for the women, the difference was significant. Hindson had observed earlier (182) that vitamin C had a therapeutic effect in cases of prickly heat. He suggested that the vitamin may be necessary "in larger quantities in the tropics to ensure normal functioning of hyperactive sweat glands." He also suggested, that, whether or not this was the reason for the decreased levels in the white blood cells, dietary supplements of vitamin C might benefit European men living in the tropics.

Studies with controlled intakes of vitamin C, however, have not shown significant benefits resulting from high ascorbic acid intakes in hot environments. Henschel et al. (178) conducted three series of experiments with a total of 44 young men exposed to hot dry environments (44° to 50° by day, 29° to 32° by night) for periods varying from 2 hours to 3.5 days. The men ate a basal diet providing 20 to 40 mg vitamin C/day or a freely chosen diet from which sources of vitamin C had been eliminated. Half of the men received a supplement of 500 mg vitamin C/day. They found that there was no difference between the two groups of men in rate of sweat excretion. The amount of vitamin C excreted in the sweat was very small and did not differ between the two groups (0.059 and 0.060 mg/100 cc). These observations were in agreement with others whose findings indicated that sweat is not an important excretory pathway for vitamin C (287, 362, 395). Urinary ascorbic acid excretion determined on the last day of the 3.5-day periods was much higher (161 to 513 mg/ 24 hours) for the men with the high vitamin C intake than for those eating the unsupplemented diet (4.3 to 9.9 mg/24 hours). Plasma ascorbic acid levels were also higher with the supplemented group (0.43 to 1.48 mg/100 cc) than with the unsupplemented group (0.22 to 1.23 mg/ 100 cc). Pulse rates, rectal temperatures, and the results of stability tests, psychomotor tests and strength tests however were not significantly different between the two groups. Heat exhaustion occurred as frequently among the men with the high vitamin C intakes as among those with the low intakes.

The effect of atmospheric pressure on vitamin C requirements is not clear. Decreased urinary ascorbic acid excretion has been reported both with the reduced pressure of a simulated altitude of 18,000 feet (52) and with increased pressure up to 2.2 atmospheres in underwater studies (50). On the other hand, Russian investigators observed increased urinary ascorbic acid excretion in deep sea divers studied in decompression chambers or immediately after actual diving tests (403). Whether these changes in excretion reflect changes in requirement is not clear.

Physical exertion

In vitro studies with frog muscle have shown that vitamin C enhances contraction and delays the onset of fatigue (35). The evidence for a dietary requirement for vitamin C for muscular work in human subjects, however, is not clear. In some studies biochemical indices such as urinary ascorbic acid excretion and blood ascorbic acid levels have been used (19, 271, 302, 369, 375). In other studies, tests of physical endurance and efficiency, vital capacity, breath holding time and the like have been used to evaluate the need for ascorbic acid during work (21, 37, 79, 127, 160, 209, 211, 219, 227, 272, 329, 375, 417).

When biochemical parameters were used, the data were usually interpreted as indicating an increased need for vitamin C during vigorous physical exertion. Namysłowski (302), for instance, observed decreased urinary ascorbic acid excretion and blood serum ascorbic acid levels in athletes while they were engaged in normal activities at the Academy of Physical Culture in Warsaw and when they were at ski camp. The athletes had a vitamin C intake of about 100 mg/day. When the intake was raised to 300 mg/day, both urinary ascorbic acid excretion and blood ascorbic acid levels increased. Based on these observations, Namysłowski recommended daily vitamin C intakes of 100 to 150 mg during normal athletic activities and 200 to 250 mg during ski camps. Senger et al. (369), on the other hand, observed significant increases in blood serum ascorbic acid levels of cycling athletes during and shortly after exercise. They reported great variations among the 33 athletes studied, however, and they noted that athletes, who had engaged in strenuous competition just before the experiment, had lower blood ascorbic acid levels than those who began the study in a well rested condition. In another study with students of physical culture, and with less active medical students, Bachinsky (19) reported that people engaged in systematic physical activity excreted less ascorbic acid in the urine during rest periods than did those not engaged in such activity. These observations indicated to Bachinsky that athletes should receive vitamin C supplements particularly during spring time when, presumably, fresh vegetables are scarce.

Maksjutinskaya et al. (271), on the other hand, could find no indication that the amount of activity influenced urinary ascorbic acid excretion. In their study with 20 school boys at summer camp, 10 boys received daily supplements of 75 mg ascorbic acid, 4,950 IU vitamin A and 3 mg thiamin. The other 10 boys served as controls, eating only the camp diet. The boys swam from 1,000 to 5,000 m daily. Their urinary ascorbic acid excretion was not significantly related to the distance they swam. The boys who received the vitamin supplement excreted only slightly more ascorbic acid in their urine (26.5 to 31.2 mg/day) than the control boys (20.1 to 23.6 mg/day). Maksjutinskaya et al. recommended that higher amounts of vitamins should be provided.

In a study in which both biochemical and physical tests were used, differences between subjects receiving vitamin C supplements and those receiving placebos were shown with the biochemical tests but not with the physical tests. Snigur (375), in two successive years, studied 65 boarding school children divided into two groups. The children in one group received a supplement of 100 mg vitamin C/day during winter and spring. The other children served as controls. Tests for fatigability as measured by the strength of the wrist muscles and for vital capacity revealed no differences between the two groups. Serum alkaline phosphatase and urinary mucoprotein excretion rose in the controls during winter and spring. Snigur recommended therefore that children should be given supplemental vitamin C throughout the year.

There is lack of agreement among the studies in which physiological indices were studied. A few investigators have found evidence of a greater requirement for vitamin C with activity (37, 160, 272). Basu and Ray (37), for instance, studied four persons of whom three received vitamin C supplements and one served as the control. The fatigue curve of the finger muscle was studied on days 1 through 6, and on days 9 and 11 of the experiment. A dose of 600 mg vitamin C was given only on days 2 through 5 (a total of 4 days). The data showed that with vitamin C supplementation, the duration of the fatigue curve and the number of contractions before fatigue set in increased. The fatigue curve remained lengthened even after supplementation had ceased and urinary ascorbic acid excretion had dropped to pre-test levels. Basu and Ray concluded from their observations that the contractibility and fatigability of a muscle depends on its vitamin C saturation status.

In a more subjective type of study with workers performing strenuous physical work in a hot, humid, noisy environment, Margolis (272), reported that fatigue at the end of the day decreased and muscular endurance and productivity improved when the workers were given a dose of 100 mg vitamin C each day before commencing work. The English abstract of this report gives no information on the vitamin C content of the workers' diet.

Harper et al. (160) studied the effect of vitamin supplementation with a group of 69 military cadets eating their meals in a university dining facility. One group (35 cadets) received, daily, 50 mg vitamin C, 6,000 IU vitamin A and 1,000 IU vitamin D. The other group (34 cadets) received placebos. At the end of 10 weeks, the treatments were reversed and the study continued for an additional 11 weeks. Physioligical measurements were made at the beginning of the study, at the end of 10 weeks and at the end of the study. The results of these tests indicated that the group receiving supplemental vitamins showed a greater increase in vital capacity, breath-holding time and endurance time than the group receiving placebos. The resting heart rate also was higher in the supplemented group than in the control group. The investigators noted that, though the number of subjects studied was small, the groups were fairly homogeneous. Furthermore the reversal of treatments midway through the study resulted in a reversal of the behavior of the groups. They concluded, therefore, that the results were a valid indication of suboptimal previous diets. The report did not indicate the amount of vitamin C supplied in the customary diet nor the total intake of vitamin C that might be considered to be optimal.

In a similar study with 178 boys and girls, 11 and 12 years old, Jenkins and Yudkin (209) found no evidence of a significant difference in vital capacity, breath-holding time or endurance between children who received a vitamin supplement at school for 1 year and those who did not. The vitamin supplement provided daily 25 mg vitamin C, 5,000 IU vitamin A, 500 IU vitamin D and 1 mg thiamin. Jenkins and Yudkin suggested that the lack of change in physiological function may have been because the children had adequate intakes of the administered vitamins before the study began.

Other studies have not shown a beneficial effect of administration of supplemental vitamin C with or without other vitamins on physiological performance. Keys and Henschel (219) studied 26 soldiers receiving either a vitamin supplement or a placebo in a total of 256 experiments. The vitamin supplement provided daily 100 or 200 mg vitamin C with 5 to 17 mg thiamin chloride, 100 mg nicotinamide, 20 mg calcium pantothenate, 10 mg riboflavin and 10 mg pyridoxine. The customary diet to which this supplement was added provided 70 mg vitamin C, 1.7 mg thiamin and 2.4 mg riboflavin/day. In some experiments energy intake was curtailed. The exercise consisted of marching for 15, 90 or 120 minutes on a treadmill at a speed of 3.85 mph and an angle of climb of 10% or 12.5%. Response to the supplementation was measured in terms of the effect on pulse rate, heart size, stroke output of the heart, oxygen consumption, respiratory quotient, urinary excretion of nitrogen and ketone bodies, and blood levels of lactate, sugar, hemoglobin and ketone bodies. The data collected showed no effects of vitamin supplementation on muscular ability, endurance, resistance to disease or recovery from exertion. Keys and Henschel concluded that the army diets then in use would not be improved by supplements of vitamins. Whether or not less nutritious diets would benefit from vitamin supplementation was not indicated.

This problem was studied by Johnson et al. (211) with 24 men in a Civilian Public Service Camp. During an 8-week period, eight men ate a diet devoid of vitamin C but adequate in all other nutrients (the deficient diet); eight men ate the deficient diet supplemented with 75 mg vitamin C; four men ate a "good normal diet" supplemented with 75 mg vitamin C. During the 8-week period, physical efficiency was measured weekly by a "pack test" of fitness for hard work (90). The data obtained from this test revealed no deterioration in physical efficiency even though blood and urine analysis indicated that the vitamin C stores of men eating the unsupplemented deficient diet were depleted. The biochemical analyses indicated that an intake of 75 mg ascorbic acid/day was sufficient to maintain or increase the body stores of vitamin C.

Furthermore, Fox et al. (116) reported that Bantus with a mean intake of about 15 mg vitamin C/day were not significantly benefited by a daily supplement of 40 mg vitamin C. Two groups of 950 laborers, each, were studied. Both groups ate the regular diet providing 12 to 25 mg vitamin C/day. One group served as the control group and the other, the treated group, received the vitamin C supplement. At the end of 7 months, no significant differences between the two groups were noted in physical efficiency, general health or resistance to infectious diseases. Twelve cases of scurvy occurred in the control group whereas only one mild case was diagnosed in the treated group.

Subsequent studies with athletes or soldiers in training (21, 127, 227, 417) have also shown no physiological evidence of improved physical performance with vitamin C supplementation. Nor has vitamin C been found in two double-blind tests to be effective in relieving or preventing muscular stiffness and pain after unaccustomed vigorous physical exertion (79, 329).

Tobacco smoking

There are reports in the literature that suggest that smokers may have different vitamin C requirements compared to nonsmokers. This assumption is based on the observation of lower blood ascorbic acid levels in smokers than in nonsmokers (51, 105, 415). Calder et al. (65) concluded that smoking had a long-term rather than an immediate effect on plasma ascorbic acid level and that there was no difference between the effect of moderate smoking (less than 14 cigarettes/day) and that of heavy smoking (15 or more cigarettes/day). Brook and Grimshaw (60) reported that smoking was associated with reduced levels of ascorbic acid in leukocytes as well as plasma and that plasma ascorbic acid

levels were also reduced with age. They concluded that the effect of smoking on the plasma ascorbic acid levels was similar to that of an increase of 40 years in chronological age. Pelletier (316–318) found that when nonsmokers and smokers were saturated, they became desaturated at the same rate when fed a diet low in vitamin C. This observation suggested that there was no impairment in the smokers' metabolism of vitamin C. Having also ascertained from statistical treatment of the data that lower vitamin C intakes were not responsible for the smokers' lower blood ascorbic acid levels, Pelletier (316, 318) suggested that vitamin C absorption may have been impaired in the smokers. He also concluded that smokers may require about twice as much vitamin C as nonsmokers require to maintain similar blood levels (317).

Another clue that may help to explain the lower blood ascorbic acid levels in smokers as compared with those of nonsmokers was provided by Saindelle et al. (360). They found with in vitro studies that certain components of cigarette smoke inhibit the reduction of dehydroascorbic acid to ascorbic acid. The most active ingredient appeared to be acrolein.

In contrast to these studies, Bailey et al. (22) reported a double-blind experiment with 20 smokers and 20 nonsmokers, all of whom were physically active young men (average age, 24.5 years). All subjects were exercised vigorously on a treadmill, then, for 5 days, 10 smokers and 10 nonsmokers were given 2 g vitamin C/day. The rest of the subjects received placebos. Plasma ascorbic acid levels measured before the 5-day period were within the normal range and there was no difference between smokers and nonsmokers. After the 5-day period the plasma levels of those subjects fed vitamin C rose to saturation levels and were significantly higher than those of the subjects fed placebos. In neither smokers nor nonsmokers did saturation have a significant effect on the physiological parameters studied (heart rate, minute ventilation, tidal volume/vital capacity, oxygen uptake and oxygen pulse).

Wound healing

In animal studies, vitamin C deficiency has been associated with impaired collagen formation. The biochemical defect appears to stem from the inability of the animal to hydroxylate a prolyl residue to hydroxyproline. In vitamin C deficiency there is reduced hydroxyproline concentration in repair tissues but this cannot be demonstrated in intact tissue (146, 226, 352). Kirchheiner (226) has suggested that because of the relative stability of connective tissue formed during normal growth as compared with that of repair tissues, the studies with animals may not have been long enough to demonstrate reduced hydroxyproline in intact tissues.

In man, there is conflicting evidence on the need for vitamin C in wound healing. Early observations with patients undergoing surgery showed that blood ascorbic acid levels decreased immediately after surgery without an accompanying increase in urinary ascorbic acid excretion (33, 83, 84, 264, 370). Administered doses of vitamin C were cleared from the plasma more quickly in patients following surgery than in well subjects (33). Browne (61), in addition, observed increased ascorbic acid retention in patients undergoing healing of wounds, bone fractures or burns. He interpreted these observations as indicating a marked destruction or utilization of vitamin C immediately after surgery, fracture or burns. Shukla (370) suggested that, in the postoperative period, there is a rapid utilization of vitamin C for the synthesis of collagen at the site of the wound. He proposed that the administration of vitamin C postoperatively might hasten healing. Crandon et al. (83, 84) also observed a drop in blood ascorbic acid values (17% in plasma, 20% in white blood cells and platelets) after surgery. In addition, in observations on about 875 patients over a 10-year period, they noted that deficient blood ascorbic acid levels were frequently associated with wound dehiscence. In 26 patients (83) they found that intakes of 100 to 300 mg vitamin C/day were needed to maintain blood ascorbic acid levels above the deficient zone. In their work, levels of less than 0.2 mg/100 ml plasma or 8 mg/100 g white blood cells and platelets were regarded as evidence of deficiency.

Coon (78) studied 150 patients undergoing major surgery that required restriction of food intake for 5 or more days. In the immediate postoperative period, the patients were divided into six groups who were given subcutaneous doses of ascorbic acid to provide a daily intake of 0, 75, 100, 150, 200 or 300 mg vitamin C. Coon found that whether or not blood ascorbic acid levels fell in the postoperative period depended on the blood ascorbic acid level in the preoperative period and on the amount of vitamin C administered postoperatively. Statistical treatment of the data indicated that at least 200 mg vitamin C/day would be required to assure that adequate blood ascorbic acid levels (>0.4 mg/100 ml) were maintained in at least 95% of a similar population group. There was, however, a great deal of variability in the responses of the patients studied. Coon noted that other investigators (236, 263) observed much variation also in the response of healthy subjects. He noted, further, that he could find no evidence that 95% confidence levels had been established for the then recommended dietary allowance of 75 mg ascorbic acid/day. He concluded therefore that "the requirement for ascorbic acid in the usual patient undergoing a major operation is probably not much greater than that expected in a comparable sample of the normal population."

Studies on the effect of ascorbic acid intake on the healing process itself have yielded little evidence of a specific vitamin C requirement over and above the intake necessary to maintain health. Crandon et al. (86) found that an experimentally inflicted wound healed normally in their subject who had been deprived of vitamin C for 3 months. At the time the incision was made, blood analysis had revealed no detectable plasma ascorbic acid for 44 days. Another incision was made at the end of 182 days of depletion. At this time indications of scurvy had appeared and plasma and white blood cell levels of ascorbic acid had been undetectable for 141 and 61 days respectively. The wound on the skin surface appeared to heal normally, but 10 days after the incision was made, biopsy examination showed that no healing had taken place beneath the skin. Histological examination showed a lack of intercellular substance at the wound site. The subject was given 1,000 mg vitamin C intravenously.

doesn't talk about wound strength

After 10 days, another biopsy showed good healing.

In a more recent study of experimental scurvy, Hodges et al. (186) reported that surgical incisions were made on the thighs of their four subjects after they had been deprived of vitamin C for 100 days. With subsequent administration of 4, 8, 16 or 32 mg ascorbic acid/day no differences were noted in rate of healing. Punch biopsies, taken 1 and 2 weeks after the incisions were made, revealed no histological differences in the healing.

In neither of these studies was there a comparison with nondepleted control subjects. Wolfer et al. (441) reported a study in which nine young men were maintained with diets containing very little vitamin C (0 to 10 mg/day) for 7 months while five other young men ate the same diet supplemented with 75 to 150 mg vitamin C/day. At the end of the 7-month period, surgical incisions were made in the subjects' thighs, were sutured and were allowed to heal. Biopsy samples were removed from the wound sites of both deprived and control subjects at intervals over a 14-day period. The biopsy samples were subjected to a standardized tensile strength test and then were examined histologically. The data obtained indicated that until day 11, healing progressed more slowly in the deprived subjects than in the controls. From day 11 on, healing progressed at the same rate in both groups. Histological tests showed less reticulum and collagen in skin and fascia of deficient subjects than of controls. Saturation tests (based on plasma ascorbic acid levels and urinary excretion after load doses of ascorbic acid) showed some correlation between tensile strength and degree of saturation. The degree of saturation or the minimum level of vitamin C intake that would be accompanied by healing, however, was not indicated.

Early reports of low blood ascorbic acid levels in patients with gastric or duodenal ulcers (14, 204, 332) led to the conclusion that ulcer patients utilize more vitamin C than normal healthy subjects (422). More recent studies (77), in which diet histories of ulcer patients were compared with those of other patients and of healthy subjects, have indicated that the low blood levels of ulcer patients are due to a dietary deficiency rather than to increased utilization. Other investigators (106, 435) suggest malabsorption as a cause.

Vitamin C has been reported to promote healing of burns as well as other types of wounds. Klasson (235) for example observed five male subjects ranging in age from 2 to 56 years. All had severe burns. Doses of 500 to 800 mg vitamin C/day were given orally and solutions of 1% or 2% ascorbic acid were applied with the dressings to the burns. Klasson concluded that the ascorbic acid treatment helped to alleviate pain, hastened the healing period and reduced the time interval necessary for grafting. He suggested that 1,000 mg ascorbic acid be given intravenously in an electrolyte solution during the first 24 hours after burns occur.

Andreae and Browne (9), on the other hand, in a study with seven burned patients and three normal controls could find no indication that high ascorbic acid intakes influenced the clinical progress of the patients. They did find, however, reduced urinary ascorbic acid excretion in the burned patients as compared with normal subjects when both groups were receiving controlled vitamin C intakes. Blood ascorbic acid levels fell in the burned patients in spite of the administration of 250 or 500 mg of vitamin C. The data did not reveal whether the vitamin C that was apparently "retained," was utilized or destroyed. Similar data were obtained by Lund et al. (265) who observed six children (4 to 14 years old) and 11 adults with minor and severe burns. They interpreted the observed low urinary ascorbic acid excretions and low plasma ascorbic acid levels as indications of alterations in ascorbic acid metabolism. The extent of the alterations paralleled the severity of the burns. Lund et al. suggested that severely burned patients should be given 1 to 2 g of ascorbic acid daily.

Infection

The early literature reviewed by Faulkner and Taylor (113) and Perla and Marmorston (322) showed correlations between the incidence of infection and scurvy in both humans and guinea pigs. These observations led to suggestions that (a) vitamin C deficiency is manifested in diseases such as rheumatic fever, (b) there is an increased requirement for vitamin C during infection, and (c) an increased intake of vitamin C helps to prevent or alleviate infection.

The suggestion that vitamin C deficiency is a causative factor in the etiology of rheumatic fever or rheumatoid arthritis (343, 345) found no support in the work of Perry (323), Faulkner (112) or Schultz (366). In their studies, the administration of large doses of vitamin C did not alter the course of the disease.

The evidence for an increased requirement for vitamin C during infection was provided by observations of lower than normal blood ascorbic acid levels during illnesses such as rheumatic fever (113, 346), rheumatoid arthritis (155, 344, 359), pneumonia (245), tuberculosis (147, 361) and hepatitis (238). Lower than normal urinary ascorbic acid excretion levels during such infections were also observed (1–3, 63, 159, 173, 175, 273, 323, 368). Gounelle and Vallette (147) estimated that tuberculous patients should receive about 250 mg vitamin C/day to assure saturation as indicated by blood levels. They noted that there was much variation in requirements among their subjects. Heise and Martin (175) also found much variation in requirements of tuberculous patients. Their estimates of requirements based on urinary excretion in response to doses of orange juice ranged from 55 to 138 mg vitamin C/day. By their method, the requirement of healthy subjects was estimated to be 15 to 20 mg/day. In additional work, Martin and Heise (273) concluded that the average vitamin C requirement of tuberculous patients is about 110 mg/day. Studies with vitamin C administered both orally and intravenously suggested to them that ascorbic acid absorption was impaired and that, in addition, there was increased destruction of the vitamin in the tissues. They also found that the degree of hypovitaminosis paralleled the extent and activity of the tuberculosis involvement.

Various reasons for the apparent increase in vitamin C requirement as indicated by lowered blood values and decreased urinary excretion have been proposed. Rinehart et al. (345) suggested that some patients may have some derangement in metabolism such as a lowered renal threshold. Abbasy et al. (1) concluded that "with infection . . . there is a greatly increased metabolic use of (and need for) vitamin C, and a correspondingly lowered degree of 'saturation' of the body tissues." Similarly, Bullowa et al. (63) finding evidence of vitamin C deficiency during fever, suggested that the deficiency was due to increased metabolism associated with increased destruction of vitamin C during hyperthermia.

Evidence for an increased requirement for vitamin C due to hyperthermia was reported by Daum et al. (91) and Zook and Sharpless (449). Daum et al. (91) observed a reduction in both blood and urinary ascorbic acid levels after patients were subjected to electrically induced artificial fever. Zook and Sharpless (449) observed decreased urinary ascorbic acid excretion but no change in blood ascorbic acid levels with artificial fever. They suggested that the apparent lack of response in blood ascorbic acid levels may have been due to changes in hemoconcentration. Osborne and Farmer (312), however, observed no significant change in blood ascorbic acid levels and no change in hemoconcentration. Falke (111) observed depressed ascorbic acid levels in both blood and urine with artificially induced fever. By means of a vitamin C balance study he estimated that the consumption of vitamin C was increased by about 100 mg/day during fever.

Heinemann (173) found evidence of increased requirement in tuberculous patients even when no fever was present. More recently Sahud and Cohen (359) found that patients with rheumatoid arthritis had low levels of ascorbic acid in the blood platelets as well as in blood serum. Their data indicated that the low ascorbic acid levels accompanied high aspirin dosage. Similar evidence in patients treated with indomethacin suggested that the observed low blood ascorbic acid levels might be due to anti-inflammation agents in general.

The results of studies carried out during the past 40 years have been equivocal on whether vitamin C helps to prevent or alleviate infections. One problem in estimating the need for vitamin C in infection has been that of finding suitable objective measurements of occurrence and severity of the disease. In some studies, the number of reported cases has been used; in others, the duration of illness has been recorded; and in still others, the alleviation of signs and symptoms has been estimated. Such criteria leave much room for variation in interpretation from subject to subject as well as from investigator to investigator.

Another problem is that vitamin C has been fed either alone or in combination with bioflavonoids or with other vitamins. When it is fed with other nutrients, the effect due primarily to vitamin C cannot be measured with certainty. Furthermore, fed alone or with other substances, the effectiveness of the administered dose will depend partly on the vitamin C status of the subject prior to the study.

Another problem that arises in interpreting the data is that the amount of supplemental vitamin C provided has varied from study to study. In investigations on the common cold, for instance, supplements ranging from 200 to 1,000 mg/day have been fed. In these studies, a number of investigators reported that vitamin C reduced the incidence, severity, or duration of colds (29, 30, 44, 82, 267, 348, 436). Other investigators observed no significantly beneficial results from the administration of the vitamin (81, 117, 126, 135, 394, 420).

Although Anderson et al. (8) observed no significant effect of massive doses of vitamin C (1–4 g) on the incidence of the common cold, they did observe a significant decrease in the number of days the treated subjects missed from work due to illness as compared with the control subjects. This reduction in the number of days of disability seemed to be due mainly to a decrease in the severity of nonspecific symptoms such as chills, fever and severe malaise. Because of the economic as well as the health aspects of these findings, Anderson et al. concluded that further research is warranted.

Hypersensitiveness

In 1938 Walzer (421) wrote that "with the new developments in the knowledge of vitamins has come a flood of reports dealing with the relationship of vitamin C to various forms of hypersensitiveness." In reviewing these reports, Walzer found little firm evidence to suggest that vitamin C had any significant effect on hypersensitiveness in animals or man. He concluded that "for the present, except in cases where there is a definite vitamin deficiency, the use of cevitamic acid in the various allergic illnesses may be considered as empiric."

In subsequent studies, the effect of vitamin C on hypersensitiveness has been evaluated by the extent to which the vitamin decreased or prevented symptoms, by the level of ascorbic acid in the blood and the amount of the vitamin necessary to maintain desired blood ascorbic acid levels, and by the excretion of ascorbic acid in the urine. In a study with 25 asthmatics, for instance, Hunt (200) found no evidence of improvement in the amount of wheezing, the incidence of attacks or the general condition of the subjects when they were given injections of 500 to 800 mg vitamin C or oral doses of 100 mg/day for 8 weeks. Goldsmith et al. (142) also found, with five patients, that the administration of vitamin C had no effect on the symptoms of asthma. In two other patients, however, they observed an apparent relationship between blood ascorbic acid levels and frequency and severity of asthma attacks. When plasma ascorbic acid levels of 29 bronchial asthmatics were examined, the investigators found that the mean level (0.410 mg/100 ml) was lower than that of a control group (0.602 mg/100 ml). After saturation, six of seven asthmatic patients could not maintain a plasma ascorbic acid level of 1.0 mg/100 ml with a standardized diet that was adequate for the control group. Goldsmith et al. interpreted these observations as indicating an increased requirement for vitamin C in asthmatic patients.

In a number of studies with patients exhibiting hypersensitiveness to ragweed pollen (195, 320) various foods (192), sulfonamides (193, 194, 319, 365) or arsphenamines (80, 96, 405), allergic reactions were either prevented or reduced in severity when relatively large doses of vitamin C were administered. Both Friend and Marquis (119) and Vail (405) observed that sensitivity to arsphenamines was commonly associated with low blood ascorbic acid levels. Friend and Marquis concluded that the low blood levels were the result of the toxic reaction rather than a predisposing factor to such reaction. Vail, on the contrary, concluded from his observations that the amount of arsenical treatment did not influence the blood ascorbic acid levels, that blood ascorbic acid levels could be raised by relatively small dietary vitamin C supplements (50 to 100 mg/day), and that, as the blood levels rose, the symptoms of arsenical sensitivity disappeared. Delp (96) similarly found no evidence of depressed plasma ascorbic acid levels with routine arsenical treatment. He reported, in addition, that, contrary to a suggestion by Cormia (80), he found no evidence that the administration of vitamin C with the arsenical compounds interfered with the effect of the latter.

McCormick (282) suggested that the toxic effects of sulfonamides might be manifestations of a latent vitamin C deficiency aggravated by a febrile condition. Evidence of a sulfonamide effect per se, on vitamin C status however, was provided by Holmes (193) who administered 30 grains of sulfathiazole daily to 10 healthy subjects for 4 days. Urinary ascorbic acid excretion increased to two or three times the normal level during the days of administration. Holmes calculated that the increased loss could be balanced by an increased daily intake of 100 mg or more of vitamin C.

Hormonal function

Because women tend to have higher blood ascorbic acid levels than men have (99), an interaction between vitamin C and endocrine function has been suggested. The information in the literature at present, however, is conflicting. In studies of blood ascorbic acid levels during the menstrual cycle, some investigators (286) reported increases midway through the cycle, others (120, 168) noted no change, whereas Kofoed et al. (237) observed an increase in dehydroascorbic acid and a decrease in ascorbic acid. In studies of urinary ascorbic acid excretion, Loh and Wilson (261) reported sharp increases about 3 days before ovulation, Hauck (168) observed no change during the menstrual cycle, and Paeschke and Vasterling (314) reported distinct decreases at the time of ovulation. Recently, Rivers and Devine (349) studied plasma ascorbic acid levels during the menstrual cycles of four young women who were taking oral contraceptives. The four experimental subjects and two control subjects who had a history of normal menstrual cycles were saturated with vitamin C throughout the 110-day study. The experimental subjects had lower plasma ascorbic acid and plasma total ascorbic acid levels than the controls had. In the control subjects, the plasma ascorbic acid levels were highest at the time of ovulation and lowest during the menses and late secretory stage. In the women taking oral contraceptives, the reverse pattern was observed, lowest levels at the time of ovulation and highest during the menses when the drugs were not being administered. Rivers and Devine (349) suggested, therefore, that oral contraceptives depress plasma ascorbic acid concentration and prevent a rise in plasma ascorbic acid at the time of ovulation.

White blood cell ascorbic acid concentrations have also been reported to be affected by oral contraceptives. Briggs and Briggs (59) examined leukocyte-platelet ascorbic acid levels in 85 women, of whom 39 were taking oral contraceptives, 18 were pregnant and 31 were untreated and nonpregnant. They reported that the ascorbic acid levels in both leukocytes and platelets were significantly lower in women taking oral contraceptives than in the pregnant or untreated nonpregnant women. They suggested that the oral contraceptive steroids "increase the breakdown of ascorbic acid, perhaps by their stimulant action on liver release of ceruloplasmin." They suggested, furthermore, that many women taking oral contraceptives may be in an "induced hypovitaminotic C condition" and that they may require vitamin C supplements.

Recently, however, McLeroy and Schendel (283) found that vitamin C supplements did not change the leucocyte ascorbic acid level significantly in women taking oral contraceptives. They measured leukocyte ascorbic acid levels in 126 healthy, premenopausal nonpregnant women. Of these women 63 had been taking oral contraceptives for at least 1 year (the test group). The other 63 women, none of whom had taken oral contraceptives during this period, served as the control group. The mean leukocyte level of the test group (19.0 mg/100 g) was significantly lower than that of the control group (25.7 mg/100 g). Within the test group, the mean leukocyte level of the women taking vitamin C supplements (19.4 mg/100 g) was not significantly different from the mean of those not taking supplements (19.0 mg/100 g). In the control group, on the other hand, the mean leukocyte ascorbic acid level of those taking vitamin C supplements (35.2 mg/100 g) was significantly higher than the mean of those not taking supplements (24.1 mg/100 g). In speculating on the reasons for the difference in response, McLeroy and Schendel suggested possible changes in intestinal absorption, in metabolism and utilization, or in excretion of vitamin C under the influence of sex hormones.

Observations of vitamin C deficiency in patients with Addison's disease (177, 434) suggested a relationship between ascorbic acid and adrenal function. Studies with animals reviewed by Sayers and Sayers (363) indicated that, under conditions of stress, or when adrenocorticotrophic hormone (ACTH) was administered, the adrenal was promptly depleted of ascorbic acid. In some types of stress there was a correlation between the degree of stress and the degree of depletion. Other investigators (190, 382) reported the occasional appearance of symptoms of vitamin C deficiency when ACTH was being administered to patients for therapeutic reasons. Beck et al. (41) noting a sharp increase in urinary ascorbic acid excretion after the administration of ACTH to patients, suggested that the renal threshold might have been lowered or that there might have been a "rapid and continued release of ascorbic acid from the adrenal" or "a general release from some other organ or tissue."

As yet, no quantitative effect of adrenal function on vitamin C requirement has been reported. Various hypotheses, however, have been offered to explain the apparent relationship between ascorbic acid and adrenal function. Andreae and Browne (9), for instance, suggested that vitamin C might participate in some way in the synthesis of "cortical hormone." However, Kark et al. (213, 214) reported that scorbutic patients showed normal adrenal response to injections of ACTH. Pirani (327) suggested that the function of ascorbic acid in the adrenal might be related to cellular respiration and metabolism. He suggested also that other substances might be able to substitute for ascorbic acid in this function.

Smolyanskii (373), in a study with 144 older people, found that the administration of vitamin C (500 mg/day) was accompanied by a significant increase in the level of 17-hydroxycorticosteroids in the blood and in the urinary output of 17-ketosteroids. Similarly Vakhtina and Zaretsky (404), studying 93 patients with atherosclerosis, found low adrenal function and impaired response to ACTH as indicated by low urinary excretion of 17-hydroxycorticosterone and dehydroepiandrosterone. Both basal excretion and response to ACTH rose when 0.3 g ascorbic acid was given thrice daily. Smolyanskii (373) suggested that the increased synthesis of adrenal steroids indicated by his observations might be due to a direct effect of ascorbic acid on the adrenal or it might be a "manifestation of the cortical response to ascorbic acid activation of the oxidation-reduction reactions of the body as a whole." Kitabchi (233) and Kitabchi and Duckworth (234), on the other hand, suggest that ascorbic acid may inhibit steroidogenesis in the adrenal, and that, under stimulation by ACTH, the adrenal first releases its ascorbic acid before steroidogenesis can take place.

Mental health

There is some evidence of a relationship between vitamin C intake and mental health. Poor vitamin C status observed in patients in mental hospitals (197, 249) may have been the consequence, in part at least, of low dietary intake. Maas et al. (266), however, noted that schizophrenic and neurotic patients with anxiety had lower plasma ascorbic acid levels than those without anxiety. Furthermore, observations by Briggs (57) and Briggs et al. (58) of high ceruloplasmin levels together with a low ratio of free ascorbic acid to ascorbic acid metabolites in the urine of schizophrenics led to the hypothesis that the fundamental biochemical lesion in schizophrenia might be a disorder in ascorbic acid metabolism coupled with a defect in copper metabolism. Briggs (57) suggested that the condition in its early stages might possibly be controlled by high vitamin C intakes (about 500 mg/day). Corroborating evidence was provided by Milner (289). He found, in a controlled blind study with 40 psychiatric patients, that there were significant improvements in depressive, manic and paranoid symptom-complexes following saturation with vitamin C. He suggested that psychiatric patients have an unusually high demand for vitamin C.

In studies with healthy subjects Grosz (151) found that hypnotically induced anxiety was not accompanied by significant changes in serum ascorbic acid levels. Baker et al. (24) and Hodges et al. (185, 186), however, in their study of experimental scurvy with four prison inmates, found that one subject during a period of intense anxiety excreted more ascorbic acid in his urine than he was ingesting. When the cause for anxiety was removed, the man began to retain the vitamin. In a subsequent study (25, 188) the investigators depleted five prison inmates of ascorbic acid and then repleted them by feeding varying levels of vitamin C. Psychological testing was done near the beginning, at midpoint and at the end of the depletion period, at midpoint of the repletion period and after 15 days of load dosing (225). The tests covered four behavioral areas: mental function, psychomotor performance, physical fitness and personality. The most significant changes were observed in personality as measured by the Minnesota Multiphasic Personality Inventory (MMPI). During the course of depletion, four MMPI scales (Hypochondriasis, Hysteria, Depression and Social Introversion) showed significant increases. These changes occurred when the body ascorbic acid pool (normally about 1,500 mg) had been depleted to levels ranging from 761 to 562 mg, at which time the whole blood ascorbic acid levels ranged from 1.21 to 1.17 mg/100 ml. These personality changes were reversed during the repletion stage. In two subjects, intakes of 6.5 mg ascorbic acid/day were sufficient to effect the reversal. In view of these observations, the lack of a statistically significant serum response to hysteria in Grosz's study (151) is not surprising.

STUDIES ON REQUIREMENTS OF SPECIFIC POPULATION GROUPS
Premature and full-term infants
(Appendix table 2)

Scurvy in infants, though not unknown, did not become a matter of great concern until artificial feeding and the use of pasteurized milk became prevalent. Then it was frequently misdiagnosed as rheumatism, rickets, colic, etc. In 1883, Barlow (31) described several cases of "acute rickets" and concluded from his analysis of them that the symptoms were not due to rickets but to scurvy. He suggested, therefore, that the condition should be called "infantile scurvy" not "acute rickets." For dietary treatment, he recommended raw meat juice, fresh milk, orange juice or other fresh raw vegetables.

In attempts to determine the cause of infantile scurvy, a committee of the American Pediatric Society examined reports of 379 cases (7). The committee concluded in its report of 1898 that infantile scurvy was dietary rather than infectious in origin. The conclusions did not suggest that there was something essential to health missing from the diet but rather that there was something present that was "unsuitable to the individual child." Hutchison (201) a few years later observed that scurvy could be cured simply by adding fruit juice to an otherwise unchanged diet. He concluded "that the fault in the diet of scurvy is one of omission and not of commission, in that fruit juice contains something which the blood in this disease lacks. . . ." His subsequent attempts to identify the curative ingredient were not successful. Hess (180), on the other hand, concluded that infantile scurvy was not "a simple dietary disease" but that it was due to "intestinal intoxication" or "autointoxication" due to "overgrowth of harmful bacteria." The diet was "at fault in allowing the intestinal bacteria to elaborate toxins." The suggestion that infantile scurvy was caused by something missing from the diet was made again by Kato (217) in 1932. An examination of the dietary patterns showing a lack of fresh vegetables suggested to him that infantile scurvy was a vitamin deficiency disease. Two years later Svensgaard (388) reported that she had cured two cases of infantile scurvy by administering 30 mg of ascorbic acid daily. Shortly thereafter, Goettsch (137) reported that the administration of ascorbic acid was "at least as effective . . . as orange juice therapy."

In metabolic studies with seven scorbutic infants, Ingalls (202) found that the patients needed vitamin C intakes totalling at least 1,000 mg before an increase in urinary excretion was noted. Intakes totalling 2,000 mg of vitamin C were needed to achieve "partial saturation." Earlier Rohmer et al. (354, 355) had suggested that infants could synthesize vitamin C. Ingalls found no evidence to support this hypothesis.

More recently, Grewar (149) concluded that infantile scurvy is a problem of greater magnitude than commonly believed because it still is being incorrectly diagnosed. He suggested that, until more precise diagnostic measures become available, 20 mg or more of ascorbic acid should be provided for every infant and growing child.

There is some evidence that premature infants may be more vulnerable to vitamin C deficiency or may have higher requirements than full-term infants (315, 398, 443). Indications of a metabolic defect in premature infants were reported in 1939 by Levine et al. (254) when they observed five premature infants excreting hydroxyphenyl compounds in the urine. This aberrant excretion was reduced when 50 to 200 mg ascorbic acid was administered parenterally. Additional work showed that tyrosinemia and tyrosyluria were more prevalent in premature infants than in full-term infants and that the incidence was greater with a high protein diet (about 5 g/kg body weight) than with a moderate protein diet (about 2.5 g/kg) (89, 253, 443). Among premature infants this incidence was greater in smaller than in larger infants (17, 256). As yet there is no clear evidence that the condition is harmful (17). Observations indicating that the administration of vitamin C prevented or alleviated the condition (17, 89, 253, 254, 256, 279, 443) led to recommendations of vitamin C allowances of 75 mg/day (17) and of 75 to 120 mg/day (179) for premature infants.

In studies with 121 healthy premature infants and 98 full-term infants, Wiesener (432) found additional evidence that the premature infant requires more vitamin C than the full-term infant does. He measured blood ascorbic acid levels and urinary ascorbic acid excretion with various levels of intake and after load doses of vitamin C. He concluded that the premature infant's formula should contain at least 10 mg ascorbic acid/100 ml in order to meet his needs. By the time the infant is 3 weeks old, supplements of 25 and 50 mg vitamin C/day should be provided with formulas containing less than 10 and 5 mg ascorbic acid/100 ml, respectively. He suggested that if a high protein formula is used, the supplement should be raised to 100 mg/day. In contrast, he found that full-term infants could satisfy their vitamin C requirements with breast milk or formulas containing 6 mg ascorbic acid/100 ml. A supplement of only 30 mg/day was suggested for 3-week-old, full-term infants receiving diets containing 5 mg or less of ascorbic acid/100 ml.

Studies of capillary fragility of healthy breast-fed infants by Braestrup (54) indicated, however, that in the first 24 hours of life the vitamin C status of 35 premature infants was similar to that of 90 full-term babies. At 10 to 15 days of age, a slightly higher proportion of premature infants than of full-term infants showed signs of vitamin C deficiency. The difference was not significant and disappeared when the study included infants 15 days to 1 month of age.

Intradermal tests on 30 premature infants also indicated that their vitamin C status was similar to that of full-term infants (372). In 10 premature infants, followed for 8 weeks after birth, good concentrations of vitamin C were maintained in the tissues when supplements of 25 to 100 mg vitamin C/day were given. The intradermal tests did not indicate increased benefit from supplements higher than 25 mg/day. Observations on weight gains, however, though not statistically significant, suggested that a supplement of 50 mg/day promoted better development than the 25 mg dose did (372).

In studying vitamin C requirements of infants, whether premature or full-term, various methods have been used. These include estimates of the vitamin C available from breast milk (203, 367, 418), intradermal tests (372), plasma ascorbic acid measurements (55, 56, 156, 290, 374), saturation tests based on urinary excretion (246, 305, 429), and observations on growth and development with emphasis on the incidence of signs of scurvy (46, 157).

Breast milk contains more vitamin C than does cow's milk (165, 247, 298, 419). Average values calculated by Lawrence et al. (247) for human milk and cow's milk were 5 mg/100 ml and 2 mg/100 ml, respectively. A summary of the information on the vitamin C content of human milk compiled by Munks et al. (298) showed average values ranging from 0.8 to 6.6 mg ascorbic acid/100 ml. Munks et al. (298) determined the vitamin C content of 329 samples of breast milk. They found that the average ascorbic acid content of immature milk (secreted during the first 10 days postpartum) was 7.2 mg/100 ml and that of mature milk (including samples collected as late as month 12 of lactation) was 5.2 mg/100 ml. Selleg and King (367) observed that the vitamin C content of breast milk increased slightly as the mother's intake of vitamin C increased and that when the mother was eating a good diet the normal vitamin C content of her milk was about 6.0 to 8.0 mg/100 ml. This amount, they concluded, should meet the requirements of her infant. On this basis, and calculating a daily milk intake of 21 ounces (about 621 ml), they suggested that the infant's vitamin C requirement is about 40 to 50 mg/day during the first few weeks of life.

Ingalls (203) used a similar type of reasoning to arrive at a recommended vitamin C intake for infants. Assuming, on the basis of information in the literature, that human milk contains 4 mg ascorbic acid/100 ml and that an infant during the first 3 months of life would consume 500 to 1,000 ml of milk daily, he calculated that a normal baby would ingest about 20 to 40 mg of vitamin C daily. Because both cow's milk and pooled pasteurized human milk contain much less vitamin C than freshly expressed human milk, Ingalls suggested that the young artificially fed infant should receive a daily supplement of 20 to 30 mg vitamin C starting early in the neonatal period. Corroborating data were provided by Vitolin and Hesselvik (418) who determined the vitamin C content of freshly expressed human milk (5.08 mg/100 ml),

pooled human milk from a milk bank (1.31 mg/100 ml) and various infant formulas based on cow's milk (0.49 to 1.40 mg/100 ml). They concluded that artificially fed infants should receive a dietary supplement of 4 mg vitamin C/kg body weight.

Serum studies by Braestrup (56) indicated that the baby is born with a higher serum ascorbic content than his mother has at parturition. In Braestrup's studies, the mean serum ascorbic acid level of 23 infants at birth was 0.69 mg/100 ml. Within 22 to 26 hours the mean level had dropped to 0.39 mg/100 ml. During the next 4 days there was a further decline to a level (0.25 mg/100 ml) similar to that of the mothers at parturition (0.26 mg/100 ml). At 10 days of age the mean level was 0.27 mg/100 ml. Braestrup found that when the babies were fed cow's milk formulas their serum ascorbic acid levels remained at this low level for at least 4 to 5 weeks. If, however, daily supplements of 20 mg vitamin C were fed, the plasma ascorbic acid level gradually increased to approach the mean level observed at birth. Braestrup noted that this amount of vitamin C (20 mg/day) was approximately equivalent to the difference between the amount supplied daily by breast milk and that supplied by cow's milk. He concluded that all infants not given human milk should have a supplement of at least 20 mg vitamin C daily for the first few months of life. Because the vitamin C content of human milk varies with the mother's diet, he suggested also that breast-fed babies should be given extra vitamin C in winter and spring.

Hamil et al. (156) also observed that the plasma ascorbic acid levels of newborn infants declined during the first week of life. Urinary excretion of ascorbic acid was high during the first 2 days of life but declined to low levels by day 4. Hamil et al. suggested that these declines in plasma and urinary levels of vitamin C might be part of the physiological adjustment to life outside the womb.

Both Mindlin (290) and Snelling and Jackson (374) observed, however, that breast-fed infants had higher serum ascorbic acid levels than formula-fed babies had during the first month of life. In Mindlin's study 21 breast-fed infants, 12 to 14 days old, had plasma levels of 0.6 to 1.6 mg ascorbic acid/100 ml, with a mean of 1.0 mg/100 ml. Nineteen formula-fed infants, receiving no vitamin C, had serum ascorbic acid levels ranging from 0.1 to 0.7 mg with a mean of 0.3 mg/100 ml, a value similar to that observed by Braestrup (56) in 5- and 10-day-old infants. Bottle-fed infants who were given vitamin C supplements had serum levels ranging from 0.4 to 0.8 mg/100 ml. Observing that the longer a child was without vitamin C supplements, the lower its serum ascorbic acid level became, Mindlin recommended that formula fed infants should receive daily supplements of ascorbic acid beginning with the first day of feeding. Similarly, Snelling and Jackson (374) advised that the formula-fed baby should receive vitamin C supplements at least from the time he is 2 weeks old. Snelling and Jackson (374) also observed that serum ascorbic acid levels of breast-fed babies were related to the level of vitamin C in the breast milk. They therefore recommended that, if there was a possibility that the mother's vitamin C intake might be low, the breast-fed baby should receive vitamin C supplements.

In saturation studies with infants the urinary response to load doses of various sizes was measured. Neuweiler (305) studied infants about 9 to 10 days old who were fed breast milk, cow's milk formula, or a combination of breast milk and cow's milk. The infants' urinary excretions reflected their intakes. Test doses of 30 mg vitamin C/kg body weight were injected into 17 babies. Neuweiler calculated from the urinary excretion data obtained that the infants' mean requirement was about 6 mg vitamin C/kg body weight. In other saturation tests with infants ranging from 2 weeks to 12 months of age, both Laurin (246) and Widenbauer (429) observed that breast-fed infants were usually saturated with vitamin C. The intakes of the breast-fed infants observed by Laurin (246) were calculated to range from 2.5 to 10 mg/kg body weight. Formula-fed infants in her study showed evidence of vitamin C deficiency (delayed urinary response in the saturation test) as early as the first month of life. Widenbauer (429) also observed that his formula fed infants,

all of whom were sick, were vitamin C deficient as indicated by urinary response to a load dose. He concluded that supplements of 20 to 40 mg vitamin C/day were indicated for infants fed the customary formulas that contain little ascorbic acid.

In growth and development studies (46, 157), relatively low requirements for vitamin C were estimated. Hamil et al. (157) observed 427 infants during their first year of life. The average age of the infants at the beginning of the study was 5.5 weeks. The babies who lived in their own homes were supplied with an evaporated milk formula supplemented to provide about 10 mg vitamin C/day. Most of the children were examined monthly for at least 9 months. The examinations included blood counts, anthropometric measurements and roentgenological exposures. Some capillary resistance tests were made also.

None of the 427 infants showed roentgenological evidence of scurvy. Twenty-one infants, however, developed a condition identified as mild scurvy. They recovered spontaneously without any dietary change. Of these 21 infants, 14 received an average of 9 mg vitamin C/day. Seven of the 21 infants consumed less than 9 mg/day. Hamil et al. (157) concluded that since the mild scurvy healed spontaneously, it was not due to inadequate supply but to inefficient absorption "or to predisposition caused by some concurrent factor." They concluded, in addition, that "the minimal requirement of the average healthy infant lies near 10 mg of vitamin C daily."

A similar but slightly smaller requirement was estimated by Bischoff and Müller (46) in a 5-month study with 17 infants who ranged in age from 4 to 17 months. All children received a standard diet containing no fruit or vegetables. The children were divided into two groups, one group receiving a daily supplement of 100 to 200 mg vitamin C, and the other group a serving of carrots providing an average total intake of 7.48 mg vitamin C/day. No symptoms of scurvy or subclinical scurvy were observed, nor were there significant differences between the two groups in the incidence of infections. Bischoff and Müller (46) concluded that the infant does not require more than 8 mg vitamin C/day. Whether the much lower estimates resulting from these two studies as compared with those discussed previously, are due to the age of the children or to the difference in methodology is not clear.

Preschool children (2 to 5 years old) (Appendix table 3)

With the exception of one study on capillary fragility (240), most of the estimates of vitamin C requirements of preschool children have been based on studies of saturation as indicated by urinary ascorbic acid excretion. Everson and Daniels (108), for instance, measured urinary output of three boys, 39, 57 and 59 months old, in twelve 15-day periods with vitamin intakes ranging from 2.7 to 7.5 mg/kg and from 10.7 to 12.7 mg/kg. Assuming that all excess of vitamin C intake was excreted through the kidneys, Everson and Daniels calculated retention as the difference between intake and urinary excretion (intake − urinary excretion = retention). Retention, which ranged from 1.7 to 4.3 mg/kg, rose as intake increased up to 7.5 mg/kg. With intakes between 10.7 and 12.7 mg/kg, the retentions were not higher than those observed with intakes between 6.4 and 7.5 mg/kg. Everson·and Daniels suggested therefore that 7.5 mg/kg is the minimum requirement for children of this age group. The total daily intake at this level (7.5 mg/kg) was about 118 mg vitamin C. This estimate is considerably higher than those of other investigators working with this age group. Meyer and Robinson (285), for instance, in a study of the vitamin C intakes, blood levels and urinary excretions of about 228 healthy infants and young children, concluded that the latter required approximately 30 to 45 mg vitamin C/day.

Similarly, Hathaway and Meyer (167) found, in a study with four preschool children, that an intake of 31 mg/day was "marginal" for saturation. In a later study with eight children, Meyer and Hathaway (284) found the intakes of 23 to 25 mg vitamin C/day were insufficient to maintain saturation. In their studies, a child was assumed to be saturated when he excreted 50% of a load dose of 200 mg ascorbic acid within 24 hours of its administration. Hathaway and Meyer (167) reported, in addition, that the vitamin C requirement did not appear to be related to sex, age, or body weight.

In other saturation studies with preschool children, Snisarenko (376) measured the urinary ascorbic acid excretion 4 hours before and 4 after a load dose of 100 mg. The reported data indicated that an intake of 35 to 50 mg vitamin C/day is required to maintain the children in a saturated state.

Even lower estimates were made by Widenbauer (430) who, by the method previously described (page 832), found with one 2- to 3-year-old boy that an intake of 21 to 22 mg vitamin C/day was sufficient to allow an excretion just slightly above the so-called "baseline" (excretion with a very low vitamin C intake).

In studies on capillary fragility of 30 children, carried out by Kosenko and Krajko (240), no change in capillary fragility was noted when diets containing 5 to 18 mg vitamin C were supplemented with varying amounts (50 to 200 mg) of the vitamin. The English summary of this report did not indicate that a vitamin C requirement had been estimated.

School children (6 to 12 years old) (Appendix table 3)

The vitamin C needs of school children have been studied by measuring blood levels of ascorbic acid. In addition, data on urinary excretion with varying intakes have been used as a basis for estimates of requirements. Some observations have been made also on vitamin C retention, capillary resistance and physical growth as influenced by vitamin C intake.

When blood levels were used to determine vitamin C requirements, the estimates were based on the ascorbic acid content of plasma, serum or white blood cells. Holmes et al. (191) observed a wide range of plasma ascorbic acid levels in apparently healthy children. They suggested, therefore, that vitamin C status could not be adequately estimated from a single determination of plasma ascorbic acid. Bessey and White (45) also found much variation in plasma ascorbic acid levels at any one level of intake and they noted that low plasma levels were not accompanied by vitamin C deficiency symptoms. In their study with 93 children, 5 to 13 years old, they measured plasma ascorbic acid levels and they calculated vitamin C intake from 24-hour dietary histories. Plasma ascorbic acid values were plotted against vitamin C intake in order to assess the minimum intake required to give the average maximum postabsorptive plasma ascorbic acid level. A curve drawn through the average plasma values increased to about 1.0 mg/100 ml at an intake of about 45 mg/day and then leveled. Bessey and White concluded that the vitamin C "requirement may be placed at 40 to 50 mg daily."

Roberts and Roberts (351) studied plasma ascorbic acid levels of five children, 7 to 12 years old, with varying levels of vitamin C intake. In this study and in a subsequent investigation with 30 girls (350), plasma levels, with much variation among subjects, increased as vitamin C intakes increased. Roberts and Roberts (351) reported that the plasma levels of their five children, initially 0.5 to 0.6 mg/100 ml, increased to a plateau at 1.15 to 1.29 mg/100 ml. The lowest intakes at which maximum plasma levels were observed were 105 to 125 mg/day. Daily intakes of 65 to 95 mg were needed to maintain plasma levels at 0.9 mg/100 ml and intakes of 55 to 65 mg/day were needed for plasma levels of 0.7 mg/100 ml. Similarly, Roberts et al. (350) found with 30 girls that intakes of 52 to 72 mg vitamin C/day were needed to maintain a plasma ascorbic acid level of 0.7 mg/100 ml. More recently, Ritchey (347) observed that 12 girls, 7 to 10 years old, were able to maintain plasma concentrations of about 0.7 mg/100 ml with vitamin C intakes of 66 to 68 mg/day.

Nicol (307) studied vitamin C metabolism in 40 pairs of Nigerian children, 9 to 15 years old. The children were paired by sex, age and height. One member of each pair was given a vitamin C supplement; the other child received a placebo. The supplement provided 33 mg vitamin C/day during the mango season and 21 mg/day when mangos were not in season. The normal diet provided 208 mg/day vitamin C during the mango season and 58 to 70 mg/day at other times. Cooking losses reduced the intakes to 175 mg in mango season and to 14 to 18 mg/day during the rest of the year. When mangos were unavailable, plasma ascorbic acid levels were 0.49 mg/100 ml in the supplemented group and 0.25 mg/100 ml in the unsupplemented group. During mango season these levels rose to 0.97 and 0.73 mg/100 ml, respectively. Intake and plasma levels were correlated in the untreated group but not in the supplemented group during mango season. Nicol suggested that the latter group might have been saturated. The supplemented group had significantly greater gains in height than the unsupplemented group but weight gains were not significantly different. Nicol interpreted this observation as indicating that the unsupplemented children's average intake of vitamin C was not sufficient to maintain the maximum rate of growth otherwise possible with the diet.

In a study in which serum ascorbic acid was measured, Dallyn and Moschette (88) found in data obtained from 7-day dietary records and blood analyses of 463 children, 8 to 11 years old, that there was a significant linear relationship between vitamin C intake and serum ascorbic acid levels until intakes above 110 mg/day or serum ascorbic acid levels above 1.1 mg/100 were reached. The graphical presentation of their data indicated that they were in agreement with Moyer et al. (297) who found with four children that "a daily intake of about 60 mg of vitamin C was consistent with a serum vitamin C concentration of 0.7 mg or more/100 cc."

The relationship of white blood cell content of ascorbic acid to intake of vitamin C was studied by Wilson and Lubschez (437) in a study with 76 healthy children, 2 to 14 years old and 40 rheumatic patients 6 to 15 years old. With intakes below 0.5 to 1.9 mg/kg body weight (15 to 40 mg/day) the white blood cell content of ascorbic acid was usually less than 25 mg/100 g. With intakes of 1.5 to 2.9 mg/kg (50 to 75 mg/day) the white blood cell content was usually 25 mg/100 g or more. With higher intakes (100 to 200 mg/day), the white blood cell content did not increase. In fact, with vitamin C intakes greater than 9 mg/kg (200 to 300 mg/day), most of the white blood cell ascorbic acid levels decreased to less than 25 mg/100 g. Wilson and Lubschez concluded that to ensure a white blood cell ascorbic acid level of 25 mg/100 g or more, an intake of 100 mg vitamin C/day is necessary. They also suggested that large intakes of 200 to 300 mg/day are unnecessary and inadvisable.

Russian studies (280) have also shown a relationship between white blood cell ascorbic acid levels and vitamin C intake. In studies with 20 children 8 to 14 years old Matsko et al. (280) found that the lowest vitamin C intake at which the maximal phagocytic reaction could be obtained was 50 mg/day. As intakes increased from 50 mg to 80 mg/day the white blood cell ascorbic acid content increased. Children who had intakes of 120 mg/day, however, had lower white blood cell ascorbic acid levels than children with intakes of 80 mg/day. There was no indication that intakes between 80 and 120 mg/day were studied.

When urinary excretion was studied, the daily ascorbic acid output uninfluenced by load doses (the "resting" excretion) was measured in some investigations. In others, the urinary response to saturation doses of vitamin C was used as the basis for estimates of requirements. Roberts and Roberts (351) reported that the "resting" urinary ascorbic acid excretion of their five children varied in direct relationship to the intake. They found that the average excretion increased from 16 to 91 mg/day when the vitamin C intake increased from 55 to 135 mg. An ascorbic acid excretion of 40 mg, assumed to indicate saturation (411), occurred in one subject with an intake of 75 mg and in the other four with intakes of 85 mg/day. Excretion increased as intake increased but vitamin C retention (intake minus urinary excretion) did not vary greatly. Roberts and Roberts reported that "the lowest intake on which each subject 'retained' an amount of ascorbic acid equivalent to the average 'retention value' ranges from 55 mg for two of the children to 75 mg for the other three."

In subsequent work, Roberts et al. (350) studied 30 children divided into six groups of five subjects each. Their diet provided approximately 22 mg vitamin C daily. The groups of children received supplements ranging from 10 to 60 mg ascorbic acid/day. Mean urinary ascorbic acid excretions increased from 8 mg to 31 mg/day as intakes increased from 32 to 72 mg/day. An additional increase in intake to 82 mg/day

was not accompanied by an increase in excretion. Only two children, with daily intakes of 72 and 82 mg, excreted more than 40 mg ascorbic acid/day. Bumbalo (64) found that among healthy children, there was wide variation in the level of daily excretion. With 16 healthy children 5 to 13 years old, 24-hour urinary ascorbic acid excretions varying from 11 to 71 mg/day were observed. The dietary intakes of these children were not analyzed. Kosenko and Krajko (240), also finding that daily urinary ascorbic acid excretion was highly variable, reported that the hourly excretion rate was a better guide in evaluating vitamin C status. Konovalova and Medvedeva (239) studied a group of 8- to 10-year-old children whose diet supplied 3.5 to 9 mg vitamin C/day. With this intake, the fasting urinary ascorbic acid varied from 0.2 to 0.5 mg/hour. A daily supplement of 50 mg vitamin C brought the urinary excretion up to 0.7 mg/hour, which the investigators considered to be the "normal" rate. Growth rates and hemoglobin levels also improved. Konovalova and Medvedeva recommended that 50 to 75 mg vitamin C should be provided daily for school children in western Siberia.

In another Russian study with 67 boarding school children in Omsk, Yakutina (445) found that the diets, after cooking, provided only 19 to 23 mg vitamin C in autumn and 5 to 10 mg in spring. When the diets were supplemented with 50 to 100 mg vitamin C, urinary ascorbic acid excretion rose from low levels to about 0.75 mg/hour. Capillary resistance which was 90 to 150 mg Hg before supplementation was increased to 130 to 180 mg Hg after supplementation. Yakutina recommended that children should receive supplements of 75 to 100 mg vitamin C in fall and at least 100 mg in spring.

Urinary response to test doses of ascorbic acid has been the basis for some estimates of requirements. Pemberton (321), for instance, studied 62 orphan boys 10 to 14 years old. The boys were divided into two groups, one of whom ate the customy institution diet providing 35 mg vitamin C/day. This estimate of dietary content was reached by calculating the vitamin content of "gross quantities of uncooked food before it was supplied to the children." The second group received dietary supplements that increased their calculated vitamin C intake to 63 mg/day. Urinary ascorbic acid excretion was measured before and for 4 hours after a test dose of about 7.9 mg vitamin C/kg body weight. The concentration of ascorbic acid in the urine of the supplemented group was much higher after the test dose (34.0 mg/100 ml) than before it (1.66 mg/100 ml). In the group of boys eating the unsupplemented diet, there were no significant changes in concentration of urinary ascorbic acid after the test dose (1.00 vs 1.07 mg/100 ml). Pemberton (321) suggested on the basis of these observations that 35 mg/day was probably close to "the minimum physiological requirement" whereas 63 mg/day represented an adequate intake.

Harris (161), in a study with 35 boys, used a procedure developed earlier by Harris and Abbasy (163). By this procedure, a test dose of 11.0 mg vitamin C/kg body weight was given in the morning and a 2.25-hour sample of urine was collected about 5 hours later. This procedure was repeated each day until the 2.25-hour urine specimen contained at least 0.8 mg ascorbic acid/kg body weight. When this occurred, the subject was assumed to be saturated. Harris divided the boys into three groups. Group 1 ate the institution diet, providing 20 to 25 mg vitamin C/day, with no supplement. Groups 2 and 3 ate the same diet supplemented with 15 and 25 mg vitamin C, respectively. The urinary excretions showed that all of the boys in group 3 (with daily intakes of 45 to 50 mg) were saturated on the first day of dosing, and all the boys in group 2 (daily intakes of 35 to 40 mg) were saturated after the second day of dosing. The boys in group 1 required 3 days of dosing. Harris concluded that intakes of 35 to 40 mg vitamin C/day were sufficient to maintain the boys in a state of "near saturation."

Roberts and Roberts (351) assumed that a subject was saturated with vitamin C when he excreted 50% or more of a 300 mg test dose within 24 hours of its administration. By this criteria, the youngest of their five 7- to 12-year-old subjects was saturated with a daily intake of 55 mg vitamin C. The other four required intakes of 65 or 75 mg/day for saturation. When the

method of Belser et al. (43) was used (see page 833), requirements for saturation were estimated as 65 to 95 mg/day. In a later study with 30 girls, 6 to 12 years old (350), daily intakes of 52 to 72 mg vitamin C were sufficient to permit excretion of 50% of the test dose. More recently, Verbinets (416) in a study with 30 boarding school children, 10 to 12 years old, living in a region where goitre is endemic, estimated a vitamin C requirement of 130 mg/day. The English abstract of this report did not describe the procedures that were used.

Adolescents (12 to 18 years old) (Appendix table 3)

Adolescents' requirements for vitamin C have been estimated principally by measuring the response of blood plasma and white blood cells to varying levels of vitamin C intake. Urinary response has been measured in only a few studies.

Oldham et al. (309) suggested that healthy children eating a good diet would have plasma ascorbic acid levels of 0.6 mg/100 ml or more. In their study with boarding school children, they found that the customary diet provided approximately 49 mg vitamin C/day for the adolescents. With this diet, over 40% of all of the children had plasma ascorbic acid levels below 0.6 mg/100 ml. The diet was supplemented with pineaple juice to provide 97 mg vitamin C/day for the adolescent pupils. At the end of 6 months only 8% of the children had plasma levels below 0.6 mg/100 ml and none had a level below 0.5 mg/100 ml. The proportion of the children having plasma levels above 0.8 mg/100 ml increased from 28% to 62% after the pineapple juice was added to the diet.

Storvick et al. (385, 386) suggested that it was probably desirable "during the strain of adolescent growth to maintain all children near saturation." In their studies, plasma levels above 0.8 mg/100 ml were considered to be near saturation levels. They studied four boys and four girls, 12 to 14 years old, during three 7-day periods. In period 1, the children ate their customary diets which provided the boys with 59 to 62 mg vitamin C/day and the girls with 41 to 50 mg daily. Plasma ascorbic acid levels ranged from 0.73 to 0.78 mg/100 ml for the boys and from 0.20 to 0.47

mg/100 ml for the girls. During period 2, the investigators saturated the children by supplementing their diets with 200 mg vitamin C/day. Plasma levels increased to range from 1.10 to 1.37 mg/100 ml for the boys and from 1.03 to 1.35 mg/100 ml for the girls. During period 3, the diets were adjusted to provide the then current recommended allowances of 75 and 90 mg vitamin C for the boys, and 80 mg for the girls (303). Plasma ascorbic acid levels declined to range from 0.84 to 0.98 mg/100 ml for the boys and 0.86 to 1.21 mg/100 ml for the girls. Storvick et al. (385) suggested that these plasma levels, which were associated with "good" but not saturated stores of ascorbic acid, indicated that adolescents require more vitamin C than either younger children or adults. In a Japanese study, however, Nagai (299) was able to maintain 12- to 14-year-old boys and girls in a saturated state with intakes (1.6 to 1.8 mg/kg body weight) similar to or lower than those of Storvick et al. (385) (1.9 to 2.1 mg/kg for boys and 1.3 to 1.7 mg/kg for girls).

In a subsequent study with older adolescents, eight boys and eight girls, 16 to 19 years old, Storvick et al. (383, 384) found that the then recommended allowances of vitamin C (100 mg/day for the boys and 80 mg/day for the girls) were sufficient to maintain high but not saturated plasma ascorbic acid levels (0.67 to 0.91 mg/100 ml for the boys and 0.83 to 1.07 mg/100 ml for the girls). Intakes reduced by 10 mg/day (90 mg for the boys and 70 mg for the girls) were as effective as the recommended allowances in maintaining adequate plasma levels in most of the subjects. These intakes (1.1 to 1.5 mg/kg for boys and 1.0 to 1.4 mg/kg for girls) were lower than those that maintained similar blood ascorbic acid levels in the younger adolescents (386) but were similar to the intakes of a group of apprentices studied by Wirths (439). In this study (439), the mean intake of 25 apprentices was 91 mg/day (1.55 mg/kg). The boys' mean plasma ascorbic acid concentration was 1.06 mg/100 ml.

Storvick's suggestion that adolescent children should be maintained near the saturation level, has received support from the data collected in a nutritional status study by Hard et al. (158). They found that the average vitamin C intakes of boys and girls, 15 to 16 years old, in two counties of the State of Washington were 82 and 83 mg/day (boys) and 79 and 59 mg/day (girls). Serum ascorbic acid levels varied from 0.64 to 0.86 mg/100 ml. In spite of these apparently adequate intakes, some clinical evidence of gingival lesions and hyperemia of the upper arm suggested a slight deficiency of vitamin C.

Wilcox and Grimes (433) found that the vitamin C content of white blood cells and platelets was lower in Navajo boarding school students with gingivitis than in those with normal gingiva. Four groups of subjects, 12 to 22 years old, were studied upon their arrival at the school. Two groups (186 subjects) had gingivitis; the other two groups (control) had normal gingiva. The boarding school diet provided 78 mg vitamin C/day for the boys and 62 mg/day for the girls. Mean white cell-platelet vitamin C contents initially were 12.2 and 14.0 mg/100 g for groups 1 and 2 (gingivitis) and 15.9 and 17.2 mg/100 g for groups 3 and 4 (normal gingiva). Groups 1 and 3 received a supplement of 300 mg vitamin C/day for 3 weeks. At the end of this period, white cell-platelet vitamin C levels had risen to 25.0 and 25.6 mg/100 g in groups 1 and 3 (supplemented) and to 17.2 and 17.9 mg/100 g in groups 2 and 4 (unsupplemented). Further increases to a mean of 32.9 mg/100 g were observed in group 2 when, during weeks 4 to 6, these subjects received a supplement of 300 mg vitamin C/day. At the end of 6 months with no additional supplementation, all four groups had mean values ranging from 23.2 to 27.4 mg/100 g, indicating that the amount of vitamin C contributed by the diet (78 mg for boys; 62 mg for girls) was sufficient to raise mean levels from low normal to high normal (83) and to maintain levels that were already in the high normal range. Khaustova (221) on the other hand, concluded, from a study with 14- to 17-year-old boys in a Russian boarding school, that the daily requirement was 100 mg vitamin C. In this study, the phagocytic index and proportion of phagocytes in total white cells reached satisfactory levels only after 100 mg vitamin C/day had been added to the diet for 2.5 months. The boarding school diet provided only 4 to 9 mg vitamin C/day. The English abstract of this paper did not indicate what Khaustova considered to be satisfactory levels for the phagocytic index.

When urinary response to known vitamin C intakes was measured, Glazebrook and Thomson (135) concluded that intakes of 60 to 65 mg vitamin C/day were needed to maintain normal urinary ascorbic acid excretion (13 to 15 mg/day). They studied boys, 15 to 20 years old, whose customary diet provided 10 to 15 mg vitamin C daily. When some of these boys who showed clinical signs of vitamin C deficiency were dosed with 200 mg ascorbic acid/day, their urinary excretion gradually increased until, by day 23, it indicated that saturation had been achieved. The dose was then reduced to 50 mg/day. With this level of supplementation, normal urinary ascorbic acid excretion was maintained.

Much higher intakes were recommended by Hoske (198) who studied the concentration of ascorbic acid in the urine. The concentration of ascorbic acid was determined daily in morning samples of urine collected under controlled conditions over a period of approximately 3 weeks. The average rate of excretion of boys and girls 14 to 18 years old was 2.0 mg/100 ml when consuming their customary diet providing 79 mg vitamin C/day or 45 mg when corrected for cooking losses. When this same diet was supplemented with 64.5 mg, thus providing an ascorbic acid intake of 109 mg/day, urinary excretion increased to about 5 mg/100 ml. Based on earlier reports that a vitamin C deficiency exists when the rate of excretion is less than 5 mg/100 ml, Hoske suggested that adolescents, 14 to 18 years old, require about 125 mg vitamin C/day.

Pregnant women (Appendix table 4)

Early studies with guinea pigs (94) indicated that the pregnant organism was highly sensitive to vitamin C deficiency. Later studies with human subjects (122, 124, 304) suggested that ascorbic acid stores were smaller in pregnant than in nonpregnant women. Neuweiler (304), for instance, studied 21 nonpregnant, 23 pregnant and 22 lactating women. After each subject was given 200 mg vitamin C intravenously, urinary ascorbic acid excretion was measured for 3 days. The nonpregnant women excreted more ascorbic acid than the pregnant women did. The lactating women excreted the least. Gaehtgens and Werner (122, 124) estimated the vitamin C status of 26 healthy pregnant women by measuring the number of days required to achieve saturation when a dose of 300 mg ascorbic acid was administered intravenously each day. A subject was assumed to be saturated when she excreted at least 50% of the test dose within 12 hours of its administration. In nonpregnant healthy women, saturation normally occurred within 4 days. Seventeen of the 26 pregnant women required more than 4 days for saturation. Gaehtgens and Werner (122) attributed the assumed deficits to the accumulation of vitamin C in the fetus and placenta. That the fetus is not completely parasitic, however, was suggested by evidence of a relationship between low serum ascorbic acid levels in the mother and the incidence of anencephaly in the fetus (402) and of perinatal death and premature rupture of the fetal membranes (428). Studies by Javert and Stander (208) and by King (224) also suggested that the administration of vitamin C to pregnant women was beneficial in preventing spontaneous abortion. In addition, Chernous (71) reported that the ascorbic acid level in the placenta and adrenals of fetuses and neonates who died of asphyxia was reduced as compared with that of normal infants. The English summary of this paper did not suggest which condition was the cause and which the effect of the other. Martin et al. (274), however, found few significant relationships between the maternal serum ascorbic acid levels and the outcome of pregnancy. They pointed out that causal relationships could not be established from their data gathered in a study of 2,046 women during pregnancy.

Numerous investigators have reported that blood ascorbic acid levels decreased during the course of pregnancy (208, 269, 274, 278, 374). Others (93, 184, 293, 448) have reported no significant changes. The reason for the decreases that have been reported is not clear. Martin et al. (274) noted that a group of subjects with consistently high intakes (80–100 mg/day) maintained essentially the same average serum vitamin C throughout pregnancy in contrast to the decrease observed with pregnancy in the subjects receiving lower intakes. In general, however, they found that the correlation between serum ascorbic acid levels and vitamin C intake was not high.

Observations that the vitamin C content of umbilical cord blood and fetal blood was higher than that of the maternal blood (32, 55, 220, 292, 372) suggest the possibility of placental synthesis of ascorbic acid. The evidence however is contradictory. Barnes (32) reported that his in vitro experiments with placental slices did not indicate that the placenta could synthesize vitamin C. Rajalakshmi et al. (340), on the other hand, reported "tentative" data indicating that in 27 out of 40 cases, studied in vitro, placental synthesis of ascorbic acid took place. Khattab et al. (220) have suggested that the higher ascorbic acid levels in fetal blood as compared to maternal blood may be because the vitamin is transferred as dehydroascorbic acid across the placenta. It is then reduced to ascorbic acid in the fetus and is retained there. They suggested further that the extent of the placental transfer of dehydroascorbic acid would depend on the level of ascorbic acid in the maternal blood.

Vitamin C requirements in pregnancy have been estimated in a few studies from measurement of blood ascorbic acid levels. In other studies, urinary response to test doses of vitamin C was observed.

Javert and Stander (208) studied the plasma ascorbic acid levels over the course of pregnancy. A total of 376 blood samples was obtained from 246 patients. They found, as noted previously, that plasma ascorbic acid levels fell progressively during pregnancy. In 100 deficient pregnant women, however, they were able to effect a rise in plasma levels to normal nonpregnant levels. This was accomplished by administering 100 mg vitamin C and 100 ml orange juice daily to each patient. They concluded, therefore, that the pregnant woman needs about 200 mg vitamin C daily.

Martin et al. (274) grouped the subjects of their study according to their daily vitamin C intakes: consistently high (80 mg or more; 193 cases), consistently intermediate (40–80 mg; 262 cases) or consistently low (under 40 mg; 166 cases). They found that the women with the high intakes maintained their serum ascorbic acid at about the same level throughout pregnancy. Those with intermediate intakes maintained their serum levels during trimester 1. During trimesters 2 and 3, however, they experienced a decrease in serum levels. The women with low intakes had low serum levels early in pregnancy. As pregnancy progressed their serum levels declined further. During the postpartum period all groups had lower levels than those observed antepartum. Martin et al. (274) concluded that vitamin C intakes of 80 to 100 mg/day supported high serum ascorbic acid levels in pregnancy. The median serum levels reported for the high intake group varied between 0.46 and 0.76 mg/100 ml during the first 33 weeks of pregnancy.

Estimates similar to that of Martin et al. (274) resulted from observations of urinary response to load doses of vitamin C. Widenbauer (430) estimated by his method, described previously (page 832), that the minimum requirement of a nonpregnant woman was 28 mg vitamin C/day. With a pregnant woman the estimated requirement was 71 mg/day in month 3 and 67 mg/day in month 8 of gestation. Gaehtgens (121), using a similar method, studied the requirements of 10 women in months 8 and 9 of pregnancy. Observing that the estimates of requirement ranged from 33 to 64 mg/day, he suggested that a safe allowance during pregnancy might be 100 mg vitamin C/day.

Toverud (399, 400) studied 8 normal nongravid women, 12 pregnant women and 10 lactating women living in a home where the diet provided about 30 mg vitamin C/day. The women were given 500 ml orange juice containing about 250 mg vitamin C (423) and urinary ascorbic acid excretion was measured during the next 24 hours. The nongravid women excreted at least 50% of the test dose; the pregnant women excreted less than 26%; the lactating women excreted 10% or less. The home diet was then supplemented with 200 ml of rose hip juice which raised the ascorbic acid content of the diet to at least 75 mg/day in winter and possibly to 100 mg/day in summer. With this diet, four of seven women tested were saturated (excreted 50% of a 250 mg test dose of pure ascorbic acid) in summer but only two of nine pregnant women were saturated in winter. When an additional dose of 100 mg vitamin C was added each day to the winter diet, the women gradually became saturated over a 3-week period. Toverud concluded that the vitamin C intake of the pregnant woman should not fall below 75 mg/day. There was no indication in her reports of a change in requirement over the course of pregnancy.

In Toverud's study (400) analysis of blood samples taken 2 hours after the test dose of ascorbic acid was given indicated that blood ascorbic acid levels rose as the women approached saturation. Although most of the women had blood ascorbic acid levels above 0.6 mg/100 ml, there was a considerable range in the values (0.3 to 1.3 mg/100 ml) when they were in a saturated state as indicated by urinary excretion. Toverud concluded that "a blood analysis is of great value but does not, according to these experiments, give a more precise indication of saturation of the organism than repeated urine analyses following a large test dose."

Lactating women (Appendix table 4)

The natural source of vitamin C for the young infant is his mother's milk. The vitamin C content of breast milk, however, varies widely depending principally on the vitamin C status of the lactating women. In literature summarized by Munks et al. (298) and in other papers (247, 250, 268), values ranging from 0.5 to 9.0 mg vitamin C/100 ml milk were reported. The vitamin C content of milk can be raised by increasing the mother's vitamin C intake (42, 76, 97, 123, 367, 431). There is, however, apparently an upper limit to which the level of ascorbic acid can be raised in milk. Baumann (39), in studies on three wet nurses with varying vitamin C intakes, found that as the intake increased, blood and milk ascorbic acid values increased until saturation was achieved. After the subject became saturated, the ascorbic acid level remained at about 1.4 mg/100 ml in the blood and at 8 mg/100 ml in the milk. With further increases in intake, urinary ascorbic acid excretion increased. Baumann (39) reported that blood ascorbic acid levels under 1.0 mg/100 ml were associated with milk values under 3.5 to 4 mg/100 ml. Blood levels lower than 0.8 to 1.0 mg/100 ml and milk values under 3.5 to 4.0 mg/100 ml indicated that the lactating woman's body was being depleted of vitamin C. Additional observations led Baumann and Rappolt (40) to conclude that the vitamin C content of milk depends on the vitamin C content of the mother's body which, in turn, depends on the vitamin C content of her diet and on the amount of milk produced. There was no indication in the literature that the mother's vitamin C intake per se affected the amount of milk she secreted.

Martin et al. (274) analysed the data on vitamin C intake and serum ascorbic acid levels of 827 lactating and 637 nonlactating women. They found a lower median serum level in the lactating group (0.16 mg/100 ml) than in the nonlactating group (0.29 mg/100 ml) when women with similar intakes were compared. They concluded that the low values in lactation were a reflection of lactation rather than the result of a preexisting difference between those who lactated and those who did not. They found that, even with high intakes (120 mg vitamin C or more/day), the lactating women had serum ascorbic acid levels of only 0.3 mg/100 ml. No information was given on the vitamin C concentration in the milk.

Baumann (39) and other investigators (409, 438) have reported seasonal variations in the vitamin C content of breast milk. These have usually been attributed to seasonal variations in the dietary intake. Martin et al. (274), however, noting seasonal variation in serum ascorbic acid levels, suggested that there could possibly be a seasonal variation in vitamin C requirements.

The concentration of vitamin C in breast milk varies over the course of lactation. Both Selleg and King (367) and Lembrych and Lika (250) found that the concentration rose during the first 10 days postpartum. Macy (268) and Munks et al. (298), however, found little difference between the mean concentration of vitamin C in colostrum secreted during the first 5 days postpartum (7.2 mg/100 ml) and that of "transitional" milk secreted during days 6 through 10 postpartum (7.1 mg/100 ml). In their study, they determined the ascorbic acid content of sixty 24-hour collections of immature milk secreted in the first 10 days postpartum and of 269 samples of mature milk collected throughout lactation. The mean vitamin C concentration of the mature milk (5.2 mg/100 ml) was lower than that of the immature milk. Whether the difference in concentration was due to changes in dietary intake or perhaps to changes in milk volume was not clear. Munks et al. (298) also reported that the concentration fluctuated throughout the 24-hour collection period. They suggested that accurate values for vitamin C secretion in milk could be obtained only by analysis of the complete 24-hour collection.

In estimating vitamin C requirements for lactating women the total amount or the concentration of ascorbic acid secreted in the milk has been the main criterion. Balance studies, saturation tests and measurements of serum ascorbic acid have also been used. Neuweiler (304) in early studies deduced that lactating women had higher vitamin C requirements than either nonpregnant or pregnant women because, with comparable intakes, they had lower urinary ascorbic acid outputs. Gaehtgens and Werner (123) observed that 10 nursing mothers during the first 10 days postpartum did not secrete enough ascorbic acid to meet the assumed needs of their infants (25 mg/day). Even when 100 mg vitamin C was administered daily to 20 women the ascorbic acid secretion did not increase enough to meet the infants' needs. Gaehtgens and Werner suggested, therefore, that infants should be provided with vitamin C supplements early in life.

Widenbauer and Kuhner (431) with six nursing women found that they could raise the milk ascorbic acid concentration from a range of 0.5 to 2.2 mg/100 ml to a range of 3.8 to 7.8 mg/100 ml by saturating the women with vitamin C. They observed that with a total daily consumption of 53 to 135 mg vitamin C the women secreted from 33 to 67 mg ascorbic acid/day in their milk. Widenbauer and Kuhner (431) deduced therefore that, in order to provide their infants with optimal intakes of 40 to 50 mg vitamin C/day, lactating mothers should consume 80 to 100 mg vitamin C/day.

A similar requirement was suggested by Toverud (399, 400). She found that the milk of 15 lactating women, whose customary diet provided 75 mg vitamin C/ day, had a mean vitamin C content of about 3.9 mg/100 ml. Saturation tests indicated that the women were quite depleted of vitamin C. As the women were gradually saturated by supplemental doses of 100 mg vitamin C/day the milk ascorbic acid gradually increased. Toverud calculated that, in order to provide the infant with about 25 to 30 mg vitamin C/day, the mother's milk should contain 5 to 6 mg ascorbic acid/100 ml. To achieve this concentration, she said, the lactating women needed about 100 mg vitamin C/day.

Deodhar et al. (97) and Rajalakshmi et al. (339), however, have reported that, in studies with Indian women, they found that some women were apparently secreting more vitamin C in the milk than they were ingesting in their daily diet. Clinical examinations during the lactation period (6 to 7 months) revealed no evidence of scurvy in the mothers or infants. They recognized that the possibility of underestimation of intake and overestimation of milk secretion (determined by weighing the infant before and after feeding) did exist, but they decided that the deficit was too great to be thus accounted for. After finding additional evidence in the literature of apparently negative vitamin C balances in lactation, they suggested that human ascorbic acid requirements during pregnancy, lactation and infancy be reviewed with the possibility of endogenous synthesis of the vitamin in mind.

The elderly (Appendix table 5)

The elderly, in general, are reputed to be in poor vitamin C status (125, 150, 336, 338, 393). The evidence for this poor status has been acquired principally through measurement of blood ascorbic acid levels. Studies by Trier (401), Difs (98) and Hagtvet (152, 153) summarized by Kirk and Chieffi (231) indicated that serum ascorbic acid levels tended to decrease with age although a statistically significant correlation between age and ascorbic acid level was not always shown. Kirk and Chieffi (231) studied whole blood ascorbic acid levels of 81 men and 61 women, 40 to 103 years old, whose daily diet supplied about 45 mg vitamin C. The actual dietary intakes were not measured. The blood values for the men decreased from 0.59 mg/100 ml (40 to 59 years old) to 0.33 mg/100 ml (80 to 103 years old). The values for the women fell from 0.48 mg/100 ml (40 to 59 years old) to 0.40 mg/100 ml (80 to 87 years old). There was a significant negative correlation between age and blood ascorbic acid levels in the men but not in the women.

Roderuck et al. (353) also found no major changes with age in whole blood serum, or plasma ascorbic acid concentration in women. They studied 569 women, 20 to 99 years of age, in five midwestern states of the U.S.A. The mean vitamin C intakes of the women ranged from 60 to 104 mg/day. Mean whole blood ascorbic acid studied in 49 women was 0.88 mg/100 ml; mean serum ascorbic acid ranged from 0.89 to 1.20 mg/100 ml for 217 women; and mean plasma ascorbic acid ranged from 0.76 to 0.84 mg/100 ml for 371 women.

Milne et al. (288), on the other hand, found that leukocyte ascorbic acid concentrations decreased significantly with age in women but not in men. Their data were obtained in a study with 215 men and 272 women, 69 to 94 years old, whose mean vitamin C intakes were about 32 mg/day for the men and 31 mg/day for the women. The mean leukocyte ascorbic acid levels decreased with age for men from 17.7 $\mu g/10^8$ cells to 14.6 $\mu g/10^8$ cells and for women, from 26.4 $\mu g/10^8$ cells to 16.5 $\mu g/10^8$ cells. Loh and Wilson (259) also found that the fall in leukocyte ascorbic acid levels was greater in elderly women than in elderly men.

In studies in which blood ascorbic acid levels of the elderly have been compared with those of young or middle aged adults, the elderly frequently have had lower levels in whole blood (231, 232), serum (270), plasma (53, 216, 426), and in leukocytes (10, 53, 207, 216, 259). Kirk (230) noted that differences in blood ascorbic acid levels between the aged and the young usually showed up with low or moderate intakes but not with very low or very high intakes.

The prevalence of low blood ascorbic acid concentrations in the elderly suggested to Kirk (229) that they might be a physiological characteristic of old age. In a subsequent study with 19 elderly patients, Kirk and Chieffi (232) were able to raise the whole blood ascorbic acid levels of 16 subjects from below 0.3 mg/100 ml to approximately 1.15 mg/100 ml by administering 100 mg vitamin C/day orally. When the supplement was withdrawn, the blood levels dropped quickly to their initial values. Because the low levels were not associated with signs of scurvy, Kirk and Chieffi questioned the desirability of raising the blood ascorbic acid values of the elderly to the levels found in normal young adults. Other investigators have suggested that some attributes, frequently ascribed to old age, such as lack of vitality and susceptibility to infection (125), vague aches and pains, purpuric spots and indolent ulcers (216), multiple bruises and normocytic anemia (291) may be manifestations of latent vitamin C deficiency. Attempts to relate blood ascorbic acid levels in the elderly to clinical signs of scurvy, however, have not been notably successful (10, 12, 15).

Impaired absorption or utilization has been suggested as a cause of low blood ascorbic acid levels in a few cases (232, 336). Inadequate dietary intake, however, has been the principal cause suggested (11, 230, 313, 337). Other investigators have reported seasonal variations in blood levels (38, 288, 401) and variation with economic status (75, 294, 313). These two factors are, of course, closely related to dietary intake.

Elderly men tend to have lower blood ascorbic acid levels than do elderly women (6, 150, 288, 294, 440, 442) even when their intakes are similar. This observation suggested to Morgan et al. (294) that the vitamin C requirement of men beyond the age of 50 years may be significantly greater than that of women. Kirk and Chieffi (231) noted that the elderly men in their study were more debilitated than the elderly women. Therefore, they suggested that the degree of debilitation should be considered as a possible factor promoting a sex difference in vitamin C status.

Estimates of the vitamin C requirements of the elderly have been based on studies of blood and urinary response to varying intakes. Bowers and Kubik (53) studied 100 men and women, 56 to 92 years old. At the beginning of the study their mean ascorbic acid concentration was 0.22 mg/100 ml in plasma and 12 μg/10^8 cells in leukocytes. When 120 mg vitamin C/day was given over a 4-week period, plasma ascorbic acid levels rose to 1.21 to 1.39 mg/100 ml and leukocyte levels increased to 29 to 35 μg/10^8 cells. Saturation was achieved with a total intake of about 1,680 mg vitamin C. Bowers and Kublik noted that Lowry et al. (263) had observed that plasma ascorbic acid rose from 0.2 to 0.95 mg/100 ml in young adults with a total intake of about 1,500 mg vitamin C. They concluded therefore that the vitamin C requirements of the aged are not greater than those of younger people. Roderuck et al. (353) who, it was noted previously (p. 861), observed no significant changes with age in blood ascorbic acid levels of women, reported that vitamin C intakes of 1.1 mg/kg body weight were associated with blood ascorbic acid levels of 0.8 mg/100 ml and with daily urinary excretions of more than 15 mg ascorbic acid. They concluded that "an ascorbic acid intake of 1.1 mg or more per kilogram of body weight from self-selected diets provides women with apparently satisfactory amounts of this vitamin." They noted, however, that individual intakes lower than 1.1 mg/kg body weight occurred frequently in the group studied (569 women).

Gander and Niederberger (125) on the basis of the results of saturation studies involving measurement of urinary response to load doses, concluded that, to prevent vitamin C deficiency, young people require 25 to 32 mg vitamin C per day whereas older people require about 50 mg. They suggested that elderly people who are ill might need even more than 50 mg. Similarly Kirchmann (228) on the basis of previous work concluded that elderly people require about 50% more vitamin C than do young people. She suggested intakes of 50 mg/day for young adults and 75 mg/day for the elderly.

Rafsky and Newman (335) concluded that elderly people have high requirements for vitamin C. In their study with 25 men and women, 66 to 83 years old, they attempted to saturate the subjects by giving them oral doses of vitamin C gradually increasing from 100 to 200 mg to 900 or 1,000 mg/day. Saturation was assumed to have been attained when a sharp drop in retention (intake minus urinary excretion) occurred. With seven subjects, retention continued to increase throughout the study and with 14 subjects the drop in retention occurred only after very large doses had been administered. Similar blood response to both oral and intravenous doses indicated that impaired absorption was not the reason for the high apparent requirements. Both Mitra (291) and O'Sullivan et al. (313) found that saturation tests based on urinary response were not satisfactory in work with elderly people. They suggested that this method be abandoned in clinical practice.

COMMENTS

The data summarized in the appendix tables show that the estimated vitamin C requirements for most population groups vary widely from one study to another. Part of the variation is due to the criteria used. In some studies the minimum intake necessary to prevent the appearance of scurvy was sought. In others, the intake needed to keep the blood or urinary ascorbic acid levels within the normal range was measured. In still others, the intake necessary to keep the body saturated with ascorbic acid was regarded as the requirement. It is clear that the vitamin C intake necessary to prevent scurvy is very small. What is not clear, at present, is how much more than the minimum amount necessary to prevent scurvy is needed to assure good health. Are saturation levels of special benefit, or are they merely wasteful, or perhaps even harmful?

The studies of Ginter and his associates (128–131, 133) have shown that, for satisfactory cholesterol metabolism, guinea pigs need more vitamin C to prevent the accumulation of cholesterol in their blood and livers than they need to prevent scurvy. Whether man has similar needs is not clear. Some investigators have reported, however, that large daily doses of ascorbic acid have beneficial effects in conditions apparently quite unrelated to scurvy (132, 189, 333, 377, 378). Others (244, 276) have suggested, mainly on the basis of studies with animals, that such high intakes may not be completely innocuous. Mašek (276) for instance, has suggested that adaptation to hypersaturation may result in "lowered resistance" to vitamin C deficiency. In other words the high rate of vitamin C catabolism observed with high intakes may continue even when the intake is lowered greatly, thus, precipitating a state of vitamin C deficiency. Hellman and Burns (176), in studies with [1-¹⁴C]ascorbic acid, found that the turnover rate of vitamin C in man was much lower than in the guinea pig and that the metabolic pathways in the two species were apparently different. Application to man of data obtained with guinea pigs or other animals, therefore, may be of questionable validity.

Another source of variation lies in the methods by which vitamin C status has been evaluated. For instance, the daily vitamin C requirement for saturation ranged from 50 to 77 mg when estimated from data on whole blood ascorbic acid levels, from 70 to 131 mg when plasma levels were determined, and from less than 22 to 83 mg when white blood cell ascorbic acid levels were assayed (Appendix table 1). An even wider range of 26 to 125 mg was observed when saturation was judged by urinary ascorbic acid excretion.

The requirement estimates based on acceptable blood ascorbic acid levels cover ranges similar to, and sometimes higher than those of the estimates based on blood saturation levels. This observation suggests that the data obtained from studies of blood ascorbic acid levels should be used with caution.

The small number of subjects studied in any age group, no doubt, has contributed to the imprecision of the requirement estimates (Appendix tables 2 to 5). Few data were found on requirements of infants 18 to 24 months old. Preschool children, with whom such older infants might be grouped, have also received little attention. In the other population groups the studies involving large numbers of subjects usually were carried out without fully controlled dietary intakes. Vitamin C intake was estimated from diet histories. (45, 274) or it

was manipulated by adding known amounts of the vitamin to the subjects' self-selected diets (53, 208).

Reports of studies in which labeled ascorbic acid was used (16, 23–28, 176, 397) suggest a promising approach to solving some of the difficulties in determining vitamin C requirements of man. With the increased availability of such techniques as mass spectrometry, or nuclear magnetic resonance, studies using stable isotopes (16) should become feasible. Isotope studies which, at present, are usually restricted to adult male subjects could then be carried out with other groups, particularly with children and pregnant women. With such studies, more precise information on utilization, turnover rates, side reactions, the interaction of various environmental and physiological conditions with vitamin C metabolism, and possible information on vitamin C synthesis would be available.

More accurate measurements of vitamin C requirements must await the use of these new techniques to obtain a better understanding of the functions of this vitamin and to develop criteria which reflect more accurately human needs.

ACKNOWLEDGMENTS

The authors wish to thank Charlotte Slayton Nace for invaluable assistance in searching the literature and collecting pertinent documents.

The Nutrition Institute thanks Dr. Mildred Adams for accepting the responsibility for the final version of the Conspectus.

LITERATURE CITED

1. Abbasy, M. A., Gray Hill, N. & Harris, L. J. (1936) Vitamin C and juvenile rheumatism with some observations on the vitamin-C reserves in surgical tuberculosis. Lancet 2, 1413–1417.
2. Abbasy, M. A., Harris, L. J. & Ellman, P. (1937) Vitamin C and infection. Excretion of vitamin C in pulmonary tuberculosis and in rheumatoid arthritis. Lancet 2, 181–183.
3. Abbasy, M. A., Harris, L. J. & Gray Hill, N. (1937) Vitamin C and infection. Excretion of vitamin C in osteomyelitis. Lancet 2, 177–180.
4. Abbasy, M. A., Harris, L. J., Ray, S. N. & Marrack, J. R. (1935) Diagnosis of vitamin-C subnutrition by urine analysis. Quantitative data—experiments on control subjects. Lancet 2, 1399–1405.

5. Ahmad, B. (1936) Observations on the excretion of vitamin C in human urine. Biochem. J. 30, 11–15.
6. Allen, M. A., Andrew, J. & Brook, M. (1969) A sex difference in leucocyte vitamin C status in the elderly. Nutrition 21, 136–137.
7. American Pediatric Society (1898) The American Pediatric Society's collective investigation on infantile scurvy in North America. Arch. Pediatr. 15, 481–508.
8. Anderson, T. W., Reid, D. B. W. & Beaton, G. H. (1972) Vitamin C and the common cold: a double-blind trial. Can. Med. Assoc. J. 107, 503–508.
9. Andreae, W. A. & Browne, J. S. L. (1946) Ascorbic acid metabolism after trauma in man. Can. Med. Assoc. J. 55, 425–432.
10. Andrews, J. & Brook, M. (1966) Leucocyte-vitamin-C content and clinical signs in the elderly. Lancet 1, 1350–1351.
11. Andrews, J., Brook, M. & Allen, M. A. (1966) Influence of abode and season on the vitamin C status of the elderly. Geront. Clin. 8, 257–266.
12. Andrews, J., Letcher, M. & Brook, M. (1969) Vitamin C supplementation in the elderly: a 17-month trial in an old persons' home. Br. Med. J. 2, 416–418.
13. Anonymous (1948) Vitamin-C requirement of human adults. Experimental study of vitamin-C deprivation in man. A preliminary report by the Vitamin C Subcommittee of the Accessory Food Factors Committee, Medical Research Council. Lancet 254, 853–858.
14. Archer, H. E. & Graham, G. (1936) The subscurvy state in relation to gastric and duodenal ulcer. Lancet 2, 364–366.
15. Arthur, G., Monro, J. A., Poore, P., Rilwan, W. B. & Murphy, E. LaC. (1967) Trial of ascorbic acid in senile purpura and sublingual haemorrhages. Br. Med. J. 1, 732–733.
16. Atkins, G. L., Dean, B. M., Griffin, W. J. & Watts, R. W. E. (1964) Quantitative aspects of ascorbic acid metabolism in man. J. Biol. Chem. 239, 2975–2980.
17. Avery, M. E., Clow, C. L., Menkes, J. H., Ramos, A., Scriver, C. R., Stern, L. & Wasserman, B. P. (1967) Transient tyrosinemia of the newborn: dietary and clinical aspects. Pediatrics 39, 378–384.
18. Aykroyd, W. R. (1970) Conquest of deficiency diseases. Achievements and prospects. FFHC Basic Study No. 24, pp. 44–49. World Health Organization, Geneva.
19. Bachinsky, P. P. (1959) Vlijanie fizičeskih upražnenij na obespečnnost organisma vitaminami C i B₁ v vesennij period. Vop. Pitan. 18(4), 53–56. Abstracted in Nutr. Abst. Rev. 30, 221 (1960).
20. Bachstrom, J. F. (1734) Observationes circa Scorbutum; ejusque Indolem, Causas, Signa et Curam. Leyden: C. Wishof. Cited by: Chick, H. (1953) Early investigations of scurvy and the antiscorbutic vitamin. Proc. Nutr. Soc. 12, 210–219.
21. Bailey, D. A., Carron, A. V., Teece, R. G. &

Wehner, H. (1970) Effect of vitamin C supplementation upon the physiological response to exercise in trained and untrained subjects. Int. Z. Vitaminforsch. 40, 435–441.
22. Bailey, D. A., Carron, A. V., Teece, R. G. & Wehner, H. J. (1970) Vitamin C supplementation related to physiological response to exercise in smoking and nonsmoking subjects. Am. J. Clin. Nutr. 23, 905–912.
23. Baker, E. M. III, Hammer, D. C., March, S. C., Tolbert, B. M. & Canham, J. E. (1971) Ascorbate sulfate: a urinary metabolite of ascorbic acid in man. Science 173, 826–827.
24. Baker, E. M., Hodges, R. E., Hood, J., Sauberlich, H. E. & March, S. C. (1969) Metabolism of ascorbic-1-¹⁴C acid in experimental human scurvy. Am. J. Clin. Nutr. 22, 549–558.
25. Baker, E. M. III, Hodges, R. E., Hood, J., Sauberlich, H. E., March, S. C. & Canham, J. E. (1971) Metabolism of ¹⁴C-and ³H-labeled L-ascorbic acid in human scurvy. Am. J. Clin. Nutr. 24, 444–454.
26. Baker, E. M., Levandoski, N. G. & Sauberlich, H. E. (1963) Respiratory catabolism in man of the degradative intermediates of L- ascorbic-1-C¹⁴ acid. Proc. Soc. Exp. Biol. Mcd. 113, 379–383.
27. Baker, E. M., Saari, J. C. & Tolbert, B. M. (1966) Ascorbic acid metabolism in man. Am. J. Clin. Nutr. 19, 371–378.
28. Baker, E. M., Sauberlich, H. E., Wolfskill, S. J., Wallace, W. T. & Dean, E. E. (1962) Tracer studies of vitamin C utilization in men: metabolism of D-glucuronolactone-6-C¹⁴, D-glucuronic-6-C¹⁴ acid and L-ascorbic-1-C¹⁴ acid. Proc. Soc. Exp. Biol. Med. 109, 737–741.
29. Banks, H. S. (1965) Common cold: controlled trials. Lancet 2, 790.
30. Banks, H. S. (1968) Controlled trials in the early antibiotic treatment of colds. Med. Officer 119, 7–10.
31. Barlow, T. (1883) On cases described as "acute rickets." Med. Chirurg. Trans. London 66, 159. Reprinted in Arch. Dis. Child. 10, 223–252, (1935).
32. Barnes, A. C. (1947) Placental metabolism of vitamin C. I. Normal placental content. Am. J. Obstet. Gynecol. 53, 645–649.
33. Bartlett, M. K., Jones, C. M. & Ryan, A. E. (1940) Vitamin C studies on surgical patients. Ann. Surg. 111, 1–26.
34. Bartley, W., Krcbs, H. A. & O'Brien, J. R. P. (1953) Vitamin C requirement of human adults. A report of the Vitamin C Subcommittee of the Accessory Food Factors Committe and A. E. Barnes, W. Bartley, I. M. Frankau, G. A. Higgins, J. Pemberton, G. L. Roberts and H. R. Vickers. Medical Research Council Special Report Series No. 280. H. M. Stationery Office, London.
35. Basu, N. M. & Biswas, P. (1940) The influence of ascorbic acid on contractions and the incidence of fatigue of different types of muscles. Indian J. Med. Res. 28, 405–417.
36. Basu, N. M. & Ray, G. K. (1940) The optimum requirements of vitamin C of per-

sons living on a Bengali diet. Indian J. Med. Res. 28, 133–143.

37. Basu, N. M. & Ray, G. K. (1940) The effect of vitamin C on the incidence of fatigue in human muscle. Indian J. Med. Res. 28, 419–426.

38. Batata, M., Spray, G. H., Bolton, F. G., Higgins, G. & Wollner, L. (1967) Blood and bone marrow changes in elderly patients, with special reference to folic acid, vitamin B_{12}, iron, and ascorbic acid. Br. Med. J. 2, 667–669.

39. Baumann, T. (1937) Untersuchungen über den C-vitaminstoffwechsel bei laktierenden Frauen und über den Grad der physiologischen und pathologischen C-Vitaminsättigung des menschlichen Organismus. Jahrb. Kinderheilk. 150, 193–227.

40. Baumann, T. & Rappolt, L. (1937) Untersuchungen zum C-Vitaminstoffwechsel. Z. Vitaminforsch. 6, 1–50.

41. Beck, J. C., Browne, J. S. L. & Mackenzie, K. R. (1951) The effect of adrenocorticotrophic hormone and cortisone acetate on the metabolism of ascorbic acid. In: Proceedings of the Second Clinical ACTH Conference Vol. 1 (Mote, J. R., ed.), pp. 355–369, The Blakiston Co., New York.

42. Belavady, B. & Gopalan, C. (1960) Effect of dietary supplementation on the composition of breast milk. Indian J. Med. Res. 48, 518–523.

43. Belser, W. B., Hauck, H. M. & Storvick, C. A. (1939) A study of the ascorbic acid intake required to maintain tissue saturation in normal adults. J. Nutr. 17, 513–526.

44. Bessel-Lorck, C. (1959) Erkältungsprophylaxe bei Jungendlichen in Skilager. Med. Welt 44, 2126–2127.

45. Bessey, O. A. & White, R. L. (1942) The ascorbic acid requirements of children. J. Nutr. 23, 195–204.

46. Bischoff, H. & Müller, K. (1942) Natürliches und synthetisches Vitamin C in der Säuglingsernahrung. Ein Beitrag zur Frage der Resistenzsteigerung und des Bedarfs. Deutsch. med. Wochenschr. 68, 1257.

47. Bly, C. G., Johnson, R. E., Kark, R. M., Consolazio, C. F., Swain, H. L., Laudani, A., Maloney, M. A., Figueroa, W. G. & Imperiale, L. E. (1950) Survival in the cold. U.S. Armed Forces Med. J. 1, 615–628.

48. Boiko, E. P. (1968) C-vitaminnaja obespečennost, ékipažej sudov dal'nego plavanija. Vop. Pitan. 27(3), 46–52.

49. Bond, A. D., McLelland, B. W., Einstein, J. R. & Finamore, F. J. (1972) Ascorbic acid-2 sulfate of the brine shrimp, artemia salina. Arch. Biochem. Biophys. 153, 207–214.

50. Bondarev, G. I., Mihel'son, D. A. & Aronova, E. N. (1969) Obmen nekotoryh vitaminov u lic nahodjaščihsja v uslovijah povyšennogo davlenija gazovoj sredy. Vop. Pitan. 28(4), 70–71.

51. Bourguin, A. & Musmanno, E. (1953) Preliminary report on the effect of smoking on the ascorbic acid content of whole blood. Am. J. Dig. Dis. 20, 75–77.

52. Boutwell, J. H., Cilley, J. H., Krasno, L. R., Ivy, A. C. & Farmer, C. J. (1950) Effect of repeated exposure of human subjects to hypoxia on glucose tolerance, excretion of ascorbic acid, and phenylalanine tolerance. J. Appl. Physiol. 2, 388–392.

53. Bowers, E. F. & Kubik, M. M. (1965) Vitamin C levels in old people and the response to ascorbic acid and to the juice of the acerola (Malpighia punicifolia L.) Br. J. Clin. Prac. 19, 141–147.

54. Braestrup, P. W. (1937) Studies of latent scurvy in infants. I. Capillary resistance of newly born children and during the first year of life. Acta Pediatr. 19, 320–327.

55. Braestrup, P. W. (1937) Studies of latent scurvy in infants. II. Content of ascorbic (cevitamic) acid in the blood-serum of women in labour and in children at birth. Acta Pediatr. 19, 328–334.

56. Braestrup, P. W. (1938) The content of reduced ascorbic acid in blood plasma in infants, especially at birth and in the first days of life. J. Nutr. 16, 363–373.

57. Briggs, M. H. (1962) Possible relations of ascorbic acid, ceruloplasmin and toxic aromatic metabolites in schizophrenia. New Zeal. Med. J. 61, 229–236.

58. Briggs, M. H., Andrews, E. D., Kitto, G. B., Segal, L., Graham, V. & Baillie, W. J. (1962) A comparison of the metabolism of ascorbic acid in schizophrenia, pregnancy and in normal subjects. New Zeal. Med. J. 61, 555–558.

59. Briggs, M. & Briggs, M. (1972) Vitamin C requirements and oral contraceptives. Nature 238, 277.

60. Brook, M. & Grimshaw, J. J. (1968) Vitamin C concentration of plasma and leukocytes as related to smoking habit, age, and sex of humans. Am. J. Clin. Nutr. 21, 1254–1258.

61. Browne, J. S. L. (1945) Effect of damage on vitamin metabolism. In: Conference on metabolic aspects of convalescence including bone and wound healing. Ninth Meeting, Feb. 2–5 (1945) (Reifenstein, E. C. Jr., ed.), pp. 34–44. Josiah Macy, Jr. Foundation, New York.

62. Bryan, A. H., Turner, D. F., Huenemann, R. L. & Lotwin, G. (1941) The relation between plasma and dietary ascorbic acid. Am. J. Med. Sci. 202, 77–83.

63. Bullowa, J. G. M., Rothstein, I. A., Ratish, H. D. & Harde, E. (1936) Cevitamic acid excretion in pneumonias and some other pathological conditions. Proc. Soc. Exp. Biol. Med. 34, 1–7.

64. Bumbalo, T. S. (1938) Urinary output of vitamin C of normal and of sick children. Am. J. Dis. Child. 55, 1212–1220.

65. Calder, J. H., Curtis, R. C. & Fore, H. (1963) Comparison of vitamin C in plasma and leucocytes of smokers and non-smokers. Lancet 1, 556.

66. Camcam, G. A. (1968) Ascorbic acid me-

tabolism of some Filipinos. 1. Total ascorbic acid in the blood and urine of some females. Philip. J. Nutr. *21*, 137–147.

67. Camcam, G. A. (1968) Ascorbic acid metabolism of some Filipinos. 2. Response to a test dose of the vitamin by some females. Philip. J. Nutr. *21*, 148–158.

68. Chen, K. C., Yü, T. F., Liu, S. H. & Chu, H. I. (1940) Studies on the vitamin C requirement of Chinese patients with scurvy. Chin. J. Physiol. *15*, 119–142.

69. Cheraskin, E. & Ringsdorf, W. M. (1968) A lingual vitamin C test: 1. Reproducibility. Int. Z. Vitaminforsch. *38*, 114–117.

70. Cheraskin, E. & Ringsdorf, W. M. (1968) A lingual vitamin C test: V. A study in dietary relationships. Int. Z. Vitaminforsch. *38*, 254–256.

71. Chernous, G. M. (1970) Soderzhanie askorbinovoi kisloty v platsente i organakh plodov i novorozhdennykh pri normal'noi i patologicheskoi beremennosti. Dokl. Akad. Nauk Beloruss. SSR *14(2)*, 177–179. Abstracted in: Chem. Abstr. *73*, 122 (1970).

72. Chevillard, L. & Hamon, F. (1943) Le taux de l'acide ascorbique dans les leucocytes et les plaquettes comme test de la carence en vitamine C. C. R. Soc. Biol. *137*, 307–309. Cited by: Mažek, J. (1966) Contribution to the problem of vitamin C requirement in adults. Rev. Czech. Med. *12*, 54–60.

73. Chick, H. (1953) Early investigations of scurvy and the antiscorbutic vitamin. Proc. Nutr. Soc. *12*, 210–219.

74. Chinn, H. & Farmer, C. J. (1939) Determination of ascorbic acid in feces. Its excretion in health and disease. Proc. Soc. Exp. Biol. Med. *41*, 561–566.

75. Chope, H. D. & Dray, S. (1951) The nutritional status of the aging. California Med. *74*, 105–107.

76. Chu, F.-T. & Sung, C. (1936) Effect of vitamin C administration on vitamin C of milk and urine of lactating mothers. Proc. Soc. Exp. Biol. Med. *35*, 171–172.

77. Cohen, M. M. & Duncan, A. M. (1967) Ascorbic acid nutrition in gastroduodenal disorders. Br. Med. J. *4*, 516–518.

78. Coon, W. W. (1962) Ascorbic acid metabolism in postoperative patients. Surg. Gynecol. Obstet. *114*, 522–534.

79. Corbett, J. L. & Barr, A. (1967) Muscle stiffness and vitamin C. Br. Med. J. *3*, 113.

80. Cormia, F. E. (1941) Postarsphenamine dermatitis: the relation of vitamin C to the production of arsphenamine sensitiveness, and its use as an adjunct to further arsphenamine therapy in patients with cutaneous hypersensitiveness to the arsphenamines. J. Invest. Dermatol. *4*, 81–93.

81. Cowan, D. W. & Diehl, H. S. (1950) Antihistaminic agents and ascorbic acid in the early treatment of the common cold. J. Am. Med. Assoc. *143*, 421–424.

82. Cowan, D. W., Diehl, H. S. & Baker, A. B. (1942) Vitamins for the prevention of colds. J. Am. Med. Assoc. *120*, 1268–1271.

83. Crandon, J. H., Landau, B., Mikal, S., Balmanno, J., Jefferson, M. & Mahoney, N. (1958) Ascorbic acid economy in surgical patients as indicated by blood ascorbic acid levels. New Engl. J. Med. *258*, 105–113.

84. Crandon, J. H., Lennihan, R., Jr., Mikal, S. & Reif, A. E. (1961) Ascorbic acid economy in surgical patients. Ann. New York Acad. Sci. *92*, 246–267.

85. Crandon, J. H. & Lund, C. C. (1940) Vitamin C deficiency in an otherwise normal adult. New Engl. J. Med. *222*, 748–752.

86. Crandon, J. H., Lund, C. C. & Dill, D. B. (1940) Experimental human scurvy. New Engl. J. Med. *223*, 353–369.

87. Dalldorf, G. (1933) A sensitive test for subclinical scurvy in man. Am. J. Dis. Child. *46*, 794–802.

88. Dallyn, M. H. & Moschette, D. S. (1952) Ascorbic acid nutrition of children. J. Am. Dietet. Assoc. *28*, 718–722.

89. Dann, M. (1942) The influence of diet on the ascorbic acid requirement of premature infants. J. Clin. Invest. *21*, 139–144.

90. Darling, R. C., Johnson, R. E., Pitts, G. C., Consolazio, F. C. & Robinson, P. F. (1944) Effects of variations in dietary protein on the physical well being of men doing manual work. J. Nutr. *28*, 273–281.

91. Daum, K., Boyd, K. & Paul, W. D. (1939) Influence of fever therapy on blood levels and urinary excretion of ascorbic acid. Proc. Soc. Exp. Biol. Med. *40*, 129–132.

92. Davey, B. L., Wu, M-L. & Storvick, C. A. (1952) Daily determination of plasma, serum and white cell-platelet ascorbic acid in relationship to the excretion of ascorbic and homogentisic acids by adults maintained on a controlled diet. J. Nutr. *47*, 341–351.

93. Dawson, E. B., Clark, R. R. & McGanity, W. J. (1969) Plasma vitamins and trace metal changes during teen-age pregnancy. Am. J. Obstet. Gynecol. *104*, 953–958.

94. Day, C. D. M. (1933) The effect of antiscorbutic deficiency on the pregnant organism and dental tissues. J. Am. Dental Assoc. *20*, 1745–1769.

95. De, H. N. & Chakravorty, C. H. (1948) Ascorbic-acid requirement of Indian adult. Indian J. Med. Res. *36*, 249–252.

96. Delp, M. (1941) Ascorbic acid in the treatment of arsenical dermatitis. J. Kansas Med. Soc. *42*, 519–523.

97. Deodhar, A. D., Rajalakshmi, R. & Ramakrishnan, C. V. (1964) Studies on human lactation. Part III. Effect of dietary vitamin supplementation on vitamin contents of breast milk. Acta Paediatr. *53*, 42–48.

98. Difs, H. (1940) Beiträge zur Diagnostik der Vitamin-C-Mangel-Krankheit. Acta Med. Scand. Suppl. 110. Cited by: Kirk, J. E. & Chieffi, M. (1953) Vitamin studies in middle-aged and old individuals. XI. The concentration of total ascorbic acid in whole blood. J. Gerontol. *8*, 301–304.

99. Dodds, M. L. (1969) Sex as a factor in blood levels of ascorbic acid. J. Am. Dietet. Assoc. *54*, 32–33.

100. Dodds, M. L. & MacLeod, F. L. (1944) Blood plasma ascorbic acid values resulting from normally encountered intakes of this vitamin and indicated human requirements. J. Nutr. 27, 77–87.

101. Drummond, J. C. (1920) The nomenclature of the so-called accessory food factors (vitamins). Biochem. J. 14, 660.

102. Dudley, S. (1953) James Lind: laudatory address. Proc. Nutr. Soc. 12, 202–209.

103. Dugal, L.-P. (1961) Vitamin C in relation to cold temperature tolerance. Ann. New York Acad. Sci. 92, 307–317.

104. Dugal, L.-P. & Fortier, G. (1952) Ascorbic acid and acclimatization to cold in monkeys. J. Appl. Physiol. 5, 143–146.

105. Durand, C., Audinot, M. & Frajdenrajch, S. (1962) Hypovitaminose C latente et tabac. Concours Med. 84, 4801–4806.

106. Esposito, R. & Valentini, R. (1968) Vitamin C and gastroduodenal disorders. Br. Med. J. 2, 118.

107. Evelyn, K. A., Malloy, M. T. & Rosen, C. (1938) Determination of ascorbic acid in urine with photoelectric colorimeter. J. Biol. Chem. 126, 645. Cited by: Ralli, E. P., Friedman, G. J. & Sherry, S. (1939) The vitamin C requirement of man. Estimated after prolonged studies of the plasma concentration and daily excretion of vitamin C in 3 adults on controlled diets. J. Clin. Invest. 18, 705–714.

108. Everson, G. J. & Daniels, A. L. (1936) Vitamin C studies with children of preschool age. J. Nutr. 12, 15–26.

109. Farmer, C. J. & Abt, A. F. (1936) Determination of reduced ascorbic acid in small amounts of blood. Proc. Soc. Exp. Biol. and Med. 34, 146–150.

110. Farmer, C. J. & Abt, A. F. (1938) Titration of plasma ascorbic acid as a test for latent avitaminosis C. Milbank Memorial Fund: Nutrition: The Newer Diagnostic Methods. pp. 114–137. Cited by: Fincke, M. L. & Landquist, V. L. (1942) The daily intake of ascorbic acid required to maintain adequate and optimal levels of this vitamin in blood plasma. J. Nutr. 23, 483–490.

111. Falke (1939) Über die Grösse des Vitamin C-Verbrauchs im Fieber. Klin. Wochenschr. 18, 818–821.

112. Faulkner, J. M. (1935) The effect of administration of vitamin C on the reticulocytes in certain infectious diseases. New Engl. J. Med. 213, 19–20.

113. Faulkner, J. M. & Taylor, F. H. L. (1937) Vitamin C and infection. Ann. Intern. Med. 10, 1867–1873.

114. Faulkner, J. M. & Taylor, F. H. L. (1938) Observations on the renal threshold for ascorbic acid in man. J. Clin. Invest. 17, 69–75.

115. Fincke, M. L. & Landquist, V. L. (1942) The daily intake of ascorbic acid required to maintain adequate and optimal levels of this vitamin in blood plasma. J. Nutr. 23, 483–490.

116. Fox, F. W., Dangerfield, L. F., Gottlich, S. F. & Jokl, E. (1940) Vitamin C requirements of native mine labourers. Br. Med. J. 2, 143–147.

117. Franz, W. L., Sands, G. W. & Heyl, H. L. (1956) Blood ascorbic acid level in bioflavonoid and ascorbic acid therapy of common cold. J. Am. Med. Assoc. 162, 1224–1226.

118. Friedman, G. J., Sherry, S. & Ralli, E. P. (1940) The mechanism of the excretion of vitamin C by the human kidney at low and normal plasma levels of ascorbic acid. J. Clin. Invest. 19, 685–689.

119. Friend, D. G. & Marquis, H. H. (1938) Arsphenamine sensitivity and vitamin C. Amer. J. Syphil. Gonorr. Vener. Dis. 22, 239–242.

120. Fujino, M., Dawson, E. B., Holeman, T. & McGanity, W. J. (1966) Interrelationships between estrogenic activity, serum iron and ascorbic acid levels during the menstrual cycle. Am. J. Clin. Nutr. 18, 256–260.

121. Gaehtgens, G. (1937) Der Tagesverbrauch an Vitamin C in der Schwangerschaft. Arch. Gynäkol. 164, 571–587.

122. Gaehtgens, G. & Werner, E. (1936) Das Vitamin C-Bedarf in der Gravidität. Arch. Gynäkol. 163, 475–486.

123. Gaehtgens, G. & Werner, E. (1937) Vitamin C-Belastungen bei stillenden Wöchnerinnen. Arch. Gynäkol. 165, 63–75.

124. Gaehtgens, G. & Werner, E. (1937) Zur Frage des Vitamin C-Defizits in der Gravidität und während der Lactation. Klin. Wochenschr. 16, 843–844.

125. Gander, J. & Niederberger, W. (1936) Ueber den Vitamin C-Bedarf alter Leute. Munchener Med. Wochenschr. 83, 1386-1389.

126. General Practitioner Research Group (1968) Ineffectiveness of vitamin C in treating coryza. The Practitioner 200, 442–445.

127. Gey, G. O., Cooper, K. H. & Bottenberg, R. A. (1970) Effect of ascorbic acid on endurance performance and athletic injury. J. Am. Med. Assoc. 211, 105.

128. Ginter, E. (1971) Vitamin-C deficiency and gallstone formation. Lancet 2, 1198–1199.

129. Ginter, E. (1972) Atherosclerosis and vitamin C. Lancet 2, 1233–1234.

130. Ginter, E. (1973) Cholesterol: vitamin C controls its transformation to bile acids. Scince 179, 702–704.

131. Ginter, E., Červeň, J., Nemec, R. & Mikuš, L. (1971) Lowered cholesterol catabolism in guinea pigs with chronic ascorbic acid deficiency. Am. J. Clin. Nutr. 24, 1238–1245.

132. Ginter, E., Kajaba, I. & Nizner, O. (1970) The effect of ascorbic acid on cholesterolemia in healthy subjects with seasonal deficit of vitamin C. Nutr. Metabol. 12, 76–86.

133. Ginter, E., Ondreička, R., Bobek, P. & Šimko, V. (1969) The influence of chronic vitamin C deficiency on fatty acid composition of blood serum, liver triglycerides and cholesterol esters in guinea pigs. J. Nutr. 99, 261–266.

134. Giza, T., Weclawowicz, J. & Zaionc, J. (1965) The perlingual method for evaluating vitamin C. III. The relation between the decolorisation time and the vitamin C content of the internal organs of human subjects. Int. Z. Vitaminforsch. 35, 9–12.

135. Glazebrook, A. J. & Thomson, S. (1942) The administration of vitamin C in a large institution and its effect on general health and resistance to infection. J. Hyg. 42, 1–19.

136. Glickman, N., Keeton, R. W., Mitchell, H. H. & Fahnestock, M. K. (1946) The tolerance of man to cold as affected by dietary modifications: high versus low intake of certain water-soluble vitamins. Am. J. Physiol. 146, 538–558.

137. Goettsch, E. (1935) Treatment of infantile scurvy with cevitamic acid. Am. J. Dis. Child. 49, 1441–1448.

138. Goldsmith, G. A. (1961) Human requirements for vitamin C and its use in clinical medicine. Ann. New York Acad. Sci. 92, 230–245.

139. Goldsmith, G. A. & Ellinger, G. F. (1939) Ascorbic acid in blood and urine after oral administration of a test dose of vitamin C. Arch. Intern. Med. 63, 531–546.

140. Goldsmith, G. A., Gowe, D. F. & Ogaard, A. T. (1939) Determination of vitamin C nutrition by means of a skin test. A critical evaluation. Proc. Soc. Exp. Biol. Med. 41, 370–374.

141. Goldsmith, G. A., Ogaard, A. T. & Gowe, D. F. (1941) Estimation of the ascorbic acid (vitamin C) requirement of ambulatory patients. Arch. Intern. Med. 67, 590–596.

142. Goldsmith, G. A., Ogaard, A. T. & Gowe, D. F. (1941) Vitamin C (ascorbic acid) nutrition in bronchial asthma. An estimate of the daily requirement of ascorbic acid. Arch. Intern. Med. 67, 597–608.

143. Göthlin, G. F. (1931) A method of establishing the vitamin C standard and requirements of physically healthy individuals by testing the strength of their cutaneous capillaries. Scand. Arch. Physiol. 61, 225–270.

144. Göthlin, G. F. (1934) Human daily requirements of dietary ascorbic acid. Nature 134, 569–570.

145. Göthlin, G. F., Frisell, E. & Rundqvist, N. (1937) Experimental determination of the indispensable requirements of vitamin C (ascorbic acid) of the physically healthy adult. Acta Med. Scand. 92, 1–38.

146. Gould, B. S. (1960) Ascorbic acid and collagen fiber formation. Vit. and Horm. 18, 89–120.

147. Gounelle, H. & Vallette, A. (1945) Besoins quotidiens du tuberculeux séreux en vitamine C. Confrontation entre ingesta et taux sanguins. Presse méd. 53, 491–492.

148. Greenberg, L. D., Rinehart, J. F. & Phatak, N. M. (1936) Studies on reduced ascorbic acid content of the blood plasma. Proc. Soc. Exp. Biol. Med. 35, 135–139.

149. Grewar, D. (1965) Infantile scurvy. Clin. Pediatr. 4, 82–89.

150. Griffiths, L. L., Brocklehurst, J. C., Scott, D. L., Marks, J. & Blackley, J. (1967) Thiamine and ascorbic acid levels in the elderly. Gerontol. Clin. 9, 1–10.

151. Grosz, H. J. (1961) The relation of serum ascorbic acid level to adrenocortical secretion during experimentally induced emotional stress in human subjects. J. Psychosom. Res. 5, 253–262.

152. Hagtvet, J. (1945) Blodets askorbinsyre hos sunde og syke. Det norske videnskapsakademis skrifter Matematisk-naturvidenskapelig klasse. No. 2, J. Dybvad, Oslo. Cited by: Kirk, J. E. & Chieffi, M. (1953) Vitamin studies in middle-aged and old individuals. XI. The concentration of total ascorbic acid in whole blood. J. Gerontol. 8, 301–304.

153. Hagtvet, J. (1945) Norske serumaskorbinsyrevaerdier hos friske 1940–42. Nord. med. 28, 2335–2336. Cited by: Kirk, J. E. & Chieffi, M. (1953) Vitamin studies in middle-aged and old individuals. XI. The concentration of total ascorbic acid in whole blood. J. Gerontol. 8, 301–304.

154. Haines, J. E., Klosterman, A. M., Hauck, H. M., Delaney, M. A. & Kline, A. B. (1947) Tissue reserves of ascorbic acid in normal adults on three levels of intake. J. Nutr. 33, 479–489.

155. Hall, M. G., Darling, R. C. & Taylor, F. H. L. (1939) The vitamin C requirement in rheumatoid arthritis. Ann. Intern. Med. 13, 415–423.

156. Hamil, B. M., Munks, B., Moyer, E. Z., Kaucher, M. & Williams, H. H. (1947) Vitamin C in the blood and urine of the newborn and in the cord and maternal blood. Am. J. Dis. Child. 74, 417–433.

157. Hamil, B. M., Reynold, L., Poole, M. W. & Macy, I. G. (1938) Minimal vitamin C requirements of artificially fed infants. A study of four hundred and twenty-seven children under a controlled dietary regimen. Am. J. Dis. Child. 56, 561–583.

158. Hard, M. M., Esselbaugh, N. S. & Donald, E. A. (1958) Nutritional status of selected adolescent children. III. Ascorbic acid nutriture assessed by serum level and subclinical symptoms in relation to daily intake. Am. J. Clin. Nutr. 6, 401–408.

159. Harde, E., Rothstein, I. A. & Ratish, H. D. (1935) Urinary excretion of vitamin C in pneumonia. Proc. Soc. Exp. Biol. Med. 32, 1088–1090.

160. Harper, A. A., MacKay, I. F. S., Raper, H. S. & Camm, G. L. (1943) Vitamins and physical fitness. Br. Med. J. 1, 243–245.

161. Harris, L. J. (1943) Vitamin-C saturation test: stardardisation measurements at graded levels of intake. Lancet 1, 515–517.

162. Harris, L. J. (1951) Vitamins. A digest of current knowledge. pp. 68–70, J. & A. Churchill, Ltd., London.

163. Harris, L. J. & Abbasy, M. A. (1937) A simplified procedure for the vitamin-C urine test. Lancet 2, 1429.

164. Harris, L. J., Abbasy, M. A., Yudkin, J. & Kelly, S. (1936) Vitamins in human nu-

trition. Vitamin-C reserves of subjects of the voluntary hospital class. Lancet *1*, 1488–1490.

165. Harris, L. J. & Ray, S. N. (1935) Diagnosis of vitamin-C subnutrition by urine analysis, with a note on the antiscorbutic value of human milk. Lancet *1*, 71–77.

166. Harris, L. J., Ray, S. N. & Ward, A. (1933) The excretion of vitamin C in human urine and its dependence on the dietary intake. Biochem. J. *27*, 2011–2015.

167. Hathaway, M. L. & Meyer, F. L. (1941) Studies on the vitamin C metabolism of four preschool children. J. Nutr. *21*, 503–514.

168. Hauck, H. H. (1947) Plasma levels and urinary excretion of ascorbic acid in women during the menstrual cycle. J. Nutr. *33*, 511–515.

169. Hawley, E. E., Stephens, D. J. & Anderson, G. (1936) The excretion of vitamin C in normal individuals following a comparable quantitative administration in the form of orange juice, cevitamic acid by mouth, and cevitamic acid intravenously. J. Nutr. *11*, 135–145.

170. Heinemann, M. (1936) Dietary influences on the amount of ascorbic acid and other reducing substances in urine. Acta brev. Neerl. Physiol. *6*, 67–70.

171. Heinemann, M. (1936) On human requirements for vitamin C under different conditions. Acta brev. Neerl. Physiol. *6*, 144–146.

172. Heinemann, M. (1936) 1. On the relation between diet and urinary output of thiosulphate (and ascorbic acid). 2. Human requirements for vitamin C. Biochem. J. *30*, 2299–2306.

173. Heinemann, M. (1937) Ascorbic acid-requirements in human tuberculosis. Acta brev. Neerl. Physiol. *7*, 48–51.

174. Heinemann, M. (1938) Requirements for vitamin C in man. J. Clin. Invest. *17*, 671–676.

175. Heise, F. H. & Martin, G. J. (1936) Ascorbic acid metabolism in tuberculosis. Proc. Soc. Exp. Biol. Med. *34*, 642–644.

176. Hellman, L. & Burns, J. J. (1958) Metabolism of L-ascorbic acid-1-C¹⁴ in man. J. Biol. Chem. *230*, 923–930.

177. Helve, O. (1947) A study of the metabolism in Addison's disease. II. On the metabolism of lipids, nitrogen, and minerals, and on the vitamin C household. Acta Med. Scand. *128*, 1–24.

178. Henscel, A., Taylor, H. L., Brozek, J., Mickelsen, O. & Keys, A. (1944) Vitamin C and ability to work in hot environments. Am. J. Trop. Med. *24*, 259–265.

179. Henze, H. & Bremer, H. J. (1969) Die transitorische Hypertyrosinämie junger Säuglinge und ihre Beziehung zum Vitamin C. Monatsschr. Kinderheilk. *117*, 433–436.

180. Hess, A. F. (1917) Infantile scurvy. V. A study of its pathogenesis. Am. J. Dis. Child. *14*, 337–353.

181. Hess, A. F. & Benjamin, H. R. (1934) Urinary excretion of vitamin C. Proc. Soc. Exp. Biol. Med. *31*, 855–860.

182. Hindson, T. C. (1968) Ascorbic acid for prickly heat. Lancet *1*, 1347–1348.

183. Hindson, T. C. (1970) Ascorbic acid status of Europeans resident in the tropics. Br. J. Nutr. *24*, 801–802.

184. Hoch, H. & Marrack, J. R. (1948) The composition of the blood of women during pregnancy and after delivery. J. Obstet. Gynaecol. Br. Empire *55*, 1–16.

185. Hodges, R. E. (1970) The effect of stress on ascorbic acid metabolism in man. Nutr. Today *5(1)*, 11–12.

186. Hodges, R. E., Baker, E. M., Hood, J., Sauberlich, H. E. & March, S. C. (1969) Experimental scurvy in man. Am. J. Clin. Nutr. *22*, 535–548.

187. Hodges, R. E. & Canham, J. E. (1970) Vitamin deficiencies: Studies of experimental vitamin C deficiency and experimental vitamin A deficiency in man. In: Problems of assessment and alleviation of malnutrition in the United States. (Hansen, R. G. & Munro, H. N., eds.), pp. 115–128. Proceedings of a Workshop sponsored by Vanderbilt University, Nutrition & Health Program, Regional Medical Programs Service, HSMHA, The Nutrition Study Section, Division of Research Grants, NIH, held at Nashville, Tennessee, January 13–14, 1970.

188. Hodges, R. E., Hood, J., Canham, J. E., Sauberlich, H. E. & Baker, E. M. (1971) Clinical manifestations of ascorbic acid deficiency in man. Am. J. Clin. Nutr. *24*, 432–443.

189. Hoffer, A. (1971) Ascorbic acid and toxicity. New Engl. J. Med. *285*, 635–636.

190. Holley, H. L. & McLester, J. S. (1951) Manifestations of ascorbic acid deficiency after prolonged corticotropin administration. Arch. Intern. Med. *88*, 760–761.

191. Holmes, F. E., Cullen, G. E. & Nelson, W. E. (1941) Levels of ascorbic acid in the blood plasma of apparently healthy children. J. Pediatr. *18*, 300–309.

192. Holmes, H. N. (1943) Food allergies and vitamin C. Ann. Allergy *1*, 235.

193. Holmes, H. N. (1943) The effect of sulfa drugs on the excretion of vitamin C. J. Southern Med. Surg. *105*, 393–394.

194. Holmes, H. N. (1945) Allergic sensitivity to sulfonamide drugs. Ohio State Med. J. *41*, 923–924.

195. Holmes, H. N. & Alexander, W. (1942) Hay fever and vitamin C. Science *96*, 497–499.

196. Hopkins, F. G. (1906) The analyst and the medical man. The Analyst *31*, 385–404.

197. Horwitt, M. K. (1942) Ascorbic acid requirement of individuals in a large institution. Proc. Soc. Exp. Biol. Med. *49*, 248–250.

198. Hoske, H. (1963) Das vitamin C im Jugendalter. 1. Mitteilung: Der vitamin C—Bedarf in der Jugend-Erholung. Med. Ernahrung *4*, 33–38.

199. Hsu, P.-C., Yu, H.-H. & Yi, P.-F. (1948)

The ascorbic acid (vitamin C) requirement for tissue saturation in Chinese college students. Chin. Med. J. *66*, 605–608.

200. Hunt, H. B. (1938) Ascorbic acid in bronchial asthma. Report of a therapeutic trial of twenty-five cases. Br. Med. J. *1*, 726–727.

201. Hutchison, R. (1904) Some disorders of the blood and blood-forming organs in early life. Lancet *1*, 1253–1262.

202. Ingalls, T. H. (1937) Studies on the urinary excretion and blood concentration of ascorbic acid in infantile scurvy. J. Pediatr. *10*, 577–591.

203. Ingalls, T. H. (1938) Ascorbic acid requirements in early infancy. New Engl. J. Med. *218*, 872–875.

204. Ingalls, T. H. & Warren, H. A. (1937) Asymptomatic scurvy. Its relation to wound healing and its incidence in patients with peptic ulcer. New Engl. J. Med. *217*, 443–446.

205. Ingleby-MacKenzie, A. (1953) Chairman's opening address: James Lind. Proc. Nutr. Soc. *12*, 233–237.

206. Interdepartmental Committee on Nutrition for National Defense (1963) Manual for Nutrition Surveys, Second Edition, p. 235. Interdepartmental Committee on Nutrition for National Defense, National Institutes of Health, Bethesda, Md.

207. Jacobs, A., Greenman, D., Owen, E. & Cavill, I. (1971) Ascorbic acid status in iron-deficiency anaemia. J. Clin. Path. *24*, 694–697.

208. Javert, C. T. & Stander, H. J. (1943) Plasma vitamin C and prothrombin concentration in pregnancy and in threatened, spontaneous, and habitual abortion. Surg. Gynecol. Obstet. *76*, 115–122.

209. Jenkins, G. N. & Yudkin, J. (1943) Vitamins and physiological function. Br. Med. J. *2*, 265–266.

210. Jetter, W. W. (1938) Correlation between blood ascorbic acid and the dichlorophenol-indophenol intradermal test. Proc. Soc. Exp. Biol. Med. *39*, 169–171.

211. Johnson, R. E., Darling, R. C., Sargent, F. & Robinson, P. (1945) Effects of variations in dietary vitamin C on the physical well being of manual workers. J. Nutr. *29*, 155–165.

212. Johnson, S. W. & Zilva, S. S. (1934) The urinary excretion of ascorbic and dehydroascorbic acids in man. Biochem. J. *28*, 1393–1408.

213. Kark, R. M. (1953) Ascorbic acid in relation to cold, scurvy, ACTH and surgery. Proc. Nutr. Soc. *12*, 279–293.

214. Kark, R. M., Chapman, R. E. & Consolazio, C. F. (1952) Ascorbic acid requirements in "damage" and its relationship to adrenocortical activity. J. Clin. Invest. *31*, 642–643.

215. Kark, R. M., Croome, R. R. M., Cawthorpe, J., Bell, D. M., Bryans, A., MacBeth, R. J., Johnson, R. E., Consolazio, F. C., Poulin, J. L., Taylor, F. H. L. & Cogswell, R. C.

(1948) Observations on a mobile Arctic force. The health, physical fitness and nutrition of exercise "Musk Ox," February–May 1945. J. Appl. Physiol. *1*, 73–92.

216. Kataria, M. S., Rao, D. B. & Curtis, R. C. (1965) Vitamin C levels in the elderly. Geront. Clin. *7*, 189–190.

217. Kato, K. (1932) A critique of the Roentgen signs of infantile scurvy, with report of thirteen cases. Radiology *18*, 1096–1110.

218. Kellie, A. E. & Zilva, S. S. (1939) The vitamin C requirements of man. Biochem. J. *33*, 153–164.

219. Keys, A. & Henschel, A. F. (1942) Vitamin supplementation of U.S. army rations in relation to fatigue and the ability to do muscular work. J. Nutr. *23*, 259–269.

220. Khattab, A. K., Al Nagdy, S. A., Mourad, K. A. H. & El Azghal, H. I. (1970) Foetal maternal ascorbic acid gradient in normal Egyptian subjects. J. Trop. Pediatr. *16*, 112–115.

221. Khaustova, T. N. (1964) Izucenie potrebnosti v vitamine C u podrostkov. Gig. Sanit. No. 8, 42–45. Abstracted in Nutr. Abst. Rev. *35*, 185 (1965).

222. King, C. G. (1953) The discovery and chemistry of vitamin C. Proc. Nutr. Soc. *12*, 219–227.

223. King, G. G. & Waugh, W. A. (1932) The chemical nature of vitamin C. J. Biol. Chem. *94*, 483–484.

224. King, W. E. (1945) Vitamin studies in abortions. Surg. Gynecol. Obstet. *80*, 139–142.

225. Kinsman, R. A. & Hood, J. (1971) Some behavioral effects of ascorbic acid deficiency. Am. J. Clin. Nutr. *24*, 455–464.

226. Kirchheiner, B. (1969) The influence of ascorbic acid deficiency on connective tissue. Danish Med. Bull. *16*, 73–76.

227. Kirchhoff, H. W. (1969) Über den Einfluss von Vitamin C auf Energieverbrauch, Kreislauf- und Ventilationsgrössen im Belastungsversuch. Nutritio Dieta *11*, 184–192.

228. Kirchmann, L.-L. (1939) Über die Bedeutung des Vitamin C für die Klinische Medizin. Ergebn. inn. Med. Kinderheilk *56*, 101–153.

229. Kirk, J. E. (1951) Nutrition and aging. Nutr. Rev. *9*, 321–324.

230. Kirk, J. E. (1954) Blood and urine vitamin levels in the aged. Symposium on Problems of Gerontology, Nutrition Symposium Series 9, 73–94. National Vitamin Foundation Inc., New York.

231. Kirk, J. E. & Chieffi, M. (1953) Vitamin studies in middle-aged and old individuals. XI. The concentration of total ascorbic acid in whole blood. J. Gerontol. *8*, 301–304.

232. Kirk, J. E. & Chieffi, M. (1953) Vitamin studies in middle-aged and old individuals. XII. Hypovitaminemia C. Effect of ascorbic acid administration on the blood ascorbic acid concentration. J. Gerontol. *8*, 305–311.

233. Kitabchi, A. E. (1967) Ascorbic acid in steroidogenesis. Nature *215*, 1385–1386.

234. Kitabchi, A. E. & Duckworth, W. C. (1970)

Pituitary adrenal axis evaluation in human scurvy. Am. J. Clin. Nutr. 23, 1012–1014.

235. Klasson, D. H. (1951) Ascorbic acid in the treatment of burns. New York State J. Med. 51, 2388–2392.

236. Kline, A. B. & Eheart, M. S. (1944) Variation in the ascorbic acid requirements for saturation of nine normal young women. J. Nutr. 28, 413–419.

237. Kofoed, J. A., Blumenkrantz, N., Houssay, A. B. & Yamauchi, E. Y. (1965) Cervical mucus and serum ascorbic and dehydroascorbic acid concentrations during the menstrual cycle. Am. J. Obst. Gynecol. 91, 95–101.

238. Komar, V. I. (1968) Soderzhanie askorbinovoi kisloty v krovi i mochi pri epidemicheskom gepatite u detei. Vop. Okhr. Mater. Det. 13, 88.

239. Konovalova, G. A. & Medvedeva, I. V. (1960) K voprosu o C-vitaminnoj potrebnosti detej mladšego škol, nogo vozrasta. Vop. Pitan. 19(6), 31–34. Abstracted in: Nutr. Abst. Rev. 32, 617 (1961).

240. Kosenko, S. A. & Krajko, E. A. (1958) Nekotorye materialy po izučeniju obespečennosti detskogo organizma vitaminom C. Vop. Pitan. 17, 24–28. Abstracted in: Nutr. Abst. Rev. 29, 285 (1959).

241. Krebs, H. A. (1953) The Sheffield experiment on the vitamin C requirement of human adults. Proc. Nutr. Soc. 12, 237–246.

242. Kuhl, W. J., Jr., Wilson, H. & Ralli, E. P. (1952) Measurements of adrenal cortical activity in young men subjected to acute stress. J. Clin. Endocrinol. Metabol. 12, 393–406.

243. Kyhos, E. D., Gordon, E. S., Kimble, M. S. & Sevringhaus, E. L. (1944) The minimum ascorbic acid need of adults. J. Nutr. 27, 271–285.

244. Lamden, M. (1971) Dangers of massive vitamin C intake. New Engl. J. Med. 284, 336–337.

245. Lasica, O. I. & Cubataja, I. G. (1970) Socetannoe primenenie vitaminov C, B1 i B6 pri pnevmonii u detej pervogo goda žizni Vop. Ohrany Mater. Det. 15(8), 90. Abstracted in: Nutr. Abst. Rev. 41, 620 (1971).

246. Laurin, I. (1938) Some ascorbic acid saturation tests on infants. Acta Pediatr. 20, 352–369.

247. Lawrence, J. M., Herrington, B. L. & Maynard, L. A. (1945) Human milk studies. XXVII. Comparative values of bovine and human milks in infant feeding. Am. J. Dis. Child. 70, 193–199.

248. League of Nations Technical Commission on Nutrition (1938) Quart. Bull. Hlth. Org., L. of N. 7, 460. Cited by: Krebs, H. A. (1953) The Sheffield experiment on the vitamin C requirement of human adults. Proc. Nutr. Soc. 12, 237–246.

249. Leitner, Z. A. & Church, I. C. (1956) Nutritional studies in a mental hospital. Lancet 1, 565–567.

250. Lembrych, S. & Lika, J. (1965) Poziom witaminy C w pokarmie kobiecym we exzesnym połogu. Pol. Tyg. Lek. 20, 950–953.

251. Lester, D., Buccino, R. & Bizzocco, D. (1960) The vitamin C status of alcoholics. J. Nutr. 70, 278–282.

252. Levcowich, T. & Batchelder, E. L. (1942) Ascorbic acid excretion at known levels of intake as related to capillary resistance, dietary estimates, and human requirements. J. Nutr. 23, 399–408.

253. Levine, S. Z., Gordon, H. H. & Marples, E. (1941) A defect in the metabolism of tyrosine and phenylalanine in premature infants. II. Spontaneous occurrence and eradication by vitamin C. J. Clin. Invest. 20, 209–219.

254. Levine, S. Z., Marples, E. & Gordon, H. H. (1939) A defect in the metabolism of aromatic amino acids in premature infants: the role of vitamin C. Science 90, 620–621.

255. Lewis, J. S., Storvick, C. A. & Hauck, H. M. (1943) Renal threshold for ascorbic acid in twelve normal adults. With a note on the state of tissue reserves of subjects on an intake of ascorbic acid approximating the suggested daily allowance. J. Nutr. 25, 185–196.

256. Light, I. J., Berry, H. K. & Sutherland, J. M. (1966) Aminoacidemia of prematurity: its response to ascorbic acid. Am. J. Dis. Child. 112, 226–236.

257. Lind, J. (1753) A Treatise of the Scurvy. 1st Ed. Sands, Murray and Cochran for A. Kincaid and A. Donaldson, Edinburgh. Cited by: Chick, H. (1953) Early investigations of scurvy and the antiscorbutic vitamin. Proc. Nutr. Soc. 12, 210–219.

258. Linghorne, W. J., McIntosh. W. G., Tice, J. W., Tisdall. F. F., McCreary, J. F., Drake, T. G. H., Greaves, A. V. & Johnstone, W. M. (1946) The relation of ascorbic acid intake to gingivitis. Can. Med. Assoc. J. 54, 106–119.

259. Loh, H. S. & Wilson, C. W. M. (1971) Relationship between leukocyte ascorbic acid and hemoglobin levels at different ages. Int. J. Vit. Nutr. Res. 41, 259–267.

260. Loh, H. S. & Wilson, C. W. M. (1971) Relationship between leukocyte ascorbic acid concentrations and total white blood cell count. Int. J. Vit. Nutr. Res. 41, 253–258.

261. Loh, H. S. & Wilson, C. W. M. (1971) Relationship of human ascorbic acid metabolism to ovulation. Lancet 1, 110–112.

262. Lorenz, A. J. (1953) Some pre-Lind writers on scurvy. Proc. Nutr. Soc. 12, 306–324.

263. Lowry, O. H., Bessey, O. A., Brock, M. J. & Lopez, J. A. (1946) The interrelationship of dietary, serum, white blood cell and total body ascorbic acid. J. Biol. Chem. 166, 111–119.

264. Lund, C. C. (1939) The effect of surgical operations on the level of cevitamic acid in the blood plasma. New Engl. J. Med. 221, 123–127.

265. Lund, C. C., Levenson, S. M., Green, R. W., Paige, R. W., Robinson, P. E., MacDonald, A. H., Taylor, F. H., Adams, M. A. & Johnson, R. E. (1947) Ascorbic acid, thiamine,

riboflavin and nicotinic acid in relation to acute burns in man. Arch. Surg. 55, 557–583.

266. Maas, J. W., Gleser, G. C. & Gottschalk, L. A. (1961) Schizophrenia, anxiety and biochemical factors. Arch. Gen. Psychiat. 4, 109–118.

267. Macon, W. L. (1956) Citrus bioflavonoids in the treatment of the common cold. Industrial Med. Surg. 25, 525–527.

268. Macy, I. G. (1949) Composition of human colostrum and milk. Am. J. Dis. Child. 78, 589–603.

269. Macy, I. G., Moyer, E. Z., Kelly, H. J., Mack, H. C., DiLoreto, P. C. & Pratt, J. P. (1954) Physiological adaptation and nutritional status during and after pregnancy. J. Nutr. 52, (Suppl. 1), 1–92.

270. Mäkilä, E. (1970) The vitamin status of elderly denture wearers. Int. Z. Vitaminforsch. 40, 81–89.

271. Maksjutinskaya, O. V., Pavlenko, T. K. & Snigur, O. I. (1967) Ėkskrecija vitaminov C močoj u škoľnikov pri različnyh nagruzhah po plavaniju. Gig. Sanit. 12, 82–84. Abstracted in Nutr. Abst. Rev. 38, 931 (1968).

272. Margolis, A. M. (1968) Vlijanie C-vitaminizacii na rabotosposobnosť i proizvoditeľnosť truda rabocih vrednyh professij. Vop. Pitan 27(1), 87–88.

273. Martin, G. J. & Heise, F. H. (1937) Vitamin C nutrition in pulmonary tuberculosis. Am. J. Dig. Dis. Nutr. 4, 368–374.

274. Martin, M. P., Bridgforth, E., McGanity, W. J. & Darby, W. J. (1957) The Vanderbilt cooperative study of maternal and infant nutrition. X. Ascorbic acid. J. Nutr. 62, 201–224.

275. Mašek, Josef (1962) Recommended nutrient allowances. World Rev. Nutr. Dietet. 3, 149–193.

276. Mašek, J. (1966) Contribution to the problem of vitamin C requirement in adults. Rev. Czech. Med. 12, 54–60.

277. Mašek, J. & Hrubá (1958) Zur Frage der Vitamin C-Bedarfsnormen. Ernährungsforchung 3, 425–445. Cited by: Mašek, J. (1962) Recommended nutrient allowances. World Rev. Nutr. Dietet. 3, 149–193.

278. Mason, M. & Rivers, J. M. (1971) Plasma ascorbic acid levels in pregnancy. Am. J. Obstet. Gynecol. 109, 960–961.

279. Mathews, J. & Partington, M. W. (1967) Tyrosine load tests in newborn babies. Biol. Neonat. 11, 273–276.

280. Matsko, S. N., Gorbunova, V. I., Anisova, A. A. & Zhmeido, A. T. (1962) Criteria of vitamin C requirement: studies of children. Vop. Pitan. 21(6), 52–56. Abstracted in Nutr. Abst. Rev. 33, 528 (1963).

281. McCollum, E. V. (1957) A history of nutrition. The sequence of ideas in nutrition investigations. pp. 252–264, Houghton Mifflin Co., Boston.

282. McCormick, W. J. (1945) Sulfonamide sensitivity and C-avitaminosis. Can. Med. Assoc. J. 52, 68–70.

283. McLeroy, V. J. & Schendel, H. E. (1973) Influence of oral contraceptives on ascorbic acid concentrations in healthy, sexually mature women. Am. J. Clin. Nutr. 26, 191–196.

284. Meyer, F. L. & Hathaway, M. L. (1944) Further studies on the vitamin C metabolism of preschool children. J. Nutr. 28, 93–100.

285. Meyer, L. F. & Robinson, P. (1939) Ueber Vitamin-C-Haushalt des gesunden und kranken Kindes. Ann. Paediatr. 152, 283–301.

286. Mickelsen, O., Dippel, A. L. & Todd, R. L. (1943) Plasma vitamin C levels in women during the menstrual cycle. J. Clin. Endocrinol. 3, 600–602.

287. Mickelsen, O. & Keys, A. (1943) The composition of sweat, with special reference to vitamins. J. Biol. Chem. 149, 479–490.

288. Milne, J. S., Lonergan, M. E., Williamson, J., Moore, F. M. L., McMaster, R. & Percy, N. (1971) Leucocyte ascorbic acid levels and vitamin C intake in older people. Brit. Med. J. 4, 383–385.

289. Milner, G. (1963) Ascorbic acid in chronic psychiatric patients—a controlled trial. Br. J. Psychiat. 109, 294–299.

290. Mindlin, R. L. (1938) The relation between plasma ascorbic acid concentration and diet in the newborn infant. J. Pediatr. 13, 309–313.

291. Mitra, M. L. (1970) Vitamin-C deficiency in the elderly and its manifestations. J. Am. Geriat. Soc. 18, 67–71.

292. Mohan Ram, M. (1965) Studies on ascorbic acid nutrition. Indian J. Med. Res. 53, 891–896.

293. Moore, M. C., Purdy, M. B., Gibbens, E. J., Hollinger, M. E. & Goldsmith, G. (1947) Food habits of women during pregnancy. J. Am. Dietet. Assoc. 23, 847–853.

294. Morgan, A. F., Gillum, H. L. & Williams, R. I. (1955) Nutritional status of the aging. III. Serum ascorbic acid and intake. J. Nutr. 55, 431–448.

295. Morse, E. H., Potgieter, M. & Walker, G. R. (1956) Ascorbic acid utilization by women. Response of blood serum and white blood cells to increasing levels of intake. J. Nutr. 58, 291–298.

296. Morse, E. H., Potgieter, M. & Walker, G. R. (1956) Ascorbic acid utilization by women. Response of blood serum and white cells to increasing levels of intake in two groups of women of different age levels. J. Nutr. 60, 229–239.

297. Moyer, E. Z., Harrison, A. P., Lesher, M. & Miller, O. N. (1948) Nutritional status of children. III. Blood serum vitamin C. J. Am. Dietet. Assoc. 24, 199–204.

298. Munks, B., Robinson, A., Williams, H. H. & Macy, I. G. (1945) Human milk studies. XXV. Ascorbic acid and dehydroascorbic acid in colostrum and mature human milk. Am. J. Dis. Child. 70, 176–181.

299. Nagai, A. (1960) Studies on the dietary allowance of vitamin C in infancy and childhood. Shikoku Acta Med. 16, 157–170.

300. Najjar, V. A., Holt, L. E., Jr. & Royston, H.

A. (1944) A note on the minimum requirements of man for vitamin C and certain other vitamins. Bull. Johns Hopkins Hosp. 75, 315–318.

301. Nakamura, M., Kawagoe, T., Ogino, Y., Nishiyama, K., Ichikawa, H. & Sugahara, K. (1967) Experimental study on the effect of vitamin C on the basal metabolism and resistance to cold in human being. Tohoku J. Exp. Med. 92, 207–219.

302. Namysłowski, L. (1956) Spostrzezenia nad zapotrzebowaniem na witaminę C u sportów-ców w zależności od wysiłku fizycznego. Rocz. Państwow. Zakl. Hig. 7, 97–122.

303. National Research Council, Food and Nutrition Board (1945). Recommended dietary allowances, revised 1945. NRC Reprint and Circular Series No. 122, Washington, D.C.

304. Neuweiler, W. (1935) Über den Bedarf an Vitamin C während Gravidität und Lactation. Klin. Wochenschr. 14, 1793–1794.

305. Neuweiler, W. (1937) Vitamin C-Stoffwechsel bei Neugeborenen. Z. Vitaminforsch. 6, 75–82.

306. Neuweiler, W. (1939) Bemerkungen zur Frage des Vitamin C-Bedarfes. Klin. Wochenschr. 18, 769–772.

307. Nicol, B. M. (1956) The nutrition of Nigerian children, with particular reference to their ascorbic-acid requirements. Br. J. Nutr. 10, 275–285.

308. O'Hara, P. H. & Hauck, H. M. (1936) Storage of vitamin C by normal adults following a period of low intake. J. Nutr. 12, 413–427.

309. Oldham, H., Roberts, L. J. & Young, M. (1945) Results of providing a liberally adequate diet to children in an institution III. Blood and urinary excretion studies before and after dietary improvement. J. Pediatr. 27, 418–427.

310. Olivová, E. (1969) Sledování změn askorbémie u člověka při púsobeni zátěže horkem. Ces Hygiena 14, 20–23.

311. Ošancová, K. & Hejda, S. (1965) Cs. Gastroenterol. Výž. 19, 4, 232. Cited by: Mažek, J. (1966) Contribution to the problem of vitamin C requirement in adults. Rev. Czech. Med. 12, 54–60.

312. Osborne, S. L. & Farmer, C. J. (1942) Influence of hyperpyrexia on ascorbic acid concentration in the blood. Proc. Soc. Exp. Biol. Med. 49, 575–578.

313. O'Sullivan, D. J., Callaghan, N., Ferriss, J. B., Finucane, J. F. & Hegarty, M. (1968) Ascorbic acid deficiency in the elderly. Irish J. Med. Sci. 1(4), 151–156.

314. Paeschke, K.-D. & Vasterling, H.-W. (1968) Photometrischer Ascorbinsäure- Test zur Bestimmung der Ovulation, verglichen mit anderen Methoden der Ovulationstermin-bestimmung. Zentrabl. Gynäkol. 90, 817–820.

315. Parks, E. A., Guild, H. G., Jackson, D. & Bond, M. (1935) The recognition of scurvy with especial reference to the early X-ray changes. Arch. Dis. Child. 10, 265–294.

316. Pelletier, O. (1968) Smoking and vitamin C levels in humans. Am. J. Clin. Nutr. 21, 1259–1267.

317. Pelletier, O. (1970) Cigarette smoking and vitamin C. Nutr. Today 5(3), 12–15.

318. Pelletier, O. (1970) Vitamin C status of cigarette smokers and nonsmokers. Am. J. Clin. Nutr. 23, 520–524.

319. Pelner, L. (1943) Sensitivity to sulfonamide compounds probably avoided by combined use with ascorbic acid. Preliminary report. New York State J. Med. 43, 1874.

320. Pelner, L. (1944) The importance of vitamin C in bodily defenses. 1. The antianaphylactic effect of vitamin C in the prevention of pollen reactions. Ann. Allergy 2, 231–232.

321. Pemberton, J. (1940) A rapid method of differentiating children with large or small reserves of vitamin C. Br. Med. J. 2, 217–219.

322. Perla, D. & Marmorston, J. (1937) Role of vitamin C in resistance. Arch. Pathol. 23, 543–575.

323. Perry, C. B. (1935) Rheumatic heart disease and vitamin C. Lancet 2, 426–427.

324. Pierce, H. B., Newhall, C. A., Merrow, S. B., Lamden, M. P., Schweiker, C. & Laughlin, A. (1960) Ascorbic acid supplementation. 1. Response of gum tissue. Am. J. Clin. Nutr. 8, 353–362.

325. Pijoan, M. & Lozner, E. L. (1944) The physiologic significance of vitamin C in man. New Engl. J. Med. 23, 14–21.

326. Pijoan, M. & Lozner, E. L. (1944) Vitamin C economy in the human subject. Bull. Johns Hopkins Hosp. 75, 303–314.

327. Pirani, C. L. (1952) Review: relation of vitamin C to adrenocortical function and stress phenomena. Metabolism 1, 197–222.

328. Plough, I. C. & Bridgforth, E. B. (1960) Relations of clinical and dietary findings in nutrition surveys. Public Health Repts. (U.S.) 75, 699–706.

329. Pollitt, N. T. (1967) Muscle stiffness and vitamin C. Br. Med. J. 3, 372–373.

330. Poncher, H. G. & Stubenrauch, C. H. (1938) Intradermal dye test for vitamin C deficiency. J. Am. Med. Assoc. 111, 302–304.

331. Popov, V. A. & Osetrov, G. G. (1962) Vitamin C content in the blood of healthy persons and some surgical patients in Arctic regions. Vop. Pitan. 21, 60–62. Abstracted in: Nutr. Abst. Rev. 33, 529 (1963).

332. Portnoy, B. & Wilkinson, J. F. (1938) Vitamin C deficiency in peptic ulceration and haematemesis. Brit. Med. J. 1, 554–560.

333. Prauer, H. W. (1971) Vitamin C and tests for diabetes. New Engl. J. Med. 284, 1328.

334. Purinton, H. J. & Schuck, C. (1943) A study of normal human requirements for ascorbic acid and certain of its metabolic relationships. J. Nutr. 26, 509–518.

335. Rafsky, H. A. & Newman, B. (1941) Vitamin C studies in the aged. Am. J. Med. Sci. 201, 749–756.

336. Rafsky, H. A. & Newman, B. (1947) Nu-

tritional aspects of aging. Geriatrics 2, 101–104.

337. Rafsky, H. A. & Newman, B. (1948) A quantitative study of diet in the aged. Geriatrics 3, 267–272.

338. Rafsky, H. A. & Newman, B. (1949) Interrelationship among the vitamins in the aged. Geriatrics 4, 358–361.

339. Rajalakshmi, R., Deodhar, A. D. & Ramakrishnan, C. V. (1965) Vitamin C secretion during lactation. Acta Paediatr. Scand. 54, 375–382.

340. Rajalakshmi, R., Subbalakshmi, G., Ramakrishnan, C. V., Joshi, S. K., Bhat, R. V. Biosynthesis of ascorbic acid in human placenta. Curr. Sci. 36(2), 45–46.

341. Ralli, E. P., Friedman, G. J. & Rubin, S. S. (1938) The mechanism of the excretion of vitamin C by the human kidney. J. Clin. Invest. 17, 765–770.

342. Ralli, E. P., Friedman, G. J. & Sherry, S. (1939) The vitamin C requirement of man. Estimated after prolonged studies of the plasma concentration and daily excretion of vitamin C in 3 adults on controlled diets. J. Clin. Invest. 18, 705–714.

343. Rinehart, J. F. (1935) Studies relating vitamin C deficiency to rheumatic fever and rheumatoid arthritis: experimental, clinical, and general considerations. I. Rheumatic fever. Ann. Intern. Med. 9, 586–599.

344. Rinehart, J. F., Greenberg, L. D. & Baker, F. (1936) Reduced ascorbic acid content of blood plasma in rheumatoid arthritis. Proc. Soc. Exp. Biol. Med. 35, 347–350.

345. Rinehart, J. F., Greenberg, L. D., Baker, F., Mettier, S. R., Bruckman, F. & Choy, F. (1938) Metabolism of vitamin C in rheumatoid arthritis. Arch. Intern. Med. 61, 537–551.

346. Rinehart, J. F., Greenberg, L. D. & Christie, A. U. (1936) Reduced ascorbic acid content of blood plasma in rheumatic fever. Proc. Soc. Exp. Biol. Med. 35, 350–353.

347. Ritchey, S. J. (1965) Metabolic patterns in pre-adolescent children. XV. Ascorbic acid intake, urinary excretion and serum concentration. Am. J. Clin. Nutr. 17, 78–82.

348. Ritzel, G. (1961) Kritische Beurteilung des Vitamins C als Prophylacticum und Therapeuticum der Erkältungskrankheiten. Helv. Med. Acta 28, 63–68.

349. Rivers, J. M. & Devine, M. M. (1972) Plasma ascorbic acid concentrations and oral contraceptives. Am. J. Clin. Nutr. 25, 684–689.

350. Roberts, V. M., Brookes, M. H., Roberts, L. J., Koch, P. & Shelby, P. (1943) The ascorbic acid requirements of school-age girls. J. Nutr. 26, 539–547.

351. Roberts, V. M. & Roberts, L. J. (1942) A study of the ascorbic acid requirements of children of early school age. J. Nutr. 24, 25–39.

352. Robertson, W. van B. (1961) The biochemical role of ascorbic acid in connective tissue. Ann. New York Acad. Sci. 92, 159–167.

353. Roderuck, C., Burrill, L., Campbell, L. J., Brakke, B. E., Childs, M. T., Leverton, R., Chaloupka, M., Jebe, E. H. & Swanson, P. P. (1958) Estimated dietary intake, urinary excretion and blood vitamin C in women of different ages. J. Nutr. 66, 15–27.

354. Rohmer, P. & Bezssonoff, N. (1935) Investigations into the pathogenesis of scorbutic dystrophy. Arch. Dis. Child. 10, 319–326.

355. Rohmer, P., Sanders, U. & Bezssonoff, N. (1934) Synthesis of vitamin C. by the infant. Nature 134, 142–143.

356. Rotter, H. (1937) Determination of vitamin C in the living organism. Nature 139, 717.

357. Ryer, R., III, Grossman, M. I., Friedemann, T. E., Best, W. R., Consolazio, C. F., Kuhl, W. J., Insull, W., Jr. & Hatch, F. T. (1954) The effect of vitamin supplementation on soldiers residing in a cold environment. 1. Physical performance and response to cold exposure. J. Clin. Nutr. 2, 97–132.

358. Ryer, R., III, Grossman, M. I., Friedemann, T. E., Best, W. R., Consolazio, C. F., Kuhl, W., Jr. & Hatch, F. T. (1954) Vitamin supplementation on soldiers residing in a cold environment. Part II. Psychological, biochemical, and other measurements. J. Clin. Nutr. 2, 179–194.

359. Sahud, M. A. & Cohen, R. J. (1971) Effect of aspirin ingestion on ascorbic-acid levels in rheumatoid arthritis. Lancet 1, 937–938.

360. Saindelle, A., Arhan, P., Gazave, J. M., Dechy, J. P. & Santais, M. C. (1969) Antagonisme in vitro entre le facteur vitaminique C₂ extrait du jus d'orange et certains constituants de la fumée de cigarette. Thérapie 24, 581–588.

361. Sakurai, K. (1970) Studies on the vitamin C level in blood of the patients of pulmonary tuberculosis. Shikoku Acta med. 26, 319–333. Abstracted in: Nutr. Abst. Rev. 41, 618.

362. Sargent, F., Robinson, P. & Johnson, R. E. (1944) Water-soluble vitamins in sweat. J. Biol. Chem. 153, 285–294.

363. Sayers, G. & Sayers, M. A. (1946) The pituitary-adrenal system. Recent Prog. Horm. Res. 2, 81–115.

364. Scheunert, A. (1949) Der Tagesbedarf des Erwachsenen an Vitamin C. Int. Z. Vitaminforsch. 20, 374–386.

365. Schropp, J. H. (1943) Sulfapyridine sensitivity checked by ascorbic acid. Can. Med. Assoc. J. 49, 515.

366. Schultz, M. P. (1936) Studies of ascorbic acid and rheumatic fever. II. Test of prophylactic and therapeutic action of ascorbic acid. J. Clin. Invest. 15, 385–391.

367. Selleg, I. & King, C. G. (1936) The vitamin C content of human milk and its variation with diet. J. Nutr. 11, 599–606.

368. Sendroy, J., Jr. & Schultz, M. P. (1936) Studies of ascorbic acid and rheumatic fever. L. Quantitative index of ascorbic acid utilization in human beings and its applicaton to

the study of rheumatic fever. J. Clin. Invest. 15, 369–383.

369. Senger, H., Neumann, G. & Baasch, G. (1969) Verlaufsuntersuchungen des Askorbinsäurespiegels im Blutserum vor, während und nach sportlicher Belastung. Deutsch. Gesundheits. 24, 2099–2102.

370. Shukla, S. P. (1969) Plasma and urinary ascorbic acid levels in the postoperative period. Experientia 25, 704.

371. Sigurjonsson, J. (1949) Dietary intakes of vitamin C in Iceland. Br. J. Nutr. 2, 275–281.

372. Slobody, L. B., Benson, R. A. & Mestern, J. (1947) A comparison of vitamin C in mothers and their premature newborn infants. J. Pediatr. 31, 333–337.

373. Smolyanskii, B. L. (1963) Effect of ascorbic acid on functional state of adrenal cortex in elderly persons. Terapeutich. Arkh. 35(1), 71. Translated in: Federation Proc. 22, T 1173–T 1176 (1963).

374. Snelling, C. E. & Jackson, S. H. (1939) Blood studies of vitamin C during pregnancy, birth, and early infancy. J. Pediatr. 14, 447–451.

375. Snigur, O. I. (1966) Pokazateli utomlenija ucascihsja pri različnom obespečenii organizma askorbinovoj kislotoj. Gig. Sanit. No. 7, 117–119. Abstracted in: Nutr. Abst. Rev. 37, 203 (1967).

376. Snisarenko, L. I. (1959) K voprosu o potrebnosti detej doskol'nogo vozrasta v vitamine C. Vop. Pitan 18(1), 50–53. Abstracted in: Nutr. Abst. Rev. 29, 1002 (1959).

377. Sokoloff, B., Hori, M., Saelhof, C., McConnell, B. & Imai, T. (1967) Effect of ascorbic acid on certain blood fat metabolism factors in animals and man. J. Nutr. 91, 107–118.

378. Spittle, C. R. (1971) Atherosclerosis and vitamin C. Lancet 2, 1280–1281.

379. Srikantia, S. G., Mohanram, M. & Krishnaswamy, K. (1970) Human requirements of ascorbic acid. Am. J. Clin. Nutr. 23, 59–62.

380. Steele, B. F., Hsu, C-H., Pierce, Z. H. & Williams, H. H. (1952) Ascorbic acid nutriture in the human. I. Tyrosine metabolism and blood levels of ascorbic acid during ascorbic acid depletion and repletion. J. Nutr. 48, 49–59.

381. Steele, B. F., Liner, R. L., Pierce, Z. H. & Williams, H. H. (1955) Ascorbic acid nutriture in the human. II. Content of ascorbic acid in the white cells and sera of subjects receiving controlled low intakes of the vitamin. J. Nutr. 57, 361–368.

382. Stefanini, M. & Rosenthal, M. C. (1950) Hemorrhagic diathesis with ascorbic acid deficiency during administration of anterior pituitary corticotropic hormone (ACTH). Proc. Soc. Exp. Biol. Med. 75, 806–808.

383. Storvick, C. A., Davey, B. L., Nitchals, R. M., Coffey, R. E. & Fincke, M. L. (1949) Ascorbic acid metabolism of older adolescents. J. Nutr. 39, 1–11.

384. Storvick, C. A., Davey, B. L., Nitchals, R. M.,

Coffey, R. E. & Fincke, M. L. (1950) Ascorbic acid requirements of older adolescents. Oregon Agr. Exp. Sta. Tech. Bull. No. 18, pp. 1–67.

385. Storvick, C. A., Fincke, M. L., Quinn, J. P. & Davey, B. L. (1947) A study of ascorbic acid metabolism of adolescent children. J. Nutr. 33, 529–539.

386. Storvick, C. A., Fincke, M. L., Quinn, J. P. & Davey, B. L. (1947) A study of ascorbic acid metabolism of adolescent children. Oregon Agr. Exp. Sta. Bull. 12, pp. 1–35.

387. Storvick, C. A. & Hauck, H. M. (1942) Excretion and plasma concentration of ascorbic acid in normal adults. J. Nutr. 23, 111–123.

388. Svensgaard, E. (1934) Infantile scurvy treated with ascorbic acid. Lancet 1, 22–23.

389. Svirbely, J. L. & Szent-Györgi, A. (1932) The chemical nature of vitamin C. Biochem. J. 26, 865–870.

390. Sydenstricker, V. P. (1953) The impact of vitamin research upon medical practice. Proc. Nutr. Soc. 12, 256–269.

391. Szent-Györgyi, A. & Haworth, W. N. (1933) "Hexuronic acid" (ascorbic acid) as the antiscorbutic factor. Nature 131, 24.

392. Tani, Z. (1959) Studies on the dietary allowance of vitamin C. 2. On the assessment of vitamin C allowance. Shikoku Acta Med. 15, 369–374.

393. Taylor, G. (1966) Diet of elderly women. Lancet 1, 926.

394. Tebrock, H. E., Arminio, J. J. & Johnston, J. H. (1956) Usefulness of bioflavonoids and ascorbic acid in treatment of common cold. J. Am. Med. Assoc. 162, 1227–1233.

395. Tennent, D. M. & Silbert, R. H. (1943) The excretion of ascorbic acid, thiamine, riboflavin, and pantothenic acid in sweat. J. Biol. Chem. 148, 359–364.

396. Todhunter, E. N. & Robbins, R. C. (1940) Observations on the amount of ascorbic acid required to maintain tissue saturation in normal adults. J. Nutr. 19, 263–270.

397. Tolbert, B. M., Chen, A. W., Bell, E. M. & Baker, E. M. (1967) Metabolism of L-ascorbic-4-³H acid in man. Am. J. Clin. Nutr. 20, 250–252.

398. Toverud, K. U. (1935) The vitamin C content of the liver of newborn infants. Arch. Dis. Child. 10, 313–318.

399. Toverud, K. U. (1939) The vitamin-C need in pregnant and lactating women. Acta Paediatr. 24, 332–340.

400. Toverud, K. U. (1939) The vitamin C requirements of pregnant and lactating women. Z. Vitaminforsch. 8, 237–248.

401. Trier, E. (1940) C-vitaminstudier hos syge og sunde. E. Munksgaard, Copenhagen. Cited by: Kirk, J. E. & Chieffi, M. (1953) Vitamin C studies in middle-aged and old individuals. XI. The concentration of total ascorbic acid in whole blood. J. Gerontol. 8, 301–304.

402. Tünte, W. (1968) Zur Frage der jahreszeitlichen Häufigkeit der Anencephalie. Humangenetik 6, 225–236.

403. Umanskij, S. S., Hejfec-Tetel'baum, B. A. & Rozov, E. E. (1968) Sekrecija želudka u vodolazovglubokovodnikov v obyčnyh uslovijah i pod vodoj. Fiziol. Ž. SSSR Sečenova 54, 365–369.

404. Vakhtina, T. I. & Zaretsky, M. M. (1969) Vlijanie vitaminov C, B_1 i B_6 na funkcional'noe sostojanie kory nadpočečnikov i bol'nyh aterosklerotičeskim kardiosklerozom. Vop. Pitan. 28(5), 27–30. Abstracted in: Nutr. Abstr. Rev. 40, 605 (1970).

405. Vail, A. D. (1941) Influence of vitamin C therapy on arsenical sensitivity. J. Missouri Med. Assoc. 38, 110–120.

406. van der Merwe, A. le R. (1962) Die voorsiening en verbruik van askorbiensuur by die Suid-Afrikaanse Antarktiese basis, 1960. S. Afr. Med. J. 36, 751–754.

407. van Eekelen, M. (1935) On the metabolism of ascorbic acid (Vitamin C) Acta brev. Neerl. Physiol. 5, 165–167.

408. van Eekelen, M. (1936) On the amount of ascorbic acid in blood and urine. The daily human requirements for ascorbic acid. Biochem. J. 30, 2291–2298.

409. van Eekelen, M. (1953) The occurrence of vitamin C in foods. Proc. Nutr. Soc. 12, 228–232.

410. van Eekelen, M., Emmerie, A., Josephy, B. & Wolff, L. K. (1933) Vitamin C in blood and urine? Nature 132, 315–316.

411. van Eekelen, M., Emmerie, A. & Wolff, L. K. (1937) Ueber der Diagnostik der Hypovitamenosen A und C durch die Bestimmung dieser Vitamine im Blut. Z. Vitaminforsch. 6, 150–162.

412. van Eekelen, M. & Heinemann, M. (1938) Critical remarks on the determination of urinary excretion of ascorbic acid. J. Clin. Invest. 17, 293–299.

413. van Eekelen, M., Heinemann, M. & van Wersch, H. J. (1936) On the daily requirements for ascorbic acid of man. Acta brev. Neerl. Physiol. 6, 107.

414. van Wersch, H. J. (1936) Determination of the daily requirements for ascorbic acid of man. Acta brev. Neerl. Physiol. 6, 86–87.

415. Venulet, F. (1953) Tabakrauch und Askorbinsäure. Endokrinologie 30, 345–351.

416. Verbinets, A. V. (1970) Gigieničeskaja ocenka pitanija i stepeni obespečennosti vitaminami C i B2 detej, proživajuščih v gornyh uslovijah Prikarpat'ja. Vop. Pitan. 29(4), 22–25. Abstracted in: Nutr. Abst. Rev. 41, 617 (1971).

417. Vinařický, R. (1954) Pokus o zlepšeni výkonnosti v běhu na strední vzdálenost vitaminy B_1, B_2 a C. Scripta med. 27, 1–18.

418. Vitolin, I. & Hesselvik, L. (1947) C-vitamin i spädbarnäldern. Nord. Med. 33, 323–325.

419. Wachholder, K. (1936) Die Versorgung des Säuglings mit Vitamin C. Klin. Wochenschr. 15, 593–596.

420. Walker, G. H., Bynoe, M. L. & Tyrrell, D. A. J. (1967) Trial of ascorbic acid in prevention of colds. Br. Med. J. 1, 603–606.

421. Walzer, M. (1938) A critical review of the recent literature on the dust atopen and on vitamin C in relation to hypersensitiveness. J. Allergy 10, 72–94.

422. Warren, H. A., Pijoan, M. & Emery, E. S., Jr. (1939) Ascorbic acid requirements in patients with peptic ulcer. New Engl. J. Med. 220, 1061–1063.

423. Watt, B. K. & Merrill, A. L. (1963) Composition of foods, raw, processed, prepared. Agricultural Handbook No. 8, Consumer and Food Economics Research Division, ARS, U.S. Department of Agriculture, Washington, D.C.

424. Waugh, W. A. & King, C. G. (1932) Isolation and identification of vitamin C. J. Biol. Chem. 97, 325–331.

425. Weir, C. E. (1971) An evaluation of research in the United States on human nutrition. Report No. 2. Benefits from nutrition research 129 pp. Science & Education Staff, U.S. Department of Agriculture, Washington, D.C.

426. Westergaard, F. (1940) Staseprøven og dens Kliniske Betydning. E. Munksgaard, Copenhagen. Cited by: Kirk, J. E. & Chieffi, M. (1953) Vitamin studies in middle-aged and old individuals. XI. The concentration of total ascorbic acid in whole blood. J. Gerontol. 8, 301–304.

427. Whitacre, J., McLaughlin, L., Futrell, M. F. & Grimes, E. T. (1959) Human utilization of ascorbic acid. J. Am. Dietet. Assoc. 35, 139–145.

428. Wideman, G. L., Baird, G. H. & Bolding, O. T. (1964) Ascorbic acid deficiency and premature rupture of fetal membranes. Am. J. Obstet. Gynecol. 88, 592–595.

429. Widenbauer, F. (1936) Ascorbinsäurestudien an Säuglingen. Klin. Wochensch. 15, 815–817.

430. Widenbauer, F. (1937) Der Vitamin C-Haushalt des Menschen unter verschiedenen Verhältnissen. Klin. Wochensch. 16, 600–602.

431. Widenbauer, F. & Kühner, A. (1937) Ascorbinsäurestudien an stillenden Frauen. Z. Vitaminforsch. 6, 50–75.

432. Wiesener, H. (1966) Untersuchungen zum Vitamin C-Bedarf junger Säuglinge. Med. Ernährung 7, 120–125.

433. Wilcox, E. B. & Grimes, M. (1961) Gingivitis-ascorbic acid deficiency in the Navajo. I. Ascorbic acid in white cell-platelet fraction of blood. J. Nutr. 74, 352–356.

434. Wilkinson, J. F. & Ashford, C. A. (1936) Vitamin-C deficiency in Addison's disease. Lancet 2, 967–970.

435. Williamson, J. M., Goldberg, A. & Moore, F. M. L. (1967) Leucocyte ascorbic acid levels in patients with malabsorption or previous gastric surgery. Br. Med. J. 2, 23–25.

436. Wilson, C. W. M. & Low, H. S. (1969) Ascorbic acid and upper respiratory inflammation. Acta Allergologica 24, 367–368.

437. Wilson, M. G. & Lubschez, R. (1946) Studies in ascorbic acid with especial refer-

ence to the white layer. II. The relation of intake to blood levels in normal children and the effect of acute and chronic illness. J. Clin. Invest. 25, 428–436.

438. Winter, S. T., Muammar, S. & Boxer, J. (1966) Vitamin C nutrition of Israeli infants. Israel J. Med. Sci. 2, 204–207.

439. Wirths, W. (1969) Vitamin C intake and vitamin C supply of apprentices in an apprentice home in Cologne. Int. Z. Vitaminforsch. 39, 259–268.

440. Wirths, W. (1970) Über die Zufuhr von Thiamin und Ascorbinsäure bei Alten- und Lehrlings-Heiminsassen. Int. Z. Vitaminforsch. 40, 617–627.

441. Wolfer, J. A., Farmer, C. J., Carroll, W. W. & Manshardt, D. O. (1947) An experimental study in wound healing in vitamin C depleted human subjects. Surg. Gynecol. Obstet. 84, 1–15.

442. Woodhill, J. M. & Nobile, S. (1971) Vitamin C (L-ascorbic acid and dehydro-L-ascorbic acid). A contribution to the Captain Cook bicentennial celebrations. Med. J. Australia 1, 1009–1014.

443. Woolf, L. I. & Edmunds, M. E. (1950) The metabolism of tyrosine and phenyl-

alanine in premature infants: the effect of large doses. Biochem. J. 47, 630–639.

444. Wright, I. S. (1938) Cevitamic acid (ascorbic acid; crystalline vitamin C); a critical analysis of its use in clinical medicine. Ann. Intern. Med. 12, 516–528.

445. Yakutina, E. V. (1965) Ob obespečecennosti vitaminom C učaščihsja školy-internata Omska. Pediatrija No. 6, 21–25. Abstracted in: Nutr. Abst. Rev. 35, 1104 (1965).

446. Youmans, J. B., Corlette, M. B., Akeroyd, J. H. & Frank, H. (1936) Studies of vitamin C excretion and saturation. Am. J. Med. Sci. 191, 319–333.

447. Young, E. G. (1964) Dietary standards. In: Nutrition, a comprehensive treatise, Vol. 11. Vitamins, nutrient requirements, and food selection. (Beaton, G. H. & McHenry, E. W., eds.), pp. 299–350, Academic Press, New York.

448. Young, J., King, E. J., Wood, E. & Wootton, I. D. P. (1946) A nutritional survey among pregnant women. J. Obstet. Gynaecol. Brit. Empire 53, 251–259.

449. Zook, J. & Sharpless, G. R. (1938) Vitamin C nutrition in artificial fever. Proc. Soc. Exp. Biol. Med. 39, 233–236.

APPENDIX TABLE 1

Studies on maintenance requirements for vitamin C

Kind of study	Number of subjects	Number of studies	Suggested daily requirements	References
Scurvy	34 men 3 women	5	6.5 to 45 mg	13, 24, 25, 34, 85, 86, 186 188, 241, 325, 326
Capillary fragility	3 men 3 women	2	23 to 35 mg	143, 145
Whole blood levels Saturation	3 men 1 woman	4	50 to 77 mg	170, 171, 392, 407, 414
Acceptable	13 women	1	55 to 70 mg	66, 67
Blood plasma levels Saturation	74 persons	4	70 to 131 mg 1.7 to 2.0 mg/kg	62, 115, 141, 342
Acceptable	67 men 6 women	4	38 to 100 mg 0.8 to 1.2 mg/kg	115, 197, 243, 396
White blood cell levels Saturation	19 men 47 women	2	<22 to 83 mg	295, 296, 379
Acceptable	>101 persons	3	60 to 100 mg	92, 263, 275
Urinary excretion Saturation	99 persons	8	26 to 125 mg 0.6 to 2.2 mg/kg	36, 43, 68, 95, 218 236, 334, 430
Acceptable	7 persons	2	15 to 25 mg	164, 218
Morbidity		1	125 mg	364
Health surveys		4	30 to 70 mg	258, 276, 328, 371

APPENDIX TABLE 2

Studies on vitamin C requirements of infants (0 to 24 months old)

Kind of study	Description of subjects	Number of subjects	Number of studies	Suggested daily requirement	References
Infantile scurvy				20 mg	149
Tyrosyluria and tyrosinemia	Premature		7	75 to 120 mg	17, 89, 179, 253, 254, 256, 279, 443
Intake from breast milk			2	20 to 50 mg	203, 367
Intradermal	Premature	10	1	25 to 50	372
Blood levels	Full-term formula fed	41	2	20 mg plus formula	56, 290
Urinary excretion Saturation	Premature	121	1	10 mg/kg	432
	Full-term breast fed & formula fed	137	3	6 mg/kg 20 to 40 mg	305, 429, 432
Growth	0 to 17 months old	444	2	8 to 10 mg	46, 157

APPENDIX TABLE 3

Studies on vitamin C requirements of children (2 to 18 years old)

Age group	Kind of study	Number of subjects	Number of studies	Suggested daily requirements	References
Preschool children 2–5 years	Urinary excretion	16	5	21 to 50 mg	108, 167, 284, 285, 376, 430
	Saturation			7.5 mg/kg	
School children 6–12 years	Blood plasma levels				
	Saturation	98	2	45 to 125 mg	45, 351
	Acceptable	47	3	52 to 72 mg	347, 350, 351
	Blood serum levels Acceptable	4	1	60 mg	297
	White blood cell levels Saturation	>76	2	50 to 100 mg	280, 437
	Urinary excretion Saturation	132	5	35 to 130 mg	161, 321, 350, 351, 416
	Acceptable	>35	4	50 to 100 mg	239, 350, 351, 445
Adolescents 13–18 years	Blood plasma levels Saturation		1	1.6 to 1.8 mg/kg	299
	Acceptable	>24	3	70 to 97 mg	30, 383–386
	White blood cell levels Acceptable		2	62 to 100 mg	221, 433
	Urinary excretion Saturation		1	125 mg	198
	Acceptable		1	60–65	135

APPENDIX TABLE 4

Studies on vitamin C requirements of pregnant and lactating women

Subjects	Kind of study	Number of subjects	Number of studies	Suggested daily requirement	References.
Pregnant women	Blood plasma levels acceptable	100	1	200	208
	Blood serum levels Acceptable	621	1	80–100	274
	Urinary excretion saturation	23	3	67–100	121, 399, 400, 430
Lactating women	Milk secretion	21	2	80–100	399, 400, 431

APPENDIX TABLE 5

Studies on vitamin C requirements of the elderly

Kind of study	Number of subjects	Number of studies	Suggested daily requirements	References
Whole blood levels Acceptable	184	1	1.1 mg/kg	353
Plasma and leukocyte levels Saturation	100	1	Same as younger people	53
Urinary excretion	39	3	50 to 75 mg	125, 228

A CONSPECTUS OF RESEARCH ON IRON REQUIREMENTS OF MAN

by

JEAN BOWERING AND ANN MACPHERSON SANCHEZ

Division of Nutritional Sciences
Cornell University
Ithaca, New York 14853

AND

M. ISABEL IRWIN [1]

Nutrition Institute
Agricultural Research Service
United States Department of Agriculture
Beltsville, Maryland 20705

THE JOURNAL OF NUTRITION

VOLUME 106, NUMBER 7, JULY 1976

(Pages 985-1074)

TABLE OF CONTENTS

INTRODUCTION

The importance of iron to health has been recognized for centuries. Studies directly relating to requirements however, have appeared only recently in the history of iron in medicine and nutrition. The purpose of this conspectus is to present research which has led to the present understanding of human requirements for iron. The investigations cited fall into several broad categories. The first category includes studies which have as a major objective the acquisition of data directly related to estimating requirements. In this category, all of the research which appeared to be valid within the limits of existing methodology has been included. The second category includes research related to factors which influence the amount of iron absorbed from the diet. In this category there was some selectivity of factors included. Also, animal studies have been cited where they offer information on relative availabilities of different iron sources. The third category of research focuses on the etiology and treatment of iron deficiency and anemia. This category is voluminous and, because the studies do not address the issue of iron requirements directly, a considerable amount of selectivity has been employed.

It is not the purpose of the conspectus to provide new estimates of human iron requirements or to provide criticism of the individual studies which have provided data for these estimates. Rather, it is the objective of this conspectus to present what kind of work has been done, the age groups and number of persons from whom existing information has been obtained, and to indicate areas in need of future research.

The earliest medical writings relating clearly to iron are on the disease syndrome called chlorosis from the Greek word meaning "green". Because of the vagueness of the early descriptions of the disease, historians disagree on the time of the earliest allusions to chlorosis (225). However, since the 16th century descriptions of a disease commonly afflicting adolescent girls and characterized by pallor, fatigue, poor appetite, and gastrointestinal, neurological and menstrual disturbances have appeared in the literature (225, 515). By 1895, the

gastric and neurological disorders included in the descriptions of chlorosis were mentioned less frequently and Stockman (639) reported case studies characterized by poor appetite and low iron intake and often by excessive menstrual blood loss. About the time that many persons were suggesting that early descriptions of chlorosis in young women had probably encompassed a variety of disorders in addition to iron deficiency, it was also realized that chlorosis affected men as well as women (225). However, as recently as 1936, two reviews appeared presenting conflicting answers to the question of whether chlorosis is a disappearing disease, a view held by Fowler (225) or a nutritional deficiency continuing to manifest itself, a view held by Patek and Heath (515). Today, the prevalence and significance of mild iron deficiency remains controversial.

Interest in iron can also be traced through the history of hematology. In the 17th century, soon after the invention of the microscope had provided a basis for modern hematology, the nature of the red blood cell under conditions of health and of many diseases was described (619). The watery consistency of the blood seen in chlorosis, however, was ascribed to hydremia and it was not until the 1890's that the decrease in the size of the red cell and reduction of its iron content in chlorosis were noted (619).

Boussingault (96) is often recognized as the first to regard iron as an essential nutrient for animals. In the 1860's, he determined the iron content of the carcasses and food sources of many species and calculated the quantity of iron required in the feed of animals from the size of a mouse to that of large farm animal.

Major steps in understanding the significance of nutrients other than iron for maintenance of normal red blood cells and hemoglobin levels were provided by Whipple and Robscheit-Robbins (714) and Robscheit-Robbins (563) in the first quarter of this century. The early 20th century was also a time of interest in iron absorption and in elimination of iron from the body (563). This interest raised questions about the content, chemical form and

Received for publication July 21, 1975.
[1] Dr. Irwin died March 25, 1975.

availability of iron from foods and iron salts (563). Although much of the conflict remains unresolved today, there is a consensus that milk contains little iron (111, 294). Since the 1920's, milk diets have been used to induce iron deficiency anemia in rats (294) for the study of iron availability (192, 569). Research on the quantitative iron requirement of man is relatively recent. Early studies (in the 1930's) on the human iron requirement were conducted with balance experiments in which iron intake and excretion were determined by chemical analysis. More recently (in the 1950's), the introduction of two radioisotopes of iron has improved the ability of researchers to detect and quantitate iron. Radioisotopes have not eliminated all of the problems inherent in nutritional studies. Their use, however, has provided new approaches to the task of estimating man's need for iron. In addition, combinations of new chemical and isotopic methodologies are providing tools for expanding the knowledge of the biological mechanisms involved in extracting iron from food and regulating its passage across the intestinal wall.

This conspectus of research on human requirements for iron begins with a review of the world literature dealing with research on requirements of the adult human, on iron absorption and availability from foods. This discussion is followed by a brief description of iron deficiency, its diagnosis and means for assessing iron status of population groups. That section is followed by a review of the literature on research on iron requirements of children from birth through adolescence, of pregnant and lactating women, and of the aged. As in the preceding conspectuses in the series (283, 338–340, 564), the objective is not to estimate requirements but rather to show what work has been done, how it has been done, and where additional research is most needed.

STUDIES ON IRON REQUIREMENTS FOR MAINTENANCE

Iron balance

In balance studies, iron losses from feces and urine are subtracted from dietary iron intake while losses from skin, hair and sweat are often not measured. It is assumed that if intake and output are equal the subject is in equilibrium, if intake exceeds loss the subject is retaining iron and is in positive balance, and if loss exceeds intake the subject is in negative balance. The critical factor influencing iron balance is the absorption of dietary iron because, once iron has entered the body, losses are normally very small. Consequently, iron balance depends primarily on small differences between two large values—dietary intake and fecal output. The advantages of the balance procedure are that nearly normal food sources and dietary patterns can be maintained and that the subject is not exposed to radiation—an especially important consideration in studying pregnant women, infants and children (93). One disadvantage is that lengthy collection periods are required. In addition, the inability to collect all losses provides a bias towards positive balance (93). Because balance studies are expensive and time consuming, comprehensive data on iron intake and iron loss have been obtained from studies with relatively few individuals.

Reports of studies on iron balances in men include 47 observations on intakes of 7.2 to 48.4 mg iron/day (table 1) (50, 51, 119, 177, 211, 434, 556, 722, 723). The number of subjects studied at any one level of intake was small (3 to 8 men). In most of the studies, the diets contained mixtures of foods from animal and·plant sources supplying 7 to 25 mg iron/day. Higher levels of intake were studied by De (177) whose Indian diets, containing whole wheat, rice and sago, provided 9 to 48 mg iron/day. The 47 balances were −1.4 to 11.3 mg/day. With intakes above 10 mg/day, positive balances only were observed. Though the data are sparse, they suggest that, with intakes of 35 mg iron/day or less, balance is related to intake. De's data (177) suggest a plateau in balance with intakes above 35 mg/day. His balance periods, however, were short (6 days) and the number of subjects studied (3 or 4 men) was small.

In most studies with women of reproductive age (table 2), controlled diets composed of foods from animal and plant sources were used. In a study by Leverton and Marsh (399), women ate self-selected diets that were carefully measured. In 11

TABLE 1

Controlled studies on iron retention of men

Daily intake	Subjects	Studies	Length of study	Daily retention	References
mg	*No.*	*No.*	*days*	*mg*	
7.2 to 8.6	8	3	5 to 14	−1.08 to 0.9	211, 434, 722
9.3 to 11.4	7	4	6 to 12	−1.4 to 2.7	51, 177, 556, 722
14.3 to 16.8	3	3	8 to 63	1.4 to 3.4	51, 556, 723
18.5 to 20.1	6	5	5 to 63	0.7 to 11.4	50, 51, 177, 556, 723
21.1 to 25.3	5	5	5 to 49	0.5 to 7.8	50, 51, 119, 177, 723
27.2 to 30.9	3	1	6	5.3 to 7.4	177
33.1 to 34.6	3	1	6	6.8 to 10.7	177
38.1 to 39.8	4	1	6	7.0 to 11.1	177
41.2 to 45.8	4	1	6	7.1 to 8.8	177
46.0 to 48.4	4	1	6	7.0 to 11.3	177

studies of 6 to 94 days with a total of 178 observations, individual daily intakes were 0.96 to 17.3 mg iron and individual balances ranged from −0.8 to >4.5 mg of iron/day (211, 336, 356, 359, 398, 399, 402, 434, 672, 722, 723). Average menstrual losses reported in several studies (211, 357, 359, 402, 722, 723) were 8 to 18 mg iron/menstrual period. These losses were not included in the balance calculations. In a study by Ohlson and Daum (501), menstrual losses were included in the balance calculation but the individual losses (fecal, urinary and menstrual) were not reported separately. In this study (501) with three women whose average iron intake was 13.8 mg/day, the iron balance was −3.4 to 2.4 mg/day.

Average balance values calculated for various intake levels (tables 1 and 2) suggest a trend toward higher retentions with higher intakes. There was, however, a wide range of balances at all intake levels. Furthermore, when the data from several studies were scrutinized, no clear patterns associated with individual response to long periods receiving the same dietary iron level could be discerned. There appeared to be no obvious means for compensating for large periodic losses. For example, Leverton and Roberts (402) studied four premenopausal women for 110 to 140 consecutive days with controlled iron intakes from animal and plant sources. The major iron sources were lean beef, salmon, and whole wheat bread and the diets also contained eggs and orange juice which may have influenced iron availability. In all four women, hemoglobin levels rose by at least 1 g/100 ml during the study from initial levels of 11.1 to 13.0 g/100 ml (401). The continuous balance study was divided into 5-day collection periods. All blood losses including menses, nose bleeds and venipuncture were recorded. With iron intakes exceeding 12.5 mg/day, only positive balances (intake minus fecal and urinary loss)

TABLE 2

Controlled studies on iron retention of women

Daily intake	Subjects	Studies	Length of studies	Daily retention	References
mg	*No.*	*No.*	*days*	*mg*	
0.96 to 5.8	29	3	6 to 94	−2.0 to 1.5	336, 398, 672
5.9 to 7.9	26	6	7 to 28	−0.58 to 2.7	356, 359, 398, 399 434, 722
8.0 to 9.9	35	4	7 to 20	−0.51 to 3.9	211, 398, 399, 402
10.0 to 11.9	56	5	7 to 42	−0.12 to 2.5	356, 359, 399, 402 723
12.0 to 13.9	20	2	7 to 28	0.47 to 1.9	399, 402
14.0 to 17.3	12	3	7 to 70	−0.61 to >4.5	399, 402, 723

were observed. With intakes of 9 to 12 mg/day, both negative and positive balances were observed. There was no apparent pattern relating iron intake to negative and positive balances even when menstrual cycles were taken into consideration.

The average menstrual losses were 11 to 14 mg iron/menstrual period for three women. Woman four lost about 23 mg/period. When menstrual as well as fecal and urinary losses were subtracted from intake, two of the women were in negative balance when their iron intakes were 13.6 and 11.7 mg. The other two were in equilibrium when their average intakes were 11.8 and 10.0 mg.

For 45 days (nine 5-day periods) in the middle of this study one woman received a daily supplement of 5 mg iron; this raised her total iron intake to 17 to 18 mg/day. Negative balances of −7.63 to −1.71 mg/day occurred in three of periods 1 to 4; retention of 7.87 mg/day occurred in period 5, and equilibrium was achieved during periods 7 to 9. These observations suggest that 25 to 30 days may be required to adjust to new levels of iron intake.

The average daily fecal and urinary iron excretion for the entire study was 0.193 mg/kg body weight. Using this value as an indication of minimum requirement, and 56 kg as the average body weight, Leverton and Roberts calculated the minimum iron requirement to be 10.8 mg/day. They proposed that this amount be increased by 50% to 16.2 mg/day for an optimal iron allowance (402).

Leverton and Roberts (402) noted that equilibrium usually occurred with a daily intake of 12 mg of iron but they suggested that the response to lower intakes was unclear. Leverton (398), using the same design (402) described previously (p. 989) studied four young women with daily iron intakes of 3.06 to 4.46 mg (mean = 3.50 mg) for periods of 25 to 94 days. All balances (intake minus fecal, urinary and menstrual losses) were negative (mean = −0.33 mg/day); serum iron fell to low normal levels (50–80 μg/100 ml); and hemoglobin decreased by about 1 g/100 ml from starting levels of 13 to 15 g/100 ml. Three of the women, after 50 to 60 days of the low iron intake were given diets providing 6.43 to 6.76 mg iron/day. The

women retained iron (2.26–3.13 mg/day) with this intake. In a subsequent 15-day period, two of the women ate diets providing 9.17 and 9.58 mg iron/day. One woman's iron balance increased from 2.8 to 4.3 mg/day but there was no change in the balance (2.9 mg/day) of the second woman.

Johnston et al. (356, 357) investigated iron absorption and retention from diets providing approximately 7 and 10 mg iron/day. In their study, five young women ate a basal diet of animal (beef, eggs and milk) and plant foods supplying 7 mg iron/day for 6 weeks (2 weeks adjustment and 4 weeks experimental). During a succeeding 4-week period, beef was added to the diet to raise its iron content to 10.4 mg. Iron retention (intake minus fecal and urinary losses) with a mean intake of 7 mg/day was 0.26 to 1.33 mg/day. With a mean intake of 10.4 mg iron, the retention was 1.77 to 2.53 mg/day. Menstrual iron losses were 10.94 to 20.14 mg/menstrual period. Johnston et al. (357) calculated that iron retentions of 0.50 to 0.62 mg/day were needed to cover the menstrual losses. In addition, they pointed out that other small losses such as those from the integument had not been measured. They concluded, therefore, that with an intake of 7 mg iron/day, "the retentions were too low for safety," but that with an intake of 10.4 mg/day "the retentions were more than adequate to satisfy the needs of the subjects."

Leverton and Marsh (399), by increasing the number of observations, attempted to minimize the effect of error introduced by short study periods, atypical behavior of subjects and inaccurate separation of fecal collections. They conducted 99 7-day balance studies on 69 young women, 17 of whom were observed two, three or four times. The women ate self-selected diets that were weighed, sampled and analyzed. Their individual iron intakes were 5.94 to 16.71 mg/day. The average daily intake and balance (intake minus fecal and urinary iron) for the 99 observations were 10.44 and 1.37 mg respectively. The observations were organized into five groups according to level of intake. The proportion of negative balances decreased from 40% in the group with intakes of 5.94 to

7.99 mg/day to 13% in the group with intakes of 12.00 to 13.99 mg/day. There were no negative balances with intakes above 14.00 mg/day. Leverton and Marsh noted that the mean iron retention of the group with intakes of 10.00 to 11.99 mg/day was 1.34 mg/day, an amount that they considered to be ample to replace the menstrual losses. They also pointed out, however, that 19% of the individual balances in this group were negative. When the intakes of other nutrients were examined, Leverton and Marsh found that, in the group with the lowest iron intakes (5.94 to 7.99 mg), the women who were in positive iron balance had higher intakes of nitrogen, calcium and phosphorus than the women in negative iron balance. They concluded that emphasis should be placed "upon obtaining diets optimum in other essential nutrients which have been shown to function in efficient iron absorption and utilization." Iron balance studies are rarely performed today because present research techniques may be simpler and more accurate. Nevertheless, it should be noted that recent isotopic techniques have provided estimates of iron requirements very similar to those obtained from the earlier balance studies.

Iron turnover

Iron turnover, or the rate of iron loss from the whole body is determined by estimating radioactivity in the whole body or in red blood cells after an oral or intravenous dose of labeled iron. After the tracer dose is administered, a few months are required for mixing of the isotope in all of the iron containing compartments of the body with the exception of hemosiderin (705). Estimates of whole body or red cell incorporation of the radioactive iron have been obtained at intervals for up to 4 years to determine the iron turnover rate. The iron turnover rate is expressed as a percentage of the body iron pool lost each day. The actual daily iron loss is determined from the turnover rate and an estimate of the miscible iron pool. Both whole body and red cell counting for determining the daily obligatory iron loss have the advantage of minimizing small daily variations that hinder the interpretation of balance studies and assessment of iron absorption. However, both whole body counting and red blood cell uptake approaches to iron turnover, in addition to requiring lengthy periods of time for completion, do not permit assessment during a nonsteady state. Hence, the response to changes in dietary level or sources of iron cannot be measured.

Whole body iron losses were determined for 91 nonanemic men (89, 217, 267, 306, 441, 537, 554, 585, 708, 731), 19 postmenopausal women (217, 306, 554), 33 premenopausal women (217, 306, 554), and 4 menorrhagic women (554) (table 3). Whole body counters employing either sodium iodide crystals or liquid scintillation detection devices yielded similar estimates of iron turnover. The results obtained by whole body counting on 44 men

TABLE 3

Studies on iron turnover and iron loss from the body

Subjects	Method	Subjects	Studies	Length of studies	Daily iron turnover[1]	Daily iron loss[2]	References
		No.	*No.*	*weeks*	%	*mg*	
Nonanemic men	Radioiron incorporation	31	4	25 to 55	0.006 to 0.086	0.2 to 3.8	89, 306, 441, 585
	whole body[3]	13	5	9 to 39	0.04 to 0.57	—	441, 537, 554, 708, 731
	Red blood cells	47	4	68 to 216	0.015 to 0.058	0.49 to 1.63	217, 267
		19 (Bantu)	1	94 to 215	0.031 to 0.088	1.06 to 4.4	267
Postmenopausal women	Radioiron incorporation whole body	7	2	12 to 39	0 to 0.299	0.45 to 1.8	306, 554
	red blood cells	12	1	216		0.64	217
Premenopausal women	Radioiron incorporation whole body	27	2	7 to 55	0 to 1.16	0.5 to 3.5	306, 554
	red blood cells	6	1	184	—[4]	1.22	217
Menorrhagic women	Radioiron incorporation whole body	4	1	6 to 12	0.129 to 4.4	—	554

[1] Percentage of miscible iron pool lost each day. Range of individual values. [2] References 89, 441, 537, 554, 708, 731 contained no estimate of miscible pool size; therefore estimation of daily iron loss could not be made. [3] Whole body counting with sodium iodide crystal, references 89, 441, 537, 554, 585, 731 with liquid scintillation counter, references 306, 708. [4] Turnover rates determined on group data; no individual values.

fall into two groups based on high and low iron turnover rates. Four studies on 31 men conducted for 25 to 55 weeks revealed a range of average daily turnover rates of 0.03% to 0.032% of the body iron pool (89, 306, 441, 585). A second group of values obtained by the same procedures carried out on 13 men for 9 to 39 weeks showed a range of average daily turnover rates of 0.13% to 0.24% of the body pool (441, 537, 554, 708, 731). Most of the studies in the group with the lower turnover rates were carried out longer than the studies in the higher turnover rate group. There was, however, no relationship between individual turnover rates and duration of the study. There was a wide range of individual values in both groups. Individual values were 0.006% to 0.086%/day in the group with the lower turnover rates and 0.04% to 0.57% in the group with the higher turnover rates. Estimates of average daily iron losses, available only from the group with the lower turnover rates, were 0.89 to 1.22 mg.

Finch (217) and Green et al. (267) used the decline in red blood cell radioactivity from 68 to 216 weeks after an intravenous injection of labeled iron to assess whole body iron loss. Their average estimates of daily iron turnover rate which was 0.023% to 0.039% of the body pool were similar to the lower range obtained by whole body counting. The range of individual turnover rates was 0.015% to 0.058%. Daily iron loss, calculated from the turnover rates and an estimated miscible iron pool of about 41 mg/kg body weight, was 0.61 to 1.02 mg (217, 267). The range of individual losses was 0.49 to 1.63 mg/day. Bothwell and Finch (94) recalculated the data of Green et al. (267) and found that the iron loss from studies in several geographical locations was 12 to 16 μg/kg/day. The study by Green et al. (267) was a collaborative study on men including white North Americans, Venezuelan Mestizos and South African Indians and Bantu. The daily turnover rates among 19 Bantu men who had enlarged iron stores was 0.031% to 0.088% which was within the range of values found in other studies (table 3). Their daily iron loss, based on a miscible body iron estimate of 50 to 60 mg/kg was 1.06 to 4.4 mg. Because of the probable existence of iron overload in the Bantu, with considerable iron stored in the forms of (non-miscible) hemosiderin, estimates of miscible iron severely underestimates the total body iron content of these subjects.

The values for daily iron loss (0.61 and 1.02 mg) calculated by Finch (217) and Green et al. (267) were about 20% to 25% lower than values obtained by investigators using whole body counters. This difference was not due so much to differences in estimates of iron turnover rates as to differences in estimates of the miscible iron pool. The estimate of miscible iron (41 mg/kg) used by Finch (217) and Green et al. (267) was derived, by a procedure described by Bothwell and Finch (93), from the sum of total red cell iron (based on an assumed blood volume of 64 ml/kg) and miscible tissue iron calculated from the early stages of the iron turnover studies (217). Saito et al. (585) assumed a value of 42 mg/kg based on hemoglobin, blood volume, and the estimate of tissue iron (600 mg) reported for men by Finch (217). Heinrich (306), on the other hand, assumed a value of 55 mg/kg body weight for the miscible iron pool.

The rate of iron turnover in women was determined in three studies using whole body (306, 554) and red blood cell counts (217) (table 3). Postmenopausal women had iron turnover rates similar to those of men. The average turnover rates for these women were 0.030% to 0.142% of the body iron pool per day (217, 306, 554). Premenopausal women had average daily turnover rates between 0.052% and 0.324% of the body pool (217, 306, 554). In one study of four menorrhagic women (554), the mean daily iron turnover rate was 1.37% with an individual range of 0.129% to 4.4% of the body pool. In calculating the total daily iron loss, two different factors for determining total body iron were used. Heinrich (306) assumed a body iron content of 45 mg/kg and estimated daily iron losses at 0.45 to 1.8 mg and 0.5 to 3.5 mg for postmenopausal and premenopausal women, respectively. Finch (217) assumed a body iron content of 36 mg/kg and estimated the daily iron loss as 0.64 mg and 1.22 mg in postmenopausal and premenopausal women, respectively.

Factorial assessment of iron requirement

By the factorial method, the iron requirement is assumed to be the amount of iron that will equal the sum of the iron losses from the body. These losses occur through the intestinal tract (endogenous loss), kidney (urinary loss), integument (skin, sweat, hair and fingernails) and, in women, through menstruation. The factorial procedure does not take into account the possibility that large losses through one route may be compensated for by a reduction in losses by other routes.

Intestinal loss. It is difficult to differentiate between iron excreted from the body and unabsorbed iron. Endogenous iron losses arise from sloughed mucosal cells, red blood cells liberated into the intestinal tract and from iron containing secretions, particularly bile. Two techniques have been used to estimate the amount of iron actually lost from the body through the intestinal tract. In the first procedure, very low levels of iron are fed on the assumption that, with extremely low intakes, the loss approaches the minimum obligatory loss from the body. The second technique for estimating intestinal iron excretion is to inject radioiron intravenously and measure the activity appearing in the feces. Using the first procedure, Ingalls and Johnston (336) studied eight women with daily intakes of 1.0 to 3.2 mg iron and found that fecal output was directly related to intake. Assuming that endogenous iron loss did not vary with intake, they extrapolated to zero intake and estimated a residual (endogenous) iron loss of about 0.2 mg/day. Green et al. (267) using intravenous ^{59}Fe injections found an initial peak in fecal radioactivity of 2 to 8 days after the injection. Thereafter, the activity plateaued. They reported a range of 0.36 to 0.71 mg/day and an average endogenous iron loss of 0.51 mg/day by two Bantu women, seven Bantu men, one white woman and three white men. Dubach et al. (186) using a similar technique, reported daily endogenous iron losses of four normal men, and one normal woman of 0.33 to 0.52 mg/day. Three women with hypochromic anemia lost 0.032 to 0.061 mg iron/day (186).

McCance and Widdowson (433) were the first to suggest that the capacity of the human body to excrete iron was extremely limited. They reported (722) that after reaching balance with an intake of 7 to 9 mg iron/day, subjects receiving orally approximately 1,000 mg iron/day, retained between 37 and 160 mg/day. Upon returning to their initial low iron intake, the subjects were again in equilibrium and showed no indication of excreting through the intestine or kidney the iron they had assimilated previously during the high intake period (722).

Urinary loss. The contribution of urinary iron loss to total iron balance is small enough to be within the limits of error in determining dietary and fecal iron. Small as it is, urinary loss is not independent of physiological influences. Women have been shown to excrete more iron in urine than men (47, 49, 167, 422, 739) and to excrete less iron in the urine immediately after their menstrual period than at any other time (422). There appears to be considerable day to day fluctuation in the amounts of iron excreted by the same individual as well as considerable variation between individuals (422).

Recently, Man and Wadsworth (422) reported average urinary iron excretions of 93 μg/24 hours for 11 men and 121 μg/24 hours for 13 women. Between 4 and 30 observations were recorded for each individual. The range of individual values for men was 23 to 396 μg/24 hours and for women 16 to 440 μg/24 hours. In earlier studies, urinary iron losses were reported for normal subjects either as part of balance studies or independently of calculations of iron balance. The meaning of these data is somewhat obscured by the different methods of reporting results. In some studies, the group mean value was based on the mean values obtained for the same individuals over a series of 24-hour periods. In other studies, the group mean values were obtained by averaging the values for a single day's iron output. The same confusion exists in reporting ranges of values. Furthermore, the term "individual value" has been used for a value that is the average of an individual subject as well as for the value from a single observation. In addition, it appears that some of the very high losses have a pathologic origin but these subjects are not clearly identified.

In balance studies in which 44 observations were made on 17 men, the mean values for urinary iron excretion were 100 to 1,020 μg/24 hours and individual values 80 to 11,500 μg/24 hours (177, 211, 434, 723). Balance studies provided 46 observations on 21 women with means of 68 to 350 μg/24 hours and individual values of 60 to 430 μg/24 hours (357, 359, 398, 434, 722). Studies on urinary iron excretion not conducted as part of iron balance studies included 223 observations on 169 men in which the mean values were 46 to 395 μg/24 hours and individual values were 11 to 1,290 μg/24 hours (45, 47, 49, 124, 167, 267, 290, 425, 739). Similar studies in which 138 observations were made on 138 women showed mean values of 74 to 489 μg/24 hours and individual values of 13 to 1,630 μg/24 hours (47, 49, 167, 739). Some investigators found elevated urinary iron with increased iron intake (177, 398, 422) but others did not (357, 359). Neither Dagg et al. (167) nor Green et al. (267) found a difference attributable to physiological condition in urinary iron loss among 24 normal, 18 sideropenic, and 32 iron deficient individuals. Dagg et al. (167) observed an increased excretion in five patients with idiopathic hemochromatosis.

Integumental losses. In nutritional balance studies, integumental losses of iron have usually been ignored because of the difficulty in measuring them. Many techniques have been used to assess integumental loss. Methods which provide information on the amount of iron contained in skin include chemical analysis of skin removed at autopsy (267), isotopic analysis of skin removed at surgery after injection of ^{59}Fe (267) and loss of iron after intradermal injection of radioiron (55, 129–131, 708). Other procedures have been performed to determine the amount of iron lost through the skin and recovered in perspiration (4, 22, 26, 143, 147, 327, 328, 358, 455, 535, 681, 682, 708). None of the procedures provides a practical or direct means of quantitating dermal iron loss from the whole body. The isotopic procedures appear to have an advantage over chemical determination where contamination of skin or hair with environmental iron may produce erroneously high values.

The iron content of skin was reported by Green et al. (267) who chemically assayed samples of eccrine skin obtained at 17 necropsies. They extrapolated from their sample to the total body surface to estimate the iron content of the total skin to be 22.5 mg, but they did not suggest a value for daily iron loss from the skin. There was no relationship between the iron contents of skin and liver. Green et al. (267) also found that the iron uptake of eccrine skin in 21 surgical patients who had received ^{59}Fe intravenously was 0.35% of the tracer dose per square meter of body surface. The seven predominantly apocrine areas studied showed an uptake of 2.14%/square meter. Since apocrine areas represent less than 5% of the total skin area, the daily iron uptake was extrapolated from eccrine skin data. The daily iron uptake averaged 0.24 mg/day and was related to the transferrin saturation. Skin iron uptake was 0 to 0.26 mg/day in 13 patients with normal transferrin saturation and 0.48 to 0.64 mg/day in four subjects with artificially elevated transferrin saturation.

Weintraub et al. (708) used a small animal whole body counter to determine radioactivity in the forearms of six iron replete subjects after intradermal injections of ^{59}Fe. There was a 75% to 85% reduction in activity in 2 days followed by a second phase with a half-life of 54 to 110 days. Autoradiographs of cells from skin excised from the site of injection showed selective localization in the epithelial cells of the epidermis and skin glands.

Several experiments on 75 normal and 14 iron deficient subjects conducted by Beamish and Jacobs (55), Cavill and Jacobs (129, 130), and Cavill et al. (131) showed that transferrin-bound iron was cleared from the skin in a manner that fits a 2-compartment model. The lymphatic or interstitial fluid compartment with a half-life of about 24 hours accounted for about 67% of an intradermally injected dose of ^{59}Fe while a cellular component with a half-life of about 67 days accounted for the remainder.

Cavill and Jacobs (129) observed that the pattern of removal of iron from skin was similar in normal and iron deficient individuals. However, in deficient subjects, iron was cleared less rapidly from the lymphatic compartment, and a greater proportion of the injected iron was retained in the epidermis. Cavill and Jacobs (130) later found that the rate of entry of iron into skin cells from interstitial fluid was 50% greater in iron deficient than in control subjects. However, because the serum iron was reduced in the iron deficient subjects, the actual amount of iron entering the skin cells was only 0.55 μg/hour compared with 1.55 μg/hour in normal individuals. The rate of iron leaving the skin cells was approximately 10% of the entry rate in both normal and iron deficient subjects.

None of the reports by Cavill and co-workers suggested a range of values for the iron loss from skin. Their most recent work (130), however, indicated that the rate of iron uptake by skin cells during iron deficiency could be reduced to 33% of that observed under normal conditions.

The iron content of sweat is most frequently used to assess the loss of iron from the skin. There are several difficulties and assumptions inherent in estimating dermal iron loss from sweat. Many investigators have reported only the iron concentration per volume of sweat or per unit of time without attempting to estimate daily iron loss by this route. The assumptions necessary to relate sweat losses collected experimentally to average daily losses are that a) total iron loss is independent of sweat volume, b) iron is lost at a constant rate throughout a 24-hour period, and c) iron is lost from all areas of skin at the same rate.

Because sweating is usually induced to produce sufficient material for analysis, it is important that the first assumption be valid. The information available in the literature indicates that is true. For instance, Apte and Venkatachalam (26) studied the same men during two seasons and found that although the volume of sweat was higher in hot weather (33°–35°) than in cool weather (22°–24°), the iron concentration of sweat decreased. Green et al. (267) showed also that men working under extremely hot, humid conditions did not have excessive iron loss when the volume of sweat was great. Furthermore Wheeler

et al. (713) found that moderate increases in activity in a hot climate did not raise the total amount of iron lost in sweat.

The remaining assumptions probably are not valid. Consolazio et al. (147) for instance, showed that, when three men were housed at constant temperature for 27 hours, the iron loss during sleep was about 50% of that incurred while the men were awake. Apte and Venkatachalam (26) found that the rate of iron loss varied with the part of the body from which the iron was collected. The iron concentration was about 6 times greater in sweat collected from the back and forehead than in a simultaneous collection from the extremities.

Iron is lost through insensible perspiration (328) as well as through active sweating where desquamation of the superficial layer of the epidermis contributes iron to the fluid collected. The contribution of cell debris to the total iron content of sweat is difficult to assess. Many studies have shown that cell-rich sweat contains more iron than cell-free sweat (4, 26, 327, 328, 535, 681). Therefore, scrubbing of the skin prior to measuring iron content of the sweat, a necessity for removing environmental contamination, may remove skin cells which contribute to dermal iron loss.

Estimates of daily iron loss through the skin have ranged from 0.07 to 6.5 mg (22, 186, 455, 535). Hourly losses have been reported to be 0.04 to 0.8 mg (22, 328, 358, 455, 681, 682). Iron losses have been based most often on the volume of sweat collected with averages of 15 to 46 μg/100 ml of cell-free sweat (4, 26, 143, 147, 327, 328, 358, 535, 681, 682) and of 30 to 161 μg/100 ml of whole (cell-free and cell-rich) sweat (22, 26, 327, 328, 535, 681).

Several groups found that anemic individuals lost less iron through the skin than did normal individuals studied under the same conditions (129, 130, 327, 535). Hussain and Patwardhan (327) found that 17 women with microcytic hypochromic anemia had no iron in their cell-free sweat and that they had lower iron concentrations in the cell-rich portion than six normal women had. After either 28 or 42 days of therapy, the iron contents of both the cell-free and cell-rich components reached the normal range. With normal healthy subjects, however, neither Johnston et al. (358) nor Vellar (682) found that iron loss in the sweat was influenced when oral iron supplements were administered. Similarly, Wheeler et al. (713) found no decrease in the average amount of iron lost in sweat (0.35 mg/day) when the iron intake was reduced from 36 mg to 17.5 mg/day. They determined 3-day balances with six healthy young men who were adapted to a hot climate and who normally performed a moderate amount of activity. When their activity was increased by 2 hours of rhythmic stepping, the mean iron loss in sweat was unchanged (0.35 mg/day) in spite of an increase in loss of cutaneous plus respiratory water from 5.5 liters to 7.9 liters.

Additional routes of iron loss include hair, fingernails, saliva and bile. Few investigators have made quantitative estimates of these losses. Data on the iron content of hair and fingernails, however, have been found.

Estimates of the iron content of hair range from 1 to 19 mg/100 g hair (187, 265, 266, 355, 596). Green and Duffield (265) after studying 358 normal people, found that most values ranged between 1 and 10 mg iron/100 g hair, regardless of color. Dutcher and Rothman (187) reported from a total of 15 observations, the following ranges in mg iron/100 g hair: red, 6.7 to 13.2; blond, 2.2 to 2.9; white, 1.8 to 4.4 and black, 0.9 to 4.9. Although individual values were not reported, Schmidt (596) found higher amounts in blond hair than in red or brown hair, in a group of 56 people. Green and Duffield found that the iron content of hair of individuals with either anemia or iron overload was similar to that of normal individuals (266). Annual losses of iron from hair were calculated as 1 mg/year by Johnston (355) and 7.3 mg/year by Schmidt (596).

Jacobs and Jenkins (348) studied the iron content of fingernails in 100 persons of 0 to 84 years. The iron content of fingernails was very high in infancy and dropped to adult levels (0–400 $\mu g/g$) by age 15. Although there was considerable overlapping of individual values, the average value for anemic individuals was lower than that for normal subjects. There was no relationship however, between the severity of the anemia and the iron content of fingernails. No other reports were found.

Menstrual iron loss (table 4). Menstrual iron loss has been expressed as mg iron/menstrual period or as ml blood/period. Iron loss has been determined directly by chemical analysis of iron (28, 30, 46, 48, 202, 333, 357, 359, 402, 451, 465, 501, 592, 722, 723) and indirectly by analysis of alkaline hematin (56, 279–281, 492, 579, 613), activity of ^{51}Cr in red blood cells (346, 547) and activity of ^{59}Fe in red blood cells (40). The average iron losses determined in 19 studies of 459 normal women were 8 to 38 mg/period (28, 30, 40, 46, 56, 202, 211, 253, 258, 281, 333, 357, 402, 451, 501, 592, 722, 723). The range of individual values was from 0.3 to 110 mg/period. Be-

TABLE 4

Studies on menstrual iron loss

Subjects	Subjects	Studies	Menstrual periods/ subject	Iron loss	References
	No.	*No.*	*No.*	*mg/menstrual period*	
Normal					
Studies covering more than one menstrual period	196	15	1 to 13	0.6 to 110	28, 30, 40, 46, 56, 202, 281, 332, 357, 359, 402, 451, 592, 722, 723
Studies of one menstrual period	263	7	1	0.3 to 84	30, 46, 56, 211, 253, 258, 501
Menorrhagia[1]	25	3	1 to 4	6 to 220	40, 48, 332
Hypochromic anemia	11	1	1	10 to 182	226

[1] Classification based on subjective evaluation by the patient.

TABLE 5

Studies on menstrual blood loss

Subjects	Subjects	Studies	Menstrual periods/ subject	Blood loss[1]	References
	No.	*No.*	*No.*	*ml/menstrual period*	
Normal					
Studies covered more than one menstrual period	216	10	1 to 12	2 to 307	28, 30, 40, 46, 281, 332, 402, 492, 579, 613
Studies of one menstrual period	816	8	1	3 to 460	30, 46, 211, 258, 279, 280, 346, 465
Menorrhagia[2]	31	4	1 to 4	9 to 970	40, 48, 547, 613
Hypochromic anemia	26	2	1 to 2	21 to 922	226, 346

[1] Blood volume was calculated from estimates of menstrual iron loss and hemoglobin level.   [2] Classification based on subjective evaluation by the patient.

cause of the wide range of apparently normal menstrual losses, distribution of values rather than averages may be more useful. Hallberg and Nilsson (281) made 144 observations on 12 women and found that 18.5% of the losses exceeded 20 mg/period while 49.5% of the losses were less than 10 mg/period. Beaton et al. (56) reported 42 observations on nine women and found that losses exceeded 20 mg/period in 38% of the periods and were less than 10 mg/period in 36% of the periods. The average losses of 25 women who considered themselves to be menorrhagic were 29 to 108 mg iron/period with individual values of 6 to 220 mg/period (40, 48, 333). One study (226) showed that the average iron loss for 11 women with hypochromic anemia was 68 mg/period with individual values of 10 to 182 mg/period.

An important factor in estimating menstrual iron loss is the variation in individual loss from one period to the next. Widdowson and McCance (723) measured menstrual loss in three women for 8 to 13 consecutive periods and concluded that an individual's loss was quite constant but that loss varied greatly among individuals. Hallberg and Nilsson (281) also showed that the differences among 144 observations on 12 women were primarily attributable to inter- rather than intra-individual variation. However, their results showed that some women's losses varied considerably more than others. For instance, in their 12-month study with 12 women, the five

women with the lowest losses never deviated from their own individual averages by more than 5 mg, but four of the 12 women deviated from their own averages by more than 11 mg at least one time. Other investigators found that there was considerable variation between periods in the same individual (28, 30, 40, 234) and that the amount of this interperiod variability differed among women (46, 451).

In many other studies, the volume of blood lost, rather than the amount of iron lost was reported. In these studies, the volume was determined indirectly because menstrual losses include other secretions as well as blood. Blood loss was estimated from the iron loss and the woman's hemoglobin level. The average blood loss reported in 16 studies of 1,032 nonanemic women who considered their menstrual flow to be normal ranged from 22 to 69 ml/period (28, 30, 40, 46, 211, 258, 279–281, 333, 346, 402, 465, 492, 579, 613) (table 5). Individual blood losses were 2 to 460 ml/period. The average losses of 31 women who considered themselves to be menorrhagic were 126 to 363 ml blood with individual values of 9 to 970 ml/period (40, 48, 333, 547, 613) (table 5). In two studies on 26 women with hypochromic anemia, the average blood loss per period was 121 ml (346) and 264 ml (226). Individual losses varied from 21 to 922 ml/period.

In an attempt to determine the volume of normal menstrual blood losses, Hallberg et al. (279) studied a random sample of 476 women of whom 357 considered themselves to be healthy and capable of working and to have normal menstrual losses. The average loss, based on one period per person was 38.5 ml of blood. A few women had losses greater than 90 ml. When data for the women with hemoglobin levels of less than 12 g/100 ml were excluded, the average blood loss for the remaining 183 women was reduced to 33.2 ml/period.

The length of the menstrual period as well as the volume of blood lost was reported in several studies (40, 46, 48, 402, 451, 578). Since several early investigators found that the duration of the period was an unreliable index of the quantity of blood lost, this factor was not reported routinely. Rybo (578) recently found that, in general, women with longer periods have a greater average loss than women with shorter periods. The frequency of the menstrual cycle is an important consideration in attempting to relate the relatively heavy iron losses incurred for a few days to an appropriate daily estimate for iron intake. Arey (31) analyzed 20,000 calendar records of 1,500 women reported in the literature and found that 27-, 28- and 29-day cycles were the most prevalent. A range of 7 to 256 days was found, with the length of most of the cycles between 25 and 31 days. If the average iron losses reported for normal women in table 4 were distributed over a 28-day cycle, the average daily iron loss through menstruation would range from 0.29 mg to 1.35 mg.

The effect of age, parity and contraceptive agents on menstrual iron loss is obscured by the wide range of normal values. Hallberg et al. (280) found a greater loss in older women but in their study parity was significant only among the women of age 25 years or less. Their hypothesis, that recent delivery may have increased the blood loss in the younger women, was not confirmed after a more thorough analysis of their data (579). Other studies by the same workers showed no statistically significant relationships between menstrual loss and age (279), parity (578, 579), or recency of childbirth (578). Cole (141) however, found a clear relationship between menstrual loss and parity but not between menstrual loss and age in a group of 378 women.

Studies of women using oral contraceptive drugs have shown that their average iron loss was lower than that of other women (490–492, 613, 659). The use of intrauterine contraceptive devices, however, may increase menstrual blood (722). Recently, Guttorm (275) reported that average menstrual blood loss doubled in a group of 20 women after insertion of intrauterine devices. All women reported an increased blood loss. Guttorm (275) also reported that, in a group of 90 women, the incidence of hemoglobin levels below 12 g/100 ml increased four- to fivefold within a 2- to 16-month period after insertion of the device. Tejuja (658) and Zadeh et al. (748) found slight declines in hemoglobin levels of women who had used intrauterine devices for about 1 year. However, a subsequent rise to original levels was observed in 2 to 4 years (658, 748).

Taymor et al. (655) concluded that chronic iron deficiency could cause menorrhagia. In their study of 83 patients with idiopathic menorrhagia, 74 women reported improvement in their condition after they had been given iron therapy (0.3 g ferrous gluconate twice daily) for at least 2 months. The degree of menorrhagia and the degree of improvement were both evaluated subjectively by the patients. Jacobs and Butler (346) however, disagreed with Taymor's conclusion. They (346) measured menstrual blood loss of 17 healthy women and of 15 women with iron deficiency anemia. The anemic women had a significantly higher blood loss than the healthy women. After their anemia had been corrected by iron therapy, the menstrual blood loss was even higher in 13 of the 15 women. Jacobs and Butler suggested that these higher blood losses were probably the women's normal losses and that while they were anemic, their flow from the endometrium was reduced to compensate for the deficiency in iron intake. When the anemia was corrected, their menstrual flow returned to normal high levels. Jacobs and Butler suggested further that iron deficiency anemia is "likely to occur when menstrual losses are above 40 ml, but, if the intake of iron is inadequate, deficiency may develop when menstrual loss is less than this."

The results of other studies also have suggested a negative relationship between large menstrual blood losses and the levels of circulating hematological indices (141, 202, 211, 226, 279, 280). Because most of the studies included only one menstrual period per woman, individuals with occasionally high losses could not be distinguished from those with chronically high losses. Elwood et al. (202) found a significant negative correlation between hemoglobin level and menstrual blood loss in a study on 440 women. Hallberg et al. (279) found that women with blood losses greater than 80 ml/period had significantly lower hemoglobin levels than women with losses less than 60 ml. Cole (141) reported lower hemoglobin, hematocrit, mean corpuscular hemoglobin concentration and serum iron among women whose menstrual blood loss exceeded 45 ml/period. Fowler and Barer (226), on the other hand, found no relationship between blood losses and hemoglobin levels of 11 women with hypochromic anemia. In their study, the menstrual blood losses were 49 to 452 ml (10–182 mg iron), and the hemoglobin levels were 4.7 to 12.4 g/100 ml.

Beaton et al. (56) recorded iron intake and measured menstrual iron loss and various hemotological indices of iron nutriture in 97 apparently healthy women. Complete data were obtained for 80 women. These data were organized into quartiles on the basis of iron intake. Each quartile was divided again into quartiles on the basis of menstrual loss. No significant relationship of hemoglobin level or mean corpuscular hemoglobin concentration to menstrual iron loss was observed at any level of iron intake. At the lowest intake level only (5.6–10.6 mg/day) plasma iron levels decreased significantly and there was a trend toward lower transferrin saturation levels as menstrual iron loss increased. These observations suggested to Beaton et al. (56) that "with iron intakes below about 11 mg/day, menstrual loss may not be compensated by intake and iron-depletion results."

STUDIES ON IRON RESERVES

Iron is stored in tissues as ferritin and hemosiderin. Ferritin, which does not stain by the Prussian Blue reaction, is composed of an iron-free protein moiety called apoferritin and micelles of a colloidal iron complex (705). Hemosiderin, which does stain with the Prussian Blue reaction, has a variable and rather poorly understood chemical composition (705). The major proportion of iron storage compounds occurs in liver, bone marrow and spleen and is found in both parenchymal cells and reticuloendothelial cells. Both ferritin and hemosiderin can be mobilized for hemoglobin formation although ferritin appears to be more readily available. Hemosiderin is not usually considered to be part of the body's miscible iron pool (705).

Ferritin, usually considered an intracellular protein, also appears in serum (349). The serum concentration has been reported to be directly related to iron stores (349, 405, 538, 631, 699). This relationship may provide a sensitive measure of the status of iron stores and may allow for detection of iron deficiency prior to the development of anemia (349).

The stores have been estimated by histological evaluation of tissue hemosiderin (39, 43, 235, 244, 423, 461, 550, 605, 649, 704, 706), chemical assay of tissue non-heme iron (136, 235, 244, 615, 649, 704, 706) and by phlebotomy, a technique used to determine the amount of stored iron that can be mobilized for hemoglobin synthesis (39, 219, 296, 331, 504, 541, 605, 630).

Comparison of chemical and histological assessment in the same sample of marrow (244) or liver (235, 706) has shown good correlation between the two techniques. However, there was a marked overlapping of chemical values at each histochemical grade. Weinfeld (704) found a good correlation between the nonheme iron contents of bone marrow and liver. The positive correlation was heavily dependent, however, on four very high liver nonheme iron values. Among the 35 people he studied there was rather wide scatter among low values.

Shoden et al. (615) reported that the relative amounts of ferritin and hemosiderin varied with the total tissue iron level. At normal physiological levels, there was slightly more ferritin than hemosiderin in liver and spleen. As the total iron concentration increased, the ferritin increased only slightly and the hemosiderin content predominated.

Phlebotomy procedures vary among different laboratories, but they all involve the removal of a relatively large volume of blood at several intervals (for example, 500 ml/week for 1 or 2 months). The ability of the body to regenerate hemoglobin from endogenous iron gives an indication of the body iron stores. Estimation of iron stores is based on hemoglobin concentrations before and after removal of blood, the quantity of hemoglobin iron removed and an estimate of the contribution of dietary iron toward replenishing hemoglobin between the periods of blood removal (296, 504, 541, 605). When iron absorption is not measured during the phlebotomy procedure, partition between dietary and endogenous iron can only be calculated.

There is disagreement on whether or not there is a correlation, between liver or bone marrow estimates of iron stores and values obtained by phlebotomy. Balcerzak et al. (39) found no correlation but Scott and Pritchard (605) found a good correlation in a group of women. Based on the phlebotomy technique, estimates of endogenous iron available for hemoglobin synthesis in 19 normal men was 130 to 1,900 mg iron with the middle 50% ranging between 550 and 800 mg (39, 296, 331, 541). For 21 premenopausal women the range was 20 to 743 mg with the middle 50% between 100 and 350 mg (541, 605). These estimates are in reasonable agreement with the average values for miscible iron of 600 mg for men and 380 mg for premenopausal women estimated by Finch (217) from the mixing of radioiron with tissue iron. Postmenopausal women showed higher values for miscible iron than premenopausal women (217, 267). Other studies in which iron stores in both men and women were measured have confirmed the observation that women generally have less storage iron than men (43, 136, 244, 638, 649, 677, 704, 706, 715). Estimates based on histological assessment of bone marrow, a technique frequently employed clinically, indicated that 67% or more of most groups of women had little or no hemosiderin (43, 461, 605, 706).

Iron stores in different population groups have been assessed by analyzing liver specimens of people dying from trauma or acute disease (43, 136, 649). Banerji et al. (43), using histological grading with a possible range of 0 to 5 reported lower values from India and Mexico (mean score 0.45–0.53) than from the United Kingdom, United States and Venezuela (mean score 0.69–0.80). Scores for liver samples from South Africa ranged from 0.41 for Indians to 2.61 for Bantu (43). No sex distinction was made because many records lacked this information. Charlton et al. (136) chemically assayed specimens from all over the world. They reported a similar range of median liver iron values in 30 to 33 groups studied. The range of median values for men was 111 to 277 μg/g and for women 103 to 213 μg/g. The men had significantly greater liver iron stores than premenopausal but not postmenopausal women. The Bantu from South Africa and Rhodesia had decidedly elevated liver iron stores with values of 776 to 946 μg/g for men and 268 to 283 μg/g for women. Average iron stores increased with age in the Bantu men but not in other population groups. The only groups with median values below 100 μg/g liver were from India and New Guinea (68–93 μg/g).

Iron stores are believed to be exhausted prior to development of anemia (218, 550). Although some investigators have looked for a relationship between iron stores and hemoglobin levels none has been found even among persons with low hemoglobin levels. In some studies, when the highest and lowest quartiles of hemoglobin levels were compared, there was no relationship between hemoglobin levels and iron stores in the liver or bone marrow (39, 704, 706). In the few individual data available for comparison there was no apparent relationship between hematocrit or hemoglobin level and iron mobilized by phlebotomy (39, 331, 541).

Once iron stores are depleted, they do not seem to be replaced readily by dietary iron and generally, therapeutic doses of iron are required (541, 704). Pritchard and Mason (541) found that when a daily oral supplement of 110 mg iron from ferrous gluconate was given to three men and three women, hemosiderin appeared in the bone marrow within 4 months or less.

STUDIES ON IRON ABSORPTION

The amount of dietary iron required to meet the body's needs is much greater than the sum of the obligatory iron losses because iron is relatively poorly absorbed (222, 463, 478, 745). The physiological and physical-chemical mechanisms involved in iron absorption, though not completely understood, have been reviewed thoroughly elsewhere (21, 91, 92, 224, 666). The literature pertinent to human requirements for iron shows much variation in the data on iron absorption. This lack of agreement is partly due to differences in primary research objectives of these studies and partly to the wide variation among normal individuals (149).

The objectives of studies on iron absorption generally fall into three broad classes. They are (a) assessment of behavior of gut mucosa as an indication of iron status or means of diagnosing iron deficiency, (b) estimation of availability of iron from foods and interactions of dietary factors, and (c) evaluation of iron sources as prophylactic and therapeutic agents for prevention and treatment of iron deficiency. With differing objectives, the experimental protocol has varied also. Therefore, comparisons drawn between studies and extrapolation of results from one study to another for the purpose of estimating the iron requirements of healthy individuals are not always appropriate.

Another source of variation in the data on absorption lies in differences in methodology and in indices of absorption. Both stable and radioactive iron isotopes have been used in balance studies. In addition the percentage of iron absorbed has been estimated by whole body counting and by counting the activity of red blood cells after the oral administration of labeled iron. Observations on the relative rise in serum iron or hemoglobin levels after the ingestion of iron-containing compounds have been employed less frequently.

In determining iron absorption in balance studies, the difference between the amount of iron ingested in food and the amount excreted in feces is assumed to be the amount absorbed. It is usually a very small amount when related to the amount of either ingested iron or fecal iron. As a result, relatively small errors in iron analysis or fecal collection are reflected in marked changes in the estimated absorption. Feeding radioactive iron and measuring radioactivity in the stools may reduce

the analytical problems but not the collection problems. Relatively poor agreement has been found between the results of the balance method using radioactive iron and those obtained by counting activity in red blood cells (138, 637) or the whole body (85, 412, 678).

Iron has two commonly available radioisotopes, ^{55}Fe, an X-ray emitter with a half-life reported as 2.6 and 2.94 years and ^{59}Fe a beta and gamma ray emitter with a half-life of 45 days (112). Detection equipment that distinguishes between the two isotopes is available. In the red cell counting procedure, iron absorption is estimated from a measurement of the radioactivity in blood and an estimate of blood volume 10 to 14 days after administration of labeled iron (102, 138, 383). The generally held assumption that all of the assimilated iron appears in red cells is probably true only for iron deficient subjects (745). In many studies with normal subjects, a correction is made for the 20% of absorbed radioiron which localizes in non-erythroid tissue. In some studies with red cell counting, one isotope was given intravenously while the other was given orally to allow correction for assimilated iron not appearing in red cells (589). Recently, with the interest in interaction between iron ingested from different sources, the two isotopes have been given orally (79, 150, 277, 388, 392, 427, 428). When a whole body counter is used, calculation of the percentage of iron absorbed is based on an initial value obtained immediately after ingestion of the test dose and the activity remaining 10 to 14 days later (58, 318, 412, 487, 678). Comparison of the results from red cell and whole body counting in the same subjects showed close agreement between the two techniques (412, 487).

The absorption of iron seems to be affected by many conditions. These can be roughly classified as physiological factors and factors affecting the availability of iron from its source.

Physiological factors affecting iron absorption

Increased iron absorption with poor iron status has been reported in many studies with patients with iron deficiency anemia or with iron depleted subjects. These observations have been made in studies using test doses of iron fed alone (85, 103, 146, 282, 291, 310, 312, 319, 320, 601, 637, 678), or fed in test meals (58, 95, 197, 524, 525) and in studies with mixed food sources (138, 329, 390, 392) or with purified iron-containing proteins (115, 146, 197, 667). A few studies, however, have failed to show increased absorption among iron deficient subjects (427, 464).

In studies designed to detect iron deficiency, a test dose of iron is given to fasting subjects either as a single labeled food or as an iron salt (85, 102–104, 146, 168, 297, 318–320, 383, 600, 601, 678) or as a labeled iron compound incorporated into a test meal (58, 95, 101, 138, 412, 524, 525). Several investigators have reported that a greater proportion of the iron test dose was absorbed when it was fed to fasting subjects than when it followed a meal (101, 152, 297).

Reports on the effect of the level of dietary iron prior to administration of the test dose are conflicting. Norrby and Solvell (474) found that 10 normal subjects absorbed 20% of a test dose after they had eaten an "iron rich" diet (20–30 mg iron/day) for a week. After they had eaten an "iron poor" diet (10 mg/day) for a week they absorbed 30% of the test dose. On the other hand, Rush et al. (576) observed no consistent increase in iron absorption after a period of feeding an "iron poor" diet. Most investigators have found that the proportion of iron absorbed is inversely related to the size of the test dose (95, 312, 524).

There is evidence that iron absorption is increased in blood donors (103, 277, 282, 319, 396, 421, 667), phlebotomized subjects (95, 146, 525), and individuals with reduced marrow iron stores (297, 312, 383, 524, 678). A significant correlation has been shown also between iron absorption and semi-quantitative assessment of marrow iron (297, 312), and between iron absorption and serum iron or saturation of iron binding capacity (297, 320, 423) and serum ferritin level (151, 631).

The results of some studies indicated that women absorbed more iron than men did from test doses (318, 383) and from bread (58, 521, 723). Other studies (297, 312), however, did not show a difference in iron absorption between men and women. The apparently greater absorptive ability of women reported by some investigators may be the result of depletion due to menstrual iron losses and lower dietary iron intake.

There is some evidence also that the amount of iron absorbed is related to age. In a group of children, 7 to 10 years old, Darby et al. (171) observed a strong trend toward increased iron absorption as the age of the children increased. Schulz and Smith (600), however, found that children under 3 years old old absorbed more naturally occurring iron from milk than children 3 to 10 years old. Both groups absorbed more iron from milk than did adults (600). Bonnet et al. (88) reported a slight decline in iron absorption in men and women between the ages of 20 and 34 years. Freiman et al. (233), however, found no evidence for an impairment of iron absorption with age in a group of 69 to 87-year old men and women.

Factors affecting iron availability

Bing (73) has suggested that the availability of iron from a food source or iron salt is not an inherent characteristic of the substance being assayed but an experimentally obtained value that indicates the absorption or utilization of the iron source under a particular set of test conditions.

The relative availability of iron from different sources has been studied with in vitro tests, experimental animals, and human subjects. The in vitro tests for iron availability include chemical determination of the ionizable iron in foods (192, 295, 347, 395, 546, 660) and quantitation of the iron liberated by in vitro digestion with pepsin and hydrochloric acid (295, 347, 546). Extrapolation from these studies to human in vivo situations should be made with caution (691).

Several investigators have suggested that the total iron content of foods obtained after ashing may be a poor indicator of the value of the food as a dietary source of iron. Some research groups have proposed that the ionizable iron determined with α-α'-dipyridyl (192, 231, 395, 610, 660), or tripyridyl triazine (295, 347) might give an indication of potential biological availability. Most of the analyses for ionizable iron were performed on bread (enriched and unenriched) in which 50% to 100% of the iron was in an ionizable form (192, 231, 395). By this method, iron in flour and dough was about 80% as available as iron in enriched or unenriched bread (395).

A few chemical studies have been performed on a variety of foods (347, 610, 660). Commercial quick freezing increased the ionizable iron content slightly whereas canning in glass effected no change (660). Treatment with pepsin-HCl mixtures has been done in attempts to simulate, in vitro, gastric digestion conditions (295, 347, 546). Under these conditions, Hart (295) found that more iron was in an ionizable form from enriched white bread than from whole wheat bread. Ranhotra et al (546) found that estimates of the relative availability of iron from bread enriched with reduced iron, sodium iron pyrophosphate and ferric orthophosphate after digestion with pepsin HCl were similar to estimates obtained in rat bioassays. Jacobs and Greenman (347) evaluated the availability of iron in 25 common cooked foods. They showed that the proportion of total iron that was in soluble form after peptic digestion ranged from 17.8% for eggs to 70% for potatoes with most values falling between 30% and 50%.

In biological systems, iron absorption may be limited not only by the availability of iron from the test source but also by physiological factors that influence the demand for iron by the test organism. The ability of the test sources of iron to maintain or regenerate hemoglobin levels has been compared with the response to a standard iron salt such as ferrous sulfate or ferric chloride. To maximize the physiological need for iron, rapidly growing or anemic experimental animals have been used. References have been made to chemical and animal assays when they augment the discussion of human studies on availability of iron from various foods and iron salts.

Iron availability has been studied in human subjects with radioactive tracers and with balance studies. Radiolabeled iron has been introduced into food biologically and by mixing an iron salt with the food before cooking. Both the red blood cell and whole body counting procedures

have been used to detect the radiolabel. Most of the iron availability studies in humans have been conducted with fasting subjects given either a test dose of iron or a tracer dose incorporated into a simple, well-defined, test meal.

Recently, several investigators have provided evidence for common pools of either nonheme iron (78–80, 150, 277, 389, 390, 588) or heme iron (277, 388) in the intestinal lumen to which all food sources and iron salts consumed in a meal contribute. Evidence for the existence of a common pool of nonheme iron in the intestinal lumen has been obtained from experiments in which iron absorption from biosynthetically labeled foods (intrinsic label) was shown not to differ significantly from absorption of a tracer dose of labeled soluble iron salt (extrinsic label) fed in the same meal (80, 150, 389). Heme iron sources labeled extrinsically and intrinsically also appear to be absorbed in the same proportions. The ratio of the percentage of iron absorbed from the extrinsic label to the percentage of iron absorbed from the intrinsic label (E/I ratio) was found to vary the least when the extrinsic label was fed in the food rather than immediately after the meal. Cook et al. (150) suggested that the level of iron in each of the labels was also an important factor influencing the E/I ratio. Layrisse and Martinez-Torres (388) found an E/I ratio of 1.1 fairly consistently when they fed an extrinsic label of 0.1 mg iron from ferric chloride with an intrinsic label of 4 mg iron. If these observations continue to be supported, the task of evaluating the availability of iron from mixed diets should be simplified.

There is considerable information currently available on the absorption of iron from numerous biologically labeled food sources. In 1951, Moore and Dubach (462, 464) reported results of iron absorption studies conducted on foods which had been biologically labeled during the growing period. Since then, biologically labeled foods have been fed individually, with simple test meals or incorporated into mixed diets or mixtures containing substances suspected of enhancing or inhibiting iron absorption. Studies have been conducted on biologically labeled wheat flour

(79, 118, 200, 329, 382, 387, 421), corn (79, 382, 387, 392), rice (587), blackbeans (phaseolus vulgaris) and broad beans (387, 392, 421, 427), soybeans (382, 387), greens (138, 388, 454), egg (79, 116, 138, 140), veal (387, 392, 428, 429), pork (311), fish (387, 392), chicken (464), hemoglobin (115, 146, 282, 309, 329, 521) and ferritin (329, 382).

Plant sources. Whole wheat products contain relatively large amounts of iron but much of the iron may be unavailable biologically. In 1942, Widdowson and McCance (723) with eight adult subjects conducted long term balance studies (42–91 days) which showed that more iron was absorbed from bread made with white flour than with whole wheat flour. Bread, which provided from 40% to 50% of the energy, was made from either white flour (1.4 mg iron/100 g) or whole wheat flour (3.5 mg iron/100 g). The percentage of iron absorbed from white bread was 8.6% to 13.8% for women and 2.3% to 14.0% for men. The percentage of iron absorbed from brown bread was 0 to 4.2% for women and 0 to 2.5% for men. Vellar et al. (683) reported corroborating evidence. They found that the rise in serum iron after subjects had consumed bread enriched with ferrous sulfate was greater if the bread was made with white flour than with whole wheat flour. Bjorn-Rasmussen (76) found that addition of bran significantly reduced iron absorption from rolls made with ferrous sulfate-enriched white flour. Iron absorption was reduced by about 20% with the addition of 1.7% bran and by about 50% with the addition of 10% bran. Senchak et al. (609) performed a balance study in which the iron intake (23.1–28.7 mg/day) was derived from 16.5 mg ferrous sulfate and various combinations of wheat, rice and milk. Iron absorption was 7.5% to 25.6% and was lower when the diets were high in wheat than when the content of rice was high. Sayers et al. (587) found that the percentage of iron absorbed from biologically labeled rice fed in a rice-vegetable soup mixture was 2.0% (0–4.1%) and increased to 11.8% (0.9–38.8%) by feeding of 100 mg ascorbic acid with the meal. When the rice was supplemented with ferrous sulfate (4 mg iron/100 g dry rice) and with 60 mg ascorbic

acid, the percentage of iron absorbed increased to 11.9% (1.0–31.4%).

Four studies (79, 329, 382, 421) have been conducted in which iron absorption from bread made of biologically labeled wheat flour was compared by the red blood cell incorporation technique to a ferrous ascorbate standard and to other labeled foods. Iron from wheat was better absorbed than iron from corn (79, 382) or eggs (79), but less well absorbed than iron from ferrous ascorbate, broadbeans, chickpeas or okra (421), soybeans (382) and ferritin or hemoglobin (329). The mean percentage of iron absorbed from wheat was 27% to 29% in five normal subjects (79), 4.5% in 21 normal and 7.8% in 21 iron deficient subjects (329) and 15% in a group of nine individuals who were either normal or iron deficient (421). When absorption of iron from wheat was related to absorption of iron from a ferrous ascorbate reference standard, iron from wheat was found to be 27% to 44% as well absorbed as iron from ferrous ascorbate (79, 382, 387).

Absorption of iron from flour has also been measured by whole body counting. Several investigators have shown that iron from low extraction flour was less available than iron from more highly refined flour (118, 200, 521). Elwood et al. (200) found that 21 Indian women absorbed 4.0% of the iron from chapatti made with white flour and 2.2% from chapatti made of whole wheat flour. When labeled ferric ammonium citrate was incorporated into the chapatti, about 2% of the iron was absorbed regardless of the kind of flour used. Callender and Warner (118) found that four women consuming an average of 12.5 to 14.2 mg iron from brown bread absorbed 1.3% to 18.6% of the iron. When they were given 5 mg of iron from ferrous sulfate, they absorbed 1.7% to 54.7% of the iron. Petrov et al. (521) reported that 81 anemic women absorbed less iron from labeled rye flour than from hemoglobin.

Layrisse et al. (392) found the percentage of iron absorbed from blackbeans, corn and ferrous ascorbate to be 2.3%, 2.1% and 13.9%, respectively, in normal subjects and 7.1%, 7.9% and 40.3%, respectively, in iron deficient subjects. In a group of 131 iron deficient and normal subjects, Layrisse et al. (387) observed relatively low iron absorption (1.7%–7.9%) from wheat, corn, blackbeans, lettuce and spinach and relatively high absorption (15%–20%) from soybeans, fish, veal, and hemoglobin. When absorption of iron from vegetable sources was related to absorption from ferrous ascorbate, the relative absorption percentages were 11% to 46%. Iron from soybeans was the most available and iron from spinach and corn was the least available (387). Absorption values of iron from other vegetables were 0.8% to 43% (79, 138, 421, 443, 464). Again, iron from greens was least available, and iron from beans, chickpeas and okra was the most readily absorbed.

One of the factors most commonly suspected of depressing the availability of iron from cereal grains and some other vegetable sources is their phytate content. The effect of phytate on iron absorption in humans has been studied by the balance method (27, 326, 612) and by red blood cell and whole body counting after feeding radiolabeled foodstuffs (230) and iron salts (282). Phytate has been introduced in its naturally occurring form (27, 326, 612) and as sodium phytate (27, 230, 282, 326, 612, 667). In two balance studies, Apte and Venkatachalam (27) and Hussain and Patwardhan (326) found that the inclusion of phytate phosphorus as 40% of the total phosphorus (typical of many Indian diets) depressed iron absorption. When the dietary phytate phosphorus level was increased from 8% to 40% of the total phosphorus, the mean iron absorption was reduced from 10% to less than 3% (326). Apte and Venkatachalam (27) suggested that with the higher level of phytate, an Indian diet should contain at least 16 mg iron, and preferably 17 to 21 mg, to maintain iron equilibrium in men.

The effect of phytate on the absorption of both labeled inorganic iron and heme iron has been studied with red blood cell incorporation procedures. Phytate was reported to depress absorption of inorganic iron (282, 612, 667) but not heme iron (282, 667). Turnbull et al. (667) reported that the addition of 4 g of sodium phytate to a 5 mg dose of iron from ferrous ascorbate depressed absorption when the iron was ingested either alone or with a meal. However, the inclusion of sodium phytate (either 4 or 10 g) actually improved absorption of hemoglobin iron. Foy et al. (230) observed no consistent depression in the percentage of absorption of iron from $^{59}FeCl_3$ mixed with whole meal bread when the test meal included 3 g sodium phytate. Sharpe et al. (612) found that absorption of iron from ferric chloride was reduced by rolled oats which contain considerable phytate, by milk which contains no phytate and by 0.2 g phytic acid added to milk. Reducing the content of rolled oats in the diet did not improve iron absorption. The investigators concluded that naturally occurring phytate did not reduce iron absorption and suggested that other factors such as increasing the bulk of the meal were more influential than phytate in reducing the rate of iron absorption.

Animal studies have suggested that iron from wheat and other cereal grains may be more available to rats than to humans. Cowan et al. (161) reported that iron absorption in the anemic rat was not impaired by phytate. In other studies, iron was as available from wheat and other grains as from ferrous sulfate· or ferric chloride for maintenance and regeneration of hemoglobin levels in growing rats (7, 231, 544, 569, 673). Ferric phytate, however, was less effective than ferric chloride for hemoglobin regeneration (477). Patwardhan (517) reported the presence of a phytase in the intestinal mucosa of the rat which might explain the difference in the ability of rats and humans to utilize iron from phytate containing sources. Recently, however, Bitar and Reinhold (75) observed phytase activity in extracts of human small intestinal mucosa.

Animal sources. Iron from animal food sources, with the exception of eggs, appears to be somewhat better absorbed than iron from plant sources. Eggs seem to be a relatively poor dietary source of iron despite their high iron content. Absorption of iron from biologically labeled eggs has been shown to be <1% to 20% (79, 116, 138, 464). Moore and Dubach (464) found that a group of 15 normal and anemic subjects absorbed 1.1% to 8.4% of the iron from egg yolks and that absorption was not enhanced by anemia. Chodos et al. (138) reported that absorption was 0.5% to 5% in seven normal subjects and 0.6%

to 20.5% in three iron deficient subjects. Bjorn-Rasmussen et al. (79) reported a mean iron absorption from eggs of 1.5% (0.3–3.6%) by seven normal subjects. Callender et al. (116) observed a mean iron absorption of 3.7% (range 0.4%–15.4%) from eggs in 26 elderly subjects; this was about 10% of the absorption of iron from ferrous sulfate. Furthermore, the inclusion of eggs in test meals inhibited the absorption of iron from bread enriched with either labeled ferric ammonium citrate or ferrous sulfate (197, 201). The poor availability of iron from egg yolk has been attributed to the presence of the phosphoprotein, phosvitin, which binds tightly nearly all of the inorganic iron in egg yolk (269, 444, 651).

Several animal studies (236, 467, 569, 614, 662) have confirmed the poor availability of iron from egg yolk shown in human studies. Iron from egg yolk was approximately 30% as available as the reference iron source in growing nonanemic rats (467) and anemic rats (236) and was not well incorporated into the carcasses of growing mice (662). Early work had suggested that additional dietary copper could improve the availability of iron from egg yolk (569, 614), but this observation was not confirmed in recent experiments on rats fed purified diets containing adequate copper (467).

Studies with rats in which animal tissues were evaluated as sources of iron showed that liver iron was as well retained as iron from ferric chloride (544) or whole wheat (567). Rose and Kung (567) reported, however, that rats did not utilize iron from liver as well as iron from whole wheat for hemoglobin formation. Amine and Hegsted (10) by radioactive labelling techniques, reported that iron from cooked muscle (rat carcass) was not as well retained (absorbed) by rats as iron from corn. Pye and MacLeod (544), determining retention by whole carcass analysis found that iron from dried beef muscle was not as well retained as iron from wheat or ferric chloride. Oldham's observations on hemoglobin regeneration (502) suggested that iron from heat treated (oven dried) beef muscle was better absorbed than iron from vacuum dried beef.

Recent studies with normal human subjects fed radiolabeled meat showed that absorption of iron from meat was comparable to absorption of iron from standard ferrous salts (311, 329, 387, 392, 428, 429, 464). The percentages of iron absorbed from chicken, fish, veal, and pork muscle and liver ferritin were 2% to 28%, with iron from chicken least available (464) and iron from pork most available (311). When some of the meat iron sources were fed to iron deficient subjects, iron absorption increased by 155% to 450% over the amount absorbed by nonanemic subjects, whereas the absorption from iron salts rose by 315% to 510% (311, 329). A recent study (391) has confirmed a previous observation (329) that iron from purified ferritin is poorly absorbed. The mean percentage of iron absorbed by a group of 108 normal and anemic adults was 1.9% with a range of 0.1% to 13.5% (391).

Because iron in meat occurs predominantly in heme compounds (428, 429), a number of investigators have studied iron absorption from purified hemoglobin (115, 146, 282, 309, 667). Iron from hemoglobin appears to be more available to human subjects than nonheme iron from food sources and it seems to be unaffected by iron valence (309), phytate (282) or ascorbate (282, 428, 667).

In 1957, Callender et al. (115), using biologically labeled hemoglobin, dispelled the commonly held belief (264) that iron present in heme compounds was biologically unavailable to humans. By comparing the absorbtion of hemoglobin iron with that of a 5 mg dose of iron from ferrous sulfate in 11 nonanemic patients, they found that the mean iron absorption from hemoglobin and ferrous sulfate was respectively, 10% (1%–21%) and 25% (11%–68%). Eleven anemic patients absorbed from hemoglobin and ferrous sulfate, respectively, 22% (0–40%) and 58% (24–96%) of the iron.

In subsequent studies, in which labeled hemoglobin or ferrous iron was fed and red cell uptake determined, heme iron was as well absorbed (4.3%–12.7%) as ferrous iron by normal subjects and slightly better absorbed (11.2%–21.4%) by anemic subjects (282, 311, 667). Hallberg and Bjorn-Rasmussen (277) fed a homogenate of foods patterned after an average Swedish diet containing 11.1 mg iron to four blood donors and four normal men who were not blood donors. The mixture was extrinsically labeled with ^{59}Fe hemoglobin and ^{55}FeCl$_3$. The blood donors absorbed 12.2% of the heme iron and 14.8% of the nonheme iron; the nondonors absorbed 6.7% of the heme iron and 2.6% of the nonheme iron.

In studies using a whole body counter, Petrov et al. (521) found that iron absorption was 6% to 34% in 32 normal individuals receiving 3 to 4 mg iron from hemoglobin. Heinrich et al. (311) reported that 7.5% of the iron was absorbed from hemoglobin by nonanemic subjects and that there was a 140% increase in absorption with iron deficiency. Conrad et al. (146), comparing iron absorption from several heme preparations, found that a combination of heme dialysate and degraded globin was as well absorbed (23%) as hemoglobin but iron from either chemically prepared hemin or heme dialysate alone was only 2.5% to 3.3% absorbed. The investigators proposed that heme was split from globin in the intestinal lumen and absorbed as an intact metalloporphyrin from which iron was split within the intestinal cell. They suggested that amino acids from degraded globin increased iron absorption by binding the coordination bonds of heme and preventing polymerization of heme molecules. Heinrich et al. (309) showed that, unlike absorption of nonheme iron, the heme iron absorption was not influenced by the iron valance. Hemoglobin samples with iron in either the ferrous or ferric states were about 8% absorbed by normal individuals and about 16% absorbed by iron depleted individuals.

Although most investigators have found that rats absorb heme iron relatively poorly, Bannerman (44) found that iron from hemoglobin was absorbed reasonably well (mean 39%) but not as well as iron from ferrous sulfate (mean 81%). Other investigators studying the uptake of labeled iron from hemoglobin (10, 707) and hemoglobin regeneration in rats (236) demonstrated that iron from hemoglobin was only about 20% (707) or 35% (236) as available as iron in ferrous sulfate and less available than iron in meat or corn (10). Weintraub et al. (709) reported that the dog appeared to be similar to man in its ability to utilize hemoglobin iron efficiently.

Mixed foods or diets. Most of the preceding discussion of iron availability from foods has emphasized single food sources, whereas, in fact, iron in most diets comes from a mixture of food sources. Interactions among foods have been observed by feeding a labeled food in the presence of other foods (labeled or unlabeled) and by adding an extrinsic radiolabel to mixtures of foods. Layrisse et al. (392), for instance, showed that inclusion of veal muscle in a meal increased absorption of iron from lebeled corn and that either corn or blackbeans decreased the absorption of labeled iron from veal mucle. Fish or a mixture of amino acids present in fish also enhanced the absorption of iron from corn.

Martinez-Torres and Layrisse (427) reported that absorption of iron from black beans was increased by adding either fish or a mixture of sulfur-containing amino acids to the meal. Martinez-Torres and Layrisse (428) also showed that a meat source of iron (veal muscle) could improve the absorption of iron from hemoglobin when the 2 sources were combined. Hemoglobin, however, had no influence on the rate of absorption of iron from veal muscle. The authors concluded that their data supported the observations of Conrad et al. (146) that suggested that protein degradation products enhanced the absorption of heme iron.

The enhancing effect on iron absorption of diets containing meat on iron absorption was verified recently by Layrisse et al. (389) by use of an extrinsic label. They found that the availability of iron from a mixture of maize and ferric chloride was increased by including meat in meals containing 0.5 to 60 mg iron from ferric chloride. Martinez-Torres et al. (429) recently observed that the percentage of iron absorbed from maize was doubled when subjects ingested veal liver in the same meal. Addition of maize to the meal, however, reduced iron absorption from either liver or ferric chloride. Cook et al. (152) showed that the inclusion of meat in a meal could offset the depressing effect of the meal itself on the absorption of labeled ferrous sulfate. More recently Layrisse et al. (390)

reported a study in which they fed meals typical of different regions of Venezuela. An extrinsic label, 0.1 mg iron from ferric chloride labeled with either [55]Fe or ^{59}Fe, was incorporated into the meals. Iron was better absorbed from the meals containing moderate amounts (50–100 g) of meat or fish than from meals containing little or no meat or fish.

Cook et al. (150) fed 0.1 mg ^{59}Fe from ferric chloride as an extrinsic label with either biologically labeled ([55]Fe) wheat, corn, soybeans or blackbeans in meals containing 2 to 4 mg iron. They found that when the intrinsic label was introduced in nonheme iron, compounds that influenced absorption of inorganic iron such as ascorbic acid, desferrioxamine or hemoglobin, did not alter the E/I ration (see p. 1003) although they influenced the overall rate of iron absorption. Others have shown that the E/I ratio stayed near unity when the mean rats of absorption was 0.5% to 29% and when the intrinsic label was provided in corn, eggs, white wheat flour (79) or from wheat bran or soybeans (277).

Layrisse and Martinez-Torres (388) studied the interactions among corn, veal muscle and rabbit hemoglobin by using an extrinsic tag of 0.1 mg iron from $FeCl_3$ labeled with [59]Fe. Despite observing some variation in E/I ratio among subjects, the investigators concluded that the percentageage of the extrinsic label absorbed was indicative of the absorption of nonheme iron (fed in this case with corn), in the presence of heme iron. Although the percentage of iron absorbed from heme and from nonheme sources was different, the presence of a nonheme iron source (corn) had no effect on the absorption of heme iron.

Other factors affecting iron absorption

In addition to the food source of iron and the phytate content of foods (19, 27, 230, 282, 326, 612), other dietary factors have been suggested as having an effect on iron absorption. Among these factors are protein, amino acids, ascorbic acid and carbohydrates.

Studies on the effect of dietary protein intake on iron absorption in humans have produced conflicting results (2, 356, 710).

Johnston et al. (356) in a balance study with five women found that increasing the iron content of a mixed diet from 7 mg to 10.4 mg by adding beef increased iron absorption from 11% (5%–20%) to 21% (18%–27%). Although they calculated the absorption of the beef iron to be 57%, they suggested that the inclusion of beef had stimulated the absorption of iron from the entire diet.

Abernathy et al. (2), however, in balance studies with 36 preadolescent girls having iron intakes of 6.8 to 12.3 mg, found no better iron absorption with higher protein intakes. Protein intake was 22 to 88 g and with the removal of milk from some of the diets, mean iron absorption actually increased 12.2% to 19.4%.

Studies on the interrelationship between protein level and iron absorption in rats have also yielded conflicting results (8, 10, 236, 381). Klavins et al. (378) found that the iron content of liver and carcass was increased by raising the dietary protein level 5% to 18%. Increasing the protein level 18% to 25% did not increase further the iron stores. Fritz et al. (236) showed that hemoglobin regeneration was improved when the dietary protein level was increased 10% to 20% in rats receiving either a poorly absorbed (ferrous carbonate) or well absorbed (ferrous sulfate) iron source. Contrary findings were reported by Ahlstrom et al. (8) who found no influence on either hemoglobin level or liver iron content in growing rats receiving diets containing 4.3% to 15.2% meat. Amine and Hegsted (10) also found that increasing the dietary protein level stepwise from 5% to 40% had no influence on the absorption of labeled iron.

Studies with rats have also demonstrated an enhancing effect of amino acids on iron absorption (380, 381, 674, 675). In the animal studies, loops of proximal intestine were perfused, in vivo, with solutions of labeled iron and selected amino acids (380, 381, 675), or amino acid analogs (674). Van Campen (674) and Van Campen and Gross (675) demonstrated a positive role in enhancing iron absorption for histidine, lysine and cysteine which was dependent on the presence of ionizing groups on the amino acids. Both L- and D-isomers were equally effective (674). Others have shown a positive role for histidine (380) and for glutamine (380, 381), glutamic acid (381) and asparagine (380).

Van Campen and Gross (675) and Van Campen (674) found no positive effect of glutamine, glutamic acid, methionine, glycine, serine or alanine. They suggested, as did Kroe et al. (380), that amino acids form chelates with inorganic iron prior to absorption. Van Campen (674) also suggested that active transport of L-amino acids is of little quantitative importance in enhancing iron absorption. An enhancing effect of amino acids on iron absorption has been suggested in several studies with humans (146, 392, 427).

Ascorbic acid has been shown to increase absorption of non-heme iron (77, 95, 104, 116, 117, 150, 201, 282, 383, 390, 464, 524, 587, 588, 637) but not of heme iron (282, 428, 429, 667). The postprandial rise in serum iron in five children was enhanced by feeding ascorbic acid (110). However, in a group of six children, 6 months to 2 years old, fed a test dose of labeled ferrous sulfate, simultaneous ingestion of orange juice decreased iron absorption 16% to 7% (601).

The amount of ascorbic acid needed to effect an increase in iron absorption was greater (200–1,000 mg) when a simple test meal containing an iron salt was fed (95, 105, 524, 637) than when more complete meals containing iron from a combination of salts and natural sources were fed (29, 116, 117, 201, 464, 637). Apte and Venkatachalam (29) found that adding 100 mg ascorbic acid to mixed diets containing from 9 to 28 mg iron increased iron retention in both men and women. Several studies showed that the inclusion of a glass of orange juice with a test meal enhanced absorption of iron from enriched bread (117, 201) and from eggs (116, 201, 464). Ascorbic acid has also been reported to increase absorption of iron from corn (150, 382, 390), rice (587), wheat (382), ferritin (382) and liver (464). Bjorn-Rasmussen (77) observed a systematic increase in the percentage of iron absorbed from maize meal supplemented with ferrous sulfate and ascorbic acid. Addition of 25 mg or more of ascorbic acid produced statistically significant increases in iron absorption. Absorption was two to six times as great as

that from control meals containing no added ascorbic acid. The beneficial effects of ascorbic acid on iron absorption were not observed when high cooking temperatures were employed to prepare wheat bread and soya biscuits (588).

Although ascorbic acid has been shown to increase iron absorption in controlled laboratory settings, no positive effect of added ascorbic acid on hemoglobin levels in clinical trials has been demonstrated (194, 602). Schulze and Morgan (602) found that the ingestion of 100 mg iron daily from ferric pyrophosphate brought about a significant increase in the hemoglobin levels of 36 children aged 7 to 12 years, and the inclusion of 100 mg ascorbic acid provided no additional benefit. Elwood (194) found that a group of women receiving enriched bread plus 50 mg ascorbic acid daily for 2 months had a slightly greater rise in hemoglobin level than had women who received only enriched bread. However, neither change in hemoglobin was significantly different from that of women who received unenriched bread.

Animal studies have provided conflicting evidence on the effect of ascorbic acid on iron absorption. Morris and Greene (467) found a marked improvement in availability of iron in egg yolk for hemoglobin syntheses in growing rats when the molar ratio of ascorbic acid to iron was 20 to 1 or greater. Fritz et al. (236), in tests with rats, found no effect of ascorbic acid on the utilization of either good or poor iron sources, when the molar ratio of ascorbic acid to iron was about 8 to 1. Greenberg et al. (268) found that ascorbic acid improved iron utilization for hemoglobin regeneration, but not to the same extent as a combination of ascorbic acid and vitamin E. Fritz et al. (236) observed no beneficial effect of vitamin E.

The influence of dietary carbohydrate on iron absorption has not been thoroughly studied in humans. Brodan et al. (105) found that in seven healthy men and women, the postprandial rise in serum iron was significantly greater when a test dose of 132 mg iron was fed with 50 g fructose than when the iron was fed alone. This reducing sugar has also been shown to enhance the absorption of iron in rats (530). The physical properties of a fructose-iron complex have been studied (135). Recently Heinrich et al. (310) found no evidence that fructose enhanced the availability of either ferrous or ferric iron. Amine and Hegsted (10) found that, with rats, when starch was the only carbohydrate (60% of the diet) the uptake of labeled iron was inhibited. Maximum absorption was obtained when either lactose or a 1:2 mixture of lactose and starch provided 60% of the diet.

STUDIES ON IRON SUPPLEMENTATION

Since the early 1940's, numerous iron preparations for the alleviation and prevention of iron deficiency have become available (20, 144). In many countries, iron enrichment of flour and bread has been made mandatory to assure adequate dietary iron intake. There is, however, very little documentation on the effectiveness of iron enrichment of flour and bread in population groups. Somewhat more information from field studies is available on the effect of iron supplements given in tablet form to various population groups. Studies which contained a large proportion of subjects with either normal hemoglobin levels or with only mild anemia showed less dramatic group response to iron supplementation than studies which included many anemic subjects. In addition to including subjects of different initial hematologic status, studies on iron supplementation have differed in duration, in the manner of administering additional iron (bread enrichment or tablets) and in the amount and form of iron given.

Much information on the relative availabilities of different iron sources has been provided by controlled studies with human subjects and by animal studies which will be discussed where appropriate. In fact, the relative biological availability of various iron salts has been far better studied in the diets of laboratory animals than in bread products consumed by man.

Enrichment of bread

Reports of five field trials lasting from 12 weeks to 12 months were found. These studies provided inconclusive evidence on the hematologic benefits of enrichment of bread with iron. Two studies showed significant increases in average hemoglobin levels (641, 683) when iron was provided as ferrous sulfate. None of the field studies (194, 204, 683) suggested that an iron salt added to bread was as well utilized as might have been anticipated from balance studies (263, 292) or radioisotope studies (117, 191, 637).

Stott (641) fed 124 prison inmates bread enriched with ferrous sulfate to provide 10 mg additional iron/day for 4 months. There was no untreated control group. During the treatment period, the mean hemoglobin level increased from 14.6 to 16.0 g/100 ml and fell to original pretreatment levels 6 months after cessation of therapy. At the beginning of the study, 15% of the men had hemoglobin levels below 13.3 g/100 ml. This proportion fell to 3% after 4 months of treatment with iron but increased to 27%, 6 months after cessation of therapy. In reviewing these results, Elwood (197) estimated that the increase in hemoglobin level reported by Stott (641) would have required about 30% of the supplementary iron to have been utilized for hemoglobin synthesis. He suggested that this much iron absorption was unlikely to have occurred in a group of men with a mean hemoglobin level of 14.7 g/100 ml. Vellar et al. (683) found that enrichment of bread with ferrous sulfate to provide 0.8 to 1.1 mg iron/100 g bread for 12 weeks produced a slight but significant rise (0.36 g/100 ml) in the hemoglobin levels of 77 women compared with that in 20 controls who ate unenriched bread. The distribution of hemoglobin values in the group receiving enriched bread shifted toward slightly higher values and two out of five women moved out of the group with hemoglobin level below 12.5 g/100 ml.

In other trials, hemoglobin levels did not increase when bread was enriched with iron despite the fact that all groups under study contained some individuals with hemoglobin levels in the "low-normal" range (194, 204, 415). Furthermore, when groups of children, 6 months to 5 years old, were fed bread enriched with ferrous carbonate to provide 12 to 21 mg iron/day for 6 months, their average hemoglobin levels did not change (415). Animal studies have shown that iron from ferrous carbonate is considerably less available than iron from ferrous sulfate (11, 236, 526).

In some studies, reduced iron was fairly well utilized by humans (152, 292, 637) and animals (11, 84, 232, 314). Elwood (194), however, found that reduced iron was not effective in raising the hemoglobin levels of moderately anemic female patients in a mental hospital. One hundred twenty-four patients received about 80 mg iron/day for 6 months and neither the entire group nor a subgroup with initial hemoglobin levels below 12.5 g/100 ml responded with a change in mean hemoglobin levels. Elwood et al. (204) reported a field study in which 237 women received bread enriched to provide an additional intake of 1 mg iron/day from either reduced iron or ferric ammonium citrate. This study included anemic women with hemoglobin levels above 8 g/100 ml. No change in average hemoglobin levels was observed after the women had received bread enriched with either iron source for 6 months. In a second study (204), 322 women received for 9 months either bread enriched with ferric ammonium citrate, a tablet containing an iron salt (specific source not reported), or a placebo. Prior to this study, the women had received oral iron therapy to increase their mean hemoglobin level by 0.8 g/100 ml. The enriched bread and iron tablet each provided 2.7 mg iron/day, but neither treatment was more successful than the placebo in maintaining hemoglobin levels. Studies in which the hematologic response of infants fed iron enriched commercial formula was compared with the response to unenriched formula are discussed on page 1034 (12, 426).

Supplementation with iron tablets

Field studies on the effectiveness of iron tablets in raising the hemoglobin levels have been carried out among groups containing a high proportion of subjects with iron deficiency anemia (97, 247, 604, 641) and among groups in which the average hemoglobin level was in the normal range (203, 246, 247, 249, 481, 484, 679). Children, adolescents and adults have been observed. The supplementary iron was fed in amounts of 5 to 80 mg/day and was provided by ferrous fumarate (203, 247, 481, 484, 679), or ferrous sulfate (97, 246, 249, 641). The duration of the studies ranged from 1 month to 3 years with most studies lasting from 2 to 6 months.

In studies on groups containing a large proportion of anemic individuals, there was some evidence that the hematinic effect of the supplement was related to the size of the dose and to the degree of iron deficiency as indicated by the low hemoglobin levels. For instance, Bradfield et al. (97) gave 15 mg iron/day to a group of 144 prepubertal Peruvian children of whom 30% had hemoglobin levels below 10 g/100 ml. There was a small hematinic effect but the increase in hemoglobin level was not statistically significant. There was no difference in the mean change in hemoglobin levels between the group of children receiving antihelminthic treatment and the group receiving no treatment. Vartiainen et al. (679) found that the mean hemoglobin level in a group of teenage Swedish girls who received a supplement of 15 mg iron daily for 2 months increased only slightly compared with that of a group of controls. In the group receiving the iron treatment, 60% of the hemoglobin values increased by 0.5 to 1.5 g/100 ml while 26% increased by more than 1.5 g/100 ml. In the untreated control group only 25% of the values increased by 0.5 to 1.5 g/100 ml and 2% increased by more than 1.5 g/100 ml. Most of the increased values occurred among girls with initial hemoglobin levels in the range of 10 to 12 g/100 ml. In Stott's studies of about 900 Mauritian children (641), however, when severely anemic children received 80 mg iron daily for about 1 month, mean hemoglobin levels increased by about 3 g/100 ml. Daily supplements of either 40 mg or 6.6 mg iron were associated with small increases in the average hemoglobin level and with marked increases in those levels that were very low initially. Similarly in a study with severely anemic adults, Stott (641) reported a mean increase in levels of 3.5 g/100 ml after 1 month of supplementation with 90 mg iron/day. Furthermore, Scott and Heller (586) gave a daily supplement of 6.5 mg iron from ferrous sulfate to 120 adult Eskimos. There was a significant increase in the hemoglobin levels of the women who had initial levels below 11.7 g/100 ml.

The hemoglobin levels of the men and the women with initial levels of 11.7 g/100 ml or greater, however, were unchanged by the supplement.

On the other hand, Garby et al. (247) gave a daily supplement of 60 mg iron to a group of Swedish women with a mean initial hemoglobin level of 10.8 g/100 ml. After 3 months there was a significant rise in the mean hemoglobin and serum iron levels. The increase in one or both parameters occurred, however, in only 30% of the women and the magnitude of change was not related to their initial levels.

In studies conducted with groups of subjects whose average hemoglobin levels were in the normal range, relatively little effect of iron supplementation was seen; Natvig et al. (482), for example, found no effect on hemoglobin levels attributable to a 30 mg iron supplement provided to 10- to 13-year-old Norwegian children for 1 year. Over a 3-year period, however, during which Elwood et al. (203) gave 30 mg of iron/day from ferrous fumarate to Welsh girls, 14 years old at the beginning of the test period, significant increases in hemoglobin and hematocrit levels were observed. In girls receiving 10 mg iron/day in the same study a slight hematinic effect was observed but the increases in hemoglobin and hematocrit levels were not significant.

Elwood et al. (203) also conducted a study in which women, 20 to 64 years old, were given tablets providing 0, 5, 10 or 30 mg iron daily for 6 months. All of the women had initial hemoglobin levels of at least 12.0 g/100 ml. Some of them, however, previously had received iron therapeutically to reach the minimum level for inclusion in the study. The hemoglobin levels of the women not given supplementary iron fell by 0.8 to 1.0 g/100 ml. The iron supplements of 10 and 30 mg/day prevented such a decrease but did not promote an increase over the initial mean hemoglobin levels. Neither Garry et al. (249) nor Garby et al. (246) found significant changes in average hemoglobin values after supplementation for 3 to 6 months with 28 mg iron/day (249) or 60 mg/day (246). The subjects of these studies were a group of college men and women (246) and a group of young women selected at random from a normal population (249). Both studies included untreated controls. The iron was provided in ferrous sulfate tablets. In shorter studies (1–3 months), Natvig and Vellar (484) also found no effect on hemoglobin levels when men and women under 40 years old were given a 60 mg iron supplement daily. Women over 40 years old, similarly treated, showed small increases in hemoglobin levels.

Addition of iron salts to human diets

Controlled studies have been performed to test the availability to human subjects of iron from ferrous sulfate, ferrous gluconate, ferrous lactate, ferric phosphate, reduced iron, sodium iron pyrophosphate, ferric orthophosphate and ferric ammonium citrate.

Schulz and Smith (601) reported a mean iron absorption of 16% (4%–28%) of a 30 mg test dose of labeled iron from ferrous sulfate in a study with six children, 6 months to 2 years old. A similar value was observed by White and Gynne (716) in a balance study with nine women. In this study (716), the subjects received diets of mixed foods and bread fortified with ferrous sulfate to provide a total daily iron intake of 22 mg. The percentage of iron absorbed was 16.3% (6%–33%). Seven women with no marrow iron stores absorbed more iron than the two women with either trace or adequate amounts of iron stores.

Gram and Leverton (263) provided 83 women consuming self-selected diets with an additional 100 mg iron/day as either ferrous gluconate, ferrous lactate, or ferrous sulfate. There was no significant difference in percentage of absorption which ranged from 9% to 13% among the three compounds. Harrill et al. (292), in 28-day balance studies with apparently healthy young women, found no significant differences in absorption of iron from bread enriched with ferric phosphate, ferrous sulfate or reduced iron. The bread was added to diets containing about 5.47 mg iron. The total iron intake when the supplemental iron was added was about 12.82 mg/day. The investigators calculated that only about 3% of the added iron was absorbed while about 10% of the total dietary iron (diet plus supplement) was absorbed.

Steinkamp et al. (637), with 32 normal subjects, compared the availability of iron from four radiolabeled salts fed alone and incorporated into bread. Twenty-eight of the 32 subjects absorbed 1% to 12% of the iron from ferrous sulfate, reduced iron, sodium ferric pyrophosphate and ferric orthophosphate when the supplement was baked into bread. The other four subjects who were suspected of having suboptimal iron stores absorbed 2% to 38% of the iron fed under similar conditions. With the exception of ferrous sulfate which was less well absorbed when based into bread than when fed alone, the method of feeding the iron salts did not influence absorption.

Using labels of ^{55}Fe and ^{59}Fe, Cook et al. (152) recently compared the absorption of doses of 3 mg of reduced iron, ferric orthophosphate or sodium iron pyrophosphate with that of 3 mg of ferrous sulfate when the iron compounds were baked into bread. Each of the three comparisons was made with eight subjects (a total of 22 women and 2 men, 19–49 years old). In addition, the absorption of a standard reference dose of 3 mg iron as ferrous sulfate-59 with ascorbic acid was determined in all 24 subjects. The absorption of the ferrous sulfate varied widely when it was baked in bread (0.9%–48.9%) and when it was in solution in the reference standard (2.1%–100.4%). When the absorption of iron in ferrous sulfate baked in bread was related to the absorption of iron in the reference standard, a mean absorption ratio of 0.26 was calculated. Cook et al. (152) interpreted this observation to mean that "the absorption of ferrous sulfate baked into rolls was therefore one-fourth of the level observed when ferrous sulfate was given as a solution of inorganic iron." The mean absorption ratios of the other three iron compounds to ferrous sulfate baked into bread were as follows: reduced iron, 0.95; ferric orthophosphate, 0.31; and sodium iron pyrophosphate, 0.05.

In tests of the relative availability of iron salts fed in test meals, Callender and Warner (117) found ferric ammonium sulfate and reduced iron to be less well absorbed than ferrous sulfate. Elwood

(197) found reduced iron to be less well absorbed than either ferrous sulfate or ferric ammonium citrate. Vellar et al. (683) used the postprandial rise in serum iron as a means of comparing iron absorption from different salts. In a series of studies in which each of 54 subjects served as his own control, ferrous sulfate appeared to be more available than reduced iron. Studies in which reduced iron has been incorporated into dietary components of human subjects have produced conflicting results with respect to the relative availability of this source of iron. Reduced or elemental iron is produced by several different processes which yield iron sources of different density, porosity and particle size (197, 315, 471). The extent to which these factors influence availability to humans has not been evaluated systematically but animal studies suggest that smaller particles may be absorbed more readily than larger particles (471, 528).

In a study of iron absorption from salts of organic acids, Brise and Hallberg (103) showed that ferrous iron was more available than ferric iron. In comparison with ferrous sulfate, the succinate, lactate, fumarate, glycine sulfate, glutamate and gluconate salts were well absorbed but the citrate, tartrate, and pyrophosphate salts were relatively poorly absorbed (103).

Animal studies

The biological availability of iron salts has been evaluated by testing the ability of various compounds to regenerate hemoglobin in young anemic rats or to maintain hemoglobin levels in non-depleted growing rats, chicks (11, 236, 527) and pigs (17). In the hemoglobin regeneration studies the rats were fed a milk diet (83, 84, 192, 232, 314, 477, 643) or a purified diet low in iron (236) to make them anemic. Studies conducted with anemic rats, non-anemic rats and chicks have generally yielded similar results on the relative levels of availability among different salts (11, 236, 527). Recently, however, it has been reported that reduced iron was utilized better by chicks than by rats (471, 528). In the study by Pla et al. (528), the relative biological value of reduced iron (with $FeSO_4$ as the standard) was 50.5 for chicks and 32.3 for rats. Motzok et al. (471) found that chicks utilized reduced iron 2 to 4 times better than rats and that the magnitude of difference depended on particle size. Estimates of availability obtained when iron salts used to enrich bread were incorporated directly into the animal diets (11, 83, 84, 236, 477, 526, 643) were similar to estimates obtained when the salts were baked into bread before being included in the diets (83, 84, 172, 232, 314, 527). Both ferrous sulfate (11, 17, 83, 84, 236, 314, 526, 527, 643) and ferric chloride (192, 232, 477) have been used as standards for comparing the relative availability of other iron salts. When the two compounds (ferrous sulfate and ferric chloride) were tested in the same study in rats and chicks (83, 84), comparable results were obtained. With a few exceptions, other compounds when compared with a ferrous sulfate standard have been rated in approximately the same order of iron availability as when compared with a ferric chloride standard. More consistent data have been obtained with ferrous sulfate and ferric chloride than with other iron salts. Bing suggested that the failure of investigators to report physical properties of the salts and method of preparation could account for many of the discrepancies in the literature (73).

As indicated on page 1013, one of the most variable iron sources is reduced iron, also known as ferrum reductum or elemental iron. This source of iron, which varies considerably in particle size, is produced by reduction under carbon monoxide and by electrolytic and hydrogen reduction (144). In several animal studies, reduced iron was as readily available as ferrous sulfate or ferric chloride (11, 84, 232, 314, 477, 629). Other investigators have reported reduced iron to be less available than ferrous sulfate or ferric chloride (17, 236, 526). In most cases, investigators either did not report particle size or did not attempt to relate particle size to biological availability. Motzok et al. (471), however, found that particle size and availability were inversely related in studies with both rats and chicks. Ferric ammonium citrate was reported to be as available to anemic rats as was ferrous sulfate or ferric chloride (236, 314, 526, 527). Ferric orthophosphate, a water insoluble form of iron, has been used to

enrich bread wafers and flour (144). Two animal experiments (236, 629) showed this salt to be a relatively good iron source, but most studies showed it to be a rather poorly available source (11, 84, 85, 236, 526). Results of studies with sodium iron pyrophosphate were conflicting. Three studies (192, 314, 477) showed availability comparable to or only slightly lower than ferrous sulfate whereas other studies showed relatively poor availability (11, 17, 84, 232, 236, 526, 527, 643). Ferrous carbonate ore has proved to be poorly absorbed in all animal studies reported (11, 236, 526). In studies with salts of organic acids, Pla and Fritz (526) found the tartrate, gluconate and fumarate salts to be good iron sources for anemic rats.

ASSESSMENT OF IRON NUTRITIONAL STATUS

Most estimates of human iron requirements have included estimates of iron intake, absorption, excretion, turnover and, occasionally, iron storage. Much of the understanding of factors that influence iron utilization in the normal human, however, has come from studies of iron deficiency.

Iron deficiency

Finch (218) has suggested that iron deficiency progresses in 3 successive stages that are 1) iron depletion, 2) iron deficient erythropoiesis and 3) iron deficiency anemia. He has characterized the criteria for evaluating iron status according to whether emphasis is placed on assessing adequacy of iron stores or on maintaining a normal rate of erythropoiesis (218). Heinrich (306) has suggested that iron status can be evaluated reliably by measuring absorption of standardized doses of iron-59 with a whole body counter. Based upon iron absorption measurements, Heinrich proposed four categories of iron status: normal iron stores, prelatent iron deficiency, latent iron deficiency and manifest iron deficiency (306). Iron absorption was found to be inversely related to iron stores on the basis of histological assessment of bone marrow (306, 631). In the classification schemes proposed by both authors (218, 306), the range of values for a given measurement shows considerable overlap between a particular stage and the adjacent stages of deficiency.

Using the criteria established by Finch (218), stage 1 of iron deficiency, iron depletion, is marked by a reduction in ferritin and hemosiderin, the reserve forms of iron found in muscle, liver and reticuloendothelial cells (244, 296, 638, 663, 704). The magnitude of iron stores has been determined quantitatively by phlebotomy (296). More often, however, in clinical situations, less quantitative estimates have been made from histological or chemical assessment of samples aspirated from bone marrow (244, 550, 638, 704). In addition, indirect evidence for a reduction of storage iron is seen in decreased marrow sideroblast count (36, 70, 369), increased iron absorption (306) and a reduction in serum iron levels (622). The optimal level of stored iron is not known (148). Some investigators have suggested, however, that the iron reserves are exhausted by the time stage 2 of iron deficiency, iron deficient erythropoiesis, is observed (36, 70, 218).

Recently it has been observed that, in healthy adults, the serum ferritin concentration is directly related to the level of available storage iron (345, 349, 350). Ferritin, the major iron storage protein, occurs mainly intracellularly in the liver and reticuloendothelial system. The physiological significance of circulating ferritin is uncertain. The range of average serum ferritin values in six studies with about 300 men was 53 to 112 ng/ml (5, 151, 349, 350, 538, 631). The range of average values in five studies with about 300 women was 27 to 43 ng/ml (5, 151, 349, 350, 538). Serum ferritin values in the range of 12 to 300 ng/ml are considered normal (349) and the distribution among healthy persons in most studies has been skewed positively (349). Serum ferritin levels decrease with iron deficiency (5, 349, 405) and increase with iron overload (5, 349, 405, 538).

Direct relationships have been observed between serum ferritin levels and iron stores assessed by phlebotomy (349, 699) and by histological evaluation of marrow iron (405, 538, 631). Serum ferritin is inversely related to iron absorption which increases when iron stores are depleted (151, 631). Serum ferritin levels have been shown to rise in the first few weeks of life

(617, 618), to decline in the period of 2 to 6 months (588, 617, 618) and to remain relatively constant in childhood (617).

Other indices of an adequate supply of iron to the erythroid marrow include normal serum (or plasma) iron levels, normal saturation of transferrin (the iron transport protein), and normal levels of erythrocyte free protoporphyrin. Serum iron, a small pool regulated mainly by release of iron from the reticuloendothelial system, has normal levels in the range of 50 to 180 μg/100 ml (36, 133, 162, 168, 738). Higher normal values have been reported for men than for women (368, 523, 625, 670). In addition, there is a diurnal variation in serum iron levels of adults (286, 516, 625, 736) and children (430, 603, 711) and possibly, individual variations throughout the menstrual cycle (168, 625, 750). Some investigators (133, 523, 625) but not others (398, 534) have shown that serum iron levels decrease with age.

The normal range of serum transferrin (or total iron binding capacity) has been reported to be 300 to 400 μg/100 ml (531, 551, 590). Serum transferrin is increased in iron deficiency, pregnancy and acute hemorrhage, and is reduced by infection, pernicious anemia and hemochromatosis (63, 531, 751). The normal range for the proporation of transferrin that is saturated with iron has been reported to be 18% to 50% (36, 63).

During the stage of iron deficient erythropoiesis, the level of the heme precursor, protoporphyrin, rises in the red cells. This rise indicates an insufficient supply of iron for the synthesis of heme. Normal average values ranging from 15 to 36 μg/100 ml of red blood cells have been reported (125, 165, 513, 676). Generally, values greater than 80 μg/100 ml red cells are indicative of iron deficiency anemia. Beutler (65) suggested that the reduction in hemoglobin level that precedes the reduction in number of red cells occurs at this stage of iron deficiency. The hemoglobin content of the red blood cells or mean corpuscular hemoglobin concentration (MCHC) is calculated from the ratio of hemoglobin to packed cell volume (738). Wintrobe (738) reported the normal range of the MCHC to be 32% to 36%. Although the MCHC has been proposed as a means for identifying iron deficient individuals before anemia has developed (65, 195, 376), several investigators have found the index to be rather insensitive (561), especially during pregnancy (123, 385).

Stage 3 of iron deficiency, iron deficiency anemia, occurs when the supply of iron to the erythroid marrow is sufficiently restricted to reduce the number of cells in circulation and to cause the appearance of hypochromic microcytic cells (218). Usually, several months of iron deficient erythropoiesis are necessary to produce a significant proportion of abnormal red cells in peripheral circulation. Although iron deficiency is probably the most common cause of anemia, a reduction of blood hemoglobin concentration, per se, can occur under any condition in which the supply of precursors is restricted (65, 692), or when an expansion in plasma or blood volume occurs without a concomitant increase in hemoglobin formation (692, 735).

In addition to causing hematological abnormalities, iron deficiency has been shown to elicit tissue changes, although the relationship between the two factors is not clear. Waldenstrom (693) reported clinically detectable alteration in epithelial tissue of subjects with latent iron deficiency in the absence of anemia. Most of the studies on the effects of iron deficiency have included measurements of the activity of enzyme systems that contain the heme molecule or require iron as a cofactor. In 1934, Cohen and Elvehjem (140) reported a decrease in the cytochrome c and cytochrome oxidase contents of rat tissue. This observation was repeated in iron deficient rats (64) and extended to include reductions in aconitase and succinic dehydrogenase (66). Catalase activity has been shown to be unaffected by iron deficiency in rats (66).

In humans, the studies on tissue effects of iron deficiency and anemia have included determinations of cytochrome oxidase (166, 344, 476), succinic dehydrogenase (476), catalase (38, 67), aconitase (71, 654) and delta-amino-levulinic acid dehydrase (575). Cytochrome oxidase in the buccal mucosa was assayed histochemically by Dagg et al. (166) and by Jacobs

(344) in 37 normal, 16 iron deficient, and 52 anemic subjects. In both studies, enzyme activity was reduced in many, but not all, of the iron deficient and anemic subjects (166, 344). Beutler found cytochrome oxidase activity of leucocytes to be moderately reduced in iron deficient subjects (66). Naiman et al. (476) reported no loss in the activities of either cytochrome oxidase or succinic dehydrogenase in the duodenal mucosa of 14 severely anemic children, 9 to 32 months old. Beutler and Blaisdell (67) found no decrease in the activity of catalase in red blood cells of anemic subjects but Balcerzak et al. (38) found a reduction when the enzyme activity was related to hemoglobin. The results of two studies (71, 654) showed that seven iron deficient subjects had normal leucocyte aconitase activity. Rubino et al. (575) found a reduction in delta-amino-levulinic acid dehydrase activity in the red cells of iron deficient individuals.

It is difficult to determine the exact stage of iron deficiency at which enzyme levels are affected, although it is generally felt that iron stores are depleted first (66). Most of the studies have reported only hemoglobin level which, as indicated previously, is a rather poor indicator of iron status. Beutler (66) observed that tissue enzyme changes appear only in a minority of patients and often bear little relationship to the severity of clinical symptoms.

In the later stages of iron deficiency, there is a reduction in the level of circulating hemoglobin (218, 245, 247). There is, however, considerable evidence suggesting that assessment of hemoglobin level is a poor means of detecting iron deficiency (218, 248). First of all, hemoglobin levels do not fall until iron deficiency has progressed relatively far (218); secondly, a low hemoglobin level is not specifically attributable to iron deficiency (738), thirdly, there is considerable individual variation among each age and sex segment of the population in the normal levels (248, 650, 692) and finally, there is a question about the clinical significance of moderately reduced hemoglobin levels (799). Despite the inappropriateness of using hemoglobin levels to detect iron deficiency, the measurement is useful in assessing the severity of anemia (218, 248).

Normal hemoglobin levels

A large number of investigators have reported averages for normal values for men and women, during various stages of the life cycle and under various stressful conditions. A summary of hemoglobin values obtained in 26 studies on approximately 12,000 men showed a range of average normal values of 13.7 to 16.6 g/100 ml (61, 122, 176, 249, 302, 304, 353, 415, 437, 445, 449, 474, 475, 480, 482, 483, 485, 506, 510, 522, 543, 586, 627, 670, 732, 737). In all but four studies (413, 543, 586, 627), the range of average values was 14.3 to 16.2 g/100 ml. In 34 studies that included approximately 20,000 women the range of average normal values was from 12.5 to 15.5 g/100 ml (61, 122, 133, 176, 179, 249, 285, 298, 302, 353, 368, 413, 420, 445, 449, 468, 475, 480, 485, 502, 509, 510, 522, 543, 566, 586, 627, 664, 670, 686, 698, 717, 732, 737). All but four investigators (413, 522, 543, 732) reported a range of normal average values of 12.8 to 14.5 g/100 ml.

Hemoglobin values in the healthy population have been found to be distributed normally for men (122, 376, 437, 506, 586) but not for women (122, 302, 400, 509, 586). Several studies have shown that the distribution of hemoglobin levels in groups of women is skewed toward low values (61, 195, 376, 449). This skewness has been attributed to the presence of iron deficiency anemia in groups of otherwise healthy women (195, 376, 449). Normal hemoglobin levels vary with altitude (18, 252, 298, 474, 572). Three studies indicated that about 200 men normally residing at elevations of 1,500 to 2,300 meters had average hemoglobin levels ranging from 16.5 to 17.7 g/100 ml (18, 252, 474). Four studies on about 300 women living at similar altitudes showed a range of hemoglobin values of 14.5 to 15.2 g/100 ml (18, 252, 474, 572). This represents an increase of about 11% over normal values observed at lower altitudes. Ross (572) found mean hemoglobin levels of 13.4 g/100 ml at 30 weeks and 14.3 g/100 ml at term in a study of 497 pregnant women living at 2,300 meters above sea level.

The influence of age on normal hemoglobin levels has been widely studied. There is general agreement that the normal level rises slowly but progressively from age 2 until puberty. During this time, there appears to be no difference in the levels of males and females (1, 205, 299, 300, 373, 393, 449, 473, 507, 580, 732). Sex differences in hemoglobin levels begin to appear in adolescence. Some investigators reported that girls show only a slight increase over their final childhood values and others suggested that childhood values are maintained (205, 474, 518, 582, 727, 730, 732); one group, however, showed a decline between ages 18 and 21 years (299). In boys during adolescence, the progressive rise which began in childhood appears to continue until age 16 or 17 resulting in higher adult values for men than for women (205, 257, 341, 373, 473, 508, 518, 581, 727, 730, 732). The reports of the effect of advanced age on hemoglobin levels are conflicting. Several investigators reported no change in old age (133, 254, 324, 367), while others found a slight decrease after age 60 years (198, 228, 316, 400, 406, 450, 452, 486, 624, 732). Some data on women have indicated a slight postmenopausal rise in hemoglobin after a decline in old age (239, 324).

Hematocrit, or packed cell volume, determined for men in 6 studies was 42.4% to 46.6% (479, 485, 543, 627). In seven studies with women, the range of average values was 38.8% to 42.4% (246, 436, 479, 485, 543, 627).

STUDIES ON FACTORS AFFECTING IRON NUTRITIONAL STATUS

No reports were found on the effect of stress on iron requirements per se. There are, however, some kinds of environmental stresses and forms of muscular activity that may be related to blood volume and hemoglobin level and thus indirectly perhaps to iron requirements.

Environmental stress

Although the effects of changes in temperature, humidity, and altitude on the need for iron have not been studied, these factors have been shown to influence hemoglobin levels and hematocrit. The influence of temperature appears to be related primarily to the effect on blood volume which, in turn, depends on relative humidity, state of hydration, rate of sweating, and vascular tone (650). In hot, dry climates hemoglobin concentrations were observed to increase due to increased sweating, (650) whereas, in hot, moist conditions hemoglobin and hematocrit levels either decreased (6, 652) or did not change (223). The relationship between iron losses through sweating and iron requirements is discussed under skin losses on page 995. In cold climates a rise in hematocrit (145, 632) but no change in hemoglobin concentration (632) was observed.

Elevated hemoglobin and hematocrit values were observed in both men and women at altitudes greater than 1,600 meters (18, 229, 252, 474, 572). In a study of the effect of altitude on iron absorption, Reynafarje (555) found that persons fully acclimated to either sea level or an elevation of 5,000 meters absorbed the same percentage of iron. However, a change in altitude in either direction greatly influenced iron absorption. When subjects acclimated to sea level were moved to 5,000 meters, iron absorption of a test dose of 100 mg ^{59}Fe increased from 3.6% to 16.3% during an 8-day period. After 30 days, there was a downward trend toward the percentage of iron that had been absorbed at sea level. When subjects, acclimated to high altitudes, were taken to sea level, iron absorption decreased from 4.8% to about 1% of a dose of 100 mg ^{59}Fe. An upward trend toward the initial percentage of iron absorption appeared in 2 months. Changes in the proportion of the absorbed iron that was used for hemoglobin synthesis occurred with changes in altitude. With the move to high altitude the amount of iron utilized for hemoglobin synthesis increased from 86% to 100%, but with the move to low altitude, iron utilization decreased from about 92% to 60%.

Exercise

Several research teams have reported increases in hemoglobin concentration due to sweating and to movement of water from blood to extravascular spaces during physical exercise (90, 183, 596). In addition to changes in blood volume associated with exercise, the possibility of a relationship between hemoglobin level and physi-

cal performance has been investigated. An adequate tissue oxygen supply is essential for efficient muscular energy expenditure. Since hemoglobin is the compound that transports oxygen between the lungs and other tissues, it seems logical to look for an association between hemoglobin levels and exercise. The pertinent studies generally included three kinds of test situations. Some investigators related work capacity to hemoglobin levels in normal subjects (163, 304, 684). Others attempted to show a relationship between impaired physical performance and either moderate anemia (14, 15, 69, 159, 684) or severe anemia (14, 69, 634). Finally, several investigators observed the effect of blood donation on work capacity of healthy subjects (42, 371, 574). Work was assessed with a treadmill (42, 69, 304, 574, 634), bicycle ergometer (14, 15, 159, 371, 560, 684) and with tests of endurance and muscular strength (163). Physical performance or work capacity has often been related to assessment of cardiopulmonary function under strenuous exercise conditions requiring maximal oxygen consumption (574, 634, 684). In situations where strenuous exercise was inadvisable or impractical, cardiopulmonary function (heart rate, oxygen uptake, carbon dioxide output, respiratory frequency) was assessed under conditions of submaximal energy expenditure (14, 15, 42, 69, 159, 163, 560). Andersen and Barkve (14) also determined the length of time for recovery of cardiopulmonary function to pre-exercise levels.

Reports of a few studies suggest an interrelationship between hemoglobin levels and physical performance. In five subjects, Andersen and Barkve (14) found an inverse relationship between hemoglobin level and length of recovery time for several parameters of cardiopulmonary function. Andersen and Stavem (15) reported prolonged recovery time from strenuous exercise, a decrease in blood pH, and an increase in nonvolatile acid end products of anaerobic metabolism in two anemic subjects when the values following exercise were compared with their own post treatment values or with values from non-anemic controls. Sproule et al. (634), studied nine severely anemic men including three with sickle cell anemia and two with pernicious anemia. When the patients were subjected to severe physical exercise, there was reduced oxygen uptake, but no decrease in blood pH or symptoms of distress. Cullumbine (163), in physical fitness tests with 200 school children, found that hemoglobin level was positively correlated with performance in moderate prolonged exercise, but not with ability to do moderate or severe short-term exercise.

Reports of other studies have provided little evidence for an impairment of work capacity attributable to low hemoglobin levels. Heath (304), Vellar and Hermansen (684), found no relationship in about 300 normal subjects between hemoglobin level and work capacity. Studies with 22 moderately anemic nonpregnant women (69, 159), two severely anemic women (69), 19 pregnant women with hemoglobin of 7.3 to 10.3 g/100 ml at 36 weeks of gestation (560), and 97 college students (684) showed no impairment in physical performance when values were with those for compared post treatment performance or with those for nonanemic controls.

Studies on blood donation (phlebotomy) in healthy subjects have provided conflicting evidence on the relationship between hemoglobin level and work capacity. The studies differed in the type of exercise, the length of time following phlebotomy when exercise was undertaken, and the magnitude of hemoglobin reduction caused by phlebotomy. Karpovich and Millman (371) found that the performance of five athletes who had donated blood was impaired in endurance tests but not in exercise requiring brief periods of intense activity when oxygen debt was high. Balke et al. (42) found an impairment in the physical performance of 14 subjects 1 hour after blood donation but not 48 or 72 hours later. Andersen and Barkve (14), with 16 subjects, reported that the recovery time for cardiopulmonary function increased only if blood donation had effected a decline in hemoglobin of 1.5 g/100 ml. Rowell et al. (574) however, found no decrease in performance of severe exercise by five subjects following blood donations which reduced hemoglobin by 2 g/100 ml. Although some investigators found apparent relationship between hematological parameters and various indices of cardiopulmonary function (14, 15, 163, 634), others showed that the circulatory system could compensate for wide variations in hemoglobin levels to deliver an adequate supply of oxygen to the tissues (69, 159, 304, 560, 684).

STUDIES ON IRON REQUIREMENTS OF SPECIFIC POPULATION GROUPS

Infants, 0 to 24 months old

Estimates of iron requirements of infants have been based on data obtained by iron balance studies (table 6), by calculating the amount of iron required to meet the increase in body iron content between birth and some later age (242, 305, 366, 584, 598, 645), and by determining the iron intakes that allow maintenance of normal hematological values. In determining the increase in body iron, some of the information on body iron content has been obtained directly by analysis of the bodies of fetuses and stillborn or older infants (table 7). Most of it, however, has been obtained indirectly. Indirect estimates have been based on the sum of factors for iron in liver and spleen (storage iron), in functional tissues (myoglobin), and in blood (hemoglobin and serum iron). Hemoglobin provides a major part of the total body iron of the newborn infant. The iron contributed by hemoglobin was estimated in one study by chemical analysis of the hemoglobin removed by perfusion from the bodies of dead infants (591). Most frequently it has been calculated from estimates of blood volume and of hemoglobin concentration in cord blood or in either capillary or venous blood (table 8). Blood volume has been estimated indirectly by using CO_2 (438) brilliant vital red dye (409, 562), Evans blue dye (100, 181, 460, 621), radioactive phosphorus (460), or ^{125}I-labeled albumen (746).

At birth, both full-term and premature infants have a high level of circulating hemoglobin which falls quite dramatically during the first few weeks of life. The iron contained in RBC hemoglobin removed from circulation returns to iron stores from which it is available for synthesis of new hemoglobin molecules as the infant grows. The major determinant of the amount of iron available to be returned to storage is

TABLE 6

Controlled balance studies with healthy infants and children

Subjects	Subjects	Balance periods			Daily iron intake	Daily iron balance	References
		Number	Number per subject	Length			
	No.	No.	No.	days	mg	mg	
Premature infants							
0 to 3 months	21	44	1 to 6	3 to 10	0.25 to 1.11	−0.48 to 0.53	403, 628, 697
3 to 6 months	11	32	1 to 11	4 to 10	0.9 to 0.42 mg/kg	−0.10 to 0.10 mg/kg	363
					0.17 to 2.08	−0.97 to 0.33	403, 697
6 to 8 months	3	7	2 to 3	7 to 10	0.18 to 0.27 mg/kg	0.04 to 0.11 mg/kg	363
					0.33 to 2.95	−0.19 to 0.56	697
Full-term infants							
0 to 3 months	47	133	1 to 11	1 to 6	0.15 to 1.07	−3.60 to 0.35	362, 635, 696
					0.06 to 11.1 mg/kg	2.34 to 2.60 mg/kg	128, 363, 364, 636
3 to 6 months	31	111	1 to 13	4 to 10	0.07 to 0.82	−0.27 to 0.39	362, 696
					0.05 to 8.3 mg/kg	−0.46 to 4.7 mg/kg	363, 364, 636
6 to 12 months	23	61	1 to 9	3 to 6	0.12 to 12.4 mg/kg	−0.63 to 3.3 mg/kg	363, 364, 636
15 days to 9 months	29	76	1 to 12	3 to 6	0.19 to 0.77	−0.11 to 0.52	595
12 to 24 months	8	16	1 to 4	3 to 5	0.03 to 1.08 mg/kg	0.0 to 0.86 mg/kg	213, 214
					0.79 to 7.9 mg/kg	0.09 to 2.0 mg/kg	364, 636
Preschool children							
2 to 5 years	23 (10 girls) 47	87	1 to 9	3 to 8	4.47 to 14.15	−1.56 to 4.32	33, 170, 394, 533, 570
					0.22 to 0.75 mg/kg	0.0 to 0.25 mg/kg	33, 70, 533
School children	(40 girls) (7 boys)	323	6 to 56	4 to 6	6.05 to 16.40	−1.00 to 3.132	2, 418
Adolescents							
13 to 18 years	48 (6 girls 13 and 14 years old)	8	8	7	8.0 to 13.3	0.33 to 2.22	592

TABLE 7

Studies on the iron content of the bodies of infants and children

Sample	Subjects	Subjects	Results	References
		No.	mg/100 g analyzed tissue[1]	
Total body	Infants			
	Fetal and premature	61	3.6 to 9.3	24, 107, 325, 337, 591, 725
	Full-term	32	3.3 to 14.4	24, 120, 121, 325, 591, 720, 725
	Children			
	Preschool	1	4.9	724
Liver	Infants (newborn)			
	Fetal and premature	65	16.6 to 73.7	255, 337, 343
	Full-term	58	7.6 to 76.8	108, 255, 343, 591, 725
	Children			
	Preschool	1	8.8	724
		9	30 to 100 (dry weight)	545
Liver and spleen	Infants (newborn)			
	Fetal and premature	21	6.8 to 30.0	725
			2.5 to 22.6 mg/total liver & spleen	591
	Full-term	12	9.1 to 37.0	404, 725

[1] Wet weight except where otherwise noted.

the size of the infant at birth; consequently, a premature infant with small blood volume has a smaller total hemoglobin concentration than a full-term infant. The requirement of the infant for iron during the first few months of life is met largely from stores. Whether or not this is adequate to maintain normal hemoglobin levels depends upon the relationships between the size of the infant at birth (magnitude of actual and potential stores), the rate of growth (rate of depletion of stores), and the amount of iron absorbed from the infants' diets. Because of the clear difference between premature and full-term infants with regard to the size of stores and the rate at which iron stores are utilized during the first few months of life, the two categories of infants are discussed separately.

To translate iron requirements calculated from changes in total body iron content into dietary iron requirements, an allowance must be made for the incomplete absorption of iron into the body. In determining the iron intake required to maintain normal hematologic values, the blood constituent most frequently measured has been hemoglobin. The hemoglobin level accepted as normal, however, has varied from one study to another as investigators have sought either simply to prevent anemia or to promote the highest hemoglobin level consistent with health. Even the level at which anemia is diagnosed has varied from 8 to 11 g/100 ml. In addition, comparison of the findings of one laboratory with those of another has been complicated by differences in analytical methodology and technique and in the terms in which the data have been expressed (32, 185, 193).

Premature infants. Iron balances of 22 prematurely born infants observed during their first 8 months of life have been reported (363, 403, 628, 697) (table 6). The babies were studied in a total of 83 balance periods of 3 to 10 days. The number of infants studied by any one investigator varied from three to eight. All of the studies were intended to obtain information on the anemia commonly observed in premature infants during their first 2 or 3 months of life. Although the data obtained did not show that iron balance was clearly related to iron intake or to age, the proportion of negative balances decreased somewhat as the age of the infants increased. Negative balances, however, were found with both low and high intakes in all age groups.

In the earliest of the balance studies

TABLE 8

Studies on blood volume and hemoglobin concentration in infants and children

Determination	Subjects	Subjects	Results	References
		No.		
Blood volume (ml)	Infants (neonatal):			
	Premature	74	109 to 260	599, 622
	Full-term	>250	198 to 857	100, 181, 409, 597, 621
			70 to 100 ml/kg	460, 562, 746
	Children:			
	Preschool	26	1,200 to 1,300	469, 577
	School-age	80	1,500 to 2,500	100, 469, 577
	Adolescent boys	65	2,500 to 6,000	100, 469, 577
	Adolescent girls	6	2,500 to 3,500	100
Hemoglobin concentration (g/100 ml)	Infants (neonatal):			
	Premature	593	9.8 to 25.2	32, 190, 261, 270, 287, 552, 599
	Full-term	1,100	9.8 to 23.2	139, 212, 243, 259, 271, 323, 606, 616, 621, 702
	Children:			
	Preschool	> 4,000	11.0 to 13.4	173, 174, 185, 208, 271–273, 373, 379, 416, 445, 473, 508, 512, 519, 522, 732
	School-age	>13,000	11.2 to 13.7	1, 6, 61, 173, 174, 178, 298–300, 302, 373, 384, 413, 416, 431, 445, 470, 473, 482–484, 495, 508, 522, 644, 665, 669, 718, 727, 728
	Adolescent boys	3,700	13.2 to 15.4	61, 257, 291, 299, 300, 302, 373, 384, 413, 445, 481, 496, 518, 522, 581, 607, 627, 640, 664, 669, 701, 727, 729
	Adolescent girls	4,000	12.2 to 1.40	291, 299, 300, 302, 303, 367, 373, 384, 393, 413, 445, 496, 518, 522, 581, 593, 627, 640, 664, 669, 701, 726, 727, 729

Lichtenstein (403) studied four premature infants at various times between the ages of 3 weeks and 5 months. With their customary intake of breast milk, all infants were in negative iron balance. Positive balance in one infant was effected by adding $FeCl_3$ to the milk to provide about 50 mg Fe/day. These findings suggested that anemia in young premature infants was due to negative iron balance and was mitigated by iron supplementation.

Snelling (628), cognizant of Lichtenstein's studies, observed seven premature babies 2 to 11 weeks old in a total of 12 balance periods of 3 to 6 days. Two infants were formula-fed and five were breast-fed. In the 12 studies, three negative and nine positive iron balances were calculated. Negative balances occurred with both the lowest and the highest daily intakes. Snelling suggested that the anemia commonly associated with prematurity was not due to negative iron balance or to inadequate iron intake but to failure to utilize the available iron supplies. This failure, he suggested further, might be due to an inadequate amount of bone marrow, a condition that would be corrected as the child grew.

Wallgren (697) in later studies with eight premature infants, 1 to 8 months old, (38 7-to-8-day balance periods) concluded, as had Snelling, that neither inadequate iron intake nor negative iron balance was responsible for the anemia occurring during the first 2 or 3 months of the premature infant's life. He concluded, however, that immature bone marrow function was not responsible either. He pointed out that in the premature infant the blood volume must increase much more rapidly than in the full-term infant. Hematopoietic function cannot always keep up with the increased blood volume with the result that hemoglobin levels in the premature infant may not be maintained at the same level as in the full-term infant. In addition, he suggested that the premature infant is more sensitive than the full-term baby to external stresses that are reflected in low hemoglobin values.

Josephs (363) studied three premature infants 6 days to 3 months old in a total of 11 balance periods of 3 to 5 days duration. One of the infants was studied again when it was 3 to 5 months old in an additional series of 10 balance periods. Of the 21 iron balances that were calculated, only one was negative. Josephs concluded that "the observations in this work indicate that prematurity has no influence on iron retention. The cases that were studied, however, cannot be considered to settle the question because of the relatively good birthweight (over 2.2 kg)." In comparing his work with that of others, Josephs noted that it was in essential agreement with that of Snelling (628) and Wallgren (697). Furthermore, he attributed the preponderance of negative balances observed by Lichtenstein (403) to the method of iron analysis which he considered to be "grossly inaccurate for small amounts of iron."

The total body iron content of premature infants has been estimated by chemical analysis of the bodies of human fetuses of various size and gestational age. In six studies reported in the literature (24, 107, 325, 337, 591, 725), data were obtained on 61 fetuses of 14 to 2,700 g and of approximately 11 to 36 weeks gestational age. In one of the earliest of these studies, Hugounenq (325) analyzed six fetuses of 4.5 to 6 months gestational age and two full-term fetuses. Noting that the fetus laid down twice as much iron in the last 3 months of pregnancy as in the preceding months, Hugouneng suggested that the infant is born with iron stores to protect against iron deficiency during the first few months of postnatal life. Other studies (24, 107, 337, 591, 725), however, showed that the total iron content of the fetal body increased with increasing bodyweight but that there were only slight increases in the concentration of iron as the fetus developed. Widdowson and Spray (725) concluded, therefore, that no large store of iron is accumulated by the fetus shortly before birth. Similarly, Schairer and Rechenberger (591) concluded that the total body iron content in relation to body weight in the premature infant is similar to that in the full-term infant; the absolute amount of iron is, however, considerably less. Apte and Iyengar (24) in a recent study of the body composition of 23 fetuses of 230 to 1,570 g (20–30 weeks of gestational age) and 18 full-term infants of 1,800 to 3,340 g, found that there were wide variations in the total body iron content among fetuses of similar weight. There was, nevertheless, a significant linear relationship between total body iron and body weight. Apte and Iyengar (24) observed also that, even in fetuses of similar body weight, the iron content of the fetuses in their study, from mothers belonging in poor socioeconomic Indian groups, was about 20% lower than that reported by Widdowson (719) for fetuses born of presumably adequately nourished Western mothers. They suggested, therefore, that "chemical composition and nutrient stores of the developing foetus can be considerably influenced by the state of maternal nutrition" (24).

The content of iron in the liver has been studied in fetuses and in premature infants who died after birth. Iob and Swanson (337) analyzed the liver of 14 fetuses of 162 to 4,030 g, ranging from lunar month 3 to term. Their data indicated that the concentration of iron in the liver increased during fetal development but that the total body iron concentration as related to fat free tissue did not increase. In earlier and later studies (255, 343), however, no evidence was found for a significant increase in concentration of iron in the liver. Iyengar and Apte (343), for instance, in 38 fetuses weighing 733 to 2,635 g, found that liver weight varied with body weight and that the total iron content of the liver increased with increasing liver weight. The concentration of iron in the liver, however, remained fairly constant. Furthermore, the proportion of total liver iron that was nonheme iron (storage iron) remained constant also.

Widdowson and Spray (725) analyzed both liver and spleen of six immature fetuses and five stillborn full-term infants for iron and found that the liver and spleen always contained the same proportion (about 12.5%) of the total body iron regardless of their size. The concentration of iron in the liver and spleen was about twice the concentration in the whole body. Similarly Schairer and Rechenberger (591) reported that the amount of iron in the liver and spleen depended upon gestational age. Infants born prematurely had less iron, though not a lower concentration of iron, in their livers than full-term babies. After birth, in both premature and full-term babies, the amount of iron in the liver and spleen rose rapidly for about 2 months and then declined during the next 22 months. Schairer and Rechenberger concluded that in the newborn infant, whether premature or full term, iron stores are mostly in hemoglobin. After birth, with the beginning of respiration and the change from oxygen poor to oxygen rich blood, hemoglobin is broken down and releases iron. At least part of the released iron is stored in the liver and spleen from where it may be drawn when hematopoiesis begins.

No reports were found on the content of myoglobin or functional tissue iron per se in premature infants. Schairer and Rechenberger (591), however, analyzed the bodies of stillborn infants after removing the hemoglobin (by perfusion), the liver and spleen, and the gut contents. The iron thus determined, they called "Resteisen" or residual iron. In four premature infants, 6 to 9 months in gestational age, the "Resteisen", 16.5 to 77 mg/body, made up 29% to 43% of the total body iron. (Total body iron equals the sum of hemoglobin iron, depot iron in liver and spleen and "Resteisen".) There was no indication of the proportion of the "Resteisen" that was composed of functional tissue iron.

The smaller body size and blood volume of the premature infant offers a potentially smaller iron store than that of the full-term infant. The smaller blood volume provides a smaller hemoglobin mass contributing iron to stores during the first few weeks of life. This factor is combined with a more rapid growth rate with a concomitant enlargement of blood volume in comparison with the full-term infant. The premature infant, therefore, will probably have a higher dietary requirement per kilogram of body weight than the full-term infant and may be at greater risk of having a low hemoglobin level. The ranges of hemoglobin levels observed during the first 2 years of life among premature infants and the effects of iron supplementation are discussed.

In the four premature infants studied by Schairer and Rechenberger (591), the amount of iron in the hemoglobin removed by perfusion varied from 31 to 96 mg/body (27.7–56.9 mg/kg body weight) making up about 51% to 61% of the total body iron. In living children, hemoglobin iron is usually calculated from estimates of blood volume and hemoglobin concentration.

Blood volume determinations in a total of 89 premature infants were reported from two studies (599, 622). In both studies, the blood volume was calculated from plasma volume determined with Evan's blue dye. Schulman and Smith (599) studied 38 infants, 1 to 94 days old (one blood volume estimate per child). They reported that, as indicated by their data, the premature infant "begins life with a relatively high blood volume (108 ml/kg) which falls steadily to about 73 ml per kilogram at the seventh week of postnatal life". Thereafter, until week 14 there was no significant change in blood volume. Sisson et al. (622) reported 145 estimates of blood volume in 51 infants, 38 of whom were studied two to six times between birth and 1 year of age. Mean values at various ages during the first year of life showed that blood volume declined "moderately" from 109 ml/kg at birth to about 97 ml/kg at 6 weeks. Thereafter, with some fluctuation, there was a gradual drop to about 73 ml/kg at 52 weeks. Sisson et al. pointed out, however, that the mean values were unreliable because of wide variation among infants particularly in the first 5 months of life. Furthermore, some of the infants "had relatively stable blood volumes as they aged whereas others . . . had fluctuating blood volumes." They recommended that, because of this variation and because of the limitations in estimating blood volume from plasma volume, such estimated values be used with caution. Both groups of investigators noted that the blood volume (ml/kg) of the premature infant at birth was slightly higher than that of the full-term newborn. Schulman and Smith (599) concluded that this difference was "related to relative excess of plasma volume" rather than to red cell mass.

Hemoglobin concentrations reported for individual premature babies at birth were about 12 to 25 g/100 ml (32). Mean levels for groups of newborn premature infants were 15 to 21 g/100 ml (32, 106, 190, 261, 270, 287, 552, 599). These data are in the same range as values for cord blood (14.5–20.5 g/100 ml) reported for premature infants (114, 270, 417, 565).

Arthurton et al. (32) reviewed the literature on factors that might affect the accuracy of such estimations. They pointed out that because analytical methods were not always standardized, the results obtained in one study may not be properly compared with those of another study. Furthermore during the first 2 or 3 weeks of life, particularly in the premature infant, higher hemoglobin readings are obtained from capillary blood than from venous blood. Arthurton et al. recommended that venous blood be studied whenever possible.

Another factor that may affect hemoglobin levels is the time when the umbilical cord is clamped. De Marsh et al. (180, 181) observed that the infant's hemoglobin level and hematocrit were significantly higher after birth if the clamping were delayed until the placenta had detached from the uterus than if the cord were clamped immediately after delivery. Measurement of the blood drained from the placenta after clamping indicated that the infant might be deprived of as much as 100 ml of blood by early clamping. Arthurton et al. (32) suggested that such deprivation would probably have greater significance in the premature than in the full-term baby. Gairdner (242) said that the effect of the additional placental blood on hemoglobin levels in later infancy was not clearly shown.

Serial and cross-sectional studies of infants showed that during the first 8 to 10 weeks after birth, hemoglobin dropped to 9 to 11 g/100 ml (32, 190, 260, 261, 287, 599, 622). This drop took place in infants receiving iron supplements as well as in those who received none. Arthurton et al. (32) in a study in which serial hemoglobin estimations were carried out on 22 healthy premature infants, observed that the postnatal drop in hemoglobin was less in babies whose initial level was less than 20 g/100 ml than in those with initial levels of greater than 20 g/100 ml. The hemoglobin levels did not seem to be related significantly to birth weight. Grunseit et al. (270) found that infants whose gestational age was less than 34 weeks had lower postnatal changes than those that were more mature. Because of the high variability in the data, however, there were no statistically significant differences between the mean hemoglobin levels of infants with gestational ages of less than 34 weeks and those of infants 34 to 38 weeks or of more than 38 weeks of gestational age. Guest and Brown (271) also found no significant difference in hematologic values between premature infants and full-term infants in the neonatal period. After the first 80 days of life, however, differences between the two groups were found with increasing frequency.

Hammond and Murphy (287) found that after the initial drop in the first 2 months of life, hemoglobin levels began to rise slowly. In infants receiving iron supplements, they rose faster than in unsupplemented infants. Another drop in hemoglobin level occurred between months 7 and 9 in the unsupplemented babies and between months 10 and 12 in the supplemented infants. The supplemented babies had received 100 mg of iron dextran intramuscularly during week 2 or 3 of life. Other investigators (190, 622) found that in unsupplemented infants, hemoglobin levels continued to drop but at a slower rate after the first 8 to 10 weeks of life. Gorten and Cross (261) noted that the reported mean values for unsupplemented infants tended to be skewed in the direction of higher values because as infants became anemic they were removed from the study group leaving only those with more adequate hemoglobin levels to be measured.

Mean serum iron values in premature infants observed by Gladtke and Rind (256) were not significantly different from those of full-term infants. They were, however, much more variable in premature infants than in full-term babies. This variability, Gladtke and Rind suggested, was a reflection of the variable iron provision from the mother. In their study and that of Sisson et al. (622), mean serum iron levels in premature infants were high (93 and 96 µg/100 ml) in the first week of life, rose higher during the first month (138 and 118 µg/100 ml), and then slowly declined during the rest of the first year. Full-term babies showed the same pattern. Brozovic et al. (106) reported a mean serum iron value of 78 µg/100 ml at birth which rose to 105 µg/100 ml at 2 weeks of age. Thereafter, despite the iron supplementation, serum iron levels fell to a low average value of 44 µg/100 ml when the infants were 6 months old. Nicola et al. (489) also observed a gradual decline during year 1 but found that in 2-year-old children serum iron levels were similar to those observed during months 2 to 3 of life. Gladtke and Rind (256) concluded that the observed pattern was typical and reflected iron metabolism in childhood. Sisson et al. (622) observed that the mean iron-binding capacity, nearly zero in week 1 of life, increased during the first year and iron saturation of serum decreased from 85% to between 11% and 14% in the same period. The administration of medicinal iron to the infants caused a marked rise in hemoglobin concentration but not always in serum iron concentration. These observations suggested to Sisson et al. that serum iron levels were more a reflection of tissue iron stores than of anemia.

Gorten (260) estimated iron gains in small premature infants (birth weight less than 1,600 g) during their first year of life. Assuming "that especially in premature infants the largest iron reserve for subsequent hemoglobin and tissue formation lies in the birth hemoglobin mass and not in latent stores in body tissue," he did not include calculations for storage iron in his estimates. His calculations showed that infants (receiving iron supplements), whose hemoglobin concentration was about 11.5 g/100 ml when they were 12 months old, utilized a mean total of 240 mg of iron per child for growth during their first year (0.73 mg iron/day). Schulman (598) assuming an optimal hemoglobin level of 12.3 g/100 ml calculated a similar requirement (238 mg/year or 0.65 mg/day) for

growth during the first year of life. Sturgeon (645), basing his calculations on hypothetical data for infants assumed to have been born in various states of iron nutriture, estimated yearly requirements of 105 to 286 mg to attain opimal hemoglobin levels. Saddi and Schapira (584) calculated a requirement of "35 to 45 mg/kg of newly acquired weight, of which from 4 to 7 mg goes for the functional tissue sector, 30 for the hemoglobin, and finally from 5 to 15 for the storage sector." For premature infants, they estimated an iron requirement of 280 mg for growth during the first year of life or 0.8 mg/day beginning in the second month of life. To translate these estimates into a recommendation for dietary, intake Gorten (260) noted that allowances for losses in bile, cellular debris and urine as well as for incomplete absorption would have to be made. He concluded that Schulman's recommendation (598) of an allowance of 2 mg iron/kg body weight daily by month 3, gradually decreasing to 1 mg/kg daily by the end of the first year would ensure satisfactory iron metabolism.

The largest of the allowances that must be made in recommending dietary intakes of iron is for incomplete absorption. Studies with radioactive iron have yielded widely varying estimates of iron absorption by premature infants. Oettinger et al. (499), for instance, administered by gavage a test dose of 6 ml ferrous chloride containing approximately 1 µg elemental iron and labeled with ^{59}Fe to 10 premature infants during the first week after birth. Two to 6 weeks later, they measured the incorporation of the labeled iron into the red cells and calculated that 0.29% to 6.8% (mean 2.8%) of the test dose was in the infants' blood. Similar values (0.4–8.2%, mean 3.2% of the test dose) were found with full-term infants. In addition, Oettinger et al. reported that the "mechanisms for absorption of iron from the gastrointestinal tract and its incorporation into hemoglobin are present and functioning at the time of birth".

With older infants (1–10 weeks old), variable but higher absorption than that reported by Oettinger et al. was observed. Gorten et al. (262) by gavage fed a formula labeled with ^{59}Fe to 14 premature infants. Prior to the test feeding, half of the infants had been fed a formula containing iron and the others had received no iron. Absorption of iron was calculated by comparing the amount of ^{59}Fe recovered in the stools with that ingested in the formula. In addition, iron utilization was estimated by measuring the ^{59}Fe incorporated into circulating red cells 7 to 14 days after the test feeding. The data indicated that 6.8% to 74.0% (mean 31.5%) of the test dose of iron was absorbed and 2.9% to 47.8% (mean 15.3%) of the test dose was utilized for hemoglobin formation. Absorption varied inversely with the quantity of iron in the test dose, but was not related significantly to previous iron intake, gestational age, birthweight, or weight at the time of testing. Rate of absorption was, however, significantly correlated with rate of growth.

When Heinrich et al. (307) used a whole body counter, they found that 28 premature infants, 4 to 66 days old, apparently absorbed 8.5% to 36.5% (mean 21%) of a test dose of ^{59}Fe administered with vitamin C. Seven additional infants who were iron deficient absorbed 45.6% to 81.3% of the test dose. In comparing their data with those obtained by other methods, Heinrich et al. (307) concluded that "measurement of the whole body retention of absorbed ^{59}Fe with the 4π-geometry of a whole body radioactivity detector with liquid organic scintillator is also for infants the most reliable, sensitive and considerate method for the quantitative estimation of the intestinal iron absorption."

Studies on the amount of iron required to maintain normal hematologic values in premature infants usually have involved a comparison of the hematologic responses of unsupplemented infants to those of infants receiving supplements. In some studies (190, 287), the supplemental iron was administered intramuscularly. In others, the supplement either was given as a salt providing about 39 mg (190) or about 13 mg iron/day (552) or was added to the formula to supply about 12 mg iron/quart (12.7 mg/liter) (260, 261, 426). The hemoglobin levels below which infants were judged to be anemic were 8.0 to 9.5 g/100 ml.

Both Hammond and Murphy (287) and Elliott (190) found that the administration of iron dextran intramuscularly during the neonatal period did not prevent a drop in hemoglobin levels during the first 2 months of life. It did, however, accelerate the recovery from this early anemia. Elliott observed the effects of doses of iron of 50 to 250 mg. He reported that doses smaller than 100 mg were as effective as those over 100 mg.

In Elliott's study (190), orally administered iron was not as effective as injected iron. This, Elliott suggested, might have been because the infants' mothers failed to administer the oral preparation regularly. Reedy et al. (552) found that iron administered orally in a preparation that provided approximately 13 mg/day, was effective in raising hemoglobin levels even when the treatment was carried out only during the first 3 months of life. With infants to whom the iron preparation was administered for the first 1 to 2 years, significant improvements in hemoglobin level and weight gain were observed as compared with infants who received no medicinal iron.

To avoid possible problems arising from overdosage or irregular dosage of medicinal iron, Marsh et al. (426) recommended that an iron supplement be added to the infant's formula. In their study with 42 premature infants, 16 were fed a formula enriched to provide 12 mg iron/quart (12.7 mg/liter). The others received either the same formula without added iron or an evaporated milk formula. The infants who were observed from birth to age 9 months received no solid food except a "specially-prepared cereal unenriched in iron" during the study. Hemoglobin levels fell during the first 6 weeks of life in all infants. Then, in those receiving the iron enriched formula, they began to rise, and at 3 months became significantly higher than in those receiving the unenriched foods. During the study no premature infants in the iron treated group became anemic (hemoglobin level below 8 mg/100 ml), but 16 infants who had received no iron supplements had to be changed to the iron enriched formula. Hematocrit and serum iron values gave information similar to that obtained from hemoglobin values. No signs of toxicity or lack of acceptance of the diet were observed in the infants receiving the iron enriched formula. Brozovic et al. (106) suggested that an iron supplement of 36 mg/day from ferrous sulfate was not sufficient to maintain normal hemoglobin levels in premature infants. In their study, the supplement was administered daily from age 5 weeks to 9 months but there was no unsupplemented control group. Although the mean hemoglobin level was 11.4 g/100 ml when infants were 6 months old and 11.5 g/100 ml when they were 9 months old, the authors concluded that "the provision of therapeutic doses of oral iron in preterm low birthweight infants does not prevent the development of iron deficiency and even iron deficiency anemia."

Gorten and Cross (261) studied 145 premature infants whose pediatric treatment included strained foods at age 3 months and a full diet (cereals, eggs, fruit, vegetables, and meat) by age 6 months. Of these infants, 69 (study group) were fed a formula containing 12 mg ferrous iron/quart (12.7 mg/liter). The other 76 infants (control group) received a similar formula with no added iron. As in other studies, the hemoglobin levels of the two groups were similar for the first 10 weeks of life. Then, the hemoglobin levels and hematocrit values of the iron supplemented group began to rise, and from 14 weeks old on, that group had significantly higher values than the control group. The mean gain in hemoglobin iron was 0.39 mg/day in the supplemented group and 0.30 mg/day in the control group. No infant in the supplemented group developed anemia. Of the 76 infants in the control group, however, 25 became anemic, and their treatment was changed to include the iron-containing formula. When this was done, the mean utilization of iron for hemoglobin formation by these infants increased from 0.15 mg/day to 0.62 mg/day.

When Gorten (260) examined the data of the smallest infants (birth weight under 1,600 g) in the study, he found that they were able to utilize iron as well as the larger infants did. During their first year of life, the smallest infants in the study group utilized 240 mg iron for growth (0.73 mg/day, 0.08 mg/kg daily) to achieve a body iron content of 35 mg/kg and a hemoglobin level of 11.5 g/100 ml. During the same period the smallest infants in the control group utilized only 167 mg iron for growth (0.52 mg/day, 0.07 mg/kg daily) and achieved a body iron content of 29 mg/kg and a hemoglobin concentration of 9.4 g/100 ml. When the smallest infants who became anemic (hemoglobin less than 9 g/100 ml) were changed to the iron-containing formula, their rate of iron utilization increased from 0.09 mg/kg daily to 0.18 mg/kg daily within 12 weeks. Their rate of iron utilization remained higher than that of the other infants for the rest of the study. Gorten calculated that for each gram of body tissue gained daily, the infant must gain 0.036 to 0.039 mg/iron day to maintain a "stable body iron status at 0.035 mg per gm of body mass". He concluded that this rate of gain could be maintained by providing a formula supplemented to contain 12 mg iron/quart (12.7 mg/liter).

Full-term infants. Iron balance in the full-term infant has been studied from the first day of life. Cavell and Widdowson (128) analyzed the meconium secreted by six newborn infants during their first 24 hours of life and found that the infants excreted 0.13 to 0.19 mg iron/kg body weight (mean 0.16 mg/kg) by this route. Ten other breast-fed neonates, 5 to 8 days old and weighing 2.63 to 4.47 kg were studied in 3-day balance periods. The iron content of the breast milk ranged from 0.033 to 0.145 mg/100 ml. The babies ingested daily 0.044 to 0.176 mg iron/kg body weight (mean 0.100 mg/kg). Analyses of the feces and urine showed that all of the infants were in negative balance. In fact, the feces contained 4 to 30 times as much iron as the diet. The average daily iron loss was slightly more than 1 mg/kg. Furthermore the amount of iron in the feces bore no apparent relationship to the amount of iron in the food. Cavell and Widdowson calculated that the babies were getting daily from breast milk an amount of iron equivalent to 0.1% of their body iron but were excreting more than 1% of their body iron. Losses as large as this, they suggested, "must be a temporary phenomenon, peculiar to the neonatal period." In speculating on how the iron was excreted into the intestine, they concluded that "whether the bile of the young baby contains a particularly large amount of iron or whether the baby is less able than the adult to re-absorb this iron, or whether some other intestinal secretion is a more important source of the iron in the infant's faeces still remains to be discovered."

With five older breast-fed infants (3 weeks to 2 months old) Wallgren (696) found positive balances in 17 of 21 balance periods. The milk supplied to the infants provided 0.044 to 0.098 mg iron/100 ml (mean 0.064 mg/100 ml). The negative balances that did occur coincided with very low iron levels in the mother's milk. Wallgren concluded that small as it is in quantity, the iron in mother's milk is sufficient to cover the needs of the infant for exogenous iron for maintenance. He pointed out, however, that it is not enough for the total needs for blood building but that the infant can use not only the iron contained in the internal organs at birth but also that released as a consequence of the physiological wear and tear of the red cells. Stearns and Stinger (636) also found that the iron provided in breast milk (0.06 to 0.08 mg iron/kg body weight) was sufficient to meet the needs of one infant 9 to 15 weeks old. The infant was in equilibrium or in positive balance (0.03 mg/kg) with an average retention of 0.01 mg/kg. Additions of egg and cow's milk to the human milk diet increased the intake (0.12 mg/kg) and also the retention of iron (0.05 mg/kg). When cow's milk and egg were fed without human milk, however, retention decreased (0.02 mg/kg) even though the iron intake was increased (0.25 mg/kg).

In most of the balance studies with infants, the diets were based on cow's milk with or without other additives (213, 214, 330, 363, 364, 595, 635, 636). Stearns and Stinger (636), for instance, having observed that "although the iron content of human milk is also low, much more iron is retained by infants fed human milk than by those fed cow's milk," attempted to simulate the mineral relationships of human milk by adding potassium chloride or carbonate to cow's milk. In other experiments, they increased the iron content of the diet by adding egg yolk, spinach, iron-rich cereal or ferric ammonium citrate. They observed 14 healthy infants, 7 to 25 weeks old, weighing 4.2 to 6.6 kg at the beginning of the study. There was wide varia-tion in the response to diets in which cow's milk without additives supplied the iron. With iron intakes averaging 0.19 mg/kg, there was an average loss of about 0.01 mg/kg. The addition of potassium salts, egg yolk or spinach did not improve retention. With the addition of iron-rich cereal or iron salts, retention rose as iron intake increased. Stearns and Stinger concluded that an intake of 0.5 mg iron/kg body weight was necessary to insure iron retention "and an intake of 1–1.5 mg per kilogram permits ample retention."

Other investigators (595, 635) also found that when the dietary iron was provided only by cow's milk, balances were usually negative and that the addition of such foods as apricots or spinach, did not appreciably improve retention. Stearns and McKinley (635) concluded that the formula-fed infant in the first 2 months of life might be expected to lose 1.25 mg iron/day with a total iron loss of about 50 to 75 mg. Josephs (363) was dubious of the validity of this conclusion. He pointed out that the analytical procedures used by Stearns and McKinley were open to question. Furthermore he reasoned that with such a loss, the iron stores in the body would be exhausted so that the rise in hemoglobin concentration that normally begins spontaneously in about month 3 of life could not occur.

Josephs (363, 364) studied iron retention in infants fed cow's milk formulas supplemented with either cereal or ferric ammonium citrate. When cereal was fed the daily iron intakes were 0.05 to 0.28 mg/kg. Higher intakes of 2.3 to 12.4 mg/kg were achieved when the iron salt was provided. Calculation of the regression of retention (intake minus output) on intake indicated that, with the milk and cereal diet, equilibrium could be achieved with an average daily intake of 0.17 mg/kg body weight in infants less than 3 months old. With infants over 3 months old, lower intakes were sufficient. The slope of the regression lines indicated that about 60% of the dietary iron was absorbed (363). When the milk formula was supplemented with iron salts (364), infants under 3 months old showed wide variation in retention. With infants over 3 months old, calculation of the regression of retention on intake showed that intakes of 2.0 mg/kg were needed to assure equilibrium. Josephs (364), in considering these observations and others reported in the literature, concluded that retention of iron is enhanced when the intake is above 2.0 mg/kg body weight, equilibrium is maintained at 0.1 to 2.0 mg/kg, and the balance tends to become negative with intakes below 0.1 mg/kg. Anemic infants tended to retain iron better than nonanemic children. Age in these studies appeared to have little influence on retention. Similar data were obtained by Feuillen (213) who, with 19 formula-fed infants, 15 days to 9 months old, observed a mean daily intake of 0.37 mg iron/kg and a mean daily retention of 0.19 mg/kg (53%). Feuillen, noting that formula-fed infants ingested and absorbed more iron than breast-fed infants, concluded that the anemia found more frequently in bottle-fed than in breast-fed infants is not due to deficient iron intakes. Other nutrients such as copper (364) and vitamin C (214) were reported to influence the utilization of iron (in hemoglobin formation) but not the absorption or retention of iron.

The whole body iron content was determined for 32 full-term infants who were either stillborn or who died shortly after birth. The earliest of these analyses, carried out by Hugounenq (325) on two bodies yielded values of 89.1 and 98.5 mg iron/kg body tissue. Widdowson and Dickerson (720) observed that when these values were corrected for the "presumed amount of fat in the fetal bodies" they agreed "extraordinarily well" with those obtained 50 years later by Widdowson and Spray (725) when they determined the body composition of six full-term infants (58.5 to 123 mg iron/kg fat free tissue). Schairer and Rechenberger (591), analyzing three bodies, also obtained values (mean 82 mg/kg body tissue) in reasonable agreement with those of Widdowson and Spray (725). Widdowson and Dickerson (720) suggested, as did Söldner (629), that much higher values reported by Camerer (120, 121) were probably the result of contamination during analysis. Lower values (33–64 mg iron/kg body tissue) were found by Apte and Iyengar (24) when they analyzed the bodies of 18 full-term infants born to poor Indian women. As noted earlier (p. 1023) they suggested that these lower values might reflect the nutritional status of the mothers. Widdowson and Dickerson (720) suggested that "had the bodies of children up to 2 years old been analyzed, they would probably have been found to contain a lower concentration of iron, for a reduction in hemoglobin concentration in the blood and of iron in the liver seems to be the normal course of events at this time of life." Data obtained by Schairer and Rechenberger (591) from the analyses of the bodies of one 6-months-old child (33 mg iron/kg) and one 1-year-old child (41.7 mg iron/kg) support this hypothesis.

Analytical data show wide variation in the iron content of the livers and spleens (storage iron) of newborn full-term infants. The iron concentration in the livers of 53 stillborn or newborn infants less than 1 day old was 7.6 to 76.8 mg/100 g and the total liver iron content was 5.9 to 144.7 mg (108, 255, 343, 404, 545). Widdowson and Spray (725) found that the concentration of inorganic iron in the livers and spleens of five stillborn infants was 10.4 to 37.0 mg/100 g, and that 5% to 19% of the total body iron was found in the liver and spleen. Lintzel et al. (404) found similar concentrations (9.1–30.4 mg/100 g) in the livers and spleens of seven infants. The total iron content of the livers and spleens in their infants was 16.4 to 43.3 mg.

Liver and spleen iron stores increase rapidly in the full-term infant for about 10 weeks after birth (255, 404, 545, 591). Gladstone (255) in 1932 reported histological data that indicated this increase. At that time, the hypothesis was generally held that the infant is born with large liver stores of iron that are withdrawn during the first few months of life when the diet is deficient in iron (111). Because his histological observations were so divergent from this hypothesis, Gladstone carried out chemical analyses on the livers of fetuses and young infants. His chemical analyses corroborated his histological observations. Later reports by Ramage et al. (545), Schairer and Rechenberger (591), and Lintzel et al. (404) agreed with Gladstone's findings. The rise in liver and spleen iron content coincided with a period of hemoglobin destruction (255, 591). Studies with older infants showed that after the initial rise, there was a gradual decrease in storage iron (108, 545, 626) which coincided with the time when the hemoglobin was rising again (626). Smith et al. (626) observed that the highest incidence of iron deficiency anemia occurs during the period when liver iron stores are lowest and are unable to compensate for dietary deficiencies or blood loss (year 2 of life).

Gairdner (242) noted the wide variation in liver and spleen iron observed by Widdowson and Spray (725) and Lintzel et al. (404) in their analyses of the bodies of newborn infants. In his estimates of total body iron content by the factorial method, Gairdner used a value of 10 mg iron/kg body weight as representative of the storage iron in newborns. By his calculations a baby whose birth weight was 3.4 kg would have 34 mg of storage iron. Within 6 weeks this storage iron would be augmented to 79 mg by the transfer of iron from hemoglobin. Thereafter the store would be gradually depleted so that (assuming no absorption of dietary iron) the infant, at age 4 months, would have stores just slightly less (29 mg) than those at birth. Sturgeon (645) and Schulman (598), using a similar type of calculation estimated that all stores would be exhausted by the time the baby was 1 year old. Saddi and Shapira (584) calculated that, without an external iron supply, liver stores would be completely depleted by the time the infant was 6–8 months old.

Estimates of functional tissue iron (myoglobin) in full-term infants have been based mainly on studies with animals. Josephs (361) found that "nonhemoglobin" iron (presumed to be functional tissue iron) in rats was maintained at the expense of hemoglobin iron and "when hemoglobin concentration was reduced to its lowest point, the tissue iron was maintained at the expense of the growth of the animal." In his studies the lowest permissible level of "nonhemoglobin" iron in young rats appeared to be about 5 mg/kg body weight. In piglets, Venn et al. (685) found that the "iron in the remainder of the body" (total body iron minus the iron in blood, liver and spleen) varied with the age and treatment of the piglets from 0.26

mg/kg body weight at birth to 2.58 to 15.0 mg/kg at 3 weeks and 7.33 mg/kg at 8 weeks. Sturgeon (645) calculated from Biorck's estimations of the myoglobin content of muscle in young infants (74) that "total parenchymal iron is 4.0 mg and 7.0 mg/kg of body weight at birth and 1 year of age respectively." Other calculations of functional tissue iron based either on Sturgeon's estimates or on the work with rats (361) or piglets (685) have ranged from 7.0 to 7.5 mg/kg body weight (242, 305, 365, 584, 598). The assumption has usually been made that the proportion of functional tissue iron to total body weight is the same in the 1-year-old infant as in the newborn. There is, however, no experimental data to support this assumption.

The full-term infant, like the premature infant, experiences an accumulation of iron stores with the rapid fall of the hemoglobin level early in life. Because of the larger initial body weight, greater blood volume and slower growth rate, the full-term infant may not be in as precarious a position as the premature infant with respect to inadequate iron reserves.

As discussed previously (p. 1024), the amount of iron contributed by hemoglobin to total body iron depends on the volume of blood and the concentration of the hemoglobin in it. Blood volume has been estimated in over 400 full-term infants ranging in age from a few hours to 2 years. In some of the infants, two or more serial observations were made (603). In the earlier studies CO_2 (438) or brilliant vital red dye (37, 172, 409, 562) was used in the indirect estimate of either plasma volume or total blood volume. In later studies, Evan's blue dye (T-1824) (100, 181, 460, 621) or radioactive tracers, ^{32}P (460) or ^{125}I-labeled albumen (746), were used. Of these, Sisson et al. (621) declared that the Evan's blue dye (T-1824) method was the most reproducible, least dangerous and simplest to use.

Blood volume determinations by these indirect methods have varied greatly from one infant to another and from one study to another. In very young infants, part of the variation was found to be related to the time at which the umbilical cord was clamped (181, 597, 746). Comparison between studies is complicated by different methods of expression (for instance, total blood volume vs ml blood/kg body weight) and by different methods for estimating whole blood volume. In some studies, blood volume itself was estimated whereas in others blood volume values were derived from estimates of plasma volume, red blood cell volume or both. Sisson et al. (621) in reviewing the various methods concluded that "the use of body weight is an adequate means of expression for comparing the blood volume of infants," and "the volumes derived from the total circulating plasma, though perhaps higher than those calculated from red blood cell volume, have no greater error."

Data on blood volume of neonates are most numerous. Records of more than 250 observations were found with values of 52 to 195 ml/kg body weight (100, 181, 409, 460, 562, 597, 621, 746). Russell (577) found that as a child grew older, total blood volume increased and blood volume as related to height or surface area increased, but blood volume as related to body weight did not change. Sisson et al. (621) determined blood volume serially in 20 infants, 1 day to 1 year, (three or more observations per child) and found a wide range of values within individual infants and among children of the same age. They concluded that "infants, both individually and collectively, up to 1 year of age demonstrate a lack of consistency in the measured plasma, erythrocyte and total blood volumes. No completely reliable average value was shown during the first year of life insofar as this might refer to an individual baby."

In estimating hemoglobin levels in early infancy, the hemoglobin concentration in the umbilical cord blood has been taken by some investigators as indicative of the concentration in the infant's blood at birth (424, 473, 645, 702). Analyses on over 3,000 samples of cord blood have yielded estimates of 11.1 to 23.8 g/100 ml. In 21 studies, the number of specimens analyzed varied from 12 to 863 and the mean hemoglobin values ranged from 14.5 to 17.9 g/100 ml (113, 132, 180, 184, 243, 271, 272, 374, 417, 424, 459, 473, 529, 565, 571, 583, 645, 671, 694, 702, 752). Some of the variation has been attributed to differences in the length of pregnancy (417, 694). Other investigators, however, found no significant correlation between cord hemoglobin concentration and gestational age (424, 565). Part of the variation has been explained also by differences in analytical technique and sample selection (132, 702); some of it, however, seems inexplicable (113).

Some investigators have reported higher hemoglobin concentrations in neonates during the first few hours of life than in the cord blood (180, 220, 243, 271, 703). This has been attributed in some instances to the drainage of cord blood into the infant. Support for this hypothesis is found in reports that babies whose umbilical cords were clamped late had higher hemoglobin concentrations than those whose cords were clamped immediately after delivery (142, 180, 606, 616, 734). On the other hand, in some cases, the apparent difference between the infant's blood and his cord blood may have been due in part to differences between capillary and venous blood (498). Oettinger (498) observed in 24 infants, 1 hour old, that the hemoglobin concentration was from 0.6 to 8.2 g/100 ml higher in capillary blood than in venous blood. Findlay (220) and Andersen and Ortmann (13) also obtained data indicating that capillary blood contained a higher hemoglobin concentration than did venous blood. Gairdner et al. (243), however, reported a rise in hemoglobin concentration in babies regardless of whether the cord was clamped early or late. Furthermore, all of their determinations were carried out on venous blood.

Gairdner et al. (243) observed that "the first 3 months of life fall into three phases." The first phase, as they defined it, was the first week of life, when the hemoglobin level remained higher than the cord level. During this time, they and other investigators observed slight declines from the mean levels (15.5 to 23.4 g/100 ml) found on day 1 or 2 of life (139, 212, 243, 259, 271, 323, 606, 616, 621, 702). Others (32, 220, 423) observed the slight declines to occur during week 2 of life. In the second phase (from week 2 until week 8) Gairdner et al. (243) observed a marked steady decline in hemoglobin levels to about 11 or 12 g/100 ml. Similar declines were observed in other studies (12, 32, 54, 193,

212, 220, 272, 446, 473, 609, 621, 635, 732), with some variation in the lowest level reached. In some studies (323, 372, 488) the decline lasted until approximately week 12. Then following the second phase, Gairdner et al. suggested, is a third phase in which "the hemoglobin is maintained at 11 to 12 g." Such a period of relatively constant hemoglobin levels was observed in some studies (193, 212, 323, 372, 446, 635). In other studies additional declines at a slower rate in the hemoglobin concentrations were observed between months 3 and 5 (732), 2 and 6 (606), 2 and 16 (271, 272) and 12 and 18 (473). These additional declines were followed by gradual increases throughout the rest of the infancy period. Mean hemoglobin concentrations reported for 2-year-old children were 11 to 12.8 g/100 ml (54, 193, 237, 271, 272, 372, 458, 473).

Some investigators (212, 446) have suggested that part of the variability in hemoglobin concentrations in infants may be due to racial or ethnic factors. Moe (457), however, found little evidence to support this hypothesis. The evidence on the influence of maternal anemia and iron supplementation during pregnancy on the hemoglobin level of the infant is also unclear (623). Woodruff and Bridgeforth (742) and Sturgeon (647) studying nonanemic women found that differences in iron status during pregnancy were not reflected in the hemoglobin concentration or iron status of the offspring at birth or during infancy. Much earlier, Strauss (642) had observed that, at birth, the hemoglobin concentration of infants born of severely anemic mothers did not differ significantly from that of infants of normal mothers. One year after birth, however, infants whose mothers had been anemic, had significantly lower hemoglobin concentrations than those whose mothers were normal. Sisson and Lund (620) also found no significant differences in hemoglobin concentration at birth between infants born of anemic and nonanemic women. They found, however, that total circulating hemoglobin mass was about 20% lower in the infants of anemic women than in those of nonanemic women. They concluded that the consequential deprivation of readily available iron stores in the infants of

anemic women "may be expected to influence the production of iron deficiency anemia in later months of life."

As noted previously, (p. 1015, 1025) serum iron is thought to reflect tissue iron stores (151, 622). Serum iron concentration has been reported in the newborn full-term infant and throughout the first year of life. The serum iron concentration of 114 newborn infants varied from 53 to 299 μg/100 ml (81, 98, 164, 256, 603, 671, 711). The range of values reported for 142 infants during their first year was 55 to 150 μg/100 ml (98, 256, 603).

In estimating iron requirements of the full-term infant by the factorial method, most investigators have based their calculations on estimates of the total body iron of the infant at birth and at 1 year. The largest component in these estimates has been hemoglobin iron. It also has been the most variable component, based on hemoglobin concentration estimates of 13 to 20 g/100 ml at birth and 12 to 13 g/100 ml at 1 year. Blood volume estimates have been 80 to 95 ml/kg at birth and 75 to 85 mg/kg at 1 year. Estimates by the factorial method of iron requirements in the first year have been 0.29 to 0.8 mg/day (305, 584, 598, 645).

The amount of dietary iron needed to meet the physiological iron requirement depends on how much iron can be absorbed into the body. Various investigators have studied iron absorption in infants by administering ^{59}Fe iron salts with or without food (248, 557, 601) or as an intrinsic marker biologically incorporated into various foods (34, 35, 600). Schulz and Smith (600) found that when ^{59}Fe was given in a pharmaceutical iron preparation, the absorption was similar whether it was given in one single daily dose or in four equal doses per day. They also found that the mean absorption of ferrous iron added to milk was similar to the absorption of iron from "in vivo tagged" milk (600).

The radioisotope has been detected in the stools (248, 600, 601), in the red blood cells (499, 557, 600, 601, 743) and in the whole body (34, 35, 307). Schulz and Smith (600) reported that absorption estimated from red blood cell incorporation of the label was similar to that estimated from stool counts. Riley (557), however, suggested that blood levels of radioactive iron are reliable as a measure of absorption only if utilization for hemoglobin production is complete. In his studies that included two normal and four anemic infants, Riley found that the proportion of absorbed iron (radioactivity of the intake minus radioactivity of the feces) that appeared in the blood (red cell activity) was 5.8% and 21.7% in the normal infants and 11.1% to 40% in the anemic patients. He concluded that "the chief factor regulating the appearance of radioactive iron in the blood appears to be the degree of anemia and the chief factor regulating absorption, the state of the body stores." Total body counting presumably measures all of the radioactive iron entering and remaining in the body and estimation of absorption by this means should not be subject to the problems involved in accurate stool collection or to some of the factors affecting hemoglobin formation. As noted earlier (p. 1027) Heinrich et al. (307) recommended whole body counting as the most reliable method for estimating absorption of iron in infants.

Regardless of the method used, the estimates of iron absorption have been variable. Recently, Rios et al. (559) reported that 42, 4 to 7 month old infants absorbed 0.2% to 51.9% of a test dose of 1.44 mg iron from ferrous ascorbate and 0.7% to 23.1% of doses of iron ranging from 1.4 to 2.6 mg from ferrous sulfate added to infant formula. Rios et al. (559) also compared the availability of several radioiron sources added to infant cereals in a study with 25 healthy infants 4 to 7 months old. Each compound provided 5 mg iron/feeding and was fed for 5 consecutive days. The percentage of iron absorbed was determined by whole body counting and was, for iron orthophosphate, 0.7% (0.2%–2.8%); for sodium iron pyrophosphate, 1.0% (0.6%–1.5%); for ferrous sulfate, 2.7% (0.4%–12.1%) and for reduced iron with fine particles, 4.0% (1.2%–8.5%). Ashworth and March (35), using whole body counting, found that the mean absorption of iron from a standard solution of ferrous ascorbate was 16.7% to 63.5% when studied in five groups of infants. The absorption by individual infants was 1.7% to 100%. In other studies in which labeled iron salts were used, six nonanemic chil-

dren, 13 to 29 months old, absorbed 7% to 63% (557, 601) and four anemic children, 11 to 18 months old, absorbed 10% to 92% (557) of test doses containing 30 mg iron. When Woodruff (741) studied iron utilization in 26 anemic infants, 7 to 24 months old, he found that, with iron doses of 0.25 to 4 mg/kg body weight, 4.5% to 68.3% of the iron was utilized in hemoglobin formation. The studies using labeled iron salts showed that the proportion of iron absorbed by the infant increased in iron deficiency anemia (307, 601) and was inversely related to the size of the test dose (248, 741). In studies in which iron absorption from radiolabeled foods was determined, absorption values varied widely within any one food as well as with the type of food, the kind of iron enrichment, and with the method of food preparation (34, 35, 600).

The requirements of full-term infants for iron have been estimated also by comparing the response to iron supplemented diets with the response to unsupplemented diets. In 1931 Mackay (414) reported the results of studies on almost 1,100 infants in which she showed that the regular administration of iron salts as iron and ammonium citrate was effective in raising hemoglobin levels. Her work showed also that anemia occurring in the second half of the infant's first year was usually nutritional in origin and could be prevented by feeding a source of iron.

In subsequent studies various investigators estimated the amount of iron required to prevent anemia and to promote good health in the infant. In some studies the iron was added to cereal (459), milk (414) or formula (12, 426) and in others it was fed as iron salts (220, 238, 646, 648) or in a vitamin-mineral mixture (210). In some studies, administration of iron began when the infants were only a few days old (12, 426). In others, it began when they were 3 to 3.5 months old or older (457, 646). In most studies, observations were made over a 6 to 9-months period until the infant was 12 months old. In some studies the infants were observed until they were 18 months old although the treatment usually stopped earlier (238, 646).

The principal criterion by which adequacy of intake was judged was the hemoglobin concentration in the blood. Hemoglobin levels accepted as satisfactory were 8 to 11.9 g/100 ml. Some investigators also included other blood parameters such as hematocrit, red cell count, red cell indices (MCV, MCHC), serum iron and serum iron binding capacity (210, 220, 426, 457, 646); others observed morbidity rates (238, 414, 457) and growth rates (220, 414, 457).

Although the majority of the studies indicated beneficial results from iron administration, Findlay (220) and Fuerth (238) failed to demonstrate any difference in blood status between infants receiving iron salts and those who did not. Fuerth pointed out that the subjects of his study were healthy infants who started to eat iron rich foods such as cereals and meat early in life and that his results might not apply to less privileged infants. Another important factor in evaluating response to supplementation is that many of the supplements are provided as salts which have relatively low availability (11, 17, 84, 152, 197, 232, 236, 526, 527, 559, 643).

The estimates of iron requirements derived from studies on iron supplementation varied from 0.9 to 1.5 mg/kg body weight daily or from 10 to 12 mg/day. The lowest of these, 0.9 mg/kg or 10 mg/day was suggested by Moe (457) who fed three groups of 67 to 85 healthy infants cereal fortified with three levels of iron (5, 12.5 and >20 mg/100 g). The infants were 3 months old when they began receiving the cereal. Group 4 of infants who received no iron supplements was studied also. When the infants were 8 to 12 months old, the total daily iron intakes were 3.4 to 7 mg for the unsupplemented group and 5.2 to 8.4 mg, 8.6 to 13.5 mg and greater than 20 mg for the three supplemented groups. Blood analysis showed that none of the infants receiving 10 ± 1.9 mg iron/day developed signs of iron deficiency anema. When the iron intakes were related to body weight, the data showed that the infants with intakes of 0.90 to 0.99 mg/kg had a mean hemoglobin level (11.84 g/100 ml) that was among the highest observed in the study. Moe concluded that the apparent iron requirements of infants under 1 year old (10 mg/day, 0.9 mg/kg) could be met if they were fed iron fortified cereal

(12.5 mg iron/100 g cereal) twice daily from the age of about 3.5 months.

The highest estimate of iron requirement (1–1.5 mg/kg) was calculated by Sturgeon (646) from data obtained when infants from low income and high income families received iron salts either orally at 3 to 18 months or intramuscularly at 9 months. More than 245 infants were studied. They were tested at ages 6, 12 and 18 months. Differences in hemoglobin levels indicated that with daily oral iron intakes of 1 to 1.5 mg/kg, a maximum mean hemoglobin concentration of 11.4 g/100 ml was achieved by age 6 months. There was no "secondary fall" during the remainder of the first year. When the infants reached 18 months, their mean hemoglobin levels increased to approximately 11.6 to 12 g/100 ml. Sturgeon concluded that "a daily dietary allowance of 1 to 1.5 mg/kg will achieve optimal iron nutrition for a substantial majority of the infant population." He suggested that this allowance could be attained with iron intakes of 6 to 9 mg/day for infants of 0 to 3 months, increasing to 8 to 12 mg by 6 months, and 10 to 15 mg/day by 12 months with no further increase after 1 year of age.

Farquhar (210) suggested that Sturgeon's higher estimate (1.5 mg/kg) should be preferred. He studied 44 infants who, in addition to their regular diets, were given a multivitamin preparation with or without 5 mg iron/day. The infants began to receive the vitamin preparation at 1 month of age. The mean hemoglobin and hematocrit levels of the infants receiving iron were significantly higher than those of infants not treated with iron at ages 3, 6 and 9 months but not at age 12 months. There was no difference in height or weight between the 2 groups. Farquhar estimated that the infants were getting about 1.0 mg iron/kg body weight daily from their diet and that the addition of 5 mg/day would increase the intake to 1.5 mg/kg.

Both Marsh et al. (426) and Andelman and Sered (12) added iron salts to formulas. Marsh et al. studied 74 infants fed from age 3 days a formula with or without the addition of 12.7 mg iron/liter (12 mg/quart). By age 3 months, the infants receiving iron had higher hemoglobin and serum iron levels than those whose diets were unenriched. The difference became more pronounced by age 9 months. No iron supplemented infant had a hemoglobin concentration of less than 8 g/100 ml. Similarly Andelman and Sered (12) studied 1,048 infants who received customary pediatric care with or without the addition of 12 mg Fe/day to their formulas. In their study only 9% of the supplemented infants became anemic (hemoglobin <10 g/100 ml) whereas 76% of the unsupplemented group became anemic. Furthermore, infants who were fed the iron enriched formula before leaving the hospital had, between ages 12 and 18 months, significantly higher hemoglobin levels than those who began to receive it after their first visit to the Child Welfare Clinic (usually during the first month). Andelman and Sered (12) concluded from this observation that infants are able "to absorb iron at a very early age for later utilization in hemoglobin synthesis."

Reports of food intake surveys (54, 216, 274) show that there is great variation in the iron intake of healthy young infants. Beal et al. (54) studied the food intake records of infants ("middle class children of European extraction") from birth to age 24 months. Their median daily iron intake rose to nearly 1.2 mg/kg between months 6 and 9 and then declined to 0.5 mg/kg by age 2 years. Individual variation, however, was wide "with a range from 0.43 to 2.20 mg/kg/day from diet alone at the peak intake ages between 6 and 9 months." Furthermore, intakes, as related to body weight in fast growing children were not appreciably different from those in slow growing children. When the average daily intake was related to hemoglobin levels, the data showed that for 96% of the children (57 infants), daily intakes of 0.5 mg/kg or more were enough to maintain hemoglobin levels at or about 10 g/100 ml. During the first year of life whether iron intake was near 0.5 mg/kg or above 2.0 mg/kg made no apparent difference in hemoglobin level. The median daily iron intake during year 1 of life by Beal's infants was 0.83 mg/kg. This is reasonably close to the median iron intake (0.9 mg/kg, 7.2 mg/day) calculated by Filer and Martinez (216) in their study of the dietary intake of 4,310 infants representative of the

infant population at age 6 months in the United States. In both studies, cereal was the principal source of iron in the infants' diets. In 40 older infants, 9 to 24 months old, studied by Guthrie (274) cereal also provided most of the dietary iron. The mean intakes in her study declined from 7.7 mg/day in 9 to 11-months-old infants to 5.3 mg/day in 21 to 24-months-old children. She noted that all children whose iron intake met the then currently recommended allowance (7 mg/day) (479) ate highly enriched cereal products. In view of the lack of relationship between iron intake and hemoglobin levels and the great variability in their study, Beal et al. (54) cautioned against indiscriminate supplementation with iron. Filer and Martinez (216) suggested that when iron supplementation is provided, it should be furnished in the principal dietary energy carrier which for younger infants would be milk.

Preschool children, 2 to 5 years old

Estimates of iron requirements of preschool children have been based primarily on data obtained from iron balance studies (table 6), from studies on iron supplementation, and from food consumption surveys. Some information on body iron content (hemoglobin, serum iron, liver iron) has been obtained also (tables 7 and 8).

In the early iron balance studies, the investigators assumed that when a subject was in negative balance, his iron excretion would reflect his minimum requirements. Rose et al. (570), for instance, studied one 31-month-old girl in a series of three 3-day periods. The child was in negative iron balance with intakes of 4.58 to 4.70 mg/day. Her mean iron excretion was 5.74 mg/day. Rose et al. concluded, therefore, that the subject's minimum iron requirement was probably about 5.70 mg/day (0.5 mg/100 kcal). Allowing a 50% margin for growth, they suggested that her daily allowance should be about 8.50 mg iron/day (0.76 mg/100 kcal). Furthermore, they recommended that children 2 to 3 years old, receive at least 0.75 mg iron/100 kcal.

Using a similar approach, Leichsenring and Flor (394) studied three girls and one boy, 35 to 56 months old, in two 5-day periods. In period 1, the children received

3.25 mg iron/day; in period 2 they received 6.50 mg/day. All four children were in positive balance at each level of intake. Assuming that the mean excretion with the lower intake reflected the maintenance requirement (2.1 mg/day or 0.12 mg/kg) and that the iron retention with the higher level reflected the requirement for growth (0.2 mg/kg), Leichsenring and Flor calculated a total minimum requirement of 0.32 mg/kg. To this they added a 50% margin for safety to suggest a "standard allowance of 0.48 milligrams per kilogram." When this standard was applied to the children in their study, they calculated the total daily iron requirement to be 8.23 mg or 0.62 mg/100 kcal, in reasonably close agreement with the recommendation of Rose et al. (570). In later work, four children, 4 and 5 years old, studied by Macy (418) were able to retain about 10% of iron intakes (0.42 and 0.44 mg/kg) that were similar to the proposed "standard allowance."

Daniels and Wright (170) and Ascham (33) suggested a higher requirement of about 0.60 mg iron/kg body weight. In their studies with a total of five girls and nine boys, 3 to 6 years old, the intakes were higher (0.55–0.75 mg/kg; 8.2–14.1 mg/day), but the retentions were no higher than those observed by Leichsenring and Flor (394) with intakes of about 0.40 mg/kg. The mean iron retention reported by Daniels and Wright (170) from 15 balance periods was 0.18 mg/kg (0.12–0.25 mg/kg), and the mean retention reported by Ascham (33) from six balance periods was 0.07 mg/kg (0.01–0.15 mg/kg).

Similar average retentions (0.06 and 0.07 mg/kg) to those found by Ascham (33) were observed by Porter (533) in a study with one girl and three boys, 3 and 5 years old. In her study, the mean intakes (0.29–0.33 mg/kg; 5.4–5.9 mg/day) were much lower than those of Daniels and Wright (170) and lower also than the standard proposed by Leichsenring and Flor (394). During this study which consisted of nine 7-day periods, all of the children remained in positive balance. Most of the iron loss was by way of the feces and that, Porter noted, varied little from one child to another. She suggested, in view of the work by Widdowson and McCance (722) indicating that the adult body does not excrete appreciable amounts of iron through the gut, that even with low intakes, levels of iron excretion were not an adequate basis for estimating iron requirements. In comparing her retention data with those of other investigators, Porter noted that there was considerable variation in retention of the individual subjects without any obvious relationship to intake (533). She suggested that retention at any one time may reflect the metabolic needs of the moment. On the other hand, the uniform average retentions of the children in her study suggested to her that the children probably were utilizing as much iron as the nature of the diet permitted. She recommended that future studies on dietary allowances of iron should "include data on utilization of iron within the body." She also suggested that "measures of blood changes correlated with balance studies" might be informative on iron utilization.

Such information on total body iron content of preschool children has been obtained directly by iron analysis at autopsy and indirectly by estimating the amount of iron circulating in blood. Widdowson et al. (724) reported that the whole body iron content of a 4.5-year-old boy weighing 14 kg was 64.2 mg/kg fat-free tissue. Since fat-free tissue comprised 22.7% of this child's total body weight, his total body iron could be estimated as about 694 mg. The total liver iron of this child was 40 mg or about 6% of the total body iron. The only other data found on liver iron content of preschool children was reported by Ramage et al. (545). In nine autopsies, the mean total iron content was 95 mg/liver with a range of 39 to 244 mg/liver. The deaths of all of these children were due to pathological conditions.

The amount of iron in blood has been calculated from estimates of blood volume and hemoglobin concentration. Morse et al. (469) and Russell (577) estimated blood volume in 26 children aged 2 to 5 years. The values were about 900 ml in the 2-year-old group and rose to between 1,200 and 1,300 ml in the 5-year-olds. The values obtained by Morse et al. (469) were generally 70 to 85 ml/kg. Russell (577) found most mean values to be 80 to 90 ml/kg body weight.

Hemoglobin determinations on over 4,000 children 2 to 5 years old have been reported. The means calculated in 17 studies were 11.0 to 13.4 g/100 ml (173, 174, 193, 208, 271–273, 373, 379, 416, 445, 473, 508, 512, 519, 522, 732). All but three of the averages (273, 416, 473) were between 11.6 and 12.7 g/100 ml. In five studies on about 9,500 children, the mean packed cell volume was 34% to 37% (99, 273, 512, 519, 520).

None of the reports of blood volume or hemoglobin included any calculations on total body iron or daily iron requirement. However, assuming the average hemoglobin value to be 12.2 g/100 ml and the iron content of hemoglobin to be 0.34%, one may calculate that a 2-year-old child with a blood volume of 900 ml would have about 375 mg iron and a 5-year-old child with a blood volume of 1,250 would have 520 mg iron in the red cells. Bothwell and Finch (93) suggested that two-thirds of the total body iron is found in the red blood cells. Using this estimate, one may calculate further that the total body iron content would be about 560 and 780 mg in the 2-year-old and 5-year-old child respectively.

Usually the content of iron in serum is not used in estimating total body iron. Low values are generally indicative of iron deficient erythropoiesis. Serum iron has been reported in five studies on about 140 children. The values (combination of means and individual observations) were 70 to 123 μg/100 ml (98, 256, 430, 603, 711). The diurnal variation observed in values for adults (p. 1015) was also found in values for children (151, 603, 711). In most cases, samples obtained in the evening contained 25% to 45% less iron than samples obtained in the morning.

The effects of iron supplementation on hematologic indices were reported in two studies (99, 458). Brigety and Pearson (99) gave 532 low-income preschool children dietary plus medicinal iron supplements for a 5-week period. The children were divided into two groups. All children received daily two meals calculated to provide 25 mg iron/week. In addition, one group received an iron supplement of 30 mg/day from ferrous gluconate. The mean hematocrit value of both groups increased significantly from an initial value of 35.7% with a greater mean increase observed in the group receiving the medicinal iron supplement. Two-thirds of the children in each group, however, showed no change in hematocrit.

Moe (458) observed a group of about 300 children, 18 months to 3 years old, who had received either no iron supplements or different forms of iron supplements during their first year of life. The iron supplemented children had received iron fortified cereal either with or without additional iron as ferrous sulfate. At age 18 months to 3 years, the children who had been unsupplemented during year 1 had significantly lower hemoglobin levels (11.1–11.5 g/100 ml) than the supplemented children (11.8 g/100 ml). Moe (458) concluded that children who had received at least 10 mg iron/day during year 1 and especially during months 8 to 12 of life, did not need more than 10 mg/day after 1 year of age.

Food consumption studies have indicated that the iron intakes of many preschool children lie below 10 mg/day. Three surveys based on 3- or 4-day food intake records in the United States yielded data indicating mean iron intakes of 3.9 to 10.9 mg/day. The lowest intakes (reported in 1926) were observed by McKay (440) in an orphanage in Ohio where 30 boys and girls had mean intakes of 3.9 to 5.3 mg/day. Individual intakes ranged from 3.7 to 5.4 mg/day. In the same study 25 children living in private homes had mean daily intakes of 6.8 to 10.9 mg and individual intakes of 5.3 to 13.2 mg. In later studies of 115 children in Minnesota (182) and 479 children in Mississippi (511), mean daily intakes of 7.3 to 8.3 mg (Minnesota) and 7.7 to 9.0 mg (Mississippi) were reported. Individual daily intakes of the Mississippi children were 1.2 to 34.1 mg. Owen et al. (511) reported that in the total Mississippi sample (about 560 children 12 to 72 months old divided into two income groups) 62% to 75% had iron intakes of less than 8 mg/day, 12% to 24% had hemoglobin levels of less than 10 g/100 ml, and 20% to 30% had plasma iron levels of less than 45 μg/100 ml.

In the United Kingdom, Widdowson

(718) calculated iron intakes of British children from 7-day records of weighed food intake. The intakes of 94 boys and 82 girls were similar until the children were 5 to 6 years old. Individual intakes as low as 1.9 and as high as 12.8 mg/day were reported. The average iron intakes of 2- and 3-year-old children were 6.6 to 7.8 mg/day and of 4- and 5-year-old children, 8.2 to 8.8 mg/day. These values were equivalent to about 0.48 mg/kg at 2 years and 0.42 mg/kg at 5 years.

School children, 6–12 years old

Estimates of iron requirements of school children have been based on a few balance studies (table 6) and on calculations of increases in total body iron based on data on hemoglobin levels, blood volume and increases in body size (table 8). Some information has been obtained also from dietary surveys.

Very few controlled studies have been performed in which the response of children, 6 to 12 years old, to different levels of dietary iron has been observed. In one series of studies a total of 36 girls, 7 to 10 years old, participated in several balance studies conducted over a period of 5 years (2, 472, 656, 657). In study 1 which included 14 4-day balance periods, 12 girls received 7.4 mg iron/day (6.5–7.9 mg) from a mixture of animal and vegetable sources (472, 656). The average iron retention was 0.16 mg/day (−1.0–1.2 mg/day), and 5 of 12 balances were negative. The protein intake was increased from 48 to 88 g/day without influencing iron absorption or retention. In a later investigation in which 12 girls were studied for five 6-day balance periods, the iron intake was increased by about 2 mg to 9.8 mg/day by adding ferric phosphate to the bread (2, 656, 657). The average iron retention was 1.2 mg/day (range −0.7 to 1.9 mg/day). Only one subject was in negative balance. When the iron intake was increased to 10.8 mg/day and protein intake reduced from 22 to 18 g/day by removing some of the milk, average iron retention increased to 2.1 mg/day (1.0–2.7 mg/day) (2, 472). A third group of 12 girls received 10.2 to 12.3 mg iron/day and 22 to 40 g protein entirely from plant sources (2, 657). The average iron retention was 0.5 to 0.8 mg/day and

was not influenced by the amount of protein in the diet. Abernathy et al. (2), in discussing these observations suggested that the lower iron retentions noted with all plant protein diet as compared with those noted with mixed diets "may have been due to a lower general digestibility of the diet, a bulkier diet, or to a higher concentration of substances which interfere with iron absorption." During the entire series of studies, the hemoglobin levels of the 36 girls were in the range of 11.5 to 15.5 g/100 ml (2, 472).

Macy (418) performed 294 iron balance studies with 11 children, 6 to 12 years old. The average daily iron intakes were 8.2 to 12.2 mg/day (0.30–0.38 mg/kg). Iron retention was 0.2 to 3.1 mg/day (0.01–0.10 mg/kg). Retention tended to be higher among the older children.

Johnston and Roberts (360) on reviewing previous work, concluded that the balance study was not an adequate method for estimating iron requirements. In an attempt to find a more sensitive index than iron retention, they related hemoglobin levels to iron intake. They reasoned that if "a good hemoglobin level could be taken as an index of an adequate iron supply . . . the procedure would be to find the lowest level of iron intake that will produce and maintain a good hemoglobin level." They studied 21 children (12 boys, 9 girls) 8 to 11 years old. In a preliminary 2-week period, they determined the hemoglobin level of each child and estimated the mean daily iron intakes by weighing all food eaten and analyzing aliquots of the diets for iron. The children were then divided into seven matched groups of three. One child in each group received a daily supplement of 4 mg iron from ferric pyrophosphate, another received 2 mg iron from the same source and the third received none. After a treatment period of 7 months, the hemoglobin levels were determined again. The hemoglobin levels, which initially ranged from 11.7 to 13.8 g/100 ml (mean 12.9 g/100 ml), were not significantly changed by the iron supplementation. On examination the iron intakes estimated during the preliminary 2-week period, Johnston and Roberts concluded that "good hemoglobin levels could be maintained on 11.4 mg per day or 0.35 mg per kilogram when the rest of the diet was adequate." They pointed out, however, that "lower intakes, had they been tried, might have been found to serve just as well."

Additional information on the iron requirements of preadolescent boys and girls has been derived from estimates of the increment in total body iron occurring in children of 6 to 12 years. Total body iron has been calculated mainly from blood volume and hemoglobin levels of healthy growing children. Blood volume measurements, based on hematocrit and plasma volume (determined with Evan's blue dye) were carried out in three studies with about 80 children 6 to 12 years old (100, 469, 577). In all three studies, there was a rise from about 1,500 ml at 6 years to about 2,500 ml at 12 years. Blood volume was strongly related to body size. Brines et al. (100) found no sex difference until the age of about 11 years. Russell (165), however, reported that boys of all ages had greater blood volume than girls of similar body size.

Average hemoglobin levels for children 6 to 9 years old, were 11.6 to 13.5 g/100 ml in 2,700 observations (61, 173, 174, 298–300, 302, 445, 665, 718, 727, 728). In 10,300 observations on children, 10 to 12 years old, the mean hemoglobin levels were 12.6 to 13.7 g/100 ml (173, 174, 299, 300, 302, 431, 445, 482–484, 665, 728). In approximately 12,500 observations made on children throughout the whole age range of 6 to 12 years, mean hemoglobin values were 11.2 to 13.7 g/100 ml (15, 178, 373, 384, 413, 416, 470, 473, 495, 508, 522, 644, 669). No sex difference for hemoglobin values was reported in this age group. Many of the investigators either showed or mentioned a trend toward higher hemoglobin values with age.

Serum iron has been reported by several investigators. In observations on about 600 children 6 to 12 years old, average values of 71 to 138 μg/100 ml were reported (98, 256, 644, 669, 711, 727, 728). The diurnal variation reported for adults was observed also with children of this age group (711).

Heath and Patek (305) calculated iron requirements for both boys and girls at 6, 9 and 12 years of age to be respectively 80, 145 and 180 mg annually or 0.2, 0.4 and 0.5 mg daily of absorbed iron. These re-

quirements were based on estimates of annual gains in circulating iron (hemoglobin and other iron-containing compounds) and in non-circulating iron. These estimates, in turn, were based on values for blood volume derived from body surface area, "normal" hemoglobin levels and an arbitrary figure of 5 mg/kg body weight for extracirculatory iron.

Hawkins et al. (301) performed anthropometric measurements and hemoglobin determinations on 1,800 children aged 6 to 17 years from which they calculated body surface area, blood volume, total hemoglobin concentrations and total circulating iron. From these data they estimated that the daily requirement for absorbed iron by both sexes was about 0.4 mg at ages 6 to 7 and about 0.7 mg at age 11.

Darby et al. (171), by measuring radioiron incorporation into red blood cells, determined iron absorption in 176 children who had received ^{59}Fe. The children absorbed 7% to 16% of a 2 to 3 mg dose of iron. Absorption was not related to hemoglobin level, but was strongly related to age. Children age 7 absorbed from 7% to 9% of the dose; children age 10 absorbed 14% to 16%. The study included children from two socio-economic groups for whom slight differences in iron intake were reported (11.7 and 10.8 mg/day). The average hemoglobin levels of 12.9 to 13.2 g/100 ml, however, were in the normal range previously reported for this age group (p. 1040).

Numerous food consumption studies have been carried out with school children, and the estimated iron contents of the diets of healthy children have been suggested as guides in recommending iron allowances. In the United Kingdom, Widdowson (718) calculated iron intakes from 7-day food intake records of 163 boys and 175 girls. Average daily intakes for boys were 9.1 mg at age 6 to 13.6 mg age 12. Average daily intakes for girls were 10.0 mg at age 6 to 12.8 mg at age 12. Hemoglobin levels were 12.4 to 13.5 g/100 ml for the boys and 12.6 to 14.4 g/100 ml for the girls.

In the United States, iron intakes have been calculated from 3- or 7-day dietary records obtained in surveys of healthy children. For about 700 children 6 to 9 years old, the average iron intake varied from 9 to 12 mg/day (178, 206, 384, 665, 728, 747). No sex difference was reported for iron intake in this age range. For 2,700 children 10 to 12 years old, mean iron intakes of 10- to 12-year-old boys were about 1 mg/day higher than those of girls of the same age. For example, from data obtained in a longitudinal study of growth and development of selected children in the Denver area, Beal and Meyers (53) charted the 10th, 50th and 90th percentiles of daily intake of dietary iron by boys and girls from birth to 18 years. The chart indicated that at the 50th percentile, girls increased their average iron intake from about 7 to 9.5 mg/day between the ages of 6 and 12. During the same age interval, boys increased their iron intake from about 8 to 11 mg/day.

Adolescent, 13 to 18 years old

The iron requirements of adolescents have had very little study. Only one report was found on controlled balance studies (573) (table 6). There have been, in addition, a few studies in which blood volume was calculated and numerous studies in which hemoglobin concentrations have been determined (table 8). Also available are data from various dietary surveys.

Schlaphoff and Johnston (592) conducted two controlled iron balance studies of 4 weeks duration with six 13- to 14-year-old girls who were 1 to 3 years postmenarche. In these studies, iron was provided at two levels from customary food sources. The iron intakes were 8.0 to 9.6 mg/day (mean, 8.6 mg/day) in the first balance study and 10.9 to 13.3 mg/day (mean, 11.7 mg/day) in the second study. Menstrual losses were collected during the studies and in subsequent menstrual periods (at least four periods/girl). Menstrual iron loss was highly variable within individual subjects and from one girl to another. Schlaphoff and Johnston calculated that the daily iron retentions needed to replace the menstrual iron were 0.18 to 1.49 mg (mean 0.59 mg). They then calculated the total required daily iron retention by adding an allowance for growth to the estimated daily requirement for menstrual loss. The allowances for growth (0.40 and 0.46 mg/day) were based on estimates of yearly iron increments made

earlier by Heath and Patek (305). The total required daily iron retention thus calculated was 0.62 to 1.82 mg/day (mean, 1.0 mg/day). When the calculated required retentions were compared with the observed retentions (iron in food minus iron in urine and feces) at each level of iron intake, Schlaphoff and Johnston concluded that "a dietary intake of 12–13 mg per day is recommended for girls of this age until more cases have been studied."

Estimates of iron increments such as those developed by Heath and Patek (305) by the factorial method have been based mainly on calculations of the increment in hemoglobin mass taking place during the adolescent period. The calculations of hemoglobin mass have depended in turn on estimates of blood volume and hemoglobin concentration. For girls, an additional allowance has been made for catamenia. Information is available on the increase in blood volume during adolescence in about 65 boys (100, 469, 577) and six girls (100). For most of the boys during the period between ages 12 and 16, blood volume increased from about 2.5 to 3.0 liters to about 5 to 6 liters. For girls of the same age, blood volume increased from about 2.5 to about 3.5 liters. Most investigators reported a rise with increasing age in hemoglobin levels of adolescent boys but not of girls. Average values of 13.2 to 15.4 g/100 ml were reported in studies on about 3,700 boys (61, 257, 291, 299, 300, 302, 341, 373, 384, 413, 445, 481, 496, 518, 522, 581, 607, 627, 640, 664, 669, 701, 727, 729). In studies with about 4,000 girls, 12 to 19 years old, mean hemoglobin values were 12.2 to 14.0 g/100 ml (291, 299, 300, 302, 303, 341, 367, 371, 384, 393, 413, 445, 496, 518, 522, 581, 593, 627, 640, 664, 669, 701, 726, 727, 729). With the exception of the study by Schlaphoff and Johnston (592) teenage girls were not considered separately from adults in studies of menstrual iron loss.

Serum iron levels were reported for about 525 adolescents (169, 354, 523, 581, 593, 607, 669, 726, 727). Mean values were 45–120 μg/100 ml, with most averages above 90 μg/100 ml. No difference due to sex was reported. Schlaphoff et al. (593) observed diurnal variation in serum iron levels. The reported mean value of total iron binding capacity of boys (607) was 364 μg/100 ml (160 observations) and of girls (726) was 362 μg/100 ml (171 observations).

Reports of dietary surveys indicate that intakes such as that recommended by Schlaphoff and Johnston (12–13 mg/day) could be achieved with normal dietary patterns. In Widdowson's survey of British children 1 to 18 years old (718), for example, 201 girls 13 to 18 years old consumed 12.5 to 14.2 mg iron/day and 158 boys 13 to 18 years old had average iron intakes of 13.6 to 18.0 mg/day. Similar ranges of intakes have been reported in the United States. There, in 12 studies with approximately 1,300 girls and 1,000 boys, the average iron intakes were 9.6 to 13.5 mg/day for girls and 14.0 to 18.7 mg/day for boys (169, 206, 288, 291, 384, 497, 634, 664, 665, 712, 728, 747). Recently Gaines and Daniel (241) and Daniel et al. (169) observed in a study of 11 to 18-year-old boys and girls of low income families that the iron intakes of the boys increased significantly as they matured sexually. The intakes of the girls, however, tended to decrease with maturation.

Pregnant women

The question of how the maternal organism compensates for the iron demands of pregnancy has not been answered satisfactorily (333, 334, 744). Assessment of iron status, which is difficult with the nonpregnant individual, is further complicated by the normal physiological changes of pregnancy. During pregnancy, the hematologic picture often suggests a state of iron deficiency. A common interpretation is that dietary iron is insufficient to meet the demands of pregnancy and that marrow iron stores of many women of childbearing age are either absent or provide an "inadequate" reserve of iron to maintain "normal" hemoglobin levels during pregnancy (322, 542).

Some of the earliest observations on maternal compensations of iron metabolism in pregnancy were made on dogs (111, 749). In 1886, Żaleski (749) found that livers of newborn puppies contained much more iron than livers of adult dogs. A few years later, Bunge (111) compared the ash content of a newborn puppy with that of its mother's milk. Of the seven mineral ele-

ments analyzed, six occurred in very nearly the same proportion in the milk as in the puppy carcass. The iron concentration in the milk, however, was only 16% of the iron concentration in the carcass. Applying these observations to humans, Bunge questioned the ability of a pregnant woman to assimilate enough food iron to meet the demands of pregnancy. He suggested that girls begin to acquire iron stores in adolescence as a reserve for future pregnancy and that the withdrawal of iron from circulation might contribute to the prevalence of chlorosis among young girls.

The research on iron requirements in human pregnancy has been carried out by balance studies, by factorial analysis including assessment of iron absorption and iron reserves, and by measuring response to therapeutic doses of iron.

Iron balance studies. The adequacy of dietary iron for maintaining iron balance during pregnancy was studied by Coons and co-workers (153–156). Nine healthy, pregnant Chicago women were the subjects of studies carried out in the homes with freely chosen diets of customary foods (153–155). At each meal, investigators weighed the food consumed and prepared a composite sample for analysis. Twenty-two balances of 4 days duration were performed during early and late phases of pregnancy (154). Five women were studied for three or more periods. The iron intakes ranged from 9.69 to 19.45 mg/day, but 67% of the intakes were between 12.1 mg and 16.9 mg. With one exception, balances were positive, 0.88 to 6.97 mg/day, and tended to be directly proportional to intake. Individual balance, however, tended to be related not to intake, but to physiological differences, such as prepregnancy anemia, nausea, altered appetite, and digestive disturbances. In general, iron retention tended to be higher in the first 20 weeks of pregnancy than in the last trimester and was, hypothetically, not sufficient to meet the elevated fetal demands. Nevertheless, Coons (154) concluded that "under fairly ideal conditions of diet and well being," it would be possible for the maternal organism to assimilate sufficient iron from her diet during pregnancy to meet the demands of the fetus.

A similar study on six Oklahoma women

was reported by Coons et al. (156) in 1935. Twenty-two balances were carried out with all but two occurring in the last trimester. Three of the women were studied for four or more periods. The iron intakes from freely chosen foods were 9.45 to 34.88 mg/day with 67% of the intakes between 11 and 17 mg. The balances were 0.03 to 6.88 mg/day with six balances less than 1 mg/day. Again, the daily iron retention during the last trimester was well below the calculated demands of the fetus, and less than the retention during the first 20 weeks. The authors suggested that the poorer retention of iron in this study compared with that in the previous study (154) was not due to a low total iron intake, but to low intakes of other dietary factors that promote iron utilization.

Factorial analysis. In the factorial approach to estimating iron needs in pregnancy, the calculated iron content of the increased blood volume, of the placenta and fetus, and of blood loss at delivery are added to the estimated iron loss of non-menstruating women.

Assessment of the increase in blood volume has included measurements of both plasma and red cell volumes. In 12 studies (3, 127, 157, 293, 335, 407, 411, 442, 573, 661, 668, 687), the plasma volumes of 612 pregnant women were compared with those of 199 nonpregnant women. The mean values in pregnancy were 3.34 to 4.13 liters or 53 to 67 ml/kg body weight. When related to the average values for nonpregnant women plasma volume in pregnancy rose by 21% to 63% but most of the mean increases were between 39% and 50%. The red cell volume in pregnancy was determined in six studies (60, 82, 127, 293, 539, 687) on 155 pregnant and 102 nonpregnant women. The mean values for red cell volume late in pregnancy were 1.53 to 1.84 liters which represented a 17% to 40% increase over values for nonpregnant women. Chesley (137) calculated a weighted average from the above values and reported a mean increase of 350 ml or 24% over values for nonpregnant women. Hytten and Leitch (334) proposed a value of 250 ml as representative of the average increase in red blood cell volume in pregnancy.

In reviewing the literature, Hytten and Duncan (333), Hytten and Leitch (334), and DeLeeuw et al. (179) compared hemoglobin levels of nonpregnant women with those of pregnant women. The mean hemoglobin levels of nine groups containing a total of 1,525 nonpregnant healthy women were 11.9 to 14.3 g/100 ml (179, 285, 420, 445, 514, 566, 647, 686, 698). The mean hemoglobin level in all but one group of 35 nonpregnant women was 13.3 g/100 ml or greater. Approximately 5,000 observations were made in 16 studies during all stages of pregnancy. Except in two studies (134, 179), average hemoglobin levels did not fall below 11 g/100 ml and several group averages did not fall below 12 g/100 ml (59, 189, 285, 410, 445, 466, 514, 549, 647, 686, 698, 733). The averages reported by DeLeeuw et al. (179) and Chanarin et al. (134) fell, late in pregnancy, to 10.4 to 10.9 g/100 ml. Chesley (137) concluded that, in general, the hemoglobin has fallen by about 0.4 g/100 ml by month 3 of pregnancy and reaches a minimum at 30 to 32 weeks.

In normal pregnancy, according to Hytten and Duncan (333), the hemoglobin concentration, red cell count, packed cell volume, all decrease for the first 7 or 8 months and rise slowly toward term. The mean corpuscular hemoglobin concentration (MCHC) usually does not change. There is no consensus on the most appropriate criteria for assessing iron status or on the hemoglobin concentrations below which iron deficiency anemia is indicated in pregnancy (59, 86, 175, 179, 375, 410, 514, 647, 653, 689).

Theoretically, the amount of iron necessary to maintain normal hemoglobin levels while blood volume increases in pregnancy can be calculated from estimates of hemoglobin concentration and red blood cell volume. Hytten and Leitch (334) reported that "the published evidence for the rise in total hemoglobin is so unsatisfactory that until better figures are available we will adhere to our own mean estimate of 85 g." Their dissatisfaction was based upon questionable methodology for determination of red cell volume (251, 377) and uncertainty regarding the extent of iron supplementation (410, 566, 668).

The iron content of the placenta has been determined histologically (439) and chemically (25, 28, 312, 435, 453). Histo-chemical analysis showed an increase in concentration and in total iron during tri-mester one, a leveling off during trimester 2, and a decrease in total placental iron during trimester 3 (439). Mischel (453) reported a similar pattern from chemical analysis. Studies of placental iron showed that the iron content of the placenta was unrelated to the infant's sex (313) or birth weight (313, 435), or to the number of previous pregnancies (435) but was in-creased by multiple births (453) and by a daily supplement of 200 mg iron (25). Placental iron content has been expressed in terms of the wet tissue (mg iron/100 g wet tissue) or as total iron. Differences in sampling techniques make comparison of the reported data difficult. Some investiga-tors, for instance, studied the placenta plus cord (28, 435); others analyzed the placenta without the cord (25, 453); in some reports the disposition of the cord was not indicated (313). In one study, the mothers were given various levels of supplemental iron (25). McCoy et al. (435) reported the mean iron content of 49 placentas plus cords to be 13.6 mg/100 g wet tissue (range 7.1–34.8 mg/100 g). Mischel (453) found that the mean iron content of 29 placentas without cords was 11.1 mg/100 g wet tissue or 4.1 mg/100 g of blood-free tissue. A still lower mean value of 2.4 mg/100 g wet tissue (range 1.2–3.7 mg/100 g) was reported by Hilgenberg (313) from a study of 35 pla-centas. He did not indicate whether the cords had been included in the samples. Apte et al. (25) studied the placentas from women who had been receiving iron sup-plements. From analyses of 25 placentas (minus cords) they reported mean iron contents of 9.1, 9.3, and 13.3 mg/100 g wet tissue for women receiving supplements of 0, 60 and 200 mg iron, respectively. The total iron content of the placenta plus blood has been estimated at 75.5 mg (30–170 mg) (435); 63.7 mg (453); 42.1 mg (29–82 mg) (28); and as 32.6, 35.1, and 57.0 mg for women receiving supplements of 0, 60 or 200 mg iron respectively (25).

At one time, it was believed that iron was transferred to the fetus only upon degradation of red blood cells that had been sequestered by the placenta (317). Fletcher and Suter (221) and Pommerenke

et al. (532) showed, however, that iron is transferred across the human placenta ex-tremely rapidly. Fletcher and Suter (221) detected ^{59}Fe in fetal tissue within minutes after injecting ferric chloride into a woman prior to delivery of a nonviable infant. Be-cause of the rapidity with which labeled iron could be recovered from fetal tissue, the investigators concluded that iron is transferred by the plasma fraction rather than by red cells (221, 532).

Coons et al. (156), summarizing the work reported before 1932, calculated an average fetal iron content of 395 mg and a maximum content of 937 mg. Widdow-son and Spray (725) reported a mean of 273 mg for six full-term fetuses weighing over 3,000 g. Apte and Iyengar (24) re-ported a concentration of 6.4 mg/100 g fat-free tissue in fetuses weighing at least 3.3 kg. They found that while total iron content increased with body weight, the proportion of iron per 100 g fat-free body weight increased only slightly. Most of the iron in fetal tissue is in the liver and spleen (188, 343, 532, 536). Fetal liver iron con-tent has been estimated to be 3.4 to 44 mg/100 g of liver mainly as ferritin (536), 39 mg/100 g of liver (343), 31.5% of the total fetal iron (343) and 80% of fetal tissue iron (188).

Apte and Venkatachalam (28) reported the mean iron content of blood lost at par-turition by 12 women to be 50.9 mg (range 25–94 mg). Fullerton (240), in a study which included women with hypochromic anemia reported an average blood loss of 350 ml (range 75–1,050 ml). The average hemoglobin level just prior to parturition was 76% (Haldane) or 11.4 g/100 ml. Using this value and the iron content of hemoglobin of 3.38 mg/g, an iron loss of 130 mg (range 28–403 mg) may be cal-culated.

Based on evidence reported in the litera-ture, the Council on Foods and Nutrition of the American Medical Association (160), the Food and Agriculture Organization and the World Health Organization (222, 744, 745) have suggested values for the iron content of each component of the factorial equation for the estimate of iron require-ments during pregnancy. These estimates range as follows: increased red cell volume, 200 to 600 mg; placenta, 25 to 170 mg;

fetus, 200 to 370 mg; blood loss at delivery, 50 to 250 mg; iron requirement of non-menstruating women, 150 to 220 mg. The estimates for a woman's total requirement during pregnancy (maintenance plus the demands of pregnancy) are 910 to 1,285 mg of absorbed iron (160, 222, 744, 745). The iron cost of pregnancy has been expressed as a net cost as well as a total cost (160, 222). In determining the net cost, it was assumed that if reserves existed most of the iron associated with increased hemoglobin mass (200–600 mg) would be returned to maternal iron stores after parturition (160, 222).

Using the factorial approach and assuming that the demand for iron is equally distributed throughout pregnancy, daily iron requirements of about 3 to 5 mg have been calculated (160). The different components, however, acquire iron at different rates. Therefore, the validity of converting values for the iron cost of the entire gestation period into a mean daily value may be questioned.

The amount of dietary iron required to meet the pregnant woman's requirements depends on how efficiently she absorbs iron from her food. Most observations on iron absorption in pregnancy have suggested the following three generalizations: a) the rate of absorption (as in most nonpregnant individuals) is inversely proportional to the size of the dose (276), b) iron absorption tends to increase as the length of gestation increases (23, 41, 308), and c) the increase in absorption is greater in iron deficient and anemic women than in non-anemic women (23, 308).

Several studies have indicated that increased absorption of iron is one of the means by which pregnant women compensate for the increased iron demands of pregnancy (23, 41, 276, 308). The percentage of iron absorbed has been determined by whole body counting (308), incorporation of iron into red blood cells after feeding ^{59}Fe labeled salts (41, 276), and from balance studies (23, 153, 156). Heinrich et al. (308) compared iron uptake in 85 pregnant and 106 nonpregnant women. Approximately 30% of a test dose of 0.558 mg of iron was absorbed by nonpregnant women and by women who were less than 5 months pregnant and not iron

deficient as indicated by hemoglobin levels, serum iron, and cytochemical assessment. Iron absorption increased from 30% to 89% of the test dose between months 5 and 9 of pregnancy. Hahn et al. (276) also reported an increase in absorption as pregnancy progressed in a group of 466 nonanemic women. They fed between 1.8 mg and 120 mg iron from $FeCl_3$ labeled with ^{59}Fe plus ascorbic acid. In the periods of gestation when absorption was maximal, the absorption ranged from 38% of 1.8 to 9 mg doses to 8% of a 120 mg dose, or an actual absorption of 3.4 mg and 9.6 mg, respectively. Somewhat lower absorptions were observed by Balfour, et al. (41) who estimated the absorption of ^{59}Fe from the appearance of the label in circulating red blood cells in 14 patients. In most subjects only 2.2% to 4.9% of the iron ingested appeared in circulation.

In 1970, Apte and Iyengar (23) assessed the absorption of iron from foods naturally occurring in the Indian diet by chemically analyzing diets and feces for iron. Between 8 and 16 weeks of pregnancy, 12 women absorbed an average of 7.4% (2%–19%) of an intake of 22 mg of iron. In nonanemic women, absorption rose to 25.7% early in trimester 3 of pregnancy and increased only slightly thereafter. Anemic women (mean hemoglobin of 9.9 g/100 ml) absorbed an average of 37.9% (32%–38%) early in the trimester.

Iron stores. In theory, if sufficient iron is not available from the diet, the bone marrow hemosiderin stores provide a potential source of iron to maintain hemoglobin levels. The presence of iron stores at the beginning of pregnancy, however, may not prevent the development of iron deficiency. Hancock et al. (289) found that 7 of 19 patients who had "moderate to plentiful" marrow iron in the first trimester, developed iron deficiency anemia later in pregnancy.

Iron stores in the form of hemosiderin have been assessed histochemically in pregnancy (244, 550). Several investigators have found little or no stainable marrow iron in women in early pregnancy (9, 289, 322) and in many nonpregnant women of child-bearing age (461, 605). Others have observed a tendency for iron stores to decline during pregnancy in women not receiving iron supplements (9, 86, 179, 322). There is some evidence that oral or intramuscular iron therapy can prevent the diminution of stainable iron (9, 179, 322). Holly and Grund (322), for instance, found that either an oral supplement (amount not specified) for 84 to 174 days or a single intramuscular injection of 1,000 mg iron was capable of increasing stores or of preventing a possible decline in stores. Because the stores did, in fact, decline in women not given an iron supplement, the investigators concluded that marrow provides a source of iron available for hemoglobin formation during pregnancy. Hancock et al. (289), on the other hand, obtained data that suggested to them that none of the infused iron entered the body stores. In their study, normal serum iron levels were maintained throughout pregnancy in women given 1,000 mg of iron intramuscularly at 16 weeks of pregnancy. Six of these women, who had no marrow iron stores initially, had repeat marrow biopsies in the third trimester. Of the six, none had stainable marrow stores although they had normal serum iron levels.

Response to oral iron therapy. Reports of 18 studies were found (59, 62, 86, 158, 175, 179, 284, 321, 342, 375, 385, 410, 466, 514, 540, 647, 653, 689) in which the hematologic responses of groups of women receiving iron supplements were compared with those of women receiving placebos. Approximately 1,300 women received oral supplements of 12 to 240 mg iron daily and 1,050 women received placebos. Most of the studies were carried out in the United States or Western Europe and included women from all socioeconomic levels. There were differences among studies in criteria for admission to the study, in duration of supplementation and in indices used to evaluate the response. Within each study, however, control and iron supplemented groups were treated similarly. Mean initial hemoglobin levels were above either 10 g/100 ml (175, 375, 466, 514, 540, 689) or 11 g/100 ml (59, 86, 158, 175, 321, 342, 410) although anemic subjects were included in some studies (62, 86, 284, 410, 653). The period of supplementation ranged from 21 days (653) to 7 months (59, 179, 342, 466) with supplementation occurring most frequently for 3

to 4 months in the latter half of pregnancy. Several groups continued the studies for varying lengths of time postpartum (59, 62, 158, 179, 321, 385, 418, 514, 647, 653, 689). Hemoglobin levels were reported in all but one study (385). Packed cell volume, red blood cell count, serum iron and iron binding capacity were reported frequently. Marrow hemosiderin (86, 179) and erythrocyte protoporphyrin (86, 321, 647) were reported occasionally. Dietary assessment and counselling were included in some of the studies (62, 158, 375, 410, 514).

The mean change in hemoglobin level of the women receiving iron was from 0 to +2.7 g/100 ml with most of the changes ranging from +0.5 to 1.5 g/100 ml. The magnitude of the hemoglobin response to oral iron was not related to the initial hemoglobin level or to the source of supplemental iron. In women not receiving iron therapy, the average change in hemoglobin level was from −1.6 to +0.4 g/100 ml. The pattern of initial decrease followed by an increase in hemoglobin late in the third trimester was similar to that reported for unsupplemented women (333).

Most of the supplements studied provided between 100 and 200 mg iron daily and, except in two studies (179, 514), observations with more than one iron level were not made by the same investigator. Three studies, however, provide information on supplements considerably lower than the others. Paintin et al. (524) compared the response to daily supplements of 12 and 115 mg iron with that to a placebo from week 20 to week 36 of pregnancy. They studied groups of about 60 women of the same mean age, height, and weight who were delivered of infants of similar weights. The mean hemoglobin levels of the three groups of women were 11.5 to 11.7 g/100 ml at week 20 of gestation. At term, the hemoglobin levels of the unsupplemented women and the women given 12 mg iron/day were the same (10.7 and 10.8 g/100 ml respectively), and were significantly lower than the 12.0 g/100 ml of women receiving 115 mg iron. The investigators concluded that the lack of hematologic effect of the 12 mg iron supplement was a reflection of an already adequate dietary iron intake. DeLeeuw et al.

(179) compared the response of women receiving supplements of 39 mg and 78 mg iron with that of untreated controls. They selected for participation in the study only patients with initial hemoglobin levels of 12 g/100 ml or more in trimester 1 or 11 g/100 ml in trimester 2. Hemoglobin at term was similar in the two supplemented groups (12.3 and 12.4 g/100 ml) but the unsupplemented women had a mean hemoglobin level of 10.9 g/100 ml. The incidence of cases with no marrow hemosiderin at term was higher in the group receiving 39 mg iron, than in the group receiving the 78 mg supplement. Iyengar and Apte (342) found that 94% of a group of nonanemic women receiving a supplement of 30 mg iron either maintained or increased their hemoglobin level. The mean initial hemoglobin values were 12.5 to 12.8 g/100 ml during weeks 8 to 16 of gestation and 11.9 to 12.1 g/100 ml during weeks 17 to 24. No reports were found of controlled studies where the level of iron supplementation was between 12 and 30 mg/day.

In studies that were continued postpartum (59, 62, 158, 179, 321, 385, 410, 514, 647, 653, 689), the positive response to iron was apparent. The response was less pronounced, however, than during pregnancy, and, again, it was unrelated to level or duration of therapy.

Several authors have questioned the regularity with which pregnant women take the entire dose of supplementary iron (87, 514). Bonnar et al. (87) found considerably greater positive hematologic response among "treated" women whose stool iron tests verified that they ingested the prescribed iron than among women who had not taken the supplement regularly. The need for supplementation throughout the entire pregnancy was questioned by Talso and Dieckmann (653) who found increases in hemoglobin level among anemic women supplemented for only 21 days similar to increases found in other investigations continued for much longer periods.

The study of iron supplementation conducted by Paintin et al. (514) encompassed most of the aspects reported in part in other studies. An attempt was made to ascertain whether or not the iron tablets were taken. General health, tiredness and breathlessness at week 30 of pregnancy were assessed subjectively and the results showed no differences in general health among the three groups. In addition to hemoglobin, determinations of packed cell volume, serum iron and iron binding capacity, plasma volume and total red cell volume were made. The effect of the small iron supplement (12 mg) was not significant for any of the indices when compared with the effect of the placebo. The high iron supplement (115 mg) significantly increased red cell volume, serum iron, and total hemoglobin. The increase of red blood cell volume (an average of 160 ml) in the group receiving the high supplement was attributed to an iron excess, since individual increases were not relatively greater in the women with low initial hemoglobin levels. The uniformity of response was attributed to a specific stimulating effect of iron on erythropoiesis. The ability of large iron supplements to increase the hemoglobin level of nonpregnant as well as of pregnant women has been demonstrated (68, 227, 688, 722).

While acknowledging that iron deficiency anemia does occur in pregnancy, Paintin et al. (514) recommended fuller hematologic examination of women with hemoglobin levels below 11 g/100 ml in trimester 3. They considered this approach superior to routine administration of large iron supplements which may prevent iron deficiency anemia in a few women while providing unnecessary treatment for many.

Lactating women

The additional requirement for iron during lactation has been calculated from estimates of the iron content of human milk and the volume of milk secreted (250, 454, 548, 744). In 240 observations, the iron content of human milk ranged from 0.02 to 0.13 mg/100 ml (72, 215, 397, 690, 695). Higher values were reported in two studies (370, 553). Reis and Chakmakjian (553) reported a mean of 0.35 mg iron/100 ml milk and a range of 0.29 to 0.45 mg/100 ml in 14 observations. Karmarkar and Ramakrishnan (370) reported average values of 0.17 to 0.21 mg/100 ml in studies with 32 women.

No relation has been found between the lactating woman's iron intake or hemoglobin concentration and the iron content of her milk. Wallgren (695) found that the iron content of milk varied considerably between individuals and among samples from the same woman. He studied 13 women on one to seven occasions during the first 9 months of lactation and calculated a group average of 0.043 mg iron/100 ml milk among women whose average iron intakes varied from 8 to 40 mg/day. Furthermore, when Wallgren gave two women supplements providing 1 g reduced iron/day for 12 days, the iron content of their milk was not affected. Bhavani and Gopalan (72) found no relationship between hemoglobin level and iron content of milk in nine Indian women from a low socioeconomic background. When six of the women with an initial mean hemoglobin level of 10.7 g/100 ml were given iron orally (source and amount not specified) for 3 weeks, their mean hemoglobin level rose to 12.6 g/100 ml. During the same period, the iron content of their milk dropped from 0.113 mg/100 ml to 0.077 mg/100 ml.

The daily milk output during lactation has been estimated as 850 ml (744), 500 to 1,000 ml (250), 450 to 888 ml (454), and, for South Indian women, 400 to 730 ml (548). Assuming a milk secretion of 850 ml/day (744) with an iron content of 0.02 to 0.13 mg/100 ml milk (72, 215, 397, 419, 695), an iron loss of 0.17 to 1.10 mg/day in the milk may be calculated. Apte and Venkatachalam (28) used an estimate of 0.12 mg iron/100 ml milk (72) and Rao's estimate of a milk secretion of 400 to 730 mg/day (548) to calculate a daily loss in the milk of 0.48 to 0.88 mg iron.

The elderly

No reports of studies directly concerned with estimating iron requirements of the elderly were found. Two investigators studied iron absorpion (109, 233) in the aged and two reported dietary iron intakes (254, 278) in groups of elderly subjects. The remainder of the reports related to iron requirements of the elderly include attempts to define normal hematological values (122, 198, 228, 254, 302, 316, 324, 352, 367, 400, 406, 445, 450, 452, 456, 480, 486, 505, 522, 523, 608, 611, 624, 732) and to assess the prevalence of iron deficiency

anemia among the aged population (52, 57, 198, 207, 209, 228, 254, 278, 316, 386, 406, 445, 452, 480, 486, 522, 534, 608).

There has been considerable variation in the lower age limit included in the studies. Most studies included only subjects over 65 years, but some included persons in the age range of 60 to 65 years (52, 122, 254, 278, 302, 324, 352, 367, 400, 445, 450, 452, 480, 522, 534, 611, 732), and 50–59 years (122, 254, 352, 367, 522, 534, 732).

Bonnet et al. (88) suggested that with advancing age, iron absorption is impaired and iron intake is reduced. They reported that the percentage of ^{59}Fe absorbed from a test dose decreased with age. However, 36 of their 41 normal subjects were between 21 and 34 years old and the ages of the five subjects over 34 years were not given. The mean iron absorption was 46% for the six men aged 21 to 29 years, and fell to 38% for the 15 men of 30 to 34 years. For 14 women of 21 to 29 years, the mean absorption was 61% to 66%, whereas one woman between 30 and 34 years old and four women of over 34 years absorbed 54% of the test dose. No other evidence was found to support the hypothesis that iron absorption is impaired among either normal or iron deficient elderly.

Freiman et al. (233) determined the percentage of iron absorbed by a group of 45 healthy residents age 69 to 87 in a geriatrics home and by a group of 16 control subjects age 27 to 60. The controls (sex not specified) absorbed 71% of a dose of radioactive ferrous sulfate. Among the elderly, the average iron absorption was 57% (range 2%–93%) for 25 women age 70 to 79, 61% (range 26%–94%) for 11 women age 80 to 87, and 49% (range 10%–70%) for nine men age 69 to 85. The mean hemoglobin levels were 12.5, 13.2 and 13.0 g/100 ml for women age 70 to 79, women over 80 and men age 69 to 85 respectively.

Bruschke et al. (109) assessed iron absorption from the rise in serum iron after giving an oral iron load of 1 mg/kg body weight. The post absorption response of their 38 subjects, age 62 to 94 years, was considered to be good by the authors. No difference in absorption of iron was observed when the subjects were divided into four quartiles according to age.

Iron intake was determined by Gillum and Morgan (254) from 3-day or 7-day dietary recalls of 577 subjects of age 50 to over 80. The study included middle class men and women living in their own homes and men residing in a home for the aged. The noninstitutionalized men consumed more iron, protein and energy than either women or the institutionalized men. The average daily iron intake (6–6.7 mg/1,000 kcal) was 10 mg for the women, 15 mg for the men living at home, and 13 mg for men in the institution. Intakes of iron and protein were correlated significantly with hemoglobin levels. Hallberg and Hogdahl (278) reported nutrient intakes from 24-hour dietary recalls taken in a community survey of 71 women over 75 years old. The average intakes were 1,382 kcal and 7.9 mg iron (5.7 mg iron/1,000 kcal). Thirty percent of the women over 75 years old had iron intakes below 7 mg/day and 16% had intakes below 5 mg/day. Intakes of both iron and energy decreased with age, but were not related to hemoglobin level.

A few groups have attempted to assess the effect of iron supplementation among the elderly (198, 209, 448, 680). Migden et al. (448) reported that they gave 39 men and women, 71 to 89 years old, 100 mg ferric pyrophosphate/day with or without D-sorbitol for 4 weeks. The initial mean hemoglobin levels were 9.8 g/100 ml for women and 10.7 g/100 ml for men. There was a significant increase in mean hemoglobin level in all groups, but the increase in the group receiving iron with sorbitol was considerably greater than in the group receiving iron alone. Vellar (680) reported a small increase in hemoglobin levels (0.2–0.4 g/100 ml) in a group of 81 elderly men and women receiving an iron supplement of 180 mg/day for 1 month. In other studies (198, 209), the authors concluded that their results did not provide sufficient evidence to prove a beneficial effect of iron supplementation in the elderly.

The reports on normal hemoglobin levels and prevalence of anemia among the elderly can be divided for each sex into those on healthy subjects (not actively seeking medical attention) living in their own homes or homes for the aged, and those on patients seen in clinics, doctors' offices or hospitals.

In 13 surveys on about 3,700 men not actively seeking medical care, the mean hemoglobin levels were 13.4 to 15.9 g/100 ml (122, 198, 254, 302, 316, 352, 445, 450, 452, 480, 522, 680, 732). In eight studies on 559 men actively receiving medical attention, the mean hemoglobin levels were 12.6 to 15.5 g/100 ml (228, 324, 406, 486, 505, 608, 611, 624). In 14 surveys on about 4,100 women not actively receiving medical care, the average hemoglobin levels were 12.5 to 15.5 g/100 ml (122, 198, 254, 302, 316, 352, 367, 400, 445, 452, 480, 522, 680, 732). In seven studies on 463 women actively receiving medical care, the average hemoglobin levels were 11.7 to 14.6 g/100 ml (228, 406, 456, 486, 505, 608, 611).

In studies on the prevalence of anemia among the elderly, the lower hemoglobin level considered to be normal were 10.0 to 13.5 g/100 ml. In most studies, however, either 11.0 or 12.0 g/100 ml was regarded as the lower limit of normal for both sexes (52, 57, 198, 228, 254, 278, 316, 386, 406, 452, 480, 486, 522, 534, 608). Several investigators reported serum iron levels and saturation of iron binding capacity, but these indices were not used in reporting the prevalence of anemia (133, 207, 406, 456, 534). The accumulated data indicate that anemia was found somewhat more frequently among women than men and considerably more frequently among patients of either sex who were observed in hospitals or doctors' offices than among those not seeking medical care.

The prevalence of anemia when the lower limits of normal hemoglobin were 10.0 to 10.2 g/100 ml ranged from 6.4% (209) to 20% (207). When the lower limit of normal hemoglobin was either 11 or 12 g/100 ml, the percentages of subjects not actively receiving medical care reported to be anemic were 1.1% to 5% (men) and 1.5% to 16% (women) (198, 316, 445, 480, 522) and 4% to 4.4% (both sexes) (254, 452). Using the same criteria, the percentages of subjects actively seeking medical care reported to be anemic were 5% to 28% (men) and 8% to 42% (women) (386, 406, 486, 608) and 10% to 41% (both sexes) (52, 57, 228, 534). Two groups of investigators reported that the prevalence of iron deficiency anemia among the aged was no greater than among the general population (57, 198). In two other studies (207, 209), however, increased prevalence of anemia among the elderly was found. A considerable proportion of the anemia was megaloblastic and associated with low blood folate levels among the elderly. Low hemoglobin levels were associated with low marrow iron levels in two studies (52, 456).

Although strong evidence is lacking for an increased prevalence of iron deficiency anemia in the elderly, several studies have shown a small decline in the average levels of hemoglobin (198, 228, 316, 400, 406, 450, 452, 486, 624, 680, 732) and serum iron (133, 523) with advancing age. Others have not shown any reduction in hemoglobin (133, 254, 324, 367, 400, 445) or serum iron (278, 406, 534) with age. Some studies (302, 505, 522, 608) showed a decline in hemoglobin among men but not women. With two exceptions (228, 406) most studies showed that elderly women had lower normal hemoglobin levels than elderly men. Some investigators also reported that elderly women had lower serum iron values than elderly men (207, 523) but others found no difference (406, 534).

CONCLUSIONS

The wide range of iron intakes and hematological values that appear to be compatible with good health suggests that adequate nutriture is achieved through a remarkable set of compensating mechanisms in the human body. The wide ranges of iron intakes and normal hematologic values found in assessing iron status also suggest that survey data obtained from population groups are of questionable value in determining the human requirement for iron.

The literature surveyed in preparing this conspectus revealed numerous gaps in the experimental basis for determining the human requirements for iron. The survey showed, however, that there is a wealth of information already available for critical analysis and re-evaluation. Much of the published research on iron requirements has escaped integration with data that either existed prior to or became available subsequent to its publication. This conspectus is an attempt to identify the re-

search that has been done. It is not intended to be an in-depth analysis of the data from which iron requirements are calculated.

Although there is much completed research awaiting further evaluation, there are some aspects relating to iron requirements and several segments of the population for which more data are needed. In general, the areas needing further work include a) studies of individual variation, b) assessment of the same individual's response to the different procedures used determine iron requirements, and c) additional evaluation of factors influencing availability of iron from foods.

The wide range of normal values observed in the assessment of iron status emphasizes our lack of information on individual variation. Because the existing techniques for determining iron requirements are both costly and time consuming, data from carefully controlled human studies with large numbers of people will probably never be available. More information that will help in extrapolating from data obtained on small groups to large populations is needed. This information could become available through a greater knowledge of the mechanisms that control iron metabolism. It may have to be obtained from studies with experimental animals.

The major techniques for determining adult maintenance requirements for iron (i.e. iron balance, iron turnover and factorial analysis) all measure something different and all differ in their underlying assumptions about the kind of information which is needed to estimate iron requirements. Both turnover studies and factorial assessment are concerned with the amount of iron lost from the body over a period of time while the balance procedure considers, in addition to losses, the replacement of losses by the dietary intake of iron. The one common feature among the techniques seems to be the requirement for long observation periods. If more adult requirement studies are to be conducted it seems essential that more than one of the three techniques be used simultaneously to allow for further interpretation of the information yielded by each procedure. Leverton and Roberts (402) and Johnston et al. (356, 357) clearly showed that balance studies must be carried out over long periods of time. The turnover procedure, almost by definition, requires many months or even years to complete.

Iron turnover studies, so far, have been conducted only with radioisotopes of iron. Radioisotopes which have provided so much valuable information about iron requirements have the inherent drawback of subjecting humans to potentially dangerous radiation. The benefits of isotopes could be enhanced immeasurably if procedures were developed for using the stable iron isotope, ^{58}Fe, as suggested by Lowman and Krivit (408). This would not only allow for repeated studies on the same individual but would extend the use of isotopes to studies with pregnant women and children without exposing them to radiation. The factorial technique, in which values for all iron losses are determined separately has been used to determine iron requirements in infants and children as well as adults. The values for each factor, however, are usually determined independently of the other factors. Very little information is available on whether or how losses through one route are related to losses through other routes, or on whether compensation for changing needs or supply is made by varying the losses through excretory routes.

Another aspect of determining dietary iron requirements which is common to all assessment techniques and to all age groups is absorption of iron from food. There are wide variations in the amount of iron that can be absorbed from food (392, 463). The variations may depend on the physiological state of the individual and on physical factors relating to the food. New techniques, using an extrinsic isotopic iron label, i.e., one which need not be biologically incorporated into food (79, 389) should promote further progress in this area. In addition we need repeated iron absorption studies on the same subject fed different food combinations and under different physiological conditions. Again, the availability of a stable isotope of iron would greatly expand the ability of researchers to study individual variation as well as the effects of dietary alteration on iron absorption.

Iron requirements, like those of many other nutrients, have been studied far less thoroughly in some segments of the population than in others. For instance, there is very little information on the iron requirements of children, 9 to 12 years old or of adolescents. No studies were found on the relationship between iron intake and stores during the prepubertal period and the iron response during the adolescent growth spurt. The elderly also have not been widely studied. Although Freiman et al. (233) found no decrease in iron absorption among a group of elderly subjects, several studies have shown an increase in the incidence of iron deficiency anemia among the elderly. It is not clear whether this increase is due to a decrease in iron intake or assimilation or to a more generalized deterioration of diet. Pregnant women have received considerable attention from researchers interested in iron metabolism but very little work has been reported on the changes, if any, in iron requirements during pregnancy. Much more work is needed to examine the relationship between maternal dietary iron intake and iron status of the newborn.

The adequacy of the dietary iron intake in parts of both industrialized and developing countries continues to be debated. Researchers working on iron nutrition, therefore, have a major responsibility to make accurate and thorough assessment of all information available to them. It seems essential that decisions regarding future experimentation on iron requirements should rest heavily on a thorough evaluation of existing information.

ACKNOWLEDGMENTS

Preparation of the conspectus was carried out in part under Contract No. 12-14-100-10999 (61) with the United States Department of Agriculture.

The authors wish to thank the following people for their participation in preparing the conspectus: Carole Bisogni for the literature search on iron absorption, Margaret Coale for the literature search on infant requirements, Janet Schwartz for assistance in the literature search, and Eugene R. Morris and Darrell R. Van Campen for helpful advice and criticism.

LITERATURE CITED

1. Abbott, O. D., Townsend, R. O. & Ahmann, C. F. (1945) Hemoglobin values for 2,205

ural school children in Florida. Am. J. Dis. Child. *69*, 346–349.

2. Abernathy, R. P., Miller. J., Wentworth, J. & Speirs, M. (1965) Metabolic patterns in preadolescent children. XII. Effect of amount and source of dietary protein on absorption of iron. J. Nutr. *85*, 265–270.

3. Adams, J. Q. (1954) Cardiovascular physiology in normal pregnancy: Studies with the dye dilution technique. Am. J. Obstet. Gynecol. *67*, 741–759.

4. Adams, W. S., Leslie, A. & Levin, M. H. (1950) The dermal loss of iron. Proc. Soc. Exp. Biol. Med. *74*, 46–48.

5. Addison, G. M., Beamish, M. R., Hales, C. N., Hodgkins, Jacobs A. & Llewellin, P. (1972) An immunoradiometric assay for ferritin in the serum of normal subjects and patients with iron deficiency and iron overload. J. Clin. Path. *25*, 326–329.

6. Adolph, E. F. (1947) Blood changes in dehydration. In: Physiology of Man in the Desert. (Adolph, E. F., ed.) pp. 160–171, Interscience Publishers, New York.

7. Ahlström, A., Koivistoinen, P. & Sytelä, M. L. (1970) Bioevaluation of dietary iron in growing rats. V. Response of rats to different levels of meat in a simulated Finnish diet. Nutr. Metabol. *12*, 65–75.

8. Ahlström, A., Koivistoinen, P. & Tainio, R. (1969) Bioevaluation of dietary iron in growing rats. III. Response of rats to different cereals in the diet. Nutr. Diet. *11*, 251–258.

9. Allaire, B. I. & Campagna, F. A. (1961) Iron-deficiency anemia in pregnancy: Evaluation of diagnosis and therapy by bone marrow hemosiderin. Obstet. Gynecol. *17*, 605–610.

10. Amine, E. K. & Hegsted, D. M. (1971) Effect of diet on iron absorption in iron-deficient rats. J. Nutr. *101*, 927–936.

11. Amine, E. K., Neff, R. & Hegsted, D. M. (1972) Biological estimation of available iron using chicks and rats. J. Agr. Food Chem. *20*, 246–251.

12. Andelman, M. B. & Sered, B. R. (1966) Utilization of dietary iron by term infants. A study of 1,048 infants from a low socioeconomic population. Am. J. Dis. Child. *111*, 45–55.

13. Andersen, B. & Ortmann, G. (1937) On the number of erythrocytes and the content of haemoglobin in blood of new-born children. Acta Med. Scand. *93*, 410–419.

14. Andersen, H. T. & Barkve, H. (1970) Iron deficiency and muscular work performance. An evaluation of the cardio-respiratory function of iron deficient subjects with and without anaemia. Scand. J. Clin. Lab. Invest. Suppl. No. 114, 62 pp.

15. Andersen, H. T. & Stavem, P. (1972) Iron deficiency anemia and the acid-base variations of exercise. Nutr. Metabol. *14*, 129–135.

16. Anderson, R. & Sandstead, H. R. (1947) Nutritional appraisal and demonstration program of the U.S. Public Health Service. J. Am. Diet. Assoc. *23*, 101–107.

17. Anderson, T. A., Filer, L. J., Fomon, S. J., Andersen, D. W., Nixt, T. L., Rogers, R. R., Jensen, R. L. & Nelson, S. E. (1974) Bioavailability of different sources of dietary iron fed to Pitman-Moore miniature pigs. J. Nutr. *104*, 619–628.

18. Andresen, M. I. & Mugrage, E. R. (1936) Red blood cell values for normal men and women. Arch. Intern. Med. *58*, 136–146.

19. Anonymous. (1967) Effect of phytate on iron absorption. Nutr. Rev. *25*, 218–222.

20. Anonymous. (1968) Iron in flour. Lancet *2*, 495–497.

21. Anonymous. (1972) Control of iron absorption by the gastrointestinal mucosal cell. Nutr. Rev. *30*, 168–170.

22. Apte, S. V. (1963) Dermal loss of iron in Indian adults. Indian J. Med. Res. *51*, 1101–1104.

23. Apte, S. V. & Iyengar, L. (1970) Absorption of dietary iron in pregnancy. Am. J. Clin. Nutr. *23*, 73–77.

24. Apte, S. V. & Iyengar, L. (1972) Composition of the human foetus. Br. J. Nutr. *27*, 305–311.

25. Apte, S. V., Iyengar, L. & Nagarajan, V. (1971) Effect of antenatal iron supplementation on placental iron. Am. J. Obstet. Gynecol. *110*, 350–351.

26. Apte, S. V. & Venkatachalam, P. S. (1962) Factors influencing dermal loss of iron in human volunteers. Indian J. Med. Res. *50*, 817–822.

27. Apte, S. V. & Venkatachalam, P. S. (1962) Iron absorption in human volunteers using high phytate cereal diet. Indian J. Med. Res. *50*, 516–520.

28. Apte, B. V. & Venkatachalam, P. S. (1963) Iron losses in Indian women. Indian J. Med. Res. *51*, 958–962.

29. Apte, S. V. & Venkatachalam, P. S. (1965) The effect of ascorbic acid on the absorption of iron. Indian J. Med. Res. *53*, 1084–1086.

30. Arens, M. A. (1945) Study in hematopoiesis: normal blood menses in females ages fifteen through twenty-three years. Am. J. Med. Technol. *11*, 155–160.

31. Arey, L. B. (1939) The degree of normal menstrual irregularity. Am. J. Obstet. Gynecol. *37*, 12–29.

32. Arthurton, M., O'Brien, D. & Mann, T. (1954) Haemoglobin levels in premature infants. Arch. Dis. Child. *29*, 38–43.

33. Ascham, L. (1935) A study of iron metabolism with pre-school children. J. Nutr. *10*, 337–342.

34. Ashworth, A., Milner, P. F. & Waterlow, J. C. (1973) Absorption of iron from maize (*Zea mays* L.) and soya beans (*Glycine hispida* Max.) in Jamaican infants. Br. J. Nutr. *29*, 269–278.

35. Ashworth, A. & March, Y. (1973) Iron fortification of dried skim milk and maize-soya-bean-milk mixture (CSM): availability of iron in Jamaican infants. Br. J. Nutr. *30*, 577–584.

36. Bainton, D. F. & Finch, C. A. (1964) The diagnosis of iron deficiency anemia. Am. J. Med. 37, 62–70.

37. Bakwin, H. & Rivkin, H. (1924) The estimation of the volume of blood in normal infants and in infants with severe malnutrition. Am. J. Dis. Child 27, 340–351.

38. Balcerzak, S. P., Vester, J. W. & Doyle, A. P. (1966) Effect of iron deficiency and red cell age on human erythrocyte catalase activity. J. Lab. Clin. Med. 67, 742–756.

39. Balcerzak, S. P., Westerman, M. P., Heinle, E. W. & Taylor, F. H. (1968) Measurement of iron stores using deferoxamine. Ann. Intern. Med. 68, 518–525.

40. Baldwin, R. M., Whalley, P. J. & Pritchard, J. A. (1961) Measurements of menstrual blood loss. Am. J. Obstet. Gynecol. 81, 739–742.

41. Balfour, W. M., Hahn, P. F., Bale, W. F., Pommerenke, W. T. & Whipple, G. H. (1942) Radioactive iron absorption in clinical conditions: normal, pregnancy, anemia and hemochromatosis. J. Exp. Med. 76, 15–30.

42. Balke, B., Grillo, G. P., Konecci, E. B. & Luft, U. C. (1954) Work capacity after blood donation. J. Appl. Physiol. 7, 231–277.

43. Banerji, L., Sood, S. K. & Ramalingaswami, V. (1968) Geographic pathology of iron deficiency with special reference to India. I. Histochemical quantitation of iron stores in population groups. Am. J. Clin. Nutr. 21, 1139–1148.

44. Bannerman, R. (1965) Quantitative aspects of hemoglobin-iron absorption. J. Lab. Clin. Med. 65, 944–950.

45. Bannerman, R. M., Callender, S. T. & Williams, D. L. (1962) Effect of desferrioxamine and D.T.P.A. in iron overload. Br. Med. J. 2, 1573–1577.

46. Barer, A. P. & Fowler, W. M. (1936) The blood loss during normal menstruation. Am. J. Obstet. Gynecol. 31, 979–986.

47. Barer, A. P. & Fowler, W. M. (1937) Urinary iron excretion. J. Lab. Clin. Med. 23, 148–155.

48. Barer, A. P. & Fowler, W. M. (1938) The blood loss in menorrhagia. Am. J. Obstet. Gynecol. 35, 839–841.

49. Barer, A. P. & Fowler, W. M. (1949) Effect of an acid and alkaline salt on the urinary excretion of iron. J. Lab. Clin. Med. 34, 932–935.

50. Bassett, S. H., Elden, C. A. & McCann, W. S. (1932) The mineral exchanges of man. II. Effect of excess potassium and of calcium on two normal men and on an oedematous nephritic. J. Nutr. 5, 1–27.

51. Basu, K. P. & Malakar, M. C. (1940) Iron and manganese requirements of the human adult. J. Indian Chem. Soc. 17, 317–325.

52. Batata, M., Spray, G. H., Bolton, F. G., Higgins, G. & Wollner, L. (1967) Blood and bone marrow changes in elderly patients, with special reference to folic acid, vitamin B₁₂, iron, and ascorbic acid. Br. Med. J. 2, 667–669.

53. Beal, V. A. & Meyers, A. J. (1970) Iron nutriture from infancy to adolescence. Am. J. Pub. Health 60, 666–678.

54. Beal, V. A., Meyers, A. J. & McCammon, R. W. (1962) Iron intake, hemoglobin, and physical growth during the first two years of life. Pediatrics 30, 518–539.

55. Beamish, M. R. & Jacobs, A. (1968) The measurement of iron clearance from the skin. Br. J. Haematol. 15, 231–235.

56. Beaton, G. H., Thein, M., Milne, H. & Veen, M. J. (1970) Iron requirements of menstruating women. Am. J. Clin. Nutr. 23, 275–283.

57. Bedford, P. D. & Wollner, L. (1958) Occult intestinal bleeding as a cause of anaemia in elderly people. Lancet 1, 1144–1147.

58. Belle, Y. S., Kagan, A. G., Lebedev, O. V., Pokrovskaya, D. V., Rysse, E. S., Shamov, V. P., Shapiro, E. L. & Shcherba, M. M. (1967) Izuchenie vsaycaniia zheleza s pomoshech'iv schetchika vsego tela. Meditsinskaia radiologiia 12, 3–9.

59. Benstead, N. & Theobald, G. W. (1952) Iron and the "physiological" anaemia of pregnancy. Br. Med. J. 1, 407–410.

60. Berlin, N. I., Hyde, G. M., Lawrence, J. H., Parsons, R. J. & Port, S. (1952) The blood volume in pre-eclampsia as determined with P³² labeled red blood cells. Surg. Gynecol. Obstet. 94, 21–22.

61. Berry, W. T. C., Cowin, P. J. & Magee, H. E. (1952) Haemoglobin levels in adults and children. Br. Med. J. 1, 410–412.

62. Bethell, F. H., Gardiner, S. H. & MacKinnon, F. (1939) The influence of iron and diet on the blood in pregnancy. Ann. Intern. Med. 13, 91–99.

63. Beutler, E. (1957) Clinical evaluation of iron stores. New Engl. J. Med. 256, 692–697.

64. Beutler, E. (1957) Iron enzymes in iron deficiency. I. Cytochrome C. Am. J. Med. Sci. 234, 517–527.

65. Beutler, E. (1959) The red cell indices in the diagnosis of iron-deficiency anemia. Ann. Intern. Med. 50, 313–322.

66. Beutler, E. (1965) Tissue effects of iron deficiency. Ser. Haematol. 6, 41–55.

67. Beutler, E. & Blaisdell, R. K. (1958) Iron enzymes in iron deficiency. II. Catalase in human erythrocytes. J. Clin. Invest. 37, 833–835.

68. Beutler, E., Larsh, S. E. & Gurney, C. W. (1960) Iron therapy in chronically fatigued, nonanemic women: a double-blind study. Ann. Intern. Med. 52, 378–394.

69. Beutler, E., Larsh, S. & Tanzi, F. (1960) Iron enzymes in iron deficiency: VII. Oxygen consumption measurements in iron-deficient subjects. Am. J. Med. Sci. 239, 759–765.

70. Beutler, E., Robson, M. J. & Buttenwieser, E. (1958) A comparison of the plasma iron, iron binding capacity, sternal marrow iron and other methods in the clinical evaluation of iron stores. Ann. Intern. Med. 48, 60–82.

71. Beutler, E. & Yeh, M. K. Y. (1959) Aconi-

tase in human blood. J. Lab. Clin. Med. *54*, 456–460.

72. Bhavani, B. & Gopalan, C. (1959) Chemical composition of human milk in poor Indian women. Indian J. Med. Res. *47*, 234–245.

73. Bing, F. C. (1972) Assaying the availability of iron. J. Am. Diet. Assoc. *60*, 114–122.

74. Biörck, G. (1949) On myoglobin and its occurrence in man. Acta Med. Scand. Suppl. *226*, 216 pp.

75. Bitar, K. & Reinhold, J. G. (1972) Phytase and alkaline phosphatase activities in intestinal mucosae of rat, chicken, calf and man. Biochim. Biophys. Acta *268*, 442–452.

76. Björn-Rasmussen, E. (1974) Iron absorption from wheat bread. Influence of various amounts of bran. Nutr. Metabol. *16*, 101–110.

77. Björn-Rasmussen, E. & Hallberg, L. (1974) Iron absorption from maize. Effect of ascorbic acid on iron absorption from maize supplemented with ferrous sulphate. Nutr. Metabol. *16*, 94–100.

78. Björn-Rasmussen, E., Hallberg, L., Isaksson, B. & Arvidsson, B. (1974) Food iron absorption in man. Applications of the two-pool extrinsic tag method to measure heme and non-heme iron absorption from the whole diet. J. Clin. Invest. *53*, 247–255.

79. Björn-Rasmussen, E., Hallberg, L. & Walker, R. B. (1972) Food iron absorption in man. I. Isotopic exchange between food iron and inorganic iron salt added to food: studies on maize, wheat, eggs. Am. J. Clin. Nutr. *25*, 317–323.

80. Björn-Rasmussen, E., Hallberg, L. & Walker, R. B. (1973) Food iron absorption in man. II. Isotopic exchange of iron between labeled foods and between a food and an iron salt. Am. J. Clin. Nutr. *26*, 1311–1319.

81. Black, D. A. K. & Stoker, M. G. P. (1946) Plasma iron in new-born babies. Nature *157*, 658.

82. Blekta, M., Hlavaty, V., Trnkova, M., Bendl, J., Bendova, L. & Chytil, M. (1970) Volume of whole blood and absolute amount of serum proteins in the early stage of late toxemia of pregnancy. Am. J. Obstet. Gynecol. *106*, 10–13.

83. Blumberg, H. & Arnold, A. (1947) Comparative biological availabilities of various forms of iron in enriched bread. Cereal Chem. *24*, 303–314.

84. Blumberg, H. & Arnold, A. (1947) The comparative biological availabilities of ferrous sulfate iron and ferric orthophosphate iron in enriched bread. J. Nutr. *34*, 373–387.

85. Boender, C. A. & Verloop, M. C. (1969) Iron absorption, iron loss and iron retention in man: Studies after oral administration of a tracer dose of ^{59}FeSO₄ and ^{131}BaSO₄. Br. J. Haematol. *17*, 45–58.

86. Bonnar, J. & Goldberg, A. (1969) The assessment of iron deficiency in pregnancy. Scot. Med. J. *14*, 209–214.

87. Bonnar, J., Goldberg, A. & Smith, J. A. (1969) Do pregnant women take their iron? Lancet *1*, 457–458.

88. Bonnet, J. D., Hagedorn, A. B. & Owen, C. A. (1960) A quantitative method for measuring the gastrointestinal absorption of iron. Blood *15*, 36–44.

89. Bonnet, J. D., Orvis, A. L., Hagedorn, A. B. & Owen, C. A. (1960) Rate of loss of radioiron from mouse and man. Am. J. Physiol. *198*, 784–786.

90. Boothby, W. M. & Berry, F. B. (1915) Effect of work on the percentage of hemoglobin and number of red corpuscles in the blood. Am. J. Physiol. *37*, 378–382.

91. Bothwell, T. H. (1968) The control of iron absorption. Br. J. Haematol. *14*, 453–456.

92. Bothwell, T. H. & Charlton, R. W. (1970) Absorption of iron. Ann. Rev. Med. *21*, 145–156.

93. Bothwell, T. H. & Finch, C. A. (1962) Iron Metabolism. Little, Brown and Company, Boston, pp. 433.

94. Bothwell, T. H. & Finch, C. A. (1968) Iron losses in man. In: Occurrence, Causes and Prevention of Nutritional Anaemias. (Blix, G., ed.), pp. 104–112, Swedish Nutr. Found. Almquist & Wiksells, Uppsala.

95. Bothwell, T. H., Pirzio-Biroli, G. & Finch, C. A. (1958) Iron absorption. I. Factors influencing absorption. J. Lab. Clin. Med. *51*, 24–36.

96. Boussingault, J. B. (1872) Du fer contenu dans le sang et dans les aliments. Acad. Sci. Paris, Comptes Rendus *74*, 1353–1359.

97. Bradfield, R. B., Jensen, M. V., Quiroz, A., Gonzales, M. L., Garrayar, C. & Hernandez, V. (1968) Effect of low levels of iron and trace elements on hematological values of parasitized school children. Am. J. Clin. Nutr. *21*, 68–77.

98. Brenner, W. (1948) Beiträge zur Kenntnis des Eisen- und Kupferstoffwechsels im Kindesalter. 1. Die Eisen- und Kupferkurve im Serum normaler Kinder. Z. Kinderheilk. *65*, 727–748.

99. Brigety, R. E. & Pearson, H. A. (1970) Effects of dietary and iron supplementation on hematocrit levels of pre-school children. J. Pediatr. *76*, 757–760.

100. Brines, J. K., Gibson, J. G. & Kunkel, P. (1941) The blood volume in normal infants and children. J. Pediatr. *18*, 447–457.

101. Brise, H. (1962) Influence of meals on iron absorption in oral iron therapy. Acta Med. Scand. *171*, Suppl. *376*, 39–45.

102. Brise, H. & Hallberg, L. (1962) A method for comparative studies on iron absorption in man using two radioiron isotopes. Acta Med. Scand. *171*, Suppl. *376*, 7–22.

103. Brise, H. & Hallberg, L. (1962) Absorbability of different iron compounds. Acta Med. Scan. *171*, Suppl. *376*, 23–37.

104. Brise, H. & Hallberg, L. (1962) Effect of ascorbic acid on iron absorption. Acta Med. Scand. *171*, Suppl. *376*, 51–58.

105. Brodan, V., Brodanová, M., Kuhn, E., Kordac, V. & Válek, J. (1967) Influence of

fructose on iron absorption from the digestive system of healthy subjects. Nutr. Diet. 9, 263–270.

106. Brozović, B., Burland, W. L., Simpson, K. & Lord, J. (1974) Iron status of preterm low birthweight infants and their response to oral iron. Arch. Dis. Child. 49, 386–389.

107. Brubacher, H. (1890) Ueber den Gehalt an anorganischen Stoffen, besonders an Kalk, in den Knochen und Organen normaler und rhachitischer Kinder. Z. Biol. 27, 517–549.

108. Brückmann, G. & Zondek, S. G. (1939) Iron, copper, and manganese in human organs at various ages. Biochem. J. 33, 1845–1857.

109. Brüschke, G., Mehls, E. & Zschenderlein, B. (1967) Die Eisenresorption im hohen Lebensalter. Dtsch. Gesundheitswesen 22, 1639–1640.

110. Bugyi, G. (1949) Beiträge zur Wirkung der Ascorbinsäure auf den Eisenstoffwechsel. Paedit. danub. 6, 97–105.

111. Bunge, G. von (1889) Ueber die Aufnahme des Eisens in den Organismus des Saüglings. Z. Physiol. Chem. 13, 399–406.

112. Bureau of Radiological Health. (1970) Radiological Health Handbook, U. S. Dept. Health, Education and Welfare, p. 248.

113. Burman, D. (1959) The normal cord haemoglobin level. J. Obstet. Gynecol. Br. Emp. 66, 147–150.

114. Burman, D. & Morris, A. F. (1974) Cord haemoglobin in low birthweight infants. Arch. Dis. Child. 49, 382–385.

115. Callender, S. T., Mallett, B. J. & Smith, M. D. (1957) Absorption of haemoglobin iron. Br. J. Haematol. 3, 186–192.

116. Callender, S. T., Marney, S. R. & Warner, G. T. (1970) Eggs and iron absorption. Br. J. Haematol. 19, 657–665.

117. Callender, S. T. & Warner, G. T. (1968) Iron absorption from bread. Am. J. Clin. Nutr. 21, 1170–1174.

118. Callender, S. T. & Warner, G. T. (1970) Iron absorption from brown bread. Lancet 1, 546–547.

119. Calloway, D. H. & McMullen, J. J. (1966) Fecal excretion of iron and tin by men fed stored canned foods. Am. J. Clin. Nutr. 18, 1–6.

120. Camerer, W. (1900) Die chemische Zusammensetzung des Neugebornen. Z. Biol. 39, 173–192.

121. Camerer, W. (1900) Die chemische Zusammensetzung des Neugebornen. Z. Biol. 40, 529–534.

122. Campbell, H., Greene, W. J. W., Keyser, J. W., Waters, W. E., Weddell, J. M. & Withey, J. L. (1968) Pilot survey of haemoglobin and plasma urea concentration in a random sample of adults in Wales 1965–66. Brit. J. Prev. Soc. Med. 22, 41–49.

123. Carr, M. C. (1971) Serum iron/TIBC in the diagnosis of iron deficiency anemia during pregnancy. Obstet. Gynecol. 38, 602–608.

124. Cartwright, G. E., Gubler, C. J. & Wintrobe, M. M. (1954) Studies on copper metabolism. XI. Copper and iron metabolism in the nephrotic syndrome. J. Clin. Invest. 33, 685–698.

125. Cartwright, G. E., Huguley, C. M., Ashenbrucker, H., Fay, J. & Wintrobe, M. M. (1948) Studies on free erythrocyte protoporphyrin, plasma iron and plasma copper in normal and anemic subjects. Blood 3, 501–525.

126. Cartwright, G. E. & Wintrobe, M. M. (1949) The anemia of infection. Studies on the iron binding capacity of serum. J. Clin. Invest. 28, 86–98.

127. Caton, W. L., Roby, C. C., Reid, D. E., Caswell, R., Maletskos, C. J., Fluharty, R. G. & Gibson, J. G. (1951) The circulating red cell volume and body hematocrit in normal pregnancy and the puerperium. Am. J. Obstet. Gynecol. 61, 1207–1217.

128. Cavell, P. A. & Widdowson, E. M. (1964) Intakes and excretion of iron, copper, and zinc in the neonatal period. Arch. Dis. Child. 39, 496–501.

129. Cavill, I. & Jacobs, A. (1970) Skin clearance of iron in normal and iron deficient subjects. Br. J. Dermatol. 82, 152–156.

130. Cavill, I. & Jacobs, A. (1971) Iron kinetics in the skin. Brit. J. Haematol. 20, 145–153.

131. Cavill, I., Jacobs, A., Beamish, M. & Owen, G. (1969) Iron turnover in the skin. Nature 222, 167–168.

132. Chalmers, D. G., Smith, A. J. & Worssam, A. R. H. (1957) A survey of cord blood haemoglobin levels in normal infants. Guy's Hospital Rep. 106, 65–67.

133. Chaloupka, M., Leverton, R. M. & Diedrichsen, E. (1951) Serum iron and hemoglobin values of 275 healthy women. Proc. Soc. Exp. Biol. Med. 77, 677–680.

134. Chanarin, I., Rothman, D. & Berry, V. (1965) Iron deficiency and its relation to folic acid status in pregnancy: results of a clinical trial. Br. Med. J. 1, 480–485.

135. Charley, P. J., Sarkar, B., Stitt, C. F. & Saltman, P. (1963) Chelation of iron by sugars. Biochim. Biophys. Acta 69, 313–321.

136. Charlton, R. W., Hawkins, D. M., Mavor, W. O. & Bothwell, T. H. (1970) Hepatic storage iron concentrations in different population groups. Am. J. Clin. Nutr. 23, 358–370.

137. Chesley, L. C. (1972) Plasma and red cell volume during pregnancy. Am. J. Obstet. Gynecol. 112, 440–450.

138. Chodos, R. B., Ross, J. F., Apt, L., Pollycove, M. & Halkett, J. A. E. (1957) The absorption of radioiron labeled foods and iron salts in normal and iron-deficient subjects and in idiopathic hemochromatosis. J. Clin. Invest. 36, 314–326.

139. Chuinard, E. G., Osgood, E. E. & Ellis, D. M. (1941) Hematologic standards for healthy newborn infants. Am. J. Dis. Child. 62, 1188–1196.

140. Cohen, E. & Elvehjem, C. A. (1934) The relation of iron and copper to the cytochrome and oxidase content of animal tissues. J. Biol. Chem. 107, 97–105.

141. Cole, S. (1971) Menstrual blood loss and

haematological indices. J. Reprod. Fertil. *27*, 158.

142. Colozzi, A. E. (1954) Clamping of the umbilical cord. Its effect on the placental transfusion. New Engl. J. Med. *250*, 629–632.

143. Coltman, C. A. & Rowe, N. J. (1966) The iron content of sweat in normal adults. Am. J. Clin. Nutr. *18*, 270–274.

144. Committee on Iron Nutritional Deficiencies (1970) Measures to increase iron in foods and diets. Summary of Proceedings of a Workshop, Food and Nutrition Board, National Academy of Sciences, Washington, D.C., 42 pp.

145. Conley, C. L. & Nickerson, J. L. (1945) Effects of temperature change on the water balance in man. Am. J. Physiol. *143*, 373–384.

146. Conrad, M. E., Benjamin, B. I., Williams, H. L. & Foy, A. L. (1967) Human absorption of hemoglobin iron. Gastroenterology *53*, 5–10.

147. Consolazio, C. F., Matoush, L. O., Nelson, R. A., Harding, R. S. & Canham, J. E. (1963) Excretion of sodium, potassium, magnesium and iron in human sweat and the relation of each to balance and requirements. J. Nutr. *79*, 407–415.

148. Cook, J. D. & Finch, C. A. (1968) Human iron requirements. In: Proceedings, Western Hemisphere Nutrition Congress II, Puerto Rico, August, pp. 174–176.

149. Cook, J. D., Layrisse, M. & Finch, C. A. (1969) The measurement of iron absorption. Blood *33*, 421–429.

150. Cook, J. D., Layrisse, M., Martinez-Torres, C., Walker, R., Monsen, E. & Finch, C. A. (1972) Food iron absorption measured by an extrinsic tag. J. Clin. Invest. *51*, 805–815.

151. Cook, J. D., Lipschitz, D. A., Miles, L. E. M. & Finch, C. A. (1974) Serum ferritin as a measure of iron stores in normal subjects. Am. J. Clin. Nutr. *27*, 681–687.

152. Cook, J. D., Minnich, V., Moore, C. V., Rasmussen, A., Bradley, W. B. & Finch, C. A. (1973) Absorption of fortification iron in bread. Am. J. Clin. Nutr. *26*, 861–872.

153. Coons, C. M. (1930) A procedure for metabolism studies. J. Am. Diet. Assoc. *6*, 111–117.

154. Coons, C. M. (1932) Iron retention by women during pregnancy. J. Biol. Chem. *97*, 215–226.

155. Coons, C. M. & Blunt, K. (1930) Retention of nitrogen, calcium, phosphorus and magnesium by pregnant women. J. Biol. Chem. *86*, 1–16.

156. Coons, C. M., Schiefelbusch, A. T., Marshall, G. B. & Coons, R. R. (1935) Studies in metabolism during pregnancy. Oklahoma Agri. Exp. Sta. Bull. No. 223, pp. 113.

157. Cope, I. (1958) Plasma and blood volume changes in late and prolonged pregnancy. J. Obstet. Gynaecol. Br. Commonw. *65*, 877–894.

158. Corrigan, J. C. & Strauss, M. B. (1936) The prevention of hypochromic anemia in pregnancy. J. Am. Med. Assoc. *106*, 1088–1090.

159. Cotes, J. E., Dabbs, J. M., Elwood, P. C., Hall, A. M., McDonald, A. & Saunders, M. J. (1969) The response to submaximal exercise in adult females; relation to haemoglobin concentration. J. Physiol. (London) *203*, 79P–80P.

160. Council on Foods and Nutrition. (1968) Iron deficiency in the United States. J. Am. Med. Assoc. *203*, 407–412.

161. Cowan, J. W., Esfahani, M., Salji, J. P. & Azzam, S. A. (1966) Effect of phytate on iron absorption in the rat. J. Nutr. *90*, 423–427.

162. Crosby, W. H., Likhite, V. V., O'Brien, J. E. & Forman, D. (1974) Serum iron levels in ostensibly normal people. J. Am. Med. Assoc. *227*, 310–312.

163. Cullumbine, H. (1949) Hemoglobin concentration and physical fitness. J. Appl. Physiol. *2*, 274–277.

164. Custo, E. L. & Muziarelli, A. (1948) Studio sul ricambio del ferro in ostetricia e ginecologia. 6a. Il ferro serico nel sangue del funicolo ombellicale e nel neonato nei primi giorni di vita. Arch. Ital. Pediatr. Puericolt. *12*, 321–344.

165. Dagg, J. H., Goldberg, A. & Lochhead, A. (1966) Value of erythrocyte protoporphyrin in the diagnosis of latent iron deficiency (sideropenia). Br. J. Haematol. *12*, 326–330.

166. Dagg, J. H., Jackson, J. M., Curry, B. & Goldberg, A. (1966) Cytochrome oxidase in latent iron deficiency (sideropenia). Br. J. Haematol. *12*, 331–333.

167. Dagg, J. H., Smith, J. A. & Goldberg, A. (1966) Urinary excretion of iron. Clin. Sci. *30*, 495–503.

168. Dahl, S. (1948) Serum iron in normal women. Br. Med. J. *1*, 731–733.

169. Daniel, W. A., Gaines, E. G. & Bennett, D. L. (1975) Iron intake and transferrin saturation in adolescents. J. Pediatr. *86*, 288–292.

170. Daniels, A. L. & Wright, O. E. (1934) Iron and copper retentions in young children. J. Nutr. *8*, 125–138.

171. Darby, W. J., Hahn, P. F., Kaser, M. M., Steinkamp, R. C., Densen, P. M. & Cook, M. B. (1947) The absorption of radioactive iron by children 7–10 years of age. J. Nutr. *33*, 107–119.

172. Darrow, D. C., Soule, H. C. & Buchman, T. E. (1928) Blood volume in normal infants and children. J. Clin. Invest. *5*, 243–258.

173. Davidson, L. S. P., Donaldson, G. M. M., Dyar, M. J., Lindsay, S. T. & McSorley, J. G. (1942) Nutritional iron deficiency anemia in wartime. I. The haemoglobin levels of 831 infants and children. Br. Med. J. *2*, 505–507.

174. Davidson, L. S. P., Donaldson, G. M. M., Lindsay, S. T. & McSorley, J. G. (1943) Nutritional iron deficiency anaemia in wartime. II. The haemoglobin levels of 3,338 persons from birth to 55 years of age. Br. Med. J. *2*, 95–97.

175. Davis, L. R. & Jennison, R. F. (1954) Response of the "physiological anaemia" of pregnancy to iron therapy. J. Obstet. Gynaecol. Br. Commonw. 61, 103–108.

176. Davis, R. H., Jacobs, A. & Rivlin, R. (1967) Dietary iron and haematological status in normal subjects. Br. Med. J. 3, 711–712.

177. De, H. N. (1950) Iron metabolism with typical Indian dietaries and assessment of its requirement for normal Indian adult. Indian J. Med. Res. 38, 393–400.

178. Dean, W. T., Davis, B. C. & McConnell, S. L. (1954) Nutritional status of pre-adolescent boys and girls in the Blacksburg School District. Va. Agr. Exp. Sta. Tech. Bull. 122, 31 pp.

179. DeLeeuw, N. K. M., Lowenstein, L. & Hsieh, Y. S. (1966) Iron deficiency and hydremia in normal pregnancy. Medicine 45, 291–315.

180. DeMarsh, Q. B., Alt, H. L., Windle, W. F. & Hillis, D. S. (1941) The effect of depriving the infant of its placental blood. J. Am. Med. Assoc. 116, 2568–2573.

181. DeMarsh, Q. B., Windle, W. F. & Alt, H. L. (1942) Blood volume of newborn infants in relation to early and late clamping of umbilical cord. Am. J. Dis. Child. 63, 1123–1129.

182. Dierks, E. C. & Morse, L. M. (1965) Food habits and nutrient intakes of pre-school children. J. Am. Diet. Assoc. 47, 292–296.

183. Dill, D. B., Talbott, J. H. & Edwards, H. T. (1930) Studies in muscular activity; response of several individuals to a fixed task. J. Physiol. 69, 267–305.

184. Dochain, J., Lemage, L. & Lambrechts, A. (1952) Principales données hematologiques chez le nouveau-ne normal. Arch. Franc. Pédiat. 9, 274–278.

185. Drucker, P. (1924) Investigations on the normal values for the haemoglobin and cell volume in the small child. Acta Paediatr. 3, 1–56.

186. Dubach, R., Moore, C. V. & Callender, S. (1955) Studies in iron transportation and metabolism. IX The excretion of iron as measured by the isotope technique. J. Lab. Clin. Med. 45, 599–615.

187. Dutcher, T. F. & Rothman, S. (1951) Iron, copper and ash content of human hair of different colors. J. Invest. Dermatol. 17, 65–68.

188. Dyer, N. C., Brill, A. B., Glasser, S. R. & Goss, D. A. (1969) Maternal-fetal transport and distribution of ^{59}Fe and ^{131}I in humans. Amer. J. Obstet. Gynecol. 103, 290–296.

189. Edgar, W. & Rice, H. M. (1956) Administration of iron in antenatal clinics. Lancet 1, 599–602.

190. Elliott, W. D. (1962) The prevention of anemia of prematurity. Arch. Dis. Child. 37, 297–299.

191. Ellis, L. D., Jensen, W. N. & Westerman, M. P. (1964) Marrow iron: An evaluation of depleted stores in a series of 1332 needle biopsies. Ann. Intern. Med. 61, 44–49.

192. Elvehjem, C. A., Hart, E. B. & Sherman, W. C. (1933) The availability of iron from different sources for hemoglobin formation. J. Biol. Chem. 103, 61–70.

193. Elvehjem, C. A., Peterson, W. H. & Mendenhall, D. R. (1933) Hemoglobin content of the blood of infants. Am. J. Dis. Child. 46, 105–112.

194. Elwood, P. C. (1963) A clinical trial of iron-fortified bread. Br. Med. J. 1, 224–227.

195. Elwood, P. C. (1964) Distribution of haemoglobin level, packed cell volume and mean corpuscular haemoglobin concentration in women in the community. Br. J. Prev. Soc. Med. 18, 81–87.

196. Elwood, P. C. (1966) Utilization of food iron—an epidemiologist's view. Nutr. Diet. 8, 210–225.

197. Elwood, P. C. (1968) Radioactive studies of the absorption by human subjects of various iron preparations from bread. In: Iron in flour. Ministry of Health Reports on Public Health and Medical subjects. No. 117, H.M. Stationery Office, pp. 1–33.

198. Elwood, P. C. (1971) Epidemiological aspects of iron deficiency in the elderly. Gerontol. Clin. 13, 2–11.

199. Elwood, P. C. (1973) Evaluation of the clinical importance of anemia. Am. J. Clin. Nutr. 26, 958–964.

200. Elwood, P. C., Benjamin, I. T., Fry, F. A., Eakins, J. D., Brown, D. A., DeKock, P. C. & Shah, J. U. (1970) Absorption of iron from chapatti made from wheat flour. Am. J. Clin. Nutr. 23, 1267–1271.

201. Elwood, P. C., Newton, D., Eakins, J. D. & Brown, D. A. (1968) Absorption of iron from bread. Am. J. Clin. Nutr. 21, 1162–1169.

202. Elwood, P. C., Rees, G. & Thomas, J. D. R. (1968) Community study of menstrual iron loss and its association with iron deficiency anemia. Br. J. Prev. Soc. Med. 22, 127–131.

203. Elwood, P. C., Waters, W. E. & Greene, W. J. (1970) Evaluation of iron supplements in prevention of iron deficiency anaemia. Lancet 2, 175–177.

204. Elwood, P. C., Waters, W. E. & Sweetnam, P. (1971) The haematinic effect on iron in flour. Clin. Sci. 40, 31–37.

205. Englar, T. S., Blakely, R. & Wilkins, W. (1948) Hemoglobin studies on Albemarle County school children. Virginia Med. Monthly 75, 236–240.

206. Eppright, E. S., Sidwell, V. D. & Swanson, P. P. (1954) Nutritive value of the diets of Iowa school children. J. Nutr. 54, 371–388.

207. Evans, D. M. D. (1971) Haematological aspects of iron deficiency in the elderly. Gerontol. Clin. 13, 12–30.

208. Evans, D. M. D., Lewis, J. & Curran, E. (1972) Hemoglobin levels in Cardiff children of nursery-school age. Arch. Dis. Child. 47, 772–776.

209. Evans, D. M. D., Pathy, M. S., Sanerkin, N. G. & Debble, T. J. (1968) Anemia in

geriatric patients. Gerontol. Clin. *10*, 228–241.

210. Farquhar, J. D. (1963) Iron supplementation during first year of life. Am. J. Dis. Child. *106*, 201–206.

211. Farrar, G. E. & Goldhamer, S. M. (1935) The iron requirement of the normal human adult. J. Nutr. *10*, 241–254.

212. Faxen, N. (1937) The red blood picture on healthy infants. Acta Paediatr. *19*, Suppl. 1, 1–142.

213. Feuillen, Y. M. (1954) Iron metabolism in infants. II. Absorption of dietary iron. Acta Paediatr. *43*, 181–187.

214. Feuillen, Y. M. & Lambrechts, A. (1954) Iron metabolism in infants. III. The influence of vitamin C on the absorption of iron. Acta Paediatr. *43*, 188–191.

215. Feuillen, Y. M. & Plumier, M. (1952) Iron metabolism in infants. I. The intake of iron in breast feeding and artificial feeding (milk and milk foods). Acta Paediatr. *41*, 138–144.

216. Filer, L. J. & Martinez, G. A. (1963) Caloric and iron intake by infants in the United States: an evaluation of 4,000 representative six-month-olds. Clin. Pediatr. *2*, 470–476.

217. Finch, C. A. (1959) Body iron exchange in man. J. Clin. Invest. *38*, 392–396.

218. Finch, C. A. (1970) Diagnostic value of different methods to detect iron deficiency. In: Iron Deficiency (Hallberg, L., Harwerth, H. G. & Vannotti, A., eds.) pp. 409–421, Academic Press, New York.

219. Finch, S., Haskins, D. M. & Finch, C. A. (1950) Iron metabolism Hematopoiesis following phlebotomy. Iron as a limiting factor. J. Clin. Invest. *29*, 1078–1086.

220. Findlay, L. (1946) The blood in infancy. Arch. Dis. Child. *21*, 195–208.

221. Fletcher, J. & Suter, P. E. N. (1969) The transport of iron by the human placenta. Clin. Sci. *36*, 209–220.

222. Food and Agriculture Organization, report of a joint FAO/WHO Expert Group. (1970) Requirements of ascorbic acid, vitamin D, vitamin B$_{12}$, folate and iron. FAO Nutrition Meetings Report Series No. 47, WHO Technical Report Series No. 452, 76 pp.

223. Forbes, W. H., Dill, D. B. & Hall, F. G. (1940) The effect of climate upon the volumes of blood and of tissue fluid in man. Am. J. Physiol. *130*, 739–746.

224. Forth, W. & Rummel, W. (1973) Iron absorption. Physiol. Rev. *53*, 724–792.

225. Fowler, W. M. (1936) Chlorosis—an obituary. Ann. Med. Hist. *8*, 168–177.

226. Fowler, W. M. & Barer, A. P. (1937) The etiology and treatment of idiopathic hypochromic anemia. Am. J. Med. Sci. *194*, 625–635.

227. Fowler, W. M. & Barer, A. P. (1941) Some effects of iron on hemoglobin formation. Am. J. Med. Sci. *201*, 642–651.

228. Fowler, W. M., Stephens, R. L. & Stump, R. B. (1941) The changes in hematological values in elderly patients. Am. J. Clin. Pathol. *11*, 700–705.

229. Foy, H. & Kondi, A. (1957) Anaemias of the tropics. Relation to iron intake, absorption and losses during growth, pregnancy and lactation. J. Trop. Med. Hyg. *60*, 105–118.

230. Foy, H., Kondi, A. & Austin, W. H. (1959) Effect of dietary phytate on faecal absorption of radioactive ferric chloride. Nature *183*, 691–692.

231. Free, A. H. & Bing, F. C. (1940) Wheat as a dietary source of iron. J. Nutr. *19*, 449–460.

232. Freeman, S. & Burrill, M. W. (1945) Comparative effectiveness of various iron compounds in promoting iron retention and hemoglobin regeneration by anemic rats. J. Nutr. *30*, 293–300.

233. Freiman, H. D., Tauber, S. A. & Tulsky, E. G. (1963) Iron absorption in the healthy aged. Geriatrics *18*, 716–720.

234. Frenchman, R. & Johnston, F. A. (1949) Relation of menstrual losses to iron requirement. J. Am. Diet. Assoc. *25*, 217–220.

235. Frey, W. G., Gardner, M. H. & Pillsbury, J. A. (1968) Quantitative measurement of liver iron by needle biopsy. J. Lab. Clin. Med. *72*, 52–57.

236. Fritz, J. C., Pla, G. W., Roberts, T., Boehne, J. W. & Hove, E. L. (1970) Biological availability in animals of iron from common dietary sources. J. Agric. Food Chem. *18*, 647–651.

237. Fuerth, J. H. (1971) Incidence of anemia in full-term infants seen in private practice. J. Pediatr. *79*, 560–562.

238. Fuerth, J. H. (1972) Iron supplementation of the diet in full-term infants: a controlled study. J. Pediatr. *80*, 974–979.

239. Fullerton, H. W. (1936) Anaemia in poor class women, with special reference to pregnancy and menstruation. Br. Med. J. *2*, 523–528.

240. Fullerton, H. W. (1936) Hypochromic anaemias of pregnancy and puerperium. Br. Med. J. *2*, 577–581.

241. Gaines, E. G. & Daniel, W. A., Jr. (1974) Dietary intakes of adolescents. J. Am. Diet. Assoc. *65*, 275–280.

242. Gairdner, D. (1958) The haematology of infancy. In: Recent Advances in Pediatrics (Gairdner, D., ed.), pp. 50–86, Little, Brown & Company, Boston.

243. Gairdner, D., Marks, J. & Roscoe, J. D. (1952) Blood formation in infancy. II. Normal erythropoiesis. Arch. Dis. Child. *27*, 214–221.

244. Gale, E., Torrance, J. & Bothwell, T. (1963) The quantitative estimation of total iron stores in human bone marrow. J. Clin. Invest. *42*, 1076–1082.

245. Garby, L. (1970) The normal hemoglobin level. Br. J. Haematol. *19*, 429–434.

246. Garby, L., Irnell, L. & Werner, I. (1967) Iron deficiency in women of fertile age in a Swedish community. I. Distribution of packed cell volume and the effect of iron supplementation. Acta Soc. Med. Upsalien. *72*, 91–101.

247. Garby, L., Irnell, L. & Werner, I. (1969) Iron deficiency in women of fertile age in a Swedish community. II. Efficiency of several laboratory tests to predict the response to supplementation. Acta Med. Scand. 185, 107–111.

248. Garby, L. & Sjölin, S. (1959) Absorption of labelled iron in infants less than three months old. Acta Paediatr. 48, Suppl. 117, 24–28.

249. Garry, R. C., Sloan, A. W., Weir, J. B. de V. & Wishart, M. (1954) The concentration of haemoglobin in the blood of young adult men and women: the effect of administering small doses of iron for prolonged periods. Br. J. Nutr. 8, 253–268.

250. Garry, R. C. & Stiven, D. (1936) A review of recent work. Dietary requirements in pregnancy and lactation with an attempt to assess human requirements. Nutr. Abstr. Rev. 5, 855–887.

251. Gemzell, C. A., Robbe, H. & Sjöstrand, T. (1954) Blood volume and total amount of haemoglobin in normal pregnancy and the puerperium. Acta Obstet. Gynecol. Scand. 33, 289–302.

252. Gil, J. R. & Terán, D. G. (1948) Determination of the number of erythrocytes, volume of packed red cells, hemoglobin and other hematologic standards in Mexico City (altitude: 7,457 feet). Study made on two hundred healthy persons. Blood 3, 660–681.

253. Gillett, L. H., Wheeler, L. & Yates, A. B. (1918) Material lost in menstruation of healthy women. Am. J. Physiol. 47, 25–28.

254. Gillum, H. L. & Morgan, A. F. (1955) Nutritional status of the aging: I. Hemoglobin levels, packed cell volumes and sedimentation rates of 577 normal men and women over 50 years of age. J. Nutr. 55, 265–288.

255. Gladstone, S. A. (1932) Iron in the liver and in the spleen after destruction of blood and transfusions. Am. J. Dis. Child. 44, 81–105.

256. Gladtke, E. & Rind, H. (1966) Die Serumeisenkonzentration bei reifen und unreifen Kindern. Klin. Wochenschr. 44, 88–90.

257. Goldhammer, S. M. & Fritzell, A. I. (1933) A study of the red blood cell count and hemoglobin in the adolescent male. J. Lab. Clin. Med. 19, 172–177.

258. Göltner, E. & Gailer, H. J. (1964) Blutverlust bei der Menstruation. Zentr. Gynäk. 86, 1177–1187.

259. Gordon, M. B. & Kemelhor, M. C. (1933) Icterus neonatorum: a study of the icterus index in relation to the fragility, hemoglobin content and number of red blood cells. J. Pediatr. 2, 685–695.

260. Gorten, M. K. (1965) Iron metabolism in premature infants. III. Utilization of iron as related to growth in infants with low birth weight. Am. J. Clin. Nutr. 17, 322–333.

261. Gorten, M. K. & Cross, E. R. (1964) Iron metabolism in premature infants. II. Prevention of iron deficiency. J. Pediatr. 64, 509–520.

262. Gorten, M. K., Hepner, R. & Workman, J. B. (1963) Iron metabolism in premature infants. I. Absorption and utilization of iron as measured by isotope studies. J. Pediatr. 63, 1063–1071.

263. Gram, M. R. & Leverton, R. M. (1952) Iron absorption by women: comparison of three ferrous salts. J. Lab. Clin. Med. 39, 871–873.

264. Granick, S. (1954) Iron metabolism. Bull. N.Y. Acad. Med. 30, 81–105.

265. Green, P. & Duffield, J. (1956) The iron content of human hair. 1. Normals. Can. Serv. Med. J. 12, 980–986.

266. Green, P. & Duffield, J. (1956) The iron content of human hair. 2. Individuals with disturbed iron metabolism. Can. Serv. Med. J. 12, 987–996.

267. Green, R., Charlton, R., Seftel, H., Bothwell, T., Mayet, F., Adams, B., Finch, C. & Layrisse, M. (1968) Body iron excretion in man. A collaborative study. Am. J. Med. 45, 336–353.

268. Greenberg, S. M., Tucker, R. G., Heming, A. E. & Mathues, J. K. (1957) Iron absorption and metabolism. I. Interrelationship of ascorbic acid and vitamin E. J. Nutr. 63, 19–31.

269. Greengard, O., Sentenac. A. & Mendelsohn, N. (1964) Phosvitin, the iron carrier of egg yolk. Biochim. Biophys. Acta 90, 406–407.

270. Grunseit, F., Lewis, C. J. & Stevens, L. H. (1971) Haemoglobin levels in the first year of life in low birthweight babies receiving iron supplements. Med. J. Aust. 1, 79–82.

271. Guest, G. M. & Brown, E. W. (1957) Erythrocytes and hemoglobin of the blood in infancy and childhood. III. Factors in variability statistical studies. A.M.A. J. Dis. Child. 93, 486–509.

272. Guest, G. M., Brown, E. W. & Wing, M. (1938) Erythrocytes and hemoglobin of the blood in infancy and in childhood. II. Variability in number, size and hemoglobin content of the erythrocytes during the first five years of life. Am. J. Dis. Child. 56, 529–549.

273. Gutelius, M. F. (1969) The problem of iron deficiency anemia in pre-school Negro children. Am. J. Pub. Health 59, 290–295.

274. Guthrie, H. A. (1963) Nutritional intake of infants. J. Am. Diet. Assoc. 43, 120–124.

275. Guttorm, E. (1971) Menstrual bleeding with intrauterine contraceptive devices. Acta Obstet. Gynecol. Scand. 50, 9–16.

276. Hahn, P. F., Carothers, E. L., Darby, W. J., Martin, M., Sheppard, C. W., Cannon, R. O., Beam, A. S., Densen, P. M., Peterson, J. C. & McClellan, G. S. (1951) Iron metabolism in human pregnancy as studied with the radioactive isotope ^{59}Fe. Am. J. Obstet. Gynecol. 61, 477–486.

277. Hallberg, L. & Björn-Rasmussen, E. (1972) Determination of iron absorption from whole diet. A new two-pool model using two radioiron isotopes given as haem and non-haem iron. Scand. J. Haematol. 9, 193–197.

278. Hallberg, L. & Högdahl, A. M. (1971) Anaemia and old age. Observations in a

population sample of women in Göteborg. Gerontol. Clin. *13*, 31–43.

279. Hallberg, L., Högdahl, A. M., Nilsson, L. & Rybo, G. (1966) Menstrual blood loss— a population study. Variation at different ages and attempts to define normality. Acta Obstet. Gynecol. Scand. *45*, 320–351.

280. Hallberg, L., Högdahl, A. M., Nilsson, L. & Rybo, G. (1966) Menstrual blood loss and iron deficiency. Acta Med. Scand. *180*, 639–650.

281. Hallberg, L. & Nilsson, L. (1964) Constancy of individual menstrual blood loss. Acta Obstet. Gynecol. Scand. *43*, 352–359.

282. Hallberg, L. & Sölvell, L. (1967) Absorption of hemoglobin iron in man. Acta Med. Scand. *181*, 335–354.

283. Halsted, J. A., Smith, J. C. Jr. & Irwin, M. I. (1974) A conspectus of research on zinc requirements of man. J. Nutr. *104*, 345–378.

284. Hamilton, H. A. & Wright, H. P. (1942) Development of hypochromic anaemia during pregnancy. Response to iron therapy. Lancet *2*, 184–186.

285. Hamilton, H. F. H. (1950) Blood viscosity in pregnancy. J. Obstet. Gynaecol. Br. Emp. *57*, 530–538.

286. Hamilton, L. D., Gubler, C. J., Cartwright, G. E. & Wintrobe, M. M. (1950) Diurnal variation in the plasm iron levels of man. Proc. Soc. Exp. Biol. Med. *75*, 65–68.

287. Hammond, D. & Murphy, A. (1960) The influence of exogenous iron on formation of hemoglobin in the premature infant. Pediatrics *25*, 362–374.

288. Hampton, M. C., Huenemann, R. L., Shapiro, L. R. & Mitchell, B. W. (1967) Caloric and nutrient intakes of teenagers. J. Am. Diet. Assoc. *50*, 385–396.

289. Hancock, K. W., Walker, P. A. & Harper, T. A. (1968) Mobilization of iron in pregnancy. Lancet *2*, 1055–1058.

290. Hanzel, R. F. & Bing, F. C. (1934) Magnitude of urinary iron excretion in healthy men. Proc. Soc. Exp. Biol. Med. *31*, 617–618.

291. Hard, M. M. & Esselbaugh, N. C. (1956) Nutritional status of selected adolescent children. 1. Description of subjects and dietary findings. Am. J. Clin. Nutr. *4*, 261–268.

292. Harrill, I. K., Hoene, A. E. & Johnston, F. A. (1957) Iron absorbed from three preparations used to enrich bread. J. Am. Diet. Assoc. *33*, 1010–1014.

293. Harrison, K. A. (1966) Blood volume changes in normal pregnant Nigerian women. J. Obstet. Gynaecol. Br. Commonw. *73*, 717–723.

294. Hart, E. B., Steenbock, H., Elvehjem, C. A. & Waddell, J. (1925) Iron in nutrition. I. Nutritional anemia on whole milk diets and the utilization of inorganic iron in hemoglobin building. J. Biol. Chem. *65*, 67–80.

295. Hart, H. V. (1971) Comparison of the availability of iron in white bread, fortified with iron powder, with that of iron naturally present in whole meal bread. J. Sci. Food Agr. *22*, 354–357.

296. Haskins, D., Stevens, A. R., Finch, S. & Finch, C. A. (1952) Iron metabolism. Iron stores in man as measured by phlebotomy. J. Clin. Invest. *31*, 543–547.

297. Hausmann, K., Kuse, R., Sonnenberg, O. W., Bartels, H. & Heinrich, H. C. (1969) Inter-relations between iron stores, general factors and intestinal iron absorption. Acta Haematol. *42*, 193–207.

298. Hawkins, W. W., Barsky, J. & Collier, H. B. (1948) Haemoglobin levels among Saskatchewan college women. Can. Med. Assoc. J. *58*, 161–162.

299. Hawkins, W. W. & Kline, D. K. (1950) Hemoglobin levels among seven to fourteen year old children in Saskatoon, Canada. Blood *5*, 278–285.

300. Hawkins, W. W., Leeson, H. J. & McHenry, E. W. (1947) Haemoglobin levels in Canadian population groups: children and young women. Can. Med. Assoc. J. *56*, 502–505.

301. Hawkins, W. W., Leonard, V. G. & Speck, E. (1956) The total body hemoglobin in children and its relation to caloric and iron requirements. Metabolism *5*, 70–78.

302. Hawkins, W. W., Speck, E. & Leonard, V. G. (1954) Variation of the hemoglobin level with age and sex. Blood *9*, 999–1007.

303. Haworth, M., Moschette, D. S. & Tucker, C. (1951) Hemoglobin values, plasma vitamin A and carotene levels in young women on institutional diets. J. Am. Diet. Assoc. *27*, 960–964.

304. Heath, C. W. (1948) The hemoglobin of healthy college undergraduates and comparisons with various medical, social, physiologic and other factors. Blood *3*, 566–572.

305. Heath, C. W. & Patek, A. J. (1937) The anemia of iron deficiency. Medicine *16*, 267–350.

306. Heinrich, H. C. (1970) Intestinal iron absorption in man—methods of measurement, dose relationship, diagnostic and therapeutic applications. In: Iron Deficiency. (Hallberg L., Harwerth, H. G. & Vannotti, A., eds.), pp. 213–294, Academic Press, New York.

307. Heinrich, H. C., Bartels, H., Goetze, C. & Schafer, K. (1969) Normalbereich der intestinalen Eisenresorption bei Neugeborenen und Säuglingen. Klin. Wochenschr. *47*, 984–991.

308. Heinrich, H. C., Bartels, H., Heinisch, B., Hausmann, K., Kuse, R., Humke, W. & Mauss, H. J. (1968) Intestinale ^{59}Fe-resorption und prälatenter Eisenmangel wahrend der Gravidatät des Menschen. Klin. Wochenschr. *46*, 199–202.

309. Heinrich, H. C., Gabbe, E. E. & Kugler, G. (1971) Comparative absorption of ferri-haemoglobin-^{59}Fe/ferro-haemoglobin-^{59}Fe and ^{59}Fe 3+/^{59}Fe 2+ in humans with normal and depleted iron stores. Eur. J. Clin. Invest. *1*, 321–327.

310. Heinrich, H. C., Gabbe, E. E., Bruggemann,

J. & Oppitz, K. H. (1974) Effects of fructose on ferric and ferrous iron absorption in man. Nutr. Metabol. 17, 236–248.

311. Heinrich, H. C., Gabbe, E. E., Kugler, G. & Pfau, A. A. (1971) Nahrungs-Eisenresorption aus Schweine-Fleish,-Leber und Hämoglobin bie Menschen mit normalen und erschopften Eisenreserven. Klin. Wochenschr. 49, 819–825.

312. Heinrich, H. C., Gabbe, E. E. & Whang, D. H. (1969) Die Dosisabhangigheit der intestinalen Eisenresorption bei Menschen mit normalen Eisenreserven und Personen mit prälatentem/latentem Eisenmangel. Z. Naturforsch. 24, 1301–1310.

313. Hilgenberg, F. C. (1930) Über Beziehungen des Eisengehaltes der menschlichen Plazenta zur Fruchtentwicklung. Z. Geburtsch. Gynakol. 98, 291–299.

314. Hinton, J. J. C. & Moran, T. (1967) The addition of iron to flour. II. The absorption of reduced iron and some other forms of iron by the growing rat. J. Food Technol. 2, 135–142.

315. Hinton, J. J. C., Carter, J. E. & Moran, T. (1967) The addition of iron to flour. I. The solubility and some related properties of iron powders including reduced iron. J. Food Technol. 2, 129–134.

316. Hobson, W. & Blackburn, E. K. (1953) Haemoglobin levels in a group of elderly persons living at home alone or with spouse. Br. Med. J. 1, 647–649.

317. Hofbauer, J. (1905) Grundzüge einer Biologie der menschlichen Plazenta. W. Braumüller, Wien. Cited in: Fletcher, J. & Suter, P. E. N. (1969) The transport of iron by the human placenta. Clin. Sci. 36, 209–220.

318. Höglund, S. (1969) Iron absorption in apparently healthy men and women. III. Studies in iron absorption. Acta Med. Scand. 186, 487–491.

319. Höglund, S. (1970) Deficiency and absorption of iron in man. Acta Med. Scand. Suppl. 518, 1–24.

320. Höglund, S., Ehn, L. & Lieden, G. (1970) Studies in iron absorption. VII. Iron deficiency in young men. Acta Haematol. 44, 193–199.

321. Holly, R. G. (1957) Iron and cobalt in pregnancy. Obstet. Gynecol. 9, 299–306.

322. Holly, R. G. & Grund, W. J. (1959) Ferrodynamics during pregnancy. Am. J. Obstet. Gynecol. 77, 731–742.

323. Horan, M. (1950) Studies in anaemia of infancy and childhood. The haemoglobin, red cell count, and packed cell volume of normal English infants during the first year of life. Arch. Dis. Child. 25, 110–128.

324. Howell, T. H. (1948) The hemoglobin level in old age. Geratrics 3, 346–352.

325. Hugounenq, L. (1899) Recherches sur la composition minérale de l' organisme chez le foetus humain et l'enfant nouveau-né. J. Physiol. Pathol. Gen. 1, 703–711.

326. Hussain, R. & Patwardhan, V. N. (1959) The influence of phytate on the absorption of iron. Indian J. Med. Res. 47, 676–682.

327. Hussain, R. & Patwardhan, V. N. (1959) Iron content of thermal sweat in iron-deficiency anemia. Lancet 1, 1073–1074.

328. Hussain, R., Patwardhan, V. N. & Sriramachari, S. (1960) Dermal loss of iron in healthy Indian men. Indian J. Med. Res. 48, 235–242.

329. Hussain, R., Walker, R. B., Layrisse, M., Clark, P. & Finch, C. A. (1965) Nutritive value of food iron. Am. J. Clin. Nutr. 16, 464–471.

330. Hutchison, J. H. (1937) Studies on the retention of iron in childhood. Arch. Dis. Child. 12, 305–320.

331. Hynes, M. (1949) The iron reserve of a normal man. J. Clin. Pathol. 2, 99–102.

332. Hytten, F. E., Cheyne, G. A. & Klopper, A. I. (1964) Iron loss at menstruation. J. Obstet. Gynaecol. Br. Commonw. 71, 255–259.

333. Hytten, F. E. & Duncan, D. L. (1956) Iron deficiency anaemia in the pregnant woman and its relation to normal physiological changes. Nutr. Abst. Rev. 26, 855–868.

334. Hytten, F. E. & Leitch, I. (1971) The Physiology of Human Pregnancy. Blackwell Scientific Publications. 599 pp.

335. Hytten, F. E. & Paintin, D. B. (1963) Increase in plasma volume during normal pregnancy. J. Obstet. Gynaecol. Br. Commonw. 70, 402–407.

336. Ingalls, R. L. & Johnston, F. A. (1954) Iron from gastrointestinal sources excreted in the feces of human subjects. J. Nutr. 53, 351–363.

337. Iob, V. & Swanson, W. W. (1938) A study of fetal iron. J. Biol. Chem. 124, 263–268.

338. Irwin, M. I. & Hegsted, D. M. (1971) A conspectus of research on amino acid requirements of man. J. Nutr. 101, 536–566.

339. Irwin, M. I. & Hegsted, D. M. (1971) A conspectus of research on protein requirements of man. J. Nutr. 101, 385–430.

340. Irwin, M. I. & Kienholz, E. W. (1973) A conspectus of research on calcium requirements of man. J. Nutr. 103, 1019–1095.

341. Isager, H. (1974) Iron deficiency, growth, and stimulated erythropoiesis. Scand. J. Haematol. Suppl. 21, 176 pp.

342. Iyengar, L. & Apte, S. V. (1970) Prophylaxis of anemia in pregnancy. Am. J. Clin. Nutr. 23, 725–730.

343. Iyengar, L. & Apte, S. V. (1972) Nutrient stores in human foetal livers. Br. J. Nutr. 27, 313–317.

344. Jacobs, A. (1961) Iron containing enzymes in the buccal epithelium. Lancet 2, 1331–1333.

345. Jacobs, A. (1974) Erythropoiesis and iron deficiency anemia. In: Iron in Biochemistry and Medicine. (Jacobs, A. & Worwood, M., eds.), pp. 405–436, Academic Press, New York.

346. Jacobs, A. & Butler, E. B. (1965) Men-

strual blood loss in iron-deficiency anemia. Lancet 2, 407–409.

347. Jacobs, A. & Greenman, D. A. (1969) Availability of food iron. Br. Med. J. 1, 673–676.

348. Jacobs, A. & Jenkins, D. J. (1960) The iron content of finger nails. Br. J. Dermatol. 72, 145–148.

349. Jacobs, A. & Worwood, M. (1975) Ferritin in Serum: Clinical and Biochemical Implications. New Engl. Med. 292, 951–956.

350. Jacobs, A. & Worwood, M. (1975) The clinical use of serum ferritin estimation. Br. J. Haematol. 31, 1–3.

351. Jacobs, A., Miller, F., Worwood, M., Beamish, M. R. & Wardrop, C. A. (1972) Ferritin in the serum of normal subjects and patients with iron deficiency and iron overload. Br. Med. J. 4, 206–208.

352. Jefferson, D. M., Hawkins, W. W. & Blanchaer, M. C. (1953) Haematological values in elderly people. Can. Med. Assoc. J. 68, 347–349.

353. Jenkins, C. E. & Don, C. S. D. (1933) The haemoglobin concentration of normal English males and females. J. Hyg. 33, 36–41.

354. Johnston, F. A. (1947) Serum iron levels in adolescent girls. A study of three cases. Am. J. Dis. Child. 74, 716–721.

355. Johnston, F. A. (1958) The loss of calcium, phosphorus, iron and nitrogen in hair from the scalp of women. Am. J. Clin. Nutr. 6, 136–141.

356. Johnston, F. A., Frenchman, R. & Boroughs, E. D. (1948) The absorption of iron from beef by women. J. Nutr. 35, 453–465.

357. Johnston, F. A., Frenchman, R. & Boroughs, E. D. (1949) The iron metabolism of young women on two levels of intake. J. Nutr. 38, 479–487.

358. Johnston, F. A., McMillan, T. J. & Evans, E. R. (1950) Perspiration as a factor influencing the requirement for calcium and iron. J. Nutr. 42, 285–296.

359. Johnston, F. A., McMillan, T. J., Falconer, G. D. & Evans, E. (1952) Iron requirement of six young women. J. Am. Diet. Assoc. 28, 633–635.

360. Johnston, F. A. & Roberts, L. J. (1942) The iron requirement of children of the early school age. J. Nutr. 23, 181–193.

361. Josephs, H. W. (1932) Studies on iron metabolism and the influence of copper. J. Biol. Chem. 96, 559–571.

362. Josephs, H. W. (1934) Iron metabolism in infancy. Relation to nutritional anaemia. Bull. Johns Hopkins Hosp. 55, 259–272.

363. Josephs, H. W. (1939) Iron metabolism in infancy. I. Factors influencing iron retention on ordinary diets. Bull. Johns Hopkins Hosp. 65, 145–166.

364. Josephs, H. W. (1939) Iron metabolism in infancy. II. The retention and utilization of medicinal iron. Bull. Johns Hopkins Hosp. 65, 167–195.

365. Josephs, H. W. (1953) Iron metabolism and the hypochromic anemia of infancy. Medicine 32, 125–213.

366. Josephs, H. W. (1959) The iron of the newborn baby. Acta Paediatr. 48, 403–418.

367. Judy, H. E. & Price, N. B. (1958) Hemoglobin level and red blood cell count findings in normal women. J. Am. Med. Assoc. 167, 563–566.

368. Kaldor, I. (1953) Studies on intermediary iron metabolism. II. Variations of the serum iron value in blood donors and control subjects. Aust. J. Exp. Biol. Med. Sci. 31, 49–53.

369. Kaplan, E., Zuelzer, W. W. & Mouriquand, C. (1954) Sideroblasts: study of stainable non-hemoglobin iron in marrow normoblasts. Blood 9, 203–213.

370. Karmarkar, M. G. & Ramakrishnan, C. V. (1960) Studies on human lactation: relation between the dietary intake of lactating women and the chemical composition of milk with regard to principal and certain inorganic compounds. Acta Paediatr. 49, 599–604.

371. Karpovich, P. V. & Millman, N. (1942) Athletes as blood donors. Res. Quart. Am. Assoc. Hlth. Phys. Educ. 13, 166–168.

372. Kato, K. & Emery, O. J. (1933) Hemoglobin content of the blood in infancy: a study of seven hundred and eighty cases from birth to two years, with one thousand and sixty five determinations. Fol. Haematol. 49, 106–114.

373. Kaucher, M., Moyer, E. Z., Harrison, A. P., Thomas, R. U., Rutledge, M. M., Lameck, W. & Beach, E. F. (1948) Nutritional status of children. VII. Hemoglobin. J. Am. Diet. Assoc. 24, 496–502.

374. Kelsall, G. A., Vos, G. H., Kirk, R. L. & Shield, J. W. (1957) The evaluation of cord-blood hemoglobin, reticulocyte percentage and maternal antiglobulin titer in the prognosis of hemolytic disease of the newborn (erythroblastosis fetalis). Pediatrics 20, 221–233.

375. Kerr, D. N. S. & Davidson, S. (1959) The prophylaxis of iron-deficiency anaemia in pregnancy. Lancet 2, 483–488.

376. Kilpatrick, G. S. & Hardisty, R. M. (1961) The prevalence of anaemia in the community. Br. Med. J. 1, 778–782.

377. Kjellberg, S. R., Lonroth, H., Rudhe, U. & Sjostrand, T. (1950) Blood volume and heart volume during pregnancy. Acta. Med. Scand. 138, 421–429.

378. Klavins, J. V., Kinney, T. D. & Kaufman, N. (1962) The influence of dietary protein on iron absorption. Br. J. Exp. Pathol. 43, 172–180.

379. Kripke, S. S. & Sanders, E. (1970) Prevalence of iron-deficiency anemia among infants and young children seen at rural ambulatory clinics. Am. J. Clin. Nutr. 23, 716–724.

380. Kroe, K., Kaufman, N., Klavins, J. V. & Kinney, T. D. (1966) Interrelation of amino acids and pH on intestinal iron absorption. Am. J. Physiol. 211, 414–418.

381. Kroe, K., Kinney, T. D., Kaufman, N. & Klavins, J. V. (1963) The influence of

amino acids on iron absorption. Blood 21, 546–552.

382. Kuhn, I. N., Layrisse, M., Roche, M., Martinez, C. & Walker, R. B. (1968) Observations on the mechanism of iron absorption. Am. J. Clin. Nutr. 21, 1184–1188.

383. Kuhn, I. N., Monsen, E. R., Cook, J. D. & Finch, C. A. (1968) Iron absorption in man. J. Lab. Clin. Med. 71, 715–721.

384. Lantz, E. M. & Wood, P. (1958) Nutritional condition of New Mexican children. J. Am. Diet. Assoc. 34, 1199–1207.

385. Lawrence, A. C. K. (1962) Iron status in pregnancy. J. Obstet. Gynecol. Br. Commonw. 69, 29–37.

386. Lawson, I. R. (1960) Anaemia in a group of elderly patients. Gerontol. Clin. 2, 87–101.

387. Layrisse, M., Cook, J. D., Martinez, C., Roche, M., Kuhn, I. N., Walker, R. B. & Finch, C. A. (1969) Food iron absorption: a comparison of vegetable and animal foods. Blood 33, 430–443.

388. Layrisse, M. & Martinez-Torres, C. (1972) Model for measuring dietary absorption of heme iron: test with a complete meal. Am. J. Clin. Nutr. 25, 401–411.

389. Layrisse, M., Martinez-Torres, C., Cook, J. D., Walker, R. & Finch, C. A. (1973) Iron fortification of food: its measurement by the extrinsic tag method. Blood 41, 333–352.

390. Layrisse, M., Martinez-Torres, C. & González, M. (1974) Measurement of the total daily dietary iron absorption by the extrinsic tag model. Am. J. Clin. Nutr. 27, 152–162.

391. Layrisse, M., Martinez-Torres, C., Renzy, I. & Leets, I. (1975) Ferritin iron absorption in man. Blood 45, 688–698.

392. Layrisse, M., Martinez-Torres, C. & Roche, M. (1968) Effect of interaction of various foods on iron absorption. Am. J. Clin. Nutr. 21, 1175–1183.

393. Leichsenring, J. M., Donelson, E. G. & Wall, L. M. (1941) Studies of blood of high school girls. Am. J. Dis. Child. 62, 262–272.

394. Leichsenring, J. M. & Flor, I. H. (1932) The iron requirements of the pre-school child. J. Nutr. 5, 141–146.

395. Leichter, J. & Joslyn, M. A. (1967) The state of iron in flour, dough and bread. Cereal Chem. 44, 346–352.

396. Leiden, G., Hoglund, S. & Ehn, L. (1975) Changes in certain iron metabolism variables after a single blood donation. Acta Med. Scand. 197, 27–30.

397. Lesne, E., Clement, R., Zizine, P. (1930) Sur la teneur en fer du lait de femme et du lait de certain mammiferès. C. R. Soc. Biol. 105, 427–428.

398. Leverton, R. M. (1941) Iron metabolism in human subjects on daily intakes of less than 5 milligrams. J. Nutr. 21, 617–631.

399. Leverton, R. M. & Marsh, A. G. (1942) The iron metabolism and requirements of young women. J. Nutr. 23, 229–238.

400. Leverton, R. M., Pazur, J., Childs, M. T., Carver, A. F., Smith, J. M., Wilkinson, H. R., Pesek, I., Swanson, P. P., Brewer, W. D., Ohlson, M. A., Biester, A., Hutchinson, M.

B., Burrill, L. & Alsup, B. (1961) Concentration of selected constituents in the blood of healthy women 30 to 90 years of age in six north central states. Nebraska Agric. Exp. Sta. Res. Bull. 198, North Central Regional Pub. 121, 21 pp.

401. Leverton, R. M. & Roberts, L. J. (1936) Hemoglobin and red cell content of the blood of normal women during successive menstrual cycles. J. Am. Med. Assoc. 106, 1459–1463.

402. Leverton, R. M. & Roberts, L. J. (1937) The iron metabolism of normal young women during consecutive menstrual cycles. J. Nutr. 13, 65–95.

403. Lichtenstein, A. (1921–22) Der Eisenumsatz bei Frühgeborenen. Acta Paediatr. 1, 194–239.

404. Lintzel, W., Rechenberger, J. & Schairer, E. (1944) Uber den Eisenstoffwechsel des Neugeborenen und des Säuglings. Z. Ges. Exp. Med. 113, 591–612.

405. Lipschitz, D. A., Cook, J. D. & Finch, C. A. (1974) A clinical evaluation of serum ferritin as an index of iron stores. New Engl. J. Med. 290, 1213–1216.

406. Lloyd, E. L. (1971) Serum iron levels and haematological status in the elderly. Gerontol. Clin. 13, 246–255.

407. Low, J. A., Johnston, E. E. & McBride, R. L. (1965) Blood volume adjustments in the normal obstetric patient with particular reference to the third trimester of pregnancy. Am. J. Obstet. Gynecol. 91, 356–363.

408. Lowman, J. T. & Krivit, W. (1963) New in vivo tracer method with the use of iron-radioactive isotopes and activation analysis. J. Lab. Clin. Med. 61, 1042–1050.

409. Lucas, W. P. & Dearing, B. F. (1921) Blood volume in infants estimated by the vital dye method. Am. J. Dis. Child. 21, 96–106.

410. Lund, C. J. (1951) Studies on the iron deficiency anemia of pregnancy including plasma volume, total hemoglobin, erythrocyte protoporphyrin in treated and untreated normal and anemic patients. Am. J. Obstet. Gynecol. 62, 947–963.

411. Lund, C. J. & Donovan, J. C. (1967) Blood volume during pregnancy. Significance of plasma and red cell volumes. Am. J. Obstet. Gynecol. 98, 393–403.

412. Lunn, J. A., Richmond, J., Simpson, J. D., Leask, J. D. & Tothill, P. (1967) Comparison between three radioisotope methods for measuring iron absorption. Br. Med. J. 3, 331–333.

413. Mack, P. B., Smith, J. M., Logan, G. H. & O'Brian, T. (1941) Hemoglobin values in Pennsylvania mass studies in human nutrition. Milbank Mem. Fund Quart. 19, 282–303.

414. Mackay, H. M. M. (1931) Nutritional anemia in infancy with special reference to iron deficiency. Medical Research Council, Spec. Report #157, H. M. Stationery Office, London, 125 pp.

415. Mackay, H. M. M., Dobbs, R. H. & Bingham,

K. (1945) The effect of national bread, of iron medicated bread, and of iron cooking utensils on the haemoglobin level of children in war-time day nurseries. Arch. Dis. Child. 20, 56–63.

416. Mackay, H. M. M., Willis, L. & Bingham, K. (1946) Economic status and the haemoglobin level of children of men in the fighting services and of civilians. Br. Med. J. 1, 711–714.

417. MacKay, R. B. (1957) Observations on the oxygenation of the foetus in normal and abnormal pregnancy. J. Obstet. Gynecol. Br. Emp. 64, 185–197.

418. Macy, I. G. (1942) Nutrition and chemical growth in childhood. Vol. 1. Evaluation, pp. 203–205, Charles C Thomas, Springfield.

419. Macy, I. G., Kelley, H. & Sloan, R. (1950) The composition of milks. National Research Council, Bulletin No. 119, p. 23, National Academy of Sciences, Washington, D.C.

420. Magee, H. E. & Milligan, E. H. M. (1951) Haemoglobin levels before and after labour. Br. Med. J. 2, 1307–1310.

421. Mameesh, M. S., Aprahamian, S., Salji, J. P. & Cowan, J. W. (1970) Availability of iron from labelled wheat, chickpea, broad bean and okra in anemic blood donors. Am. J. Clin. Nutr. 23, 1027–1032.

422. Man, Y. K. & Wadsworth, G. R. (1969) Urinary loss of iron and the influence on it of dietary levels of iron. Clin. Sci. 36, 479–488.

423. Manchanda, S. S., Lal, H. & Khanna, S. (1969) Iron stores in health and disease. Bone marrow studies in 1134 children in Punjab, India. Arch. Dis. Child. 44, 580–584.

424. Marks, J., Gairdner, D. & Roscoe, J. (1955) Blood formation in infancy. III. Cord blood. Arch. Dis. Child. 30, 117–120.

425. Marlow, A. & Taylor, F. H. L. (1934) Constancy of iron in the blood plasma and urine in health and in anemia. Arch. Int. Med. 53, 551–560.

426. Marsh, A., Long, H. & Stierwalt, E. (1959) Comparative hematologic response to iron fortification of a milk formula for infants. Pediatrics 24, 404–412.

427. Martinez-Torres, C. & Layrisse, M. (1970) Effect of amino acids on iron absorption from a staple vegetable food. Blood 35, 669–682.

428. Martinez-Torres, C. & Layrisse, M. (1971) Iron absorption from veal muscle. Am. J. Clin. Nutr. 24, 531–540.

429. Martinez-Torres, C., Leets, I., Rienzi, M. & Layrisse, M. (1974) Iron absorption by humans from veal liver. J. Nutr. 104, 983–993.

430. Maurer, L. (152) Serumeisen-Tageskurven bein Kindern. Z. Kinderheilk. 70, 527–534.

431. McBee, J., Moschette, D. S. & Tucker, C. (1950) The hemoglobin concentrations, erythrocyte counts, and hematocrits of selected Louisiana elementary school children. J. Nutr. 42, 539–556.

432. McCance, R. A., Edgecombe, C. N. & Widdowson, E. M. (1943) Phytic acid and iron absorption. Lancet 2, 126–128.

433. McCance, R. A. & Widdowson, E. M. (1937) Absorption and excretion of iron. Lancet 1, 680–684.

434. McCance, R. A. & Widdowson, E. M. (1938) The absorption and excretion of iron following oral and intravenous administration. J. Physiol. 94, 148–154.

435. McCoy, B. A., Bleiler, R. E. & Ohlson, M. A. (1961) Iron content of intact placentas and cords. Am. J. Clin. Nutr. 9, 613–615.

436. McDonough, J. R., Hames, C. G., Garrison, G. E., Stulb, S. C., Lichtman, M. A. & Hefelfinger, D. C. (1965) The relationship of hematocrit to cardiovascular states of health in the Negro and white populations of Evans County, Georgia. J. Chron. Dis. 18, 243–257.

437. McGeorge, M. (1936) Haematological variations in fifty normal adult males. J. Path. Bacteriol. 42, 67–73.

438. McIntosh, R. (1929) The determination of the circulating blood volume in infants by the carbon dioxide method. J. Clin. Invest. 7, 203–227.

439. McKay, D. G., Hertig, A. T., Adams, E. C. & Richardson, M. V. (1958) Histochemical observations on the human placenta. Obstet. Gynecol. 12, 1–36.

440. McKay, H. (1926) The phosphorus intake of pre-school children as shown by a dietary study made by the individual method. Ohio Agr. Exp. Sta. Bull. 400, 387–423.

441. McKee, L. C., King, J. A., Hartmann, R. C. & Heyssel, R. M. (1965) Studies of human iron metabolism with a whole body counter. In: Radioactivity in Man. (Meneely, G. R. & Linde, S. M., eds.) pp. 402–416. Charles C Thomas, Springfield.

442. McLennan, C. E. & Thouin, L. G. (1948) Blood volume in pregnancy. A critical review and preliminary report of results with a new technique. Am. J. Obstet. Gynecol. 55, 189–200.

443. McMillan, T. J. & Johnston, F. A. (1951) The absorption of iron from spinach by six young women, and the effect of beef upon the absorption. J. Nutr. 44, 383–398.

444. Mecham, D. & Olcott, H. (1949) Phosvitin, the principal phosphoprotein of egg yolk. J. Am. Chem. Soc. 71, 3670–3679.

445. Medical Research Council (1945) Haemoglobin levels in Great Britain in 1943 with observations on serum protein levels. Spec. Rep. Ser. No. 252. H. M. Stationery Office, 128 pp.

446. Merritt, K. K. & Davidson, L. T. (1933) The blood during the first year of life. I. Normal values for erythrocytes, hemoglobin, reticulocytes and platelets, and their relationship to neonatal bleeding and coagulation time. Am. J. Dis. Child. 46, 990–1010.

447. Merritt, K. K. & Davidson, L. T. (1934) The blood during the first year. II. The anemia of prematurity. Am. J. Dis. Child. 47, 261–301.

448. Migden, J. (1959) The treatment of iron deficiency in the aged: a controlled study. J. Am. Geriat. Soc. 7, 928–932.

449. Milam, D. F. & Muench, H. (1946) Hemoglobin levels in specific race, age, and sex groups of a normal North Carolina population. J. Lab. Clin. Med. 31, 878–885.

450. Miller, I. (1939) Normal hematologic standards in the aged. J. Lab. Clin. Med. 24, 1172–1176.

451. Millis, J. (1951) The iron losses of healthy women during consecutive menstrual cycles. Med. J. Aust. 2, 874–879.

452. Milne, J. S. & Williamson, J. (1972) Hemoglobin, hematocrit, leukocyte count, and blood grouping in older people. Geriatrics 27, 118–126.

453. Mischel, W. (1958) Die anorganischen Bestandteile der placenta VI. Der Gesamt- und Gewebseisengehalt der reifen und unreifen normalen und pathologischen menschlichen Placenta. Arch. Gynäkol. 190, 638–652.

454. Mitchell, H. H. & Curzon, E. G. (1939) The dietary requirement of calcium and its significance. Actualites Scientifique et Industrielles, No. 771, pp. 36–101, Hermann & Co., Paris.

455. Mitchell, H. H. & Hamilton, T. S. (1949) The dermal excretion under controlled environmental conditions of nitrogen and minerals in human subjects, with particular reference to calcium and iron. J. Biol. Chem. 178, 345–361.

456. Mitchell, T. R. & Pergrum, G. D. (1971) The diagnosis of mild iron deficiency in the elderly. Geront. Clin. 13, 296–306.

457. Moe, P. J. (1963) Iron requirements in infancy. Longitudinal studies of iron requirements during the first year of life. Acta Paediatr. Suppl. 150, 67 pp.

458. Moe, P. J. (1964) Iron requirements in infancy. 2. The influence of iron-fortified cereals given during the first year of life on the red blood picture of children at 1 1/2–3 years of age. Acta Paediatr. 53, 423–432.

459. Mollison, P. L. & Cutbush, M. (1951) A method of measuring the severity of a series of cases of hemolytic disease of the newborn. Blood 6, 777–788.

460. Mollison, P. L., Veall, N. & Cutbush, M. (1950) Red cell and plasma volume in newborn infants. Arch. Dis. Child. 25, 242–253.

461. Monsen, E. R., Kuhn, I. N. & Finch, C. A. (1967) Iron status of menstruating women. Am. J. Clin. Nutr. 20, 842–849.

462. Moore, C. V. (1964) Iron nutrition. In: Iron Metabolism. (Gross, F., ed.), pp. 241–255, Springer-Verlag, Berlin.

463. Moore, C. V. (1968) The absorption of iron from foods. In: Occurrence, Causes and Prevention of Nutritional Anaemias. (Blix, G., ed.), pp. 92–103, Swedish Nutr. Found. Almquist & Wiksells, Uppsala.

464. Moore, C. V. & Dubach, R. (1951) Observations on the absorption of iron from foods

tagged with radioiron. Trans. Assoc. Am. Physicians 64, 245–256.

465. Moore, C. V., Minnich, V. & Welch, J. (1939) Studies in iron transportation and metabolism. III. The normal fluctuations of serum and "easily split-off" blood iron in individual subjects. J. Clin. Invest. 18, 543–552.

466. Morgan, E. H. (1961) Plasma-iron and haemoglobin levels in pregnancy. The effect of oral iron. Lancet 1, 9–12.

467. Morris, E. R. & Greene, F. E. (1972) Utilization of the iron of egg yolk for hemoglobin formation by the growing rat. J. Nutr. 102, 901–908.

468. Morris, F. K., Loy, V. E., Strutz, K. M., Schloesser, L. L. & Schilling, R. F. (1956) Hemoglobin concentrations as determined by a methemoglobin method. Am. J. Clin. Path. 26, 1450–1455.

469. Morse, M., Cassels, D. E. & Schultz, F. W. (1947) Blood volumes of normal children. Am. J. Physiol. 151, 448–458.

470. Moschette, D., Causey, K., Cheely, E., Dallyn, M., McBryde, L. & Patrick, R. (1952) Nutritional status of pre-adolescent boys and girls in selected areas of Louisiana. La. Agr. Exp. Sta. Tech. Bull. No. 465, 34 pp.

471. Motzok, I., Pennell, M. D., Davies, M. I. & Ross, H. U. (1975) Effect of particle size on the biological availability of reduced iron. J. Assoc. Off. Anal. Chem. 58, 99–103.

472. Moyer, E. Z. & Irwin, M. I. (1967) Basic data on metabolic patterns in 7- to 10-year-old girls in selected southern states. Home Economics Research Report No. 33. Agricultural Research Service, U.S. Department of Agriculture, 167 pp.

473. Mugrage, E. R. & Andresen, M. I. (1936) Values for red blood cells of average infants and children. Am. J. Dis. Child. 51, 775–791.

474. Mugrage, E. R. & Andresen, M. I. (1938) Red blood cell values in adolescence. Am. J. Dis. Child. 56, 997–1003.

475. Myers, V. C. & Eddy, H. M. (1939) The hemoglobin content of human blood. J. Lab. Clin. Med. 24, 502–511.

476. Naiman, J. L., Oski, F. A., Diamond, L. K., Vawter, G. F. & Shwachman, H. (1964) The gastrointestinal effects of iron-deficiency anemia. Pediatrics 33, 83–99.

477. Nakamura, F. I. & Mitchell, H. H. (1943) The utilization for hemoglobin regeneration of the iron in salts used in the enrichment of flour and bread. J. Nutr. 25, 39–48.

478. National Academy of Sciences-National Research Council (1958) Recommended Dietary Allowances. NAC-NRC Publ. 589, Washington, D.C.

479. National Health Survey (1967) Mean blood hematocrit of adults: United States—1960–1962. National Center for Health Statistics, Ser. 11, No. 24, 36 pp.

480. Natvig, H. (1963) Studies on hemoglobin values in Norway. I. Hemoglobin levels in adults. Acta Med. Scand. 173, 423–434.

481. Natvig, H., Bjerkedal, T. & Jonassen, Ø.

(1963) Studies on hemoglobin values in Norway. II. The effect of supplementary intake of ascorbic acid and iron on the hemoglobin level of school-children and men. Acta Med. Scand. *174,* 341–350.

482. Natvig, H., Bjerkedal, T. & Jonassen, Ø. (1963) Studies on hemoglobin values in Norway. III. Seasonal variations. Acta Med. Scand. *174,* 351–359.

483. Natvig, H., Bjerkedal, T. & Jonassen, Ø. (1966) Studies on hemoglobin values in Norway. IV. Hemoglobin concentrations among school children. Acta Med. Scand. *180,* 605–612.

484. Natvig, H. & Vellar, O. D. (1967) Studies on hemoglobin values in Norway. VIII. Hemoglobin, hematocrit and MCHC values in adult men and women. Acta Med. Scand. *182,* 193–205.

485. Natvig, K. (1966) Studies on hemoglobin values in Norway. V. Hemoglobin concentration and hematocrit in men aged 15–21 years. Acta Med. Scand. *180,* 613–620.

486. Newman, B. & Gitlow, S. (1943) Blood studies in the aged: the erythrocyte in the aged male and female. Am. J. Med. Sci. *205,* 677–687.

487. Newton, D., Eakins, J. D., Brown, D. A. & Owen, G. M. (1968) Radioisotope techniques in a study of the absorption of iron from bread. In: Iron in Flour. Ministry of Health. Reports on Public Health and Medical Subjects. No. 117, pp. 41–49, H. M. Stationery Office, London.

488. Niccum, W. L., Jackson, R. L. & Stearns, G. (1953) Use of ferric and ferrous iron in the prevention of hypochromic anemia in infants. J. Dis. Child. *86,* 553–567.

489. Nicola, P., Vaccino, P. & Carolei, G. (1961) Comportamento della sideremia e transferrinemia del prematuro durante il primo biennio di vita. Minerva Pediat. *13,* 230–236.

490. Nilsson, L. & Rybo, G. (1971) Treatment of menorrhagia. Am. J. Obstet. Gynecol. *110,* 713–720.

491. Nilsson, L. & Sölvell, L. (1967) Clinical studies on oral contraceptives—a randomized, double blind, crossover study of four different preparations. (Anovlar mite, Lyndiol mite, Ovulen and Volidan). Acta. Obstet. Gynecol. Scand. *46,* Suppl. 8, 1–31.

492. Norrby, A., Rybo, G. & Solvell, L. (1972) The influence of a combined oral contraceptive on the absorption of iron. Scand. J. Haematol. *9,* 43–51.

493. Norrby, A. & Solvell, L. (1972) Effect of dietary iron on iron absorption in man. Scand. J. Haematol. *9,* 396–399.

494. North Central Regional Publ. No. 59. (1955) Nutrition of 9-, 10- and 11-year old public school children in Iowa, Kansas and Ohio. I. Dietary Findings. Iowa Agr. Exp. Sta. Res. Bull. No. 434, p. 614–632.

495. North Central Regional Publ. No. 72. (1957) Nutritional status of 9-, 10- and 11-year old public school children in Iowa, Kansas, and Ohio. II. Blood findings. Ohio Agr. Exp. Sta. Res. Bull. No. 794, 63 pp.

496. Odland, L. M. & Ostle, R. J. (1956) Clinical and biochemical studies of Montana adolescents. J. Am. Diet. Assoc. *32,* 823–828.

497. Odland, L. M., Page, L. & Guild, L. P. (1955) Nutrient intakes and food habits of Montana students. J. Am. Diet. Assoc. *31,* 1134–1142.

498. Oettinger, L. & Mills, W. B. (1949) Simultaneous capillary and venous hemoglobin determinations in the newborn infant. J. Pediatr. *35,* 362–365.

499. Oettinger, L., Mills, W. B. & Hahn, P. F. (1954) Iron absorption in premature and full-term infants. J. Pediatr. *45,* 302–306.

500. Ohlson, M. A., Cederquist, D., Donelson, E. G., Leverton, R. M., Lewis, G. K., Himwich, W. A. & Reynolds, M. S. (1944) Hemoglobin concentrations, red cell counts and erythrocyte volumes of college women of the north central states. Am. J. Physiol. *142,* 727–732.

501. Ohlson, M. A. & Daum, K. (1935) A study of the iron metabolism of normal women. J. Nutr. *9,* 75–89.

502. Oldham, H. G. (1941) The effect of heat on the availability of the iron of beef muscle. J. Nutr. *22,* 197–203.

503. Oldham, H., Schultz, F. W. & Morse, M. (1937) Utilization of organic and inorganic iron by the normal infant. Am. J. Dis. Child. *54,* 252–264.

504. Olsson, K. S. (1972) Iron stores in normal men and male blood donors. Acta Med. Scand. *192,* 401–407.

505. Orchard, N. P. (1955) Blood changes in the aged. Geriatrics *10,* 459–468.

506. Osgood, E. E. (1926) Hemoglobin, color index, saturation index and volume index standards. Arch. Intern. Med. *37,* 685–706.

507. Osgood, E. E. (1935) Normal hematologic standards. Arch. Intern. Med. *56,* 849–863.

508. Osgood, E. E. & Baker, R. L. (1935) Erythrocyte, hemoglobin, cell volume and color, volume and saturation index standards for normal children of school age. Am. J. Dis. Child. *50,* 343–358.

509. Osgood, E. E. & Haskins, H. D. (1927) Relation between cell count, cell volume and hemoglobin content of venous blood of normal young women. Arch. Intern. Med. *39,* 643–655.

510. Osgood, E. E., Haskins, H. D. & Trotman, F. E. (1931–32) The value of accurately determined color, volume and saturation indexes in anemias. J. Lab. Clin. Med. *17,* 859–886.

511. Owen, G. M., Garry, P. J., Kram, K. M., Nelsen, C. E. & Montalvo, J. M. (1969) Nutritional status of Mississippi pre-school children. Am. J. Clin. Nutr. *22,* 1444–1458.

512. Owen, G. M., Nelsen, C. E. & Garry, P. J. (1970) Nutritional status of pre-school children: hemoglobin, hematocrit and plasma iron values. J. Pediatr. *76,* 761–763.

513. Pagliardi, E., Prato, V., Giangrandi, E. & Fiorina, L. (1959) Behaviour of the free erythrocyte protoporphyrins and of the

erythrocyte copper in iron deficiency anaemias. Br. J. Haematol. 5, 217–221.

514. Paintin, D. B., Thompson, A. M. & Hytten, F. E. (1966) Iron and the haemoglobin level in pregnancy. J. Obstet. Gynecol. Br. Commonw. 73, 181–190.

515. Patek, A. J. & Heath, C. W. (1936) Chlorosis. J. Am. Med. Assoc. 106, 1463–1466.

516. Paterson, J. C. S., Marrack, D. & Wiggins, H. S. (1952) Hypoferraemia in the human subject: the importance of diurnal hypoferraemia. Clin. Sci. 11, 417–423.

517. Patwardhan, V. N. (1937) The occurrence of a phytin-splitting enzyme in the intestines of albino rats. Biochem. J. 31, 560–564.

518. Peacock, P. B. (1964) Haemoglobin values among adolescents. Can. J. Pub. Health 55, 480–488.

519. Pearson, H. A., Abrams, I., Fernbach, D. J., Gyland, S. P. & Hahn, D. A. (1967) Anemia in pre-school children in the United States of America. Pediatr. Res. 1, 169–172.

520. Pearson, H. A., McLean, F. W. & Brigety, R. E. (1971) Anemia related to age. Study of a community of young black Americans. J. Am. Med. Assoc. 215, 1982–1984.

521. Petrov, V. N., Ryss, E. S., Scerba, M. M., Gurvic, M. I. & Sapiro, E. L. (1970) Vsasyvanie razlincnyh form piscevogo zeleza. Ter. Arkh. 42, 68–72.

522. Pett, L. B. & Ogilvie, G. F. (1948) Haemoglobin levels at different ages. Can. Med. Assoc. J. 58, 353–355.

523. Pirrie, R. (1952) The influence of age upon serum iron in normal subjects. J. Clin. Pathol. 5, 10–15.

524. Pirzio-Biroli, G., Bothwell, T. H. & Finch, C. A. (1958) Iron absorption. II. The absorption of radioiron administered with a standard meal in man. J. Lab. Clin. Med. 51, 37–48.

525. Pirzio-Biroli, G. & Finch, C. A. (1960) Iron absorption. III. The influence of iron stores on iron absorption in the normal subject. J. Lab. Clin. Med. 55, 216–220.

526. Pla, G. W. & Fritz, J. C. (1970) Availability of iron. J. Assoc. Off. Anal. Chem. 53, 791–800.

527. Pla, G. W. & Fritz, J. C. (1971) Collaborative study of the hemoglobin repletion test in chicks and rats for measuring availability of iron. J. Assoc. Off. Anal. Chem. 54, 13–17.

528. Pla, G. W., Harrison, B. N. & Fritz, J. C. (1973) Comparison of chicks and rats as test animals for studying bioavailability of iron, with special reference to use of reduced iron in enriched bread. J. Assoc. Off. Anal. Chem. 56, 1369–1373.

529. Poláček, K. (1955) The clinical assessment of haemolytic disease of the newborn. Arch. Dis. Child. 30, 217–223.

530. Pollack, S., Kaufman, R. M. & Crosby, W. H. (1964) Iron absorption: effect of sugars and reducing agents. Blood 24, 577–581.

531. Pollycove, M. (1966) Iron metabolism and kinetics. Sem. Haematol. 3, 235–298.

532. Pommerenke, W. T., Hahn, P. F., Bale, W. F. & Balfour, W. M. (1942) Transmission of radio-active iron to the human fetus. Am. J. Physiol. 137, 164–170.

533. Porter, T. (1941) Iron balances on four normal pre-school children. J. Nutr. 21, 101–113.

534. Powell, D. E. B., Thomas, J. H. & Mills, P. (1968) Serum iron in elderly hospital patients. Geront. Clin. 10, 21–29.

535. Prasad, A. S., Schulert, A. R., Sandstead, H. H., Miale, A. & Farid, Z. (1963) Zinc, iron and nitrogen content of sweat in normal and deficient subjects. J. Lab. Clin. Med. 62, 84–89.

536. Pribilla, W. & Gehrmann, G. (1956) Untersuchungen über die Eisenversorgung des menschlichen Föten unter besondered Berucksichtigung des Ferritins. Folia Haematol. 1, 23–29.

537. Price, D. C., Cohn, S. H., Wasserman, L. R., Reizenstein, P. G. & Cronkite, E. P. (1962) The determination of iron absorption and loss by whole body counting. Blood 20, 517–531.

538. Prieto, J., Barry, M. & Sherlock, S. (1975) Serum ferritin in patients with iron overload and with acute and chronic liver disease. Gastroenterology 68, 525–533.

539. Pritchard, J. A. & Adams, R. H. (1960) Erythrocyte production and destruction during pregnancy. Am. J. Obstet. Gynecol. 79, 750–757.

540. Pritchard, J. A. & Hunt, C. F. (1968) A comparison of the hematologic responses following the routine prenatal administration of intramuscular and oral iron. Surg. Obstet. Gynecol. 106, 516–518.

541. Pritchard, J. A. & Mason, R. A. (1964) Iron stores of normal adults and replenishment with oral iron therapy. J. Am. Med. Assoc. 190, 897–901.

542. Pritchard, J. E. & Scott, D. E. (1970) Iron demands during pregnancy. In: Iron Deficiency, (Hallberg, L., Harwerth, H.-G. & Vannotti, A., eds.), pp. 173–182, Academic Press, New York.

543. Pryce, J. D. (1960) Level of haemoglobin in whole blood and red blood cells, and proposed convention for defining normality. Lancet 2, 333–336.

544. Pye, O. F. & MacLeod, G. (1946) The utilization of iron from different foods by normal young rats. J. Nutr. 32, 677–687.

545. Ramage, H., Sheldon, J. H. & Sheldon, W. (1933) A spectrographic investigation of the metallic content of the liver in childhood. Proc. Royal Soc. Lond. B. Biol. Sci. 113, 308–327.

546. Ranhotra, G. S., Hepburn, F. N. & Bradley, W. B. (1971) Availability of iron in enriched bread. Cereal Chem. 48, 377–384.

547. Rankin, G. L. S., Veall, N., Huntsman, R. G. & Liddell, J. (1962) Measurement with ^{51}Cr of red-cell loss in menorrhagia. Lancet 1, 567–569.

548. Rao, K. S., Swaminathan, M. C., Swarup, S. & Patwardhan, V. N. (1959) Protein malnutrition in South India. W.H.O. Bull. 20,

603–639. Cited by: Apte, B. V. & Ven-katachalam, P. S. (1963) Iron losses in Indian women. Indian J. Med. Res. 51, 958–962.

549. Rath, C. E., Caton, W., Reid, D. E., Finch, C. A. & Conroy, L. (1950) Hematological changes and iron metabolism of normal pregnancy. Surg. Gynecol. Obstet. 90, 320–326.

550. Rath, C. E. & Finch, C. A. (1948) Sternal marrow hemosiderin: a method for the determination of available iron stores in man. J. Lab. Clin. Med. 33, 81–86.

551. Rath, C. E. & Finch, C. A. (1949) Chemical, clinical and immunological studies on the products of human plasma fractionation XXXVIII. Serum iron transport. Measurement of iron binding capacity of serum in man. J. Clin. Invest. 28, 79–85.

552. Reedy, M. E., Schwartz, S. O. & Plattner, E. B. (1952) Anemia of the premature infant. A two-year study of the response to iron medication. J. Pediatr. 41, 25–39.

553. Reis, F. & Chakmakjian, H. H. (1932) Determination of iron in cow's milk and human milk. J. Biol. Chem. 98, 237–240.

554. Reizenstein, P. & Brann, I. (1965) Normal and pathological radioiron excretion in man. In: Radioactivity in Man. (Meneely, G. R. & Linde, S. M., eds.) pp. 391–401, Charles C Thomas, Springfield.

555. Reynafarje, C. & Ramos, J. (1961) Influence of altitude changes on intestinal iron absorption. J. Lab. Clin. Med. 57, 848–855.

556. Reznikoff, P., Toscani, V. & Fullarton, R. (1934) Iron metabolism studies in a normal subject and in a polycythemic patient. J. Nutr. 7, 221–230.

557. Riley, I. D. (1960) Absorption of radioactive iron by anaemic infants. Arch. Dis. Child. 35, 355–359.

558. Rios, E., Lipschitz, D. A., Cook, J. D. & Smith, N. J. (1975) Relationship of maternal and infant iron stores as assessed by determination of plasma ferritin. Pediatrics 55, 694–699.

559. Rios, E., Hunter, R. E., Cook, J. D., Smith, N. J. & Finch, C. A. (1975) The absorption of iron as supplements in infant cereals and infant formulas. Pediatrics 55, 686–693.

560. Robbe, H. (1958) Total amount of haemoglobin and physical working capacity in anaemia of pregnancy. Acta Obstet. Gynecol. Scand. 37, 312–347.

561. Robertson, P. D. & MacLean, D. W. (1970) Iron deficiency without anaemia—the M.C.H.C. in screening. J. Chron. Dis. 23, 191–195.

562. Robinow, M. & Hamilton, W. F. (1940) Blood volume and extracellular fluid volume of infants and children. Am. J. Dis. Child. 60, 827–840.

563. Robscheit-Robbins, F. S. (1929) The regeneration of hemoglobin and erythrocytes. Physiol. Rev. 9, 686–709.

564. Rodriguez, M. S. & Irwin, M. I. (1972) A conspectus of research on vitamin A requirements of man. J. Nutr. 102, 909–968.

565. Rooth, G. & Sjostedt, S. (1957) Haemo-globin in cord blood in normal and prolonged pregnancy. Arch. Dis. Child. 32, 91–92.

566. Roscoe, M. H. & Donaldson, G. M. M. (1946) The blood in pregnancy. Part II The blood volume, cell volume and haemoglobin mass. J. Obstet. Gynaecol. Br. Commonw. 53, 527–538.

567. Rose, M. S. & Kung, L. (1932) Factors in food influencing hemoglobin regeneration. II. Liver in comparison with whole wheat and prepared bran. J. Biol. Chem. 98, 417–437.

568. Rose, M. S. & Vahlteich, E. M. (1932) Factors in food influencing hemoglobin regeneration. I. Whole wheat flour, white flour, prepared bran, and oatmeal. J. Biol. Chem. 96, 593–608.

569. Rose, M. S., Vahlteich, E. M. & MacLeod, G. (1934) Factors in food influencing hemoglobin regeneration. III. Eggs in comparison with whole wheat, prepared bran, oatmeal, beef liver, and beef muscle. J. Biol. Chem. 104, 217–229.

570. Rose, M. S., Vahlteich, E., Robb, E. & Bloomfield, E. M. (1930) Iron requirement in early childhood. J. Nutr. 3, 229–235.

571. Rosenfield, R. E. (1955) A-B hemolytic disease of the newborn. Analysis of 1480 blood specimens with special reference to the direct antiglobulin test and to the group 0 mother. Blood 10, 17–28.

572. Ross, S. M. (1972) Haemoglobin and haematocrit values in pregnant women on a high iron intake and living at a high altitude. J. Obstet. Gynaecol. Br. Commonw. 79, 1103–1107.

573. Rovinsky, J. J. & Jaffin, H. (1965) Cardiovascular hemodynamics in pregnancy. 1. Blood and plasma volumes in multiple pregnancy. Am. J. Obstet. Gynecol. 93, 1–15.

574. Rowell, L. B., Taylor, H. L. & Wang, Y. (1964) Limitations to prediction of maximal oxygen intake. J. Appl. Physiol. 19, 919–927.

575. Rubino, G. F., Teso, G. & Rasetti, L. (1960) Erythrocyte delta-amino laevulinic acid dehydrase in anaemia. Acta Haematol. 24, 300–310.

576. Rush, B., Figallo, M. A. & Brown, E. B. (1966) Effect of a low iron diet on iron absorption. Am. J. Clin. Nutr. 19, 132–136.

577. Russell, S. J. M. (1949) Blood volume studies in healthy children. Arch. Dis. Child. 24, 88–98.

578. Rybo, G. (1966) Menstrual blood loss in relation to parity and menstrual pattern. Acta Obstet. Gynecol. Scand. 45, Suppl. 7, 25–45.

579. Rybo, G. & Hallberg, L. (1966) Influence of heredity and environment on normal menstrual blood loss. A study of twins. Acta Obstet. Gynecol. Scand. 45, 57–78.

580. Sachs, A., Levine, V. E. & Fabian, A. A. (1936) Copper and iron in human blood. IV. Normal children. Arch. Intern. Med. 58, 523–530.

581. Sachs, A., Levine, V. E. & Griffith, W. O.

(1937) Copper and iron in human blood. V. Normal adolescent children from 14 to 19 years of age. Arch. Intern. Med. *60*, 982–989.

582. Sachs, A., Levine, V. E. & Griffith, W. O. (1937–38) Blood copper and iron in relation to menstruation. J. Lab. Clin. Med. *23*, 566–571.

583. Sachs, A., Levine, V. E., Griffith, W. O. & Hansen, C. H. (1938) Copper and iron in human blood. Comparison of maternal and fetal blood after normal delivery and after cesarean section. Am. J. Dis. Child. *56*, 787–796.

584. Saddi, R. & Schapira, G. (1969) Iron requirements during growth. In: Iron Deficiency. (Hallberg, L., Harwerth, H. G., Vannotti, A., eds.) pp. 183–198, Academic Press, New York.

585. Saito, H., Sargent, T., Parker, H. G. & Lawrence, J. H. (1964) Whole body iron loss in normal man measured with a gamma spectrometer. J. Nucl. Med. *5*, 571–580.

586. Sankaran, G. & Rajagopal, K. (1938) Haematological investigations in South India. I. The estimation of haemoglobin. Indian J. Med. Res. *25*, 741–751.

587. Sayers, M. H., Lynch, S. R., Charlton, R. W. & Bothwell, T. H. (1974) Iron absorption from rice meals cooked with fortified salt containing ferrous sulphate and ascorbic acid. Br. J. Nutr. *31*, 367–375.

588. Sayers, M. H., Lynch, S. R., Jacobs, P., Charlton, R. W., Bothwell, T. H., Walker, R. B. & Mayet, F. (1973) The effects of ascorbic acid supplementation on the absorption of iron in maize, wheat and soya. Br. J. Haematol. *24*, 209–218.

589. Saylor, L. & Finch, C. A. (1953) Determination of iron absorption using two isotopes of iron. Am. J. Physiol. *172*, 372–376.

590. Schade, A. L., Oyama, J., Reinhart, R. W. & Miller, J. R. (1954) Bound iron and unsaturated iron-binding capacity of serum; rapid and reliable quantitative determination. Proc. Soc. Exp. Biol. Med. *87*, 443–448.

591. Schairer, E. & Rechenberger, J. (1943) Über den Eisenbestand und Eisenstoffwechsel frühgeborener Kinder. Z. Kinderheilk. *64*, 255–264.

592. Schlaphoff, D. & Johnston, F. A. (1949) The iron requirement of six adolescent girls. J. Nutr. *39*, 67–82.

593. Schlaphoff, D., Johnston, F. A. & Boroughs, E. D. (1950) Serum iron levels of adolescent girls and the diurnal variation of serum iron and hemoglobin. Arch. Biochem. *28*, 165–173.

594. Schlutz, F. W., Morse, M., Cassels, D. E. & Iob, L. V. (1940) A study of the nutritional and physical status and the response to exercise of sixteen Negro boys 13 to 17 years of age. J. Pediatr. *17*, 466–480.

595. Schlutz, F. W., Morse, M. & Oldham, H. (1933) The influence of fruit and vegetable feeding upon the iron metabolism of the infant. J. Pediatr. *3*, 225–241.

596. Schmidt, G. (1958) Der Eisengehalt des menschlichen Haares. Z. Ges. Inn. Med. *13*, 189–192.

597. Schüching, A. (1879) Die Blutmenge der Neugeborener. Eine neuer Beitrag zur Abnabelungstheorie. Berlin. Klin. Wochenschr. *16*, 581–583.

598. Schulman, I. (1961) Iron requirements in infancy. J. Am. Med. Assoc. *175*, 118–123.

599. Schulman, I. & Smith, C. H. (1954) Studies on the anemia of prematurity. II. The blood volume in premature infants. Am. J. Dis. Child. *88*, 575–582.

600. Schulz, J. & Smith, N. J. (1958) A quantitative study of the absorption of food iron in infants and children. A.M.A. J. Dis. Child. *95*, 109–119.

601. Schulz, J. & Smith, N. J. (1958) Quantitative study of the absorption of iron salts in infants and children. A.M.A. J. Dis. Child. *95*, 120–125.

602. Schulze, H. V. & Morgan, A. F. (1946) Relation of ascorbic acid to effectiveness of iron therapy in children. Am. J. Dis. Child. *71*, 593–600.

603. Schwartz, E. & Baehner, R. L. (1968) Diurnal variation of serum iron in infants and children. Acta Paediatr. Scand. *57*, 433–435.

604. Scott, E. M. & Heller, C. A. (1964) Iron deficiency in Alaskan Eskimos. Am. J. Clin. Nutr. *15*, 282–286.

605. Scott, D. E. & Pritchard, J. A. (1967) Iron deficiency in healthy young college women. J. Am. Med. Assoc. *199*, 897–900.

606. Selander, P. (1944) The haemoglobin and erythrocyte values during the first year of life following different methods of clamping of the umbilical cord. Acta Paediatr. *32*, 38–57.

607. Seltzer, C. C., Wenzel, B. J. & Mayer, J. (1963) Serum iron and iron-binding capacity in adolescents. I. Standard values. Am. J. Clin. Nutr. *13*, 343–353.

608. Semmence, A. (1959) Anaemia in the elderly. Br. Med. J. *2*, 1153–1154.

609. Senchak, M. M., Howe, J. M. & Clark, H. E. (1973) Iron absorption by adults fed mixtures of rice, milk, and wheat flour. J. Am. Diet. Assoc. *62*, 272–275.

610. Shackleton, L. & McCance, R. A. (1936) The ionisable iron in foods. Biochem. J. *30*, 582–591.

611. Shapleigh, J. B., Mayes, S. & Moore, C. V. (1952) Hematologic values in the aged. J. Gerontol. *7*, 207–219.

612. Sharpe, L. M., Peacock, W. C., Cooke, R. & Harris, R. S. (1950) The effect of phytate and other food factors on iron absorption. J. Nutr. *41*, 433–446.

613. Shaw, S. T., Aaronson, D. E. & Moyer, D. L. (1972) Quantitation of menstrual blood loss—further evaluation of the alkaline hematin method. Contraception *5*, 497–513.

614. Sherman, W. C., Elvehjem, C. A. & Hart, E. B. (1934) Factors influencing the utilization of the iron and copper of egg yolk

for hemoglobin formation. J. Biol. Chem. *107*, 289–295.

615. Shoden, A., Gabrio, B. W. & Finch, C. A. (1953) The relationship between ferritin and hemosiderin in rabbits and man. J. Biol. Chem. *204*, 823–830.

616. Siddall, R. S., Crissey, R. R. & Knapp, W. L. (1952) Effect on cesarean section babies of stripping or milking of the umbilical cords. Am. J. Obstet. Gynecol. *63*, 1059–1064.

617. Siimes, M. A., Addiego, J. E. & Dallman, P. R. (1974) Ferritin in serum: Diagnosis of iron deficiency and iron overload in infants and children. Blood *43*, 581–590.

618. Siimes, M. A., Koerper, M. A., Licko, V. & Dallman, P. R. (1975) Ferritin turnover in plasma: an opportunistic use of blood removed during exchange transfusion. Pediatr. Res. *9*, 127–129.

619. Simon, J. F. (1845) Chemistry of Man. pp. 91–277, Lea & Blanchard, Philadelphia.

620. Sisson, T. R. C. & Lund, C. J. (1959) The influence of maternal iron deficiency on the newborn. Am. J. Clin. Nutr. *6*, 376–385.

621. Sisson, T. R. C., Lund, C. J., Whalen, L. E. & Telek, A. (1959) The blood volume of infants. I. The full-term infant in the first year of life. J. Pediatr. *55*, 163–179.

622. Sisson, T. R. C., Whalen, L. E. & Telek, A. (1959) The blood volume of infants. II. The premature infant during the first year of life. J. Pediatr. *55*, 430–446.

623. Smith, C. A., Cherry, R. B., Maletskos, C. J., Gibson, J. G., Roby, C. C., Caton, W. L. & Reid, D. E. (1955) Persistence and utilization of maternal iron for blood formation during infancy. J. Clin. Invest. *34*, 1391–1402.

624. Smith, J. S. & Whitelaw, D. M. (1971) Hemoglobin values in aged men. Can. Med. Assoc. J. *105*, 816–825.

625. Smith, M. D. (1952) The value of estimation of the serum iron in the investigation of anaemia. Glasgow Med. J. *33*, 309–319.

626. Smith, N. J., Rosello, S., Say, M. B. & Yeya, K. (1955) Iron storage in the first five years of life. Pediatrics *16*, 166–173.

627. Snell, F. M. (1950) Observations on the hematologic values of the Japanese. Blood *5*, 89–100.

628. Snelling, C. E. (1933) The metabolism of iron in the anemia of premature infants. J. Pediatr. *2*, 546–552.

629. Söldner (1903) Die Aschenbestandteile des neugebornen Menschen und der Frauenmilch. Z. Biol. *44*, 61–77.

630. Sood, S. K., Banerji, L. & Ramalingaswami, V. (1968) Geographic pathology of iron deficiency with special reference to India. II. Quantitation of iron stores by repeated phlebotomy in Indian volunteers. Am. J. Clin. Nutr. *21*, 1149–1155.

631. Sorbie, J., Valberg, L. S., Corbett, W. E. N. & Ludwig, J. (1975) Serum ferritin, cobalt excretion and body iron status. Can. Med. Assoc. J. *112*, 1173–1178.

632. Spealman, C. R., Newton, M. & Post, R. L. (1947) Influence of environmental temperature and posture on volume and composition of blood. Am. J. Physiol. *150*, 628–640.

633. Sprauve, M. E. & Dodds, M. L. (1965) Dietary survey of adolescents in the Virgin Islands. J. Am. Diet. Assoc. *47*, 287–289.

634. Sproule, B. J., Mitchell, J. H. & Miller, W. F. (1960) Cardiopulmonary physiological responses to heavy exercise in patients with anemia. J. Clin. Invest. *39*, 378–388.

635. Stearns, G. & McKinley, J. B. (1937) The conservation of blood iron during the period of physiological hemoglobin destruction in early infancy. J. Nutr. *13*, 143–156.

636. Stearns, G. & Stinger, D. (1937) Iron retention in infancy. J. Nutr. *13*, 127–141.

637. Steinkamp, R., Dubach, R. & Moore, C. V. (1955) Studies in iron transportation and metabolism. VIII. Absorption of radioiron from iron-enriched bread. Arch. Intern. Med. *95*, 181–193.

638. Stevens, A. R., Coleman, D. H. & Finch, C. A. (1953) Iron metabolism: clinical evaluation of iron stores. Ann. Intern. Med. *38*, 199–205.

639. Stockman, R. (1895) Observations on the causes and treatment of chlorosis. Br. Med. J. *2*, 1473–1476.

640. Storvick, C. A., Hathaway, M. L. & Nitchals, R. M. (1951) Nutritional status of selected population groups in Oregon. II. Biochemical tests on the blood of native born and reared school children in two regions. Milbank Mem. Fund Quart. *29*, 255–272.

641. Stott, G. (1960) Anaemia in Mauritius. W.H.O. Bull. *23*, 781–791.

642. Strauss, M. B. (1933) Anemia of infancy from maternal iron deficiency in pregnancy. J. Clin. Invest. *12*, 345–353.

643. Street, H. R. (1943) A study of the availability of the iron in enriched bread. J. Nutr. *26*, 187–195.

644. Sturgeon, P. (1954) Studies of iron requirements in infants and children. I. Normal values for serum iron, copper and free erythrocyte protoporphyrin. Pediatrics *13*, 107–125.

645. Sturgeon, P. (1956) Iron metabolism: a review with special consideration of iron requirements during normal infancy. Pediatrics *18*, 267–298.

646. Sturgeon, P. (1958) Studies of iron requirements in infants and children. In: Iron in Clinical Medicine. (Wallerstein, R. O. & Mettier, S. R., eds.), pp. 183–203, Univ. of California Press, Berkeley.

647. Sturgeon, P. (1959) Studies of iron requirements in infants. III Influence of supplemental iron during normal pregnancy on mother and infant. A. The mother. Br. J. Haematol. *5*, 31–44.

648. Sturgeon, P. (1959) Studies of iron requirements in infants. III. Influence of supplemental iron during normal pregnancy on mother and infant. B. The infant. Br. J. Haematol. *5*, 45–55.

649. Sturgeon, P. & Shoden, A. (1971) Total

liver storage iron in normal populations of the U.S.A. Am. J. Clin. Nutr. 24, 469–474.

650. Sunderman, F. W., MacFate, R. P., MacFadyen, D. A., Stevenson, G. F. & Copeland, B. E. (1953) Symposium on clinical hemoglobinometry. Am. J. Clin. Path. 23, 519–598.

651. Taborsky, G. (1963) Interaction between phosvitin and iron and its effect on a rearrangement of phosvitin structure. Biochemistry 2, 266–271.

652. Talbott, J. H., Edwards, H. T., Dill, D. B. & Drastich, L. (1933) Physiological responses to high environmental temperature. Am. J. Trop. Med. 13, 381–397.

653. Talso, P. J. & Dieckmann, W. J. (1948) Anemias of pregnancy. Am. J. Obstet. Gynecol. 55, 518–523.

654. Tanaka, K. R. & Valentine, W. N. (1961) Aconitase activity of human leucocytes. Acta Haematol. 26, 12–20.

655. Taymor, M. K., Sturgis, S. H. & Yahia, C. (1964) The etiological role of chronic iron deficiency in production of menorrhagia. J. Amer. Med. Assoc. 187, 323–327.

656. Technical Committee, Southern Regional Nutrition Research Project (S-28) (1959) Metabolic patterns in pre-adolescent children. I. Description of metabolic studies. Southern Cooperative Series Bull. No. 64, 94 pp.

657. Technical Committee, Southern Regional Nutrition Research Project (S-28) (1964) Metabolic patterns in pre-adolescent children. X. Description of 1962 study. Southern Cooperative Series Bull. No. 94, 54 pp.

658. Tejuja, S. (1971) Clinical significance of hemoglobin levels in users of the IUD—a 4-year study. Am. J. Obstet. Gynecol. 110, 735–737.

659. Thein, M., Beaton, G. H., Milne, H. & Veen, M. J. (1969) Oral contraceptive drugs: some observations on their effect on menstrual loss and hematological indices. Can. Med. Assoc. J. 101, 678–679.

660. Theriault, F. R. & Fellers, C. R. (1942) Effect of freezing and of canning in glass and in tin on available iron content of foods. Food Res. 7, 503–508.

661. Thomson, K. J., Hirsheimer, A., Gibson, J. G. & Evans, W. A. (1938) Studies on the circulation in pregnancy. III. Blood volume changes in normal pregnant women. Am. J. Obstet. Gynecol. 36, 48–59.

662. Tompsett, S. L. (1940) Factors influencing the absorption of iron and copper from the alimentary tract. Biochem. J. 34, 961–969.

663. Torrance, J. D., Charlton, R. W., Schmaman, A., Lynch, S. R. & Bothwell, T. H. (1968) Storage iron in "muscle". J. Clin. Pathol. 21, 495–500.

664. Tucker, R. E. & Brown, P. T. (1955) Nutrition studies in Rhode Island. R.I. Agr. Exp. Sta. Bull. No. 327, 25 pp.

665. Tucker, R. E., Chalmers, F. W., Church, H. N., Clayton, M. M., Foster, W. D., Gates, L. O., Hagan, G. C., Steele, B. F., Wertz,

A. W. & Young, C. M. (1952) Cooperative nutritional status studies in the Northeast region. IV. Dietary findings. R.I. Agr. Exp. Sta. Bull. No. 319, 24 pp.

666. Turnbull, A. (1974) Iron absorption. In: Iron in Biochemistry and Medicine. (Jacobs, A. & Worwood, M., eds.), pp. 369–403, Academic Press, New York.

667. Turnbull, A., Cleton, F. & Finch, C. A. (1962) Iron absorption. IV. The absorption of hemoglobin iron. J. Clin. Invest. 41, 1897–1907.

668. Tysoe, F. W. & Lowenstein, L. (1950) Blood volume and hematologic studies in pregnancy and the puerperium. Am. J. Obstet. Gynecol. 60, 1187–1205.

669. Vahlquist, B. (1939) Investigations on serum-iron in children. Preliminary report. Acta Paediatr. 25, 302–330.

670. Vahlquist, B. (1950) The cause of sexual differences in erythrocyte, hemoglobin and serum iron levels in human adults. Blood 5, 874–875.

671. Vahlquist, B. C. (1941) Das Serumeisen. Eine pädiatrisch-klinische und experimentelle Studie. Acta Paediatr. 28, (Suppl 5), 1–374.

672. Vahlteich, E. M., Funnell, E. H., MacLeod, G. & Rose, M. S. (1935) Egg yolk and bran as sources of iron in the human dietary. J. Am. Diet. Assoc. 11, 331–334.

673. Vahlteich, E. M., Rose, M. S. & MacLeod, G. (1936) The effect of digestibility upon the availability of iron in whole wheat. J. Nutr. 11, 31–36.

674. Van Campen, D. (1973) Enhancement of iron absorption from ligated segments of rat intestine by histidine, cysteine and lysine: effects of removing ionizing groups and of stereoisomerism. J. Nutr. 103, 139–142.

675. Van Campen, D. & Gross, E. (1969) Effect of histidine and certain other amino acids on the absorption of iron-59 by rats. J. Nutr. 99, 68–74.

676. Van Eijk, H. G., Wiltink, W. F. & Bos, G. (1974) The relation of erythrocyte porphyrins to haemoglobin, haematocrit, transferrin and serum iron. Clin. Chim. Acta 53, 35–42.

677. Van Eijk, H. G., Wiltink, W. F., Bos, G. & Goossens, J. P. (1974) Measurement of the iron content in human liver specimens. Clin. Chim. Acta 50, 275–280.

678. Van Hoek, R. & Conrad, M. E. (1961) Iron absorption. Measurement of ingested iron[59] by a human whole-body liquid scintillation counter. J. Clin. Invest. 40, 1153–1159.

679. Vartiainen, E., Widholm, O. & Tenhunen, T. (1967) Iron prophylaxis in menstruating teenage girls. Acta Obstet. Gynecol. Scand. 46, Suppl. 1, 49–54.

680. Vellar, O. D. (1967) Studies on hemoglobin values in Norway. IX. Hemoglobin, hematocrit and MCHC values in old men and women. Acta Med. Scand. 182, 681–689.

681. Vellar, O. D. (1968) Studies on sweat losses of nutrients. I. Iron content of whole body sweat and its association with other

sweat constituents, serum iron levels, hematological indices, body surface area, and sweat rate. Scand. J. Clin. Lab. Invest. *21*, 157–167.

682. Vellar, O. D. (1968) Studies on sweat losses of nutrients. II. The influence of an oral iron load on the iron content of whole body cell-free sweat. Scand. J. Clin. Lab. Invest. *21*, 344–346.

683. Vellar, O. D., Borchgrevink, C. & Natvig, H. (1968) Iron fortified bread. Absorption and utilization studies. Acta Med. Scand. *183*, 251–256.

684. Vellar, O. D. & Hermansen, L. (1971) Physical performance and hematological parameters. Acta Med. Scand. Suppl. No. 522, 40 pp.

685. Venn, J. A. J., McCance, R. A. & Widdowson, E. M. (1947) Iron metabolism in piglet anaemia. J. Comp. Pathol. *57*, 314–325.

686. Ventura, S. & Klopper, A. (1951) Iron metabolism in pregnancy: the behaviour of haemoglobin, serum iron, the iron-binding capacity of serum proteins, serum copper and free erythrocyte protoporphyrin in normal pregnancy. J. Obstet. Gynaecol. Brit. Emp. *58*, 173–189.

687. Verel, D., Bury, J. D. & Hope, A. (1956) Blood volume changes in pregnancy and the puerperium. Clin. Sci. *15*, 1–7.

688. Verloop, M. C., Blokhuis, E. W. M. & Bos, C. C. (1959) Causes of the differences in haemoglobin and serum-iron values between males and females. Acta Haematol. *21*, 199–205.

689. Verloop, M. C., Blokhuis, E. W. M. & Bos, C. C. (1959) Causes of the "physiological" anaemia of pregnancy. Acta Haematol. *22*, 158–164.

690. Vestermark, S. & Andersen, B. (1966) Iron determination in human milk. Danish Med. Bull. *13*, 8–10.

691. Waddell, J. (1974) The bioavailability of iron sources and their utilization in food enrichment. Federation Proc. *33*, 1779–1783.

692. Wadsworth, G. R. (1959) Nutritional factors in anaemia. World Rev. Nutr. Diet. *1*, 145–175.

693. Waldenström, J. (1938) Iron and epithelium. Some clinical observations. Acta Med. Scand. Suppl. No. 90, 380–397.

694. Walker, J. & Turnbull, E. P. N. (1953) Haemoglobin and red cells in the human foetus and their relation to the oxygen content of the blood in the vessels of the umbilical cord. Lancet 2, 312–318.

695. Wallgren, A. (1932) On the iron content in milk. Acta Paediatr. *12*, 153–169.

696. Wallgren, A. (1933) Le fer dans la nutrition de l'enfant. III. Recherches sur le métabolisme du fer chez les enfants nourris au sein pendant la première année de leur existence. Rev. Franc. Pédiatr. 9, 196–235.

697. Wallgren, A. (1939) Le fer dans la nutrition de l'enfant. IV. Recherches sur le métabolisme du fer chez les enfants prématurés, nourris au sein, pendent la première

année de leur existence. Rev. Franc. Pédiatr. *15*, 117–183.

698. Walsh, R. J., Arnold, B. J., Lancaster, H. O., Coote, M. A. & Cotter, H. (1953) A study of haemoglobin values in New South Wales with observations on haematocrit and sedimentation rate values. Nat. Health & Med. Res. Council, Spec. Report Ser. No. 5, Canberra. Cited in: Hytten, F. E. & Duncan, D. L. (1956) Iron deficiency anemia in the pregnant woman and its relation to normal physiological changes. Nutr. Abstr. Rev. *26*, 855–868.

699. Walters, G. O., Miller, F. M. & Worwood, M. (1973) Serum ferritin concentration and iron stores in normal subjects. J. Clin. Path. *26*, 770–772.

700. Walters, G. O., Jacobs, A., Worwood, M., Trevett, D. & Thomson, W. (1975) Iron absorption in normal subjects and patients with idiopathic haemochromatosis: Relationship with serum ferritin concentration. Gut *16*, 188–192.

701. Warnick, K. P., Bring, S. V. & Woods, E. (1956) Nutritional status of school children 15 and 16 years of age in three Idaho communities. Idaho Agr. Exp. Sta. Res. Bull. No. 33, 74 pp.

702. Waugh, T. R., Merchant, F. T. & Maughan, G. B. (1939) Blood studies on the newborn: I. Determination of hemoglobin, volume of packed red cells, reticulocytes, and fragility of the erythrocytes over a nine-day period. Am. J. Med. Sci. *198*, 646–665.

703. Wegelius, R. (1948) On the changes in the peripheral blood picture of the newborn infant immediately after birth. Acta Paediatr. *35*, Suppl. 4, p. 1–107.

704. Weinfeld, A. (1964) Storage iron in man. Acta Med. Scand. *177*, Suppl. 427, 1–155.

705. Weinfeld, A. (1970) Iron stores. In: Iron Deficiency. (Hallberg, L., Harwerth, H. G. & Vannotti, A., eds.), pp. 329–363. Academic Press, New York.

706. Weinfeld, A., Lundin, P. & Lundvall, O. (1968) Significance for the diagnosis of iron overload of histochemical and chemical iron in the liver of control subjects. J. Clin. Pathol. *21*, 35–40.

707. Weintraub, L. R., Conrad, M. E. & Crosby, W. H. (1965) Absorption of hemoglobin iron by the rat. Proc. Soc. Exp. Biol. Med. *120*, 840–843.

708. Weintraub, L. R., Demis, D. J., Conrad, M. E. & Crosby, W. H. (1965) Iron excretion by the skin. Selective localization of iron in epithelial cells. Am. J. Pathol. *46*, 121–127.

709. Weintraub, L. R., Weinstein, M. B., Huser, H. J. & Rafal, S. (1968) Absorption of hemoglobin iron: the role of a heme-splitting substance in the intestinal mucosa. J. Clin. Invest. *47*, 531–539.

710. Went, L. N., Channer, D. M., Harding, R. Y. & Clunes, B. E. (1960) The effect of iron and protein supplementations on the haemoglobin level of healthy female students. W. Indian Med. J. 9, 209–214.

711. Werner, E. & Gladtke, E. (1970) Der

zirkadiane Rhythmus des Serumeisens bei Kindern. Dtsch. Med. Wochenschr. 95, 1476–1483.

712. Wharton, M. A. (1963) Nutritive intake of adolescents. J. Am. Diet. Assoc. 42, 306–310.

713. Wheeler, E. A., El-Neil, H., Willson, J. O. C. & Weiner, J. S. (1973) The effect of work level and dietary intake on water balance and the excretion of sodium, potassium and iron in a hot climate. Br. J. Nutr. 30, 127–137.

714. Whipple, G. H. & Robscheit-Robbins, F. S. (1925) Blood regeneration in severe anemia. III. Iron reaction favorable—arsenic and germanium dioxide almost inert. Am. J. Physiol. 72, 419–430.

715. White, H. S. (1968) Iron nutriture of girls and women—a review. II. Iron stores. J. Am. Diet. Assoc. 53, 570–574.

716. White, H. S. & Gynne, T. N. (1971) Utilization of inorganic elements by young women eating iron-fortified foods. J. Am. Diet. Assoc. 59, 27–33.

717. White, H. S. & Johnson, E. E. (1969) Hemoglobin concentrations of 2,263 university women. J. Am. Coll. Health Assoc. 17, 255–256.

718. Widdowson, E. M. (1947) A study of individual children's diets. Medical Research Council, Spec. Rep. Ser. No. 257, H. M. Stationery Office, London, pp. 196.

719. Widdowson, E. M. (1968) Growth and composition of the fetus and newborn. In: Biology of Gestation. Vol. 2. The Fetus and Neonate (Assali, N. S., ed.) pp. 1–49, Academic Press, New York.

720. Widdowson, E. M. & Dickerson, J. W. T. (1964) Chemical composition of the body. In: Mineral Metabolism, an Advanced Treatise (Comar, C. L. & Bonner, F., eds.), Vol. 2, Part A, pp. 1–247, Academic Press, New York.

721. Widdowson, E. M. & McCance, R. A. (1936) Iron in human nutrition. J. Hyg. 36, 13–23.

722. Widdowson, E. M. & McCance, R. A. (1937) The absorption and excretion of iron before, during and after a period of very high intake. Biochem. J. 31, 2029–2034.

723. Widdowson, E. M. & McCance, R. A. (1942) Iron exchanges of adults on white and brown bread diets. Lancet 1, 588–591.

724. Widdowson, E. M., McCance, R. A. & Spray, C. M. (1951) The chemical composition of the human body. Clin. Sci. 10, 113–125.

725. Widdowson, E. M. & Spray, C. M. (1951) Chemical development in utero. Arch. Dis. Child. 26, 205–214.

726. Widholm, O., Vartiainen, E. & Tenhunen, T. (1967) Iron study among teen-agers. 1. On iron requirements in menstruating teen-age girls. Acta Obstet. Gynecol. Scand. 46, Suppl. No. 1, 29–46.

727. Wijn, J. F. & Pikaar, N. A. (1971) Hemoglobin, serum iron and iron binding capacity during growth from age 9 to 17. Semilongi-tudinal study of boys and girls. Nutr. Metabol. 13, 44–53.

728. Wilcox, E. B. & Galloway, L. S. (1954) Children with and without rheumatic fever. 1. Nutrient intake, physique, and growth. J. Am. Diet. Assoc. 30, 345–350.

729. Wilcox, E. B., Mangelson, F. L., Galloway, L. S. & Wood, P. (1955) Children with and without rheumatic fever. IV. Hemoglobin, packed red cells, red and white cell count, sedimentation rate, blood glucose, serum iron and copper. J. Am. Diet. Assoc. 31, 45–51.

730. Wilkins, W., Blakely, R. & Brunson, J. (1947) Hemoglobin levels in Parker High School students. J. South Carolina Med. Assoc. 43, 31–33.

731. Will, G. & Boddy, K. (1967) Iron turnover estimated by a whole body monitor. Scot. Med. J. 12, 157–162.

732. Williamson, C. S. (1916) Influence of age and sex on hemoglobin. Arch. Intern. Med. 18, 505–528.

733. Wills, L., Hill, G., Bingham, K., Miall, M. & Wrigley, J. (1947) Haemoglobin levels in pregnancy. The effect of the rationing scheme and routine administration of iron. Br. J. Nutr. 1, 126–138.

734. Wilson, E. E., Windle, W. F. & Alt, H. L. (1941) Deprivation of placental blood as a cause of iron deficiency in infants. Am. J. Dis. Child. 62, 320–327.

735. Wilson, S. J. & Boyle, P. (1952) Erroneous anemia and polycythemia. Arch. Intern. Med. 90, 602–609.

736. Wiltink, W. F., Kruithof, J., Mol, C., Bos, G. & Van Eijk, H. G. (1973) Diurnal and nocturnal variations of the serum iron in normal subjects. Clin. Chim. Acta 49, 99–104.

737. Wintrobe, M. M. (1933) Blood of normal men and women. Erythrocyte counts, hemoglobin and volume of packed red cells of 229 individuals. Bull. Johns Hopkins Hosp. 52, 118–130.

738. Wintrobe, M. M. (1961) Clinical Hematology, pp. 1186, Lea & Febiger, Philadelphia.

739. Wohler, F. (1964) Diagnosis of iron storage diseases with desferrioxamine (Desferal test). Acta Haematol. 32, 321–337.

740. Woodruff, C. W. (1958) Multiple causes of iron deficiency in infants. J. Am. Med. Assoc. 167, 715–720.

741. Woodruff, C. W. (1961) The utilization of iron administered orally. Pediatrics 27, 194–198.

742. Woodruff, C. W. & Bridgeforth, E. B. (1953) Relationship between the hemogram of the infant and that of the mother during pregnancy. Pediatrics 12, 681–685.

743. World Health Organization, Report of a Study Group (1959) Iron deficiency anaemia. W.H.O. Tech. Rep. Ser. No. 182, 15 pp.

744. World Health Organization, Report of a WHO Expert Committee. (1965) Nutri-

tion in Pregnancy and Lactation. W.H.O.
Tech. Rep. Ser. No. 302, 53 pp.

745. World Health Organization, Report of a
WHO Scientific Group. (1968) Nutritional
Anaemias. W.H.O. Tech. Rep. Ser. No. 405,
37 pp.

746. Yao, A. C., Moinian, M. & Lind, J. (1969)
Distribution of blood between infant and
placenta after birth. Lancet 2, 871–873.

747. Young, C. M. & Pilcher, H. L. (1950) Nutritional status survey, Groton Township,
New York II. Nutrient usage of families and
individuals. J. Am. Diet. Assoc. 26, 776–
781.

748. Zadeh, J. A., Karabus, C. D. & Fielding, J.
(1967) Haemoglobin concentration and
other values in women using an intrauterine
device or taking corticosteroid contraceptive
pills. Br. Med. J. 4, 708–711.

749. Zaleski, S. (1886) Studien über die Leber.
Z. Physiol. Chem. 10, 453–502.

750. Zilva, J. F. & Patston, V. J. (1966) Variations in serum-iron in healthy women.
Lancet 1, 459–462.

751. Zizza, F. & Block, M. (1961) The interrelationship of the serum iron, iron binding
capacity and tissue iron. Acta Haematol. 25,
1–21.

752. Zuelzer, W. W. & Kaplan, E. (1954) ABO
heterospecific pregnancy and hemolytic disease: study of normal and pathologic variants; hematologic findings and erythrocyte
survival in normal infants. Am. J. Dis. Child.
88, 307–338.

A CONSPECTUS OF RESEARCH ON FOLACIN
REQUIREMENTS OF MAN[1]

by

MILDRED S. RODRÍGUEZ

*Department of Home Economics, California State University at Long Beach,
Long Beach, California 90840*

THE JOURNAL OF NUTRITION

VOLUME 108, NUMBER 12, DECEMBER 1978

(Pages 1983-2103)

INTRODUCTION

The study of human folacin requirements is a relatively new field. In 1946, Watson and Castle (772) firmly established that folacin was a compound distinctly different from the one which effectively cured pernicious anemia: that is, vitamin B_{12}. Most of the studies on the quantitative requirements for folacin have been published since 1960.

In this conspectus, we have indicated what research has been done with human subjects on folacin requirements and how it was done. This information in turn, points up what further research is needed in order to complete our knowledge of human folacin needs. It is not intended to be another estimate of folacin requirements nor a critical evaluation of the individual studies, although some evaluative comments have been included. For the reader's convenience references to basic background information and critical discussions on methodology are cited. Experiments with animals have been included only when studies with humans are lacking in an important area of research.

We have incorporated some discussion of folacin metabolism because this background information is necessary for understanding the reported research and also for evaluating the sensitivity of the criteria that have been used in estimating folacin requirements. The development of more sensitive criteria for use in future studies, furthermore, is based upon our knowledge of folacin metabolism. The National Research Council has published the proceedings of a recent workshop on the biochemistry and physiology of folacin in relation to human requirements.[2]

Most of our knowledge of human folacin requirements derives from reports of the amount of supplemental folic acid—the oxidized monoglutamate—that is required to correct folacin deficiency symptoms (therapeutic studies) or the amount required to prevent clinical and biochemical signs of folacin deficiency (prophylactic studies). In most studies, the amount of folacin in the diet was either not determined or at best "ill defined." Food intake and nutritional status surveys were seldom used because accurate food tables and adequate analytical techniques for readily determining the type and amount of the different folacins in the diet are lacking (258, 791). A few investigators have measured the amount of folacin activity in the average diet of healthy people (101, 123, 365, 529, 541, 639); others have tried to estimate requirements from balance studies (185, 186) but found that this was not feasible. Some have calculated requirements from animal studies (165, 181) or compared body stores and depletion time (319, 321).

In therapeutic studies the most commonly used criterion has been the amount of folacin required to elicit an optimal hematological response (reticulocytosis; increased hemoglobin, hematocrit or number of red blood cells; and the disappearance of circulating megaloblasts) in patients with megaloblastic anemia. Criteria used in prophylactic studies include: hematological values, nuclear hypersegmentation of polymorphonuclear leukocytes, formiminoglutamic acid (FIGLU) excretion after a test load of histidine, clearance rate of folacin and serum, and red blood cell folacin activity.

The requirements of pregnant women have been studied the most intensively; young adults and infants have also been covered. But the needs of preschool children, lactating women, and the elderly have received scant attention. And we found no data on children over 6 years old or during puberty and adolescence.

A number of factors affect folacin requirements. Increases in the number of body cells or the rate of cell turnover are especially important since the folacins are required for DNA and RNA synthesis.

---

[1] Requests for reprints should be directed to USDA, Science and Education Administration, Nutrition Institute, Building 307, Beltsville, Md. 20705.

[2] Since the completion of this conspectus, the National Academy of Sciences has published the proceedings of a workshop, which was held in Washington, D.C., June 2–3, 1975, on human folacin requirements: Food and Nutrition Board, National Research Council (1977) Folic Acid. Biochemistry and Physiology in Relation to the Human Nutrition Requirement. Nat. Acad. Sci. U.S.A., Washington, D.C.

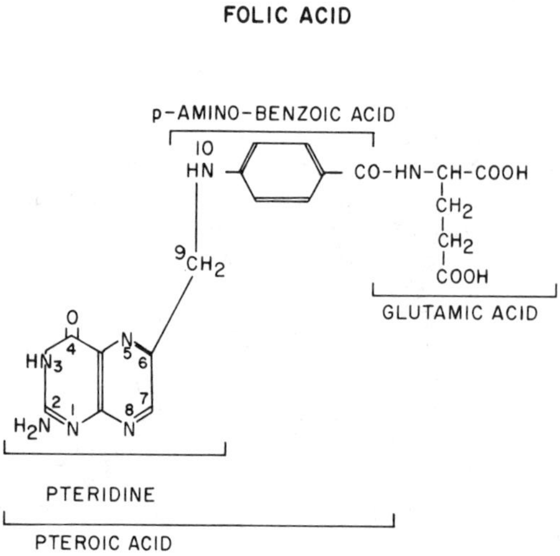

FOLIC ACID

Figure 1

Thus growth, pregnancy, and lactation, as well as innumerable pathological conditions, affect requirements.

Availability of dietary folacin is also an important factor. After the early reports of the poor availability of the conjugated forms of folacin from large amounts of yeast (60, 386, 697, 725) and inability of patients with malabsorptive disorders to utilize dietary folacin (661), some investigators (314) concluded that the polyglutamate forms were generally not available to humans. Recent research indicates that dietary polyglutamates are at least partially available (22, 729). However, the chemical structure of the folacin (mono- versus polyglutamate, oxidized versus reduced and one-carbon substitutes), cellulose content of the diet, naturally occurring antagonists, glucose, pH, and folacin deficiency itself may affect folacin absorption. There is also some evidence that compounds such as iron, oral contraceptives, ascorbic acid, cobalamin, methionine, alcohol, and certain drugs affect folacin utilization. In addition, malabsorptive diseases of the small intestine, such as tropical sprue and gluten-induced enteropathy prevent normal utilization of folacin.

The folacins—derivatives and nomenclature

There are probably more derivatives of folic acid, the fundamental unit of which

is common to a family of biologically active substances, than there are of any other vitamin (470). Baugh and Krumdieck (42) estimated that theoretically there could be at least 150 different folacins if the poly-γ-glutamyl side chain does not contain more than six residues. The early history and the chemistry of the folacins have been reviewed in detail by Stokstad and his associates (397, 710, 712).

The principal derivatives of folic acid (fig. 1), the oxidized monoglutamate, and the various names and abbreviations that have been used to identify them are summarized in table 1. The pteridine nucleus may exist in any one of three different oxidation/reduction states—folic acid, the oxidized form; 5,6-dihydrofolic acid (H_2-folic acid); or 5,6,7,8-tetrahydrofolic acid (H_4-folic acid), the reduced metabolically active parent compound. These compounds usually have any one of six different one-carbon (C_1) substituent in the N_5 and/or N_{10} position (5-methyl, 5-formyl, 10-formyl, 5,10-methylene, 5,10-methenyl, and 5-formimino) of H_4-folic acid. In the naturally occurring folacins, the glutamyl residue of H_4-folic acid is commonly linked in a γ-peptide linkage to a polyglutamyl side chain consisting of one to six γ-glutamyl residues (42). This γ-peptide linkage is readily split by the enzyme(s) γ-glutamyl carboxypeptidase (commonly referred to as "conjugase") (66). It is ubiquitous in both plant and animal tissues (73).

In this paper we have followed the tentative rules of nomenclature for vitamins recommended by the International Union of Nutrition Sciences Committee on Nomenclature and the Committee on Nomenclature of the American Institute of Nutrition (IUNS-AIN) for identifying derivatives of the monoglutamate, folic acid (368). ". . . the generic descriptor for folic acid and related compounds exhibiting qualitatively the biological activity of folic acid" is folacin (368). In the literature, folacin that can be utilized by *L. casei* without treating the sample with conjugase is referred to as "free folate." Since we are using the IUNS-AIN tentative nomenclature system, we will call it "free folacin." In those cases where we are sure that con-

TABLE 1

Folacin nomenclature

Compound[1]	Abbreviation[1]	Synonyms and common abbreviations
Oxidized folacins:		
Folic acid		Pteroylglutamic acid (PGA)(PteGlu), Vitamin B_c, folate
Folic acid glutamates		Folate conjugates
Pteroyldiglutamic acid	$PteGlu_2$	Folic acid glu_1
Pteroyltriglutamic acid	$PteGlu_3$	Folic acid glu_2, Teropterin, folyldiglutamic acid, "fermentation *L. casei* factor," γ-folyl-γ-glutamylglutamic acid, triglutamate
Pteroylheptaglutamic acid	$PteGlu_7$	Folic acid glu_6, vitamin B_c conjugate, folylhexaglutamic acid, pteroylhexa-γ-glutamylglutamic acid
10-formylfolic acid	10-CHO-folic acid	10-Formylpteroylglutamic acid (10-CHO–PteGlu)
10-Formylpteroyltriglutamic acid	10-CHO–$PteGlu_3$	10-formylfolic acid glu_2
Partially reduced folacins:		
Dihydrofolic acid	H_2-folic acid	5,7,8-Dihydropteroylglutamic acid (H_2-Pte-Glu), DHF
10-formyldihydrofolic acid	10-CHO–H_2-folic acid	10-Formyl-7,8-dihydropteroylglutamic acid (10-CHO–H_2PteGlu)
Reduced folacins:		
Tetrahydrofolic acid	H_4-folic acid	5,6,7,8-tetrahydropteroylglutamic acid (H_4PteGlu), (THFA, THF, $PGAH_4$), H_4-folate
5-formyltetrahydrofolic acid	5-CHO–H_4-folic acid	N^5-CHO–THFA, N^5-F–$PGAH_4$, citrovorum factor ("CF"), leucovorin, folinic acid, 5-formyltetrahydropteroylglutamic acid (5-CHO–H_4PteGlu)
10-formyltetrahydrofolic acid	10-CHO–H_4-folic acid	10-formyltetrahydropteroylglutamic acid (10-CHO–H_4PteGlu), N^{10}-CHO–THFA, N^{10}-F–$PGAH_4$, heat-labile citrovorum factor (HLCF), N^{10}-formyl–THFA
5,10-methylenetetrahydrofolic acid	5,10-CH_2–H_4-folic acid	5,10-Methylenetetrahydropteroylglutamic acid (5,10-CH_2–H_4PteGlu)
5-methyltetrahydrofolic acid	5-CH_3–H_4-folic acid	N^5-methyltetrahydrofolacin, N^5-CH_3–THFA, N^5-M–$PGAH_4$, "prefolic A," 5-methyltetrahydropteroylglutamic acid (5–CH_3–H_4PteGlu)
5,10-methenyltetrahydrofolic acid	5,10–CH=H_4-folic acid	5,10-Methenyltetrahydropteroylglutamic acid (5,10-CH=H_4-PteGlu), anhydroleucovorin
5-formimidoyltetrahydrofolic acid	5-HCNH–H^4-folic acid	5-Formimidoyltetrahydropteroylglutamic acid (5–HCNH–H_4–PteGlu) (formimino)

[1] Recommended by the IUNS Committee on Nonmenclature (1971) Tentative rules for generic descriptors and trivial names for vitamins and related compounds. J. Nutr. *101*, 133–140.

jugase has been used we will use the term "total folacin."

Polyglutamates are the folic acid derivatives in which the glutamic acid residue is combined through a peptide bond with another glutamic acid residue which may or may not be similarly combined with γ-glutamyl residues. In this paper polyglutamate refers to any folacin containing one or more glutamyl residues in the side chain. They will be designated as pteroyl-diglutamic acid, pteroyltriglutamic acid, etc. In the literature the terms "PteGlu$_3$, folic acid glu$_2$, and triglutamate" are used interchangeably (table 1). In many papers polyglutamates refers to those folacins that cannot be utilized by *L. casei* without prior treatment with conjugase.

Metabolic role of folacin

The folacin coenzymes are involved in the transfer of one-carbon units throughout the body. They are required for the oxidation and reduction of single carbon units; for the synthesis of purine and pyrimidine bases; and for the metabolism of amino acids such as serine-glycine interconversion, methionine methyl group biosynthesis, and the degradation of histidine. In addition, jejunal glycolytic enzymes are induced by large doses (15 mg/day) of oral folic acid (624). It may also be involved in the desaturation and hydroxylation of long-chain fatty acids in the brain (130). Our present knowledge of the enzyme reactions involving folacin coenzymes has been reviewed in detail by Stokstad and Koch (712), Blakley (73), and Rader and Huennekens (598). Nevertheless, as Baker (30) pointed out, we still have much to learn about the metabolic role of the folacins, especially the peptide derivatives which are found universally.

Identifying and quantitating the folacins

In attempting to determine the kinds and amount of folacin in biological materials, investigators have encountered a number of obstacles including: the low concentration of folacin in most biological materials; the difficulty of separating the numerous derivatives; and their extreme susceptibility to destruction or change in form by heat, light, oxygen, pH, and endogenous conjugase. These problems have been reviewed by a number of investigators (42, 145).

Scientists are trying to develop better methods of identifying and quantitating the folacin derivatives in biological material; current methods are laborious and the multiple steps required increase the prob-ability of errors. Because of its ultrasensitivity, the microbiological assay has been used in most of the studies on human folacin requirements. However, it does not provide precise information on the kind or the amount of the individual folacin derivatives in the sample. Furthermore, growth-supporting activity for bacteria does not necessarily indicate folacin activity for humans (469).

Lactobacillus casei (*L. casei*), *Streptococcus faecalis R* (*S. faecalis*), and *Pediococcus cerevisiae* (*P. cerevisiae*) all require folacin. However, *L. casei* is generally used for quantitating folacin activity since it can utilize more of the folacin derivatives (table 2). It utilizes the oxidized or the reduced form and it is the only one of the three test organisms that can use the methyl derivative, the predominant form in plasma, red blood cells, and liver (73). It has been generally accepted that *L. casei* cannot utilize folacins containing more than a total of three glutamic acids. In a recent study, Tamura et al. (728) obtained identical growth response curves with folic acid, pteroyldiglutamic acid and pteroyltriglutamic acid, which indicates that *L. casei* can use all three derivatives equally well. In addition, they found that, on a molar basis the polyglutamates, pteroyltetra-, penta-, hexa-, and heptaglu-tamic acid, are utilized by *L. casei* 65.6, 19.9, 3.5, and 2.4%, respectively, as effectively as the monoglutamate, folic acid. The early experimental results of Bird and Robbins (68) suggested that this was the case but reports of growth response due to large amounts of polyglutamates must be interpreted with caution since contamination with monoglutamates would give false values.

P. cerevisiae responds only to the fully reduced monoglutamates, while *S. faecalis* can utilize either the oxidized or the reduced form. In addition, *S. faecalis* utilizes folic acid and pteroyldiglutamic acid equally well (45). *S. faecalis* can also utilize pteroic acid, a part of the folic acid molecule (fig. 1).

The folacin activity of a compound varies according to the microorganism used for assaying, as recently demonstrated by Dong and Oace (190). In addition, the microbiological assay itself is subject to variability (627). Butterfield and Calloway (94) reported that the coefficient of variation for the *L. casei* assay was approximately 25%. The mean serum *L. casei* folacin activities of normal subjects, obtained by 17 different laboratories, ranged from 4.6 to 15.8 ng/ml (532).

As recent reviewers (145, 211), and researchers (34, 485, 732) have pointed out, numerous factors including the organism used for assaying, the standard, the source and purity of conjugase, pH, the extent of deconjugation of polyglutamates, autolysis, the degree of hemolysis of red blood cells, extraction methods, the presence of inhibitors or stimulants other than folacin, the use of reducing agents throughout the assay, incubation time, and method of storing the sample may all affect the microbiological assay. Tamura et al. (728) have found that "the forms of folate added to the inoculum broth for the growth of *L. casei* prior to the last assay" influences the "free folate" activity of the material being tested. Temperley et al. (732) have reported that prior extraction by autoclaving (a common practice) results in a 20% loss of the vitamin.

The folacins may also be measured spectrophotometrically and chemically (73, 320) but these methods are too insensitive for determining the folacin content of most natural materials. Others have used animal assays and enzymatic identification of folacin compounds (320).

Many of the folacins have been separated chromatographically on paper or on columns of DEAE- and TEAE-cellulose. Herbert and Bertino (320) concluded that these methods "can be made extremely sensitive if the compounds are detected by using bioautographic techniques. . . ." Although they have been used for determining the naturally occurring folacins, they are time-consuming and absolute resolution of all the compounds still has not been achieved (727).

Folacin derivatives in food

Due in part to the rapid changes in the C_1 moiety, the state of oxidation and the number of glutamyl residues in the peptide side chain during food preparation and

TABLE 2

Microbial utilization of folacin and related compounds[1]

	L. casei	*S. faecalis*	*P. cerevisiae*
Folacin:			
Folic acid	+	+	−
10-CHO-folic acid	+	+	−
Folic acid glu₁	+	+	−
Folic acid glu₂	+	−	−
10-CHO-folic acid glu₂	+	−	−
Folic acid glu₆	−	−	−
H₂-folic acid	+	+	−
10-CHO–H₂-folic acid	+	+	−
H₄-folic acid	+	+	+
5-CHO–H₄-folic acid	+	+	+
10-CHO–H₄-folic acid	+	+	+
5-HCNH–H₄-folic acid	+	+	+
5,10-CH₂–H₄-folic acid	+	+	+
5-CH₃–H₄-folic acid	+	−	−
5-CHO–H₄-folic acid glu₁	+	+	+
5-CHO–H₄-folic acid glu₂	+	−	+
Related compounds:			
Pteroic acid	−	+	−
10-CHO pteroic acid	−	+	−
5-CHO–H₄-pteroic acid	−	+	−

[1] Adapted from Johns, D. G. & Bertino, J. R. (1965) Folates and megaloblastic anemia: A review. Clin. Pharmacol. Therap. *6*, 372–392.

analysis, there are few data on the folacin derivatives in different foods. In addition, as much as 50 to 95% of the activity may be destroyed by cooking and/or processing (128, 363, 652).

Assays with *L. casei* indicate that about 75% (range, 50 to 97%) of the folacins in a sample meal or diet have peptide chains containing more than two glutamic acids (94, 101, 123, 353, 354, 365, 386, 441, 529, 541, 578, 637, 639). Perry (578), who recently separated the derivatives chromatographically, found that after cooking 89% of the folacins in a mixed Western type meal were polyglutamates not readily available to *L. casei* before treating with conjugase. Polyglutamates also account for 85 to 90% of the folacin activity in liver (67, 664, 785) and 95 to 97% in yeast (94, 648).

Streiff (718) and Tamura and Stokstad (729) found that most of the folacins in orange juice were "free" (caused a response by *L. casei* before conjugase treatment). Others (94, 190) have reported that one-half of the activity was not available to *L. casei* without conjugase treatment. When Tamura et al. (727) separated the folacins in orange juice by column chromatography, they found that they were predominantly reduced methylated polyglutamates; the peptide side chain of more than one-half of the folacins contained three or more glutamyl residues. Tamura et al. (727) suggested that the difference in the microbial and chromatographic assays might be due to the fact that *L. casei* is also able to utilize glutamyl peptide side chains containing more than two glutamyl residues, albeit more slowly (728).

Some of the apparent differences in polyglutamate content in foods may also be due to the action of intrinsic enzymes that degrade the γ-glutamyl peptide. They are present in most animal and plant tissues (73, 726) and they can produce large changes in the naturally occurring folacins during extraction and analysis. Chan et al. (106) and Tamura et al. (726) estimated that at least 85 to 90% of the folacins in cabbage are polyglutamates. However, if cabbage is homogenized 15 minutes before inactivating the intrinsic conjugase, then the total activity is the same but only 14% of it is not utilized by *L. casei* (726). Investigators (67, 560) have demonstrated that freezing and thawing also causes deconjugation and oxidatively alters the C_1 moiety. The methyl form is converted to the more stable 5-formyl form.

The folacins from both plant and animal sources contain formyl and methyl derivatives. Perry (578) has recently reported that in a cooked meal 60% of the folacin derivatives were methyl and 33% were formyl derivatives. Cossins and Shah (151) detected a similar pattern in whole leaf extracts of pea seedlings. Those in liver (561, 664), orange juice (190), milk (191, 663), egg (94), and cabbage (106) are predominantly methyl derivatives. But most of the folacins in yeast (648) and soybeans (663) are formyl derivatives. In the early 1960's Butterworth et al. (101) and Santini et al. (638) found three folacin derivatives in food when they separated them chromatographically: 10-CHO-folic acid (55%), 5-CHO-H$_4$-folic acid (34%), and folic acid (11%).

Recent reports in the literature indicate total folacin content of foods and the effects of plant variety, processing and storage, but few researchers have quantitated the derivatives. Many questions remain to be resolved about the kinds and amounts of the different folacins in food "as eaten."

Food composition tables

Unfortunately when Toepfer et al. (740) assayed the folacin activity of food in 1951, the importance of protecting food folacin during assay by adding ascorbic acid had not been recognized. More recent assays of the folacin in food (94, 314, 363, 578, 718) indicate that in the surveys and studies where these tables have been used, folacin intake has been underestimated. The folacin values are also underestimated in the tables compiled by McCance and Widdowson in 1960 (510). Moscovitch and Cooper (539) have found that diets analyzed in their laboratory by newer methods contained 4.1 to 4.7 times more *L. casei* folacin activity than the amount calculated from the tables of Toepfer et al. (740). Thenen (733) therefore suggested that, until it is possible to prepare new tables, dietary folacin intake should be estimated by multiplying the total folacin values of Toepfer et al. (740) by a factor of 4.4. Perloff and Butrum (577) have recently published a compilation of provisional data on the folacin in selected foods.

EARLY STUDIES OF REQUIREMENTS

Folacin deficiency was probably first recorded by Biermer in 1872 (63) when he described an anemia among pregnant women which he called "progressive pernicious anemia." But the possibility that this new type of anemia in pregnant women might be related to a dietary deficiency was not considered until 1919 (569). During the 1930's Wills and Mehta (806) found that cases of macrocytic anemia in pregnant Indian women, which were distinct from pernicious anemia, responded to treatment with either Campolon, a crude liver extract, or Marmite, an autolyzed yeast extract (802, 803). Investigators in England (750), the United States (745), and Holland (275) also reported the effectiveness of Marmite in treating patients with macrocytic anemia.

Monkeys fed a diet similar to that of the Indian women also developed a macrocytic anemia which could be cured with crude extracts of liver, yeast, or wheat germ (804). This anemia, however, did not respond to the highly purified liver extract used to treat pernicious anemia (804). Day et al. (180) reported similar experimental results with monkeys.

Early investigators also reported cases of megaloblastic anemia in infants which responded to liver preparations (23, 38, 71, 224), Brewer's yeast (38), or fresh fruits and vegetables (752). These have been reviewed by Zuelzer and Rutzky (818). The anemia was frequently preceded by a respiratory infection, diarrhea and/or vomiting (23, 38, 224). In some cases the anemia was attributed to an apparent lack of a required substance in the goat's milk formula (38, 574, 617, 752).

Later researchers have estimated that the autolyzed yeast used in the initial studies (275, 745, 750, 802) supplied 0.05 to 1.4 mg folacin activity/day, depending on the method of analysis (109, 254, 780). In treating tropical macrocytic anemia, Wills and Evans (805) frequently gave 2 ml/day of Campolon, the crude liver extract. After World War II, Girdwood (254) assayed two different batches of Campolon, which had been manufactured in Germany just before the war. One contained 0.7 μg S. faecalis folacin activity and 2.9 μg cyanocobalamin/ml, the other, 4.5 and 8.0 μg/ml, respectively (254). The report, however, did not indicate whether conjugase was used before measuring total folacin. Recent studies indicate that most of the folacins in liver are polyglutamates (73, 96, 118, 561, 664, 785) and 67 to 100% of the folacin activity is present as the methyl derivative (73, 96, 118, 561, 785). Neither of these forms is active for S. faecalis (table 2).

Meanwhile, other scientists were busy trying to isolate and identify the newly discovered metabolically active compound(s). The history of the discovery, isolation, and identification of the various folacins has been thoroughly reviewed by Jukes and Stokstad (397). In 1945, Angier et al. (9) synthesized a new compound which they said was identical with the L. casei factor from liver and determined its structure (10): N-[4-{[(2-amino-4-hydroxy-6-pteridyl) methyl] amino} benzoyl] glu-

tamic acid. Clinical investigators found that this compound, commonly referred to as folic acid, elicited a prompt and satisfactory hematological response in patients with Addisonian pernicious anemia (6, 534, 696, 756), tropical and non-tropical nutritional macrocytic anemia (169, 265, 411, 690, 691, 756), macrocytic anemia in pregnant women (51, 534), and sprue (164, 166, 534, 690, 691, 693, 694). These initial clinical experiments with folic acid have been reviewed by Darby (162). Folic acid, given orally or parenterally, also had a distinct curative effect on the megaloblastic anemia of eight infants, 4 to 12 months old (817). In those cases that were followed for 3 to 20 months after the treatment was initiated, there was no reoccurrence of the anemia.

In 1946, Spies (691) tentatively recommended an intake of 20 mg folic acid/day, parenterally or by mouth for patients with megaloblastic anemia. Later he and his associates (690) reasoned that, since 10 mg/day by mouth produced a maximum hemopoietic response in five patients with tropical sprue, the minimal amount required by these patients might be lower. Suarez et al. (721) suggested that 2.5 to 5 mg folic acid daily was probably an adequate dose for the majority of tropical sprue patients. After reviewing the early studies on sprue patients Darby (162) pointed out that there was no appreciable difference between the maximum reticulocyte response reportedly induced by daily oral doses of 5 mg folic acid and quantities 4 to 40 times this amount.

Between 1948 and 1954, numerous investigators found that the megaloblastic anemia of pregnant women, both in tropical and in temperate climates, responded satisfactorily to large doses (>5 mg/day) of folic acid. Many of these early reports have been reviewed by Lowenstein et al. (465). Others reported from the United States (692), Canada (465), England (226, 247), and Ireland (393) that supplemental iron plus 3 to 15 mg folic acid/day prevented megaloblastic anemia in pregnant women from high risk populations.

Some early investigators tried to calculate human folacin requirements from the results of animal studies. Day and Totter

(181) estimated that young monkeys receiving 325 kcal daily required 50 to 100 μg folic acid/day. So they postulated that the human requirement was between 300 and 600 μg folic acid daily. Darby et al. (165) reported that, according to a personal communication with Jukes, the chick's requirement for *L. casei* factor was one-fifth to one-tenth that of its requirement for riboflavin. Thus Darby et al. (165) calculated that "If a similar ratio holds in man, a maintenance dose would be of the order of 0.1 to 0.2 mg/day, while curative doses may well be in the magnitude of a milligram daily."

STUDIES ON ADULT MAINTENANCE REQUIREMENTS

Therapeutic studies

Soon after investigators established the effectiveness of folic acid in treating megaloblastic anemia, they began to recognize that the large amounts they were using temporarily masked vitamin B_{12} deficiency. It caused a hematological response in these patients but it did not deter the neurological degeneration (306, 757). There was, therefore, considerable interest in determining the minimal amount of folic acid required to cure folacin deficiency. In many of the studies the patients had tropical sprue. Since it has been shown that this condition impairs the absorption of both the mono- and the polyglutamyl forms of folacin (150, 346), these papers will be discussed separately.

Hematological values

Some investigators (500, 705) found that 400 μg folic acid daily by mouth produced an immediate hematological response. After observing striking reticulocytosis attended by increased hemoglobin, leukocyte and platelet counts, and symptomatic improvement, Marshall and Jandl (500) concluded that 200 to 500 μg folic acid/day should prevent folacin deficiency without endangering patients with undiagnosed pernicious anemia.

Others (272, 304, 313, 380, 385, 532, 592, 650) have found that 100 to 250 μg folic acid daily usually stimulated reticulocytosis and increased leukocyte and platelet counts, but more was required to quickly correct other signs of folacin deficiency. Jandl and Gabuzda (385) reported that daily intramuscular injections of 125 to 250 μg folic acid produced hematologic responses in two men with scurvy and associated anemia while they were maintained on a scorbutic diet which was also low in folacin. Adding vitamin C caused a second reticulocyte response but a regular diet produced no further response. Their food intake had been inadequate for about 7 months prior to hospital admission.

Gough et al. (272) reported that supplementing a low folacin diet containing "15 μg folic acid per day" with 200 μg folic acid daily produced a satisfactory reticulocyte response in two megaloblastic women within 2 weeks. Their hemoglobin values reached acceptable values within a month. They calculated from the food composition tables of McCance and Widdowson (510) that the food in their previous diet contained 13 to 14 μg "folic acid" before it was cooked. The calculated intake of five other deficient patients ranged from 20 to 30 μg daily.

Lawler et al. (449) found that treating a folacin deficient subject with 100 μg folic acid for 9 days significantly improved her bone marrow cytology and chromosomal morphology; the frequency of chromosomal breakage decreased from 60 to 4%. According to Schmid and Frick (650), 100 μg folic acid for 3 weeks effectively induced reticulocytosis and a week after treatment ended, the patient's serum iron had decreased from 300 to 61 μg/100 ml, indicating red cell synthesis. Six weeks later, however, some megaloblasts remained in the marrow and plasma folic acid clearance tests indicated that she was still deficient. After receiving 15 mg folic acid daily for 4 days, intramuscularly, her hemoglobin increased from 11.3 to 12.8 g/100 ml.

The anemia of a 45-year old woman who had been taking anti-convulsant drugs (diphenyhydantoin and phenobarbital) for 4 years did not improve after 1 week of eating a hospital diet (193). But her hematologic response to 25 μg folic acid/day was dramatic. When she was discharged 41 days after the start of folic acid therapy, her hemoglobin was 13.4 g/100 ml blood.

Druskin et al. (193) thus concluded that "man's daily requirement of folic acid needs further revision downward." It has since been shown that diphenylhydantoin and phenobarbital interfere with the utilization of folacins (259, 702).

In another severely depleted woman, 50 μg folic acid daily for 12 days was insufficient to affect reticulocytosis (352). There was, however, a marked mental change within 6 hours, soreness of mouth disappeared by day 2, papillation of tongue was normal by day 10, platelet and white cell counts by days 4 and 7, respectively, and by day 12 she had gained 3 pounds. A normal diet plus 5 mg folic acid daily produced immediate reticulocytosis, followed by increased hemoglobin, hematocrit, and red blood cell count. Hoogstraten et al. (352) suggested that 50 μg folic acid daily, given over a prolonged period of time, might have been sufficient to induce a complete hematologic response. Ten days of treatment with 30 g of Marmite/day, a liver extract containing 15 μg S. faecalis free folacin activity and 45 μg L. casei total folacin activity, produced a reticulocyte response in five of Vinke's (759) seven patients. Three of them needed no further treatment; the other two had a second response to 15 mg folic acid daily.

Blood values

The following studies indicate that although small amounts (50 to 75 μg) of folic acid may produce a complete hematological response in folacin deficient patients this does not indicate the amount of folacin or the length of time required to replete body stores and raise the blood values to normal. Izak et al. (380) injected four groups of women with 10, 100, 500, or 1,000 μg folic acid daily for 12 to 20 days and all groups except those who received the 10 μg had normal hematological responses. But even the largest dose (1,000 μg daily for 20 days) was not enough to raise the whole blood folacin activity to "normal"; only those patients who received an oral dose of 5 mg daily for 20 to 24 days attained normal values (69 ng/ml). Izak et al. (380) pointed out that it is possible that part of the increase in red cell folacin may have been due to

folic acid uptake by circulating red cells. This phenomenon had been reported when therapeutic amounts of folic acid were used (83, 278, 377). Blood values for the individual groups receiving 100, 500, or 1,000 μg parenterally were not included. The two daily food samples which Izak et al. (380) analyzed in their laboratory after they had been prepared by the patients contained 30 μg "folate"; the raw ingredients contained six times as much.

Herbert (313) reported that 250 μg folic acid produced a dramatic hematological response in one subject after he had depleted his folacin stores by consuming a diet containing "approximately" 5 μg L. casei "folate" activity/day for 4.5 months. After eating a "regular" diet for 4 weeks however, his serum folacin activity still had not returned to pre-experimental level and his erythrocyte L. casei value was still less than 20 ng/ml. The folacin content of the diet was not indicated.

Hansen and Weinfeld (304) found that 100 μg folic acid/day, injected intravenously, was enough to stimulate reticulocytosis and produce normal bone marrow in some patients but others required 200 to 400 μg/day. More was also required to correct FIGLU excretion and increase serum and whole blood levels. In most cases, FIGLU excretion decreased after injecting 200 μg for 2 to 14 days, but those patients with initially high FIGLU excretion rates (76 to 840 μmoles/hour) did not return to normal until they were treated with 15 mg folic acid for 2 to 3 days. Chanarin (109) states that normal range is reached within 6 to 10 days if excretion is "relatively high." Moderate increases in whole blood values after 10 days of therapy were observed only in the two subjects who received 400 μg folic acid daily. Similarly, except for one subject who received 400 μg daily, serum folacin values remained in the deficient range during the 10 to 25 days of therapy. Still, there was improvement and, had the experiment been continued for a longer period of time, all tissues might have been repleted. Hansen and Weinfeld (304) concluded that 100 μg folic acid daily, as a supplement to the diet, was sufficient to prevent nutritional folacin deficiency.

From the results of two studies with

two patients on controlled diets, investigators (723, 815) have suggested that the "minimal amount" of folic acid required is in the range of 50 μg daily. Zalusky and Herbert (815) studied a malnourished 60-year old man who had been existing on coffee, doughnuts, and stale hamburgers. The patient was treated with a vitamin-free diet plus a daily intravenous injection of one g of ascorbic acid for 14 days. He then received 50 μg folic acid daily, intramuscularly, and 3 days later he began receiving other vitamin therapy. Although the 50 μg folic acid daily initiated reticulocytosis within 3 days, serum iron concentration remained elevated, conversion of the bone marrow to normoblastic erythropoiesis was incomplete, and serum folacin activity remained low (2.2 ng/ml). On the 24th day he began eating a normal hospital diet in addition to the 50 μg folic acid daily. During the next 4 weeks, his serum folacin activity increased slightly (3.7 ng/ml) and FIGLU excretion slowly returned to normal.

In the second study Sullivan and Herbert (723) found that a low folacin diet ("approximately" 5 μg "total" L. casei folacin activity) plus 25 or 50 μg oral folic acid, administered for 14 and 17 days, respectively, was insufficient to elicit a complete reticulocyte response in a former alcoholic who was folacin depleted. However, 75 μg/day effected a prompt response. She continued to eat the low folacin diet plus 75 μg folic acid daily for almost 2 years (317, 318) while ingesting ethanol intermittently. The patient's serum folacin level rose above the deficient range after 50 days; macrocytosis and neutrophil nucleus hypersegmentation disappeared after 214 and 282 days, respectively. Sullivan and Herbert (723) concluded that since her tissues were apparently gradually replenished, 75 μg folic acid daily was probably more than the amount required to "sustain normality."

Sullivan and Herbert (723) also reported that, in the absence of alcohol intake, a normal hospital diet produced reticulocytosis in folacin depleted patients. The folacin content of this diet was not indicated. Similarly, Eichner et al. (198) found that a high folacin diet (216 μg

free L. casei activity) increased the serum L. casei folacin activity of two alcoholic patients from 3.8 and 2.0 to 6 and 7 ng/ml in 11 and 19 days, respectively. Initially, the bone marrow of one patient was normoblastic; the second had mild megaloblastic bone marrow changes and thrombocytopenia. These findings are frequently observed in subjects inbibing alcohol (723).

Banerjee et al. (36) investigated the minimum amount of folic acid required to maintain normal serum and red blood cell levels (not less than 4 and 100 ng/ml, respectively) in healthy adult Indians. After six subjects had eaten a low folacin diet, which contained 15 μg "folate" (480), for an average of 6 weeks their serum folacin values had decreased to 3 ng/ml or less and their red blood cell values had begun to decline. When the diet was supplemented with 25 μg folic acid daily for 1 to 3 weeks, serum values remained stationary but all red blood cell values continued to decrease. Although the serum folacin levels of four subjects receiving 50 μg daily for 1 to 3 weeks increased substantially, only three of the six had values greater than 4 ng/ml. Red blood cell folacin decreased dramatically in three of the subjects, increased slightly in two, and stayed the same in one. Supplementing the diet of three of the six subjects with 75 μg/day for 1 week increased all serum values but the red cell content remained stationary in two of them. On the basis of these data, Banerjee et al. (36) concluded that the minimum daily folic acid requirement of healthy adult Indian subjects was 75 μg.

Tropical sprue patients. Many of the studies on the folacin requirements of patients with megaloblastic anemia have been reported from areas of the world where tropical sprue and other intestinal disorder are reportedly common. Considering the abnormalities in the jejunal mucosa and the malabsorption of both folic acid and the polyglutamates in patients with tropical sprue (150, 245, 255, 565, 566, 724), studies of folacin requirements with such patients are probably of limited value (484). As Klipstein (426) pointed out in his review of tropical malabsorption, patients with tropical sprue usually have multiple nutritional deficiencies, especially folacin, vitamin B_{12} and protein. The relationship of these nutrients to folacin requirements and the absorption of folacin in tropical sprue patients are both discussed under "factors affecting folacin requirements."

Darby et al. (167) found that 260 mg supplemental folic acid, given intramuscularly, was enough to induce and maintain remission of megaloblastosis for about 200 days in one patient with tropical sprue. Darby (161) speculated from the data of Heinle et al. that the patient may have excreted half of the dose of folic acid and thus estimated that he probably utilized about 650 μg folic acid daily.

In five other studies, the amount of folic acid required to correct folacin deficiency in tropical sprue patients varied from 25 to 250 μg/day (422, 484, 531, 565, 566, 661). Previous antibiotic therapy (422, 661), severity of deficiency (565, 566, 661), and vitamin B_{12} status (484, 531) influenced the response. In some cases 200 μg folic acid daily was sufficient for complete recovery from folacin deficiency (531, 565, 566), especially if the deficiency was not severe (565). O'Brien and England (565, 566) reported that after injecting 200 μg folic acid intramuscularly for 28 days, the serum folacin activity of 16 patients averaged 32 ng/ml. But it took several months for the intestines to become completely "normal" (565).

Sheehy et al. (661) reported that 25 μg supplemental folic acid daily elicited a hematological response in 11 of their 30 patients, four of whom had previously received antibiotic therapy. Nine others responded to doses ranging from 75 to 250 μg daily; results with the remaining patients were variable. None of these 30 patients had previously responded to a hospital diet containing 50 to 75 μg free and 1,000 to 1,500 μg total S. faecalis folacin activity. It is not known how much if any of the dietary folacin they utilized.

On the other hand, none of the 19 patients of Maldonado et al. (484) responded to a regular diet plus folic acid supplements ranging from 25 to 220 μg daily. However, three others who injested 100 μg folic acid/day on an empty stomach for 10 days and a low folacin diet containing 5 μg free and 63 μg total S. faecalis activity responded well. Maldonado et al. (484) suggested that, concomitant vitamin B_{12} deficiency may have limited their response to supplemental folic acid.

The findings of Mollin and Booth (531) support this suggestion. Three single daily injections of 1 μg vitamin B_{12} produced a brisk reticulocytosis in one of their tropical sprue patients who had not responded to 50 μg supplemental folic acid daily. It did not, however, cure all symptoms of tropical sprue. After taking both vitamins for 4 weeks she was "well" but her serum folacin activity was still "subnormal" (<4 ng/ml). She continued this regimen in addition to a "good" diet but 2 years later her ability to absorb folic acid was still "marginally abnormal." And 3 years after discharge she remained mildly folacin deficient (serum, 2.5 ng/ml).

On the other hand Klipstein (422) found that a regular diet which contained 150 μg total L. casei folacin activity/day produced brisk reticulocytosis and a sharp increment in the platelet count of one folacin deficient patient with tropical sprue who had been treated with tetracycline for the previous 10 days while ingesting a diet containing 5 to 10 μg folacin activity. Thirty-eight days after she began eating the regular diet, her serum and urinary folacin levels were higher than initial values but remained "subnormal." Giant metamyelocytes and hypersegmented neutrophils were also still present in the blood. She was therefore given an oral supplement of 25 μg folic acid daily. Thirteen days later her hematocrit reading and serum folacin were normal (37% and 9.2 ng/ml, respectively). The abnormally rapid clearance of an intravenous test dose of folic acid and low urinary excretion of folic acid activity, however, indicated that her folacin stores were still not completely replenished. As Maldonado et al. (484) concluded "besides variable degrees of absorption, variations in serum and tissue stores of folic acid and vitamin B_{12} make it difficult to establish minimum requirements of folic acid . . . in patients with tropical sprue."

Prophylactic studies

Hematological values

While studying man's minimum vitamin C requirements, Najjar et al. (545) used a synthetic diet which presumably contained no folacin activity. Since the seven young healthy subjects had no hematological signs of folacin deficiency during the 18 month experimental period, Najjar et al. (545) stated that folic acid appeared not to be a dietary essential for man. Later, however, Najjar and Barrett (544) found that the dextrimaltose in the diet furnished 14 to 17 μg *S. lactis R* folacin activity/day. According to Velez et al. (754), Goldsmith was unable to produce folacin "deficiency signs" in four healthy subjects who ate a diet containing less than 5 μg "folic acid" daily for as long as 8 months; serum folacin remained around 1 ng/ml.

Formiminoglutamic acid (FIGLU) excretion

In 1961, Knowles et al. (434) found that after four normal subjects had consumed an artificial liquid diet, containing less than 0.5 μg "folic acid"/kg for 4 to 5 weeks, they excreted excess FIGLU following a load dose of histidine (20 g). But there were no hematological changes and after 10 months, one of the subjects was still not anemic (Hb. 15 g/100 ml) (433). A fifth subject ate additional food (8 oz. milk and one raw egg) which contained 2 to 5 μg folacin activity and after 3 months his FIGLU excretion was still normal (434). Thus they concluded that the minimum folacin requirement of man was about 5 μg/day (434).

Later, these workers (209) reported that the amount of folacin in the liquid formula had been estimated from the tables of Toepfer et al. (740). When they used the methods of Herbert (312) and Waters and Mollin (769) for assaying folacin activity, they found that the liquid diet contained about 25 μg *L. casei* "folic acid" activity. The supplement contained 25 to 75 μg "folic acid," making a total intake of 50 to 100 μg/day. After taking these corrections into consideration, Fleming et al.

(209) suggested that the minimum maintenance requirement was probably 10 times more than they had originally estimated, i.e., around 50 μg "folic acid"/day. There was no indication that conjugase was used in the assays.

Blood values

The work of Denko et al. (184) suggests that 22 μg *L. casei* folacin activity/day is adequate. During a 15-week study, they found no appreciable change in the mean whole blood folacin values of five subjects who ate a diet containing 22 μg *L. casei* folacin activity/day (23.2 versus 16.2 ng/ml). Nor was there "significant variation" between the blood values of these five subjects and the two controls who received additional food containing 90 μg folacin activity/day. Prior to the experiment, all seven subjects had eaten a carefully controlled "normal" diet, containing 64 μg "folic acid" for 12 weeks.

Denko et al. (184) did not indicate that they had used conjugase in the analyses. Furthermore, these determinations were made before Toennies et al. (739) discovered that folacin activity is lost during analysis unless a reducing agent is added. These factors might account for the low blood and dietary values.

Velez et al. (754) concluded from his study with six iron deficient anemic patients with hookworm infestations that less than 8 μg *L. casei* folacin activity daily was enough to prevent the development of all signs of folic acid deficiency for at least 4 months. Although their previous diets had contained more than 100 μg folacin activity/day, their bone marrows showed megaloblastic maturation. Serum folacin values ranged from 1.6 to 13.8 ng/ml. The method of estimating dietary folacin was not described.

After receiving iron injections plus the low folacin diet for 65 to 121 days (one patient), all patients had normoblastic bone marrow and four of them had normal serum folacin values (6.8 to 8.5 ng/ml). Velez et al. (754) suggested that when all dietary requirements are provided, "the normal dietary need for folacin may be so low as to make dietary deficiency extremely difficult to produce in the otherwise undiseased or undamaged host." It is possible that their initial folacin stores were higher than average. Mahmud et al. (479) and others have found increased red cell folacin levels in iron deficient patients. Recent research indicates that iron deficiency may interfere with the utilization of the body's folacin stores (328, 568, 642, 643).

On the basis of a 5- to 6-week study with three young women, Herbert et al. (321) suggested that the minimal daily adult requirement for folic acid was 50 µg. Each woman received a tablet containing 25, 50, or 100 µg folic acid daily in addition to a low folacin diet which contained "approximately" 5 µg "total" L. casei folacin activity. Their initial and terminal serum folacin values were approximately: 9 and <5; 9 and >5, and 12.5 and 9.5 ng/ml, respectively. The red cell folacin activities before and after the experiment were 135 and 110; 160 and 168; and 80 and 110 ng/ml, respectively. Hematological values were unaffected.

Only the subject who received 25 µg folic acid/day had a clear decline in serum folacin activity. Nevertheless, Herbert et al. (321) pointed out that a longer experimental period might possibly have produced a definite decline in the serum values of the other two subjects. Perry and Chanarin (579) stated that, since all three of the subjects had lower serum folacin levels at the end of the study than at the beginning, "the only conclusion that can be drawn is that the requirement was greater than 100 µg daily."

The value of serum folacin activity as an indicator of folacin status has been widely debated (700). Most researchers have found that it correlates poorly with hepatic (176), bone marrow (155, 313, 744), red cell (286, 347), and whole blood values (230) of non-anemic subjects. A few have reported good correlation between the serum and hepatic folacin values of some hospital patients (118, 452). Eichner et al. (198) suggested that there are two different plasma levels—one reflecting the immediate dietary intake and the other reflecting the folacin status. Changes in red cell folacin values of subjects eating a low folacin diet show little change for the first 40 to 50 days (198, 230).

Survey data

Although data from surveys are not precise, a comparison of nutrient intake with nutritional status in a given population provides general guidelines for estimating adequate and inadequate amounts of dietary folacin.

Estimates of the folacin content of the diet of healthy adults vary with the locale and the assay method used. Early estimates of the mean folacin intake of healthy adults ranged from 62 µg L. casei folacin activity (185) to 47 µg total S. faecalis folacin activity for a poor diet, 157 µg for a low-cost diet, and 193 µg for a high-cost diet (486). In 1962, Santini et al. (637) reported that the mean total S. faecalis folacin content of rural and urban Puerto Rican diets was 369 and 588 µg/day, respectively. Folacin deficiency is not uncommon in this population but tropical sprue, which interferes with folacin absorption, is widespread in Puerto Rico. Recent reports from Japan (529, 541), Puerto Rico (639), South Africa (365), England (123, 578),[3] Canada,[4] and the United States (101) indicate that the mean total L. casei folacin activity intake of healthy adults ranges from about 194 to 2,345 µg/day.

Jagerstad et al. (384) estimated the folacin content of the diet of healthy Swedish men (10) and women (10) with "normal" whole blood folacin values. During 7 days, the median values for free and total dietary folacin for the men were 250 and 366; for the women, 108 and 127 µg L. casei activity. On the other hand, the data of Izak et al. (378) and Levy et al. (455) suggest that this amount is insufficient for women of child-bearing age from upper Galilee. Levy et al. (455) estimated that the mean total folacin intake of 29

[3] Chanarin, I. & Perry, J. (1977) Mechanisms in the production of megaloblastic anemia. In: Folic Acid. Biochemistry and Physiology in Relation to the Human Nutrition Requirement. (Food and Nutrition Board, National Research Council) Proceedings of a workshop on human folate requirements. Washington, D.C., June 2–3, 1975. pp. 156–168, Nat. Acad. Sci. U.S.A., Washington, D.C.
[4] Hoppner, K., Lampi, B. & Smith, D. C. (1977) Data on folacin activity in foods: Availability, applications and limitations. In: Folic Acid. Biochemistry and Physiology in Relation to the Human Nutrition Requirement. (Food and Nutrition Board, National Research Council) Proceedings of a workshop on human folate requirements. Washington, D.C., June 2–3, 1975, pp. 69–81, Nat. Acad. Sci. U.S.A., Washington, D.C.

mothers from Kiryat Shmoneh was 160.2 ± 63.3 μg L. casei folacin activity/day; for 28 fathers, 265.7 ± 98.9 μg/day. Data from previous nutritional status surveys of people from this same population indicated that 47% of the 192 women examined had whole blood folacin values below normal (378). All of the 26 men had normal values (378).

Levy et al. (455) calculated the folacin content of the diets from the data of Hurdle et al. (363) and, where no food folacin values had been published, they assayed the food. However, the amount of total folacin in these diets may be underestimated. Malin (485) has reported that Hurdle made no adjustment of the extract from pH 6 to pH 7.8, the optimum pH for chicken pancreas conjugase. Malin found that in some studies correcting the pH more than doubled the total folacin activity.

In 1968, Hurdle (359) estimated that the mean folacin intake of eight young healthy British adults was 225.1 μg free L. casei folacin activity/day. That same year Chanarin et al. (123) reported that the mean folacin content of 10 separate 24-hour British hospital diets was 117 μg free and 487 μg total L. casei folacin activity. The mean values for the diets of 16 pregnant women were 160 μg free and 676 μg total L. casei folacin activity. The bone marrow of 13 of the 100 unsupplemented patients showed megaloblastic changes in both erythroid and myeloid cells (124). Perry (578), of England, found that a "typical Western type meal" (lunch or dinner) contained 53 μg free and 497 μg total L. casei folacin activity and 13 μg free and 76 μg total S. faecalis folacin activity. In 1975, however, Chanarin and Perry[3] suggested that their earlier estimate (123) of the folacin activity in the diet of pregnant women was too high. After assaying food components and complete diets "our estimate for folate content of mixed diets is 129 to 300 μg/day. . . ." At the same workshop Hoppner et al.[4] reported that a composite diet "based on the apparent per capita consumption of major foods in Canada" contained a similar amount—103 μg free and 194 μg total L. casei folacin activity. Basing their conclusions on Cooper's data, the Canadian Bureau of

Nutritional Sciences reported that "folate deficiency in Canada is unusual, and that the folate available to more than 90% of Canadians is adequate to maintain a normal level of serum folate."[5]

Body folacin stores and depletion time

Estimates of the body "stores" of a nutrient and the length of time required to deplete them is another method of estimating daily nutrient requirements. The folacins are found in all organs, tissues and body fluids—especially the liver, kidneys, spleen, bone marrow cells, erythrocytes, leukocytes, intestinal mucosal cells, cerebral spinal fluid, and brain (73, 109, 367, 588). Studies with humans and/or animals indicate that the folacin content of these tissues decreases during folacin deprivation. There are data on the amount of folacin in the liver but little is known about the total amount of "stored" as well as "functional" body folacin used during depletion studies. Herbert et al. (321) stated that the "average" tissue folacin store of the middle class New England adult male was 7.5 ± 2.5 mg while Shinton (665) estimated that the total body folacin content was approximately 70 mg. But neither investigator gave any details of how they arrived at these amounts.

Reports of the folacin activity in human liver vary from 0.69 to 17 μg/g liver (28, 118, 251, 452, 586, 616, 768, 785). Many of these values, however, were from hospitalized patients with various diseases. The mean liver folacin values for seven males hospitalized for aortic aneurysm (118) and for five patients (one male and four females) who were undergoing elective cholecystectomy or donor nephrectomy (785) were similar (7.4 and 7.44 μg/g wet liver). Using 1,500 g as the mean weight of an adult human liver (575), the mean L. casei value is approximately 11.1 mg/ liver. Romine (616) reported that the mean L. casei folacin value for 14 patients with heart disease was 5.85 μg/g wet liver.

We found three controlled studies of the hematological and clinical sequence of

5 Cooper, B. A. Report of a project supported by Health and Welfare, Canada, 1976. Cited by: Bureau of Nutritional Science (1977) Food Consumption Patterns Report, Nutrition Canada, Ottawa.

events during folacin depletion (195, 230, 313). Herbert (313) reported the folacin deficiency signs of a healthy 35-year old male who consumed a low folacin diet for 19 weeks. Gailani et al. (230) recorded the signs of folacin deficiency in seven patients with advanced neoplastic diseases who ate a semisynthetic folacin-deficient diet for varying periods of time. One of these patients, a 63-year old man with a tumor, was followed for 140 days. The man was active and "remained cheerful throughout the dietary treatment." In these two studies, the symptoms of deficiency and time of onset were similar. Since exact figures for some of the pertinent data are not given in the text of these two papers, where necessary they will be "approximated" from the charts. O'Brien (564) reported that the chronologic development of folacin deficiency is similar in patients with tropical sprue. In the third study, Eichner and Hillman (195) also recorded the clinical sequence of events during folacin deprivation but their findings will be discussed separately since alcohol suppresses hematopoiesis (723).

Gailani et al. (230) reported that the original serum folacin value of their patient was low (3.3 ng/ml) and after an initial rapid drop it slowly declined to 0.35 ng/ml by day 127. His original whole blood folacin value was "approximately" 70 ng/ml and there was no apparent decrease during the first month. A slight drop was noticed by day 40 and by the end of the study whole blood folacin had fallen by more than 60%. The folacin activity in his leukocytes declined from 37 ng/10^9 cells on day 12 to 2.75 ng/10^9 on day 137 but there was no definite change in the number of leukocytes. There was, however, some increase in the mean number of segments in the neutrophils.

By day 47 the patient's liver folacin activity was one-half the initial value ("approximately" 2.25 versus 4.5 μg/g liver) and a further marked decline took place by day 91 when it was "approximately" 300 ng/g liver. Tumor values declined similarly but at day 137 folacin activities for both the tumor and the liver had increased "slightly" compared to day 91. The marked drop in liver folacin activity by day 91 coincided with the ap-

pearance of "slight megaloblastoid changes in the erythroid series in the bone marrow." On day 137, when the study terminated, the marrow showed further increase in the abnormality but there was no "classic" megaloblastic change.

Herbert (313) also observed a rapid drop in the serum folacin activity of his subject with the first 10 days of the low folacin diet. By the end of week 3, it had decreased from >7 ng/ml to <3 ng/ml. His initial red cell folacin value was >150 ng/ml and declined to <20 ng/ml by week 17. FIGLU excretion increased at week 14; by week 7 some hypersegmentation had appeared but clearcut macroovalocytosis did not develop until week 18. True megaloblastic blood and marrow changes occurred at about day 135. Herbert (313) concluded from his study that the normal folacin reserves are adequate for a little more than 1 month. On the basis of 7.5 mg of stored folacin and the 4.5 months required for a healthy male to develop megaloblastic anemia, Herbert et al. (319, 321) calculated that the minimal folic acid requirement was approximately 50 μg/day.

Studies with experimental animals indicate that the liver (367, 547, 662, 688), kidneys (367, 547, 662, 668), and spleen (367, 547, 668) of rats injected with radioactive folacin take up a greater part of the labeled compound. Likewise, during folacin deprivation the liver (126, 279, 513) and kidneys (279, 513) are rapidly depleted. Chanarin et al. (126) found that 90% of the folacin activity in the liver and serum was depleted in 3 and 9 weeks, respectively. Rats on a sugar and water diet plus sulphathiazole, to prevent intestinal microbial synthesis, lost 50% of the folacin activity in the liver, kidneys, and serum in 6 days (513). Studies with monkeys (84) and dogs (271) also suggest that some folacin may be stored in the kidney tubular cells. Three days after administering labeled folic acid to monkeys, Brown et al. (84) found 26.4 and 0.9% of the label in the liver and kidneys, respectively. The forms of labeled folacin in the two organs were similar—mostly methylated polyglutamates.

Recent experiments indicate that intestinal mucosal cells from rats (367, 688) and monkeys (84) take up parenterally administered radioactive folacin and the label later appears in the polyglutamates (84). The large uptake of ^{14}C-folic acid by the skin and brain of folacin deprived rats indicate that these tissues have also been depleted (553). Herbert (313) reported that during his depletion study, the buccal mucosal cells of the subject "gradually and almost imperceptibly became abnormal."

Balance studies

Balance studies—a comparison of nutrient intake with the amount excreted in urine and feces—are commonly used to estimate the amount of a nutrient utilized by the body. Denko et al. (185) tried this method of estimating human folacin requirements in the 1940's. According to their findings, the mean daily L. casei folacin activity in the urine and feces of seven healthy young adults, who ate a "normal" diet containing 62 μg L. casei folacin activity/day (range, 43 to 86 μg) for 12 weeks, was 3.99 and 304 μg, respectively. Reducing or increasing dietary folacin intake had little effect on the folacin excreted (186). When five of the subjects ate a diet containing 22 μg folacin activity/day for 15 weeks, mean urinary and fecal excretions were 3 and 322 μg, respectively. Two other subjects ingested 112 μg/day for 10 weeks and excreted similar amounts. These studies demonstrated that balance studies were not a feasible method of estimating human folacin requirements.

Folacin losses from the body

Since the sources of fecal folacin activity, the metabolic end products of folacin metabolism and the method(s) of excretion are still uncertain, the factorial method of ascertaining human folacin requirements is also currently unfeasible. However, a number of investigators have contributed information about the metabolic fate of body folacins.

Urine

Numerous investigators (147, 185, 252, 253, 386, 395, 603, 605, 641, 697, 701, 703, 722, 725) have reported low urinary folacin activity (1 to 12 μg L. casei or S. fae-

calis folacin activity/day) which remains relatively constant over a wide range of dietary intake (147). Thenen et al. (734) calculated from their data that a rat lost 25 μg folacin/day from the liver, yet "the urinary excretion of folic acid by a rat on a low folate diet is less than 1 μg/day." From this they concluded that "It is apparent that the folate lost from the liver is degraded eventually either in the liver or in other tissues after redistribution." Jukes et al. (396) reached a similar conclusion 26 years earlier. Barford and Blair (37) have recently found a metabolite of folacin, 4 α-hydroxy-5-methyltetrahydrofolic acid, in the urine of rats which does not appear to be utilized by microorganisms (447).[6] (See discussion in "Bile").

After administering radiolabeled folacin, some investigators have found urinary radioactivity in the chromatographic fractions which contain ρ-amino-benzoylglutamate (394, 558) and pteridine (394). Johns et al. (394), however, pointed out that since no reducing agent was used, some of the compounds may have resulted from the breakdown of reduced folacins. Later work with rats substantiates this suggestion (72). It is not known whether other body pteridines that are ultimately excreted in the urine initially derive from folacin (231, 410), or if they are synthesized de-novo (73). Chanarin (109) suggested that "in man folate is the source of both folate coenzymes and unconjugated pteridine coenzymes and failure of supply of folate thus also affects other pteridine compounds."

Feces

Denko et al. (185) found that feces contained 5 to 15 times the amount of folacin activity ingested. Possible sources of this folacin activity include: unabsorbed dietary folacin, folacin synthesized by oral and intestinal microflora, endogenous metabolism such as that which is secreted in bile and saliva, or from the degradation of gastro-intestinal cells. There is a dearth of information on the possible metabolic end-products of folacin in feces.

---

[6] Cooper (1975) A comment on the paper presented by Barford, P. A. & Blair, J. A. In: Chem. Biol. Pteridines, Proc. Int. Symp., 5th (Pfleiderer, W., ed.), p. 427, Walter de Gruyter, New York (comment).

Bile

Bile contains a number of different "free" folacins (447, 589). ³H-folic acid, infused intravenously (447) or ingested (589), appears promptly in bile—within 30 to 45 minutes after ingestion. Lavoie and Cooper (447) found that some of the infused radioactivity appeared in bile as breakdown products of folic acid and some was associated with microbiologically active folacins. Much of it, however, appeared as an unidentified compound which contained both the pteridine and p-amino-benzoate portions of folic acid. But it did not appear to support growth of the test microorganisms. The investigators suggested that "it may be a transport form of folate or a special modification imposed on folic acid during transport across the liver." Cooper [6] later reported that this compound chromatographed in the same position as the folacin metabolite 4 α-hydroxy-5-methyltetrahydrofolic acid, that Barford and Blair (37) had found in urine. According to Blakley (73), Watanabe (767) found that rats excreted folacin cleavage products into the bile.

Reports of the concentration of folacin in bile range from 10 to 89 ng *L. casei* activity/ml (31, 316, 447, 492, 589, 605)—2 to 10 times as much as the folacin activity in serum (31, 316, 492, 589). Herbert (316) calculated from his experimental results that the daily bile secretion (about 1 liter) of an 80-year old man with pernicious anemia who had had a cholecystectomy contained about 100 µg folacin activity.

Folacin which is excreted into bile is "believed" to be reabsorbed. But both Herbert (316) and Baker et al. (31) agreed that, in the cases of diarrhea or malabsorption, folacin lost through the bile could rapidly deplete the body stores. Researchers have suggested that protein binding may facilitate folacin absorption (216–218, 375, 523, 775). Ford et al. (220) found that the bile from 10-week old piglets was able to bind 13.5 ng folic acid/ml. Retief and Huskisson (605) reported that almost half of the total folacin activity in the bile of one subject was bound (4.2 versus 9.6 ng/ml bile).

Saliva

Saliva contains folacin activity but little is known about the derivatives present, the source of origin, or their ultimate utilization. The mean values obtained with S. *faecalis*—0.1 and 0.8 ng/ml (189, 262)—are much less than mean values obtained with lactobacilli as the test organism—3.8 to 40.8 ng/ml saliva (183, 409, 481, 605). It appears that some of the folacins are in the polyglutamate form. Disraely et al. (189) found that, after treating the saliva with chick conjugase, S. *faecalis* activity increased from 0.8 to 5.04 ng/ml. And Retief and Huskisson (605) reported that about 29% of the folacin activity was protein bound.

There are data indicating that folacin is secreted from the salivary glands of humans (482) and marmosets (192). It is also synthesized by bacteria in the mouth (189, 481). Other possible sources of salivary folacin include: "food ingestion, tissue breakdown or seepage of fluids from the gingiva" (189). The data of Bruckner and Bertino (87) suggest that "leucovorin" is absorbed directly from the oral mucosa. We did not, however, find any data indicating whether salivary folacin contributes to the amount of folacin activity in the feces.

Epithelial cells

From the data on epithelial cell renewal which Weinstein (777) has recently reviewed, it appears that in humans the cells of the small intestinal mucosa are renewed every 4 to 6 days. This rapid turnover of cells would also contribute to fecal folacin activity but we are unable to find any estimates of the amount.

Dermal loss

Johnson et al. (395) found that the mean dermal loss of *L. casei* folacin activity for four subjects, during the 8 hours each day that they were kept under hot (37°) moist conditions (70% relative humidity) was 30 µg (8.8 µg/liter sweat). The S. *lactis* value was 5.3 µg/liter sweat; the ratio of dermal to urinary excretion of folacin activity was 4.9 to 1. On the other hand, Girdwood (256) reported that sweat contained 0.10 to 0.65 µg/l S. *faecalis* activity (mean, 0.31 μg). Although reviewers (205, 266, 492) have suggested that folacin may also be lost by desquamation, we have found no experimental data.

Excess folacin

We found no reports of toxicity from the intake of excess dietary folacin. A few cases of sensitivity to folic acid have been reported (117, 501, 527) but it is generally regarded as nontoxic in man. Early investigators used large amounts of folic acid (100 mg/day for 10 days) in treating patients with tropical sprue with no "apparent" ill effects (721) in patients with adequate vitamin B_{12}. Little, however, is known about the subclinical effects of excessive folic acid intake.

In 1970, Hunter et al. (358) reported that pharmacological doses of folic acid (15 mg/day) for 1 month produced mental changes, sleep disturbance, gastrointestinal symptoms, malaise, and irritability in most of their 14 healthy subjects. In double-blind placebo-controlled studies, however, neither Hellström (308) nor Richens (609) were able to confirm the findings of Hunter et al. Similarly, Sheehy (659) reported normal psychiatric analysis, electroencephelograms, small bowel mucosa and serum vitamin B_{12} values in a 62-year old doctor who had taken 15 mg folic acid/day for 3 years because of previous problems (diarrhea for 15 years and upper gastrointestinal hemorrhage).

Hunter and Barnes (356) suggested that Hellström's failure to reproduce their results might have been due "in part" to the lower serum folacin values attained by the latter's patients. The terminal mean serum values in the two studies were 120 and 50 ng/ml, respectively. Hunter et al. (357) later reported that a single large dose of folic acid (30 mg by mouth) reduced the level of the dopamine metabolite, homovanillic acid, in cerebrospinal fluid. They hypothesized that, if this is due to impaired breakdown of dopamine, an increase in dopamine concentration could account for some of the mental changes observed in patients ingesting excess folacin.

After finding that one out of eight epileptic patients who were also receiving diphenylhydantoin therapy developed seizures when they were given 7.2 mg folic

acid in a 3 minute period, Ch'ien et al. (131) cautioned that "megadoses of folic acid should be employed with great caution in all subjects" since it is not known whether it might induce seizures in certain "obstensibly normal individuals." The role of folacin in brain metabolism is still poorly understood (323).

Other reports indicate that it is unwise to give patients with megaloblastic anemia large doses of folic acid. Lawson et al. (451) reported that excessive amounts of folic acid (15 mg/day) resulted in the death of folacin depleted patients with severe megaloblastic anemia. They attributed it to "a fall in serum potassium which in the majority of cases occurred at the onset of the reticulocyte response." In 1964, Hoogstraten et al. (352) observed an unexplained seizure in a folacin deficient patient treated with 50 μg folic acid/day. And, as Katz pointed out (408), large doses ($>$400 μg/day) of folic acid can be dangerous when given to patients with undiagnosed vitamin B_{12} deficiency since it temporarily relieves the megaloblastic anemia caused by vitamin B_{12} deficiency. It does not, however, prevent the irreversible damage to the nervous system which occurs in vitamin B_{12} deficiency (306, 757).

In rats, pharmacological doses of injected folic acid (15 mg) reportedly decreased histidine catabolism (554). Massive doses—200 to 500 mg/kg body weight —caused acute renal failure (309) and renal tubule damage (540). Ford et al. (220) recently suggested that excess folic acid may have an adverse effect on the microbial population in the intestine of infants by increasing the growth of folacin-requiring bacteria but this hypothesis has not been tested.

STUDIES ON FOLACIN REQUIREMENTS DURING GROWTH

Folacin is required for cell metabolism as well as for the synthesis of purines and pyrimidines which are components of DNA and RNA. Therefore, when the total number of cells in the body or the rate of cell synthesis increases, folacin requirements also increase. In the last trimester of pregnancy and in neonates the number of new cells being synthesized is very large.

Pregnant women

More cases of folacin deficiency have been reported in pregnant or puerperal women than in any other population group (194). A number of workers have reviewed the numerous reports on the incidence of folacin deficiency in pregnancy (73, 143, 235, 465). It is more prevalent in the multiparous (73, 248, 329, 628, 789) and in those with twins (11, 33, 119, 329, 475, 628). Hibbard and Hibbard (331) reported that 73% of the folacin deficient pregnant women that they examined had shown signs of deficiency in previous pregnancy. In some countries, more than 50% of the pregnant women are folacin deficient (407). The poorer the initial nutritional status of the patients, the sooner the deficiency symptoms appear (124, 731) and the more severe they become as pregnancy progresses. The folacin requirement of pregnant women thus appears to be related to the patient's folacin status at the beginning of pregnancy.

Two investigators (140, 487) have estimated the amount of folic acid that needs to be added to the food in the diet to prevent folacin deficiency but there are no controlled studies of the dietary folacin requirements of pregnant women. In two other studies (4, 592) the patients ate a controlled diet while determining the amount of supplemental folic acid required to elicit a hematological response. Dietary folacin intake was estimated in four studies. Three groups used dietary survey information and food composition tables (144, 463, 539, 800); the fourth (124) analyzed sample diets from the experimental group. Most patients in these studies were in the third trimester. Research on the folacin requirements in the first trimester of pregnancy is lacking.

Since the diets in most studies were not controlled, one cannot be certain that the observed deficiency signs were due to pure folacin deficiency. A number of nutrients, especially vitamin B_{12} and iron, are interrelated with folacin metabolism and thus they may have an effect on apparent folacin requirement. We have therefore indicated when the diet was supplemented with these nutrients. Some investigators have "assumed" that the patients had adequate vitamin B_{12} because pregnancy is believed not to occur in vitamin B_{12} deficient women (33, 288, 381).

In addition to the criteria commonly used for evaluating folacin status, in countries where severe folacin deficiency is common, weight of the neonate and placental development have been used as criteria for estimating "minimum" folacin requirement of pregnant women. The folacin activity in fetal cord blood and liver versus the mean folacin intake of pregnant women in a given population have also been compared. Hemoglobin concentration has been measured in many of the studies (70, 93, 121, 132, 173, 247, 369, 370, 376, 520) but due to the insensitivity of the criteria, the interrelationship between iron and folacin and the common occurrence of simultaneous iron and folacin deficiency in pregnant women, studies using this criterium are of limited value for determining the folacin requirements of pregnant women. Clinicians have also debated the relationship between folacin status and congenital malformations, abortion and abruptio placentae but we did not find any reports of the mother's folacin intake.

Because of the physiological changes during pregnancy, some investigators have suggested that the "normal" values used in evaluating the folacin status of other groups are not applicable to pregnant women. Chanarin et al. (124) found that serum folacin levels were "low in pregnancy irrespective of the state of haemopoiesis." There was, however, a highly significant correlation between the dietary folacin intake of pregnant women and their red cell folacin values ($P = 0.001$). Chanarin et al. (124) therefore considered the red cell value a useful guide to body stores of folacin. The data of a number of other researchers (213, 290, 303, 382) also indicate that red cell folacin value is a better indicator of the folacin status of pregnant women than serum value. Due to the relatively slow turnover of red cells, however, it does not reflect the immediate state of hematopoiesis. Therefore, Chanarin et al. (124) concluded that there is no substitute for marrow aspiration in determining folacin status. Several critiques on the value of the various criteria for evaluating folacin status during pregnancy have been published (223, 299, 405, 419, 470, 628).

A number of studies (304, 313, 380) indicate that the folacin in the tissues of patients with megaloblastic anemia is depleted. Since this folacin must be restored before plasma and red cell values return to normal (304, 313, 380), we have divided reports on the folacin requirements of pregnant women into therapeutic (the amount required to correct the deficiency as well as meet the daily requirements of the mother and the fetus) and prophylactic (the amount required to maintain optimal folacin status) studies.

Therapeutic studies

According to Hibbard and Hibbard (333) 1.5 and 15 mg folic acid/day were equally effective in correcting the folacin deficiencies of pregnant women—hemoglobin concentration above 10.5 g/100 ml blood, normal FIGLU excretion, and serum folacin activity above 4 ng/ml. The equivalent of 1.5 mg/day also produced a reticulocyte response in all 22 patients that Chanarin and Rothman treated (120). Conversely, Dawson (173) and Luhby[7] reported that only 150 μg supplemental folic acid/day produced a hematological response in some pregnant women. Most investigators, however, have found that at least 400 μg folic acid/day is required to produce a hematological response (591, 592) or to correct megaloblastic bone marrow in pregnant women (461, 462).

The anemia of the two pregnant women whom Alperin et al. (4) treated did not respond to 100 or 200 μg folic acid/day plus a low-folacin diet containing 30 μg free L. casei folacin activity. After delivery, however, the same amounts of folacin activity produced immediate and spectacular increases in circulating leukocytes, platelets, and reticulocytes. In both subjects, after maximum reticulocyte response (6 to 10 days postpartum), the bone marrow showed no evidence of megaloblastosis. On the basis of this study and the results of other reports in the literature, Alperin et al. (4) suggested that the "minimal daily requirement for folic acid during the third trimester in women exhibiting folate deficiency is greater than 200 μg and may be 400 μg or more."

Pritchard and his associates (591, 592) found that at least 525 μg folacin activity/day was required to elicit an optimal hematological response in folacin depleted women in their 31st to 38th week of pregnancy. Some patients responded to 500 μg folic acid while consuming a low folacin diet that contained 45 μg free L. casei folacin activity (592). Others responded to a regular hospital diet, which contained 125 μg free folacin activity, plus 400 μg folic acid/day. None, however, responded to the regular hospital diet alone. If it is assumed that approximately one-fourth of the total folacin in food is "free" (101, 123) then the low folacin diet contained approximately 130 μg total folacin activity and the hospital diet, 500 μg. Since 1 mg/day supplemental folic acid produced a hematological response in all patients, Pritchard et al. (592) concluded that this amount would undoubtedly provide most pregnant women with an excess of folacin.

Lowenstein et al. (461, 462, 464) found that 200 μg folic acid/day was sufficient to reverse the megaloblastic changes in the bone marrow of some pregnant women but most of them (70%) required at least 400 μg. A few required 800 μg/day (462). Lowenstein et al. (461) observed that the oral administration of 400 μg folic acid/day resulted in a significant increase ($P < 0.05$) in the serum folacin activity of patients but the magnitude of this increase was approximately equal in patients who responded to therapy and those who did not. As Lowenstein et al. (462) pointed out, however, since dietary folacin was not considered, it is not possible to estimate the daily folacin requirements of pregnant women from these studies.

Prophylactic studies

Since the amount of supplemental folic acid required to prevent folacin deficiency during pregnancy is dependent on the initial status as well as the current daily folacin intake of the subject, these studies will be divided into two groups: (1) those that were conducted with women from

[7] Luhby, A. L., Feldman, R., Gordon, M. & Cooperman, J. M. (1967) The requirement and some aspects of folate metabolism in human pregnancy and the puerperium. Federation Proc. 26, 696 (abstr.).

populations where the people are generally well-nourished and (2) those with women from populations where symptoms of folacin deficiency are common and appear early, i.e., those with presumably low dietary folacin intake and low initial folacin stores.

Supplementation of well-nourished pregnant women. Investigators have found that 100 µg supplemental folic acid/day was adequate to maintain the antenatal whole blood (302, 303) or red cell folacin values (124) of well-nourished pregnant women. The amount to maintain serum values was, however, more variable (302, 303). Hansen and Rybo (302, 303) supplemented the diets of pregnant Swedish women with 50, 100, 200, or 500 µg folic acid/day during the last half of pregnancy. In control subjects and those who received 50 µg folic acid daily the *L. casei* activity in whole blood decreased; in those who received 100 µg, it increased significantly and the mean value at week 36 to 38 of pregnancy was equivalent to that of healthy nonpregnant women (58 ng/ml). The whole blood folacin values of 5 of the 19 women who took 200 µg daily exceeded the highest normal value for healthy nonpregnant women (95 ng/ml). In those who took 500 µg daily the mean was also above the normal range; 8 of the 17 patients had extremely high values.

Hansen and Rybo (302, 303) found that a supplement of 100 µg folic acid daily also prevented a decrease in mean serum folacin activity. Three of the 20 women thus treated, however, had values equivalent to those found in nonpregnant women with slight megaloblastic anemia (2.0 ng/ml). The mean serum value for those women taking 200 µg increased slightly from the initial level but it was still lower than the mean value for healthy nonpregnant women (6.2 ng/ml) while the mean serum value of those taking 500 µg was higher than the mean for nonpregnant women. Hansen and Rybo (303) pointed out, however, that further studies are necessary "in order to confirm to what extent the folic acid dose capable of maintaining a normal serum and whole blood concentration can also normalize the megaloblastic changes which take place in the myelopoiesis, both in bone marrow and

in peripheral blood during the final part of the pregnancy."

Fleming et al. (213) recently reported that at delivery the mean red cell and serum folacin values of Australian women who had received 500 µg supplemental folic acid during the last half of pregnancy were three and four times greater than the values for nonsupplemented women. Six weeks after delivery both values remained elevated (213).

In 1965, Chanarin et al. (122) found that 20 µg supplemental folic acid/day, beginning with week 16 of gestation, was insufficient to prevent megaloblastosis during pregnancy; there was no statistically significant difference in the mean serum values of folacin supplemented and nonsupplemented patients (5.8 versus 5.2 ng/ml). Three years later, however, Chanarin et al. (124) reported that supplementing the diets of 105 well-nourished pregnant women with 100 µg folic acid and 260 mg ferrous fumarate/day effectively reduced changes in the erythroid and myeloid cells; it also maintained normal mean serum and red cell folacin values. The mean folacin content of 111 separate 24-hour food collections from 16 of the pregnant women was 160 µg free (range, 53 to 296) and 676 µg total (range, 197 to 1,615) *L. casei* folacin activity (123).

Chanarin et al. (124) found hypersegmented neutrophils in the peripheral blood of 6% of the 101 unsupplemented women (group 1) and of only 1% of the supplemented (group 2) by week 37 of pregnancy. Megaloblastic changes in both erythroid and myeloid cells were found in the bone marrow aspirates of 13 of the 100 women in group 1 and in 5 of the 101 in group 2.

At week 15 of pregnancy there were no significant differences in serum or red cell folacin levels of the women in the two groups but thereafter the differences became highly significant ($P = 0.001$). The mean serum folacin value of the unsupplemented group declined from 6.1 ng/ml at ± 15 weeks to 4.2 ng/ml at week 38. In the supplemented group the mean serum folacin level remained constant between week 15 (6.6 ng/ml) and week 38 (6.3 ng/ml). Red cell folacin values declined continuously in group 1. In those receiving

100 μg folic acid/day there was an initial increase in the red cell folacin and this level was maintained to the end of the experiment. The mean red cell folacin value of all women at 15 weeks gestation was similar to the mean value of the nonpregnant controls—162 and 165 ng/ml, respectively. However, in the 18 pregnant women who subsequently had megaloblastic changes in the bone marrow the mean initial value was significantly lower—131 ng/ml ($P = 0.01$). The folacin intake of the unsupplemented women who did not develop any signs of folacin deficiency was not indicated.

Supplementation of patients from populations with a high incidence of folacin deficiency. Studies in populations where symptoms of folacin deficiency are prevalent indicate that 200 to 300 μg supplemental folic acid/day are required to maintain normal serum (140, 143, 800, 801) and red cell (369, 801) folacin values in pregnant women.

Dawson et al. of Britain (177) reported that eight periodic doses of folic acid (15 mg/dose) during the last trimester of pregnancy prevented megaloblastic anemia and megaloblastic bone marrow. And, according to Vanier and Tyas (747), it was also sufficient to maintain serum and red cell folacin levels in poor risk patients who had received an oral iron supplement since their first visit to the antenatal clinic. At week 38, 80% of the folic acid supplemented patients had normal serum folacin values (mean, 9.5 ng/ml). The mean red cell folacin value for the supplemented group was 379 and for the nonsupplemented, 189 ng/ml.

Vanier and Tyas (747) also reported that at 3 months postpartum, the serum folacin values of three women who had received 15 mg folic acid/dose during trimester 3 were still higher than they had been at week 28 of pregnancy and the red cell folacin activities of two of the women were higher than the values of three nonpregnant women who had received the same amount of supplemental folic acid. At 3 months postpartum the serum values of two nonsupplemented patients were lower than they had been at week 28 of pregnancy but there was little difference in red cell folacin activity. The final red

cell values of both nonsupplemented women, however, were less than those of the supplemented women. It is not known how much of the 15 mg dose of folic acid was absorbed by the patients in these studies. Several investigators have reported that as much as 75% of a large dose may be excreted into the urine (147, 394, 396).

Fleming et al. (212) found that the equivalent of 350 and 700 μg folic acid/day in trimesters 2 and 3, respectively, was sufficient to prevent low serum folacin values and hypersegmented polymorphs in 59% of the 28 Nigerian women who were also receiving antimalarial drugs and iron (600 mg ferrous sulfate/day). In trimester 2, the women took 5 mg folic acid every 2 weeks and in trimester 3, 5 mg/week. At term, only 1 of the 24 women examined had megaloblastic erythropoiesis. In the group that did not receive supplemental folic acid, 85% of the 26 patients were folacin deficient; 30% of whom had frank megaloblastic erythropoiesis.

Other British (334) and Canadian (461, 463) investigators have found that even in "bad risk" populations 500 μg folic acid/day prevented folacin deficiency during pregnancy. Hibbard and Hibbard (335) reported that 500 μg folic acid/day during the last half of pregnancy maintained serum folacin values in the normal range and all FIGLU excretion tests were negative. Lowenstein and his associates (461) compared the folacin status of Canadian women who received polyvitamin-mineral pills containing 78 mg iron (group 1) with those who also received 500 μg folic acid and 5 μg vitamin B_{12}/day (group 2). During the last trimester of pregnancy megaloblastic bone marrow changes occurred in 28% of the 130 women in group 1 whereas only 4.1% of the 65 women in group 2 showed changes. Likewise more than one-half of those in group 1 had low serum folacin activity, compared with 9.6% of group 2. A similar trend was observed in erythrocyte folacin activities.

In a second study Lowenstein et al. (463) found that at the 38th week of pregnancy 40 to 60% of their patients not receiving supplemental folic acid had low blood folacin values. The serum activity of 23% of them was less than 3.0 ng/ml. The blood values of those who received

500 μg folic acid/day, however, were generally high; more than 60% of the serum values were ≥7.0 ng/ml and 50% of the red cell folacin values exceeded 599 ng/ml. Megaloblastic bone marrow changes occurred only in 2.7% (three) of those receiving the supplement. Low serum and red cell folacin values correlated well with megaloblastosis and the marrow was normoblastic in 93% of the cases having normal blood folacin values. On the other hand, only 50% of those with low blood values had megaloblastic marrow. When 5% or more of the neutrophils were hypersegmented (had five or more lobes/cell), there was a strong correlation of the neutrophil lobe count with bone marrow megaloblastosis.

Lowenstein et al. (463) estimated from nutritional surveys that the median dietary folacin intakes of 311 subjects during trimesters 1, 2, and 3 of pregnancy were 92, 82, and 83 μg total *L. casei* folacin activity/day, respectively. These data were calculated from food composition tables for folacin activity in uncooked foods. When representative diets were cooked by methods prevalent in this population group, they contained 10 to 65% less folacin than the uncooked foods (463). Moscovitch and Cooper (539) later reported that the food tables used included those of McCance and Widdowson (510) and Toepfer et al. (740).

Although Lowenstein et al. (463) could not correlate the dietary folacin intake with the incidence of megaloblastic erythropoiesis, serum or red cell folacins, they concluded that daily folacin intakes of 82 to 93 μg were suboptimal. In view of the "supernormal" blood folacin values and the disappearance of megaloblastosis in the supplemented group, they suggested that 0.5 mg folic acid/day given during the latter half of gestation "may well be above the minimal daily requirement." Lowenstein et al. (465) attributed the low incidence of subnormal serum and red cell folacin activity and megaloblastosis among Greek women to the custom of eating liver once or twice a week.

Moscovitch and Cooper (539) have recently reported that the food eaten for 4 days by 10 pregnant women from this same Canadian population contained 206 μg free and 242 μg total *L. casei* folacin activity. When they calculated the folacin content of these diets from the food composition tables used earlier by Lowenstein et al. (463) the figures were similar in the two studies—80 ± 34.8 and 82 to 92 μg/day, respectively. Moscovitch and Cooper (539) therefore concluded from the clinical findings of Lowenstein et al. (463) that a dietary intake of 206 μg free or 242 μg total *L. casei* folacin activity was associated with a high incidence of folacin deficiency but a low incidence of frank megaloblastic anemia.

Cooper et al. (143) have found that pregnant Canadian women from the lower socio-economic level who received 200 μg supplemental folic acid daily maintained "normal" serum levels. The mean serum folacin values for 46 patients in the 38th week of gestation, 7 days postpartum, and 42 days postpartum were 7.09, 6.96, and 6.85 ng/ml, respectively. According to previous dietary surveys (464), the average "total" folacin intake of pregnant women in this population group was 66 μg/day. In view of these findings and the work of Chanarin et al. (123, 124) Cooper et al. (143) calculated that, if food folacin is absorbed one-third as efficiently as folic acid (579), a dietary intake of 500 to 600 μg "total" folacin activity/day should prevent all deficiency symptoms in pregnant women. Dawson (173), however, concluded that 150 μg supplemental folic acid/day was inadequate for those patients particularly susceptible to folacin deficiency. At term, only 12 of 20 subjects who had received 150 μg folic acid and 105 mg elemental iron/day since the 28th week of gestation had serum folacin values above 3 ng/ml.

Investigators from England (799–801), South Africa (140), and India (369) have found that 300 μg supplemental folic acid/day will prevent folacin deficiency in pregnant women from "high risk" populations. Using megaloblastic anemia and postpartum serum folacin activity as the criteria for evaluating folacin status, Willoughby and Jewell (800) concluded that pregnant women eating a low folacin diet required at least 300 μg folic acid/day. On the basis of the weekly food intake of 150 women, they estimated from the food tables of McCance and Widdowson (510) that the diet of 60% of the 350 women studied contained less than 50 μg folacin activity/day.

The women received one of the following treatments during the last 2 trimesters of pregnancy: no supplement, 105 μg iron, or 105 μg iron plus 100, 300, or 450 μg folic acid/day. The initial hemoglobin level of all subjects was at least 10 g/100 ml. Since the lowest serum folacin levels associated with pregnancy are reached during the immediate postpartum period (33, 122, 194, 685), Willoughby and Jewell (800) determined the serum L. casei folacin activity 2 to 4 days postpartum.

The mean serum value of subjects receiving iron plus 100 μg folic acid (4.1 ng/ml) was significantly higher (P < 0.05) than that of those receiving iron only (3.13 ng/ml). The mean serum folacin value of those receiving iron plus 300 μg folic acid (7.43 ng/ml) was, in turn, significantly higher (P < 0.001) than that of those receiving iron plus 100 μg folic acid. The difference in mean serum folacin values between those receiving 300 μg folic acid (7.43 ng/ml) and those receiving 450 μg folic acid (10.4 ng/ml) was also significant (P < 0.02). The median serum folacin activity of the 77 women who received 300 μg folic acid daily was the same as the median value of normal healthy nonpregnant adults (5.0 ng/ml). Megaloblastic anemia developed in 11% of the group that received no supplement, 6.2% of those who received iron alone, 2.2% of those who received iron and 100 μg folic acid, and in none of those who received iron and 300 or 450 μg daily.

Willoughby's second study (799) substantiated these findings. He determined the incidence of megaloblastic anemia among 3,599 pregnant patients, each of whom was allocated randomly to one of 5 different treatment groups (1) no supplement, (2) iron only, (3) iron plus 100 μg folate, (4) iron plus 300 μg folate and, (5) iron plus 450 μg folate at her first antenatal visit. The incidence of megaloblastic anemia in the five groups was 3.4, 1.4, 0.7, 0.3, and 0.3%, respectively. In addition to the incidence of megaloblastic anemia, Willoughby (799) also found that the mean whole blood folacin levels of

6-week old infants born to mothers in groups 4 and 5 were higher than the values of infants from mothers in groups 1, 2, and 3. The mean value of infants from mothers who received 300 μg folic acid daily (121.2 ng/ml) was significantly higher (P < 0.05) than that of infants from mothers who received 100 μg daily (105.5 ng/ml).

In a third similar study Willoughby and Jewell (801) confirmed that during trimesters 2 and 3, a supplement of 300 μg folic acid daily met the requirements of high risk pregnant women. None of their 21 patients who received iron and 330 μg oral folic acid daily during the last 2 trimesters of pregnancy had subnormal serum, whole blood or red cell folacin values and, in the peripheral blood there was no morphological evidence of megaloblastic changes, 2 to 4 days postpartum. The median whole blood value for the group (171 ng/ml) was higher than the median pretreatment value (112 ng/ml). However, by 6 weeks after delivery, the median value had decreased to 128 ng/ml.

In an "iron only" group the median and mean whole blood folacin values remained close to "normal" throughout pregnancy and the immediate puerperium. However, at 6 weeks postpartum the medium value was 48 ng/ml; 9 out of 14 determinations were less than 60 ng/ml, the lower limit of normal. In addition, immediately after delivery, the median serum folacin level of this group was lower than the median for healthy nonpregnant females—3.7 and 5.8 ng/ml, respectively. Also, 3 of the 27 unsupplemented patients developed morphological evidence of megaloblastic changes in the postpartum period.

Other investigators (303, 347, 719) have suggested that red cell folacin activity reflects the erythropoietic folacin stores at the time they are generated in the marrow some 2 or 3 months earlier, rather than the folacin stores at the time they are measured. This concept is supported by the data of Willoughby and Jewell (801) who found a significant correlation between the patient's immediate postpartum serum folacin value and her whole blood folacin level 6 weeks after delivery. On the basis of these data, Willoughby and Jewell (801) suggested that the "supranormal" median red cell folacin value at term in the folic acid supplemented group probably indicated that 330 μg folic acid/day was in excess of the daily folacin requirement during trimester 2; but the decline in whole blood folacin activity by 6 weeks postpartum indicated that this supplement just covered the average increased requirement in trimester 3. The report did not indicate whether these women were nursing their babies.

Colman et al. (140) have recently found that adding 300 μg folic acid/day to maize meal, which was then cooked into a porridge, prevented progressive folacin depletion of South African women from a poorly-nourished population who were in their last month of pregnancy. A serving of maize porridge fortified with 1,000, 500, or 300 μg folic acid or a tablet containing 300 μg folic acid/day, during the last 10 to 50 days of pregnancy, significantly increased the red cell and serum folacin values of all groups. At delivery mean serum folacin activity and mean hemoglobin concentration of the nonsupplemented (group 1) were both significantly lower than the means for each of the other four groups ($P < 0.001$). The mean serum folacin activity of group 1 was in the deficient range. All women in these studies had received supplemental iron since their first antenatal visit and none of them had hemoglobin values less than 11 g/100 ml blood when supplementation began.

The folacin activity in the diets of these South African women was not stated. In 1970, Metz et al. (522) reported that the free and total folacin activity in the two types of uncooked milled maize most commonly used in this area was 23.7 to 27 and 27.3 to 38.3 μg/kg meal, respectively. Colman et al. (139) later reported that they had assessed the individual food intake of the people in this population but they did not include their findings in the publication. The data of Margo et al. (487) indicate that more folic acid is required when it is added to bread. They reported that the rate of rise in red cell folacin activity of pregnant women from this same South African population, who ate bread made from flour which had been fortified with 900 μg folic acid, was similar to the rate for patients who received 300 μg folic acid

in tablet form or 500 μg added to maize meal.

After supplementing the diets of 95 pregnant Indian women with 60 mg elemental iron or 60 mg elemental iron plus 100, 200, or 300 μg folic acid/day from the 20th to the 24th week of pregnancy until term, Iyengar (369) also concluded that poor women whose dietary folacin was "low" required between 200 and 300 μg folic acid daily. The red cell folacin values of women receiving 200 to 300 μg folic acid increased during the last trimester of pregnancy and at 6 weeks postpartum the values remained higher. The red cell folacin activity of those who received 100 μg daily remained constant throughout the experiment. In those receiving no folic acid supplement, red cell values decreased in the last trimester and postpartum values continued to be low. In addition, the hemoglobin concentration of women taking 200 or 300 μg increased from the initial value, their babies weighed an average of 300 g more than the babies of mothers in the other groups and, at 6 weeks of age, the red cells of their babies contained significantly more folacin activity (199 and 238 ng/ml, respectively) than red cells from infants whose mothers received no supplemental folic acid (139 ng/ml).

Russell et al. (631) reported that the serum folacin levels of pregnant Iranian women were well maintained throughout pregnancy. They attributed it to the large intake (50 to 70% of their total calories) of Iranian flatbread prepared from wholemeal or from flours of high extraction rate and cooked for only 1.5 to 5 minutes. Russell et al. (632) estimated that an Iranian eats between 300 and 500 g (dry wt) of this bread/day. "The free folate content of such amounts of bread is calculated to be about 102 to 170 μg for Tanok and 213 to 355 μg for Bazari bread." Total folacin content was not determined. Gebre-Medhin et al. (238) also reported a low incidence of folacin deficiency in non-privileged multiparous pregnant Ethiopian women whose diet consists primarily of *injera* (unleavened bread baked from teff), *wat* (a sauce) and a glass of *tella* (homemade beer).

Maternal requirements for optimal fetal development

There is little information on the required maternal folacin intake for optimal development of the fetus. As Wadsworth (763) has pointed out, folacin deficiency early in pregnancy may interfere with the normal development of the placenta. We do not, however, have precise information about the intake or folacin status of mothers just before and at the onset of pregnancy. Toe (738) found a relationship between maternal red cell value at week 12 of gestation and mean placental weight. Hibbard (330) reported a relationship between red cell folacin values at week 16 of gestation and incidence of small-for-date babies.

In countries where folacin deficiency is prevalent among pregnant women, supplemental folic acid increased fetal birthweight and improved placental development (46, 369, 373, 597). Although 5 mg folic acid and 200 mg iron/day had no apparent beneficial effect on the outcome of pregnancy in well-nourished European women living in South Africa, in Bantu women it produced a significant increase in birthweight and a reduction in the number of infants born prematurely (46).

Similarly, infants born to high risk Indian mothers who received 60 mg supplemental iron and 200 or 300 μg folic acid/day weighed about 300 g more than the babies born to mothers receiving only iron or iron plus 100 μg folic acid/day (369). Investigators (373, 597) from India have recently found that babies born to mothers receiving 500 μg folic acid and 60 mg iron during the last 12 to 16 weeks of pregnancy weighed 9.1% more ($P < 0.001$) and the incidence of small-for-date babies was half that observed in the iron-only group. This improvement in birthweight of babies born to folacin supplemented mothers appears to be due to an increase in size, cell number, and protein content of the placenta (373). Garrow (234) has shown that the amount of "metabolically active" protein in the placenta is a good indicator of the normality of this organ.

Although the effect of maternal folacin intake on the folacin content of fetal liver

has not been studied, at term, the livers of fetuses of mothers from the same region of India mentioned above (371) and from Mexico (751) contained only half as much folacin activity/g liver as the livers of infants in England who died in the perinatal period [8] (2.4 and 2.54 versus 4.8 μg/g, respectively). Iyengar (369) found that in the last trimester of pregnancy 60% of the Indian women from this population had low serum (<3 ng/ml) and red cell folacin values (<90 ng/ml). The folacin status of women in England was not mentioned but severe deficiencies which affect birthweight are not common in this country (110). These data suggest that increasing maternal folacin intake increases the amount of folacin in the fetal liver but we do not know the capacity of the fetal liver to store folacin or the maternal intake required for optimal fetal stores. Human (371) and animal (651, 658) studies with poorly-nourished mothers indicate that fetal liver stores are related to fetal weight. Experiments with rats suggest that fetal hepatic folacin stores are directly related to the "adequacy" of maternal blood folacin levels and indirectly to the growth velocity of the fetus (678). In humans, however, optimal maternal and fetal blood folacin concentrations have not been clearly established (21, 25, 337, 445).

The folacin activity in neonatal blood is two to five times higher than the value in maternal blood (21, 25, 280, 337, 400, 445, 537) and maternal supplementation increases both maternal and cord blood folacin activities (188, 445). The clinical value of excessively high blood concentrations, however, has been questioned (337). As Chanarin (110) pointed out in his review of the literature, after birth, infant blood folacin values decline rapidly. The "normal" rate of decline and the biological reason for this phenomena have not been clearly established.

Landon and Hey (442) have recently found that during the first 5 days of life the amount of folacin activity excreted in the urine of neonates was more than enough to account for the observed de-

---

[8] Hussain, M. A. & Wadsworth, G. R. (1968) Liver folate of infants dying in the perinatal period. Proc. Nutr. Soc. *27,* 7A–8A (abstr.).

crease in plasma folacin activity. The mean urinary folacin activity/unit body surface area of 10 infants 31 to 40 weeks gestation was nearly eight times as high as in adult life. During this period, the plasma folacin level of the neonates halved and urinary folacin excretion approximately doubled. The effect of this high urinary excretion rate on the folacin stores of the infant is unknown. Landon and Oxley (445) found no "essential" difference in the plasma folacin activities of 6-week old infants of supplemented and unsupplemented mothers. But the whole blood (799) and red cell (369) folacin values of 6-week old infants born to mothers from high risk populations reflected the maternal folacin intake during pregnancy.

McClain et al. (511) and Herbert and Tisman (323) have reviewed some of the literature indicating the importance of "adequate" folacin intake for brain maturation. Gross et al. (276) found that 8 of the 14 African children (6 weeks to 4 years old) whose mothers had been severely deficient in folacin during pregnancy showed abnormal or delayed development in one or more of the four general areas tested. Most had developmental deficits in the gross motor area. The minimal amount of folacin required to insure proper brain development, however, has not been investigated.

The data of Hussain and Wadsworth (366) suggest that the fetal liver is depleted before the brain. In infants born to women on a "low plane" of nutrition, the ratio of brain:liver weight increased as the amount of folacin in the liver decreased. Studies with mice show that the offspring of mice that were deprived of folacin during the last week of gestation showed significant correlation on the seventh postnatal day between liver folacin and body weight and liver folacin and brain levels of DNA, RNA and protein (658). Schreiber et al. (651) observed similar results.

Investigators have suggested that folacin deficiency of pregnant women is related to the incidence of a number of complications in pregnancy such as abortion, abruptio placentae and fetal malformation. In 1964 Hibbard (329) reported that an unduly large number of his patients with abruptio placentae had evidence of folacin defi-

ciency and suggested that the deficiency might be due to a defect in folacin metabolism (329, 331).

Various investigators have reviewed the literature on the possible relationship of folacin deficiency and complications in pregnancy (13, 46, 73, 109, 249, 310, 594, 595, 713). Some of the data suggest that it may be dependent on the severity of the deficiency (46, 249, 289, 595) and/or the period in pregnancy when the deficiency occurs (335). In most studies the women were in the third trimester of pregnancy or postpartum. Wadsworth (763) and Hibbard (330) have pointed out the possible importance of looking at folacin status before or at the time of cell implantation, cell differentiation and organogenesis. Folacin deficiency has been shown to have a maximal teratogenic effect in rats between days 8 and 10 of gestation (551).

Hall (287) did not find any relationship between serum folacin activity before week 12 of gestation and malformations. On the other hand, Hibbard (330) reported that the differences in the incidence of malformations and small-for-date infants in patients with normal versus low red cell folacin values before week 16 of gestation were "highly significant." Also, four of the five patients who suffered abruption were in the folacin deficient group.

Folacin deficiency reportedly causes chromosomal abnormalities (chromosome breakage, incomplete chromosome contraction and centromere spreading) (305, 449) which can be corrected with small amounts (100 μg daily) of folic acid (449). However, it is not known whether this is related to congenital malformations in pregnant women. Hoffbrand and Pegg (348) found that the base composition of the DNA in cells with abnormal chromosomes was normal.

A number of drugs interfere with the metabolism of folacin and therefore cause fetal malformations and abortion, especially when given early in pregnancy. These include the folacin antagonists aminopterin and methotrexate and anticonvulsant drugs of the barbiturate and hydantoin group. Many of the studies on the teratogenic effects of these drugs have recently been reviewed (61, 227, 323, 689).

Folacin metabolism in pregnancy

In pregnancy, many physiological changes occur (512) which suggest that folacin metabolism in general is altered (260, 300, 332, 336). For example, both blood volume and the number of red cells increase but the proportionately greater increment in blood volume results in some diminution of hematological values. Although a comprehensive review of folacin metabolism in pregnancy is beyond the scope of this paper, in view of the importance of the effect of metabolic changes on the "acceptable" values for the criteria used in evaluating folacin status, a brief discussion has been included.

A number of the observed changes indicate that folacin is preferentially supplied to the fetus. For example, before delivery 400 to 500 μg folic acid is required to elicit a maternal reticulocyte response in megaloblastic women. But after delivery approximately 100 μg is effective (4, 47, 380, 592). This coincides with the ratio of folacin in fetal versus maternal blood (2 to 5:1) (337, 400).

Several investigators have also found that the rate of plasma folacin clearance begins to increase before week 12 of gestation, remains elevated throughout pregnancy (119, 194, 210, 300) and is most rapid at parturition (194). Although Hansen and Klewesahl-Palm (300) observed a significant correlation ($r = +0.44$) between folacin clearance rate and serum folacin activity in pregnant women and 10 days postpartum, the whole blood folacin values of these patients remained unchanged. No mention was made about whether the women were lactating. Others have also found that serum folacin activity did not appear to reflect the folacin status of pregnant women (21, 143, 491). A decrease in serum *L. casei* activity is well documented (450, 719) but the significance of a "modest" decrease (serum values >3 ng/ml) is not known. "Acceptable" serum values are controversial.

A number of researchers have suggested that a special mechanism operates to supply the fetus with the required amount of folacin (143, 280, 537). An enzyme that catalyzes the reduction of folic acid or dihydrofolic acid has been isolated from human placenta (387). Furthermore, Kamen and Caston (400) have just reported the isolation of a folacin-binding factor from normal umbilical cord serum with a strong affinity for 5-CH_3-H_4-folic acid, the predominant form in human plasma. The complexed folacin was present in concentrations equivalent to as much as 60 ng 5-CH_3-H_4-folic acid/ml serum. Free folacin activity in maternal and fetal serum was similar (6 versus 9 ng/ml) but fetal serum contained four times as much protein-bound folacin as maternal serum (15 versus 4 ng/ml). These data present a possible molecular mechanism by which the fetus can sequester and concentrate folacin across the placenta from maternal circulation. The data of Kaminetzky et al. (401) suggest that the vitamin is taken up by neonatal circulation even in the face of maternal hypovitaminemia.

Recent reports indicate that hormonal changes affect the protein binding of maternal plasma folacin (152, 498). Markkanen et al. (498) have found that in healthy humans about one-half of the serum folacin activity is bound to proteins. The majority is bound to α-2-macro-globulin, transferrin and albumin. During the reproductive years the transferrin zone of women contains more folacin activity/mg protein than in men. In middle and late phases of the menstrual cycle the binding of folacin activity to γ-globulin and albumin also increases to some extent. During pregnancy, the amount of transferrin increases and the amount of folacin activity bound to transferrin increases; after delivery it decreases rapidly (490, 493).

DaCosta and Rothenberg (152) reported an unsaturated folic acid binding protein in the serum and leukocyte lysates of some women taking oral contraceptives and some pregnant women but it was not present in samples from nonpregnant women. The significance of this unsaturated binder and why it is not found in the serum of all pregnant women is yet to be discovered. The 90% drop in the folic acid binding capacity of the leukocyte lysates from two of the women after parturition suggests that it is stimulated by the hormonal changes associated with pregnancy and oral contraceptives. DaCosta and Rothenberg (152) suggested that "hormonal induction of this protein may contribute to megaloblastosis by sequestering FH_2 an intermediary folacin coenzyme in DNA-thymine synthesis."

Although DaCosta and Rothenberg (152) did not find a definite relationship between clinical folacin deficiency and the presence of the folic acid binding protein, only 38% of the pregnant subjects with leukocyte folic acid binding protein had serum folacin activities greater than 5 ng/ml. It is possible that the concentration of this unsaturated binder might be used to indicate folacin status. Saturated folacin binding protein was not measured.

Excess FIGLU excretion during pregnancy has also been reported (194, 520, 633, 714). The cause of this phenomenon and its relationship to folacin metabolism is not clear. Metz et al. (520) and Hibbard (336) found that in most cases supplemental folic acid corrected the excess excretion yet both suggested that it indicated a metabolic change and not necessarily inadequate folacin intake. Stone et al. (714) reported that FIGLU excretion was a good indicator of folacin status but Kershaw and Girdwood (414) found no correlation between FIGLU excretion tests and serum folacin activity. Since the absorption and excretion of histidine are altered in pregnancy (125, 133), Chanarin (108) reasoned that FIGLU excretion is a poor test of folacin status. A number of factors such as iron deficiency (596), vitamin B_{12} deficiency (398), and thyrotoxicosis (530) also affect FIGLU excretion.

It appears that during pregnancy the renal tubules do not absorb folacin as well as they do normally. Landon and Hytten (443) found that healthy pregnant women excreted four times as much folacin activity as they did 6 weeks postpartum (14 versus 3.4 µg/24 hours). Fleming (210) reported similar results.

Some investigators have reported folacin malabsorption during pregnancy (113, 119, 246, 260, 790). But others have found that pregnant women absorbed folacin as well as the control subjects [9] (375, 444, 491, 516). Whitfield (790) suggested that the increased folacin requirement during pregnancy unmasked preexisting chronic conditions that impaired folacin absorption. Devi et al. (187) stressed the need for more research in this area.

Lactating women

Although some researchers have reported the amount of folacin required to maintain (521) or improve (47, 137, 523) the folacin status of the mother, most of our knowledge about the folacin requirements of lactating women has been obtained indirectly from the approximate amount of folacin secreted in the milk plus the estimated maintenance requirement of the mother.

Folacin depletion during pregnancy is not uncommon. In reviewing the reports of megaloblastic anemia due to pregnancy, Chanarin et al. (119) found that 52% of the 318 cases were diagnosed postpartum, mostly in the first few weeks after delivery. Beresford et al. (53) also found that the red cell folacin values of lactating women continued to decrease during the first 6 months postpartum but then, in the second 6 months following pregnancy, they increased slightly. The amount of folacin required to maintain optimal maternal folacin status and also provide milk containing adequate folacin for the infant therefore depends on the status of the mother at the end of pregnancy, the stage of lactation and the amount of folacin required for metabolism related to producing milk. The data of Williamson (798) suggest that the folacin requirement of female rats may be higher during lactation than in pregnancy.

Folacin in human milk

As Ramasastri (599) pointed out, before the improved methods of assaying folacin activity, investigators reported that mature human milk contained 2 to 3 µg L. casei free folacin activity/liter. More recently, however, Karlin (403) has found that the mature milk (months 4 to 9 of lactation) of healthy French women contained about 40 µg free and 60 µg total L. casei folacin activity/liter. Burland et al. (90) and Ford and Scott (219) reported similar mean values for the milk of English women—64 and 52 µg total folacin activity/liter, re-

[9] Indian Council of Medical Research (1975) National Institute of Nutrition Annual Report, Jan. 1, 1974 to Dec. 31, 1974, pp. 111–115, Hyderabad, India.

spectively. According to Kon and Mawson (435), the amount of milk produced by one English woman for 32 weeks ranged from 215 to 870 ml/day. During weeks 13 to 21, daily secretion exceeded 800 ml. These data indicate that a healthy woman secretes about 42 to 51 μg total folacin activity/day during full lactation.

Nicol and Davis (556) reported that the mean free folacin content of six samples of milk from Australian women was 14 μg/l (range, 10 to 19) but the stage of lactation was not mentioned. Human colostrum contains only about 5 μg free folacin activity/liter (403, 514, 599) but thereafter the content gradually increases until it reaches a plateau around month 4. The mean free folacin values of milk from French women at various times during lactation were as follows in μg/liter: days 2 to 7 after parturition, 5; day 8, 11; days 10 to 15, 12.9; days 15 to 30, 24; month 2, 31.6; month 3, 35.8 and months 4 to 9, about 40 μg/liter (403). In other species the folacin content of colostrum is high (217, 403). Karlin (403) suggested that women at parturition and in early lactation may not be getting adequate folacin and recommended that the effect of supplemental folacin on the amount of folacin in colostrum and early milk should be investigated.

Studies in India suggest that in general, these women secrete less milk which also contains less folacin. L. casei free folacin values for milk from "apparently" normal healthy women from the low socio-economic group were as follows in μg/liter milk: colostrum 4.4 (range 2.8 to 8.4); transitional (days 5 to 15), 8.4 (range 4.5 to 12.1) and mature milk (15 days postpartum), 16.5 (range 7.5 to 23.7) μg/liter (599). Jathar et al. (388) reported that the mean folacin content of milk from Indian mothers who were lacto-vegetarians, non-vegetarians who occasionally ate meat and non-vegetarians who frequently ate meat were 10.3, 6.6, and 10.8 μg/liter, respectively. Gopalan (267–269) found that Indian women subsisting mainly on rice secreted 400 to 600 g of milk/day. The work of Someswara Rao et al. (686) indicates that the milk yield of 148 women from the low economic level ranged between 520 and 720 ml during the first year of lactation. After 4 years, four of the women secreted an average of 340 ml/day.

According to Matoth et al. (502), the mean L. casei "total" folacin activity of breast milk from 35 Israeli mothers was 24 μg/liter. However, the mean whole blood folacin value of the lactating women (56.6 ng/ml) was significantly lower ($P < 0.001$) than the value for normal adults from this population (89 ng/ml) (379). And the mean whole blood folacin value for the 74 breast fed infants (98.8 ng/ml) was significantly higher ($P < 0.001$) than the mean value for 145 artificially fed infants (65.5 ng/ml). On the basis of a daily intake of 800 ml breast milk/day, Matoth et al. (502) calculated that the mother secreted 20 μg folacin/day. Although the investigators refer to this as "total" folacin, there is no mention of using conjugase in the assay. Matoth et al. (502) found no correlation between folacin levels in the blood and milk of individual mothers.

According to these data, the ranges of folacin activity expected to be secreted in the milk of healthy Western European (90, 219, 401, 435), Israeli (502), and Indian women from the low socio-economic group (267–269, 388, 599, 686) were as follows: 42 to 51 μg total, 20 μg "total" and 3 to 17 μg free L. casei folacin activity/day, respectively.

A number of investigators have found that folacin is preferentially supplied to the milk at the expense of the mother (521, 523, 654). Metz and Hackland (521) reported that the serum folacin values of women consuming a low folacin diet decreased rapidly but the folacin content of breast milk remained constant. About 10 days after serum folacin values began to fall, however, the folacin content of their milk also began to decrease. Small amounts of supplemental folic acid (<50 μg/day) caused an immediate increase in the folacin activity of milk but serum values failed to rise. Similar results have been observed by Metz et al. (523) in folacin deficient lactating patients. The administration of 100 μg folic acid resulted in an increase in milk folacin activity of one patient but her serum folacin and reticulocyte count remained unchanged. When a second patient was given 200 μg daily, breast milk folacin activity increased rapidly but reticulocytosis was delayed until day 10 and maternal serum folacin values remained low (523). A number of investigators have reported the presence of proteins in human milk which firmly bind folic acid (242, 496, 497, 523, 776). Waxman and Schreiber (776) recently found that the purified folic acid binding protein in human milk consisted of two basic glycoproteins which bind folacins by noncovalent bonds. Metz et al. (523) suggested that the greater affinity of the milk than of the serum protein binder for folacin may help explain why folacin concentrates in mother's milk.

Requirement studies

The results of Metz and Hackland (521) indicate that the minimum amount of folic acid required to maintain the serum folacin level of a lactating woman eating a low folacin experimental diet was 200 to 300 μg/day. Arakawa et al. (15) found that brain function maturation was delayed in infants 3 to 6 months old who were fed milk from mothers with serum folacin values less than 5.9 ng/ml (range, 3.1 to 5.8). Arakawa et al. (16) continued to examine these children and when they were 2 years old or more, the delay persisted even though their serum folacin values were then within the normal range (8.7 to 17.6 ng/ml). This change in brain function maturation may be due to folacin deficiency during pregnancy and/or lactation.

The amount of folacin activity required to elicit a hematological response in deficient patients was similar. Baumslag and Metz (47) found that three heads of lettuce daily for 6 days effected a reticulocyte response in one lactating patient with megaloblastic anemia. According to Santini et al. (638), lettuce contains 0.06 μg free and 0.2 μg total folacin activity/g. Thus her intake was approximately 250 to 300 μg/day. Colman et al. (137) studied the effects of a low folacin diet plus maize meal fortified with 100 to 500 μg folic acid. The 100 μg/day supplement (before cooking) caused a suboptimal hematological response in one of the five folacin-deficient South African lactating patients with megaloblastic anemia. A meal containing 300 to 500 μg/day produced optimal hematological responses in the other four patients.

Folic acid added to the meal is utilized less efficiently than folic acid alone (136).

Infants

The folacin requirements of premature and low birthweight infants have been studied the most extensively because of the drastic drop in blood folacin values after birth and the high incidence of megaloblastic anemia in these infants. Estimates of the folacin requirement of infants are based on the estimated folacin intake from milk, the major food in an infant's diet. However, the assay of folacin activity in milk presents several complex problems [10] (191, 543). Although the folacin content of human and cow's milk is similar (219, 403, 404), the folacin status of breast-fed babies appears to be better (502, 746). This difference may be due in part to the destruction of heat labile forms of folacin during formula preparation which breast milk does not undergo.

The criteria used in studying infant folacin requirements include: blood folacin values, blood and bone marrow cell morphology, hemoglobin, FIGLU excretion, and incidence of infection. After birth, there are physiological changes in blood folacin and hemoglobin values that need to be reviewed before discussing infant folacin requirements.

In full-term infants "erythropoiesis diminishes after birth and erythropoietin is not detected until 2 to 3 months of age as the early anemia of infants resolves" (708). In his text on infant nutrition, Fomon (214) also points out that hemoglobin concentration gradually declines and the total iron content of the liver increases from about 30 mg at birth to 100 mg at age 3 months. In premature infants, however, the fall in hemoglobin significantly exceeds that of full-term infants and there is a direct correlation between birthweight and the magnitude of the fall. The exact reason for this phenomena is not well understood. Stockman (708) has recently reviewed the "anemia of prematurity."

At birth, the plasma folacin values of

[10] Cooperman, J. M., Luhby, L. & Shimizu, N. (1972) The folic acid content of milks. Proc. Western Hemisphere Nutr. Congr. III, Aug. 30 thru Sept. 2, 1971, Miami Beach, Fla., pp. 381–382, Futura Publishing Co., Inc., Mt. Kisco (abstr.).

both premature and full-term infants are higher than "normal" adult values (746, 748). After birth, the plasma and red cell folacin values of both groups decline. However, the fall in blood folacin values of premature infants (90, 668, 720, 748) is steeper and reaches minimum values at an earlier age than those of full-term infants (502, 746). The steepest drop occurs in infants with the lowest weight at birth (612, 668, 720, 749).

The significance of this rapid decline in infant blood folacin values is not known. Some consider it physiological (576, 708); others suggest that the decline indicates folacin status (502, 503, 670, 746). Amyes et al. (7) recently reported that the red cell, plasma, and liver folacin values of various experimental animals also fall after birth. We found no controlled studies on the folacin intake and blood folacin values of healthy infants at periodic intervals.

Premature infants

Reports in the literature suggest that the folacin requirements of premature infants are related to their weight at birth[8] (243, 668, 720), rate of growth (243), and maternal folacin status (178, 338). In 1946, Zuelzer and Ogden (817) successfully treated the megaloblastic anemia of 25 infants with folic acid and suggested that in cases in which megaloblastic anemia developed during the first 3 months of life, prematurity was a contributing factor. Since then other clinicians have reported cases of megaloblastic anemia (273, 417, 748, 818) or megaloblastic changes in the bone and blood cells (243, 720) of premature infants, most of whom were 3 to 8 weeks old and weighed less than 1,700 g at birth. Ghitis and Canosa (243) found that 4 of the 10 infants with birthweights less than 1,625 g, who had gained more than 700 g by the time they were 30 to 57 days old, had megaloblastic changes in their bone marrow. These data suggest that since folacin is required for the synthesis of DNA, which is essential for cellular proliferation, rapidly growing premature, and low birthweight infants may need more folacin per unit body weight than full-term infants.

Most of the work on the folacin requirements of premature and/or low birth-weight infants has been done in the United Kingdom with infants weighing less than 1,800 g. The folacin activity in the formula was estimated in five studies (90, 243, 576, 612, 748) but the amount of formula ingested at different ages and the method of preparing the formula by the individual mothers were usually not indicated. Investigators (401, 502, 543) have found that 17 to 74% of the folacin activity in milk can be destroyed by drying, terminal sterilization, or boiling. Reheating milk leads to even greater losses (92, 502). According to Ford and Scott (219) these are common practices in the preparation of the formula of premature infants. It is also a common practice to feed premature infants skimmed or low-fat (half-cream) milk (748) but cream is reportedly a rich source of folacin (494, 497). Some investigators mentioned that "other" foods were added to the diet of 2- to 4-month old infants (338, 412, 576, 612, 613, 748) but the folacin content was not estimated. We found no studies with non-processed human breast milk. However, the effects of giving premature infants supplemental folic acid has been studied by several researchers (90, 178, 243, 412).

Infants weighing less than 1,800 g. In three studies (90, 243, 748) infants with birthweights less than 1,800 g were fed formulas containing 14 to 53 μg free *L. casei* folacin activity/liter and during months 2 and 3 all groups had some signs of folacin deficiency. Ghitis and Canosa (243) found that at day 50 of life, three of the four premature South American infants who had been fed an autoclaved powdered milk formula that provided 3 to 5 μg folacin activity/kg body weight per day (14 to 22 μg/liter) had moderately low serum folacin activities (3.2 to 4.4 ng/ml) and one was borderline (5.6 ng/ml). The serum folacin activities of three similar infants who received 50 μg supplemental folic acid/day for 35 days in addition to the folacin in the formula were 11.2, 13.3, and >20 ng/ml.

Vanier and Tyas (748) reported similar results. The mean serum folacin value of 20 premature English infants (birthweight, 1.1 to 2.0 kg; mean 1.4 kg) 2 to 3 months old, who had been fed a partially defatted powdered milk which contained 17 μg folacin activity/liter for the first 2 months was 4.8 ng/ml. Vanier and Tyas (748) calculated that "an infant weighing 2 kg might have a folate intake of as little as 7 μg/day." From month 2 forward, depending on the infant's weight, semi-solid foods and full-cream milks were gradually introduced. The folacin content, however, was not mentioned. In a previous study they (746) reported that full-cream powdered milk contained 26 μg/liter folacin activity.

By months 2 to 3 the initial mean whole blood and red cell folacin values (343 and 698 ng/ml) of these 20 infants had decreased to 41 and 164 ng/ml, respectively. Six of the infants had abnormal FIGLU excretion and hypersegmented neutrophils. At age 6 to 8 months, however, the mean serum, whole blood, and red cell *L. casei* folacin activities (8.9, 114 and 229 ng/ml, respectively) and body weights of all infants were comparable to the values of full-term infants 3 to 4 months old. On the basis of these data Vanier and Tyas (748) concluded that "low folate stores are primarily due to an inadequate intake." They suggested that with very low birthweight (<1.5 kg), infants who fail to thrive during the first few weeks and those who suffer from infection would benefit from supplemental folic acid.

Burland et al. (90) compared the folacin status of 10 low birthweight infants who received intramuscular injections of 100 μg folic acid every other day from day 5 of life to day 33 with 20 untreated low birthweight infants. All of them were fed an evaporated milk formula which contained 68 μg total and 53 μg free *L. casei* folacin activity/l. The mean folacin intake of 1-week old infants was 13.6 μg total and 10.6 μg free; at age 5 weeks, 40.8 μg total and 31.8 μg free. The food intake of each infant was carefully measured. In the unsupplemented group, the initial mean serum (26.5 ng/ml) and red cell (581 ng/ml) folacin values had dropped to 4.3 and 159 ng/ml by day 28 and month 3, respectively. By month 6, however, both blood values had increased and there was no significant difference in the red cell values of the supplemented and unsupplemented infants. At month 3 a number of subjects also had neutrophils with five lobes which "might suggest" subclinical

deficiency. Throughout the 9 month observation period, the supplemented group remained "normal" by all three criteria. Therefore, Burland et al. (90) concluded that the folacin supplied by milk alone was inadequate and recommended that low birthweight infants ($\leq$2,000 g) receive supplemental folic acid "in the early months to prevent depletion and subclinical folate deficiency."

Likewise, Strelling et al. (720) found that all six premature English infants (birthweight <1,500 g) who were fed an evaporated milk formula had megaloblastic changes in the buffy coat preparations at weeks 7 to 11. Similar changes were found in 3 of the 18 infants with birthweights of 1,500 to 1,800 g and in 2 of the 30 who weighed more than 1,800 g at birth. The more rapid depletion of folacin in the smallest babies may be partially accounted for by the fact that they have smaller livers and therefore less total folacin activity per liver [8] (371). The folacin content and method of preparing the formulas were not indicated. Ford and Scott (219), however, reported from England at about the same time that samples of seven brands of evaporated milk diluted to be equivalent to total solids content of fresh cow's milk contained 32 to 49 μg total *L. casei* folacin activity/liter. Three of the seven brands contained 27 to 39 μg/liter when they were diluted as recommended by the manufacturer for feeding 10- to 11-pound babies.

On the other hand, Pathak and Godwin (576) recently reported that at a mean age of 40 days (range, 21 to 60) the red cell folacin activities of 10 healthy premature American infants (mean birthweight, 1,339 g), fed a standard evaporated milk formula containing "130 μg/liter folic acid," exceeded 160 ng/ml and peripheral blood smears showed no oval macrocytes or hypersegmented polymorphs. Cereals were added to the diet at 4 to 6 weeks or when weight exceeded 2,500 g, vegetables at 6 to 8 weeks and meat at weeks 10 to 12. No analysis of the folacin content was given. Although three infants had serum values less than 4 ng/ml at days 28 to 42 of life, Pathak and Godwin (576) considered the drop "physiologic" and concluded that the necessity for supplemental folic acid therapy was "not definite." Vanier and Tyas (748) reported that a milk product containing more than 100 μg *L. casei* folacin activity/liter produced an immediate hematological response in a 2-month old folacin deficient infant.

Infants weighing more than 1,800 g. There are no controlled studies on the folacin requirements of premature and low birthweight infants weighing more than 1,800 g. In the four reports (178, 338, 412, 612, 613), the investigators have been primarily concerned with the effects of infant and maternal folic acid supplementation.

Roberts et al. (613) concluded from two field studies that the drastic drop in the hemoglobin concentration of premature infants could be modified by supplementing the infant's diet with folic acid. In Hospital B, 44 infants were fed boiled human breast milk containing 1.0 to 7.5 μg free folacin *L. casei* activity/liter (3 μg/day) until mixed feeding was started at about month 4. This study was reported in detail in 1969 (612). In Hospital A; 66 infants, who were mainly fed a powdered milk preparation and then "full-cream powdered milk," also received 100 μg folic acid from day 28 until they were 6 months old. All mothers had received supplemental folic acid since their first antenatal visit to the clinic (group B, 3.4 mg and group A, 0.4 mg/day).

Initially, the mean hemoglobin level of group A was "significantly" higher than the mean value of group B (19.2 versus 17.3 g/dl, respectively). For the period, days 20 to 29, the mean values of groups A and B were similar (13.4 and 14.2, respectively). At week 8, however, when the mean hemoglobin values of both groups reached their lowest levels, the mean for group A (10.3 g/dl) was higher than the mean for group B (8.3 g/dl). Thereafter, the "increase for both groups was significant, and the rates of increase were not significantly different." The mean increment for both groups was 0.023 g/dl per day. At day 180 the hemoglobin level of group B had just reached the level found in group A at day 80.

The mean red cell folacin activity of group B continued to drop throughout the study while the level for group A began increasing 10 days after supplementation, reaching a maximum at day 80 (761 ng/ml).

At 6 months of age the mean values for groups A and B were 487 and 103 ng/ml, respectively. These data indicate that folacin intake of infants in group B was inadequate (613). In the earlier study (group B), Roberts et al. (612) found a significant relationship between serum folacin activity and hemoglobin levels and between red cell folacin and hemoglobin up to the age of 6 months.

The findings of others, however, do not support the conclusion of Roberts et al. Burland et al. (90), studying babies that weighed less than 1,800 g at birth, observed no difference in the hemoglobin values of folacin supplemented and unsupplemented infants in their controlled study. Roberts et al. attribute the negative findings of Burland et al. to the time of supplementation (days 5 to 33). In the study of Burland et al. (90), initial mean hemoglobin values of supplemented and nonsupplemented infants were similar (16.7 and 16.3 g/100 ml) and the basic formula, which was fed to both groups of infants, contained more folacin than the diet of the nonsupplemented infants in the study of Roberts et al. (612, 613) (68 μg/liter versus 1.0 to 7.5 μg/liter). The folacin content of the formula which Roberts et al. fed the supplemented group (group A) was not mentioned (613).

Dawson (178) and Kendall et al. (412), who gave supplemental folic acid (1 mg/day for 3 months and 50 μg for 6 months, respectively) to newborn infants weighing more than 1,900 g, also found no difference in the hemoglobin values of supplemented and control infants. The folacin content of the diets in these two studies was not indicated. Kendall et al. (412), however, stated that they fed all infants reconstituted dried cow's milk with semi-solids added at about month 2 or 3. The data of Hibbard and Kenna (338) confirm these observations.

Three of the four investigators (178, 338, 412) of the folacin requirements of premature and low birthweight infants weighing more than 1,800 g at birth concluded that these infants did not need supplemental folic acid. They did, however, stress the importance of well-nourished mothers. In two of the three studies (178, 338) the mothers had received supplemental folic acid antenatally. Although Dawson (178) and Kendall et al. (412) found that the serum and red cell folacin values of nonsupplemented infants dropped to lower levels than those of treated infants, they were still within the "normal" range and Dawson (178) found no difference in neutrophil lobe counts. Kendall et al. (412), however, found that the mean corpuscular volume (MCV) of the control group was significantly higher at 6 months and the infants had more infections but the difference was not significant. Since all other parameters were normal they concluded that the diet contained adequate folacin. The mean red cell folacin activities of the untreated group were 472 and 590 ng/ml at 4 and 6 months of age, respectively.

Hibbard and Kenna (338) compared the serum and red cell folacin values of preterm (gestation <259 days) and small-for-date (birthweight <10th percentile for gestation age) infants from prenatally supplemented and control mothers. The infants were fed sterilized expressed breast milk or half-cream dried milk formula. Cereals and semi-solids were added at 2 to 4 months of age. The infants of antenatally supplemented mothers had higher blood folacin values at birth, but they found minor differences in the four groups at age 3 months. At age 6 months the mean red cell values for all four groups (range, 185 to 282 ng/ml) were much lower than Kendall et al. (412) reported, but there was no evidence of "deteriorating folate status."

Full-term infants

Prophylactic studies. In their field study of 373 Israeli infants from birth to 1 year of age, Matoth et al. (503) found that the mean whole blood folacin value of 8-week old infants was below the mean value for normal adults from this population (89 ng/ml) (379). From 8 weeks on mean folacin values remained below the adult mean. However, the mean for 23 breast-fed infants, 8 to 36 weeks old, was significantly higher (P < 0.001) than the mean value for all infants aged 8 weeks and above (102.9 versus 71.22 ng/ml, respectively).

The following year, Matoth et al. (502) reported that the mean whole blood folacin values of 74 breast-fed infants, attending the clinic, was significantly higher (P < 0.001) than the mean value for 146 artificially-fed infants from the previous study (503) (98.8 versus 65.5 ng/ml). The infants in both groups were 6 weeks to 6 months old. The mean folacin value for the milk of 35 of the mothers was 24 μg/liter. Assuming that an infant consumed 800 ml milk/day (435), they calculated that the folacin intake of a 5- to 6-month old nursing infant was 20 μg/day. The folacin intake of the bottle-fed infants was uncertain. Pasteurized bottled cow's milk contained 35.5 μg folacin activity/liter. However, Matoth et al. (502) pointed out that it is a common practice for Israeli mothers to boil the formula. Boiled pasteurized milk contained 11.8 μg/liter and milk sterilized in the bottle, 9.3 μg/liter.

Since the whole blood folacin values of breast-fed infants 6 weeks to 6 months old were higher than the mean value for normal adults, Matoth et al. (502) concluded that the intake of the breast-fed infants was adequate but the intake of the artificially fed was inadequate. As Matoth et al. (504) pointed out "to what extent moderately lowered blood folic acid levels reflect a state of deficiency which is detrimental to the health of the infants cannot be assessed with certainty."

Vanier and Tyas (746) also found that the mean blood folacin values of 24 artificially-fed English infants were lower than the mean values for normal healthy adults. Two breast-fed infants, moreover, had higher blood folacin values. Serum, whole blood, and red cell values gradually declined until month 8. The mean whole blood folacin value of infants 3 to 4 months old was 99 ng/ml versus 195 ng/ml for normal adults. Matoth et al. (502) reported mean values of 116.4 and 65.0 ng/ml for breast-fed and artificially-fed infants of approximately the same age. In the study of Vanier and Tyas (746) the primary source of folacin was a powdered "full-cream" milk, which contained 26 μg folacin activity/liter. The diet of two 3-month old infants contained 29.7 and 26.6 μg folacin activity/day. FIGLU excretion and neutrophil lobe count were within normal limits. On the basis of these data Vanier and Tyas (746) considered the folacin intake of these infants "marginal." Neither Matoth et al. (502) nor Vanier and Tyas (746) mentioned using conjugase in the folacin assay of milk.

Although the 35 mothers in the study of Matoth et al. (502) were apparently "healthy," the mean whole blood folacin value (56.5 ng/ml) was significantly less ($P < 0.001$) than the mean for the population (89 ng/ml) (379). We found no studies with breast-fed infants of mothers with "normal" whole blood folacin activity. Ford and Scott (219) reported that the mean total folacin activity of the breast milk of 10 British women with infants 7 days to 7 months old was 52 μg/liter; mean values for raw and pasteurized cow's milk were similar (55 and 51 μg/liter, respectively). On the basis of these data Ford and Scott (219) concluded that "20 μg/day allows little margin for safety and should be regarded as the minimal requirement." They suggested that 40 μg total folacin activity/day [52 μg/liter $\times$ 800 ml milk/day (435)] would provide "optimum" nutrition. Other investigators from France (403) and England (90) also reported higher mean folacin values for human milk (32 to 40 μg free and 60 to 64 μg total folacin activity/liter). In their survey, Guzman and Tantengco (285) found no folacin deficiency among the 78 Filipino infants, 0 to 11 months old, most of whom were breast-fed; all had serum values of 4.5 ng/ml or higher. But we found no data on the folacin content of milk from Filipino mothers.

Ek and Magnus (199) defined the optimal daily folacin requirements of infants "as the amount of folate necessary to obtain the same plasma and red cell levels as found in breast-fed infants." The mean plasma and red cell values of 1-month old breast-fed Norwegian babies were 14.5 and 262 ng/ml, respectively; and at month 6, 21.5, and 271 ng/ml. Mittal et al. (528) reported that the mean serum folacin activity of 28 Indian infants, who had been fed a formula that provided 100 to 200 μg folic acid/day, was 17.95 ng/ml. The infants, most of whom were less than 1 year old, had received the formula since birth. Although the folacin content of human milk is similar to (219) or less than (502) the amount in cow's milk, both Matoth et al. (502) and Vanier and Tyas (746), reported that the mean serum and whole blood folacin values of breast-fed infants were higher than those of bottle-fed of approximately the same age. Some of the difference may be due to the loss of folacin during the preparation of the formulas (502, 401, 543). Matoth et al. (502) and Ford (216) have suggested that factors other than quantitative folacin intake, such as absorption and intestinal microflora may also be contributing factors to the folacin status of infants.

Reports in the literature suggest that the folacin derivatives in cow's milk and human milk are similar. The ratios of "free": total L. casei folacin activity in human (403) and cow's milk (404) were 0.67 and 0.66, respectively. Shin et al. (663) recently reported that 60% of the total L. casei folacin activity in cow's milk is monoglutamates. In both human (219, 599) and cow's milk (191, 219, 241, 663) the folacin derivatives are predominantly in the methyl form. The data from two studies suggest that newborn infants utilize both the mono- (634, 669) and the polyglutamate forms of folic acid (634) but we did not find any research on the young infant's ability to absorb food folacin.

Ford (216) suggested that the protein-binding of milk folacin, which Ghitis reported in 1966 (241), may affect the folacin status of infants. He and his associates (217) found that goat colostrum is high in folacin which is firmly bound to protein. At parturition, the plasma folacin activity in kids was about 1 ng/ml but by day 2, it had increased to 28 ng/ml. Since the plasma folacin was also associated with a protein, they suggested that the folacin-protein complex might be transported intact.

The data of Ghitis (242) suggest that the "free" L. casei folacins in cow's milk are protein bound. On the other hand, Markkanen et al. (496) found that only 10% of the folacin activity in cow's milk is protein-bound but most all of the folacin activity in skimmed human milk is bound (497). The status of the folacin in cream, which contains 2 to 10 times more folacin activity per volume unit than skimmed milk (494, 497), was not mentioned. The binding capacity of cow's milk is destroyed by heating at "115° for 5 minutes" (216).

Izak et al. (375) reported that in rats weighing 100 g the absorption of tritiated folic acid bound to cow or goat milk protein was 20% less in the jejunum than that of unbound folic acid. In the ileum, on the other hand, absorption of protein-bound folic acid was almost three times that of unbound folic acid. Ford (216), however, pointed out that the effect of infant intestinal pH and enzyme activities on the protein binding of folacin in vivo is not known.

In 1969 Ford et al. (218) showed that in vitro, the protein-folacin complex disassociated at pH 3.6 but recombined when the pH was restored to pH 7. Also, the data reviewed by Fomon (214) indicate that during the first month of life, hydrochloric acid secretion/unit body weight remains low, thus suggesting a higher gastric pH. Ford (216) found that in vitro digestion of goat's colostrum reduced the binding activity to about one-half its original capacity and when further digested with trypsin, the colostrum no longer hindered the uptake of added folic acid by *Lactobacillus bifidus*.

In addition to affecting folacin absorption, Ford (216) suggested that folacin-binding proteins may affect folacin status through their influence on the microflora in the gut. He found that goat's colostrum reduced the uptake of folic acid by microbial strains that require folacin. Ghitis (241) recommended that folic acid be added to processed milk intended for infant feeding but Ford et al. (220) pointed out that if free folic acid is available to intestinal microflora it might have an adverse effect by increasing the growth of folate-requiring microbes. Conversely, in mice fed a folacin-free diet, there is a marked increase in the incidence of folacin-synthesizing microbes (429). Ford et al. (220) therefore suggested that "unsaturated binder-protein in milk, in acting to sequester the milk folate and reduce the growth of folate-dependent bacteria in the gut, would encourage the growth of bacteria that contribute to the folate nutrition of the host." It might also help retain

some of the folacin which is excreted into the bile. As Ford (216) pointed out, more research is needed in this area.

Therapeutic studies—young infants. A number of investigators [11] (50, 80, 472, 514, 808, 818) have reported megaloblastic anemia in infants fed goat's milk. As Wise et al. (808) pointed out, since it is frequently given to infants with feeding difficulties and food allergies, the folacin deficiency observed in these infants is sometimes attributed to inadequate food intake, vomiting and diarrhea. The reports of Braude (80), Becroft and Holland (50) and Sullivan et al.,[11] however, indicate that the folacin requirement of infants 3 to 5 months old exceeds the amount of *L. casei* folacin activity supplied by goat's milk— <5 to 13 µg free (50, 543, 556) and 2 to 11 µg total folacin activity/liter (217, 219). Braude's 3-month old patient had no history of diarrhea, hemorrhage, or infection and the parents were healthy. The infant had been fed exclusively boiled goat's milk since she was 2 weeks old and pallor, which became progressively worse, was first observed at month 1. Similarly, the three patients of Becroft and Holland (50), age 4.5 to 5 months, had been fed goat's milk for the last 14 to 15 weeks and "took solids poorly." They had no diarrhea, only minor infections, and some vomiting. The canned sterilized or fresh-frozen goat's milk contained less than 5 µg *L. casei* folacin activity/liter. Furthermore, the infants in both studies responded to folic acid treatment.

Therapeutic studies—older infants. In 1951, Woodruff et al. (811) suggested that the minimal effective quantity of parenterally administered citrovorum factor (5-CHO-H$_4$-folic acid) for infants may be less than 75 µg/day. They found that this amount, administered for 13 and 17 days, produced a permanent remission of megaloblastic anemia in two 10.5-month old infants.

Robinson (614) and Sullivan et al.[11] both found that the megaloblastic anemia of infants 5 to 12 months old responded to

[11] Sullivan, L. W., Luhby, A. L. & Streiff, R. R. (1966) Studies of the daily requirement for folic acid in infants and the etiology of folate deficiency in goat's milk megaloblastic anemia. Am. J. Clin. Nutr. *18*, 311 (abstr.).

50 μg folic acid intramuscularly [11] (614) or orally.[11] Although the response of the infant in Robinson's study was "delayed," he concluded that since it completely cured the megaloblastic anemia while the infant was eating a folacin-free diet, "the daily minimal requirement of free folic acid is equal to or less than this amount." Sullivan et al.[11] initially treated one of the three infants in their study with smaller amounts of folic acid (10 and 20 μg for 7 and 10 days, respectively) but there was no reticulocyte response until he was given 50 μg/day intramuscularly. All infants had previously been fed diets consisting mainly of goat's milk (500 to 800 ml/day) containing 2.6 to 15.1 μg folacin activity/liter compared to 42 μg/liter folacin activity in 7 samples of cow's milk. On the basis of these data Sullivan et al.[11] suggested that the "folic acid" requirement of infants was "in the range of 20 to 50 μg/day." Dietary folacin requirement, however, depends on how efficiently food folacin is absorbed.

Ghitis and Tripathy (244) reported that 35 and 15 μg folacin activity/day cured the megaloblastic anemia of two 9- and 12-month old infants, respectively. They also concluded that folic acid and the folacin activity in cow's milk are utilized equally well. After the 12-month old infant had been fed a milk diet containing 15 μg folacin activity for 22 days, his bone marrow became normoblastic and after 2 additional months, his anemia continued to improve but serum folacin activity remained low (1.9 ng/ml). It appears that the folacin activity in the milk diet was "free" folacin since no mention is made of assaying for the "total" folacin activity. He was then fed a "folic acid-free diet" which contained 2 μg free and 15 μg total folacin activity/liter but megaloblastosis did not develop until month 5. One month later, when megaloblastosis was moderate, he was given 15 μg folic acid/day in addition to the "folic acid-free diet." His megaloblastosis had disappeared by the end of 5 weeks. The second infant responded hematologically after being treated with milk containing 35 μg folacin activity for 45 days or to "folic acid-free" milk plus 35 μg folic acid for 4 days.

Children

We found no controlled studies on the folacin requirements of healthy children. Nutritional status surveys in California,[12] the Philippines (285), Canada (563), and India (679) indicate that the older the child, the higher the percentage of children within each age group with serum folacin values in the deficient (<2.5 to 3 ng/ml) and moderate risk (<5 and 6 ng/ml) categories. The Canadians (563) point out that although the consequences of such a prevalence of low serum folacin levels are not known (533), the finding must be viewed with concern until we have more information for interpreting the data.

Preschool (1 to 6 years old)

Most of the data on the folacin requirements of preschool age children derive from the treatment of malnourished children. They may, however, be of limited value in estimating the folacin requirements of healthy children of comparable age (645). As Kamel et al. (399) pointed out in their study, "The influence of diverse factors such as infection, heightened requirement due to recovery from protein-calorie starvation, or excessive demands for homopoiesis, cannot be assessed." Kamel et al. (399) partially corrected the general malnutrition before they initiated their study of folacin requirements.

Velez et al. (753) induced normal hematopoiesis in seven 1- to 4-year old kwashiorkor patients with 5 to 20 μg orally administered folic acid/day in addition to a diet "extremely low" in folacin. Initially, the patients were fed a formula containing skim milk and brown sugar. With improvement, they added other foods, including mashed potatoes, saltine crackers, and vegetables. "No patient received more than 10 μg of total folic 'activity' per day" from the diet. Information on the folacin content of the diet was taken from Stokstad's 1954 article (710). Sideroblast counts, which Velez et al. (753) considered a more sensitive indicator of the efficacy of a given daily dose of folic acid, and bone marrow morphology were the criteria used.

[12] California State Department of Public Health (1971) National Nutrition Survey in California, Termination of Contract Report, California State Dept. of Public Health, Berkeley.

Velez et al. (753) began treatment with folic acid on day 2 to 68 after admission (in six cases, day 2 to 21) and it was administered for 5 to 49 days. The least was required by a 3-year old child (5 μg for 5 days). The bone marrow of one 4-year old patient became normoblastic after eating a diet containing approximately 60 μg total folacin activity for 45 days. Velez et al. (753) calculated that if 10 to 20% of dietary folacin activity is absorbed the boy "received approximately 6 to 12 μg of total 'folic acid activity' per day." Since the children in this study were folacin deficient, Velez et al. (753) suggested that the minimal daily folic acid requirements of normal healthy children 1 to 4 years old should be less than 5 to 20 μg/day. Becroft and Holland (50) later commented that the requirement estimates of Velez et al. (753) may be too low "because there is no way of assessing accurately the additional folic acid supplied by concurrent changes in diet."

Halsted et al. (297) fed 27 children from Cairo, 6 months to 2 years old, who had kwashiorkor, a formula prepared from reconstituted powdered milk which contained 51 μg total and 31 μg free folacin activity/liter. During the first 2 weeks (period 1) the children ingested 36.6 to 51 μg total and 21 to 30 μg free folacin/day. Iron dextran was added during the second 2 weeks (period 2) and 75 μg folic acid/day was administered subcutaneously during the third 2 weeks (period 3). On admission, 70.3% of the patients had megaloblastic bone marrow. During period 1, one patient with megaloblastosis became normal and 4 of the normal became moderately megaloblastic and in period 2, three more developed megaloblastosis. "Megaloblastic bone marrows were uniformly corrected during the folic acid therapy" (period 3). On admission, the mean serum folacin value of 22 children was 4.4 ± 2.97 ng/ml (range, 1.7 to 12.2); when 13 of them were discharged the mean was 8.6 ± 4.57 ng/ml (3.3 to 18.5). Halsted et al. (297) concluded that the anemia of kwashiorkor in Cairo "is responsive to a combination of dietary protein with supplemental iron and folic acid."

Kamel et al. (399) fed 25 children, 9 to 34 months old, who were being treated for severe protein-calorie malnutrition, a low folacin diet, which provided 5.8 μg free and 6.3 μg total folacin activity/kg body weight per day. The diet had previously been proven suitable for use with kwashiorkor children (766). After 2 to 3 weeks, most of the clinical signs of protein-calorie malnutrition and iron deficiency disappeared but the folacin status remained stationary or became worse. Kamel et al. (399) then gave the children "folic acid by intramuscularly graded doses of 20, 30, 40, and 50 μg/day for 2 to 5 weeks" while they continued to eat the low folacin diet. There was little difference in the number who responded to 20 μg vs 50 μg/day except that hemoglobin exceeded 11 g/100 ml in more of those receiving 50 μg/day. At all levels of supplemental folic acid, mean hemoglobin values increased, polymorphonuclear neutrophil (PMN) hypersegmentation decreased, megaloblastosis in bone marrow improved and serum folacin activity increased "significantly." Data from the double reticulocyte test by Minot and Castle (526) were also similar. They, therefore, "concluded that the minimal daily requirement as assessed by these criteria is no higher than the lowest dose administered."

Assuming that one-half of the free folacin is absorbed, as suggested in a Food Agriculture Organization/World Health Organization (FAO/WHO) report (205), Kamel et al. (399) calculated that "20 to 50 μg of intramuscular folic acid would be equivalent to 40 and 100 μg of dietary folate, or in this series of patients, to 5.4 and 13 μg/kg body weight." After taking into consideration the intake from dietary folacin and minimum folic acid administered they "tentatively concluded" that approximately 11.2 μg free dietary folacin/kg body weight per day (5.8 + 5.4 μg) would have been sufficient to promote recovery from folacin deficiency in most children recovering from protein-calorie malnutrition. They reasoned, however, that during repletion folacin needs are probably greater than normal. Therefore, the minimum requirement of healthy children of comparable age would be less than 11.2 μg/kg body weight per day.

In a recent survey of the nutritional status of California preschool children 3 to

6 years old, Ruffin et al. (630) found that the serum folacin activity of 64% of the 28 children was less than 6 ng/ml; only one child's value was less than 3 ng/ml. They calculated the folacin content of the diets from Handbook No. 29 (740) with supplemental data from Hurdle et al. (363) and Santini et al. (637). The diet of the children contained less than two-thirds of the 1968 Recommended Daily Allowance (RDA) (200 μg/day) (546) which is equivalent to 134 μg/day. The diet of 29% of them contained less than one-third the RDA, or <66 μg/day. Sandstead et al. (635) reported that 16.9% of 100 preschool age children in Tennessee had serum folacin values less than 4 ng/ml. The estimated mean folacin intake of 29 of the children was 47 μg/day (median, 43 μg).

Adolescents

In both the Californian [12] and the Canadian (563) nutritional status surveys approximately 50% of the adolescents had low serum folacin values and 10 to 13% were in the high risk group. More than 40% of the adolescent Eskimos were in the high risk group (563). The results of three other recent surveys in the United States, however, indicated that the plasma (159, 160) and whole blood (159, 488) folacin values of most of the adolescents were "within the normal range" in spite of the fact that the calculated folacin intake was about one-fourth the RDA in 2 studies (160, 488) and less than one-half the RDA in the third (159). In one survey, the plasma folacin values of girls were higher than those of boys, yet the boys took in more folacin. They interpreted this as indicating an increased requirement for boys (160). Daniel et al. (160) concluded that the discrepancy in blood values and intake was due to the tables used for calculating the folacin content of the diet and pointed out the need for new ones. In all three of the surveys the researchers calculated the folacin content of the diets from USDA Handbook 29 (740).

STUDIES ON REQUIREMENTS OF THE ELDERLY

Three field studies (359–601) and three surveys (272, 476–478) of folacin intake and nutritional status of people 60 years old or more have been reported. The four studies (272, 477, 478, 601) in which folacin intake was calculated from the tables of McCance and Widdowson (510) suggest that approximately 50 μg dietary folacin activity/day is adequate. On the other hand, Hurdle (362) estimated that the typical diet of an elderly folacin deficient patient contained 60 μg free L. casei folacin activity.

Read et al. (601) reported that 40 (80%) of the 51 entrants to an "old people's home" had folacin deficiency (serum activity <6 ng/ml). Values were below 3 ng/ml in 10 of them. The serum values of the controls, a group of apparently healthy subjects of similar age, were all above 3 ng/ml (>6 ng/ml in 70%). The mean folacin intakes of the two groups were 32 and 53 μg/day, respectively. Over a 4-week period, the mean daily folacin intake of the patients was 51 μg. After 6 months in the home, FIGLU excretion returned to normal in 17 of the 23 patients but the diet did not raise the serum values.

Gough et al. (272) successfully treated the megaloblastic anemia of two patients, 62 and 82 years old, with a low "folic acid" diet containing 15 μg activity plus 200 μg folic acid/day. Their original diets contained 13 and 14 μg folacin activity/day. On the basis of hemoglobin values, MacLennan et al. (476) concluded that folacin deficiency was rare among the elderly people they studied (1% of subjects). The mean serum folacin activities of men and women with hemoglobin values ranging from <11.9 to >13 g/100 ml was 4.1 ng/ml (range 1.3 to 16.3). Seventeen of the 365 subjects had values less than 1.5 ng/ml. Mean folacin intakes varied from 33 to 51 μg/day (range, 9 to 149 μg/day). In another recent study MacLennan et al. (477, 478) found no significant difference in the red cell folacin values of patients in a long-stay geriatric hospital whose diets contained more and those whose diets contained less than 50 μg folacin activity/day. They suggested that "problems involved in measuring folate intake might account for the disappointing results. . . ." (477).

Hurdle (359) compared the folacin intake and serum values of elderly people more than 70 years old who were hospital patients or living at home with the values of healthy adults, 25 to 41 years old. The mean folacin intakes of the three groups were 101.1, 145.5, and 225.1 µg free *L. casei* folacin activity/day, respectively. Their mean serum folacin activities were 3.3, 9.6, and 9.8 ng/ml.

Hurdle (360) also investigated the long-term effect of a hospital diet on the folacin status of 17 patients. Nine of the patients, who had been in the hospital for at least 52 days, had folacin deficiency without anemia. After 100 to 133 days the folacin status of the patients remained unaltered. The mean serum and red cell folacin values of those patients consuming less than 80 µg free folacin activity/day were 4.2 and 119 ng/ml, respectively. Mean values for those who consumed more than 79 µg/day were 6.1 and 202 ng/ml. On the basis of these data he suggested that the minimum dietary folacin requirement of an adult in basal condition is 80 to 100 µg free *L. casei* folacin activity/day.

The data from a number of surveys indicate that there is no difference in the serum folacin values of healthy elderly subjects and younger people (201, 261, 359, 536). Lewi (456) suggested abnormal hydrolysis of dietary polyglutamates in the elderly but others have reported normal folacin absorption (272, 360, 749). In view of the number of reports of folacin deficiency in the elderly (39, 261, 364, 601, 749) and the problems encountered in quantitating the folacins in food and their availability, Girdwood (257) recommended a survey with adequate young controls, to see if there are regional differences in folacin status. If so, then "a close study of variations in feeding habits would be rewarding." In the recent Canadian (563) and Californian [12] surveys, serum folacin values in more than one-half of the elderly subjects were in the low and/or deficient range. Seventy-seven percent of the Eskimos surveyed had serum values in the high risk range (563).

A number of reports of mental dysfunction (dementia) in folacin deficient elderly patients have appeared in the literature (39, 225, 301, 364, 517, 585, 601, 657, 683, 716). Folic acid reportedly corrected the dementia in some patients (517, 585, 716); in others it did not (225, 657). Sneath et al. (683) found no overall correlation between mental assessment score and serum and red cell folacin activity. However, there was some correlation ($P < 0.10$) between mental assessment scores and red cell folacin in those with low red cell folacin values.

Folacin activity in the cerebral spinal fluid is normally more than double the amount in serum (109) and in folacin deficiency the activity in the brain decreases, though not as rapidly as that in serum (607). Reynolds et al. (608) and Melamed et al. (517) suggested that severity and duration of folacin deficiency are important in the development of mental symptoms. On the other hand, Sneath et al. (683) proposed that dementia led to the folacin deficiency because of poor food intake. In some of the studies cited, the patients were taking drugs—primidone, phenobarbital, phenothiazines, or trimethadione (301, 517, 657). The effects of drugs on folacin utilization and/or metabolism have been reviewed by Herbert and Tisman (323) and Stebbins et al. (702).

Recent research indicates that folacin coenzymes are involved in a number of different reactions in the brain (454, 511). Reynolds (606) recently reviewed some of the hypotheses on the metabolic role of folacin in the brain. The discovery by McClain et al. (511) that folacin is localized in the synaptic region suggests that this "might represent an important site of involvement of these coenzymes in neural metabolism and function." During aging, physiological changes take place in the central nervous system (736). It is not known whether these changes have any effect on the utilization and/or requirements for nutrients involved in brain metabolism.

Fehling et al. (206) investigated the effect of folacin deficiency on the peripheral and central nervous system of rats. They concluded that "The central nervous system is resistant to systemic folate depletion, whereas the peripheral nerves are depleted to the same degree as the extraneural tissues." Brain folacin activity was reduced by only 16% in the folacin deficient animals compared with the controls, but whole blood, liver and sciatic nerve folacin values fell by 60, 50, and 59%, respectively.

FACTORS AFFECTING DIETARY FOLACIN REQUIREMENTS

Factors that may affect human folacin requirements include: availability and absorption of dietary folacins; intestinal microbes; interrelationship of folacin utilization with other nutrients (iron, ascorbic acid, vitamin B_{12}, and methionine); ethanol intake; drugs and infection. The study of folacin utilization has been complicated by differences in the rate of absorption of various compounds, rapid tissue uptake, enterohepatic circulation, microbial synthesis of folacins in the lower bowel, inability to measure degradation products, and the rapid interconversion of compounds with folacin activity.

Absorption of folacins

Folacin absorption has been estimated by measuring urinary excretion or increased serum microbiological activity after an oral dose; perfusing a given segment of small intestine and estimating the folacin absorbed by the difference in concentration between the amount infused and withdrawn; assessing the ability of a folacin deficient patient to respond hematologically to oral doses of folic acid; and by measuring the rise in plasma, urinary and/or fecal radioactivity after an oral dose of a labeled compound (342). Methods of estimating folacin absorption have been reviewed and analyzed by a number of investigators (109, 228, 619, 771).

Although folic acid constitutes only about 1% of the dietary folacins (151, 578), it has been the most widely used derivative in absorption studies because of its clinical importance and the availability of the tritium labeled compound. It has been used as the reference standard in most studies. There is little information on the absorption and utilization of dietary folacin. This is due in part to the problem of developing a satisfactory method of quantitating the amount of dietary folacin absorbed. With the exception of yeast and liver, two concentrated sources of folacin, it is necessary to ingest large amounts of food in order to significantly change plasma or urinary values.

Synthetic monoglutamates. In 1960, Anderson et al. (8) found that the mean absorption of a 200 μg dose of ³H-folic acid by 13 healthy subjects was 79% (range, 41 to 91%); the rest of the label was recovered from the feces. Others (202, 372, 392, 436, 542) have reported similar mean values (79 to 87.7%). When Anderson et al. (8) increased the dose to 40 μg/kg body weight mean folic acid absorption for three subjects was 85% (range, 67 to 95%). Yoshino (814) found 3.5% of the labeled folic acid in the feces of 11 subjects who had been preloaded with 15 mg folic acid before ingesting 40 μg ³H-folic acid/kg body weight.

Anderson et al. (8) also found that when they injected 15 mg folic acid parenterally before giving 2 mg of ³H-folic acid orally, they recovered 41% (range, 31 to 53%) of the radioactivity in a 24 hour urine sample. With an oral dose of 200 μg they recovered 42% (range, 28 to 65%). These findings have been verified by others (228, 263, 294, 418, 421, 814). A number of reviews of folic acid absorption have recently been published (86, 149, 669).

The absorption (24, 87, 580) and hemopoietic effectiveness (465) of 5-CHO-H_4-folic acid in man has been demonstrated. Many of the early studies were reviewed by Darby (163). Its stability in the gastrointestinal tract, however, has been debated. May et al. (506) found that it was unstable at pH 1 to 2. On the basis of the experimental data of Girdwood (252), Chanarin (109) suggested that more than one-half the amount ingested may be lost due to the action of gastric acidity. Others, however, have found that it is well utilized (96, 558, 787). Butterworth (96), for example, reported an optimal response in one patient with tropical sprue who ingested 50 μg/day. Whitehead et al. (787) concluded that 5-CHO-H_4-folic acid was absorbed as well as folic acid, since the increment in plasma folacin activity after feeding 1 mg to subjects with and without gastric acid was similar to those that ingested 1 mg folic acid (589, 786). Nixon and Bertino (558) concluded from measurements of the amount of labeled folacin activity in the feces, that four subjects absorbed 90% of the amount ingested (50 μg/kg body weight).

Three groups of investigators have compared the absorption of a number of monoglutamate compounds (86, 580, 729).

Perry and Chanarin (580) found that three hours after ingesting 10 μg/kg body weight of folic acid, 5-CHO-H₄-folic acid, 5-CH₃-H₄-folic acid, H₄-folic acid, or H₂-folic acid, mean serum L. casei activities were similar (20.0, 21.5, 21.2, 16.2, and 18.6 ng/ml, respectively). Mean 24 hour urinary excretions in μg were (79.8, 47.1, 62.0, 20.5, and 14.2, respectively). Tamura and Stokstad (729) concluded that all of the crystalline compounds that they tested (5-CHO-H₄-folic acid, 3-CH₃-H₄-folic acid, H₄-folic acid, pteroyltriglutamic acid, and pteroylheptaglutamic acid) were absorbed as well as folic acid.

Brown et al. (86) reported that the mean increases in serum L. casei folacin activity were significant after the 21 normal subjects had ingested 0.68 μmole (300 μg) of any one of the nine different monoglutamates. Quantitative differences between certain of the compounds were also significant. 5,10-CH₂-H₄-folic acid and H₄-folic acid produced the smallest increase (<3 ng/ml) in serum L. casei activity; folic acid, 5-CHO-H₄-folic acid, 5-HCNH-H₄-folic acid, and 5-CH₃-H₄-folic acid exhibited a greater increase (6 to 9 ng/ml) and 10-CHO-H₄-folic acid and 5,10-CH-H₄-folic acid elicited the greatest increases (>10 ng/ml).

O'Broin et al. (567) studied the stability of six reduced monoglutamates at different pH and ion concentrations in vitro. They suggested that since CH₃-H₄-folic acid was quite unstable at a pH below neutrality, it may have less nutritional value than expected. The "nutritionally most stable" compound examined was 5-CHO-H₄-folic acid (pH 4.0 to 10). Since 10-CHO-H₄-folic acid was nutritionally more stable than expected they suggested that it may be a much more important source of dietary folacin than previously thought. This hypothesis is consistent with the findings of Brown et al. (86).

Leslie and Rowe (453) found that adding one-carbon moieties to H₄-folic acid and increasing the γ-glutamyl peptide chain length reduced the affinity of these folacins for the binding proteins in the brush border membrane of the small intestinal epithelial cells. Perry and Chanarin (581) suggested that, in vivo, the transfer of folacin polyglutamates into the intestinal

cell may represent the chief limitation to their utilization.

Synthetic polyglutamates. The utilization of the conjugated forms of dietary folacin containing more than 2 γ-glutamyl residues in the side chain has been one of the major unresolved questions (618). Although Cooperman and Luhby (146) reported that the folacins may be absorbed as polyglutamates, this finding has not been confirmed. To the contrary, most investigators agree that the glutamyl peptide side chain must be removed or contain no more than one residue before the folacins are absorbed (29, 95, 97, 263, 292, 346, 349, 579, 623).

In 1944, Binkley et al. (65) prepared a fraction from yeast which was active for folacin deficient chicks but it had relatively little potency for stimulating the growth of L. casei until it was subjected to an undescribed "enzyme digestion" which liberated folacin in a microbiologically active form. Since then γ-glutamylcarboxypeptidase(s) ("conjugase") has been found in many plant and animal tissues (73, 397) including human plasma (440, 448, 640, 644, 809), duodenal aspirate (424), bile (54), small intestinal homogenates (57, 623), and mucosal cells from the jejunum (343, 448, 637). The findings of Baker et al. (29) indicate that the jejunum is necessary for the utilization of the polyglutamates, pteroyldiglutamate and pteroyltriglutamate, but folic acid and 5-CHO-H₄-folic acid are absorbed in the absence of the jejunum. Bernstein et al. (57) found conjugase activity in all parts of the guinea pig's small intestines but the jejunum was the most active. When Rosenberg and Godwin [13] incubated human intestinal mucosal homogenates with ³H-pteroylheptaglutamic acid, medium chain polyglutamates were released first but eventually all of the substrate was converted to ³H-folic acid and glutamic acid.

The recent jejunal perfusion experiments of Halsted et al. (292) provide direct evidence of human intestinal deconjugation of pteroylheptaglutamic acid. After infusing equimolar amounts of ³H-folic acid and ¹⁴C-pteroylheptaglutamic acid along a 30

[13] Rosenberg. I. H. & Godwin, H. A. (1970) Study of intestinal metabolism of folate using synthetic tritium-labeled pteroylheptaglutamic acid. Gastroenterology 58, 990 (abstr.)

cm segment of the intestine they found that the luminal disappearance rate of ^{3}H was 1.5 times that of ^{14}C and its derivatives. The luminal concentrations of ^{3}H-folic acid and ^{14}C-pteroylheptaglutamic acid decreased progressively with passage of the solution along the jejunal segment. During the 40 minute equilibrium and 50 minute collection periods, 74.7% ^{3}H and 52.6% ^{14}C of the infused labels disappeared. More ^{3}H than ^{14}C was also recovered in the urine of one patient (51.3 versus 44.4%). "Column chromatography of intestinal aspirates demonstrated a spectrum of ^{14}C-labeled folates corresponding to chain lengths from [^{14}C]PG-1 to [^{14}C]-PG-7, with distal accumulation of derived [^{14}C]PG-1" (292). Contact with the intestinal mucosa is apparently required for hydrolysis since ^{14}C-pteroylheptaglutamate remained unchanged after in vitro incubation with intestinal juice. Halsted et al. (292) concluded that progressive mucosal hydrolysis is an integral part of the absorption of pteroylheptaglutamates in man. Experiments with dogs substantiate these findings (43, 44). In 1971, Baugh et al. (43) observed that the absorption rate of polyglutamates appeared to be inversely related to the length of the γ-glutamyl side chain. Recent experiments indicate that γ-glutamylcarboxypeptidase(s) is "either located within intestinal absorptive cells or bound to the cell surface, or both" (44). Rosenberg and Neumann (622) have found that three distinct enzymes are involved in the complete hydrolysis of pteroylheptaglutamates in chicken intestine.

Until Krumdieck and Baugh (437) synthesized radioactive pteroylpolyglutamic acids in 1969, it was not possible to evaluate quantitatively the digestion, absorption, and availability of the polyglutamates. Early reports, which have been reviewed by Darby (162), indicated that patients with pernicious anemia, sprue, and nutritional macrocytic anemia responded hematologically to pteroyldi-, tri-, and heptaglutamic acids. Girdwood (250) also found that pteroyldi- and triglutamic acids were utilized by patients with pernicious anemia. The peak serum values which Baker et al. reported (24, 26) after large doses (5 mg) of folic acid, pteroyldiglutamic acid and

pteroyltriglutamic acid indicated that they were well utilized. In fact, they suggest that the addition of the γ-glutamyl peptide improved absorption in patients with celiac disease.

Three studies with synthetic pteroylheptaglutamic acid indicate that it is well absorbed (97, 263, 729). In an absorption study with labeled folacin, Butterworth et al. (97) found that the patient who ingested 10 μmoles of ^{3}H-folic acid absorbed 90% of the test dose. The patient who ingested an equivalent amount of ^{3}H-pteroylheptaglutamic acid absorbed 75%. However, the net retention of the test doses were 46 and 66.7%, respectively. The longer the chain, the more label appeared in the feces but the shorter the γ-glutamyl peptide chain, the more appeared in the urine. He concluded that "it is clear that polyglutamates constitute a source of folate available to man and should be taken into account in calculating dietary intake." (97).

Godwin and Rosenberg (263) reported that the mean radioactivity in the urine of 11 subjects over a 48 hour period, following the ingestion of 0.6 μmoles ^{3}H-folic acid or ^{3}H-pteroylheptaglutamic acid, was 70.8 versus 56.1% of the test dose. Mean recovery of the label in the urine and feces was 94%. Based on a response curve relating folic acid intake to urinary folacin activity excretion, Tamura and Stokstad (729) found that presaturated subjects who had ingested 0.75 mg of the triglutamate or 0.75 to 2.0 mg of the heptaglutamate (equivalent to folic acid) absorbed 85.2 (range, 27 to 144) and 90.4 (range, 13 to 140) percent of the amount ingested. In a second study, Tamura et al. (727) reported 125% availability for 2.27 mg pteroylheptaglutamic acid (equivalent to 1 mg folic acid). These studies indicate that folacin derivatives are well absorbed but they do not provide information on the bioavailability of the folacins in food.

Dietary folacins—yeast. Reports of the availability of the pteroylheptaglutamates in yeast and yeast extracts vary depending on the method of preparing the extract, the status of the individual, the amount ingested and the criteria used. Early investigators (656, 802, 804) effectively treated nutritional macrocytic anemia with a crude extract of yeast but later researchers have reported that yeast and yeast extracts contain an inhibitor which interferes with the utilization of folylpolyglutamates. In 1945, Pfiffner et al. (584) isolated and in the following year they (583) identified the conjugated vitamin in yeast as a pteroylheptaglutamate. Bethell et al. (60) reported that patients with pernicious anemia exhibited little evidence of red cell regeneration when given a crude yeast concentrate but when given the purified conjugate, hematological responses, and urinary excretions were similar to those produced by an equivalent amount of folic acid activity. However, one patient with nutritional macrocytic anemia responded suboptimally to the crude extract.

Swendseid et al. (725) found that the urinary folacin excretion of healthy subjects who ingested 4 mg folic acid or an equivalent amount of the polyglutamate from purified yeast concentrate were similar. Adding 30 g of the crude yeast extract to the purified concentrate, however, decreased the urinary folacin activity to about 15% of the amount excreted when the subjects ingested folic acid. The extract had no effect on the absorption of folic acid. Since it also took more conjugase to split the polyglutamate in the crude preparation, Swendseid et al. (725) suggested that yeast contained a conjugase inhibitor.

Eleven studies on the availability of the folacins in yeast and/or yeast extract have been reported[14] (22, 27, 282, 386, 516, 579, 581, 649, 697, 729). The subjects were presaturated in three of them (22, 581, 729); test doses ranged from 0.2 to 6.8 mg. Rosenberg and Godwin[14] reported that the increment in serum folacin activity after crude yeast extract was ingested was less than 3% of that produced by an equimolar amount of folic acid. Crude yeast extract, however, had no effect on the absorption of folic acid.

The results of four studies, in which the rise in serum values and increased urinary folacin excretion of normal subjects after ingesting 1.0 to 1.5 mg folic acid or an equivalent amount of folacin from yeast extract were compared, suggest that polyglutamates are poorly absorbed (386, 579, 581, 697). Jandl and Lear (386) concluded that two subjects absorbed 25% of the

1,500 μg folacin activity which was 90% polyglutamates and 10% free folacins. After the extract had been treated with conjugase, they absorbed 60% of the test dose as compared to 95% of the folic acid.

In addition to the above-mentioned absorption experiment, Perry and Chanarin (579) also supplemented the diets of 12 healthy subjects with 0.227 μmoles (100 μg) folic acid/day for 5 months. Six other subjects received 17 tablets of yeast concentrate/day which provided 0.227 μmoles folacin activity as the heptaglutamate. In 2 months, red blood cell folacin activity was 45% above baseline in those receiving folic acid versus a 16% increment for the group that received the polyglutamate. Perry and Chanarin (579) concluded that the folacin in the yeast extract was utilized one-third as well as an equal amount of folic acid.

Schertel et al. (649) reported that 30% of the 1,350 μg S. faecalis folacin activity in 45 g yeast was available; for 6,800 μg folacin activity, the availability was 22%. As the yeast intake decreased the availability of the folacin increased. On the other hand, only 8% of the 4,750 μg folacin activity in 83.3 g yeast extract was available. Schertel et al. (648) found that more than 95% of the folacins in pure dry yeast contained more than two glutamyl residues in the side chain (i.e., more than three glutamyl residues in the molecule). The polyglutamates were all substituted and were in various oxidation states (5- or 10-formyl, 77% and 5-methyl, 20%). Baker et al. (27) reported no difference in the mean peak increment in serum folacin values after 12 healthy subjects ingested yeast, containing 1.9 mg folacin activity or an equivalent amount of folic acid (34.6 and 32.8 ng/ml, respectively).

In recent experiments, Tamura and Stokstad (729) did not find any difference in the utilization of the folacins in yeast or yeast extracts prepared by the method of Perry and Chanarin (579). The subjects absorbed the 0.75 mg folacin activity from a charcoal eluate 63% as well as an equivalent amount of folic acid; and for 1.5 mg

[14] Rosenberg, I. H. & Godwin, H. A. (1971) Inhibition of intestinal γ-glutamyl carboxypeptidase by yeast nucleic acid: an explanation of variability in utilization of dietary polyglutamyl folate. J. Clin. Invest. 50, 78a (abstr.).

folacin activity in 3 g yeast, 60%. On the other hand, Babu and Srikantia (22) reported that the mean availability of folacin activity from yeast was 10.1%. The subjects in both studies were presaturated with folic acid, and availability was calculated from a dose-response curve.

Based on serum increment, McLean et al. (516) concluded that pregnant women absorbed 200 μg from yeast extract as well as an equal amount of folic acid. Grossowicz et al. (282) compared the increment in serum folacin activity of 19 students fed 100 to 3,000 μg folacin activity from yeast extract or an equivalent amount of folic acid. When they ingested 300 μg folacin

activity from the extract (containing 30 μg "free folacin"), serum folacin values rose to a level equivalent to 300 μg folic acid. Higher intakes of yeast extract containing 1,000 and 3,000 μg folacin activity did not produce higher elevations of serum folacin than the administration of 300 μg folic acid. Grossowicz et al. (282) therefore concluded that small amounts of yeast folacin fed to healthy subjects are fully utilized. In 1969 Ford et al. (218) suggested that the observed difference in nutritional availability of the polyglutamates may be more apparent than real, if the level of folacin binder in the intestinal mucosa is only sufficient to facilitate the

TABLE 3

Availability of folacin in food

Food	Total folacin activity in food	Basal dose folic acid	Total folacin in supplement	Availability		No. subjects	No. tests
				Mean	Range		
	μg	μg	μg	%	%		
Banana[1]	192–252	400	592–652	45.6	0–148	8	
Banana[2]	250	350	600	82	0–148	—	6
Bengal gram[1]	282	400	682	68.8	29–163	7	
Cabbage (cooked)[2]	330–430	200–350	530–780	47	0–127		6
Cabbage (raw)[2]	490	200–350	690–820	47	0– 93		6
Defatted soybean[2] meal	610	350	910	46	0– 83		6
Egg (hen)[1]	210–350	400	610–750	72.4	35–137	7	
Egg yolk[2]	350	400	750	39	0–129		10
Green gram[1]	314	400	714	55.2	0–118	7	
Lima beans[2] (dry, cooked)	240	350	590	70	0–138		6
Lima beans[2] (frozen cooked)	420	350	770	96	48–181		6
Liver (Beef cooked,)[2]	670–1010	0–350	670–1360	50	22–103		12
Liver (goat)[1]	315	400	715	70.0	9–125	5	
Orange juice[2]	840	none	840	31	17– 40		14
Romaine extract[a]	500	none	500	48	38– 52		4
Romaine lettuce[2]	750	none	750	25	12– 37		13
Spinach[1]	310	400	710	62.8	26– 99	8	
Tomato[1]	300	400	700	37.2	24– 71	7	
Wheat germ[2]	730	350	1080	30	0– 64		6
Yeast (Brewers)[1]	300	400	700	10.1	0– 36	8	
Yeast (Brewers)[2]	1400	none	1400	60	55– 67		6
Yeast extract[2]	750	none	750	63	59– 69		3

[1] Babu, S. & Srikantia, S. G. (1976) Availability of folates from some foods. Am. J. Clin. Nutr. *29*, 376–379. [2] Tamura, T. & Stokstad, E. L. R. (1973) The availability of food folate in man. Brit. J. Haematol. *25*, 513–532.

uptake of a small proportion of a large dose.

Conjugated folacin from yeast extracts purified by diethylaminoethyl (DEAE) cellulose ion exchange chromatography are also well absorbed (344–346, 620). Investigators found no significant difference in the peak increase in serum *L. casei* activity when subjects ingested 200 μg folacin activity from polyglutamates or from folic acid.

Dietary folacin—other foods. The availability of folacin from a number of foods has been investigated in three studies (22, 604, 729) by comparing urinary excretion of *L. casei* folacin activity after a test meal to a response curve previously established with folic acid. In the first study, Retief (604) reported "uncontrollable fluctuations" in urinary folacin excreted. Later investigators (22, 729) avoided this problem by keeping the subjects saturated with folic acid. The results of two of the studies (22, 729) are shown in table 3.

The data from these three studies demonstrate that the availability of dietary folacin varies widely from food to food. There were also considerable differences among individuals in their ability to absorb the folacins from different foods, especially lima beans, cabbage (729), and bananas (22, 729). The availability of folacin in some foods varied between 0 and 100% (22, 729). The investigators were unable to explain an availability of more than 100% for different foods in some individuals (22, 729). All three groups pointed out that the amount of test food ingested often exceeded the amount consumed under normal conditions. Tamura and Stokstad (729) suggested that this might adversely affect the utilization of folacin. Babu and Srikantia (22) also found that the free folacin content of food was a poor indicator of the availability of total folacin content.

Retief (604) suggested that total folacin from calves liver, spinach, and peas was well absorbed but the folacin in cauliflower, pumpkin, and tomatoes was less available. The reports by other investigators (281, 315, 489) of rapid and prolonged increases in the plasma level of 5-CH$_3$-H$_4$-folic acid after ingesting liver suggest efficient absorption of liver folacins.

Tamura and Stokstad (729) and Babu and Srikantia (22) reported 50 and 70% availability, respectively. The mean availability of folacin from seven different commonly used Indian foods was more than 50% (22).

Tamura and Stokstad (729) found that of the 12 foods studied, the mean folacin availability was highest for frozen cooked lima beans (96%), followed by bananas and dried cooked lima beans. The folacin activity in egg yolk, orange juice, wheat germ, and romaine lettuce was least available. Tamura and his associates (727) later reaffirmed the poor availability of folacin from orange juice. They also found that egg yolk (729) and romaine lettuce (727) did not significantly affect the availability of added pteroylheptaglutamic acid but orange juice definitely inhibited the availability of added pteroylheptaglutamate (727, 729). On the other hand, Nelson et el. (550) recently concluded that the availability of folacin in orange juice was equivalent to that of synthetic folic acid; 60 and 58%, respectively, were absorbed during triple lumen perfusion. Colman and Herbert (138) have, however, questioned the design of their experiment.

Synthetic folacins from foods. The data of Colman and his associates (136, 140, 487) indicate that the addition of folic acid to foods decreases its bioavailability. Colman et al. (136) compared the increment in serum folacin activity 1 and 2 hours after subjects, who had been previously presaturated with folic acid, ingested folic acid alone, or folic acid added to different foods before cooking. They concluded that folic acid cooked in maize porridge, boiled rice and whole wheat bread was absorbed 52.7, 57.6, and 38.3% as well as folic acid alone. Colman et al. (140) also found that the increment in hemoglobin and serum and red cell folacin values of pregnant women who consumed a maize meal containing 500 μg folic acid/day was similar to that of women who took 300 μg folic acid in tablet form. When the folic acid in the maize was increased to 1,000 μg/day, however, only one-third of the additional amount was utilized. Margo et al. (487) reported that the mean increment in red cell folacin activity of pregnant women eating whole wheat bread fortified with 900 μg folic acid/day was similar to that observed in women studied previously (140) who took 300 μg folic acid/day in tablet form.

Folacins synthesized by intestinal microbes. The data indicate that microbes in the alimentary tract synthesize folacin but its contribution to the nutrition of humans has not been established. There is evidence of microbial synthesis of folacin in the mouth (189, 481). Disraely et al. (189) found that saliva, which had been treated with conjugase, contained little *S. faecalis* folacin activity—5.04 ng/ml. Incubating saliva with glucose, however, increased free and total folacin activity to 3.62 and 25.2 ng/ml, respectively (189). Since the number of folacin synthesizing bacteria also increased during incubation, they suggested that bacteria increased the amount of "folic acid-like compounds" in saliva. Mäkilä (481) found a difference, which approached statistical significance, in mean *L. casei* activity of resting whole saliva from edentulous denture wearers, those with teeth largely destroyed by caries and subjects with slight caries—49.5, 56.6, and 18.2 ng/ml, respectively. The compounds in saliva have not been identified. Bruckner and Bertino (87) demonstrated that 5-formyl-H_4-folic acid is absorbed from the mouth.

Bacteria, such as coliform organisms, capable of synthesizing folacin are found in the ileum (270) and in the feces of healthy humans (232, 283). Grundy et al. (283) reported that the antibiotic, phthalysulphathiazole, caused a drastic decrease in the fecal excretion of *L. casei* activity (10% of its original value) of five subjects maintained on a carefully controlled diet. The data also suggested a decrease in *L. casei* activity in the urine but it was not a "decisive drop." Thus, Grundy et al. (283) were unable to draw any firm conclusion about human utilization of folacin synthesized by intestinal bacteria. Hoffbrand et al. (350) concluded that bacteria in the distal small intestine did not affect folacin status since patients with high *E. coli* counts in the ileum had low-normal or subnormal serum folacin activity. No mention was made of dietary intake.

The results of a number of investigators suggest that the effect of folacin-synthesizing intestinal microflora on folacin status may depend on the kind of folacin derivatives synthesized, the place of synthesis and also the folacin status of the individual. Baker et al. (29) found that a patient with only the jejunum removed absorbed the monoglutamates, folic acid, and folinic acid, but not the polyglutamate forms. However, the plasma *L. casei* folacin activity of a patient with almost no small intestine did not increase when he ingested any of these folacins (29). The results of Chanarin and Bennett (114) suggest that, when large amounts of folic acid (0.5 to 5 mg) are ingested, some of it may be absorbed from the ileum. On the other hand, both Hepner et al. (311) and Sorrell et al. (687) found that folic acid was poorly absorbed from the ileum and the colon, respectively. In vitro experiments with rats indicate that protein-bound folic acid is absorbed from the ileum three times as well as folic acid (375). Folacin deficient rats also absorb more folic acid from the ileum than normal rats (374). We found no studies on the absorption of the types of folacin synthesized by microbes in the ileum.

Some data from studies with experimental animals suggest that folacin synthesized by bacteria is of nutritional importance to them (430, 466, 552). In his recent review of folacin metabolism in germ-free animals, Luckey (466) pointed out that germ-free chicks required more folate than "classic" chicks. The requirement decreased when they were associated with *E. coli*, which can synthesize folacin, and increased when they were associated with *S. faecalis*, a bacteria that requires preformed folacin. Similarly, Klipstein et al. (430) reported that the administration of a folacin deficient diet to weanling rats caused moderate depression of serum, hepatic and intestinal mucosal folacin concentration but this was followed by partial folacin repletion. The addition of 1% sulfasuxidine to the deficient diet prevented folacin repletion.

Conversely, Baugh et al. (41) suggested that folacin synthesized by intestinal microflora is not of great significance to the rat, since only a small fraction (0.02%) of the labeled ρ-aminobenzoic acid which they added to the drinking water of rats was later found in the liver. The data of Bernstein et al. (55) suggest that dogs are also unable to absorb from the ileum folacins synthesized by microbes.

The piglets studied by Ford et al. (220) had much more folacin activity in their livers than could be accounted for from their milk intake. They proposed that it derived from bacterial synthesis in the intestine. Ford (216) also suggested that the unsaturated folacin-binding protein in sows milk may strongly influence the ecology of the intestinal microflora by hindering the growth of folacin-dependent species of bacteria. The importance of a balance among the intestinal microbes is pointed out by the work of Marko et al. (499) who found that the folacin status of patients with ulcerative colitis was correlated with the degree of disturbance in microbial composition of the intestine.

Factors affecting absorption

Dietary components. Investigators have been primarily concerned with factors that affect conjugase activity. The presence of conjugase inhibitors in yeast was first suggested by Bird et al., in 1946 (69). The data of Swendseid et al. (725) supported this hypothesis. Mims et al. (524) and Rosenberg and Godwin [11] both reported that in vitro yeast nucleic acids were strong inhibitors of γ-glutamyl carboxypeptidase. Mims et al. (524), however, did not find that in vivo they had any inhibitory effect on the utilization of purified yeast folacin. Hudson (341) concluded that proteins had an inhibitory effect on conjugase. Perry and Chanarin (581), however, were unable to show that in vitro, yeast extracts had any inhibitory effect on human plasma conjugase and therefore concluded that "the view that absorption of natural folate polyglutamate is due to inhibitors is unproven."

Santini et al. (637) suggested that the food residue in Puerto Rican diets might contain an inhibitor to "glutamate conjugase" since autoclaved food samples which were filtered before incubation contained three times as much total folacin activity as unfiltered samples. Luther et al. (473) proposed that filtering the Puerto Rican diets before incubating with conjugase removed compounds that adsorbed the released monoglutamates since the diets are high in cellulose and they found that nondietary fibers bound monoglutamates. On the other hand, Russell et al. (632) did not find that the undigestible fiber in Iranian flatbread that had been cooked for 1.5 to 5 minutes interfered with the absorption of folic acid.

In 1973, Krumdieck et al.[15] reported that extracts of red kidney beans, pinto beans, black-eyed peas, lima beans, lentils, navy beans, and soybeans contained an inhibitor to conjugase. It appears that the precursor molecule is largely concentrated in the skin of the seed; less activity was found in the embryo portion and cotyledon. Butterworth et al. (100) reported that the inhibitory effect is temporarily lost when red kidney beans are stored in the cold, but boiling restores it. Furthermore, the inhibitor is absorbable by humans "and therefore capable of exerting its effect on tissues such as liver and bone marrow" (100). Butterworth et al. (100) suggested that physiological role of such inhibitors in plants may be related to dormancy.

Earlier, Butterworth (95) had suggested that in some cases dietary pteroic acid might interfere with folacin absorption by tieing up the mucosal binding sites. Butterworth et al. (99) observed that two patients with tropical sprue excreted pteroic acid while receiving folic acid therapy. He (95) suggested that it was being displaced from tissue binding sites by the folic acid. According to Leslie and Rowe (453), the pteroic acid portion of the monoglutamate appears to be the structural determinant for the binding of folacins by the folacin binding proteins in the intestinal mucosa.

The data of Tamura et al. (727) suggest that the pH of orange juice may inhibit conjugase. They found that 600 g concentrated orange juice (pH 3.7) decreased the availability of pteroylheptaglutamic acid to 54%. Solutions containing 12 and 24 g citric acid (pH 3.7) decreased the availability of the polyglutamate to 66 and 39%, respectively. Orange juice had no effect on the availability of folic acid and it was only mildly inhibited by the 12 or

---

[15] Krumdieck, C. L., Newman, A. J. & Butterworth, C. E., Jr. (1973) A naturally occurring inhibitor of folic acid conjugase (pteroylpolyglutamyl hydrolase) in beans and other pulses. Am. J. Clin. Nutr. 26, 460–461 (abstr.).

24 g citric acid solutions. Adding glucose and sucrose to the 12 g citric acid solution (pH 3.7) eliminated the inhibitory effect of citric acid on folic acid availability but it did not completely reverse the inhibitory effect on the availability of the heptaglutamate. Increasing the pH of the 12 g citric acid solution to 6.4, however, increased the availability of pteroylheptaglutamic acid to 105%.

Previous data on the effect of pH on folic acid absorption are conflicting. Based on rise in serum folacin activity after a test dose of folic acid, Benn et al. (52) concluded that 10 g sodium bicarbonate, which increased the pH of the intestinal lumen by about 1 pH unit, decreased folic acid absorption. Perry and Chanarin (581) found that it increased folic acid absorption.

Studies of folic acid absorption by jejunal perfusion indicate that glucose increases folic acid absorption in humans (149, 240). Billich et al. (64) found that absorption of folic acid decreased significantly after 5 days of fasting and activities of sucrase and maltase also decreased. The recent data of Stifel et al. (707) "suggest an intimate relationship between folate and carbohydrate metabolism."

Little is known about the effect of protein binding on the availability of food folacins. Allfrey and King (3) reported that the polyglutamate in yeast is associated with a protein and dissociation is pH dependent. As previously pointed out, some investigators (216, 375) have suggested that the folacin binders in milk may facilitate utilization. The folacin in goat's milk is firmly bound to a protein (216) and autoclaving nearly doubled L. casei folacin activity (543). Hellendoorn et al. (307) reported that autoclaving whole meals increased L. casei folacin activity 50%.

Nutritional folacin deficiency. Reports on the effect of folacin deficiency on functional and morphological changes in the epithelial cells of the intestine are controversial. It may be a matter of the degree and duration of the deficiency (62, 807). Hurdle (361) found normal jejunal mucosa and tritiated folic acid absorption in patients with mild folacin deficiency. Others also reported no structural change in the jejunal mucosa of folacin deficient patients with megaloblastic bone marrow (an early manifestation of folacin deficiency) (807) or megaloblastic anemia (344).

On the other hand, Anderson et al. (8) and Jeejeebhoy et al. (392) both observed slightly impaired absorption of tritiated folic acid in patients with nutritional megaloblastic anemia. Elsborg (203) reported that 35% of the 53 geriatric patients with nutritional folacin deficiency had folic acid maladsorption which improved significantly (P < 0.0005) after treatment with folic acid. He concluded that folacin deficiency per se can produce a malabsorption syndrome which results in further depletion of folacin.

Weir et al. (779) and Jacobson (383) reported cases of "puerperal folate deficiency resembling tropical sprue" which responded completely to parenteral and oral folic acid. Others have found extensive changes in the intestinal mucosa (174) and abnormal xylose absorption (174, 222) in patients with severe nutritional deficiency which disappeared after folic acid therapy. Davidson and Townley (170) recently reported disaccharidase deficiency and structural abnormalities in the small intestine of four Australian infants with megaloblastic anemia. When their diets, which consisted primarily of goat's milk, were supplemented with 0.5 mg folic acid/day, their intestine quickly returned to normal.

Megalocytic changes in the intestinal epithelium, in association with megaloblastic bone marrow have also been reported in alcoholics with severe folacin deficiency (62, 327). In his recent review, Halsted (291) pointed out that "more studies are needed to determine the frequency and extent of intestinal abnormality in severe folate deficiency."

Tropical sprue and celiac disease. The intestinal pathologic changes caused by tropical sprue, which appears to affect the entire gastrointestinal tract (784), have been described in detail (48, 204, 647, 724, 784). However, the exact cause of tropical sprue is not known. Bernstein et al. (56, 57) have found that in vivo and in vitro the bile salts, deoxycholic acid, and chenodeoxycholic acid, are strong inhibitors of human and guinea pig intestinal conjugase.

They (57) suggested that the bile acids produced by intestinal microbes may play a role in the development of tropical sprue. Other possible etiological mechanisms have recently been reviewed by Butterworth et al. (100).

Investigators have presented data indicating that their patients were unable to utilize the conjugated forms of folacin (346, 389, 661) and 40 to 100% of those tested had impaired absorption of pharmacological doses (40 μg/kg body weight) of crystalline folic acid (99, 245, 390, 423, 427). Reduced absorption of physiological amounts (20 to 200 μg) of folic acid in 35 to 47% of the patients has also been reported [16] (346, 392, 427). However, when glucose was added to the folic acid solution, Gerson et al. (239) and Corcino et al. (149) found that all patients with tropical sprue had impaired folic acid absorption. Using the combined techniques of luminal disappearance and subsequent urinary recovery, Corcino et al. (150) have recently shown marked malabsorption of both the mono- and the polyglutamate forms of folacin in untreated tropical sprue.

Pharmacological doses of folic acid produce clinical improvement (hematologic response and remission of megaloblastosis; decreased diarrhea, nausea and steatorrhea; increased serum folacin activity; and increased xylose and vitamin B_{12} absorption) in folic acid deficient patients (32, 432, 660) but they do not cure the disease (660, 784). Prolonged antibiotic therapy (6 months or more) appears to be the most effective treatment for tropical sprue, providing folacin intake is adequate [16] (390, 425, 784). Gregory,[16] however, found that folic acid malabsorption persisted for more than a year in two patients, despite clinical and histological improvement after tetracycline.

Klipstein (426) and Lindenbaum et al. (457) have also reviewed reports from various parts of the world, especially the tropics, of changes in intestinal morphology and reduced xylose absorption in apparently healthy people. In some asymptomatic subjects, intestinal lesions apparently persist for years before clinical signs of tropical sprue manifest themselves (427, 518). Keusch et al. (415) reported that Americans stationed in Thailand acquired xylose malabsorption and other signs of tropical malabsorption syndrome but there was no significant difference in their serum folacin activity before and after their residence in Thailand. The cause, prevalence, and significance of asymptomatic intestinal abnormalities are not known (148).

Klipstein et al. (431) concluded that, when dietary folacin intake is "adequate" mild impairment of intestinal absorption usually does not result in the development of a nutritional deficiency state. However, when dietary intake is marginal, and "the supplemental factor of impaired intestinal absorption is added, deficiencies develop in a large proportion of such individuals" (431). These data suggest that the dietary folacin requirements of people from areas where subclinical malabsorption is common may be different from those of people who reside in parts of the world where asymptomatic malabsorption is less common. Weir et al. (779) suggested that tropical sprue may also occur in a temperate climate.

Celiac disease, which is also called gluten-sensitive enteropathy, primary idiopathic steatorrhea, non-tropical sprue, and adult celiac disease (816), causes malabsorption of both the mono- and the polyglutamate forms of folacin. Chanarin (109) has reviewed the reports in the literature through 1968 and since then others (228, 344) have reported similar findings. The exact cause of the disease is unknown; however, most patients respond to a gluten-free diet. Recent reports which have been reviewed in Nutrition Reviews (14) suggest that "local cell-mediated immunity to α-gliadin is responsible for villous atrophy and crypt hyperplasia in celiac disease." In addition to malabsorption and the possible loss of endogenous folacin due to failure to reabsorb biliary folacin, there may be further losses due to excessive sloughing of the intestinal cells in celiac patients (158).

Congenital malabsorption. Congenital malabsorption of folacin, which was first reported by Luhby et al. (471) in 1961 has been confirmed by Santiago-Borrero et al. (636) and Lanskowzky et al. (446).

---

[16] Gregory, D. H. (1970) Simultaneous calcium and folic acid absorption, a new oral test. Gastroenterology 58, 1042 (abstr.).

Interrelationship of folacin utilization with other nutrients

Iron

The interrelationship between iron and folacin is complex and, as Hershko et al. (328) and Roberts et al. (611) have pointed out, many of the reports in the literature appear to be contradictory (121). A number of studies suggest that the amount of folacin used is dependent on the iron status of the individual. It appears that iron deficiency may interfere with the utilization of folacin. Investigators have found that the response of anemic patients to treatment depends on an adequate intake of both iron and folacin. Others have suggested that iron deficiency may increase folacin requirements. Little is known about the biochemical mechanisms responsible for these observations or the subclinical effect of marginal iron deficiency on folacin metabolism and requirements.

Most of our information on the effect of iron status on folacin metabolism and/or requirement has come from the treatment of patients with varying degrees of nutrient deficiency. Knowledge of their previous food intake was usually lacking and control subjects were often not included. Furthermore, dietary intake during treatment has not been included in any of the reports (328). This lack of information on the nutritional status of the patient has led to a great deal of confusion.

Since the metabolism of iron, folic acid, vitamin B_{12}, and other nutrients is interrelated, the criteria used for evaluating status often indicate "apparent" rather than "true" status for a given nutrient (611, 730). In folacin deficiency iron stores are above normal (4, 248) and in iron deficiency red cell folacin is often normal in spite of apparent signs of folacin deficiency (49, 175, 611). In vitamin B_{12} deficiency, serum folacin is increased and red cell values are low (122, 141).

Experimental data indicate that both iron and folacin status affect hemoglobin concentration. The initial status of both nutrients is especially important when treating anemic patients (420). Some investigators have found that iron or iron and folic acid are equally effective in raising hemoglobin concentration (74, 132, 370); others have reported that iron plus folic acid was much more effective than iron or folic acid alone (376). In some cases, the need for supplemental folic acid appeared to be related to the amount of iron given (369).

Recent investigators have found that iron supplementation alone effectively increased the hemoglobin concentration of anemic patients who had normal serum (611) or red cell (20, 134, 328) folacin activities. But it was less effective in those patients with low serum (175, 611) or red cell (328) values. Iron and folic acid supplements had no effect on the hemoglobin concentration of subjects who were initially moderately- or well-nourished (70, 463, 520).

A number of different studies indicate that iron therapy increases the amount of folacin used. Some investigators (75, 475, 653, 730) have reported cases of "masked" folacin deficiency. Patients with apparent simple iron-deficiency anemia (including normoblastic bone marrow) responded poorly to iron therapy and began to show signs of folacin deficiency—megaloid cells and white cell changes in peripheral blood and bone marrow—after receiving iron injections for varying periods of time. These folacin deficiency symptoms responded well to folic acid supplements. Tasker (730) suggested that folacin stores were just sufficient to prevent megaloblastic changes and that the sudden regeneration of new cells, following iron medication, quickly exhausted the available folacin. Excess iron injected into women with severe folacin deficiency is toxic (653).

Combrink et al. (141) reported that there was a marked increase in FIGLU excretion of pregnant women who received injected iron but it was not apparent in those who received oral iron. Butler (93) found that the administration of oral iron alone to pregnant women caused an overproduction of red cells and a compensatory increase in plasma volume but the administration of 3.4 mg folic acid along with 122 mg elemental iron daily prevented this problem. Weyden et al. (783) have recently presented evidence that an iron dependent enzyme functions in the conversion of ribonucleotides to deoxyribonucleotides, thus providing biochemical evidence for the established morphological findings that iron deficiency alters or masks megaloblastic maturation in appropriate conditions.

Experimental results indicate that pregnant women who receive supplemental iron use more folacin. Chanarin and Rothman (121) reported that women given supplemental iron had more megaloblastosis than the control group and the babies of women with megaloblastosis weighed more. Iyengar (369) and Aung-Than-Batu and Hla-Pe (20) found that the red cell folacin values of women receiving supplemental iron decreased during pregnancy and 4 to 6 weeks postpartum values remained low (369) or continued to fall (20). However, in the group that received no supplements, there was only a slight fall in red cell folacin during pregnancy and values remained constant at 4 weeks postpartum (20). Aung-Than-Batu and Hla-Pe (20) found that serum folacin decreased in the last trimester of pregnancy in both the supplemented and the placebo groups. During the postpartum period serum values continued to decline in the iron supplemented group but they increased significantly in the nonsupplemented group (20). Chanarin et al. (122) observed similar effects of iron supplementation on postpartum serum values. Supplemental iron administered to anemic women during the postpartum period also prevented the normal postpartum increment in serum folacin (519).

Toskes et al. (743) suggested that iron deficiency increased folacin requirements. They observed intramedullary and peripheral red cell destruction in iron deficient rats. Chanarin and Rothman (121) concluded that since supplemental iron did not reduce the frequency of megaloblastic hemopoiesis in pregnancy, iron does not have a direct effect on folacin status; the association of iron deficiency and megaloblastic anemia "is the result of poor nutrition, and . . . there is no cause-and-effect relation between them."

Recent data suggest that iron deficiency interferes with the utilization of folacin. Some investigators have reported megaloblastic changes (135, 519, 754) and low serum folacin values in iron deficient humans (122, 754) and rats (743) which improved with iron treatment. Others have found that in iron deficient children (134, 135, 596, 642) and adults (49, 175, 328, 479, 568, 611, 762) red cell folacin stores were normal (134, 135, 175, 328, 611, 642) or above normal (49, 298, 479, 568, 596) and yet most of the patients had one or more signs of folacin deficiency—low serum values (134, 175, 328, 611), giant metamyelocytes (49, 175, 611), or megaloblastic maturation of red cell precursors (135, 762) in the bone marrow, hypersegmented neutrophils (49, 135, 175, 298, 596, 611) or macrocytes (762) in peripheral blood and positive FIGLU test (49, 611). When iron was administered, red cell folacin values decreased (49, 568, 611, 642) or increased (328); serum folacin values increased (175, 328, 568), decreased (49, 611) or remained the same (596, 643); the abnormal cells in the bone marrow (135, 298, 611, 762) and peripheral blood (49, 135, 175, 611, 762) were significantly reduced or disappeared; and excess FIGLU excretion improved (49) or remained abnormal (611). Saraya et al. (642) concluded from these results that iron deficiency prevents the release of stored folacin.

There is little information on the biochemical mechanism(s) responsible for these observed results. Vitale et al. (761) found that experimental iron deficiency in rats produced low serum folacin values, megaloblastic changes in the bone marrow, excess excretion of FIGLU after a histidine load test and decreased liver glutamate formiminotransferase activity. Arakawa et al. (17) has reported a congenital defect in hepatic glutamate formiminotransferase activity in an 8-month old baby who showed evidence of folacin deficiency. Others (91, 655), however, found hepatic enzyme activity unaltered in iron deficient rats. Sharma (655) suggested that since vitamin B_{12} is reduced in iron deficient rats, excess FIGLU excretion was the result of vitamin B_{12} deficiency. But Hill et al. (339) found significant dyserythropoiesis in iron deficient patients with high serum folacin and normal B_{12} levels. They had giant granulocytes but no morphological features of megaloblastic erythropoiesis. Hill et al. (339) therefore suggested that iron plays an important role in erythroblast DNA and conceivably RNA synthesis.

Izak et al. (376) recently concluded that "it seems that the question of causal relationship of iron and folate deficiencies cannot be satisfactorily resolved on the basis of the data available today."

Ascorbic acid

The effect of ascorbic acid status on folacin requirements is uncertain. Occasionally, megaloblastic anemia occurs in patients with scurvy (19, 81, 82, 127, 156, 264, 385, 549, 709, 793, 815). In some of the patients ascorbic acid alone reportedly corrected the anemia (19, 81, 82, 264). Others required supplemental folic acid (709, 815). Zalusky and Herbert (815) concluded that the megaloblastosis found in patients with scurvy is due to folic acid deficiency. A scorbutic diet is usually also low in folacin (19, 127, 815). Asquith et al. (19) and Cox et al. (157) suggested that the difference between those responding to ascorbic acid alone and those requiring supplemental folacin may be in the degree of tissue folacin depletion.

The data of May et al. (507, 509) suggest that ascorbic acid deficiency may increase the folacin requirement of the rhesus monkey. In 1950, they (507) reported that monkeys fed boiled milk, which had also been treated with cupric ions to destroy any residual ascorbic acid, developed scurvy. Shortly thereafter they also developed megaloblastosis but it was quickly eliminated by supplemental folic acid. It could also be cured by ascorbic acid alone (509). Monkeys that received supplemental ascorbic acid in the morning feeding did not develop megaloblastic anemia. They found no difference in the amount of folacin activity excreted in the urine, but the livers of the control monkeys contained more folacin (1.42 versus 0.18 μg/g liver).

May et al. (509) later reported that monkeys receiving supplemental ascorbic acid also developed megaloblastosis after 269 days. The ascorbate deficient monkeys developed megaloblastosis in 70 to 116 days. It was concluded that ascorbic acid deficiency led to "a deficiency of, or some disturbance in the metabolism of pteroylglutamic acid."

The data of Ghitis (241) and Ford (215) indicate that boiling milk and treating it with cupric ions significantly reduces the folacin content. As Ghitis (241) pointed out, May et al. (507, 509) also fed the monkeys an "unwittingly induced low folate diet" which "resulted in a defective protection of the body folates. . . ." Ghitis (241) divided the free folacins in milk into three fractions. The first, which comprises about 44% of the total free folacin activity, cannot resist boiling but it does resist pasteurization. The second fraction is destroyed by boiling in the presence of cupric ions. And the third fraction (about 26%) resists oxidation by boiling in the presence of cupric ions. The stability of the polyglutamates was not studied.

Nichol and Welch (555) reported that ascorbic acid increased the in vitro conversion of folic acid to 5-CHO-H_4-folic acid by rat liver slices. However, Stokstad (711) pointed out in his review of the literature that there is little evidence to show that ascorbic acid is required for this reduction.

Data on the folacins in the urine of scorbutic patients before and after receiving ascorbic acid suggest that ascorbic acid deficiency affects the metabolism of folacin and may therefore affect folacin requirements (157, 709). Cox et al. (156) reported that after scorbutic patients had been treated with ascorbic acid they excreted significantly less folacin activity following 5 mg test doses of folic acid. Stokes et al. (709) found that the major folacin compound in the urine of one scorbutic patient with megaloblastic anemia was 10-CHO-folic acid. After treatment with ascorbic acid, the predominant folacin was 5-CH_3-H_4-folic acid. They reasoned that scorbutic subjects lose folacins from the body at an increased rate because, in the absence of ascorbic acid, 10-CHO-H_4-folic acid, the metabolically active form of folacin in the serum, is oxidized to the metabolically inactive form, 10-CHO-folic acid, and excreted in the urine. They therefore postulated that "the anemia of scurvy is due in part to this depletion of the folate pool and that an important role for ascorbic acid in human metabolism may well be to reduce the rate of oxidation of 10-formyl-THF and thereby keep the folate metabolic pool replete."

Carefully controlled studies are needed to clarify the metabolic relationship between ascorbic acid and folacin and the effect of ascorbic acid status on folacin requirements.

Vitamin B_{12} and methionine

The interrelationship between vitamin B_{12} and folacin is complex (112, 343). A deficiency of vitamin B_{12} interferes with the metabolism and storage of folacin. Decreased red cell (144, 347, 391, 582) and leukocyte (582, 758) folacin activity, which are indicative of folacin deficiency, have been observed in vitamin B_{12} deficient patients. Excess FIGLU excretion after a histidine load test (107, 115, 322, 347), rapid folate clearance rate (347) and an increased rate of renal excretion of 5-CH_3-H_4-folic acid or its derivatives and a decreased rate of renal metabolism of 5-CH_3-H_4-folic acid to other urinary folacin derivatives (559) have been reported. Vidal and Stokstad (755) also found that B_{12} deficient rats lost excess folacin in the urine. Although serum folacin activity is often elevated in patients with vitamin B_{12} deficiency (144, 325, 414, 642, 698, 770) decreased folacin activity in the livers of vitamin B_{12} deficient sheep (172, 681, 682), rats (794), and baboons (675) have been reported. When sheep ingested B_{12}, the liver folacin content increased (172).

The mechanism of folacin depletion in vitamin B_{12} deficiency has not been elucidated. Some investigators have hypothesized that B_{12} deficiency prevents folacin from entering the cell (737). Gawthorne and Smith (236) suggested that B_{12} may be needed to supply methionine which is required for membrane transport of folacin. However, Perry et al. (582) concluded that there was no failure to transport 5-CH_3-H_4-folic acid into the cells of B_{12} deficient patients but rather a failure to synthesize polyglutamates.

Some have found a comparatively greater depletion of polyglutamate rather than monoglutamate folacins in the red cells of patients with pernicious anemia (391) and in the livers of B_{12} deficient rats (735) and ewes (681). Others, however, did not find that the polyglutamates in rat livers were depleted to any greater degree than monoglutamates (682).

The data of a number of investigators suggest that the action of vitamin B_{12} deficiency on folacin status is mediated via methionine metabolism (236, 237, 677, 682, 755, 760). Sauer and Wilmanns (646) concluded from their studies with vitamin B_{12} deficient patients that reduced methionine synthetase activity was responsible for the secondary alterations in folacin metabolism. In 1962, Noronha and Silverman (562) reported that "dietary methionine causes a rearrangement of folic acid distribution pattern in the liver of the rat. . . ." Williams and Spray (795) recently reported a tendency for a higher concentration of either methionine or homocystine in the diet of rats to be associated with a higher concentration of both folacin and vitamin B_{12} in the liver. Methionine reportedly reduces abnormal FIGLU excretion in B_{12} and/or folacin deficient humans (322), rats (677), and ewes (682).

In vitamin B_{12} and methionine deficient rats there is decreased liver folacin (760) and decreased uptake of ^{3}H-folic acid (237, 755). Vitale and Hegsted (760) reported that supplementing the deficient diet with methionine or B_{12} caused an increase in liver folacin while Gawthorne and Stokstad (237) found that when small doses of methionine (40 mg) were given B_{12} was also necessary to increase the rate of uptake of ^{3}H-folic acid. However, large doses of methionine alone (200 mg) were effective. Buehring et al. (88) found that methionine changed the form of folacin in the liver of rats. It reduced the amount of 5-CH_3-H_4-folic acid and increased the proportion of other monoglutamates and polyglutamate forms of folacin. In addition, both Vidal and Stokstad (755) and Gawthorne and Smith (236) found that the concentration of S-adenosyl-L-methionine in the liver of B_{12} deficient rats and sheep, respectively, was about one-half of that in normal animals and either vitamin B_{12} or L-methionine restored it to normal. Some of the possible effects of excess methionine on folacin metabolism have been reviewed by Stebbins et al. (702).

Other vitamins and amino acids

Waxman et al. (774) have reviewed some of the possible interrelationships of glycine, homocysteine, serine and pyridoxine with folacin metabolism and their possible effects of folacin requirements. Studies with rats (77, 351) suggest that riboflavin deficiency interferes with the metabolism of folacin while supplemental "histidine was associated with significantly higher folate concentrations in the livers of cyanocobalamin-supplemented rats" (795). The study of the effect of amino acids and other vitamins on human folacin requirements is in its infancy.

Other factors affecting folacin utilization and requirements

Ethanol

Varying degrees of folacin deficiency are commonly encountered in chronic alcoholics (118, 171, 195, 208, 233, 326, 327, 813). Their serum (171, 195, 196, 208, 233, 340, 571) and liver (118) folacin values are often significantly less than normal and they develop megaloblastosis more quickly than healthy subjects when they eat a low folacin diet (195). It is not known, however, if the apparent decreased folacin status is primarily due to decreased dietary intake (182, 221, 797) or if alcohol itself alters dietary folacin absorption, storage and requirements.

Williams and Girdwood (797) found that the mean serum and red blood cell folacin values of alcoholics who were not undernourished and who ate regular meals did not differ significantly from the mean values of healthy adults. Deller et al. (182) reported that the serum folacin levels of subjects who drank wine and spirits were often subnormal but beer drinkers were seldom deficient. Neither group (182, 797) found that the severity of liver disease was especially related to folacin deficiency.

Although folacin deficiency was common in the alcoholics whom Wu et al. (813) examined, they concluded that alcohol intake and extent of liver damage did not affect folacin status. In fact, the red cell folacin values of alcoholics consuming more than 160 g ethanol/day were significantly higher than the values of those who drank less. They suggested that this might be partially attributed to the fact that 50% of them drank beer which is high in folacin. Carney (103, 104) found that chronic alcoholics had higher mean serum folacin

values than controls but he was unable to correlate it with beer drinking (104). Wu et al. (813) concluded that dietary folacin intake appeared to be the main factor in determining the folacin status of people who drank alcohol. Diets were classified as "adequate" if they consisted of more than one meal/day. They found good correlation between liver, serum, and red cell folacin values. The range of liver values was almost identical with that found in patients without liver disease (118).

Klipstein and Lindenbaum (428) concluded that inadequate folacin intake was of major importance in the development of folacin deficiency in liver disease. They pointed out, however, that secondary complications due to alcoholism, such as gastrointestinal bleeding, hypersplenism, and overt hemolysis, would increase folacin requirements. McGuffin et al. (513) reported that the drop in kidney and liver folacin was the same in rats fed sugar and water or with added ethanol. Serum values, however, declined much more rapidly in the rats fed ethanol.

The effect of alcohol itself on folacin absorption is not known. Halsted et al. (294) compared the amount of tritiated folic acid in the serum and urine of alcoholics with liver disease and non-alcoholics who ingested a test dose of 4.5 oz whiskey with healthy non-drinkers after labeled folic acid was administered orally. All subjects were presaturated with folic acid. Urinary excretion was similar in all groups but increment in serum ^{3}H-folic acid of alcoholics was significantly less than the values for non-alcoholics. Halsted et al. (294) therefore concluded that folic acid absorption in chronic alcoholics was impaired. Cherrick et al. (129) attributed the disparity between serum and urinary response in the alcoholics to the inability of the diseased liver to retain folacin. Data from rat experiments suggest that ethanol may directly affect the formation of liver pteroylpolyglutamates (85).

Triple lumen perfusion of the jejunum with ^{3}H-folic acid indicated decreased absorption in chronic alcoholics with a "poor diet" as compared to well-nourished alcoholics (295). Abstinence and a hospital diet for 2 weeks restored folic acid absorption to normal and, in five out of seven folacin repleted alcoholics, ingesting alcohol for 2 weeks did not affect folic acid absorption. Halsted et al. (295) suggested that the malabsorption was caused by poor nutrition rather than a toxic effect of ethanol on the jejunum. Others (62, 327) have reported changes in the intestinal mucosa of alcoholic patients with severe nutritional folacin deficiency which disappeared after folic acid therapy. The mucosal changes occurred only when folacin deficiency developed (327).

Halsted et al. (296) also found that when three former alcoholics ate a low folacin diet until they became depleted, jejunal uptake of ^{3}H-folic acid was unchanged in the subject who remained sober but in those that drank 200 g ethanol daily, uptake decreased from 32 and 40% to 19 and 12%, respectively. They therefore concluded that malabsorption was caused by a combination of folacin deficiency and prolonged ethanol intake. There was no observable difference in the jejunal "uptake of ^{3}H-folic acid among rats fed normal diet, normal diet plus ethanol, a protein-deficient diet, or a protein-deficient diet plus ethanol" (293).

Halsted et al. (293) pointed out, however, that the effects of alcohol itself on the digestion and absorption of food folacins are still undetermined. Baker et al. (27) concluded that although alcoholics with liver disease utilized folic acid, they were unable to utilize polyglutamates since their serum values did not increase 2 to 5 hours after ingesting 35 g Brewer's yeast, and after 3 weeks of abstinence there was still no improvement. Control subjects utilized folic acid and the folacin from yeast equally well.

The suppression of hematopoiesis by alcohol in healthy subjects with good folacin status suggests that it alters metabolism in the bone marrow. In 1964, Sullivan and Herbert (723) reported that during alcohol ingestion reticulocyte response to small doses of folic acid (75 μg) was impaired. Larger doses (500 μg DL-folinic acid or 150 μg folic acid) produced a brisk hematologic response in two patients but their bone marrow remained megaloblastic until alcohol was removed. Others have also reported hematopoietic suppression by alcohol (153, 154, 171, 195, 355, 458, 765,

812). A number of reports of thrombocytopenia, leucopenia, and impaired erythropoiesis in alcoholics with no apparent folacin deficiency were reviewed in 1968 (12). Wu et al. (812) also recently observed megaloblastic bone marrow and macrocytosis in alcoholics in the absence of folacin deficiency. Lindenbaum and Lieber (458) found that "hematologic alterations occurred despite the concomitant administration of pharmacologic doses of folic acid." Some investigators reported, however, that alcohol decreased serum values (195, 196, 723, 765). Others reported no effect on serum (153, 458, 812) or red cell (153, 812) values. When ethanol was withdrawn, hematopoiesis (153, 195, 723, 812) and serum values (195, 196, 765) immediately returned to normal.

The mechanism of this toxic effect of ethanol on bone marrow has not been elucidated. The in vitro studies of Bertino et al.[17] indicate that alcohol inhibits formyl-H_4-folic acid synthetase in bone marrow. This could account for the suppression of hematopoiesis mediated through the impaired biosynthesis of nucleic acids.

Folic acid increases the activity of human jejunal glycolytic enzymes (625) but small amounts (60 to 100 ml) of alcohol depresses the activity of these enzymes and inhibits the increase in enzyme activities due to folic acid (274). Pharmacologic doses (15 mg/day) of folic acid, however, reversed this inhibitory effect of ethanol. Greene et al. (274) therefore suggested that if some of the deleterious effects of ethanol are related to decreases in enzyme activities, then pharmacological amounts of folic acid might exert a protective action in individuals without irreversible liver disease.

Studies with rats (535, 587) indicate that they recover from previously induced nutritional hepatic lesions, even when alcohol contributes approximately 50% of the total calories "if the accompanying intake of all essential food factors and vitamins are abundant (super diet)" (587). The vitamin mixture contained folic acid. On the other hand, Feinman and Lieber (207) maintain that ethanol, as compared to iso-

---

[17] Bertino, J. R., Ward, J., Sartorelli. A. C. & Silber, R. (1965) An effect of ethanol on folate metabolism. J. Clin. Invest. 44, 1028 (abstr.).

energetic amounts of carbohydrate, in the diets of humans causes changes in the liver despite massive dietary supplementation with choline, minerals, vitamins and protein.

Drugs

Oral contraceptives. Oral contraceptives alter the metabolism of folacin but the biological significance of these changes, which are similar to those seen in pregnant women, has not been elucidated. The question of the net effect of oral contraceptives on folacin requirements remains unanswered.

Reports on the effect of oral contraceptives on blood folacin values are conflicting. Seven investigators [18, 19] (229, 406, 588, 673, 699) compared the serum and red cell values of women who took oral contraceptives and those who did not. None of the subjects had megaloblastic anemia and there was no mention of clinical malabsorption. Four of them [18, 19] (229, 673) found that both serum and red cell values of users were significantly lower than the values of non-users. In one study (588) only red cell values of oral contraceptive users were significantly lower than non-users and in the other two (406, 699) blood values of users and non-users were similar. In three of the studies [19] (229, 673) women taking oral contraceptives also excreted significantly more FIGLU after a histidine load test. Shojania (666) found that women taking oral contraceptives also excreted more folacin in the urine than controls for any given level of serum or red cell folacin. Pregnant women also excreted more urinary folacin activity (210).

Serum folacin values only were compared in 10 surveys [20] (98, 105, 515, 572, 593, 626, 672, 704, 781). Two investigators found a significant difference in users and non-users (672, 781). Shojania et al. (674) pointed out that in some surveys "the number studied is too small, the control subjects had not been from the same source, or the duration of oral contraceptive therapy has been too short." In the recent surveys of Paine et al. (572) and Ross et al. (626), however, the subjects had taken oral contraceptives for 3 to 96 months. Boots et al. (76) found that there was no

decrease in the serum folacin level of baboons who took oral contraceptives for 9 months. Since their endocrine parameters resemble humans and "experimental protocols can be rigidly adhered to," they recommended detailed studies with baboons to resolve some of the many unanswered questions.

In four other studies serum (615, 674, 680) and red cell (2, 680) folacin values of women taking oral contraceptives were followed for 6 months to 4 years. Blood folacin values fell significantly with duration of contraceptive use. Shojania et al. (674) found that no subjects developed megaloblastic anemia, but the number with serum folacin values less than 3 ng/ml rose progressively from 9% at less than 1 year to 21% at 2 years and 42% after 4 years. Only 2% of the controls had pathologically low folacin values. Both Gaafar et al. (229) and Shojania et al. (674) emphasized that the effect of oral contraceptives is mild and in normal women it takes a long time to see the effects of oral contraceptives on folacin status.

The 14 reports, since 1969, of 31 cases of megaloblastic anemia in patients taking oral contraceptives for 1 to 5 years have been reviewed by Lindenbaum et al. (459). In some of the cases, other factors such as malabsorption diseases, dietary deficiency and other drugs which adversely affect folacin status were present. Both Chanarin (111) and Shojania (667) pointed out that there was no definite proof that oral contraceptives were the cause of the anemia. The data of Wood et al. (810), however, suggest that they may precipitate folacin deficiency in patients with marginal deficiency due to other causes.

Butterworth et al. (98) found no difference in the absorption of 5-CHO-H$_4$-folic acid in users and non-users. However, tests with women taking oral contraceptives, who had not been presaturated with folic acid, indicated impaired absorption of folyl-

---

[18] Alperin, J. B. (1973) Folate metabolism in women using oral contraceptive agents. Am. J. Clin. Nutr. *26*, 19 (abstr.).
[19] Luhby, A. L., Shimizu, N., Davis, P. & Cooperman, J. M. (1971) Folic acid deficiency in users of oral contraceptive agents. Fed. Proc., Fed. Am. Soc. Exp. Biol. *30*, 239 (abstr.).
[20] Maniego-Bautista, L. P. & Bassano, G. (1969) Effect of oral contraceptives on serum lipid and folate levels. J. Lab. Clin. Med. *74*, 988 (abstr.)

polyglutamates (548, 704, 717). Stephens et al. (704) and Shojania and Hornady (671) found that when users and non-users were previously saturated with folic acid, there was no difference between the two groups in absorption of folic acid and polyglutamates. Moreover, synthetic sex hormones did not inhibit jejunal conjugase in vitro (704). These data suggest that the clearance rate is more rapid in women taking oral contraceptives. Stephens et al. (704) did not think that it was due to "significant tissue depletion since there is no correlation between peak rises observed and the initial fasting serum folate concentrations." They (704) found no significant difference in fasting serum folacin values of users and non-users. Shojania (666) found that during the first 5 minutes the clearance rate of women taking oral contraceptives was more rapid than controls but subsequent rates were the same in the two groups.

Recent animal experiments indicate that sex hormones (male and female) increase the activity of jejunal enzymes involved in folacin metabolism and thus affect the synthesis of folacin coenzymes (79, 483, 629, 706, 741). Castrated male rats had a reduced capacity to convert injected folic acid to the active form and therefore excreted more into the urine (78). Maxwell et al. (505) suggested that oral contraceptives may act by accelerating folacin metabolism through induction of hepatic enzymes. Laffi et al. (439) reported that estrogen caused a significant lowering of 5-CH_3-H_4-folic acid and an increase in 10-CHO-H_4-folic acid in both the uterus and the liver of castrated female rats, in comparison to untreated castrated animals (78). Sex hormones also control the amount of "free" and "total" folacin in the uterus (438). Conjugase levels and "free" folacin derivatives increased in uterine homogenates of castrated animals 12 to 18 hours after the injection of estradiol-17 β.

Lindenbaum et al. (459) and Whitehead et al. (788) found megaloblastic cells in the cervical epithelium of humans which disappeared when the women were given folic acid for 3 weeks. When they were re-examined 3 years later, the abnormal cells had reappeared (459). Whitehead et al. (788) could not relate the cytologic ab-

normalities to hematologic findings or serum folacin values. Changes in serum folacin-binding proteins similar to those observed in pregnant women have been found in some women taking oral contraceptives (152, 197, 498). On the other hand, Ross et al. (626) found no free folacin binding proteins in the serum, no increase in the amount of folacin bound to serum proteins and no megaloblastic changes in the cervical epithelium of women who had taken oral contraceptives for 9 to 72 months.

Other drugs. The number of drugs that reportedly affect folacin metabolism and in some cases induce megaloblastic anemia are rapidly increasing. These have been covered extensively in a recent symposium (58) as well as a number of recent reviews (259, 323, 702). In many cases the mechanism of action is not known; it is a very active research area. Methotrexate and aminopterin are both powerful inhibitors of the enzyme dihydrofolate reductase. The antimalarial drug, pyrimethamine, and trimethoprim, an antibacterial drug, also inhibit dihydrofolate reductase. The anticonvulsant drugs—diphenylhydantoin, primidone, and barbiturates—appear to antagonize folacin status since epileptics tend to develop folacin deficiency after taking the drugs for prolonged periods of time.

Ritland et al. (610) reported that the bile sequestering agent, polidexide, which is used in treating hyperlipoproteinemia II caused "slight transient changes in serum folic acid" values of adults who took 15 g/day for up to 18 months. Similarly, Nikkila et al. (557) reported reduced serum folacin concentration in 8 of their 20 patients who took this amount for more than 2 years. On the other hand, West and Lloyd (782) reported that prolonged treatment (18 months) of children 1 to 14 years old with 0.7 g polidexide/kg body weight twice daily produced folacin deficiency. It was overcome by administering 5 mg folic acid/day.

Alter et al. (5) suggested that aspirin caused a redistribution of folacin in the body. They observed that patients with rheumatoid arthritis who were taking aspirin had abnormally rapid plasma clearance of ³H-folic acid and a significant reduction in the "binding" of serum ³H-folic acid. Patients not taking aspirin had normal values. In normal subjects aspirin caused ^{3}H-folic acid binding and serum folacin values to decrease. In vitro, the more aspirin added to serum the greater the decrease in "binding."

Buehring et al. (89) recently reported that the administration of the carcinogen, diethylnitrosamine, to rats led to a decrease in hepatic levels of folacin.

Infection

Infection and megaloblastic anemia due to folacin deficiency are frequently associated but the effect of infection on folacin requirements has not been established. As Chanarin (109) explained, "The role of infection is difficult to evaluate and it is uncertain whether malnourished folate deficient infants are more susceptible to infections, or whether the infection itself places added stress on folate metabolism and leads to a megaloblastic form of haemopoiesis." Folacin deficiency in patients with infection has been attributed to a combination of factors including low reserves, inadequate dietary intake, loss through diarrhea and vomiting, increased granulocyte and red cell turnover, and impaired absorption or utilization of folacin due to the infection (417, 468, 474, 753, 808, 817, 818). The interrelationship between infection and folacin deficiency may depend on the kind of infection.

Many clinicians have reported megaloblastic anemia due to folacin deficiency in infants and children with diarrhea (413, 416, 468, 474, 614, 753, 808, 818), gastroenteritis (742, 764), and respiratory infections (50, 273, 413, 468, 474, 614, 753, 764, 817), especially in premature infants (273, 818) and in those less than 6 months old (468, 742, 818). Diarrhea ceased when folic acid was administered (413, 474). Others (273, 614, 764, 808) have reported that diarrhea and infections preceded the development of megaloblastic anemia, suggesting that increased folacin requirements due to infection precipitated the anemia. Luhby (468) concluded that in infants 2 to 5 months old severe infection was the principal cause of megaloblastic anemia. In older infants (8 to 12 months old), however, inadequate diet appeared to be the principal etiological factor.

Similar data have been reported for adult humans as well as other primates. Mollin and Hoffbrand (532) reported that 6 weeks after a man with marginal folacin stores developed bronchopneumonia he was anemic, thrombocytopenic and leucopenic. All signs of folacin deficiency were relieved with small doses of folic acid (200 μg/day). However, folacin intake during the illness was not mentioned.

In 1944, Day (179) reviewed the numerous reports in the early literature of vitamin "M" deficiency in rhesus monkeys and increased susceptibility to "spontaneous infections." In his laboratory he found that feeding living dysentery bacilli to monkeys receiving a normal diet did not produce diarrhea but those given a "vitamin M-deficient diet" developed cytopenia and acute clinical dysentery. May et al. (508) found that the folacin levels in the livers of monkeys with natural or experimentally induced infections were much lower than normal. Their appetite, activity and weight also declined. Siddons (676) recently reported that baboons on an experimental folacin deficient diet developed anorexia, asthenia, diarrhea, leucopenia, thrombocytopenia, and in some animals, macrocytic anemia. The administration of folic acid caused an "immediate return of appetite and well-being."

Cook et al. (142) and Areekul et al. (18) reported impaired absorption of folic acid in patients with systemic bacterial infections (lobar pneumonia and pulmonary tuberculosis) and malaria, respectively. The experimental results of Panders and Rupert (573) indicate that in vitro, incubating folic acid with a chicken liver enzyme preparation at an elevated temperature (39°) inhibits the reduction of folic acid to H$_4$-folic acid. Others have reported increased utilization of folacin due to increased red cell hemolysis in patients with malaria (18, 116) and infectious mononucleosis (102). The observed increase in hypersegmented neutrophils in the latter patients suggests folacin deficiency (102). Das and Hoffbrand (168) found that in vitro, rapidly dividing phytohaemagglutinin-stimulated transformed lymphocytes took up significantly more folacin than non-stimulated mature lymphocytes.

There is also experimental evidence that folacin deficiency causes depressed cellular-mediated immunity. In 1951, Ludovici and Axelrod (467) reported that folacin deficiency severely impaired the antibody response of rats inoculated with human erythrocytes. Others have also reported impaired cell-mediated immune response in chickens (570) and rats (1, 796). Aboko-Cole and Lee (1) concluded that folacin deficiency in rats infected with *Trypantosoma lewisi* caused a delay in the formation of the reproduction-inhibiting antibody, ablastin. The deficient rats had twice as many parasites in their blood as control animals and they also remained infected for longer periods.

On the basis of the response of folacin deficient patients with megaloblastic anemia to dinitrochlorobenzene skin tests, phytohemagglutinin-stimulated lymphocyte transformation and rosette inhibition by antilymphocyte globulin, Gross et al. (277) concluded that folacin deficiency inhibited cell-mediated immunity in humans. On the other hand, Kaplan and Basford (402) recently reported that they found "no impairment of phagocytosis-associated metabolism or microbicidal activity in the leukocytes of patients with folic acid deficiency." Herbert (313) reported that during the 4.5 months of experimental folacin deprivation the subject did not have a single cold. Every winter for the prior 17 years, however, he had had frequent episodes of coryza. The response of folacin deficient patients may depend on the type of infection. We found no controlled studies on human folacin intake and resistance to infection.

COMMENTS

The amount of supplemental folic acid—the readily available synthetic monoglutamate that comprises about 1% of the total folacin activity in the average diet—required to cure and/or prevent signs of deficiency has been studied extensively in pregnant women and to a lesser degree in adults and premature infants. Yet, we have limited knowledge concerning human requirements for dietary folacin, an essential nutrient for the synthesis and functioning of all cells. Most of our information has come from a limited number of field studies in which the general nutritional status of the subjects varied. In the few studies where dietary folacin has been quantitated total folacin activity was usually not determined and even free folacin activity was often ill-defined.

One of the major obstacles in the study of dietary folacin requirements has been the lack of information on the folacins in food and their bioavailability. In 1953, Darby (163) stressed the urgent need for "a critical systematic differential study of folic acid activity of foods—a study which will define the quantity of free folic acid, or conjugates, or thymidine and other non-folic stimulants, as well as give information on the presence of conjugase inhibitors." He also pointed out that in order to obtain meaningful information on human dietary requirements the minimal effective level of each of the folacins should then be determined. Moreover, the interrelationship of folacin with "other dietary and metabolic factors" should be considered.

Progress in fulfilling these needs has been slow. The development of a readily available method of quantitating the different folacins which is accurate, rapid and automatable continues to be a most urgent need. Development of methods to remove quantitatively folacins from their protein binders and to cleave the C^9-N^{10} bond (40, 778) along with the recently developed chromatographic methods of separating the folacin derivatives [22] (602, 715) may help fill this void.

In 1974, Baugh et al. (40) used a reductive procedure (Zn powder, 0.5 N HCl) to cleave the C^9-N^{10} bond of folylpolyglutamates. However, Maruyama et al.[21] recently found that with alkaline permanganate oxidation, which others have used, the bond in folic acid, H_4-folic acid and N^5-CHO-H_4-folic acid was cleaved but the bond in the methyl derivatives of folacin, the principal form in serum and red cells, resisted cleavage. Maruyama et al.[21] suggested cleaving the C^9-N^{10} bond in the

---

[21] Since the completion of this conspectus the following pertinent article was published: Maruyama, T., Shiota, T. & Krumdieck, C. L. (1978) The oxidative cleavage of folates: A critical study. Anal. Biochem. 84, 277–295.

methyl derivatives by acidifying the mixture after the oxidative procedure. Baugh et al. (40) did not mention the use of one-carbon substituted folacin derivatives in their experiments. Despite many shortcomings, the microbiological assay is still the principal method of estimating folacin content. Yet microbial growth does not necessarily indicate folacin activity in man.

The bioavailability of the polyglutamates has been a controversial topic. The results of some early studies (695, 722) suggested that they were utilized by man. However, the reports on conjugase inhibitors in yeast, plus the inability of microbes and patients with tropical sprue to utilize folacins containing more than two glutamyl residues in the side chain, led others to conclude that they were generally unavailable. Thus, many researchers did not bother to determine total dietary folacin activity. After 1969, when the synthesis of labeled polyglutamates made it possible to quantitate their absorption, it became apparent that physiological amounts of oxidized polyglutamates were well absorbed (97, 263, 729) and, as Butterworth (97) pointed out, they "should be taken into account in calculating dietary intake." Limited data suggest that the reduced monoglutamate derivatives are utilized equally well.

The bioavailability of dietary folacins, however, has not been resolved to any extent. The results of three studies (22, 604, 729) suggested a wide range of individual variability and it did not appear that availability correlated with mono- and polyglutamate content or the coenzyme forms present. Folic acid availability is reduced when added to food but the cause for this is uncertain. The possibility that monoglutamates may be bound by cellulose fibers has been suggested but needs further investigation (473, 632). Conjugase inhibitor(s) has been found in yeast and in legumes. To what extent it exists in other foods, however, remains to be determined. Glucose and pH also affect folacin absorption. Other dietary factors that need further study include the folacin binding proteins and intestinal microbes. Recent reports suggest that processing increases the availability of folacin in some foods. We need further studies on the availability of the natural folacins in food

and on synthetic folacins administered with natural inhibitors (100, 263).

Sensitive standardized criteria for evaluating folacin status, which are specific and adaptable to field use, are also urgently needed. As pointed out by the WHO committee on Nutritional Anaemias (791), at the present time it is difficult to quantitate "normal" folacin stores and to define "deficiency." Hypersegmented PMNs and red cell folacin content are helpful indicators. The latter, however, does not reflect the current status because of the lifetime of red cells. In the recent nutritional status surveys of Canada (563) and California,[12] low serum folacin values were found in a large proportion of the population. However, the clinical significance of these low values, especially in the absence of other hematological signs of folacin deficiency, is not known. More data are needed. The Canadians continue their search for possible relationships between the combined clinical and biochemical survey results and the dietary intake data (525). Hopefully, these analyses will help define human folacin requirements and the effects of deficient intakes of folacin on health. A sorely needed compendium of food folacin values employing more modern methods will be another valuable contribution of their work. The recently published compilation of provisional data on the folacin in selected foods by Perloff and Butrum (577) should also help meet our long-standing need for more accurate estimates of dietary folacin intake. Estimates of total folacin intake both in past and future nutritional status surveys should assist us in estimating dietary folacin requirements of various populations.

The ability to analyze survey data, however, does not diminish our need for controlled metabolic studies of sufficient duration. Considering the complex interrelationship of the folacins with other compounds, their effects on folacin requirements must also be carefully considered. As Lowe (460) noted trenchantly: "nutrient quality is dependent upon the nutrient environment, the relationship of the one nutrient to the other, and of nutrients to nonnutrient products consumed. . . ."

Studies with pregnant women and their infants are urgently needed to establish the dietary intake required to provide optimal fetal development and liver storage while at the same time maintaining the status of the mother for subsequent lactation. Deutero folic acid, labeled either in the ρ-aminobenzoic acid or glutamate moieties, which Rosenberg et al. (621) recently synthesized, should be useful in studying folacin metabolism (body pools and turnover) especially in pregnant women and infants. "Normal" postnatal blood folacin values and the dietary intake required to maintain optimal values in the infant must also be established.

The kinds and/or the ratio of the folacins in serum and in red cells may possibly be a better indicator of folacin status than total serum values (35, 176, 284, 391). Dawson and Geary (176) found that the rise in 5-CH_3-H_4-folic acid in the systemic circulation following the absorption of folic acid was directly related to the folacin content of the liver. The data of Ratanasthien et al. (600) suggest that the concentration of serum 10-CHO-H_4-folic acid, which is relatively constant in normal subjects, may indicate increased cell replication rate.

The amount of free versus protein-bound folacin, the distribution of folacin activity among the folacin binding proteins and the amount of unsaturated folacin binding protein in the serum may also be useful in evaluating folacin status (152, 400, 494, 495). Unsaturated folacin binding proteins, which are easily detected with labeled folic acid, have been found in a number of different conditions including: pregnancy, use of oral contraceptives, alcoholism, leukemia, and uremia. Their production appears to be under hormonal control but their source and significance have not been elucidated. Waxman (773) and Prefontaine (590) have recently reviewed many of these reports and the current status of folic acid radioassays. The protein bound folacins, which are more difficult to detect, have not received much attention.

Hibbard (330) pointed out recently that in order to evaluate folacin status more critically, investigators must determine what is going on at the cellular level. Hopefully, shifts in enzyme activity that are specific indicators of folacin status will be found. Hypersegmentation of the neutrophilic polymorphonuclear leukocytes is one of the first signs of folacin deficiency (313) but this is also a symptom of vitamin B_{12} deficiency. Since leukocytes and epithelial cells turn over rapidly, it is possible that subclinical changes in enzyme activity or folacin content may occur early in these cells. Gailani et al. (230) reported a decline in the folacin content of leukocytes during folacin deprivation. Ellegaard and his associates (200, 684) recently developed a method of measuring the folacin activity in isolated human lymphocytes by quantitating the rate of incorporating ^{14}C-formate into serine. It appears to be a sensitive indicator of folacin status but it is ineffective in patients with pyridoxine deficiency.

The deoxyuridine (dU) suppression test, a measure of the de novo pathway to the synthesis of DNA-thymine, is also a sensitive indicator of folacin or vitamin B_{12} deficiency. Biochemical megaloblastosis can be recognized even in the absence of morphological change in the bone marrow. (324, 792). However, bone marrow samples must be taken. Bessman and Johnson (59) recently suggested that erythrocyte size-frequency distribution curves, which can now be readily and accurately determined with the Coulter Counter, "may afford a quantitative and serial measurement of the bone marrow erythropoietic status." This may be a valuable method of monitoring bone marrow response to varying kinds and amounts of dietary folacin. In short, human dietary folacin requirements continue to be a challenging field of research.

ACKNOWLEDGMENTS

Dr. M. Isabel Irwin directed plans for this conspectus while the author was still an employee of the U.S. Department of Agriculture, Agricultural Research Service at Beltsville, Maryland; and she read the initial draft of one of the sections before her untimely death on March 25, 1975. Her editorial expertise was sorely missed.

The work was completed under Contract No. 5535-ARS-76 from the USDA. I appreciate the help and counsel of many people at Beltsville; Mrs. Judith Leinhas, likewise provided excellent technical assistance and, in particular, interpreted the literature on infant requirements. The California State University at Long Beach supported the research effort with a mini-grant that made it possible to hire a part-time technician; and the librarians at the institution helped to procure reprints of articles.

LITERATURE CITED

1. Aboko-Cole, G. F. & Lee, C. M. (1974) Interaction of nutrition and infection: Effect of folic acid deficiency on resistance to *Trypanosoma lewisi* and *Trypanosoma rhodesiense*. Int. J. Biochem. 5, 693–702.

2. Ahmed, F., Bamji, M. S. & Iyengar, L. (1975) Effect of oral contraceptive agents on vitamin nutrition status. Am. J. Clin. Nutr. 28, 606–615.

3. Allfrey, V. G. & King, C. G. (1950) An investigation of the folic acid-protein complex in yeast. J. Biol. Chem. 182, 367–384.

4. Alperin, J. B., Hutchinson, H. T. & Levin, W. C. (1966) Studies of folic acid requirements in megaloblastic anemia of pregnancy. Arch. Intern. Med. 117, 681–688.

5. Alter, H. J., Zvaifler, N. J. & Rath, C. E. (1971) Interrelationship of rheumatoid arthritis, folic acid, and aspirin. Blood 38, 405–416.

6. Amill, L. A. & Wright, M. (1946) Synthetic folic acid therapy in pernicious anemia. J. Am. Med. Assoc. 131, 1201–1207.

7. Amyes, S. J. G., Roberts, P. M., Scott, P. P. Suri, B. S. (1973) Post-natal changes in red cell, plasma and liver folate concentrations of the cat, rat, rabbit and dog. J. Physiol. 232, 23P–24P.

8. Anderson, B., Belcher, E. H., Chanarin, I. & Mollin, D. L. (1960) The urinary and faecal excretion of radioactivity after oral doses of ^{3}H-folic acid. Br. J. Haematol. 6, 439–455.

9. Angier, R. B., Boothe, J. H., Hutchings, B. L., Mowat, J. H., Semb, J., Stokstad, E. L. R., SubbaRow, Y., Waller, C. W., Cosulich, D. B., Fahrenbach, M. J., Hultquist, M. E., Kuh, E., Northey, E. H., Seeger, D. R., Sickels, J. P. & Smith, J. M., Jr. (1945) Synthesis of a compound identical with the *L. casei* factor isolated from liver. Science 102, 227–228.

10. Angier, R. B., Boothe, J. H., Hutchings, B. L., Mowat, J. H., Semb, J., Stokstad, E. L. R., SubbaRow, Y., Waller, C. W., Cosulich, D. B., Fahrenbach, M. J., Hultquist, M. E., Kuh, E., Northey, E. H., Seeger, D. R., Sickels, J. P. & Smith, J. M., Jr. (1946) The structure and synthesis of the liver *L. casei* factor. Science 103, 667–669.

11. Anonymous. (1967) Folic acid and pregnancy I. Nutr. Rev. 25, 325–328.

12. Anonymous. (1968) Ethanol and hemopoiesis. Nutr. Rev. 26, 301–305.

13. Anonymous. (1968) Folic acid and pregnancy II. Nutr. Rev. 26, 5–8.

14. Anonymous. (1975) Cell-mediated immunity to gliadin within the small-intestinal mucosa in celiac disease. Nutr. Rev. 33, 267–268.

15. Arakawa, T., Mizuno, T., Honda, Y., Tamura, T., Sakai, K., Tatsumi, S., Chiba, F. & Coursin, D. B. (1969) Brain function of infants fed on milk from mothers with low serum folate levels. Tohoku J. Exp. Med. 97, 391–397.

16. Arakawa, T., Mizuno, T., Honda, Y., Tamura, T., Watanabe, A., Komatsushiro, M., Takagi, T., Iinuma, K., Yamauchi, N., Tatsumi, S., Chiba, F. & Coursin, D. B. (1970) Longitudinal study on maturation patterns of EEG basic waves of infants fed on milk from mothers with low serum folate levels. Tohoku J. Exp. Med. 102, 81–90.

17. Arakawa, T., Ohara, K., Takahashi, Y., Ogasawara, J., Hayashi, T., Chiba, R., Wada, Y., Tada, K., Mizuno, T., Okamura, T. & Yoshida, T. (1965) Formiminotransferase-deficiency syndrome: A new inborn error of folic acid metabolism. Ann. Paediat. 205, 1–11.

18. Areekul, S., Pinyawatana, W. & Charoenlarp, P. (1974) Serum folate and folic acid absorption in patients with *Plasmodium falciparum* malaria. S. E. Asian J. Trop. Med. Pub. Hlth. 5, 353–358.

19. Asquith, P., Oelbaum, M. H. & Dawson, D. W. (1967) Scorbutic megaloblastic anaemia responding to ascorbic acid alone. Br. Med. J. 4, 402.

20. Aung-Than-Batu & Hla-Pe, U. (1972) Studies on folic acid. In: Proceedings of the First Asian Congress on Nutrition, pp. 122–133, Nutrition Society of India, Burma Medical Research Inst., Rangoon.

21. Avery, B. & Ledger, W. J. (1970) Folic acid metabolism in well-nourished pregnant women. Obstet. Gynecol. 35, 616–624.

22. Babu, S. & Srikantia, S. G. (1976) Availability of folates from some foods. Am. J. Clin. Nutr. 29, 376–379.

23. Bachman, A. L. (1936) Macrocytic hyperchromic anemia in early infancy. Report of a case and review of the literature. Am. J. Dis. Child. 52, 633–647.

24. Baker, H., Frank, O., Feingold, S., Ziffer, H., Gellene, R. A., Leevy, C. M. & Sobotka, H. (1965) The fate of orally and parenterally administered folates. Am. J. Clin. Nutr. 17, 88–95.

25. Baker, H., Frank, O., Pasher, I., Ziffer, H. & Sobotka, H. (1960) Pantothenic acid, thiamine and folic acid levels at parturition. Proc. Soc. Exp. Biol. Med. 103, 321–323.

26. Baker, H., Frank, O. & Sobotka, H. (1964) Mechanisms of folic acid deficiency in nontropical sprue. J. Am. Med. Assoc. 187, 119–121.

27. Baker, H., Frank, O., Zetterman, R. K., Rajan, K. S., Hove, W. & Leevy, C. M. (1975) Inability of chronic alcoholics with liver disease to use food as a source of folates, thiamin, and vitamin B_6. Am. J. Clin. Nutr. 28, 1377–1380.

28. Baker, H., Frank, O., Ziffer, H., Goldfarb, S., Leevy, C. M. & Sobotka, H. (1964)

Effect of hepatic disease on liver B-complex vitamin titers. Am. J. Clin. Nutr. *14*, 1–6.

29. Baker, H., Thomson, A. D., Feingold, S. & Frank, O. (1969) Role of the jejunum in the absorption of folic acid and its polyglutamates. Am. J. Clin. Nutr. *22*, 124–132.

30. Baker, S. J. (1968) Discussion of Herbert's paper. Vitamins & Hormones *21*, 537–538.

31. Baker, S. J., Kumar, S. & Swaminathan, S. P. (1965) Excretion of folic acid in bile. Lancet *1*, 685.

32. Baker, S. J. & Mathan, V. I. (1971) Tropical sprue in Southern India. In: Tropical Sprue and Megaloblastic Anaemia, Wellcome Trust Collaborative Study 1961–1969, pp. 189–260, Churchill-Livingstone, London.

33. Ball, E. W. & Giles, C. (1964) Folic acid and vitamin B_{12} levels in pregnancy and their relation to megaloblastic anaemia. J. Clin. Pathol. *17*, 165–174.

34. Banerjee, D. K. & Chatterjea, J. B. (1966) Observations on the presence of pteroyl polyglutamates in human serum. Blood *28*, 913–917.

35. Banerjee, D. K. & Chatterjea, J. B. (1971) Observations on the lability of serum whole blood and R.B.C. folates of human blood. Indian J. Med. Res. *59*, 369–376.

36. Banerjee, D. K., Maitra, A., Basu, A. K. & Chatterjea, J. B. (1975) Minimal daily requirement of folic acid in normal Indian subjects. Indian J. Med. Res. *63*, 45–53.

37. Barford, P. A. & Blair, J. A. (1975) Novel urinary metabolites of folic acid in the rat. In: Chem. Biol. Pteridines, Proc. 5th Int. Symp. (Pfleiderer, W., ed.), pp. 413–427, Walter de Gruyter, New York.

38. Bass, M. H. (1944) Deficiency anemia in infants. Report of two cases, with associated temporary deficiency of antianemic factor in one and allergy and abnormal digestion of protein in the other. Am. J. Dis. Child. *67*, 341–347.

39. Batata, M., Spray, G. H., Bolton, F. G., Higgins, G. & Wollner, L. (1967) Blood and bone marrow changes in elderly patients, with special reference to folic acid, vitamin B_{12}, iron, and ascorbic acid. Br. Med. J. *2*, 667–669.

40. Baugh, C. M., Braverman, E. & Nair, M. G. (1974) The identification of poly-γ-glutamyl chain lengths in bacterial folates. Biochemistry *13*, 4952–4957.

41. Baugh, C. M., Braverman, E. & Nair, M. G. (1975) Poly-γ-glutamyl chain lengths in some natural folates and contributions of folic acid synthesized by intestinal microflora to rat nutrition. In: Chem. Biol. Pteridines, Proc. 5th Int. Symp. (Pfleiderer, W., ed.), pp. 465–474, Walter de Gruyter, New York.

42. Baugh, C. M. & Krumdieck, C. L. (1971) Naturally occurring folates. Ann. N.Y. Acad. Sci. *186*, 7–28.

43. Baugh, C. M., Krumdieck, C. L., Baker, H. J. & Butterworth, C. E., Jr. (1971) Studies on the absorption and metabolism of folic acid. I. Folate absorption in the dog after exposure of isolated intestinal segments to

synthetic pteroylpolyglutamates of various chain lengths. J. Clin. Invest. *50*, 2009–2021.

44. Baugh, C. M., Krumdieck, C. L., Baker, H. J. & Butterworth, C. E., Jr. (1975) Absorption of folic acid poly-γ-glutamates in dogs. J. Nutr. *105*, 80–99.

45. Baugh, C. M., Stevens, J. C. & Krumdieck, C. L. (1970) Studies on γ-glutamyl carboxypeptidase. I. The solid phase synthesis of analogs of polyglutamates of folic acid and their effects on human liver γ-glutamyl carboxypeptidase. Biochim. Biophys. Acta *212*, 116–125.

46. Baumslag, N., Edelstein, T. & Metz, J. (1970) Reduction of incidence of prematurity by folic acid supplementation in pregnancy. Br. Med. J. *1*, 16–17.

47. Baumslag, N. & Metz, J. (1964) Response to lettuce in a patient with megaloblastic anaemia associated with pregnancy. S. Afr. Med. J. *38*, 611–613.

48. Bayless, T. M., Swanson, V. L. & Wheby, M. S. (1971) Jejunal histology and clinical status in tropical sprue and other chronic diarrheal disorders. Am. J. Clin. Nutr. *24*, 112–116.

49. Beard, M. E. J. & Weintraub, L. R. (1969) Hypersegmented neutrophilic granulocytes in iron deficiency anaemia. Br. J. Haematol. *16*, 161–163.

50. Becroft, D. M. O. & Holland, J. T. (1966) Goat's milk and megaloblastic anaemia of infancy: a report of three cases and a survey of the folic acid activity of some New Zealand milks. N. Zeal. Med. J. *65*, 303–307.

51. Benjamin-Allan, A. (1946) A case of aplastic anaemia of pregnancy treated with folic acid. J. Assoc. Med. Women in India *34*, 9–10.

52. Benn, A., Swan, C. H. J., Cooke, W. T., Blair, J. A., Matty, A. J. & Smith, M. E. (1971) Effect of intraluminal pH on the absorption of pteroylmonoglutamic acid. Br. Med. J. *1*, 148–150.

53. Beresford, C. H., Milner, P. F., Gurney, M. & Fox, H. (1972) Haemoglobin, iron, folate, and vitamin B_{12} levels in pregnant and lactating women in Jamaica. West Indian Med. J. *21*, 70–76.

54. Bernstein, L. H. & Gutstein, S. (1969) Folate conjugase in bile. N. Engl. J. Med. *281*, 565.

55. Bernstein, L. H., Gutstein, S., Efron, G. & Wager, G. (1972) Experimental production of elevated serum folate in dogs with intestinal blind loops: Relationship of serum levels to location of the blind loop. Gastroenterology *63*, 815–819.

56. Bernstein, L. H., Gutstein, S. & Weiner, S. (1969) Folic acid conjugase: inhibition by unconjugated dihydroxy bile acids. Proc. Soc. Exp. Biol. Med. *132*, 1167–1169.

57. Bernstein, L. H., Gutstein, S. & Weiner, S. V. (1970) Gamma glutamyl carboxypeptidase (conjugase), the folic acid-releasing enzyme of intestinal mucosa. Am. J. Clin. Nutr. *23*, 919–925.

58. Bertino, J. R., ed. (1971) Folate Antago-

nists As Chemotherapeutic Agents. Ann.
N.Y. Acad. Sci. Vol. 186.

59. Bessman, J. D. & Johnson, R. K. (1975) Erythrocyte volume distribution in normal and abnormal subjects. Blood 46, 369–380.

60. Bethell, F. H., Meyers, M. C., Andrews, G. A., Swendseid, M. E., Bird, O. D. & Brown, R. A. (1947) Metabolic function of pteroylglutamic acid and its hexaglutamyl conjugate. I. Hematologic and urinary excretion studies on patients with macrocytic anemia. J. Lab. Clin. Med. 32, 3–22.

61. Biale, Y., Lewenthal, H. & Aderet, N. B. (1975) Congenital malformations due to anticonvulsive drugs. Obstet. Gynecol. 45, 439–442.

62. Bianchi, A., Chipman, D. W., Dreskin, A. & Rosensweig, N. S. (1970) Nutritional folic acid deficiency with megaloblastic changes in the small-bowel epithelium. N. Engl. J. Med. 282, 859–861.

63. Biermer, A. (1872) Gesellschaft der Aerzte des Kantons Zurich. Correspondenz Schweiz. Artze 2, 14–22.

64. Billich, C., Bray, G. A., Gallagher, T. F., Hoffbrand, A. V. & Levitan, R. (1972) Absorptive capacity of the jejunum of obese and lean subjects. Arch. Intern. Med. 130, 377–380.

65. Binkley, S. B., Bird, O. D., Bloom, E. S., Brown, R. A., Calkins, D. G., Campbell, C. J., Emmett, A. D. & Pfiffner, J. J. (1944) On the vitamin Bc conjugate in yeast. Science 100, 36–37.

66. Bird, O. D., Binkley, S. B., Bloom, E. S., Emmett, A. D. & Pfiffner, J. J. (1945) On the enzymic formation of vitamin Bc from its conjugate. J. Biol. Sci. 100, 413–414.

67. Bird, O. D., McGlohon, V. M. & Vaitkus, J. W. (1965) Naturally occurring folates in the blood and liver of the rat. Anal. Biochem. 12, 18–35.

68. Bird, O. D. & Robbins, M. (1946) The response of Lactobacillus casei and Streptococcus faecalis to vitamin Bc and vitamin Bc conjugate. J. Biol. Chem. 163, 661–665.

69. Bird, O. D., Robbins, M., Vandenbelt, J. M. & Pfiffner, J. J. (1946) Observations on vitamin Bc conjugase from hog kidney. J. Biol. Chem. 163, 649–659.

70. Bjerre, B. (1967) Study of the haematological effect of profylactic folic acid medicamentation in pregnancy. Acta Obstet. Gynecol. Scand. 46, Suppl. 7, 71–85.

71. Blackfan, K. D. & Diamond, L. K. (1944) Atlas of the Blood in Children. Commonwealth Fund, New York.

72. Blair, J. A. & Dransfield, E. (1971) The urinary excretion of orally administered pteroyl-L-glutamic acid by the rat. Biochem. J. 123, 907–914.

73. Blakley, R. L. (1969) The Biochemistry of Folic Acid and Related Pteridines, Frontiers of Biology, Vol. 13, North-Holland Pub. Co., Amsterdam-London.

74. Boer, C. H. de (1959) Folic-acid deficiency in pregnancy. Lancet 2, 1145.

75. Bonnar, J. (1965) Anaemia in obstetrics:

An evaluation of treatment by iron-dextran infusion. Br. Med. J. 2, 1030–1033.

76. Boots, L., Cornwell, P. E. & Beck, L. R. (1975) Effect of ethynodiol diacetate and mestranol on serum folic acid and vitamin B12 levels and on tryptophan metabolism in baboons. Am. J. Clin. Nutr. 28, 354–362.

77. Bovina, C., Landi, L., Pasquali, P. & Marchetti, M. (1969) Biosynthesis of folate coenzymes in riboflavin-deficient rats. J. Nutr. 99, 320–324.

78. Bovina, C., Tolomelli, B., Rovintetti, C. & Marchetti, M. (1972) Acute effects of testosterone propionate on folate coenzyme synthesis in the rat. J. Endocrinol. 54, 457–464.

79. Bovina, C., Tolomelli, B., Rovinetti, C. & Marchetti, M. (1972) Effects of testosterone on folate coenzymes in the rat. Proc. Soc. Exp. Biol. Med. 140, 176–178.

80. Braude, H. (1972) Megaloblastic anaemia in an infant fed on goat's milk. S. Afr. Med. J. 46, 1288–1289.

81. Bronte-Stewart, B. (1953) The anaemia of adult scurvy. Quart. J. Med. 22, 309–329.

82. Brown, A. (1955) Megaloblastic anaemia associated with adult scurvy: Report of a case which responded to synthetic ascorbic acid alone. Br. J. Haematol. 1, 345–351.

83. Brown, J. P., Davidson, G. E. & Scott, J. M. (1973) Thin-layer chromatography of pteroylglutamates and related compounds. Application to transport and metabolism of reduced folates in blood. J. Chromatogr. 79, 195–207.

84. Brown, J. P., Davidson, G. E. & Scott, J. M. (1974) The identification of the forms of folate found in the liver, kidney and intestine of the monkey and their biosynthesis from exogenous pteroylglutamate (folic acid). Biochim. Biophys. Acta 343, 78–88.

85. Brown, J. P., Davidson, G. E., Scott, J. M. & Weir, D. G. (1973) Effect of diphenylhydantoin and ethanol feeding on the synthesis of rat liver folates from exogenous pteroylglutamate [3H]. Biochem. Pharmacol. 22, 3287–3289.

86. Brown, J. P., Scott, J. M., Foster, F. G. & Weir, D. G. (1973) Ingestion and absorption of naturally occurring pteroylmonoglutamates (folates) in man. Gastroenterology 64, 223–232.

87. Bruckner, H. W. & Bertino, J. R. (1975) Absorption of leucovorin (NSC-3590) from a mouthwash. Cancer Chemother. Rep., Part 1 59, 575–576.

88. Buehring, K. U., Batra, K. K. & Stokstad, E. L. R. (1972) The effect of methionine on folic acid and histidine metabolism in perfused rat liver. Biochim. Biophys. Acta 279, 498–512.

89. Buehring, Y. S. S., Poirier, L. A. & Stokstad, E. L. R. (1976) Folate deficiency in the livers of diethylnitrosamine-treated rats. Cancer Res. 36, 2775–2779.

90. Burland, W. L., Simpson, K. & Lord, J. (1971) Response of low birthweight infants to treatment with folic acid. Arch. Dis. Child. 46, 189–194.

91. Burns, D. G. & Spray, G. H. (1969) Normal folic acid metabolism in iron-deficient rats. Br. J. Nutr. 23, 665–670.

92. Burton, H., Ford, J. E., Franklin, J. G. & Porter, J. W. G. (1967) Effects of repeated heat treatments on the levels of some vitamins of the B-complex in milk. J. Dairy Res. 34, 193–197.

93. Butler, E. B. (1968) The effect of iron and folic acid on red cell and plasma volume in pregnancy. J. Obstet. Gynaecol. Br. Commonw. 75, 497–510.

94. Butterfield, S. & Calloway, D. H. (1972) Folacin in wheat and selected foods. J. Am. Dietet. Assoc. 60, 310–314.

95. Butterworth, C. E., Jr. (1968) Absorption and malabsorption of dietary folate. Am. J. Clin. Nutr. 21, 1121–1127.

96. Butterworth, C. E., Jr. (1968) The availability of food folate. Br. J. Haematol. 14, 339–343.

97. Butterworth, C. E., Jr., Baugh, C. M. & Krumdieck, C. (1969) A study of folate absorption and metabolism in man utilizing carbon-14-labeled polyglutamates synthesized by the solid phase method. J. Clin. Invest. 48, 1131–1142.

98. Butterworth, C. E., Jr., Krumdieck, C. L., Stinson, H. N. & Cornwell, P. E. (1975) A study of the effect of oral contraceptive agents on the absorption, metabolic conversion, and urinary excretion of a naturally-occurring folate (citrovorum factor). Ala. J. Med. Sci. 12, 330–335.

99. Butterworth, C. E., Jr., Nadel, H., Perez-Santiago, E., Santini, R., Jr. & Gardner, F. H. (1957) Folic acid absorption, excretion, and leukocyte concentration in tropical sprue. J. Lab. Clin. Med. 50, 673–681.

100. Butterworth, C. E., Jr., Newman, A. J. & Krumdieck, C. L. (1975) Tropical sprue: A consideration of possible etiologic mechanisms with emphasis on pteroylpolyglutamate metabolism. In: Transactions of the American Clinical and Climatological Assoc., The Eighty-Seventh Annual Meeting (Am. Clin. Climatol. Assoc., ed.), Vol. 86, pp. 11–22, Am. Clin. Climatol. Assoc., Nashville.

101. Butterworth, C. E., Jr., Santini, R., Jr. & Frommeyer, W. B., Jr. (1963) The pteroylglutamate components of American diets as determined by chromatographic fractionation. J. Clin. Invest. 42, 1929–1939.

102. Cantow, E. F. & Kostinas, J. E. (1967) Studies on infectious mononucleosis. V. The arneth count (preliminary observations). Am. J. Med. Sci. 253, 221–224.

103. Carney, M. W. P. (1967) Serum folate values in 423 psychiatric patients. Br. Med. J. 4, 512–516.

104. Carney, M. W. P. (1970) Serum folate and cyanocobalamin in alcoholics. Quart. J. Studies. Alc. 31, 816–822.

105. Castrén, O. M. & Rossi, R. R. (1970) Effect of oral contraceptives on serum folic acid content. J. Obstet. Gynaecol. Br. Commonw. 77, 548–550.

106. Chan, C., Shin, Y. S. & Stokstad, E. L. R. (1973) Studies of folic acid compounds in nature. III. Folic acid compounds in cabbage. Can. J. Biochem. 51, 1617–1623.

107. Chanarin, I. (1963) Urocanic acid and formimino-glutamic acid excretion in megaloblastic anaemia and other conditions: The effect of specific therapy. Br. J. Haematol. 9, 141–157.

108. Chanarin, I. (1964) Studies on urinary formimino-glutamic acid excretion. Proc. Roy. Soc. Med. 57, 384–388.

109. Chanarin, I. (1969) The Megaloblastic Anaemias, Blackwell Scientific Publications, Oxford.

110. Chanarin, I. (1973) Folate metabolism in pregnancy. Nutrition 27, 7–11.

111. Chanarin, I. (1973) Recent advances in megaloblastic anaemia. In: Ninth Symposium on Advanced Medicine (Walker, G., ed.), pp. 272–280, Pitman Med., London.

112. Chanarin, I. (1974) Vitamin B_{12}-folate interrelations. In: Advances in Haematology (Huntsman, R. G. & Jenkins, G. C., eds.), pp. 87–107, Butterworth, London.

113. Chanarin, I., Anderson, B. B. & Mollin, D. L. (1958) The absorption of folic acid. Br. J. Haematol. 4, 156–166.

114. Chanarin, I. & Bennett, M. C. (1962) Absorption of folic acid and D-xylose as tests of small-intestinal function. Br. Med. J. 1, 985–989.

115. Chanarin, I., Bennett, M. C. & Berry, V. (1962) Urinary excretion of histidine derivatives in megaloblasitc anaemia and other conditions and a comparison with the folic acid clearance test. J. Clin. Path. 15, 269–273.

116. Chanarin, I., Dacie, J. V. & Mollin, D. L. (1959) Folic acid deficiency in haemolytic anemia. Br. J. Haematol. 5, 245–256. Cited by: Strickland, G. T. & Kostinas, J. E. (1970) Folic acid deficiency complicating malaria. Am. J. Trop. Med. Hyg. 19, 910–915.

117. Chanarin, I., Fenton, J. C. B. & Mollin, D. L. (1957) Sensitivity to folic acid. Br. Med. J. 1, 1162–1163.

118. Chanarin, I., Hutchinson, M., McLean, A. & Moules, M. (1966) Hepatic folate in man. Br. Med. J. 1, 396–399.

119. Chanarin, I., MacGibbon, B. M., O'Sullivan, W. J. & Mollin, D. L. (1959) Folic-acid deficiency in pregnancy. The pathogenesis of megaloblastic anaemia of pregnancy. Lancet 2, 634–639.

120. Chanarin, I. & Rothman, D. (1965) Response to folic and folinic acid in megaloblastic anaemia in pregnancy. J. Obstet. Gynaecol. Br. Commonw. 72, 374–375.

121. Chanarin, I. & Rothman, D. (1971) Further observations on the relation between iron and folate status in pregnancy. Br. Med. J. 2, 81–84.

122. Chanarin, I., Rothman, D. & Berry, V. (1965) Iron deficiency and its relation to folic-acid status in pregnancy: results of a clinical trial. Br. Med. J. 1, 480–485.

123. Chanarin, I., Rothman, D., Perry, J. & Stratfull, D. (1968) Normal dietary folate, iron, and protein intake, with particular

reference to pregnancy. Br. Med. J. 2, 394–397.

124. Chanarin, I., Rothman, D., Ward, A. & Perry, J. (1968) Folate status and requirement in pregnancy. Br. Med. J. 2, 390–394.

125. Chanarin, I., Rothman, D. & Watson-Williams, E. J. (1963) Normal formiminoglutamic acid excretion in megaloblastic anaemia in pregnancy. Studies on histidine metabolism in pregnancy. Lancet 1, 1068–1072.

126. Chanarin, I., Smith, G. N. & Wincour, V. (1969) Development of folate deficiency in the rat. Br. J. Haematol. 16, 193–195.

127. Chazen, J. A. & Mistilis, S. D. (1963) The pathophysiology of scurvy. Am. J. Med. 34, 350–358.

128. Cheldelin, V. H., Woods, A. M. & Williams, R. J. (1943) Losses of B vitamins due to cooking of foods. J. Nutr. 26, 477–485.

129. Cherrick, G. R., Baker, H., Frank, O. & Leevy, C. M. (1965) Observations on hepatic avidity for folate in Laennec's cirrhosis. J. Lab. Clin. Med. 66, 446–451.

130. Chida, N., Hirono, H. & Arakawa, T. (1972) Effects of dietary folate deficiency on fatty acid composition of myelin cerebroside in growing rats. Tohoku J. Exp. Med. 108, 219–224.

131. Ch'ien, L. T., Krumdieck, C. L., Scott, C. W., Jr. & Butterworth, C. E., Jr. (1975) Harmful effect of megadoses of vitamins: Electroencephalogram abnormalities and seizures induced by intravenous folate in drug-treated epileptics. Am. J. Clin. Nutr. 28, 51–58.

132. Chisholm, M. (1966) A controlled clinical trial of prophylactic folic acid and iron in pregnancy. J. Obstet. Gynaecol. Br. Commonw. 73, 191–196.

133. Chisholm, M. & Sharp, A. A. (1964) Formimino-glutamic acid excretion in anaemia of pregnancy. Br. Med. J. 2, 1366–1369.

134. Choudhry, V. P., Ghai, O. P. & Saraya, A. K. (1973) Hemopoietic nutrients in anemia of infancy and childhood with suggestive vitamin B_{12} and folic acid deficiency. Indian Pediatr. 10, 435–442.

135. Choudhry, V. P., Saraya, A. K. & Ghai, O. P. (1972) Morphological changes in relation to haemopoietic nutrient deficiency in nutritional macrocytic anaemia in infancy and childhood. Indian J. Med. Res. 60, 1764–1773.

136. Colman, N., Green, R. & Metz, J. (1975) Prevention of folate deficiency by food fortification. II. Absorption of folic acid from fortified staple foods. Am. J. Clin. Nutr. 28, 459–464.

137. Colman, N., Green, R., Stevens, K. & Metz, J. (1974) Prevention of folate deficiency by food fortification. VI. The antimegaloblastic effect of folic acid-fortified maize meal. S. Afr. Med. J. 48, 1795–1798.

138. Colman, N. & Herbert, V. (1976) Bioavailability of folate. Am. J. Clin. Nutr. 29, 235–236.

139. Colman, N., Larsen, J. V., Barker, M., Barker, E. A., Green, R. & Metz, J. (1974) Prevention of folate deficiency by food fortification. Part V. A pilot field trial of folic acid-fortified maize meal. S. Afr. Med. J. 48, 1763–1766.

140. Colman, N., Larsen, J. V., Barker, M., Barker, E. A., Green, R. & Metz, J. (1975) Prevention of folate deficiency by food fortification. III. Effect in pregnant subjects of varying amounts of added folic acid. Am. J. Clin. Nutr. 28, 465–470.

141. Combrink, P. B., Turchetti, L. C., Pannell, P. & Metz, J. (1966) Nutritional anaemia in early pregnancy in the South African Bantu: Therapeutic considerations with special reference to intramuscular iron and the effect of iron therapy on tests of folate nutrition. S. Afr. Med. J. 40, 234–237.

142. Cook, G. C., Morgan, J. O. & Hoffbrand, A. V. (1974) Impairment of folate absorption by systemic bacterial infections. Lancet 2, 1416–1417.

143. Cooper, B. A., Cantlie, G. S. D. & Brunton, L. (1970) The case for folic acid supplements during pregnancy. Am. J. Clin. Nutr. 23, 848–854.

144. Cooper, B. A. & Lowenstein, L. (1964) Relative folate deficiency of erythrocytes in pernicious anemia and its correction with cyanocobalamin. Blood 24, 502–521.

145. Cooperman, J. M. (1971) Microbiological assay of folic acid activity in serum and whole blood. In: Methods in Enzymology, Vol. XVIII, Vitamins and Coenzymes, Part B. (McCormick, D. B. & Wright, L. D., eds.), pp. 629–642, Academic Press, New York.

146. Cooperman, J. M. & Luhby, A. L. (1965) The physiological fate in man of some naturally occurring polyglutamates of folic acid. Isr. J. Med. Sci. 1, 704–707.

147. Cooperman, J. M., Pesci-Bourel, A. & Luhby, A. L. (1970) Urinary excretion of folic acid activity in man. Clin. Chem. 16, 375–381.

148. Corcino, J. J. (1975) Recent advances in tropical sprue. In: Intestinal absorption and malabsorption. International Symposium, Lexington, Ky., May 28–30, 1974. (Csáky, T. Z., ed), pp. 285–299, Raven Press, New York.

149. Corcino, J. J., Coll, G. & Klipstein, F. A. (1975) Pteroylglutamic acid malabsorption in tropical sprue. Blood 45, 577–580.

150. Corcino, J. J., Reisenauer, A. M. & Halsted, C. H. (1976) Jejunal perfusion of simple and conjugated folates in tropical sprue. J. Clin. Invest. 58, 298–305.

151. Cossins, E. A. & Shah, S. P. J. (1972) Pteroylglutamates of higher plant tissues. Phytochemistry 11, 587–593.

152. Costa, M. da & Rothenberg, S. P. (1974) Appearance of a folate binder in leukocytes and serum of women who are pregnant or taking oral contraceptives. J. Lab. Clin. Med. 83, 207–214.

153. Cowan, D. H. & Hines, J. D. (1971) Thrombocytopenia of severe alcoholism. Ann. Intern. Med. 74, 37–43.

154. Cowan, D. H. & Hines, J. D. (1974) Al-

cohol, vitamins, and platelets. In: Drugs and Hematologic Reactions (Dimitrov, N. V. & Nodine, J. H., eds.), pp. 283–295, Grune & Stratton, New York.

155. Cox, E. V., Matthews, D. M., Meynell, M. J., Cooke, W. T. & Gaddie, R. (1960) Cyanocobalamin, ascorbic acid and pteroylglutamates in normal and megaloblastic bone marrow. Blood 15, 376–387.

156. Cox, E. V., Meynell, M. J., Cooke, W. T. & Gaddie, R. (1962) Scurvy and anaemia. Am. J. Med. 32, 240–250.

157. Cox, E. V., Meynell, M. J., Northam, B. E. & Cooke, W. T. (1967) The anaemia of scurvy. Am. J. Med. 42, 220–227.

158. Croft, D. N., Loehry, C. A. & Creamer, B. (1968) Small-bowel cell-loss and weight-loss in coeliac syndrome. Lancet 2, 68–70.

159. Daniel, W. A., Jr., Gaines, E. G. & Bennett, D. L. (1975) Dietary intakes and plasma concentrations of folate in healthy adolescents. Am. J. Clin. Nutr. 28, 363–370.

160. Daniel, W. A. Jr., Mounger, J. R. & Perkins, J. C. (1971) Obstetric and fetal complications in folate-deficient adolescent girls. Am. J. Obstet. Gynecol. 111, 233–238.

161. Darby, W. J. (1947) The physiological effects of the pteroylglutamates in man—with particular reference to pteroylglutamic acid (PGA). Vitam. Horm. 5, 119–161.

162. Darby, W. J. (1948) The treatment of nutritional anemias with folic acid. In: Nutritional Anemia, Vol. 1, pp. 61–78, Robert Gould Research Foundation, Cincinnati.

163. Darby, W. J. (1953) Folic acid and citrovorum factor in human nutrition. Nutr. Symp. Ser. No. 7, pp. 85–99, Nat. Vitam. Found., Inc., New York.

164. Darby, W. J. & Jones, E. (1945) Treatment of sprue with synthetic L. casei factor (folic acid, vitamin M). Proc. Soc. Exp. Biol. Med. 60, 259–260.

165. Darby, W. J., Jones, E. & Johnson, H. C. (1946) Effect of synthetic Lactobacillus casei factor in treatment of sprue. J. Am. Med. Assoc. 130, 780–786.

166. Darby, W. J., Jones, E. & Johnson, H. C. (1946) The use of synthetic L. casei factor in the treatment of sprue. Science 103, 108.

167. Darby, W. J., Kaser, M. M. & Jones, E. (1947) The influence of pteroylglutamic acid (a member of the vitamin M group) on the absorption of vitamin A and carotene by patients with sprue. J. Nutr. 33, 243–250.

168. Das, K. C. & Hoffbrand, A. V. (1970) Studies of folate uptake by phytohaemagglutinin-stimulated lymphocytes. Br. J. Haematol. 19, 203–221.

169. Das Gupta, C. R. & Chatterjea, J. B. (1946) The role of synthetic folic acid (L. casei factor) in the treatment of nutritional macrocytic anaemia. Indian Med. Gazette 81, 402–410.

170. Davidson, G. P. & Townley, R. R. W. (1977) Structural and functional abnormalities of the small intestine due to nutritional folic acid deficiency in infancy. J. Pediat. 90, 590–594.

171. Davis, R. E. & Smith, B. K. (1974) Pyridoxal and folate deficiency in alcoholics. Med. J. Aust. 2, 357–360.

172. Dawbarn, M. C., Hine, D. C. & Smith, J. (1958) Folic acid activity in the liver of sheep. 3. The effect of vitamin B_{12} deficiency on the concentration of folic acid and citrovorum factor. Aust. J. Exp. Biol. Med. Sci. 36, 541–546.

173. Dawson, D. W. (1966) Microdoses of folic acid in pregnancy. J. Obstet. Gynaecol. Br. Commonw. 73, 44–48.

174. Dawson, D. W. (1971) Partial villous atrophy in nutritional megaloblastic anaemia corrected by folic acid therapy. J. Clin. Pathol. 24, 131–135.

175. Dawson, D. W. & Buckley, A. L. (1969) Vitamin B_{12}, serum folate, and hypochromic anaemia. Br. Med. J. 2, 187.

176. Dawson, D. W. & Geary, C. (1971) Hepatic and serum folates in patients fasting and after oral folic acid. J. Clin. Pathol. 24, 129–130.

177. Dawson, D. W., More, J. R. S. & Aird, D. C. (1962) Prevention of megaloblastic anaemia in pregnancy by folic acid. Lancet 2, 1015–1018.

178. Dawson, K. P. (1972) Folic acid and low birth weight infants. Scot. Med. J. 17, 371–373.

179. Day, P. L. (1944) The nutritional requirements of primates other than man. VII. Nutritional cytopenia in the monkey-Vitamin M. Vitam. Horm. 2, 91–105.

180. Day, P. L., Langston, W. C. & Darby, W. J. (1938) Failure of nicotinic acid to prevent nutritional cytopenia in the monkey. Proc. Soc. Exp. Biol. Med. 38, 860–863.

181. Day, P. L. & Totter, J. R. (1946) Reported at the AAAS Conference on Vitamins, Gibson Island, July 31, 1946. Cited by: Darby, W. J. (1947) The physiological effects of the pteroylglutamates in man—with particular reference to pteroylglutamic acid (PGA). Vitamins & Hormones 5, 119–161.

182. Deller, D. J., Kimber, C. L. & Ibbotson, R. N. (1965) Folic acid deficiency in cirrhosis of the liver. Am. J. Digest. Dis. 10, 35–42.

183. Denko, C. W. (1952) Some B-complex vitamins and tryptophane in saliva. Med. Nutr. Lab. Report No. 90, MRDB Project No. 6-60-11-001, Chicago. Cited by: Mäkilä, E. (1968) Salivary vitamins. Int. Z. Vitaminforsch. 38, 260–269.

184. Denko, C. W., Grundy, W. E. & Porter, J. W. (1947) Blood levels in normal adults on a restricted dietary intake of B-complex vitamins and tryptophan. Arch. Biochem. 13, 481–484.

185. Denko, C. W., Grundy, W. E., Porter, J. W., Berryman, G. H., Friedemann, T. E. & Youmans, J. B. (1946) The excretion of B-complex vitamins in the urine and feces of seven normal adults. Arch. Biochem. 10, 33–40.

186. Denko, C. W., Grundy, W. E., Wheeler, N. C., Henderson, C. R. & Berryman, G. H.

(1946) The excretion of B-complex vitamins by normal adults on a restricted intake. Arch. Biochem. *11*, 109–117.

187. Devi, P. K., Mehta, S. K. & Manchanda, S. (1973) Vitamin B$_{12}$ and folate status in the normal puerperium. Indian J. Med. Res. *61*, 454–460.

188. Diez-Ewald, M., Fernández, G., Velásquez, N. & Molina, R. (1973) Importancia de la administracion prenatal de acido folico en el estado hematologico de la madre y el recien nacido. Invest. Clin. *14*, 58–73.

189. Disraely, M. N., Shiota, T. & Caplow, M. (1959) The occurrence and origin of certain vitamins in human saliva. Arch. Oral Biol. *1*, 233–240.

190. Dong, F. M. & Oace, S. M. (1973) Folate distribution in fruit juices. J. Am. Dietet. Assoc. *62*, 162–166.

191. Dong, F. M. & Oace, S. M. (1975) Folate concentration and pattern in bovine milk. J. Agric. Food Chem. *23*, 534–538.

192. Dreizen, S. & Hampton, J. K. (1969) Radioisotopic studies of the glandular contribution of selected B vitamins in saliva. J. Dent. Res. *48*, 579–582.

193. Druskin, M. S., Wallen, M. H. & Bonagura, L. (1962) Anticonvulsant-associated megaloblastic anemia. Response to 25 microgm. of folic acid administered by mouth daily. N. Engl. J. Med. *267*, 483–485.

194. Edelstein, T., Stevens, K., Brandt, V., Baumslag, N. & Metz, J. (1966) Tests of folate and vitamin B$_{12}$ nutrition during pregnancy and the puerperium in a population subsisting on a suboptimal diet. J. Obstet. Gynaecol. Br. Commonw. *73*, 197–204.

195. Eichner, E. R. & Hillman, R. S. (1971) The evolution of anemia in alcoholic patients. Am. J. Med. *50*, 218–232.

196. Eichner, E. R. & Hillman, R. S. (1973) Effect of alcohol on serum folate level. J. Clin. Invest. *52*, 584–591.

197. Eichner, E. R., Paine, C. J., Dickson, V. L. & Hargrove, M. D., Jr. (1975) Clinical and laboratory observations on serum folate-binding protein. Blood *46*, 599–609.

198. Eichner, E. R., Pierce, H. I. & Hillman, R. S. (1971) Folate balance in dietary-induced megaloblastic anemia. N. Engl. J. Med. *284*, 933–938.

199. Ek, J. & Magnus, E. (1974) Folic acid levels in infancy. Int. Congr. Pediatria, 14th, pp. 49–51, Editorial Medica Panamericana, Buenos Aires.

200. Ellegaard, J. & Esmann, V. (1973) Folate activity of human lymphocytes determined by measurement of serine synthesis. J. Clin. Lab. Invest. *31*, 9–19.

201. Elman, A., Einhorn, J., Olhagen, B. & Reizenstein, P. (1970) Metabolic studies of folic acid in non-malignant diseases. Acta Med. Scand. *187*, 347–352.

202. Elsborg, L. (1975) A modified fecal excretion test for assaying intestinal absorption of ^{3}H-folic acid. Scand. J. Gastroenterol. *10*, 207–208.

203. Elsborg, L. (1976) Reversible malabsorption of folic acid in the elderly with nutritional folate deficiency. Acta Haematol. *55*, 140–147.

204. England, N. W. J. (1968) Intestinal pathology of tropical sprue. Am. J. Clin. Nutr. *21*, 962–975.

205. FAO/WHO Expert Group. (1970) Requirements of ascorbic acid, vitamin D, vitamin B$_{12}$, folate, and iron. FAO Nutr. Meet. Report Series no. 47, Rome. WHO Tech. Report Series no. 452, Geneva.

206. Fehling, C., Jagerstad, M., Lindstrand, K. & Elmquist, D. (1976) Reduction of folate levels in the rat: Difference in depletion between the central and the peripheral nervous system. Z. Ernährungswiss. *15*, 1–8.

207. Feinman, L. & Lieber, C. S. (1973) Fibrogenic effect of alcohol in rat liver: role of diet. Science *179*, 407.

208. Fennelly, J., Frank, O., Baker, H. & Leevy, C. M. (1964) Peripheral neuropathy of the alcoholic: I. Aetiological role of aneurin and other B-complex vitamins. Br. Med. J. *2*, 1290–1292.

209. Fleming, A., Knowles, J. P. & Prankerd, T. A. J. (1963) Pregnancy anaemia. Lancet *1*, 606.

210. Fleming, A. F. (1972) Urinary excretion of folate in pregnancy. J. Obstet. Gynaecol. Br. Commonw. *79*, 916–920.

211. Fleming, A. F., Comley, L. & Stenhouse, N. S. (1971) Assay of serum whole blood folate by a modified aseptic addition technique. Am. J. Clin. Nutr. *24*, 1257–1264.

212. Fleming, A. F., Hendrickse, J. P. de V. & Allan, N. C. (1968) The prevention of megaloblastic anaemia in pregnancy in Nigeria. J. Obstet. Gynaecol. Br. Commonw. *75*, 425–432.

213. Fleming, A. F., Martin, J. D., Hahnel, R. & Westlake, A. J. (1974) Effects of iron and folic acid antenatal supplements on maternal haematology and fetal well being. Med. J. Aust. *2*, 429–435.

214. Fomon, S. J. (1974) Infant Nutrition. W. B. Saunders Co., Philadelphia.

215. Ford, J. E. (1967) The influence of the dissolved oxygen in milk on the stability of some vitamins towards heating and during subsequent exposure to sunlight. J. Dairy Res. *34*, 239–247.

216. Ford, J. E. (1974) Some observations on the possible nutritional significance of vitamin B$_{12}$- and folate-binding proteins in milk. Br. J. Nutr. *31*, 243–257.

217. Ford, J. E., Knaggs, G. S., Salter, D. N. & Scott, K. J. (1972) Folate nutrition in the kid. Br. J. Nutr. *27*, 571–583.

218. Ford, J. E., Salter, D. N. & Scott, K. J. (1969) The folate-binding protein in milk. J. Dairy Res. *36*, 435–446.

219. Ford, J. E. & Scott, K. J. (1968) The folic acid activity of some milk foods for babies. J. Dairy Res. *35*, 85–90.

220. Ford, J. E., Scott, K. J., Sansom, B. F. & Taylor, P. J. (1975) Some observations on the possible nutritional significance of vitamin B$_{12}$- and folate-binding proteins in milk. Absorption of [^{58}Co]cyanocobalamin by suckling piglets. Br. J. Nutr. *34*, 469–492.

221. Forshaw, J. (1965) Nutritional deficiency of folic acid. Br. Med. J. 2, 1061.
222. Forshaw, J. (1969) Effect of vitamin B₁₂ and folic acid deficiency on small intestinal absorption. J. Clin. Pathol. 22, 551–553.
223. Forshaw, J. & Harwood, L. (1971) Diagnostic value of the serum folate assay. J. Clin. Pathol. 24, 244–249.
224. Fouts, P. J. & Garber, E. (1942) Nutritional anemia in an infant responding to purified liver extract. Am. J. Dis. Child. 64, 270–273.
225. Fox, J. H., Topel, J. L. & Huckman, M. S. (1975) Dementia in the elderly—a search for treatable illnesses. J. Gerontol. 30, 557–564.
226. Francis, H. H. & Scott, J. S. (1959) Folic-acid deficiency in pregnancy. Lancet 2, 1033–1034.
227. Fraumeni, J. F., Jr. (1974) Chemicals in human teratogenesis and transplacental carcinogenesis. Pediatrics 53, 807–812.
228. Freedman, D. S., Brown, J. P., Weir, D. G. & Scott, J. M. (1973) The reproducibility and use of the tritiated folic acid urinary excretion test as a measure of folate absorption in clinical practice: Effect of methothrexate on absorption of folic acid. J. Clin. Pathol. 26, 261–267.
229. Gaafar, A., Toppozada, H. K., Hozayen, A., Abdel-Malek, A. T., Moghazy, M. & Youssef, M. (1973) Study of folate status in long-term Egyptian users of oral contraceptive pills. Contraception 8, 43–52.
230. Gailani, S. D., Carey, R. W., Holland, J. F. & O'Malley, J. A. (1970) Studies of folate deficiency in patients with neoplastic diseases. Cancer Res. 30, 327–333.
231. Gál, E. M. & Roggeveen, A. E. (1973) Cerebral hydroxylases: stimulation by a new factor. Science 179, 809–811.
232. Gall, L. S. (1970) Normal fecal flora of man. Am. J. Clin. Nutr. 23, 1457–1465.
233. Gardner, A. J. (1971) Folate status of alcoholic in-patients. Br. J. Addict. 66, 183–184.
234. Garrow, J. S. (1970) The relationship of foetal growth to size and composition of the placenta. Proc. Roy. Soc. Med. 63, 498–500.
235. Gatenby, P. B. B. & Lillie, E. W. (1960) Clinical analysis of 100 cases of severe megaloblastic anaemia of pregnancy. Br. Med. J. 2, 1111–1114.
236. Gawthorne, J. M. & Smith, R. M. (1974) Folic acid metabolism in vitamin B₁₂-deficient sheep. Biochem. J. 142, 119–126.
237. Gawthorne, J. M. & Stokstad, E. L. R. (1971) The effect of vitamin B₁₂ and methionine on folic acid uptake by rat liver. Proc. Soc. Exp. Biol. Med. 136, 42–46.
238. Gebre-Medhin, M., Killander, A., Vahlquist, B. & Wuhib, E. (1976) Rarity of anaemia of pregnancy in Ethiopia. Scand. J. Haematol. 16, 168–175.
239. Gerson, C. D., Cohen, N., Brown, N., Lindenbaum, J., Hepner, G. W. & Janowitz, H. D. (1971) Interrelationships of glucose, galactose, and folic acid (H³PGA) absorption in sprue. Clin. Res. 19, 391. Cited by: Gerson, C. D. (1971) Glucose and intestinal absorption in man. Am. J. Clin. Nutr. 24, 1393–1398.
240. Gerson, C. D., Cohen, N., Hepner, G. W., Brown, N., Herbert, V. & Janowitz, H. D. (1971) Folic acid absorption in man: Enhancing effect of glucose. Gastroenterology 61, 224–227.
241. Ghitis, J. (1966) The labile folate of milk. Am. J. Clin. Nutr. 18, 452–457.
242. Ghitis, J. (1967) The folate binding in milk. Am. J. Clin. Nutr. 20, 1–4.
243. Ghitis, J. & Canosa, C. (1965) Folate and B₁₂ serum levels in premature infants. With a note on milk folate. J. Pediatr. 67, 701–702.
244. Ghitis, J. & Tripathy, K. (1970) Availability of milk folate. Studies with cow's milk in experimental folic acid deficiency. Am. J. Clin. Nutr. 23, 141–146.
245. Ghitis, J., Tripathy, K. & Mayoral, G. (1967) Malabsorption in the tropics. Am. J. Clin. Nutr. 20, 1206–1211.
246. Giles, C. (1966) An account of 335 cases of megaloblastic anaemia of pregnancy and the puerperium. J. Clin. Pathol. 19, 1–11.
247. Giles, C. & Burton, H. (1960) Observations on prevention and diagnosis of anaemia in pregnancy. Br. Med. J. 2, 636–640.
248. Giles, C. & Shuttleworth, E. M. (1958) Megaloblastic anaemia of pregnancy and the puerperium. Lancet 2, 1341–1347.
249. Giles, P. F. H., Harcourt, A. G. & Whiteside, M. G. (1971) The effect of prescribing folic acid during pregnancy on birth-weight and duration of pregnancy. A double-blind trial. Med. J. Aust. 2, 17–21.
250. Girdwood, R. H. (1951) Vitamin B₁₂ and folic acid in the megaloblastic anaemias. Edinburgh Med. J. 58, 309–335.
251. Girdwood, R. H. (1952) The occurrence of growth factors for Lactobacillus leichmanni, Streptococcus faecalis and Leuconostoc citrovorum in the tissues of pernicious anaemia patients and controls. Biochem. J. 52, 58–63.
252. Girdwood, R. H. (1953) A folic-acid excretion test in the investigation of intestinal malabsorption. Lancet 2, 53–60.
253. Girdwood, R. H. (1953) Some aspects of the metabolism of antimegaloblastic substances in man. Blood 8, 469–485.
254. Girdwood, R. H. (1954) Some aspects of disordered folic acid metabolism in man. In: Chemistry Symposium on Biology of Pteridines (Wolstenholme, G. E. W. & Cameron, M. P., eds.), pp. 385–405, Churchill, London.
255. Girdwood, R. H. (1956) Absorption in sprue of vitamins of the B complex. Lancet 2, 700–703.
256. Girdwood, R. H. (1960) Folic acid deficiency in man. In: Proc. 7th Congr. European Soc. Haematol., London, 1959. part II, pp. 40–51, S. Karger, Basel.
257. Girdwood, R. H. (1969) Folate depletion in old age. Am. J. Clin. Nutr. 22, 234–237.
258. Girdwood, R. H. (1971) Problems in the assessment of vitamin deficiency. Proc. Nutr. Soc. 30, 66–73.
259. Girdwood, R. H. (1974) Drug induced

megaloblastic anaemia. In: Blood Disorders Due To Drugs and Other Agents (Girdwood, R. H., ed.), pp. 49–82, Excerpta Medica, Amsterdam.

260. Girdwood, R. H. & Delamore, I. W. (1961) Observations on tests of folic acid absorption and clearance. Scot. Med. J. 6, 44–59.

261. Girdwood, R. H., Thomson, A. D. & Williamson, J. (1967) Folate status in the elderly. Br. Med. J. 2, 670–672.

262. Glavind, J., Granados, H., Hansen, L. A., Schilling, K., Kruse, I. & Dam, H. (1948) The presence of vitamins in the saliva. Int. Z. Vitaminforsch. 20, 234–238.

263. Godwin, H. A. & Rosenberg, I. H. (1975) Comparative studies of the intestinal absorption of [³H]pteroylmonoglutamate and [³H]pteroylheptaglutamate in man. Gastroenterology 69, 364–373.

264. Goldberg, A. (1963) The anaemia of scurvy. Quart. J. Med. 32, 51–64.

265. Goldsmith, G. A. (1946) The treatment of macrocytic anemia with Lactobacillus casei factor (pteroylglutamic acid). J. Lab. Clin. Med. 31, 1186–1200.

266. Goldsmith, G. A. (1975) Vitamin B complex. Thiamine, niacin, folic acid (folacin), vitamin B_{12}, biotin. Prog. Food Nutr. Sci. 1, 559–609.

267. Gopalan, C. (1956) Protein intake of breast-fed poor Indian infants. J. Trop. Pediatr. 2, 89–92.

268. Gopalan, C. (1958) Effect of protein supplementation and some so-called "Galactogogues" on lactation of poor Indian women. Indian J. Med. Res. 46, 317–324.

269. Gopalan, C. (1958) Studies on lactation in poor Indian communities. J. Trop. Pediatr. 4, 87–95.

270. Gorbach, S. L., Banwell, J. G., Jacobs, B., Chatterjee, B. D., Mitra, R., Sen, N. N. & Mazumder, D. N. Guha (1970) Tropical sprue and malnutrition in West Bengal. I. Intestinal microflora and absorption. Am. J. Clin. Nutr. 23, 1545–1558.

271. Goresky, C. A., Watanabe, H. & Johns, D. G. (1963) The renal excretion of folic acid. J. Clin. Invest. 42, 1841–1849.

272. Gough, K. R., Read, A. E., McCarthy, C. F. & Waters, A. H. (1963) Megaloblastic anaemia due to nutritional deficiency of folic acid. Quart. J. Med. 32, 243–256.

273. Gray, O. P. & Butler, E. B. (1965) Megaloblastic anaemia in premature infants. Arch. Dis. Child. 40, 53–56.

274. Greene, H. L., Stifel, F. B., Herman, R. H., Herman, Y. F. & Rosensweig, N. S. (1974) Ethanol-induced inhibition of human intestinal enzyme activities: reversal by folic acid. Gastroenterology 67, 434–440.

275. Groen, J. & Snapper, I. (1937) Dietary deficiency as a cause of macrocytic anemia. Am. J. Med. Sci. 193, 633–646.

276. Gross, R. L., Newberne, P. M. & Reid, J. V. O. (1974) Adverse effects on infant development associated with maternal folic acid deficiency. Nutr. Rep. Int. 10, 241–248.

277. Gross, R. L., Reid, J. V. O., Newberne, P. M., Burgess, B., Marston, R. & Hift, W.

(1975) Depressed cell-mediated immunity in megaloblastic anemia due to folic acid deficiency. Am. J. Clin. Nutr. 28, 225–232.

278. Grossowicz, N., Aronovitch, J., Rachmilewitz, M., Izak, G., Sadovsky, A. & Bercovici, B. (1962) Clearance of parenterally administered folic acid in healthy and anemic subjects. J. Lab. Clin. Med. 60, 375–384.

279. Grossowicz, N., Izak, G. & Rachmilewitz, M. (1964) Experimental folic acid deficiency. Proc. 9th Congr. Europ. Soc. Haemat. Lisbon, 1963, pp. 394–397, S. Karger, Basel/New York.

280. Grossowicz, N., Izak, G. & Rachmilewitz, M. (1966) The effect of anemia on the concentration of folate derivatives in paired fetal-maternal blood. Isr. J. Med. Sci. 2, 510–512.

281. Grossowicz, N., Rachmilewitz, M. & Izak, G. (1972) Absorption of pteroylglutamate and dietary folates in man. Am. J. Clin. Nutr. 25, 1135–1139.

282. Grossowicz, N., Rachmilewitz, M. & Izak, G. (1975) Utilization of yeast polyglutamate folates in man. Proc. Soc. Exp. Biol. Med. 150, 77–79.

283. Grundy, W. E., Freed, M., Johnson, H. C., Henderson, C. R. & Berryman, G. H. (1947) The effect of phthalylsulfathiazole (sulfathalidine) on the excretion of B-vitamins by normal adults. Arch. Biochem. 15, 187–194.

284. Gupta, O. P., Dube, M. K. & Mehta, K. (1969) Serum folate levels in anaemia of pregnancy. J. Indian Med. Assoc. 53, 288–291.

285. Guzman, V. B. & Tantengco, V. O. (1972) Malnutrition problems of infants and preschool children in Victoria, Laguna: Protein-calorie, vitamin A, iron and folic acid deficiencies. Acta Medica Philippina 8, 22–32.

286. Hall, C. A., Bardwell, S. A., Allen, E. S. & Rappazzo, M. E. (1975) Variation in plasma folate levels among groups of healthy persons. Am. J. Clin. Nutr. 28, 854–857.

287. Hall, M. (1972) Folic acid deficiency and congenital malformation. J. Obstet. Gynaecol. Br. Commonw. 79, 159–161.

288. Hall, M. & Davidson, R. J. L. (1968) Prophylactic folic acid in women with pernicious anaemia pregnant after periods of infertility. J. Clin. Pathol. 21, 599–602.

289. Hall, M. H. (1972) Folic acid deficiency and abruptio placentae. J. Obstet. Gynaecol. Br. Commonw. 79, 222–225.

290. Hall, M. H., Pirani, B. B. K. & Campbell, D. (1976) The cause of the fall in serum folate in normal pregnancy. Br. J. Obstet. Gynaecol. 83, 132–136.

291. Halsted, C. H. (1975) The small intestine in vitamin B_{12} and folate deficiency. Nutr. Rev. 33, 33–37.

292. Halsted, C. H., Baugh, C. M. & Butterworth, C. E., Jr. (1975) Jejunal perfusion of simple and conjugated folates in man. Gastroenterology 68, 261–269.

293. Halsted, C. H., Bhanthumnavin, K. & Mezey, E. (1974) Jejunal uptake of tritiated folic acid in the rat studied by in vivo perfusion. J. Nutr. 104, 1674–1680.

294. Halsted, C. H., Griggs, R. C. & Harris, J. W. (1967) The effect of alcoholism on the absorption of folic acid (H³-PGA) evaluated by plasma levels and urine excretion. J. Lab. Clin. Med. 69, 116–131.

295. Halsted, C. H., Robles, E. A. & Mezey, E. (1971) Decreased jejunal uptake of labeled folic acid (³H-PGA) in alcoholic patients: roles of alcohol and nutrition. N. Engl. J. Med. 285, 701–706.

296. Halsted, C. H., Robles, E. A. & Mezey, E. (1973) Intestinal malabsorption in folate-deficient alcoholics. Gastroenterology 64, 526–532.

297. Halsted, C. H., Sourial, N., Guindi, S., Mourad, K. A. H., Kattab, A. K., Carter, J. P. & Patwardhan, V. N. (1969) Anemia of kwashiorkor in Cairo: deficiencies of protein, iron, and folic acid. Am. J. Clin. Nutr. 22, 1371–1382.

298. Hansen, H. A. (1964) On the Diagnosis of Folic Acid Deficiency, Almqvist & Wiksell, Stockholm. Cited by: Roberts, P. D., St. John, D. J. B., Sinha, R., Stewart, J. S., Baird, I. M., Coghill, N. F. & Morgan, J. O. (1971) Apparent folate deficiency in iron-deficiency anaemia. Br. J. Haematol. 20, 165–176.

299. Hansen, H. A. (1968) Occurrence of folic acid deficiency in pregnancy. In: Symposia Swedish Nutr. Found. VI. Occurrence, Causes and Prevention of Nutritional Anaemias (Blix, G., ed.), pp. 50–65, Almqvist & Wiksells, Uppsala.

300. Hansen, H. A. & Klewesahl-Palm, H. V. (1963) Blood folic acid levels and clearance rate of injected folic acid in normal pregnancy and puerperium. Scand. J. Clin. Lab. Invest. 15, Suppl 69, 78–99.

301. Hansen, H. A., Nordqvist, P. & Sourander, P. (1964) Megaloblastic anemia and neurologic disturbances combined with folic acid deficiency. Acta Med. Scand. 176, 243–251.

302. Hansen, H. A. & Rybo, G. (1966) Folsyraprofylax under graviditet. Särtryck ur Nordisk Medicin 76, 867–871.

303. Hansen, H. & Rybo, G. (1967) Folic acid dosage in profylactic treatment during pregnancy. Acta Obstet. et Gynecol. Scand. 46, Suppl 7, 107–112.

304. Hansen, H. A. & Weinfeld, A. (1962) Metabolic effects and diagnostic value of small doses of folic acid and B₁₂ in megaloblastic anemias. Acta Med. Scand. 172, 427–443.

305. Heath, C. W. (1966) Cytogenetic observations in vitamin B₁₂ and folate deficiency. Blood 27, 800–815.

306. Heinle, R. W. & Welch, A. D. (1947) Folic acid in pernicious anemia. Failure to prevent neurologic relapse. J. Am. Med. Assoc. 133, 739–741.

307. Hellendoorn, E. W., Groot, A. P. de, Mijill Deukker, L. P. van der, Slump, P. & Willems, J. J. L. (1971) Nutritive value of canned meals. J. Am. Dietet. Assoc. 58, 434–441.

308. Hellström, L. (1971) Lack of toxicity of folic acid given in pharmacological doses to healthy volunteers. Lancet 1, 59–61.

309. Helmchen, U., Kneissler, U., Fischbach, H., Reifferscheid, P. & Schmidt, U. (1972) Plasma renin activity in folic acid induced acute renal failure. Klinische Wochenschrift 50, 797–798. Cited in: Nutr. Abst. Rev. 43, 291 (1973).

310. Henry, G. R. (1968) The aetiology of abruptio placentae with special reference to folate metabolism. Irish J. Med. Sci. 7, 509–515.

311. Hepner, G. W., Booth, C. C., Cowan, J., Hoffbrand, A. V. & Mollin, D. L. (1968) Absorption of crystalline folic acid in man. Lancet 2, 302–306.

312. Herbert, V. (1961) The assay and nature of folic acid activity in human serum. J. Clin. Invest. 40, 81–91.

313. Herbert, V. (1962) Experimental nutritional folate deficiency in man. Trans. Assoc. Am. Physicians 75, 307–320.

314. Herbert, V. (1963) A palatable diet for producing experimental folate deficiency in man. Am. J. Clin. Nutr. 12, 17–20.

315. Herbert, V. (1964) Studies of folate deficiency in man. Proc. Roy. Soc. Med. 57, 377–384.

316. Herbert, V. (1965) Excretion of folic acid in bile. Lancet 1, 913.

317. Herbert, V. (1966) Nutritional requirements for vitamin B₁₂ and folic acid. In: Proceedings of the Plenary Sessions, XI Congress of the International Society of Haematology, pp. 109–119, Blight, Sydney.

318. Herbert, V. (1968) Nutritional requirements for vitamin B₁₂ and folic acid. Am. J. Clin. Nutr. 21, 743–752.

319. Herbert, V. (1971) Predicting nutrient deficiency by formula. New Engl. J. Med. 284, 976–977.

320. Herbert, V. & Bertino, J. R. (1967) Folic acid. In: The Vitamins. Chemistry, Physiology, Pathology, Methods (György, P. & Pearson, W. N., eds.), Vol. VII, 2nd ed., pp. 243–269, Academic Press, New York.

321. Herbert, V., Cunneen, N., Jaskiel, L. & Kapff, C. (1962) Mineral daily adult folate requirement. Arch. Intern. Med. 110, 649–652.

322. Herbert, V. & Sullivan, L. W. (1963) Formiminoglutamicaciduria in humans with megaloblastic anemia: Diminution by methionine or glycine. Proc. Soc. Exp. Biol. Med. 112, 304–305.

323. Herbert, V. & Tisman, G. (1973) Effects of deficiencies of folic acid and vitamin B₁₂ on central nervous system function and devolpment. Biol. Brain Dysfunction 1, 373–392.

324. Herbert, V., Tisman, G., Go, L. T. & Brenner, L. (1973) The dU suppression test using ¹²⁵I-UdR to define biochemical megaloblastosis. Br. J. Haematol. 24, 713–723.

325. Herbert, V. & Zalusky, R. (1962) Interrelations of vitamin B₁₂ and folic acid metabolism: Folic acid clearance studies. J. Clin. Invest. 41, 1263–1276.

326. Herbert, V., Zalusky, R. & Davidson, C. S.

(1963) Correlation of folate deficiency with alcoholism and associated macro-cytosis, anemia, and liver disease. Ann. Intern. Med. *58*, 977–988.

327. Hermos, J. A., Adams, W. H., Liu, Y. K., Sullivan, L. W. & Trier, J. S. (1972) Mucosa of the small intestine in folate-deficient alcoholics. Ann. Intern. Med. *76*, 957–965.

328. Hershko, C., Grossowicz, N., Rachmilewitz, M., Kesten, S. & Izak, G. (1975) Serum and erythrocyte folates in combined iron and folate deficiency. Am. J. Clin. Nutr. *28*, 1217–1222.

329. Hibbard, B. M. (1964) The role of folic acid in pregnancy. With particular reference to anaemia, abruption and abortion. J. Obstet. Gynaecol. Br. Commonw. *71*, 529–542.

330. Hibbard, B. M. (1975) Folates and the fetus. S. Afr. Med. J. *49*, 1223–1226.

331. Hibbard, B. M. & Hibbard, E. D. (1966) Recurrence of defective folate metabolism in successive pregnancies. J. Obstet. Gynaecol. Br. Commonw. *73*, 428–430.

332. Hibbard, B. M. & Hibbard, E. D. (1968) Folate metabolism and reproduction. Br. Med. Bull. *24*, 10–14.

333. Hibbard, B. M. & Hibbard, E. D. (1969) The treatment of folate deficiency in pregnancy. Acta Obstet. Gynecol. Scand. *48*, 349–356.

334. Hibbard, B. M. & Hibbard, E. D. (1969) The prophylaxis of folate deficiency in pregnancy. Acta Obstet. Gynecol. Scand. *48*, 339–348.

335. Hibbard, B. M., Hibbard, E. D. & Jeffcoate, T. N. A. (1965) Folic acid and reproduction. Acta Obstet. Gynecol. Scand. *44*, 375–400.

336. Hibbard, E. D. (1967) FIGLU excretion in pregnancy. Acta Obstet. Gynecol. Scand. *46*, Suppl 7, 61–69.

337. Hibbard, E. D. (1973) Plasma and erythrocyte folate concentrations in normal mature infants. Arch. Dis. Child. *48*, 743–745.

338. Hibbard, E. D. & Kenna, A. P. (1974) Plasma and erythrocyte folate levels in low-birth-weight infants. J. Pediatr. *84*, 750–753.

339. Hill, R. S., Pettit, J. E., Tattersall, M. H. N., Kiley, N. & Lewis, S. M. (1972) Iron deficiency and dyserythropoiesis. Br. J. Haematol. *23*, 507–512.

340. Hines, J. D. (1974) Metabolic abnormalities of vitamin B₆ and magnesium in alcohol-induced sideroblastic anemia. In: Progress in Clinical and Biological Research. Erythrocyte Structure and Function. Proceedings of the Third International Conference (Brewer, G., ed.), Vol. 1, pp. 621–640, Alan R. Liss, Inc., New York.

341. Hodson, A. Z. (1948) Inhibitory effect of pure and semipurified proteins on the activity of hog kidney conjugase. Arch. Biochem. *16*, 309–311.

342. Hoffbrand, A. V. (1971) Folate absorption. J. Clin. Pathol. *24*, Suppl. 5, 66–76.

343. Hoffbrand, A. V. (1971) The megaloblastic anaemias. In: Recent Advances in Haematology (Goldberg, A. & Brain, M. C., eds.), pp. 1–76, Churchill Livingstone, London.

344. Hoffbrand, A. V., Douglas, A. P., Fry, L. & Stewart, J. S. (1970) Malabsorption of dietary folate (pteroylpolyglutamates) in adult coeliac disease and dermatitis herpetiformis. Br. Med. J. *4*, 85–89.

345. Hoffbrand, A. V. & Necheles, T. F. (1968) Mechanism of folate deficiency in patients receiving phenytoin. Lancet *2*, 528–530.

346. Hoffbrand, A. V., Necheles, T. F., Maldonado, N., Horta, E. & Santini, R. (1969) Malabsorption of folate polyglutamates in tropical sprue. Br. Med. J. *2*, 543–547.

347. Hoffbrand, A. V., Newcombe, B. F. A. & Mollin, D. L. (1966) Method of assay of red cell folate activity and the value of the assay as a test for folate deficiency. J. Clin. Pathol. *19*, 17–28.

348. Hoffbrand, A. V. & Pegg, A. E. (1972) Base composition of normal and megaloblastic bone marrow DNA. Nature New Biol. *235*, 187–188.

349. Hoffbrand, A. V. & Peters, T. J. (1969) The subcellular localization of pteroyl polyglutamate hydrolase and folate in guinea pig intestinal mucosa. Biochim. Biophys. Acta *192*, 479–485.

350. Hoffbrand, A. V., Tabaqchali, S., Booth, C. C. & Mollin, D. L. (1971) Small intestinal bacterial flora and folate status in gastrointestinal disease. Gut *12*, 27–33.

351. Honda, Y. (1968) Folate derivatives in the liver of riboflavin-deficient rats. Tohoku J. Exp. Med. *95*, 79–86.

352. Hoogstraten, B., Cuttner, J. & Natovitz, B. (1964) Sequence of recovery from multiple manifestations of folic acid deficiency. J. Mt. Sinai Hosp. *31*, 10–16.

353. Hoppner, K., Lampi, B. & Perrin, D. E. (1972) The free and total folate activity in foods available on the Canadian market. J. Inst. Can. Sci. Technol. Aliment. *5*, 60–66.

354. Hoppner, K., Lampi, B. & Perrin, D. E. (1973) Folacin activity of frozen convenience foods. J. Am. Dietet. Assoc. *63*, 536–539.

355. Hourihane, D. O'B. & Weir, D. G. (1970) Suppression of erythropoiesis by alcohol. Br. Med. J. *1*, 86–89.

356. Hunter, R. & Barnes, J. (1971) Toxicity of folic acid. Lancet *1*, 755.

357. Hunter, R., Barnes, J., Curzon, G., Kantamaneni, B. D. & Duncan, C. (1971) Effect of folic acid by mouth on cerebrospinal fluid homovanillic acid and 5-hydroxyindoleacetic acid concentration. J. Neurol. Neurosurg. Psychiat. *34*, 571–575.

358. Hunter, R., Barnes, J., Oakeley, H. F. & Matthews, D. M. (1970) Toxicity of folic acid given in pharmacological doses to healthy volunteers. Lancet *1*, 61–33.

359. Hurdle, A. D. F. (1968) An assessment of the folate intake of elderly patients in hospital. Med. J. Aust. *2*, 101–104.

360. Hurdle, A. D. F. (1968) The influence of hospital food on the folic-acid status of long-stay elderly patients. Med. J. Aust. *2*, 104–110.

361. Hurdle, A. D. F. (1970) Folic acid

([3]HFA) absorption and jejunal biopsy in mild nutritional folic acid deficiency. Pathology 2, 193–198.

362. Hurdle, A. D. F. (1973) The assay of folate in food. Nutrition 27, 12–16.

363. Hurdle, A. D. F., Barton, D. & Searles, I. H. (1968) A method for measuring folate in food and its application to a hospital diet. Am. J. Clin. Nutr. 21, 1202–1207.

364. Hurdle, A. D. F. & Williams, P. (1966) Folic-acid deficiency in elderly patients admitted to hospital. Br. Med. J. 2, 202–205.

365. Huskisson, Y. J. & Retief, F. P. (1970) Folaatinhoud van voedsel. S. Afr. Med. J. 44, 362–363. Cited in: Nutr. Abstr. Rev. 41, 188 (1971).

366. Hussain, M. & Wadsworth, G. R. (1967) Nutritional status of Asian infants. Proc. Nutr. Soc. 26, 212–218.

367. Ishida, H. (1973) Studies on the fate of tetrahydrofolic acid. Shika Igaku 36, 501–515. Cited in: Chem. Abstr. 81, 265 (1974).

368. IUNS-AIN Committee on Nomenclature (1976) Nomenclature policy: Generic descriptors and trivial names for vitamins and related compounds. J. Nutr. 106, 8–14.

369. Iyengar, L. (1971) Folic acid requirements of Indian pregnant women. Am. J. Obstet. Gynecol. 111, 13–16.

370. Iyengar, L. & Apte, S. V. (1970) Prophylaxis of anemia in pregnancy. Am. J. Clin. Nutr. 23, 725–730.

371. Iyengar, L. & Apte, S. V. (1972) Nutrient stores in human foetal livers. Br. J. Nutr. 27, 313–317.

372. Iyengar, L. & Babu, S. (1975) Folic acid absorption in pregnancy. Br. J. Obstet. Gynaecol. 82, 20–23.

373. Iyengar, L. & Rajalakshmi, K. (1975) Effect of folic acid supplement on birth weights of infants. Am. J. Obstet. Gynecol. 122, 332–336.

374. Izak, G., Galevski, K., Grossowicz, N., Jablonska, M. & Rachmilewitz, M. (1972) Studies on folic acid absorption in the rat. II. The absorption of crystalline pteroylglutamic acid from selected small intestine segments. Am. J. Dig. Dis. 17, 599–602.

375. Izak, G., Galewski, K., Rachmilewitz, M. & Grossowicz, N. (1972) The absorption of milk-bound pteroylglutamic acid from small intestine segments. Proc. Soc. Exp. Biol. Med. 140, 248–250.

376. Izak, G., Levy, S., Rachmilewitz, M. & Grossowicz, N. (1973) The effect of iron and folic acid therapy on combined iron and folate deficiency anaemia: The results of a clinical trial. Scand. J. Haematol. 11, 236–240.

377. Izak, G., Rachmilewitz, M., Grossowicz, N., Galewski, K. & Kraus, Sh. (1968) Folate activity in reticulocytes and the incorporation of tritiated pteroylglutamic acid into red cells. Br. J. Haematol. 14, 447–452.

378. Izak, G., Rachmilewitz, M., Levy, S., Hershko, C. & Grossowicz, N. (1971) Anemia in pregnant women and children in Kiryat Shmoneh. Harefuah 80, 67. Cited by: Levy, S., Rachmilewitz, M., Grossowicz, N.,

Reshef, Y. & Izak, G. (1975) Nutritional survey in an iron- and folate-deficient population. Am. J. Clin. Nutr. 28, 1454–1457.

379. Izak, G., Rachmilewitz, M., Sadovsky, A., Bercovici, B., Aronovitch, J. & Grossowicz, N. (1961) Folic acid metabolites in whole blood and serum in anemia of pregnancy. Am. J. Clin. Nutr. 9, 473–477.

380. Izak, G., Rachmilewitz, M., Zan, S. & Grossowicz, N. (1963) The effect of small doses of folic acid in nutritional megaloblastic anemia. Am. J. Clin. Nutr. 13, 369–377.

381. Jackson, I. M. D., Doig, W. B. & McDonald, G. (1967) Pernicious anaemia as a cause of infertility. Lancet 1, 1159–1160.

382. Jacob, M., Hunt, I. F., Dirige, O. & Swendseid, M. E. (1976) Biochemical assessment of the nutritional status of low-income pregnant women of Mexican descent. Am. J. Clin. Nutr. 29, 650–656.

383. Jacobson, R. J. (1972) Puerperal folate deficiency resembling tropical sprue. S. Afr. Med. J. 46, 1103.

384. Jägerstad, M., Lindstrand, K. & Westesson, A. K. (1971) Folsyra i födan och dess absorption. Läkartidningen 68, 4024–4026, 4030. Cited in: Nutr. Abstr. Rev. 44, 17 (1974).

385. Jandl, J. H. & Gabuzda, G. J., Jr. (1953) Potentiation of pteroylglutamic acid by ascorbic acid in anemia of scurvy. Proc. Soc. Exp. Biol. Med. 84, 452–455.

386. Jandl, J. H. & Lear, A. A. (1956) The metabolism of folic acid in cirrhosis. Ann. Intern. Med. 45, 1027–1044.

387. Jarabak, J. & Bachur, N. R. (1971) A soluble dihydrofolate reductase from human placenta: Purification and properties. Arch. Biochem. Biophys. 142, 417–425.

388. Jathar, V. S., Kamath, S. A., Parikh, M. N., Rege, D. V. & Satoskar, R. S. (1970) Maternal milk and serum vitamin B₁₂, folic acid, and protein levels in Indian subjects. Arch. Dis. Child. 45, 236–241.

389. Jeejeebhoy, K. N., Desai, H. G., Borkkar, A. V., Deshpande, V. & Pathare, S. M. (1968) Tropical malabsorption syndrome in West India. Am. J. Clin. Nutr. 21, 994–1006.

390. Jeejeebhoy, K. N., Desai, H. G., Noronha, J. M., Antia, F. P. & Parekh, D. V. (1966) Idiopathic tropical diarrhea with or without steatorrhea (tropical malabsorption syndrome). Gastroenterology 51, 333–344.

391. Jeejeebhoy, K. N., Pathare, S. M., & Noronha, J. M. (1965) Observations on conjugated and unconjugated blood folate levels in megaloblastic anemia and the effects of vitamin B₁₂. Blood 26, 354–359.

392. Jeejeebhoy, K. N., Ramanath, P., Mehan, K. P., Pathare, S. M., Parekh, D. V., Nadkarni, G. D. & Ganatra, R. D. (1967) A simple method of estimating folic acid absorption (a modified faecal excretion method). J. Nucl. Med. 8, 40–49.

393. Jessop, J. D. (1962) The efficacy of folic acid in preventing megaloblastic anaemia in twin pregnancy. Irish J. Med. Sci. 6, 317–320.

394. Johns, D. G., Sperti, S. & Burgen, A. S. V.

(1961) The metabolism of tritiated folic acid in man. J. Clin. Invest. *40*, 1684–1695.

395. Johnson, B. C., Hamilton, T. S. & Mitchell, H. H. (1945) The excretion of "folic acid" through the skin and in the urine of normal individuals. J. Biol. Chem. *159*, 425–429.

396. Jukes, T. H., Franklin, A. L., Stokstad, E. L. R. & Boehne, J. W. III. (1947) The urinary excretion of pteroylglutamic acid and certain related compounds. J. Lab. Clin. Med. *32*, 1350–1355.

397. Jukes, T. H. & Stockstad, E. L. R. (1948) Pteroylglutamic acid and related compounds. Physiol. Rev. *28*, 51–106.

398. Kahn, S. B. & Brodsky, I. (1968) Metabolic interrelationship between vitamin B_{12} and ascorbic acid in pernicious anemia. Blood *31*, 55–65.

399. Kamel, K., Waslien, C. I., El-Ramly, Z., Guindy, S., Mourad, K. A., Khattab, A. K., Hashem, N., Patwardhan, V. N. & Darby, W. J. (1972) Folate requirements of children. Response of children recovering from protein-calorie malnutrition to graded doses of parenterally administered folic acid. Am. J. Clin. Nutr. *25*, 152–165.

400. Kamen, B. A. & Caston, J. D. (1975) Purification of folate binding factor in normal umbilical cord serum. Proc. Nat. Acad. Sci. U.S.A. *72*, 4261–4264.

401. Kaminetzky, H. A., Baker, H., Frank, O. & Langer, A. (1974) The effects of intravenously administered water-soluble vitamins during labor in normovitaminemic and hypovitaminemic gravidas on maternal and neonatal blood vitamin levels at delivery. Am. J. Obstet. Gynecol. *120*, 697–703.

402. Kaplan, S. S. & Basford, R. E. (1976) Effect of vitamin B_{12} and folic acid deficiencies on neutrophil function. Blood *47*, 801–805.

403. Karlin, R. (1967) Etude sur les taux d'acide folique du lait humain et du lait bovin. Int. Z. Vitaminforsch. *37*, 334–342.

404. Karlin, R. (1969) Sur la teneur en folates des laits de grand mélange. Effects de divers traitements thermiques sur les taux de folates, B_{12} et B_6 de ces laits. Int. Z. Vitaminforsch. *39*, 359–371.

405. Karlin, R. (1971) Sur le dépistage des carences en acide folique par la détermination de l'activité, folique *L. casei* dans le sérum sanguin, le sang total et les globules rouges. Ann. Nutr. Alim. *25*, 77–90.

406. Karlin, R. & Bourgeay, M. (1976) Étude de l'action de contraceptifs oraux sur les taux sanguins des folates. Pathol. Biol. *24*, 251–255.

407 Karthigaini, S., Gnanasundaram, D. & Baker, S. J. (1964) Megaloblastic erythropoiesis and serum vitamin B_{12} and folic acid levels in pregnancy in South Indian women. J. Obstet. Gynaecol. Br. Commonw. *71*, 115–122.

408. Katz, M. (1973) Potential danger of self-medication with folic acid. N. Engl. J. Med. *289*, 1095.

409. Kauffman, S. L., Kasai, G. J. & Koser, S. A. (1953) The amounts of folic acid and

vitamin B_6 in saliva. J. Dent. Res. *32*, 840–849.

410. Kaufman, S. (1967) Pteridine cofactors. Annu. Rev. Biochem. *36*, 171–184.

411. Kemp, T. A. (1947) Liver and folic acid in the treatment of nutritional macrocytic anaemia. Lancet *2*, 350–353.

412. Kendall, A. C., Jones, E. E., Wilson, C. I. D., Shinton, N. K. & Elwood, P. C. (1974) Folic acid in low birthweight infants. Arch. Dis. Child. *49*, 736–738.

413. Kende, G., Ramot, B. & Grossowicz, N. (1963) Blood folic acid and vitamin B_{12} activities in healthy infants and in infants with nutritional anaemias. Br. J. Haematol. *9*, 328–335.

414. Kershaw, P. W. & Girdwood, R. H. (1964) Some investigations of folic-acid deficiency. Scot. Med. J. *9*, 201–212.

415. Keusch, G., Plant, A. G. & Troncale, F. J. (1972) Subclinical malabsorption in Thailand. II. Intestinal absorption in American military and Peace Corps personnel. Am. J. Clin. Nutr. *25*, 1067–1073.

416. Khalil, M., Tanios, A., Moghazy, M., Aref, M. K., Mahmoud, S. & El Lozy, M. (1973) Serum and red cell folates, and serum vitamin B_{12} in protein calorie malnutrition. Arch. Dis. Child. *48*, 366–369.

417. Kho, L-K. & Odang, O. (1959) Megaloblastic anemia in infancy and childhood in Djakarta. A. M. A. J. Dis. Child. *97*, 209–218.

418. Kinnear, D. G., Johns, D. G., MacIntosh, P. C., Burgen, A. S. V. & Cameron, D. G. (1963) Intestinal absorption of tritium-labeled folic acid in idiopathic steatorrhea: effect of a gluten-free diet. Can. Med. Assoc. J. *89*, 975–979.

419. Kitay, D. Z. (1969) Folic acid deficiency in pregnancy. On the recognition, pathogenesis, consequences, and therapy of the deficiency state in human reproduction. Am. J. Obstet. Gynecol. *104*, 1067–1107.

420. Kitay, D. Z. & Marshall, J. S. (1968) Remission of folic acid deficiency in pregnancy. Am. J. Obstet. Gynecol. *102*, 297–303.

421. Klipstein, F. A. (1963) The urinary excretion of orally administered tritium-labeled folic acid as a test of folic acid absorption. Blood *21*, 626–639.

422. Klipstein, F. A. (1964) Antibiotic therapy in tropical sprue. The role of dietary folic acid in the hematologic remission associated with oral antibiotic therapy. Ann. Intern. Med. *61*, 721–728.

423. Klipstein, F. A. (1964) Tropical sprue in New York City. Gastroenterology *47*, 457–470.

424. Klipstein, F. A. (1967) Intestinal folate conjugase activity in tropical sprue. Am. J. Clin. Nutr. *20*, 1004–1009.

425. Klipstein, F. A. (1969) Absorption of physiologic doses of folic acid in subjects with tropical sprue responding to tetracycline therapy. Blood *34*, 191–203.

426. Klipstein, F. A. (1970) Recent advances in tropical malabsorption. Scand. J. Gastroenterol. Suppl. *6*, 93–114.

427. Klipstein, F. A. & Falaiye, J. M. (1969) Tropical sprue in expatriates from the tropics living in the continental United States. Medicine (Balt.) 48, 475–491.

428. Klipstein, F. A. & Lindenbaum, J. (1965) Folate deficiency in chronic liver disease. Blood 25, 443–456.

429. Klipstein, F. A. & Lipton, S. D. (1970) Intestinal flora of folate-deficient mice. Am. J. Clin. Nutr. 23, 132–140.

430. Klipstein, F. A., Lipton, S. D. & Schenk, E. A. (1973) Folate deficiency of the intestinal mucosa. Am. J. Clin. Nutr. 26, 728–737.

431. Klipstein, F. A., Rubio, C., Montas, S., Tomasini, J. T. & Castillo, R. G. (1973) Nutritional status and intestinal function among rural population of the West Indies. III. Barrio Cabreto, Dominican Republic. Am. J. Clin. Nutr. 26, 87–95.

432. Klipstein, F. A., Samloff, I. M., Smarth, G. & Schenk, E. A. (1969) Treatment of overt and subclinical and malabsorption in Haiti. Gut 10, 315–322.

433. Knowles, J. P. & Prankerd, T. A. J. (1961) Megaloblastic anaemias of gastrointestinal origin. Postgrad. Med. J. 37, 755–760.

434. Knowles, J. P., Prankerd, T. A. J. & Westall, R. G. (1961) Folic acid requirements in man. J. Physiol. 157, 24P–25P.

435. Kon, S. K. & Mawson, E. H. (1950) Human Milk. Wartime Studies of Certain Vitamins and Other Constituents. Medical Research Council Special Report Series no. 269, H. M. Stationery Office, London, 188 p.

436. Kremenchuzky, S., Musso, A. M., Hoffbrand, V. & Rochna Viola, E. M. (1967) Tritiated folic acid (^{3}H F.A.). Excretion tests for the study of folic acid absorption. J. Nucl. Biol. Med. 11, 89–95.

437. Krumdieck, C. L. & Baugh, C. M. (1969) The solid-phase synthesis of polyglutamates of folic acid. Biochemistry 8, 1568–1572.

438. Krumdieck, C. L., Boots, L. R., Cornwell, P. E. & Butterworth, C. E., Jr. (1975) Estrogen stimulation of conjugase activity in the uterus of ovariectomized rats. Am. J. Clin. Nutr. 28, 530–534.

439. Laffi, R., Tolomelli, B., Bovina, C. & Marchetti, M. (1972) Influence of short-term treatment with estradiol-17β on folate metabolism in the rat. Int. J. Vitam. Nutr. Res. 42, 196–204.

440. Lakshmaiah, N. & Ramasastri, B. V. (1975) Folic acid conjugase from plasma. I. Partial purification and properties. Int. J. Vitam. Nutr. Res. 45, 183–193.

441. Lakshmaiah, N. & Ramasastri, B. V. (1975) Folic acid conjugase from plasma. III. Use of the enzyme in the estimation of folate activity in foods. Int. J. Vitam. Nutr. Res. 45, 262–272.

442. Landon, M. J. & Hey, E. N. (1974) Renal loss of folate in the newborn infant. Arch. Dis. Child. 49, 292–296.

443. Landon, M. J. & Hytten, F. E. (1971) The excretion of folate in pregnancy. J. Obstet. Gynaecol. Br. Commonw. 78, 769–775.

444. Landon, M. J. & Hytten, F. E. (1972) Plasma folate levels following an oral load of folic acid during pregnancy. J. Obstet. Gynaecol. Br. Commonw. 79, 577–583.

445. Landon, M. J. & Oxley, A. (1971) Relation between maternal and infant blood folate activities. Arch. Dis. Child. 46, 810–814.

446. Lanzkowsky, P., Erlandson, M. E. & Bezan, A. I. (1969) Isolated defect of folic acid absorption associated with mental retardation and cerebral calcification. Blood 34, 452–465.

447. Lavoie, A. & Cooper, B. A. (1974) Rapid transfer of folic acid from blood to bile in man, and its conversion into folate coenzymes and into a pteroylglutamate with little biological activity. Clin. Sci. Mol. Med. 46, 729–741.

448. Lavoie, A., Tripp, E. & Hoffbrand, A. V. (1975) Sephadex-gel filtration and heat stability of human jejunal and serum pteroylpolyglutamate hydrolase (folate conjugase). Evidence for two different forms. Biochem. Med. 13, 1–6.

449. Lawler, S. D., Roberts, P. D. & Hoffbrand, A. V. (1971) Chromosome studies in megaloblastic anaemia before and after treatment. Scand. J. Haematol. 8, 309–320.

450. Lawrence, C. & Klipstein, F. A. (1967) Megaloblastic anemia of pregnancy in New York City. Ann. Intern. Med. 66, 25–34.

451. Lawson, D. H., Murray, R. M. & Parker, J. L. W. (1972) Early mortality in the megaloblastic anaemias. Quart. J. Med. 41, 1–14.

452. Leevy, C. M., Baker, H., Hove, W. Ten, Frank, O. & Cherrick, G. R. (1965) B-complex vitamins in liver disease of the alcoholic. Am. J. Clin. Nutr. 16, 339–346.

453. Leslie, G. I. & Rowe, P. B. (1972) Folate binding by the brush border membrane proteins of small intestinal epithelial cells. Biochemistry 11, 1696–1703.

454. Levi, R. N. & Waxman, S. (1975) Schizophrenia, epilepsy, cancer methionine, and folate metabolism. Pathogenesis of schizophrenia. Lancet 2, 11–13.

455. Levy, S., Rachmilewitz, M., Grossowicz, N., Reshef, Y. & Izak, G. (1975) Nutritional survey in an iron- and folate-deficiency population. Am. J. Clin. Nutr. 28, 1454–1457.

456. Lewi, S. (1974) L'activiteté folique du sérum sanguin chez les sujets agés. Observations personnelles et discussion des données de la littérature. Nouv. Rev. Fr. Hématol. 14, 29–44.

457. Lindenbaum, J., Gerson, C. D. & Kent, T. H. (1971) Recovery of small-intestinal structure and function after residence in the tropics. I. Studies in Peace Corps volunteers. Ann. Intern. Med. 74, 218–222.

458. Lindenbaum, J. & Lieber, C. S. (1969) Hematologic effects of alcohol in man in the absence of nutritional deficiency. N. Engl. J. Med. 281, 333–338.

459. Lindenbaum, J., Whitehead, N. & Reyner, F. (1975) Oral contraceptive hormones,

folate metabolism, and the cervical epithelium. Am. J. Clin. Nutr. 28, 346–353.

460. Lowe, C. U. (1972) Research in infant nutrition: The untapped well. Am. J. Clin. Nutr. 25, 245–254.

461. Lowenstein, L., Brunton, L., Cooper, B. A., Milad, A. A. & Hsieh, Yang-Shu (1964) The relation of erythrocyte and serum L. casei folate activity to folate deficiency in certain megaloblastic anaemias. In: Proc. 9th Congr. Europ. Soc. Haemat., Lisbon, 1963, pp. 364–375, S. Karger, Basel/New York.

462. Lowenstein, L., Brunton, L. & Hsieh, Y. S. (1966) Nutritional anemia and megaloblastosis in pregnancy. Can. Med. Assoc. J. 94, 636–645.

463. Lowenstein, L., Cantlie, G., Ramos, O. & Brunton, L. (1966) The incidence and prevention of folate deficiency in a pregnant clinic population. Can. Med. Assoc. J. 95, 797–806.

464. Lowenstein, L., Leeuw, N. K. M. de, Cantlie, G. S. D. & Brunton, L. (1968) Iron and folate deficiency in pregnancy. Med. Times 96, 563–574.

465. Lowenstein, L., Pick, C. & Philpott, N. (1955) Megaloblastic anemia of pregnancy and the puerperium. Am. J. Obstet. Gynecol. 70, 1309–1337.

466. Luckey, T. D. (1970) Vitamin metabolism in germfree animals: folic acid. In: Proc. 8th Int. Congr. Nutr., Prague, 1969 (Josef Masek et al., eds.), pp. 399–407, Excerpta Medica, Amsterdam.

467. Ludovici, P. P. & Axelrod, A. E. (1951) Circulating antibodies in vitamin-deficiency states. Pteroylglutamic acid, niacin-tryptophan, vitamins B₁₂, A, and D deficiencies. Proc. Soc. Expt. Biol. Med. 77, 526–530.

468. Luhby, A. L. (1959) Megaloblastic anemia in infancy. III. Clinical considerations and analysis. J. Pediatr. 54, 617–632.

469. Luhby, A. L. & Cooperman, J. M. (1963) Folic acid content of milk and milk substitutes. Pediatrics 32, 463–464.

470. Luhby, A. L. & Cooperman, J. M. (1964) Folic acid deficiency in man and its interrelationship with vitamin B₁₂ metabolism. Adv. Metab. Disorders. 1, 263–334.

471. Luhby, A. L., Eagle, F. J., Roth, E. & Cooperman, J. M. (1961) Relapsing megaloblastic anemia in an infant due to a specific defect in gastrointestinal absorption of folic acid. Am. J. Dis. Child. 102, 482–483.

472. Luhby, A. L. & Wheeler, W. E. (1949) Megaloblastic anemia of infancy: II—Failure of response to vitamin B₁₂ and the metabolic role of folic acid and vitamin C. Ohio State Univ., Health Center J. 3, 1–20.

473. Luther, L., Santini, R., Brewster, C., Perez-Santiago, E. & Butterworth, C. E., Jr. (1965) Folate binding by insoluble components of American and Puerto Rican diets. Ala. J. Med. Sci. 2, 389–393.

474. Mac Iver, J. E. & Back, E. H. (1960) Megaloblastic anaemia of infancy in Jamaica. Arch. Dis. Child. 35, 134–145.

475. MacKenzie, A. & Abbott, J. (1960) Megaloblastic erythropoiesis in pregnancy. Br. Med. J. 2, 1114–1116.

476. MacLennan, W. J., Andrews, G. R., MacLeod, C. & Caird, F. I. (1973) Anaemia in the elderly. Quart. J. Med. 42, 1–13.

477. MacLennan, W. J., Coombe, N. B., Martin, P. & Mason, B. J. (1975) The relationship of laboratory parameters to dietary intake in a long-stay hospital. Age Aging 4, 189–194.

478. MacLennan, W. J., Martin, P. & Mason, B. J. (1975) Causes for reduced dietary intake in a long-stay hospital. Age Aging 4, 175–180.

479. Mahmud, K., Kaplan, M. E., Ripley, D., Swaim, W. R. & Doscherholmen, A. (1974) The importance of red cell B₁₂ and folate levels after partial gastrectomy. Am. J. Clin. Nutr. 27, 51–54.

480. Maitra, A., Banerjee, D. K. & Basu, A. K. (1972) Preparation of folic acid deficient diet. Bull. Calcutta School Trop. Med. 20, 50–51.

481. Mäkilä, E. (1965) Salivary folic acid activity in various conditions of the human mouth. Arch. Oral Biol. 11, 839–844.

482. Mäkilä, E. & Kirveskari, P. (1967) Salivary folic acid activity after oral administration of folic acid. Int. Z. Vitaminforsch. 37, 487–491.

483. Makulu, D. R., Smith, E. F. & Bertino, J. R. (1973) Effects of steroids, folate deprivation and protein deprivation upon tetrahydrofolate dehydrogenase levels in mammalian tissues. Biochim. Biophys. Acta 304, 526–532.

484. Maldonado, N., Fradera, J., Santini, R., Horta, E. & Pérez-Santiageo, E. (1969) Hematologic response to physiologic doses of folic acid in tropical sprue. Am. J. Clin. Nutr. 22, 733–739.

485. Malin, J. O. (1974) Implications of pH in the assay of total folate activity. J. Sci. Food Agric. 25, 1051.

486. Mangay Chung, A. S., Pearson, W. N., Darby, W. J., Miller, O. N. & Goldsmith, G. A. (1961) Folic acid, vitamin B₆, pantothenic acid, and vitamin B₁₂ in human dietaries. Am. J. Clin. Nutr. 9, 573–582.

487. Margo, G., Barker, M., Fernandes-Costa, F., Colman, N., Green, R. & Metz, J. (1975) Prevention of folate deficiency by food fortification. VII. The use of bread as a vehicle for folate supplementation. Am. J. Clin. Nutr. 28, 761–763.

488. Mark, M. S. van de & Wright, A. C. (1972) Hemoglobin and folate levels of pregnant teen-agers. J. Am. Dietet. Assoc. 61, 511–516.

489. Markkanen, T. (1968) Absorption tests with natural folate material in controls and in gastrectomized patients. Am. J. Clin. Nutr. 21, 473–481.

490. Markkanen, T., Himanen, P., Pajula, R. L., Ruponen, S. & Castrén, O. (1973) Binding of folic acid to serum proteins. I. The effect of pregnancy. Acta Haematol. 50, 85–91.

491. Markkanen, T., Levanto, A. & Castrén, O. (1969) Folate metabolism in connection with parturition. Int. Z. Vitaminforsch. 39, 37–43.

492. Markkanen, T. & Mäkilä, E. (1965) Assessment of postoperative renal function. Lancet 1, 1118–1119.

493. Markkanen, T., Pajula, R. L., Himanen, P. & Virtanen, S. (1973) Serum folic acid activity (L. casei) in Sephadex gel chromatography. J. Clin. Pathol. 26, 486–493.

494. Markkanen, T. & Peltola, O. (1970) Binding of folic acid activity by body fluids. Acta Haematol. 43, 272–279.

495. Markkanen, T., Peltola, O. & Himanen, P. (1971) Metabolic aspects of serum PGA in megaloblastic states. Int. J. Vitam. Nutr. Res. 41, 457–463.

496. Markkanen, T., Pajula, R. L., Himanen, P. & Virtanen, S. (1974) Binding of folic acid to serum proteins IV in some animal species. Int. J. Vitam. Nutr. Res. 44, 347–356.

497. Markkanen, T., Pajula, R. L., Virtanen, S. & Himanen, P. (1974) Binding of folic acid activity (FAA) to protein in mother's milk. Int. J. Vitam. Nutr. Res. 44, 195–202.

498. Markkanen, T., Virtanen, S., Pajula, R. L. & Himanen, P. (1974) Hormonal dependence of folic acid protein binding in human serum. Int. J. Vitam. Nutr. Res. 44, 81–94.

499. Marko, O. P., Bolotin, S. M. & Levitan, M. Kh. (1969) Correlation of the folic acid content and the nature of intestinal microflora in nonspecific ulcerous colitis. Sovet. Med. 11, 24–27.

500. Marshall, R. A. & Jandl, J. H. (1960) Responses to "physiologic" doses of folic acid in the megaloblastic anemias. Arch. Intern. Med. 105, 352–360.

501. Mathur, B. P. (1966) Sensitivity of folic acid. A case report. Indian J. Med. Sci. 20, 133–134.

502. Matoth, Y., Pinkas, A. & Sroka, C. (1965) Studies on folic acid in infancy. III. Folates in breast fed infants and their mothers. Am. J. Clin. Nutr. 16, 356–359.

503. Matoth, Y., Pinkas, A., Zamir, R., Mooallem, F. & Grossowicz, N. (1964) Studies on folic acid in infancy. I. Blood levels of folic and folinic acid in healthy infants. Pediatrics 33, 507–511.

504. Matoth, Y., Zamir, R., Bar-Shani, S. & Grossowicz, N. (1964) Studies on folic acid in infancy. II. Folic and folinic acid blood levels in infants with diarrhea, malnutrition, and infection. Pediatrics 33, 694–699.

505. Maxwell, J. D., Hunter, J., Stewart, D. A., Ardeman, S. & Williams, R. (1972) Folate deficiency after anticonvulsant drugs: an effect of hepatic enzyme induction? Br. Med. J. 1, 297–299.

506. May, M., Bardos, T. J., Barger, F. L., Lansford, M., Ravel, J. M., Sutherland, G. L. & Shive, W. (1951) Synthetic and degradative investigations of the structure of folic acid. J. Am. Chem. Soc. 73, 3067–3075.

507. May, C. D., Nelson, E. N., Lowe, C. U. & Salmon, R. J. (1950) Pathogenesis of megaloblastic anemia in infancy. Am. J. Dis. Child. 80, 191–206.

508. May, C. D., Stewart, C. T., Hamilton, A. & Salmon, R. J. (1952) Infection as cause of folic acid deficiency and megaloblastic anemia. Experimental induction of megaloblastic anemia by turpentine abscess. Am. J. Dis. Child. 84, 718–728.

509. May, C. D., Sundberg, R. D., Schaar, F., Lowe, C. U. & Salmon, R. J. (1951) Experimental nutritional megaloblastic anemia: relation of ascorbic acid and pteroylglutamic acid. I. Nutritional data and manifestations of animals. Am. J. Dis. Child. 82, 282–309.

510. McCance, R. A. & Widdowson, E. M., eds. (1960) The Composition of Foods, Medical Research Council Special Report Series no. 297, H. M. Stationery Office, London.

511. McClain, L. D., Carl, G. F. & Bridgers, W. F. (1975) Distribution of folic acid coenzymes and folate dependent enzymes in mouse brain. J. Neurochem. 24, 719–722.

512. McFee, J. G. (1973) Anemia in pregnancy—a reappraisal. Obstet. Gynecol. Survey 28, 769–793.

513. McGuffin, R., Goff, P. & Hillman, R. S. (1975) The effect of diet and alcohol on the development of folate deficiency in the rat. Br. J. Haematol. 31, 185–192.

514. McKellar, M. (1963) The diagnostic and experimental uses of microbiological assays of vitamin B_{12} and folic acid in hospital laboratory practice. M. D. Thesis, University of Otago, Dunedin, New Zealand. Cited by: McKellar, M. (1966) Nutritional anaemia in New Zealand. New Zealand Med. J., Haematol. Suppl. 65, 897–903.

515. McLean, F. W., Heine, M. W., Held, B. & Streiff, R. R. (1969) Relationship between the oral contraceptive and folic acid metabolism. Am. J. Obstet. Gynecol. 104, 745–747.

516. McLean, F. W., Heine, M. W., Held, B. & Streiff, R. R. (1970) Folic acid absorption in pregnancy: Comparison of the pteroylpolyglutamate and pteroylmonoglutamate. Blood 36, 628–631.

517. Melamed, E., Reches, A. & Hershko, C. (1975) Reversible central nervous system dysfunction in folate deficiency. J. Neurol. Sci. 25, 93–98.

518. Menendez-Corrada, R. (1968) Current views on tropical sprue and a comparison to nontropical sprue. Med. Clin. N. Am. 52, 1367–1385.

519. Metz, J., Edelstein, T., Divaris, M. & Zail, S. S. (1967) Effect of total dose infusion of iron-dextran on iron, folate, and vitamin B_{12} nutrition in postpartum anaemia. Br. Med. J. 3, 403–406.

520. Metz, J., Festenstein, H. & Welch, P. (1965) Effect of folic acid and vitamin B_{12} supplementation on tests of folate and vitamin B_{12} nutrition in pregnancy. Am. J. Clin. Nutr. 16, 472–479.

521. Metz, J. & Hackland, P. (1968) Folate metabolism during lactation. Congr. S. Afr. Soc. Haematol., Cape Town, July. Cited by: Metz, J. (1970) Folate deficiency con-

ditioned by lactation. Am. J. Clin. Nutr. 23, 843–847.

522. Metz, J., Lurie, A. & Konidaris, M. (1970) A note on the folate content of uncooked maize. S. Afr. Med. J. 44, 539–541.

523. Metz, J., Zalusky, R. & Herbert, V. (1968) Folic acid binding by serum and milk. Am. J. Clin. Nutr. 21, 289–297.

524. Mims, V., Swendseid, M. E. & Bird, O. D. (1947) The inhibition of pteroylglutamic acid conjugase and its reversal. The effect of nucleic acid- and sulfhydryl-combining reagents. J. Biol. Chem. 170, 367–377.

525. Ministry of National Health and Welfare (Canada) Bureau of Nutritional Sciences (1975) Saskatcheway Survey Report: Nutrition Canada. Information Canada. Ottawa, Canada.

526. Minot, G. R. & Castle, W. B. (1935) The interpretation of reticulocyte reactions. Their value in determining the potency of therapeutic materials, especially in pernicious anaemia. Lancet 2, 319–330.

527. Mitchell, D. C., Vilter, R. W. & Vilter, C. F. (1949) Hypersensitivity to folic acid. Ann. Int. Med. 31, 1102–1105.

528. Mittal, V. S., Agarwal, K. N. & Taneja, P. N. (1967) Studies on the serum B₁₂ and folic-acid levels in Indian infants under optimal nutritional conditions. Indian J. Med. Res. 55, 558–566.

529. Miyamoto, T., Murata, K. & Kawamura, M. (1973) Folic acid contents of some fermented soybean products and vegetables. Vitamins 47, 233–237. Cited in: Chem. Abstr. 79, 344, (1973).

530. Mohamed, S. D. & Roberts, M. (1965) Abnormal histidine metabolism in thyrotoxicosis in man. Lancet 2, 933–935.

531. Mollin, D. L. & Booth, C. C. (1971) Chronic tropical sprue in London. In: Tropical Sprue and Megaloblastic Anaemia, Wellcome Trust Collaborative Study, 1961–1969, pp. 61–127, Churchill-Livingstone, London.

532. Mollin, D. L. & Hoffbrand, A. V. (1965) The diagnosis of folate deficiency. Ser. Haematol. 3, 1–18.

533. Mollin, D. L. & Waters, A. H. (1968) Nutritional megaloblastic anaemia. In: Symposia Swedish Nutr. Found. VI. Occurrence, Causes and Prevention of Nutritional Anaemias (Blix, G., ed.), pp. 121–134, Almqvist & Wiksells, Uppsala.

534. Moore, C. V., Bierbaum, O. S., Welch, A. D. & Wright, L. D. (1945) The activity of synthetic Lactobacillus casei factor ("folic acid") as an antipernicious anemia substance. I. Observations of four patients: Two with Addisonian pernicious anemia, one with nontropical sprue and one with pernicious anemia of pregnancy. J. Lab. Clin. Med. 30, 1056–1069.

535. Moretti, A., Ciceri, C. & Suchowsky, G. K. (1969) Effect of a combination of B complex vitamins and ascorbic acid on liver lipid content in rats intoxicated with ethyl alcohol. Arzneim.-Forsch. 19, 1742–1743.

536. Morgan, A. G., Kelleher, J., Walker, B. F., Losowsky, M. S., Droller, H. & Middleton,

R. S. W. (1973) A nutritional survey in the elderly: Haematological aspects. Int. J. Vitam. Nutr. Res. 43, 461–471.

537. Morgan, S. K. (1968) Newborns and folic acid. J. S. Carolina Med. Assoc. 64, 499–502.

538. Morse, E. E. & Maxwell, B. (1976) Clinical interpretations of the measurement of folic acid and vitamin B₁₂ in neuromuscular disease. Ann. Clin. Lab. Sci. 6, 137–141.

539. Moscovitch, L. F. & Cooper, B. A. (1973) Folate content of diets in pregnancy: Comparison of diets collected at home and diets prepared from dietary records. Am. J. Clin. Nutr. 26, 707–714.

540. Mullin, E. M., Bonar, R. A. & Paulson, D. F. (1976) Acute tubular necrosis. An experimental model detailing the biochemical events accompanying renal injury and recovery. Invest. Urol. 13, 289–294.

541. Murata, M. & Miyamoto, T. (1974) Folic acid contents of foods and the amount of intake. Vitamins 48, 205–206. Cited in: Chem. Abstr. 81, 331, (1974).

542. Musso, A. M., Kremenchuzky, S. & Rochna Viola, E. M. (1970) Simultaneous study of the absorption of tritiated pteroylglutamic acid and ⁶⁰Co-vitamin B₁₂. J. Nucl. Med. 11, 569–575.

543. Naiman, J. L. & Oski, F. A. (1964) The folic acid content of milk: Revised figures based on an improved assay method. Pediatrics 34, 274–276.

544. Najjar, V. A. & Barrett, R. (1945) The synthesis of B vitamins by intestinal bacteria. Vitam. Horm. 3, 23–48.

545. Najjar, V. A., Holt, L. E., Jr. & Royston, H. M. (1944) A note on the minimum requirements of man for vitamin C and certain other vitamins. Bull. Johns Hopkins Hosp. 75, 315–318.

546. National Research Council Food and Nutrition Board (1968) Recommended Dietary Allowances. Seventh revised edition, publication 1694, National Academy of Sciences, Washington, D.C.

547. Neal, G. E. & Williams, D. C. (1965) The fate of intravenously injected folate in rats. Biochem. Pharmacol. 14, 903–914.

548. Necheles, T. F. & Synder, L. M. (1970) Malabsorption of folate polyglutamates associated with oral contraceptive therapy. N. Engl. J. Med. 282, 858–859.

549. Neilson, J. M. (1960) Megaloblastic anemia in scurvy. Report of a case. Scot. Med. J. 5, 42–44.

550. Nelson, E. W., Strieff, R. R. & Cerda, J. J. (1975) Comparative bioavailability of folate and vitamin C from a synthetic and a natural source. Am. J. Clin. Nutr. 28, 1014–1019.

551. Nelson, M. M. (1960) In: Ciba Foundation Symposium on Congenital Malformations, p. 151, Churchill, London. Cited by: Nelson, M. M. & Forfar, J. O. (1971) Associations between drugs administered during pregnancy and congenital abnormalities of the fetus. Br. Med. J. 1, 523–527.

552. Nelson, M. M. & Evans, H. M. (1948) The effect of succinylsulfathiazole on pteroylglu-

tamic acid deficiency during lactation in the rat. Arch. Biochem. *18*, 153–159.

553. Newbold, P. C. (1974) Distribution of methotrexate in rat tissues. Br. J. Dermatol. *90*, 669–677.

554. Ngo, T. M. & Winchell, H. S. (1969) Alterations in histidine catabolism in normal rats given pharmacological doses of folic acid and cyanocobalamin. Proc. Soc. Exp. Biol. Med. *132*, 168–170.

555. Nichol, C. A. & Welch, A. D. (1950) Synthesis of citrovorum factor from folic acid by liver slices; augmentation by ascorbic acid. Proc. Soc. Exp. Biol. Med. *74*, 52–55.

556. Nicol, D. J. & Davis, R. E. (1967) The folate and vitamin B_{12} content of infant milk foods with particular reference to goat's milk. Med. J. Aust. *54*, 212–214.

557. Nikkila, E. A., Miettinen, T. A. & Lanner, A. (1976) Treatment of hypercholesterolemia with Secholex. A long-term clinical trial and comparison with cholestyramine. Atherosclerosis *24*, 407–419.

558. Nixon, P. F. & Bertino, J. R. (1972) Effective absorption and utilization of oral formyltetrahydrofolate in man. N. Engl. J. Med. *286*, 175–179.

559. Nixon, P. F. & Bertino, J. R. (1972) Impaired utilization of serum folate in pernicious anemia. J. Clin. Invest. *51*, 1431–1439.

560. Noronha, J. M. & Aboobaker, V. S. (1963) Studies on the folate compounds of human blood. Arch. Biochem. Biophys. *101*, 445–447.

561. Noronha, J. M. & Silverman, M. (1962) Distribution of folic acid derivatives in natural material. I. Chicken liver folates. J. Biol. Chem. *237*, 3299–3302.

562. Noronha, J. M. & Silverman, M. (1962) On folic acid, vitamin B_{12}, methionine and formiminoglutamic acid metabolism. In: Vitamin B_{12} und Intrinsic Factor 2. Europaisches Symposion (Heinrich, H. C., ed.), pp. 728–736, Stuttgart.

563. Nutrition Canada (1973) Nutrition Canada National Survey. Information Canada, Ottawa.

564. O'Brien, W. (1968) Acute military tropical sprue in Southeast Asia. Am. J. Clin. Nutr. *21*, 1007–1012.

565. O'Brien, W. & England, N. W. J. (1964) Folate deficiency in acute tropical sprue. Br. Med. J. *2*, 1573–1575.

566. O'Brien, W. & England, M. W. J. (1966) Military tropical sprue from South-east Asia. Br. Med. J. *2*, 1157–1162.

567. O'Broin, J. D., Temperley, I. J., Brown, J. P. & Scott, J. M. (1975) Nutritional stability of various naturally occurring monoglutamate derivatives of folic acid. Am. J. Clin. Nutr. *28*, 438–444.

568. Omer, A., Finlayson, N. D. C., Shearman, D. J. C., Samson, R. R. & Girdwood, R. H. (1970) Plasma and erythrocyte folate in iron deficiency and folate deficiency. Blood *35*, 821–828.

569. Osler, W. (1919) The severe anaemias of pregnancy and the post-partum state. Br. Med. J. *1*, 1–3.

570. Pagnini, P., Compagnucci, M. & Biondi, E. (1969) Fattori alimentari e malattie infettive aviarie. Ricerche sull' importanza della dieta priva di acido folico nella produzione degli anticorpi inibenti l'E.A. da virus pseudo-pestoso aviario. Acta Med. Vet. *15*, 447–463.

571. Paine, C. J., Eichner, E. R. & Dickson, V. (1973) Concordance of radioassay and microbiological assay in the study of the ethanol-induced fall in serum folate level. Am. J. Med. Sci. *266*, 135–138.

572. Paine, C. J., Grafton, W. D., Dickson, V. L. & Eichner, E. R. (1975) Oral contraceptives, serum folate, and hematologic status. J. Am. Med. Assoc. *231*, 731–733.

573. Panders, J. T. & Rupert, M. S. E. (1965) The effect of temperature on folic acid metabolism. Br. J. Haematol. *11*, 518–524.

574. Parsons, L. G. (1933) Studies in the anaemias of infancy and early childhood. Arch. Dis. Child. *8*, 85–144.

575. Passmore, R. & Robson, J. S., eds. (1968) A Companion to Medical Studies, Vol. 1: Anatomy, Biochemistry, Physiology and Related Subjects, Blackwell Scientific Publications, Oxford.

576. Pathak, A. & Godwin, H. A. (1972) Vitamin B_{12} and folic acid values in premature infants. Pediatrics *50*, 584–589.

577. Perloff, B. P. & Butrum, R. R. (1977) Folacin in selected foods. J. Am. Dietet. Assoc. *70*, 161–172.

578. Perry, J. (1971) Folate analogues in normal mixed diets. Br. J. Haematol. *21*, 435–441.

579. Perry, J. & Chanarin, I. (1968) Absorption and utilization of polyglutamyl forms of folate in man. Br. Med. J. *4*, 546–549.

580. Perry, J. & Chanarin, I. (1970) Intestinal absorption of reduced folate compounds in man. Br. J. Haematol. *18*, 329–339.

581. Perry, J. & Chanarin, I. (1972) Observations on folate absorption with particular reference to folate polyglutamate and possible inhibitors to its absorption. Gut *13*, 544–550.

582. Perry, J., Lumb, M., Laundy, M., Reynolds, E. H. & Chanarin, I. (1976) Role of vitamin B_{12} in folate coenzyme synthesis. Br. J. Haematol. *32*, 243–248.

583. Pfiffner, J. J., Calkins, D. G., Bloom, E. S. & O'Dell, B. L. (1946) On the peptide nature of vitamin B_c conjugate from yeast. J. Amer. Chem. Soc. *68*, 1392.

584. Pfiffner, J. J., Calkins, D. G., O'Dell, B. L., Bloom, E. S., Brown, R. A., Campbell, C. J. & Bird, O. D. (1945) Isolation of an antianemia factor (vitamin B_c conjugate) in crystalline form from yeast. Science *102*, 228–230.

585. Pincus, J. H., Reynolds, E. H. & Glaser, G. H. (1972) Subacute combined system degeneration with folate deficiency. J. Am. Med. Assoc. *221*, 496–497.

586. Pitney, W. R. & Onesti, P. (1961) Vitamin B_{12} and folic acid concentrations of human liver with reference to the assay of needle biopsy material. Aust. J. Exp. Biol. 39, 1–8.

587. Porta, E. A., Koch, O. R. & Hartroft, W. S. (1972) Recovery from chronic hepatic lesions in rats fed alcohol and a solid super diet. Am. J. Clin. Nutr. 25, 881–896.

588. Prasad, A. S., Lei, K. Y., Oberleas, D., Moghissi, K. S. & Stryker, J. C. (1975) Effect of oral contraceptive agents on nutrients. II. Vitamins. Am. J. Clin. Nutr. 28, 385–391.

589. Pratt, R. F. & Cooper, B. A. (1971) Folates in plasma and bile of man after feeding folic acid-^{3}H and 5-formyltetrahydrofolate (folinic acid). J. Clin. Invest. 50, 455–462.

590. Prefontaine, M. (1976) A review of folic acid radioassays. Can. J. Med. Technol. 38, B-126, B-128, B-130.

591. Pritchard, J. A. (1962) Megaloblastic anemia during pregnancy and the puerperium. Am. J. Obstet. Gynecol. 83, 1004–1020.

592. Pritchard, J. A., Scott, D. E. & Whalley, P. J. (1969) Folic acid requirements in pregnancy-induced megaloblastic anemia. J. Am. Med. Assoc. 208, 1163–1167.

593. Pritchard, J. A., Scott, D. E. & Whalley, P. J. (1971) Maternal folate deficiency and pregnancy wastage. Am. J. Obstet. Gynecol. 109, 341–346.

594. Pritchard, J. A., Scott, D. E., Whalley, P. J. & Haling, R. F., Jr. (1970) Infants of mothers with megaloblastic anemia due to folate deficiency. J. Am. Med. Assoc. 211, 1982–1984.

595. Pritchard, J. A., Whalley, P. J. & Scott, D. E. (1969) The influence of maternal folate and iron deficiencies on intrauterine life. Am. J. Obstet. Gynecol. 104, 388–396.

596. Purugganan, G., Leikin, S. & Gautier, C. (1971) Folate metabolism in erythroid hyperplastic and hypoplastic states. Am. J. Dis. Child. 122, 48–56.

597. Qureshi, S., Rao, N. P., Madhavi, V., Mathur, Y. C. & Reddi, Y. R. (1973) Effect of maternal nutrition supplementation on the birth weight of the newborn. Indian Pediat. 10, 541–544.

598. Rader, J. I. & Huennekens, F. M. (1973) Folate coenzyme-mediated transfer of one-carbon groups. In: Enzymes (Boyer, P. D., ed.), 3rd ed, pp. 197–223, Academic Press, New York.

599. Ramasastri, B. V. (1965) Folate activity in human milk. Br. J. Nutr. 19, 581–586.

600. Ratanasthien, K., Blair, J. A., Leeming, R. J., Cooke, W. T. & Melikian, V. (1974) Folates in human serum. J. Clin. Pathol. 27, 875–879.

601. Read, A. E., Gough, K. R., Pardoe, J. L. & Nicholas, A. (1965) Nutritional studies on the entrants to an old people's home, with particular reference to folic-acid deficiency. Br. Med. J. 11, 843–848.

602. Reed, L. S. & Archer, M. C. (1976) Separation of folic acid derivatives by high-performance liquid chromatography. J. Chromatography 121, 100–103.

603. Register, U. D. & Sarett, H. P. (1951) Urinary excretion of vitamin B_{12} folic acid, and citrovorum factor in human subjects on various diets. Proc. Soc. Exp. Biol. Med. 77, 837–839.

604. Retief, F. P. (1969) Urinary folate excretion after ingestion of pteroylmonoglutamic acid and food folate. Am. J. Clin. Nutr. 22, 352–355.

605. Retief, F. P. & Huskisson, Y. J. (1970) Folate binders in body fluids. J. Clin. Pathol. 23, 703–707.

606. Reynolds, E. H. (1976) Folate and epilepsy. In: Biochem. Neurol. Proc. Conf. (Bradford, H. F. & Marsden, C. D., eds.), pp. 247–252, Academic, London.

607. Reynolds, E. H., Gallagher, B. B. & Mattson, R. H. (1972) Relationship between serum and cerebrospinal fluid folate. Nature 240, 155–157.

608. Reynolds, E. H., Rothfeld, P. & Pincus, J. H. (1973) Neurological disease associated with folate deficiency. Br. Med. J. 2, 398–400.

609. Richens, A. (1971) Toxicity of folic acid. Lancet 1, 912.

610. Ritland, S., Fausa, O., Gjone, E., Blomhoff, J. P., Skrede, S. & Lanner, A. (1975) Effect of treatment with a bile-sequestering agent (Secholex) on intestinal absorption, duodenal bile acids, and plasma lipids. Scand. J. Gastroenterol. 10, 791–800.

611. Roberts, P. D., St. John, D. J. B., Sinha, R., Stewart, J. S., Baird, I. M., Coghill, N. F. & Morgan, J. O. (1971) Apparent folate deficiency in iron-deficiency anaemia. Br. J. Haematol. 20, 165–176.

612. Roberts, P. M., Arrowsmith, D. E., Rau, S. M. & Monk-Jones, M. E. (1969) Folate state of premature infants. Arch. Dis. Child. 44, 637–642.

613. Roberts, P. M. M., Arrowsmith, D. E., Lloyd, A. V. C. & Monk-Jones, M. E. (1972) Effect of folic acid treatment on premature infants. Arch. Dis. Child. 47, 631–634.

614. Robinson, M. G. (1965) Megaloblastic anemia of infancy. Response to a minimal dose of pteroylglutamic acid. Minn. Med. 48, 1623–1628.

615. Roetz, R. & Nevinny-Stickel, J. (1973) Serumfolat, Serumeisen und totale Eisenbindungskapazität des Serums unter hormonaler Kontrazeption. Ergebnisse einer prospektiven Untersuchung. Geburtsh. u. Frauendeilk 33, 629–635.

616. Romine, M. K. (1960) The folic acid activity of human livers as measured with Lactobacillus casei. J. Vitaminol. 6, 196–201.

617. Rominger, E., Meyer, H. & Bomskov, C. (1933) Anämiestudien am wachsenden Organismus. Über die Pathogenese der Ziegenmilchanämie. Ztschr. ges. exper. Med. 89, 786–803. Cited by: Zuelzer, W. W. & Rutzky, J. (1953) Megaloblastic anemia of infancy. Adv. Pediatr. 6, 243–306.

618. Rosenberg, I. H. (1975) Folate absorption and malabsorption. N. Engl. J. Med. 293, 1303–1308.

619. Rosenberg, I. H. & Godwin, H. A. (1971) The digestion and absorption of dietary folate. Gastroenterology 60, 445–463.

620. Rosenberg, I. H., Godwin, H. A., Streiff, R. R. & Castle, W. B. (1968) Impairment of intestinal deconjugation of dietary folate. A possible explanation of megaloblastic anaemia associated with phenytoin therapy. Lancet 2, 530–532.

621. Rosenberg, I. H., Hachey, D. L., Beer, D. E. & Klein, P. D. (1973) Deuterium labeled folic acid: synthesis and applications to studies in man. In: Proc. 1st Int. Conf. Stable Isotop. Chem., Biol., Med. (Klein, P. D., ed.), pp. 421–427, NTIS, Springfield.

622. Rosenberg, I. H. & Neumann, H. (1974) Multi-step mechanism in the hydrolysis of pteroylpolyglutamates by chicken intestine. J. Biol. Chem. 249, 5126–5130.

623. Rosenberg, I. H., Streiff, R. R., Godwin, H. A. & Castle, W. B. (1969) Absorption of polyglutamic folate: participation of deconjugating enzymes of the intestinal mucosa. N. Engl. J. Med. 280, 985–988.

624. Rosensweig, N. S. (1975) Diet and intestinal enzyme adaptations: implications for gastrointestinal disorders. Am. J. Clin. Nutr. 28, 648–655.

625. Rosensweig, N. S., Herman, R. H., Stifel, F. B. & Herman, Y. F. (1969) Regulation of human jejunal glycolytic enzymes by oral folic acid. J. Clin. Invest. 48, 2038–2045.

626. Ross, C. E., Stone, M. K., Reagan, J. W., Wentz, W. B. & Kellermeyer, R. W. (1976) Lack of influence of oral contraceptives on serum folate, hematologic values, and uterine cervical cytology. Semin. Hematol. 13, 233–237.

627. Rothenberg, S. P., da Costa, M. & Rosenberg, Z. (1972) A radioassay for serum folate: Use of a two-phase sequential-incubation, ligand-binding system. N. Engl. J. Med. 286, 1335–1339.

628. Rothman, D. (1970) Folic acid in pregnancy. Am. J. Obstet. Gynecol. 108, 149–175.

629. Rovinetti, C., Bovina, C., Tolomelli, B. & Marchetti, M. (1972) Effects of testosterone on the metabolism of folate coenzymes in the rat. Biochem. J. 126, 291–294.

630. Ruffin, M., Calloway, D. H. & Margen, S. (1972) Nutritional status of preschool children of Marin County welfare recipients. Am. J. Clin. Nutr. 25, 74–84.

631. Russell, R. M., Ismail-Beigi, F., Alfrasiabi, K., Rahimifar, M., Pourkamal, D. & Ronaghy, H. (1976) Folate levels among various populations in central Iran. Am. J. Clin. Nutr. 29, 794–798.

632. Russell, R. M., Ismail-Beigi, F. & Reinhold, J. G. (1976) Folate content of Iranian breads and the effect of their fiber content on the intestinal absorption of folic acid. Am. J. Clin. Nutr. 29, 799–802.

633. Sacco, O., Ferrarese, R., Colavita, D. & Gilardi, G. (1973) Folic acid metabolism in third-trimester gestoses. Ann. Fac. Med. Chir. Univ. Studi Perugia Atti Accad. Anat.-Chird, 64, 5–10. Cited in: Chem. Abstr. 82, 374 (1975).

634. Samuel, P. D., Burland, W. L. & Simpson, K. (1973) Response to oral administration of pteroylmonoglutamic acid or pteroylglutamate in newborn infants of low birth weight. Br. J. Nutr. 30, 165–169.

635. Sandstead, H. H., Carter, J. P., House, F. R., McConnell, F., Horton, K. B. & Zwaag, R. V. (1971) Nutritional deficiencies in disadvantaged preschool children. Am. J. Dis. Child. 121, 455–463.

636. Santiago-Borrero, P. J., Santini, R., Jr., Pérez-Santiago, E. & Maldonado, N. (1973) Congenital isolated defect of folic acid absorption. J. Pediatr. 82, 450–455.

637. Santini, R., Jr., Berger, F. M., Berdasco, G., Sheehy, T. W., Aviles, J. & Davila, I. (1962) Folic acid activity in Puerto Rican foods. J. Am. Dietet. Assoc. 41, 562–567.

638. Santini, R., Brewster, C. & Butterworth, C. E., Jr. (1964) The distribution of folic acid active compounds in individual foods. Am. J. Clin. Nutr. 14, 205–210.

639. Santini, R. & Corcino, J. J. (1974) Analysis of some nutrients of the Puerto Rican diet. Am. J. Clin. Nutr. 27, 840–844.

640. Santini, R., Perez-Santiago, E., Walker, L. & Butterworth, C. E., Jr. (1966) Folic acid conjugase in normal human plasma and in the plasma of patients with tropical sprue. Am. J. Clin. Nutr. 19, 342–344.

641. Santini, R., Jr., Sheehy, T. W., Aviles, J. & Davila, I. (1962) Daily urinary excretion of folic acid in normal subjects and in patients with tropical sprue. Am. J. Trop. Med. Hyg. 11, 421–422.

642. Saraya, A. K., Choudhry, V. P. & Ghai, O. P. (1973) Interrelationships of vitamin B_{12}, folic acid, and iron in anemia of infancy and childhood: effect of vitamin B_{12} and iron therapy on folate metabolism. Am. J. Clin. Nutr. 26, 640–646.

643. Saraya, A. K., Tandon, B. N. & Ramachandran, K. (1971) Folic acid deficiency: Effects of iron deficiency on serum folic acid levels. Indian J. Med. Res. 59, 1796–1802.

644. Sastry, B. V. R. & Lakshmaiah, N. (1970) Some studies on folyl-γ-glutamyl carboxypeptidase from human plasma and its use in the estimation of folic acid content of foods. J. Sci. Indian Res. 29, S51–S54.

645. Satoskar, R. S., Kulkarni, B. S., Mehta, B. M., Sanzgiri, R. R. & Bamji, M. S. (1962) Serum vitamin B_{12} and folic acid (P.G.A.) levels in hypoproteinaemia and marasmus in Indian children. Arch. Dis. Child. 37, 9–16.

646. Sauer, H. & Wilmanns, W. (1977) Cobalamin dependent methionine synthesis and methyl-folate-trap in human vitamin B_{12} deficiency. Br. J. Haematol. 36, 189–198.

647. Schenk, E. A., Samloff, M. & Klipstein, F. A. (1968) Morphology of small bowel biopsies. Am. J. Clin. Nutr. 21, 944–961.

648. Schertel, M. E., Boehne, J. W. & Libby, D. A. (1965) Folic acid derivatives in yeast. J. Biol. Chem. 240, 3154–3158.

649. Schertel, M. E., Libby, D. A. & Loy, H. W. (1965) Yeast folate availability to man determined microbiologically on human bioassay samples. J. Assoc. Off. Agric. Chem. 48, 1224–1230.

650. Schmid, J. R. & Frick, P. G. (1965) Alimentäre Folsaruemangelanämie, Untersuchungen mit H^3-Folsäure, Co^{58}-Vitamin B_{12}, Fe^{59} und H^3-Thymidin. Schweiz. Med. Wochenschr. 95, 589–595. Cited in: Nutr. Abstr. Rev. 36, 195 (1966).

651. Schreiber, R. A., Shaw, W. & Zemp, J. W. (1973) The effects of folic acid deficiency on some aspects of development in DBA/2J and C57BL/6J mice. Nutr. Rep. Int. 8, 229–236.

652. Schweigert, B. S., Pollard, A. E. & Elvehjem, C. A. (1946) The folic acid content of meats and the retention of this vitamin during cooking. Arch. Biochem. Biophys. 10, 107–111.

653. Scott, J. M. (1963) Iron-sorbitol-citrate in pregnancy anaemia. Br. Med. J. 2, 354–357.

654. Shapiro, J., Alberts, H. W., Welch, P. & Metz, J. (1965) Folate and vitamin B_{12} deficiency associated with lactation. Br. J. Haematol. 11, 498–504.

655. Sharma, D. C. (1973) Histidine catabolism in iron-deficient rats. Br. J. Nutr. 30, 447–450.

656. Sharp, E. A., Vonder Heide, E. C. & Wolter, B. S. (1944) Preliminary clinical observations on the antianemia vitamin B_c (yeast concentrate). J. Am. Med. Assoc. 124, 734.

657. Shaw, D. M., MacSweeney, D. A., Johnson, A. L., O'Keeffe, R., Naidoo, D., MacLeod, D. M., Jog, S., Preece, J. M. & Crowley, J. M. (1971) Folate and amine metabolites in senile dementia: a combined trial and biochemical study. Physiol. Med. 1, 166–171.

658. Shaw, W., Schreiber, R. A. & Zemp, J. W. (1973) Perinatal folate deficiency: effects on developing brain in C57BL/6J mice. Nutr. Rep. Int. 8, 219–228.

659. Sheehy, T. W. (1973) Folic acid: lack of toxicity. Lancet 1, 37.

660. Sheehy, T. W., Baggs, B., Perez-Santiago, E. & Floch, M. H. (1962) Prognosis of tropical sprue. A study of the effect of folic acid on the intestinal aspects of acute and chronic sprue. Ann. Intern. Med. 57, 892–908.

661. Sheehy, T. W., Rubini, M. E., Perez-Santiago, E., Santini, R., Jr. & Haddock, J. (1961) The effect of "minute" and "titrated" amounts of folic acid on the megaloblastic anemia of tropical sprue. Blood 18, 623–636.

662. Shin, Y. S., Buehring, K. U. & Stokstad, E. L. R. (1974) Studies of folate compounds in nature. Folate compounds in rat kidney and red blood cells. Arch. Biochem. Biophys. 163, 211–224.

663. Shin, Y. S., Kim, E. S., Watson, J. E. & Stokstad, E. L. R. (1975) Studies of folic acid compounds in nature. IV. Folic acid compounds in soybeans and cow milk. Can. J. Biochem. 53, 338–343.

664. Shin, Y. S., Williams, M. A. & Stokstad, E. L. R. (1972) Identification of folic acid compounds in rat liver. Biochem. Biophys. Res. Commun. 47, 35–43.

665. Shinton, N. K. (1972) Vitamin B_{12} and folate metabolism. Br. Med. J. 1, 556–559.

666. Shojania, A. M. (1975) The effect of oral contraceptives on folate metabolism. III. Plasma clearance and urinary folate excretion. J. Lab. Clin. Med. 85, 185–190.

667. Shojania, A. M. (1975) Vitamins and oral contraceptive use. Lancet 1, 1198.

668. Shojania, A. M. & Gross, S. (1964) Folic acid deficiency and prematurity. J. Pediatr. 64, 323–329.

669. Shojania, A. M. & Hornady, G. (1970) Folate metabolism in newborns and during early infancy. I. Absorption of pteroylglutamic (folic) acid in newborns. Pediatr. Res. 4, 412–421.

670. Shojania, A. M. & Hornady, G. (1970) Folate metabolism in newborns and during early infancy. II. Clearance of folic acid in plasma and excretion of folic acid in urine by newborns. Pediatr. Res. 4, 422–426.

671. Shojania, A. M. & Hornady, G. J. (1973) Oral contraceptives and folate absorption. J. Lab. Clin. Med. 82, 869–875.

672. Shojania, A. M., Hornady, G. & Barnes, P. H. (1968) Oral contraceptives and serum folate level. Lancet 1, 1376–1377.

673. Shojania, A. M., Hornady, G. & Barnes, P. H. (1969) Oral contraceptives and folate metabolism. Lancet 1, 886.

674. Shojania, A. M., Hornady, G. J. & Barnes, P. H. (1971) The effect of oral contraceptives on folate metabolism. Am. J. Obstet. Gynecol. 111, 782–791.

675. Siddons, R. C. (1974) The experimental production of vitamin B_{12} deficiency in the baboon (Papio cynocephalus). A 2-year study. Br. J. Nutr. 32, 219–228.

676. Siddons, R. C. (1974) Experimental nutritional folate deficiency in the baboon (Papio cynocephalus). Br. J. Nutr. 32, 579–587.

677. Silverman, M. & Pitney, A. J. (1958) Dietary methionine and the excretion of formiminoglutamic acid by the rat. J. Biol. Chem. 233, 1179–1182.

678. Singh, M. (1975) Interaction between protein and folate status on the cellular development in the fetal rat. Indian J. Med. Res. 63, 545–557.

679. Singla, P. N., Saraya, A. K. & Ghai, O. P. (1970) Vitamin B_{12} and folic acid deficiency in nutritional megaloblastic anaemia of infancy and childhood. Indian J. Med. Res. 58, 599–604.

680. Smith, J. L., Goldsmith, G. A. & Lawrence, J. D. (1975) Effects of oral contraceptive steroids on vitamin and lipid levels in serum. Am. J. Clin. Nutr. 28, 371–376.

681. Smith, R. M. & Osborne-White, W. S. (1973) Folic acid metabolism in vitamin B_{12}-deficient sheep. Depletion of liver folates. Biochem. J. 136, 279–293.

682. Smith, R. M., Osborne-White, W. S. & Gawthorne, J. M. (1974) Folic acid metab-

olism in vitamin B_{12}-deficient sheep. Biochem. J. *142*, 105–117.

683. Sneath, P., Chanarin, I., Hodkinson, H. M., McPherson, C. K. & Reynolds, E. H. (1973) Folate status in a geriatric population and its relation to dementia. Age Ageing *2*, 177–182.

684. Sölling, H., Ellegaard, J. & Esmann, V. (1973) A clinical evaluation of a rapid method for determination of folate deficiency by ^{14}C-formate incorporation into serine of lymphocytes. Scand. J. Clin. Lab. Invest. *31*, 453–457.

685. Solomons, E., Lee, S. L., Wasserman, M. & Malkin, J. (1962) Association of anaemia in pregnancy and folic acid deficiency. J. Obstet. Gynaecol. Br. Commonw. *69*, 724–728.

686. Someswara Rao, K., Swaminathan, M. C., Swarup, S. & Patwardhan, V. N. (1959) Protein malnutrition in South India. Bull. Wld. Hlth. Org. *20*, 603–639.

687. Sorrell, M. F., Frank, O., Thomson, A. D., Aquino, H. & Baker, H. (1971) Absorption of vitamins from the large intestine *in vivo*. Nutr. Rep. Int. *3*, 143–148.

688. Sotobayashi, H. (1974) Folic acid in organs. Vitamins *48*, 202–203. Cited in: Chem. Abstr. *81*, 331 (1974).

689. Speidel, B. D. (1973) Folic acid deficiency and congenital malformation. Dev. Med. Child Neurol. *15*, 81–83.

690. Spies, T. (1946) Effect of folic acid on persons with macrocytic anemia in relapse. J. Am. Med. Assoc. *130*, 474–477.

691. Spies, T. D. (1946) Treatment of macrocytic anaemia with folic acid. Lancet *1*, 225–228.

692. Spies, T. D. (1949) Observations on the macrocytic anemia associated with pregnancy. Surg. Gynecol. Obstet. *89*, 76–78.

693. Spies, T. D., Lopez, G. G., Menendez, J. A., Minnich, V. & Koch, M. B. (1946) The effect of folic acid on sprue. S. Med. J. *39*, 30–32.

694. Spies, T. D., Milanes, F., Menéndez, A., Koch, M. B. & Minnich, V. (1946) Observations on the treatment of tropical sprue with folic acid. J. Lab. Clin. Med. *31*, 227–241.

695. Spies, T. D. & Stone, R. E. (1947) Some recent experiences with vitamins and vitamin deficiencies. S. Med. J. *40*, 46–55.

696. Spies, T. D., Vilter, C. F., Koch, M. B. & Caldwell, M. H. (1945) Observations of the anti-anemic properties of synthetic folic acid. So. Med. J. *38*, 707–709.

697. Spray, G. H. (1952) The utilization of folic acid from natural sources. Clin. Sci. *11*, 425–428.

698. Spray, G. H. (1964) Microbiological assay of folic acid activity in human serum. J. Clin. Path. *17*, 660–665.

699. Spray, G. H. (1968) Oral contraceptives and serum-folate levels. Lancet *2*, 110–111.

700. Spray, G. H. (1969) Estimation of red cell folate activity. J. Clin. Pathol. *22*, 212–216.

701. Spray, G. H., Fourman, P. & Witts, L. J. (1951) The excretion of small doses of folic acid. Br. Med. J. *2*, 202–205.

702. Stebbins, R., Scott, J. & Herbert, V. (1973) Drug-induced megaloblastic anemias. Semin. Hematol. *10*, 235–251.

703. Steinkamp, R., Shukers, C. F., Totter, J. R. & Day, P. L. (1946) Urinary excretion of orally administered pteroylglutamic acid. Proc. Soc. Exp. Biol. Med. *63*, 556–558.

704. Stephens, M. E. M., Craft, I., Peters, T. J. & Hoffbrand, A. V. (1972) Oral contraceptives and folate metabolism. Clin. Sci. *42*, 405–414.

705. Stevens, K. & Metz, J. (1964) The absorption of folic acid in megaloblastic anaemia associated with pregnancy. Trans. Roy. Soc. Trop. Med. Hyg. *58*, 510–516.

706. Stifel, F. B., Herman, R. H. & Rosenweig, N. S. (1970) Dietary regulation of glycolytic enzymes. X. The effect of oral intramuscular and conjugated sex steroids on jejunal folate-metabolizing enzyme activities in normal and castrated male and female rats. Biochim. Biophys. Acta *222*, 71–78.

707. Stifel, F. B., Taunton, O. D., Greene, H. L., Lufkin, E. G., Hagler, L. & Herman, R. H. (1974) Hormonal regulation of hepatic and jejunal formiminotransfearse activity in man and rat. Biochim. Biophys. Acta *354*, 194–205.

708. Stockman, J. A. III (1975) Anemia of prematurity. Semin. Hematol. *12*, 163–173.

709. Stokes, P. L., Melikian, V., Leeming, R. L., Portman-Graham, H., Blair, J. A. & Cooke, W. T. (1975) Folate metabolism in scurvy. Am. J. Clin. Nutr. *28*, 126–129.

710. Stokstad, E. L. R. (1954) Pteroylglutamic acid. In: The Vitamins. Chemistry, Physiology, Pathology (Sebrell, W. H. & Harris, R. S., eds.), Vol. III, pp. 87–217, Academic Press, New York.

711. Stokstad, E. L. R. (1968) Experimental anemias in animals resulting from folic acid and vitamin B_{12} deficiencies. Vitam. Horm. *26*, 443–463.

712. Stokstad, E. L. R. & Koch, J. (1967) Folic acid metabolism. Physiol. Rev. *47*, 83–116.

713. Stone, M. L. (1968) Effects on the fetus of folic acid deficiency in pregnancy. Clin. Obstet. Gynecol. *11*, 1143–1153.

714. Stone, M. L., Luhby, A. L., Feldman, R., Gordon, M. & Cooperman, J. M. (1967) Folic acid metabolism in pregnancy. Am. J. Obstet. Gynecol. *99*, 638–648.

715. Stout, R. W., Cashmore, A. R., Coward, J. K., Horvath, C. G. & Bertino, J. R. (1976) Separation of substituted pteroyl monoglutamates and pteroyl oligo-γ-L-glutamates by high pressure liquid chromatography. Anal. Biochem. *71*, 119–124.

716. Strachan, R. W. & Henderson, J. G. (1967) Dementia and folate deficiency. Quart. J. Med. *36*, 189–204.

717. Streiff, R. R. (1970) Folate deficiency and oral contraceptives. J. Am. Med. Assoc. *214*, 105–108.

718. Streiff, R. R. (1971) Folate levels in citrus and other juice. Am. J. Clin. Nutr. 24, 1390–1392.

719. Streiff, R. R. & Little, A. B. (1967) Folic acid deficiency in pregnancy. N. Engl. J. Med. 276, 776–779.

720. Strelling, M. K., Blackledge, G. D., Goodall, H. B. & Walker, C. H. M. (1966) Megaloblastic anaemia and whole-blood folate levels in premature infants. Lancet 1, 898–900.

721. Suárez, R. M., Spies, T. D. & Suárez, R. M., Jr. (1947) The use of folic acid in sprue. Ann. Intern. Med. 26, 643–677.

722. Suárez, R. M., Welch, A. D., Heinle, R. W., Suárez, R. M., Jr. & Nelson, E. M. (1946) Effectiveness of conjugated forms of folic acid in the treatment of tropical sprue. J. Lab. Clin. Med. 31, 1294–1304.

723. Sullivan, L. W. & Herbert, V. (1964) Suppression of hematopoiesis by ethanol. J. Clin. Invest. 43, 2048–2062.

724. Swanson, V. L., Wheby, M. S. & Bayless, T. M. (1966) Morphologic effects of folic acid and vitamin B_{12} on the jejunal lesion of tropical sprue. Am. J. Pathol. 49, 167–191.

725. Swendseid, M. E., Bird, O. D., Brown, R. A. & Bethell, F. H. (1947) Metabolic function · of pteroylglutamic acid and its hexaglutamyl conjugate. II. Urinary excretion studies on normal persons. Effect of a conjugase inhibitor. J. Lab. Clin. Med. 32, 23-27.

726. Tamura, T., Buehring, K. U. & Stockstad, E. L. R. (1972) Enzymatic hydrolysis of pteroylpolyglutamates in cabbage. Proc. Soc. Exp. Biol. Med. 141, 1022–1025.

727. Tamura, T., Shin, Y. S., Buehring, K. U. & Stokstad, E. L. R. (1976) The availability of folates in man: Effect of orange juice supplement on intestinal conjugase. Br. J. Haematol. 32, 123–133.

728. Tamura, T., Shin, Y. S., Williams, M. A. & Stokstad, E. L. R. (1972) Lactobacillus casei response to pteroylpolyglutamates. Anal. Biochem. 49, 517–521.

729. Tamura, T. & Stokstad, E. L. R. (1973) The availability of food folate in man. Br. J. Haematol. 25, 513–532.

730. Tasker, P. W. G. (1959) Concealed megaloblastic anaemia. Trans. Roy. Soc. Trop. Med. Hyg. 53, 291–295.

731. Temperley, I. J., Meehan, M. J. M. & Gatenby, P. B. B. (1968) Serum folic acid levels in pregnancy and their relationship to megaloblastic marrow change. Br. J. Haematol. 14, 13–19.

732. Temperley, I. J., O'Broin, J. D. & Scott, J. M. (1975) An explanation of the decreased serum folate values found using methods that involve prior extraction of the serum. Isr. J. Med. Sci. 144, 395–398.

733. Thenen, S. W. (1975) Food folate values. Am. J. Clin. Nutr. 28, 1341–1342.

734. Thenen, S. W., Shin, Y. S. & Stokstad, E. L. R. (1973) The turnover of rat-liver folate pools. Proc. Soc. Exp. Biol. Med. 142, 638–641.

735. Thenen, S. W. & Stokstad, E. L. R. (1973) Effect of methionine on specific folate co-enzyme pools in vitamin B_{12} deficient and supplemented rats. J. Nutr. 103, 363–370.

736. Timiras, P. S. & Vernadakis, A. (1972) Structural, biochemical, and functional aging of the nervous system. In: Developmental Physiology and Aging (Timiras, P. S., ed.), pp. 502–526, Macmillan Co., New York.

737. Tisman, G. & Herbert, V. (1973) B_{12} dependence of cell uptake of serum folate: An explanation for high serum folate and cell folate depletion in B_{12} deficiency. Blood 41, 465–469.

738. Toe, T. (1972) Ph.D. Thesis. Univ. London. Cited by: Wadsworth, G. R. (1973) Some historical aspects of knowledge about folate deficiency. Nutrition 27, 17–22.

739. Toennies, G., Usdin, E. & Phillips, P. M. (1956) Precursors of the folic acid-active factors of blood. J. Biol. Chem. 221, 855–863.

740. Toepfer, E. W., Zook, E. G. & Orr, M. L. (1951) Folic acid content of foods, Agr. Handbook no. 29, U.S.D.A. U. S. Govt. Printing Office, Washington, D.C.

741. Tolomelli, B., Rovinetti, C., Bovina, C. & Marchetti, M. (1972) Studies on folate metabolism in castrated rats and those treated with testosterone. Experientia 28, 197–198.

742. Torregrosa, M. V. de & Carceres de Costas, M. (1964) Megaloblastic anemia of infancy. Etiology and diagnosis based on a study of 56 cases in childhood. Clin. Pediatr. 3, 348–354.

743. Toskes, P. P., Smith, G. W., Bensinger, T. A., Giannella, R. A. & Conrad, M. E. (1974) Folic acid abnormalities in iron deficiency: The mechanism of decreased serum folate levels in rats. Am. J. Clin. Nutr. 27, 355–361.

744. Trubowitz, S., Frank, O. & Baker, H. (1974) Survey of vitamin B_{12} and folate in the serum and marrow tissue of hospitalized patients. Am. J. Clin. Nutr. 27, 580–583.

745. Ungley, C. C. (1933) The effect of yeast and wheat embryo in anaemias. 1. Marmite, Yestamin, and Bemax in megalocytic and nutritional hypochromic anaemias. Quart. J. Med. 2, 381–405.

746. Vanier, T. M. & Tyas, J. F. (1966) Folic acid status in normal infants during the first year of life. Arch. Dis. Child. 41, 658–665.

747. Vanier, T. M. & Tyas, J. F. (1966) The effect of prophylactic folic acid on serum and whole blood levels during the last trimester of pregnancy. J. Obstet. Gynaecol. Br. Commonw. 73, 934–939.

748. Vanier, T. M. & Tyas, J. F. (1967) Folic acid status in premature infants. Arch. Dis. Child. 42, 57–61.

749. Varadi, S. & Elwis, A. (1967) Folate deficiency in the elderly. Br. Med. J. 3, 112–113.

750. Vaughan, J. M. & Hunter, D. (1932) The treatment by marmite of megalocytic hyperchromic anaemia. Occurring in idiopathic steatorrhoea (coeliac disease). Lancet 1, 829–834.

751. Vaz Pinto, A., Torras, V., Sandoval, J. F. F., Dillmann, E., Mateos, C. R. & Córdova, M. S. (1975) Folic acid and vitamin B₁₂ determination in fetal liver. Am. J. Clin. Nutr. 28, 1085–1086.

752. Veeneklaas, G. M. H. (1942) Über megalozytäre Mangelanämien bei Kleinkindern. Folia haemat. 65, 303–330. Cited by: Zuelzer, W. W. & Rutzky, J. (1953) Megaloblastic anemia of infancy. Adv. Pediatr. 6, 243–306.

753. Velez, H., Ghitis, J., Pradilla, A. & Vitale, J. J. (1963) Cali-Harvard Nutrition Project. I. Megaloblastic anemia in kwashiorkor. Am. J. Clin. Nutr. 12, 54–65.

754. Velez, H., Restrepo, A., Vitale, J. J. & Hellerstein, E. E. (1966) Folic acid deficiency secondary to iron deficiency in man. Am. J. Clin. Nutr. 19, 27–36.

755. Vidal, A. J. & Stokstad, E. L. R. (1974) Urinary excretion of 5-methyltetrahydrofolate and liver S-adenosylmethionine levels of rats fed a vitamin B₁₂-deficient diet. Biochim. Biophys. Acta 362, 245–257.

756. Vilter, C. F., Spies, T. D. & Koch, M. B. (1945) Further studies on folic acid in the treatment of macrocytic anemia. S. Med. J. 38, 781–785.

757. Vilter, C. F., Vilter, R. W. & Spies, T. D. (1947) The treatment of pernicious and related anemias with synthetic folic acid. I. Observation on the maintenance of a normal hematologic status and on the occurrence of combined system disease at the end of one year. J. Lab. Clin. Med. 32, 262–273.

758. Vilter, R. W., Will, J. J., Wright, T. & Rullman, D. (1963) Interrelationships of vitamin B₁₂, folic acid and ascorbic acid in megaloblastic anemias. Am. J. Clin. Nutr. 12, 130–144.

759. Vinke, B. (1964) The action of Marmite in nutritional megaloblastic anaemia. Trans. Roy. Soc. Trop. Med. Hyg. 58, 503–509.

760. Vitale, J. J. & Hegsted, D. M. (1969) Effects of dietary methionine and vitamin B₁₂ deficiency on folate metabolism. Br. J. Haematol. 17, 467–475.

761. Vitale, J. J., Restrepo, A., Velez, H., Riker, J. B. & Hellerstein, E. E. (1966) Secondary folate deficiency induced in the rat by dietary iron deficiency. J. Nutr. 88, 315–322.

762. Voolen, G. A. van & Yu, N. L. (1971) Iron deficiency and RBC morphology. N. Engl. J. Med. 284, 108–109.

763. Wadsworth, G. R. (1973) Some historical aspects of knowledge about folate deficiency. Nutrition 27, 17–22.

764. Walt, F., Holman, S. & Hendrickse, R. G. (1956) Megaloblastic anaemia of infancy in kwashiorkor and other diseases. Br. Med. J. 1, 1199–1203.

765. Wardrop, C. A. J., Tennant, V. B., Heatley, R. V. & Hughes, L. E. (1975) Acute folate deficiency in surgical patients on amino acid/ethanol intravenous nutrition. Lancet 2, 640–642.

766. Waslien, C. I., Kamel, K., El-Ramly, Z., Carter, J. P., Mourad, A., Khattab, A. K. & Darby, W. J. (1972) Folate requirements of children. I. A formula diet low in folic acid for study of folate deficiency in protein-calorie malnutrition. Am. J. Clin. Nutr. 25, 147–151.

767. Watanabe, H. (1962) M. Sc. Thesis, Department of Physiology, McGill University, Montreal. Cited by: Blakley, R. L. (1969) The Biochemistry of Folic Acid and Related Pteridines, Frontiers of Biology, Vol. 13, p. 386, North-Holland Pub. Co., Amsterdam-London.

768. Waters, A. H. (1963) Folic acid metabolism in the megaloblastic anaemias. Ph.D. thesis. Univ. London. Cited by: Chanarin, I. (1969) The Megaloblastic Anaemias, p. 328, Blackwell Scientific Publications, Oxford.

769. Waters, A. H. & Mollin, D. L. (1961) Studies on the folic acid activity of human serum. J. Clin. Path. 14, 335–344.

770. Waters, A. H. & Mollin, D. L. (1963) Observations on the metabolism of folic acid in pernicious anaemia. Br. J. Haematol. 9, 319–327.

771. Waters, A. H., Newmark, P. A., Child, J. A., Cowan, J. D. & Mollin, D. L. (1975) Intestinal absorption of water-soluble vitamins. In: Pharmacology of Intestinal Absorption: Gastrointestinal Absorption of Drugs, International Encyclopedia of Pharmacology and Therapeutics, Section 39B (Forth, W. & Rummel, W., eds.), Vol. II, pp. 403–446, Pergamon Press Inc., New York.

772. Watson, J. & Castle, W. B. (1946) Nutritional macrocytic anemia, especially in pregnancy. Response to a substance in liver other than that effective in pernicious anemia. Am. J. Med. Sci. 211, 513–530.

773. Waxman, S. (1975) Folate binding proteins. Br. J. Haematol. 29, 23–29.

774. Waxman, S., Corcino, J. & Herbert, V. (1970) Aggravation or initiation of megaloblastosis by amino acids in the diet. J. Am. Med. Assoc. 214, 39–42.

775. Waxman, S. & Schreiber, C. (1974) The role of folic acid binding proteins (FABP) in the cellular uptake of folates. Proc. Soc. Exp. Biol. Med. 147, 760–764.

776. Waxman, S. & Schreiber, C. (1975) The purification and characterization of the low molecular weight human folate binding protein using affinity chromatography. Biochemistry 14, 5422–5428.

777. Weinstein, W. M. (1974) Epithelial cell renewal of the small intestinal mucosa. Med. Clin. North Am. 58, 1375–1386.

778. Weir, D. G. (1974) The pathogenesis of folic acid deficiency in man. Isr. J. Med. Sci. 143, 3–20.

779. Weir, K., Bank, S., Novis, B. & Marks, I. N. (1972) Puerperal folate deficiency resembling tropical sprue. S. Afr. Med. J. 46, 505–507.

780. Welch, A. D. & Heinle, R. W. (1951) Hematopoietic agents in macrocytic anemias. Pharmacol. Rev. 3, 345–411.

781. Wertalik, L. F., Metz, E. N., LoBuglio, A. F. & Balcerzak, S. P. (1972) Decreased serum B₁₂ levels with oral contraceptive use. J. Am. Med. Assoc. 221, 1371–1374.

782. West, R. J. & Lloyd, J. K. (1975) The effect of cholestyramine on intestinal absorption. Gut 16, 93–98.

783. Weyden, M. van der, Rother, M. & Firkin, B. (1972) Megaloblastic maturation masked by iron deficiency: a biochemical basis. Br. J. Haematol. 22, 299–307.

784. Wheby, M. S., Swanson, V. L. & Bayless, T. M. (1971) Comparison of ileal and jejunal biopsies in tropical sprue. Am. J. Clin. Nutr. 24, 117–123.

785. Whitehead, V. M. (1973) Polygamma-glutamyl metabolites of folic acid in human liver. Lancet 1, 743–745.

786. Whitehead, V. M. & Cooper, B. A. (1967) Absorption of unaltered folic acid from the gastro-intestinal tract in man. Br. J. Haematol. 13, 679–686.

787. Whitehead, V. M., Pratt, R., Viallet, A. & Cooper, B. A. (1972) Intestinal conversion of folinic acid to 5-methyl-tetrahydrofolate in man. Br. J. Haematol. 22, 63–72.

788. Whitehead, N., Reyner, F. & Lindenbaum, J. (1973) Megaloblastic changes in the cervical epithelium. Association with oral contraceptive therapy and reversal with folic acid. J. Am. Med. Assoc. 226, 1421–1424.

789. Whitfield, C. R. (1966) A study of megaloblastic pregnancy anaemia in Singapore. J. Obstet. Gynaecol. Br. Commonw. 73, 586–593.

790. Whitfield, C. R. (1970) Obstetric sprue. J. Obstet. Gynaecol. Br. Commonw. 77, 577–586.

791. WHO Expert Group (1972) Nutritional anaemias. WHO Tech. Report Series no. 503, Geneva.

792. Wickramasinghe, S. N. & Saunders, J. (1976) Correlations between the deoxyuridine-suppressed value and some conventional haematological parameters in patients with folate or vitamin B₁₂ deficiency. Scand. J. Haematol. 16, 121–127.

793. Will, G. & Murdoch, W. R. (1960) Megaloblastic anaemia associated with adult scurvy. Postgrad. Med. J. 36, 502–504.

794. Williams, D. L. & Spray, G. H. (1970) Observations on folate metabolism in rats on a vitamin B₁₂-deficient diet. Br. J. Haematol. 19, 353–360.

795. Williams, D. L. & Spray, G. H. (1976) The effects of dietary histidine, methionine and homocystine on vitamin B₁₂ and folate levels in rat liver. Br. J. Nutr. 35, 299–307.

796. Williams, E. A. J., Gross, R. L. & Newberne, P. M. (1975) Effect of folate deficiency on the cell-mediated immune response in rats. Nutr. Rep. In. 12, 137–148.

797. Williams, I. R. & Girdwood, R. H. (1970) The folate status of alcoholics. Scot. Med. J. 15, 285–288.

798. Williamson, M. B. (1949) Increased requirement for pteroyl glutamic acid during lactation. Proc. Soc. Exp. Biol. Med. 70, 336–339.

799. Willoughby, M. L. N. (1967) An investigation of folic acid requirements in pregnancy. II. Br. J. Haematol. 13, 503–509.

800. Willoughby, M. L. N. & Jewell, F. J. (1966) Investigation of folic acid requirements in pregnancy. Br. Med. J. 2, 1568–1571.

801. Willoughby, M. L. N. & Jewell, F. G. (1968) Folate status throughout pregnancy and in postpartum period. Br. Med. J. 4, 356–360.

802. Wills, L. (1931) Treatment of "pernicious anaemia of pregnancy" and "tropical anaemia." With special reference to yeast extract as a curative agent. Br. Med. J. 1, 1059–1064.

803. Wills, L. (1934) Studies in pernicious anaemia of pregnancy. Part VI. Tropical macrocytic anaemia as a deficiency disease, with special reference to the vitamin B complex. Indian J. Med. Res. 21, 669–681.

804. Wills, L., Clutterbuck, P. W. & Evans, B. D. F. (1937) A new factor in the production and cure of macrocytic anaemias and its relation to other haemopoietic principles curative in pernicious anaemia. Biochem. J. 31, 2136–2147.

805. Wills, L. & Evans, B. D. F. (1938) Tropical macrocytic anaemia: its relation to pernicious anaemia. Lancet 2, 416–421.

806. Wills, L. & Mehta, M. M. (1930) Studies in "pernicious anaemia" of pregnancy. Part I. Preliminary report. Indian J. Med. Res. 17, 777–792.

807. Winawer, S. J., Sullivan, L. W., Herbert, V. & Zamcheck, N. (1965) The jejunal mucosa in patients with nutritional folate deficiency and megaloblastic anemia. N. Engl. J. Med. 272, 892–895.

808. Wise, G. A., Lovric, V. A. & Hughes, D. W. O. (1963) Some experiences with the syndrome of megaloblastic anaemia in infancy. Med. J. Austral. 2, 877–880.

809. Wolff, R., Drouet, L. & Karlin, R. (1949) Occurrence of vitamin Bc conjugase in human plasma. Science 109, 612–613.

810. Wood, J. K., Goldstone, A. H. & Allan, N. C. (1972) Folic acid and the pill. Scand. J. Haematol. 9, 539–544.

811. Woodruff, C. W., Peterson, J. C. & Darby, W. J. (1951) Citrovorum factor and folic acid in treatment of megaloblastic anemia in infancy. Proc. Soc. Exp. Biol. Med. 77, 16–18.

812. Wu, A., Chanarin, I. & Levi, A. J. (1974) Macrocytosis of chronic alcoholism. Lancet 1, 829–830.

813. Wu, A., Chanarin, I., Slavin, G. & Levi, A. J. (1975) Folate deficiency in the alcoholic—its relationship to clinical and haematological abnormalities, liver disease and folate stores. Br. J. Haematol. 29, 469–478.

814. Yoshino, T. (1968) The clinical and experimental studies on the metabolism of folic acid using tritiated folic acid. I. Absorption tests of tritiated folic acid in man. J. Vitaminol. *14*, 21–34.

815. Zalusky, R. & Herbert, V. (1961) Megaloblastic anemia in scurvy with response to 50 microgm. of folic acid daily. N. Engl. J. Med. *265*, 1033–1038.

816. Zamcheck, N. & Broitman, S. A. (1973) Nutrition in diseases of the intestines. In: Modern Nutrition in Health and Disease (Goodhart, R. S. & Shils, M. E., eds.), pp. 785–818, Lea & Febiger, Philadelphia.

817. Zuelzer, W. W. & Ogden, F. N. (1946) Megaloblastic anemia in infancy. A common syndrome responding specifically to folic acid therapy. Am. J. Dis. Child. *71*, 211–243.

818. Zuelzer, W. W. & Rutzky, J. (1953) Megaloblastic anemia of infancy. Adv. Pediatr. *6*, 243–306.

490

A CONSPECTUS OF RESEARCH ON COPPER METABOLISM AND REQUIREMENTS OF MAN [1]

by

KARL E. MASON [2]

*Consultant—NIAMDD, National Institutes of Health,
Bethesda, Maryland 20014*

THE JOURNAL OF NUTRITION

VOLUME 109, NUMBER 11, NOVEMBER 1979

(Pages 1979-2066)

TABLE OF CONTENTS

INTRODUCTION

The discovery of copper, following that of gold and silver, goes back to the postglacial epoch in southwestern Asia, especially the semi-arid regions of Central Anatolia and Iran, during the period 6000 to 3000 B.C. (834). The later Bronze Age (3000–1000 B.C.) takes its name from the use during this period of bronze, an alloy of copper and tin. The word copper is derived from the Latin *cuprum*, a corruption of cyprium, named after the island of Cyprus which was an important source of copper about 3000 B.C. Thus, aside from gold and silver, which were employed chiefly for ornamental purposes, copper represents the first metal to be used by mankind for more practical purposes. The alloys of copper and tin (bronze), copper and zinc (brass), and of copper, zinc and nickel (nickel silver or German silver), have had a tremendous impact upon human development over many past centuries.

Beginning about the time of Hippocrates (400 B.C.) copper compounds were commonly prescribed in the treatment of mental, pulmonary and other diseases. During the 19th century many different copper compounds came into use in the unsuccessful treatment of a wide variety of human diseases (447). Copper amulets were also in vogue. Not until about 150 years ago was copper recognizd as a normal constituent of blood. And as early as 1900, Abderhalden (1) recorded that animals kept on a whole milk diet developed an anemia that could not be prevented by additions of inorganic iron, and recognized the fact that some other mysterious substance, probably organic, was wanting. But the thought that copper should ever be considered an important component of the diet for either animals or man was quite remote until the second decade of this century, following closely on the heels of the discovery of vitamins A, B, C, D and E. At this time there appeared the reports of Hart et al. (311, 312) and Waddell et al. (812) corroborating the observations of Abderhalden and indicating that either extracts or the ash of dried cabbage, corn meal and chlorophyll, all essentially iron-free, definitely favored assimilation and utilization of iron in hemoglobin building in rabbits fed a whole milk diet. Also, at about this same time, McHargue (507) recorded results of studies on rats fed purified diets deficient in copper, zinc and/or manganese in which he employed improvised glass-lined cages. This represents the first known use of cages of this type. McHargue concluded that manganese in particular, and possibly copper and zinc, have important functions in animal metabolism.

There followed the classic studies of Hart, Steenbock, Waddell and Elvehjem (313) demonstrating that rats fed exclusively on milk developed an anemia which was responsive to iron only after the addition of copper; also, that the same relationships prevailed in chicks fed diets of milk and rice (187). Later came evidence from experimental studies with pigs (188) that whereas impure organic salts of iron cured nutritional anemia, the pure salts failed to do so unless supplemented with small amounts of copper. Recognition of the clinical importance of these early observations was first given by Mills (520, 521) and Josephs (389) who reported that copper supplements accelerated hemoglobin synthesis in hypochromic anemia of infants treated with iron salts. Although several investigators were not in agreement (274, 275, 476), others confirmed these findings (186, 399, 455, 799) and extended them to hypochromic microcytic anemia of adults (521). The early history and later developments are detailed in several reviews (99, 540, 693). During this same period appeared Tompsett's report (785) of the first copper balance study carried out on 17 human subjects, indicating that the normal daily intake appeared to vary from 2.0 to 2.5 mg/day. In the same

Received for publication October 16, 1978.
[1] Requests for reprints should be directed to Nutrition Institute, Science and Education Administration, Building 307, Room 217, USDA, Beltsville, Maryland 20705.
[2] Deceased December 8, 1978.

year Daniels and Wright (142) reported the first balance study on young children (4–6 years old) indicating an average intake of 1.48 mg/day and a requirement not less than 0.10 mg/kg/day. These estimates are in remarkably good agreement with those recorded in the later literature (see p. 2032). Thus, the stage was set for an extensive exploration of the metabolism, deficiencies, excesses and requirements of copper in man witnessed during the past half century.

An overview of what has transpired during this period should include: 1) a vast number of studies on copper depletion and effects of copper supplementation in laboratory animals; 2) recognition of naturally occurring deficiency of copper in farm animals, especially cattle and sheep, in geographic areas where there exists a deficiency of copper in the soil and vegetation; 3) exhaustive analyses of the copper content of plant and animal tissues, including those of man; 4) recognition of states of copper deficiency in the human infant reared on diets similar to those employed in inducing copper deficiency states in experimental animals, combined with states of protein calorie malnutrition, infection and other metabolic disorders; 5) the effects of parenteral alimentation, especially in infants suffering from developmental anomalies of the alimentary tract and post-surgical stresses; 6) recognition of two genetically determined abnormalities of copper metabolism in man (Menkes' kinky-hair, or steely-hair, syndrome affecting primarily young infants and Wilson's disease, affecting the adolescent and adult, together with therapeutic measures for the same; and 7) exhaustive studies of the many copper-containing proteins distributed throughout the blood and other tissues, and their role in metabolic processes of man and lower animals.

In the present review it is not possible to consider the first three categories of research mentioned above, other than to make reference to certain observations which have particular relevance to the understanding of copper metabolism and requirements of man. For additional information on the first areas of research mentioned the reader is referred to a rather extensive series of reviews (6, 7, 32, 71, 99, 139, 140, 185, 211, 257, 319, 461, 493, 779, 798).

COPPER IN THE HUMAN BODY

Many opinions have been expressed concerning the total copper content of the human body. More than 40 years ago Chou and Adolph (115), in studies based upon analyses of nine organs from two adults at autopsy, in which they found an average of about 116 mg, estimated that the human body contained between 100 and 150 mg of copper. Since then estimates have been reduced. Cartwright and Wintrobe (105) considered 80 mg of copper to be a more reasonable estimate for a 70-kg man. Sass-Kortsak (666), on the basis of data of Tipton and Cook (781), calculated a mean of 75 mg, with a range of 50 to 120 mg. A slightly lower estimate of 70 mg has been given recently by Sumino et al. (762), based upon analyses of 18 different organs and tissues of 30 Japanese subjects, victims of accidental deaths, 28 of whom ranged in age from 20 to more than 60 years. These investigators also estimated that about one-third of body copper was in the liver and brain combined, one-third in the musculature, and the remaining third dispersed in other tissues. The mean content of copper in human liver is about 15% of total body copper (668).

It has long been recognized that the liver and brain contain a much higher concentration of copper than other organs and tissues, amounting to about 8 mg in each of these organs (105). The liver content is, in large part, related to its function as a storage organ for copper and also as the only site of synthesis and release of ceruloplasmin. Copper is unevenly distributed in the brain. While some investigators report very little difference in the copper content of grey and white matter of the cerebral cortex (102, 138, 613), others have found a considerably higher content in the grey than in the white matter (134, 138, 178, 780, 828). The substantia nigra and locus ceruleus, both components of the grey matter, are exceptionally rich in copper (134, 178). Possible relationships of the pigmented nerve cells of the locus ceruleus to their content of melanin and to tyrosinase have been suggested and explored by in vitro studies with no positive results, possibly due to the use of necropsy material rather than fresh tissue (178). Gubler et al. (285) record mean copper values (in terms of $\mu g/g$ wet weight) of 6.3, 6.5, 5.7, 4.2, 2.6 and 1.7, repsectively, for whole brain, cerebellum, basal ganglia, cerebral cortex, brain stem and cervical spinal cord. These data are based on five adult males who died following traumatic injuries.

Compared to the liver and brain, lesser levels of copper are found in the heart, kidney, pancreas, spleen, lungs, bone and skeletal muscle, diminishing generally in the order mentioned (102, 115, 182, 208, 285, 397, 509, 691, 762, 786). Gubler et al. (285) give mean values ($\mu g/g$ wet weight) of 5.3, 3.2, 2.2, 1.0 and 0.9, respectively, for liver, heart, kidney, spleen and skeletal muscle. The total copper content of the whole liver, brain, kidney, heart and spleen, respectively, is estimated to be 8.0, 8.0, 1.2, 0.9 and 0.1 mg (105).

In the fetus and infant, the distribution of copper is quite different from that in the adult. During fetal life there is a progressive increase in percentage of copper and iron in the body, while that of zinc remains relatively constant (704), such that at birth the liver and spleen contain about 1/2 the copper, 1/4th the zinc and 1/8th the iron in the whole body (846). Liver of the newborn has an exceptionally high concentration of copper, approximately 6 to 10 times that of adult man (538, 844, 846). After the first few months of life these concentrations decrease rapidly to those of the adult (69, 565, 845). During the transition from infancy to the early years of life, there is a decrease in copper concentration in kidney, heart and spleen and an increase in brain (69, 845), which is relatively low in the newborn (780).

On the basis of analyses of major organs of man in different geographic areas Forssen (222) states that the Finns have somewhat lower copper levels than Americans, and that peoples of Africa and the Near and Far East have levels 1.5 to 2 times those of the Finns. Whether these observations may or may not reflect differences in soils, dietary habits or ethnic factors is not clear. They are in accord with earlier observations of Schroeder et al. (691) who found that other races have larger mean amounts of copper in aorta, kidney, liver, lung and spleen than do Americans, Swiss and African Caucasoids, and that Orientals have especially high values.

The levels of copper in human hair have been the subject of numerous studies in the hope that such information might provide some measure of the copper status of the body, especially states of copper deficiency. Wide individual variations with respect to age and sex (415), to hair pigmentation (357) and to exogenous contamination (298) have indicated that copper levels in hair have little meaningfulness in evaluating the status of copper in man (798). However, a recent report (378) states that determination of copper in hair may be useful in evaluating total liver content of copper.

COPPER PROTEINS

Many proteins in tissues have the capacity to form copper complexes. Some of these do not occur in mammalian species, but appear only in lower animal forms and plants (e.g., hemocyanin, laccase, ascorbic acid oxidase, polyphenol oxidases, turacine). There have come to be recognized a large number of cuproproteins of mammalian species in which copper is part of the molecular structure and in which there is a characteristic ratio between moles of protein and atoms of associated copper. By virtue of these characteristics and the fact that the contained copper does not dissociate during isolation of the protein, these cuproproteins function as enzymes and are often grouped with other metal-containing enzymes, all of which are referred to as "metalloproteins." Those accepted in this category include ceruloplasmin, superoxide dismutase, cytochrome c oxidase, lysyl oxidase, tyrosinase and dopamine β-hydroxylase. One other important metalloprotein, metallothionein, lacks enzymic properties but is capable of binding copper as well as certain other heavy metals. Several plasma and connective tissue oxidases isolated from mammalian organs and tissues are at least copper dependent (monoamine oxidase, spermine oxidase, diamine oxidase, benzylamine-oxidase, etc.) but their significance in human metabolism is rather obscure. These proteins will be discussed in the general order mentioned. It may be noted that this panorama of cuproproteins has been subject to frequent changes in identification, description, terminology and functional attributes over recent years. Hence, some statements and views expressed may be considered in a state of flux subject to considerable revision as new advances are made.

Ceruloplasmin (ferroxidase I)

The classic studies of Holmberg and Laurell (346, 347) described a blue plasma copper-containing protein which they named "ceruloplasmin." They reported that it was an α-globulin representing almost all the copper present in mammalian plasma, and differed remarkably from all other such proteins in its molecular weight of about 151,000 daltons, its copper content of about 0.32% and its content of eight atoms of copper per molecule. Human ceruloplasmin has been highly purified and crystallized as tetragonal crystals (537). According to Scheinberg and Morell (676), who provide an excellent review of the subject, its molecular weight may vary from 132,000 to 160,000, depending upon the method employed. More recently, it has been reported that its molecular weight is 134,000 ± 3,000, and that the number of copper atoms varies from 6 to 6.6 (653). Of these, about one-half are in the cupric and the other half in the cuprous state (395). The nature of the copper-protein bond is not known. It is also recognized that ceruloplasmins from different animals show some cross-reactivity (395) and that they differ in p-phenylenediamine oxidase activity (502). Two other blue oxidases, ascorbate oxidase and laccase are enzymes found only in the plant world, where ceruloplasmin does not exist. An excellent comparison of the chemical structure and physiological properties of these three oxidases is given by Dawson et al. (151).

Ceruloplasmin contains about 8% carbohydrate, composed principally of glucosamine, mannose and galactose. Almost, if not all, of its oligosaccharide side chains are terminated by a sialic acid residue, apparently essential for its survival in the circulation (550). Copper is incorporated into ceruloplasmin only at the time of its synthesis in the liver and the liver is its only site of synthesis (439, 742, 824). In the blood stream ceruloplasmin does not exchange its copper with other copper complexes in the serum or blood cells. In vitro, copper is released from ceruloplasmin only after acidification, indicating strong protein binding of copper. Ceruloplasmin is heterogeneous, existing in several forms depending upon its prosthetic carbohydrate groups (65, 535).

A moderate oxidase activity of ceruloplasmin toward a variety of substrates, of which p-phenylenediamine is the best, was recognized by Holmberg and Laurell (348) in 1951. This enzyme reaction, as employed in the method of Ravin (629), has provided a useful means of qualitatively measuring ceruloplasmin in body fluids. There has also been developed an immunological method using highly purified human ceruloplasmin as an antigen to incite specific antibody, usually in rabbits (339, 490, 674). Careful studies of Rosenberg et al. (644) demonstrate that both methods yield comparable results. Although ceruloplasmin is primarily a plasma protein, it is found also in synovial, ascitic and cerebrospinal fluids (744).

Much interest has centered around this protein not only because of the mystery surrounding its true physiological functions but also because of impairment of its synthesis and other possible derangements in Wilson's disease (p. 2009) and its low plasma levels associated with Menkes' kinky-hair (steely-hair) syndrome, a genetically determined copper-deficiency disease in children (p. 2005). It is of interest that in the early studies of Holmberg and Laurell, who were aware of recent evidence of abnormalities of copper metabolism in Wilson's disease, ceruloplasmin plasma levels were found to be normal in a patient said to have Wilson's disease but who, several years later, was found not to be a victim of that disease. Hence, as stated by Scheinberg (671), "The capstone of physiological significance to these discoveries ironically and undeservedly eluded them." This same type of study carried out by

Scheinberg and Gitlin (674) laid the basis of the concept that Wilson's disease is usually characterized by a lifelong deficiency or absence of ceruloplasmin, and that this deficiency is autosomal recessive in nature.

Advances in knowledge concerning ceruloplasmin, as well as the role of copper in human metabolism, have in large part been the consequence of intensive research on the nature, cause and treatment of Wilson's disease, resulting in truly voluminous literature. In contrast, investigations concerning Menkes' disease have focused largely on the role of metallothionein-like cuproproteins and defects in intestinal absorption of copper. Here also, in the interim since its first recognition in 1962 (513), an extensive literature has evolved. On the other side of the ledger are advances made during the past 12 years in elucidating the role of copper in iron metabolism. These have, in large part, resolved questions in the minds of those investigators of 50 years ago (311, 313) who first recognized the important role of copper in nutrition.

The role of ceruloplasmin in biological processes began to receive some rational explanation about 1960, with evidence that in vitro it catalyzed the oxidation of ferrous iron (141). Further investigation of this oxidase activity of ceruloplasmin provided indications that it represented an enzyme in human plasma responsible for oxidation of ferrous iron, and that the latter was the substrate for its greatest activity (504, 583, 585). Based on these findings, Osaki et al. (583) proposed that the name ferroxidase may be more useful than designating this enzyme as a "sky-blue substance from plasma." Since then, ceruloplasmin and ferroxidase I have become synonymous terms. However, in the discussion to follow the more common designation "ceruloplasmin" will be used.

The hypothesis proposed was that by this mechanism ceruloplasmin may play an important biological role in the release and transfer of iron from storage cells to plasma transferrin. This concept was promptly supported by studies on copper-deficient swine (445, 446, 625), and by liver perfusion studies on dogs and swine (584).

The studies on copper-deficient swine clearly demonstrated the effectiveness of ceruloplasmin in counteracting the defective movement of iron from hepatic cells, reticuloendothelial cells and the intestinal mucosa to the plasma. This general subject has been extensively discussed and reviewed elsewhere (211, 226–230, 390, 446).

The current concept of ceruloplasmin function in iron metabolism appears to be as follows. For normal hemoglobin synthesis iron must be transported from storage sites in the liver, reticuloendothelial system and intestine to the bone marrow by transferrin. In the storage sites iron is present in the ferric state, as ferritin. This iron can be reduced by reduced riboflavin and riboflavin derivatives, liberating ferrous iron from the ferritin. This ferrous iron is then oxidized catalytically back to ferric iron by virtue of the ferroxidase activity of ceruloplasmin, allowing the Fe^{3+} to combine with apotransferrin, as the initial step in the mobilization of stored iron.

The mechanism of iron transfer from the storage cell to transferrin has not been clearly established. It is possible that Fe^{2+} and ceruloplasmin interact to form a ferric intermediate that transfers iron to apotransferrin by a specific ligand exchange reaction (850). In any case, Fe^{3+} combines with transferrin and provides the progenitors of the erythrocytes in the bone marrow with the necessary iron for hemoglobin synthesis. As has been expressed (230), the life cycle of the copper in ceruloplasmin is a one-time journey to the tissues or a return to the liver for resynthesis.

Ceruloplasmin is a multifunctional protein involved not only in the mobilization of plasma iron but also in copper transport and in regulation of biogenic amines. The suggestion of Broman (65) that it functions as a copper-transport protein has been well substantiated by animal studies indicating that its copper atoms are transferred to cytochrome c oxidase and probably to other copper-containing proteins of body tissues (230, 365). Close correlations between low serum ceruloplasmin and low cytochrome c oxidase in leucocytes in Wilson's disease (715) suggest that the same is true in man. Ceruloplas-

min also has the capacity to oxidize naturally occurring substances such as serotonin, melatonin, epinephrine and norepinephrine, and may possibly play an
important role in the control of blood and
tissue levels of biogenic amines (585).
There are also suggestions that abnormalities in copper metabolism may be involved
in Parkinson's disease (34). For further
details concerning the multifunctional nature of ceruloplasmin, its biological functions and catalytic activity the reader is
referred to the recent reviews of Frieden
and Hsieh (230) and of Sass-Kortsak and
Bearn (668).

Ceruloplasmin is not the only compound
with ferroxidase-like activity in human
plasma. In 1969, Lee et al. (444) reported
the presence of citrate, differing from
ceruloplasmin in that it is not inhibited by
azide and yet has the same capacity to
accelerate oxidation of ferrous ion to ferric
ion and, possibly, to accelerate the rate of
reaction of ferric ion with transferrin. Additional mechanisms, perhaps not involving
copper directly, have been implicated in
iron translocation (56a). A deterrent to
recognition of a role of ceruloplasmin in
hematopoietic functions of man has been
the finding that many subjects suffering
from Wilson's disease may have no demonstrable plasma ceruloplasmin and yet show
no evidence of iron-deficiency anemia.
This anomaly seems now to have a reasonable explanation with the isolation of another cuproprotein from human serum by
Topham and Frieden (788) which normally accounts for about 7% of the total
ferroxidase activity. It has a molecular
weight of about 800,000 daltons and contains approximately 0.8% copper. Its designation as ferroxidase II seems quite appropriate. It is a lipoprotein with a cholesterol
and phosphatidylcholine content of approximately 20%. It differs from ceruloplasmin also in its yellow color and its lack
of p-phenylenediamine oxidase activity,
and may be responsible for the maintenance of near-normal iron metabolism,
despite low-levels or absence of plasma
ceruloplasmin, in Wilson's disease. Whether
citrate plays a comparable role is still a
question. Furthermore, most of the new
postulations with respect to the roles of the

ferroxidases and citrate are based upon in
vitro studies on human blood and observations on experimental animals. Their applicability to man seems reasonable but remains to be established.

Other intriguing aspects of ceruloplasmin are: 1) its increased plasma levels in
response to estrogenic hormones, as in
users of oral contraceptives and pregnant
women; 2) its very low levels in plasma
of the fetus and newborn; 3) its rapid
synthesis by the newborn infant through
utilization of a special neonatal hepatomitochondrocuprein not found at any other
stage of life; 4) its stabilization at adult
plasma levels at or about puberty; 5) its
low serum levels in the genetically determined Wilson's and Menkes' diseases;
and 6) suggestions that copper is incorporated into cytochrome c oxidase only if
it is presented to the cell as ceruloplasmin
(3, 65). These topics will be considered
later.

Superoxide dismutase

Almost 40 years ago, Mann and Keilin
(486) isolated two blue copper proteins
from bovine erythrocytes and liver which
they designated *hemocuprein* and *hepatocuprein*, respectively. Both proteins had
molecular weights of about 35,000 daltons
and contained 0.34% copper. Similar proteins were later isolated from human erythrocytes (*erythrocuprein*) by Markowitz et
al. (490), from human brain (*cerebrocuprein*) by Porter and Ainsworth (612)
and from adult human liver (*hepatocuprein*) by Porter et al. (616).

Subsequently, Carrico and Deutsch (95)
clearly demonstrated that these copper
proteins were identical and proposed the
term cytocuprein to encompass them. They
later considered the term inappropriate,
since the protein also contained 2-g atoms
of zinc per mole (96). On the basis that
these cuproproteins catalyze the dismuta-
tion of superoxide-free radical ions, and
thus have true enzymatic function, the
designation "superoxide dismutase" was
proposed by McCord and Fridovich (500,
501), and is now in common usage. The
primary function of superoxide dismutase
appears to be that of scavenging the intermediates of oxygen reduction in aerobic

organisms, namely superoxide anion radical (500). Superoxide dismutase catalyzes the conversion of the superoxide radical to hydrogen peroxide plus oxygen and the hydrogen peroxide is removed by catalyses and peroxidases. Thus, superoxide dismutase helps protect the cell from the damaging effects of oxygen toxicity.

Cytochrome c oxidase

Although cytochrome c oxidase has been recognized as a copper and heme containing protein for almost 40 years, the state and function of its copper component have been very difficult to clarify. The history of these explorations, up to 1966, has been well reviewed by Beinert (43) and Wharton and Gibson (837). It has not yet been possible to clearly establish its molecular weight, or whether it contains one or two copper ions and one or two heme groups. This enzyme is found in all aerobic cells and is mainly responsible for the introduction of oxygen into the oxidative machinery that produces energy for biochemical synthesis and for physical activity. As the terminal enzyme in the electron transport chain, it catalyzes the oxidation of reduced cytochrome c by molecular oxygen and, in the process, oxygen is reduced to water. It represents an enzyme vital to essentially all forms of life, by virtue of serving as the terminal enzyme in the oxidative phosphorylation process of living cells.

A significant decrease in cytochrome c oxidase activity is considered a major cause of neural and cardiac abnormalities observed in the offspring of different animal species fed diets deficient in copper. Neural lesions varying from defective myelination to necrosis occur in lambs and goats (361, 798), in the guinea pig (201, 202) and in the rat (92, 401). Myocardial abnormalities ranging from focal failure of tissue respiration to myocardial hypertrophy and acute cardiac failure occur in cattle (798), swine (707) and rats (3, 92, 241, 316).

Lysyl oxidase

This copper-containing enzyme, lysyl oxidase, is one of the amine oxidases (308) but is given separate consideration here because of its well established status and special importance. It has now been partially purified from several sources (308, 601, 648a, 650, 716). Its major function appears to be to catalyze the oxidative deamination of ε-amino groups of peptidyl lysine or hydroxylysine to form α-amino-adipic-δ-semialdehyde derivatives as a first step in the cross-linking of immature elastin and collagen into stabile fibrils. In collagen, the cross-links are derived from either lysine or hydroxylysine. In elastin, however, hydroxylysine and hydroxylysine-derived cross-links are not present.

The story of lysyl oxidase goes back to early studies of experimental copper-deficiency in the chick (331, 571, 734) and pigs (93, 94, 129, 707) in which dissecting aneurisms and sometimes rupture of the aorta and large vessels were noted. These vascular defects were ascribed to abnormalities of the elastic component of the vascular wall and to low tissue levels of copper. These observations coincided in time with the demonstration by Partridge et al. (594) that the vital crosslinking groups in elastin, which they named "desmosine" and "isodesmosine," were formed from lysine. Other studies on copper-deficient chicks (117) gave evidence of a role of copper in crosslinking of collagen. It is now clear that the basis for these observations was the role of copper as a cofactor for lysyl oxidase (648a).

Further, a foundation was laid for the development of current concepts related to the role of copper with respect to biochemical and structural abnormalities seen in collagen and elastin in experimental animals, livestock (798) and non-domestic animals (219). Furthermore, one can observe an example of application of knowledge gained from experimentally induced deficiency in the chick and lower animals to a better understanding of human disorders, since many of the manifestations of Menkes' kinky-hair syndrome (513), a congenital state of copper-deficiency in young children, are also characterized by vascular and skeletal defects. For further details, the reader is referred to several recent reviews (93, 130, 568–570, 648a, 650) and to p. 2009.

Tyrosinase (phenoloxidase)

This cuproprotein enzyme contains about 0.2% copper, or 1 atom per molecule (68), and has a molecular weight of about 33,000 daltons. Actually it may represent a series of cuproproteins which catalyze a series of reactions that convert tyrosine to melanin (213, 479). The enzymatic activity is thought to be associated with the mitochondrial component of cells. The skin and uveal tissues of the eye in human albinos have no demonstrable tyrosinase activity; hence, the absence of melanin. Decreased production of tyrosinase is responsible for the loss of hair pigmentation in animals deficient in copper and in infants with Menkes' steely-hair syndrome.

Dopamine β-hydroxylase

This cuproprotein (3,4-dihydroxyphenyl-ethylamine β-hydroxylase) is an oxidase containing 4 to 7 copper atoms per molecule and having a molecular weight of about 290,000 daltons (232). It was originally isolated from beef adrenals and later from cattle brain and hearts. In experimental animals it appears to serve a function in catalyzing the conversion of dopamine to form norepinephrine (568, 570). A comparable role in man may be assumed but has not been proven.

Metallothionein

The rather tortuous history of identification and nomenclature of copper proteins leading up to the proper recognition of superoxide dismutase has been somewhat paralleled by the history of metallothionein. This designation was given by Kagi and Vallee (392, 393) to a protein isolated from equine and human kidney, with a molecular weight of about 10,000 daltons, a content of 26 sulfhydryl groups per mole, and a capacity to bind zinc and cadmium as well as copper. Metallothionein is not an enzyme. By virtue of its high content of sulfhydryl groups it binds copper by forming mercaptides. In fact, it may represent a family of metallothioneins specifically designed for the binding of either one metal or specific groups of metals such as copper, zinc and cadmium.

Accumulating knowledge of metallothionein or metallothionein-like proteins, with variable affinities for copper, especially as they occur and function in the intestinal mucosa and liver, may well add greatly to our understanding of the two clinical disorders of copper metabolism in man; namely, Wilson's disease and Menkes' steely-hair syndrome. For example, one recognized and basic defect in Menkes' disease is an inadequate transport of copper across the intestinal mucosa (145, 147). It is possible that the retention of abnormal amounts of copper in the intestinal mucosa involves increased affinity of a mucosal metallothionein or of another protein not normally involved in copper transport (351). Furthermore, there is evidence that the usual metallothionein concerned with storage and release of absorbed copper in the liver may, in Wilson's disease, be of an abnormal type with a binding constant about four times greater than normal (197).

An unusual variant of metallothionein, referred to as neonatal hepatomitochondrocuprein, has been isolated from immature bovine liver and from human newborn liver (615). It contains 25% cystine and about 4% copper, which is at least 10 times that of adult hepatocuprein. It increases just before birth and decreases rapidly during the first few months of postnatal life, as it is released for synthesis of ceruloplasmin, which is present in plasma in small amounts at birth. It is thought to represent a special storage type of protein to tide the newborn infant over the early period of life when breast milk does not meet normal requirements (610). Although concentrated in the heavy mitochondrial fraction, it is not a true mitochondrial constituent in that some of it may be localized in lysosomes of a "heavy" type, and probably represents a polymer of metallothionein (614).

Other cuproproteins

Since the identification and characterization of a sulfhydryl-rich cuproprotein in human liver with a molecular weight of 8,000 to 10,000 daltons, designated L-6D (536, 703), there have been described similar cuproproteins derived from chick intestine (733), rat liver (856), rat intestine (198), adult human liver (74) and human fetal liver (654). These proteins differ somewhat with respect to estimated molecular weight, copper content and amino-acid components, especially cysteine and thionein, which may reflect differences in methods employed in isolation and analysis as well as species differences in composition. There is good reason to believe that they have important functions in copper-homeostatic mechanisms such as storage, transport and detoxification, especially in the intestine and liver. Unquestionably, future research will clarify many of these differences and delineate more clearly the physiological and biochemical role(s) of these low-molecular weight cuproproteins.

Monoamine oxidases. Aside from lysyl oxidase, there are other amine oxidases that are present in connective tissues (116, 330, 334, 335). It is now presumed that these oxidases serve in deamination of norepinephrine, serotonin and histamine. Amine oxidases, presumably containing copper, derived from beef and swine plasma have been highly purified and crystallized (73, 308, 649, 807, 867). A monoamine oxidase from human plasma has also been purified (505) and is said to increase in states of congestive heart failure and parenchymal liver disease (506). However, whether or not this enzyme is copper dependent is not clear.

Diamine oxidase. Purification of diamine oxidase from pig kidney· has been carried out by many investigators since 1943. Its crystallization was first reported by Yamada et al. (866) who described it as a pink copper-protein containing 2.17 atoms of copper per molecule, capable of oxidizing histamine, cadaverine, putrescine and other like substances. The identity of this enzyme with histiminase had previously been proposed by Mondovi et al. (534). Whether this enzyme plays a role in human metabolism remains to be determined.

Albocuprein I and II. These two colorless cuproproteins, neither of which possess enzyme activity or undergo alterations in pathological states, have been isolated from human brains (238). Both contain hexoses. Albocuprein II may be the primary copper-containing protein of the brain (550).

Uricase (urate oxidase). This cuproprotein, found in the kidney and liver of lower mammals, has a molecular weight of about 110,000, a copper content of 0.6% and is involved in the catabolism of uric acid. There are no recognized effects of its deficiency or excess in animals. It does not occur in primates (478).

Tryptophan-2,3-dioxygenase. This heme protein with a molecular weight of 167,000 daltons and 2 cuprous atoms per molecule, isolated from rat liver cytosol (694), is said to catalyze the insertion of molecular oxygen into the pyrrole ring of L-tryptophan (58).

Pink copper protein. A pink copper protein with a molecular weight of about 32,000 has been isolated from human erythrocytes (631). The biological function of this protein still remains to be demonstrated.

Mitochondrial monoamine oxidase. This enzyme, previously obtained in highly purified form from many sources (beef and hog plasma, human plasma, rabbit serum, liver and kidney of several animal species, and human placenta) has been isolated from human liver, and identified as a flavoprotein with a molecular weight of 64,000 (563). It is said to have the ability to oxidize epinephrine and serotonin. On the other hand, its status as a cuproenzyme has since been questioned (730).

The large number of cuproproteins and the multiplicity of their enzymatic functions, as well as the homeostatic mechanisms involved in normal metabolism of copper, emphasize its great importance in mammalian nutrition. For further aspects of cuproproteins, the reader is referred to a series of reviews (191–195, 211, 308, 309, 350, 458, 550, 568–570, 634, 650, 663, 671, 676).

ABSORPTION OF COPPER

As is true of most metals, absorption of copper is regulated at the level of the intestinal mucosa and excretion is predominantly through the intestinal tract, either via the bile or as nonabsorbed copper. Urinary excretion is negligible in normal healthy man, amounting to about 1 to 2% of the intake.

Although the site of maximal absorption of copper varies among different mammalian species, in man absorption occurs primarily in the stomach and duodenum. This conclusion is based upon observations that after oral administration of radio-active copper the isotope appears rapidly in the blood, reaching maximum levels within 1 to 3 hours, as further discussed below. Concepts of the processes of absorption of copper from dietary sources in man are based in large part upon studies of experimental animals.

Animal studies indicate that at least two mechanisms are concerned in copper absorption (132, 256). One of these, presumably an energy-dependent one, involves the absorption of complexes of copper and amino acids. There is also evidence that L-amino acids facilitate the absorption of copper, and that absorption progressively decreases with increasing molecular size of copper-amino acid complexes (408). The other mechanism is an enzymatic one involving the binding of copper to, and successive release from, macromolecular proteins.

Studies of experimental animals indicate that mechanisms of copper storage and transfer involve not only metallothionein as first identified in the chick intestinal mucosa (733), but that there also may exist a variety of metallothioneins, differing slightly in amino-acid content and metal-binding characteristics (518, 562). There is real need for better determination of the extent to which findings in experimental animals have application to the problem of copper absorption and metabolism in man.

This applies also to the many factors in animals which are known to interfere with copper absorption through various mechanisms (competition for binding sites by zinc, perhaps to a much lesser extent by cadmium; interactions between molybdenum, sulphates and copper; the effects of dietary phytates, and the influence of ascorbic acid intake). In the case of the latter, dietary deficiency results in increased liver and plasma copper (337), whereas increased oral intake decreases the absorption and retention of copper in the chick (333), rabbit (370), pig (254) and rat (199). Moreover, in the pig, high intake of ascorbic acid can overcome the effects of excess copper either by interfering with copper absorption or by increasing the absorption and utilization of iron (254). Such evidence raises questions

as to whether due consideration has been given to the secondary effects that may be related to the somewhat astronomical human intakes of ascorbic acid currently in vogue. It is also important to note that the type, configuration and degree of polymerization of amino acids present in the intestine can influence the absorption of copper (798). Moreover, little is known regarding the chemical forms of copper in foods, and the influence of different methods of cooking upon its availability.

The great difficulty in determining that portion of dietary copper which is absorbed becomes apparent when one considers the many variable factors affecting copper absorption such as: competition for protein-binding sites in the intestinal lumen and mucosa; inhibition of binding at these sites; difficulties in measuring the amount of copper secreted by the bile, by accessory glands of the digestive tract and by the intestinal mucosa; and possible reabsorption by the intestinal mucosa of some of the secreted copper. Excellent reviews of this subject have been presented by Dowdy (169), Evans (192), Hambidge and Walravens (301) and Van Campen (804).

Mechanisms

The general concept of the mechanism involved in copper absorption is as follows: from ingested foodstuff copper is released either as ionic copper or as a copper-amino acid complex. In the intestinal lumen there exists a high molecular weight protein which binds copper and preferentially releases it to the plasma membranes on the luminal side of the absorptive cells of the mucosa. Within the absorptive cells is metallothionein (or metallothionein-like proteins) rich in sulfhydryl groups, which binds copper through formation of mercaptide bonds. Since this cuproprotein serves as a storage depot and also releases copper to the plasma cell membrane on the serosal side, it is considered to provide one of the protective and regulatory mechanisms in copper homeostasis. However, it is not quite that simple, since its binding to copper is constantly in competition with other trace elements and can also be influenced by other dietary components such as the sulphate radical, phytates, fiber and ascorbic acid.

Dynamic studies with radioactive copper have yielded important information. In man, oral administration of ^{64}Cu or ^{67}Cu is followed by a prompt appearance of the isotope in the blood serum, indicating at least major absorption from the stomach and duodenum (40, 42, 80, 179, 387, 832). Within 1 or 2 hours the isotope is bound to serum albumin and amino acids (41, 80). There follows a sharp decline as the isotope is taken up by the liver. Subsequently, there occurs increased activity of the serum for 48 to 72 hours as the liver incorporates the radioisotope into newly synthesized ceruloplasmin and releases it into the blood (40, 41, 80, 179). That not immediately extracted by the liver remains in the serum attached to albumin or amino acids, or is used to maintain erythrocyte copper levels.

Amount

The proportion of dietary copper that is actually absorbed is very important in the making of judgments on balance studies and their bearing upon normal human requirements for copper. Unfortunately the information currently available is both meager and somewhat inconclusive. Van Ravensteyn (805) estimated that about 25% of copper (as $CuSO_4$) added to the diet of normal men, is absorbed. Later, Cartwright and Wintrobe (105) stated that about 32% of ingested copper is absorbed.

Early studies employing oral and intravenous administration of ^{64}Cu to small numbers of control subjects in investigations primarily designed to determine whether or not there is an absorption defect in Wilson's disease gave quite variable results, in terms of the percentage of the dose recovered in the feces over periods of 3 to 4 days (41, 80, 498). Furthermore, since radio-copper is both excreted into and absorbed by the gastrointestinal tract, fecal excretion provides a measure of retention but not of true absorption. Assuming that after 48 hours the serum concentration of ^{64}Cu is proportional to either an intravenous dose or to a certain fraction of an oral dose absorbed, Sternlieb (736) estimates that on the basis of studies on 49 normal subjects the mean absorption of an oral dose of 2 mg of copper daily, is

0.8 mg, or 40%. Weber et al. (832), employing similar methodology, concluded that the net absorption of orally administerred copper varies from 15 to 97%, with a mean of about 60%. A more sophisticated approach by Strickland et al. (752), involving four normal adults given ^{64}Cu orally and ^{67}Cu intravenously, with copper absorption calculated by whole body counting and by plasma ^{64}Cu and ^{67}Cu concentrations, gave a mean copper absorption value of 56% (range 40–70%). It was their opinion that if Sternlieb (736) had made allowance for a 20% fecal excretion of copper (753), the three studies mentioned would have been in close agreement. Quite recently King et al. (407) reported an overall copper absorption of 57% based upon balance studies with the stable isotope ^{65}Cu. On the basis of the evidence presented above, it seems reasonable to assume an absorption of 40 to 60% of the oral intake of copper, accepting the fact that there is wide individual variation.

Copper absorption may be significantly impaired in states of severe, diffuse disease of the small bowel produced by sprue, lymphosarcoma, or scleroderma (739), or protein calorie malnutrition (474). In Menkes' steely-hair syndrome defects in intestinal transport and release constitute one of the primary bases for this disorder (p. 2007). Information concerning the role of the lymphatics in the absorption of copper is sadly lacking. Sternleib et al. (748) report that in the dog and man the amount of an oral dose of ^{64}Cu absorbed by the intestinal lymphatics is negligible. On the other hand, Trip et al. (789) found concentrations of copper (non-ceruloplasmic) in the thoracic duct of three patients equivalent to or higher than in serum. It must be noted that these subjects suffered from carcinoma and Hodgkin's disease and cannot be considered normal. Regrettably, the impossibility of obtaining thoracic duct lymph from normal healthy subjects offers little hope of determining the role of the intestinal lymphatics in absorption of copper.

TRANSPORT OF COPPER

Intestine to liver

Following release from the intestinal mucosa, copper becomes bound to albumin and to amino acids in the portal blood. In the form of these complexes it can be measured colorimetrically following reaction with diethyldithiocarbamate, a copper chelator. It is referred to as "direct reacting" or "labile" copper. By virtue of its homeostatic mechanisms the liver allows a portion of these loosely bound copper complexes to pass directly to the systemic circulation, where they constitute about 7% of plasma copper. Upon arrival at the liver, copper is released from albumin to hepatocyte cell membrane receptors from which it is transferred to the cytosol where it is bound to metallothionein (or metallothionein-like cuproproteins).

Metabolism and distribution

Copper apparently binds also to proteins other than metallothionein in the hepatocytes, as revealed by analyses of subcellular fractions of the liver of laboratory animals. How applicable these findings are to man is not clear. In a review of the subject Evans (192) lists four different fractions as follows: 1) microsomal fraction containing about 10% of liver copper, most of which is probably located in newly synthesized cuproproteins being prepared for transport to other sites; 2) nuclear fraction, with about 20% of total liver copper, which may represent a temporary site of storage; 3) large granule fraction, with about the same amount of copper, containing both mitochondria and lysosomes, the latter being especially involved in sequestering copper prior to biliary excretion; and 4) the cytosol, containing about one-half of total liver copper, in which a small percentage is in copper-dependent enzymes and the predominant portion in the form of a copper-binding protein similar to metallothionein. Evans (192) also describes interesting differences in the copper content of these cell fractions in the newborn and during postnatal development, and also changes observed in animals given dietary excess of copper. The latter studies indicate that in metallothionein there is preferential binding, after which excess copper is distributed to other fractions. He notes that the binding capacity of metallothionein is limited, and that the lysosomes and

nuclear proteins assist in maintaining copper homeostasis.

Marceau and Aspin (488, 489) have shown that when rats are given [^{67}Cu]-ceruloplasmin intravenously the ^{67}Cu is taken up by all tissues, but primarily by the liver where it appears in a specific protein fraction of the hepatocyte cytosol having a molecular weight of 30,000 to 40,000 daltons and exhibiting superoxide dismutase activity. It also becomes tightly bound to cytochrome c oxidase in the mitochondria. Since no [^{67}Cu]ceruloplasmin is demonstrable in the cell, it is assumed that copper is released at or within the cell membrane. In contrast, the ^{67}Cu of [^{67}Cu]-albumin complexes with proteins of about 10,000 daltons in the soluble cell fraction and becomes loosely bound to cytochrome c oxidase. Similar distribution of the two plasma proteins is observed in the rat brain and spleen.

In addition to serving as the major pathway of copper excretion via the biliary tract, the liver releases copper to maintain the labile pool of copper in the serum and blood cells. This pool provides copper for incorporation into superoxide dismutase and into the many other copper-containing enzymes of body tissues, some of which may be synthesized in the liver itself. However, a major function of the liver is the synthesis of ceruloplasmin. This form of tightly bound copper is referred to as "indirect reacting" copper, since it requires acidification to release its 0.3% copper which can then be measured, as in the case of "direct reacting" copper, by the diethyldithiocarbamate reaction. Its more reliable measurement by enzymatic and immunological methods has been discussed earlier (p. 1984). Once synthesized, ceruloplasmin is released by the liver such that it comprises approximately 93% of plasma copper. In healthy adult humans this level is remarkably constant. There is no interchange in the blood stream between ceruloplasmin copper and other forms of copper (742). Animal studies (741) indicate that the liver microsomes are the site of ceruloplasmin synthesis. Despite evidence that almost 0.5 mg of copper is incorporated into ceruloplasmin daily, close to the estimated daily absorption from the diet (742), the physiological role of ceruloplasmin has only recently begun to be clarified (pp. 1984–1986).

Copper in blood

The first evidence of the presence of copper in blood, that of the ox, was recorded in 1830 by Sarzeau (665). The first demonstration of copper in human serum was reported almost 100 years later by Warburg and Krebs (827) and Krebs (426), who employed a catalytic method developed by Warburg. Although the values obtained were somewhat below those currently accepted, they did recognize lower levels in normal males (aver. 0.82 μg/100 ml) than in females (aver. 0.98 μg/100 ml), and also increased levels in pulmonary tuberculosis (aver. 1.55 μg/100 ml) and in the later stages of pregnancy (aver. 2.07 μg/100 ml). Quite comparable values were reported by Locke et al. (464), who were among the first to employ diethyldithiocarbamate as a reagent for the detection and estimation of copper. While not recognized at the time, the routine acidification of samples necessary for release and measurement of copper in ceruloplasmin did not make it possible to recognize that the increased levels in pregnancy and infectious states were due primarily to increases in ceruloplasmin.

Because of the diversity of chemical, biophysical and immunological methods for the estimation of copper and ceruloplasmin in blood and other tissues for over more than 50 years, the values presented in the literature for whole blood, plasma, serum and red cells show considerable variation. An excellent description and appraisal of methods used up to 1965 has been presented by Sass-Kortsak (666). There has not come to the author's attention a comparable review and critique of methods developed since that time. Even with the employment of a single method such as atomic absorption spectrometry values obtained for copper levels in serum, plasma and urine vary considerably, due in large part to differences in preparation of the sample (763).

Blood levels of copper are commonly expressed either as serum or plasma levels, with little or no distinction made between the two. Cartwright (100) states that since the ratio of the volume of erythrocytes to leukocytes and platelets in normal blood is about 47/0.7, failure to separate the latter from erythrocytes results in an insignificant difference in copper values obtained. It must be recognized, however, that white blood cells do contain a small amount of copper (about 1/4th the concentration in erythrocytes) even though they represent a rather small component of total blood cells. A recent report (646) records significant differences between serum and plasma copper levels in 28 adult subjects studied on the same day, mean values being 119 and 127 μg/100 ml, respectively. These findings require confirmation. Investigators suggest that copper might be released from platelets, leukocytes or erythrocytes during coagulation and clot reaction.

Heilmeyer et al. (319) summarized 10 prior studies on adult humans employing six different methods and proposing normal values ranging from 65 to 200 μg/100 ml in blood serum. Their own studies yielded mean values of 106.2 μg/100 ml for 15 males and 106.9 μg/100 ml for 15 females, thus failing to reveal the sex differences reported in later studies. In a review of the literature up to 1950, Cartwright (100) gives data from seven different studies involving a total of 184 males and 274 females from which can be calculated average mean values of 106 and 114 μg/100 ml for plasma of males and females, respectively. Neale et al. (551) report corresponding mean serum levels of 100 and 108 μg/100 ml for 53 normal subjects of each sex. Wintrobe et al. (857) record plasma copper values of 105 ± 16 and 116 ± 16 μg/100 ml for males and females, respectively. An increase in serum copper with age is said to occur in males but not in females (871), but no adequate explanation is offered.

In plasma (or serum) most of the copper is bound to ceruloplasmin as indirect reacting copper (119, 286). In man it was first estimated that this represents 96% of total plasma copper (286). There are later estimates of 93% (105) and of 90% (75, 321). Most investigators now accept 93%. The remaining copper, constituting the labile pool, is less firmly bound in large part to albumin and in smaller part to amino acids (553), especially to histidine, threonine and glutamine (554). The smaller portion of "free" copper bound to amino acids, the existence of which was first demonstrated by Neumann and Sass-Kortsak (553, 554) and Sakar and Kruck (658), may be important as a transport form of copper in the blood, capable of actively diffusing across cell membranes such as those of erythrocytes, whereas albumin-bound copper preferentially releases its copper to receptor proteins of the plasma membrane of hepatocytes and other cells. After exposure of human serum to a centrifugal force greater than necessary to sediment albumin, copper may be demonstrated in serum in the form of mixed amino acid-complexes consisting of one atom of copper and two different amino acids, predominantly complexes of copper with histidine, threonine and glutamine (553, 554). Moreover, in ultrafiltrates of human serum there can be identified not only these complexes but also a mixed complex of histidine-copper-threonine (554).

In the red blood cells copper exists both in a labile pool, much like that in the plasma but proportionately much larger, and also in a firmly bound form, almost entirely as erythrocuprein (superoxide dismutase). Total erythrocyte copper in normal man is about 89 ± 11.4 $\mu g/100$ ml of packed red cells (492). The labile pool represents copper complexed with amino acids, freely dialyzable and probably involved in providing copper for superoxide dismutase. It contains about 40% of the erythrocyte copper. The remaining 60% is almost entirely bound to erythrocuprein, a cuproprotein first isolated by Markowitz et al. (490), described more fully by Kimmel et al. (406), and later identified as superoxide dismutase by McCord and Fridovich (501). In addition, a small amount of copper is thought to be bound to a pink copper-binding protein isolated by Reed et al. (631). This may correspond to the non-erythrocuprein copper fraction observed in human red blood cells by Shields, et al. (708). This protein has no amine oxidase or superoxide dismutase activity, and its

biological function remains to be demonstrated.

It is apparent that neither whole blood, blood cell nor blood plasma levels of copper provide useful information regarding nutritional copper status in man. The erythrocyte copper of both compartments is remarkably stable regardless of dietary intake, and is not involved in transport of copper to tissues. The latter function is mainly ensured by the small compartment of plasma copper (about 7% of the total) bound largely to albumin and to a lesser degree to amino acids, the latter complexes being essential for active transport of copper across cell membranes. The albumin and amino acid-bound forms of plasma copper, together with minute amounts of free ionic copper, represent the direct reacting copper of serum which may increase with intake only temporarily before liver homeostasis comes into play. The much larger compartment of ceruloplasmin copper is generally not influenced by dietary intake of copper but does react to a great variety of conditions responsible for states of hypocupremia and hypercupremia, as discussed later (pp. 2014–2020). A small diurnal variation in plasma copper has been reported (434, 460).

EXCRETION OF COPPER

As previously stated (p. 1991) in normal man perhaps up to 40 to 60% of dietary copper is actually absorbed, with the gastric and duodenal mucosa playing the major role. Such estimates are, in large part, based upon differences between oral and intravenous intake and fecal excretion, since urinary excretion of copper plays a very minor role. Therefore, the real problem in evaluating these differences lies in determining what fecal excretion truly represents. Presumably, it represents unabsorbed dietary copper plus copper excreted via the biliary tract (a major factor), salivary glands and gastric and intestinal mucosae, minus copper which may be reabsorbed by the gastrointestinal tract in the course of transit. Aside from these considerations are losses of copper via sweat and the menses, which are measurable with a limited degree of accuracy. It is hoped that the discussion to follow may

Biliary excretion

delineate the state and lack of current knowledge concerning many of the physiological mechanisms mentioned.

Sheldon and Ramage (705) were the first to note the presence of copper in bile and to suggest that this represents a channel of excretion. They also hypothesized, on the basis of the high values obtained from gall bladder bile, that the body may attempt to conserve its supply of copper by reabsorption through the highly vascular wall of the gall bladder. The latter remains an unsettled question. An isolated report of phenomenally high concentration in pigment gall stones (689) seems not to have been confirmed.

In 1944 Van Ravensteyn (805) stated that "We could not find in the medical literature any data on copper excretion with the bile or via the intestinal wall in man after administration of copper by mouth or by intravenous injection of copper compounds." In his studies he found that, unlike iron, oral copper had little effect upon blood levels, but caused a marked increase in bile and feces. He also discussed the possible reabsorption of biliary copper by the small intestine and of fecal copper by the colon. For the latter there is little or no evidence. This suggestion was based upon his observations that biliary excretion and fecal excretion did not run parallel, following intravenous injections of a non-toxic organic salt of copper. For the duodenal bile of eight normal subjects, Van Ravensteyn found the average copper content to be 0.118 mg/100 ml (range 0.03–0.20 mg/100 ml). These may be compared to an average content of 0.2 mg/100 ml (range 0.06–0.32 mg/100 ml) for common duct bile in three subjects, and of 0.48 mg/100 ml (range 0.09–1.07 mg/100 ml) in gall bladder bile from 19 cases of chronic cholecystitis, obtained at the time of operation for bladder stones, as reported the same year by Judd and Dry (391).

As noted by the next investigators to contribute to this subject (105), a number of factors makes it very difficult to determine with a reasonable degree of accuracy the amount of copper excreted via the biliary tract. The daily outflow is intermittent and may vary from 250 to 1,100 ml/day. Bile cannot be collected quantitatively from normal subjects, even those with exterioration of the bile duct or indwelling T-tube, since in these situations the volume of bile flow is not normal. Moreover, copper in bile aspirated from the gall bladder during surgery or postmortem is considerably concentrated as compared to liver bile or duodenal bile, and the latter is subject to contamination by duodenal contents and the tubes used for the collection. It is reported (105) that copper in gall bladder bile obtained postmortem from six normal subjects ranged from 0.024 to 0.54 mg/100 ml, with an average value of 0.329 mg/100 ml. One subject with a cutaneous bile fistula following complete obstruction of the common duct excreted an average of 0.46 mg/100 ml copper per day. Another subject with primary biliary cirrhosis and T-tube drainage, gave an average value of 0.05 mg/100 ml (range 0.03–0.95 mg/100 ml) in bile collected daily for 17 days. No data on total daily output of copper were obtained.

In their conclusions, Cartwright and Wintrobe (105) state that assuming a daily intake of 2.0 to 5.0 mg of copper, 0.6 to 1.6 mg (32%) is absorbed. From 0.01 to 0.06 mg is excreted in urine, 0.1 to 0.3 mg passes directly into the bowel, and 0.5 to 1.3 mg is excreted in the bile. The latter estimate is in reasonable accord with a later report of Frommer (235) indicating that in 10 control subjects biliary excretion approximated 1.2 mg/day, based upon bile aspirated from the duodenum after overnight fasting. Walshe (822) states that in subjects with external biliary drainage up to 10% of ingested labeled copper can be recovered in the bile within 24 hours.

Human bile is said to contain copper-binding complexes of low and high molecular weight, the former predominating in hepatic bile and the latter in gall bladder bile (263, 266). However, the high molecular weight fractions may represent artifacts in chromatographic procedures, and essentially all of the copper may be bound to complexes of low molecular weight (4,000–8,000 daltons) (236), as observed in bile of the rat (196) which, by the way, possesses no gall bladder. The question of an enterohepatic circulation of copper, considered unlikely on the basis of the macromolecular complexes of copper predominating in the gall bladder bile (266), now justifies more critical study.

More recently evidence has been found that the mechanism of copper excretion may involve its complexing with taurochenodeoxycholate in the liver, thereby preventing its reabsorption from the upper intestine, with subsequent splitting of the complex in the lower intestine where reabsorption of the bile acid but not of copper may take place (454). Other evidence, also based upon bile from T-tubes, suggests that orally administered ^{64}Cu becomes combined with conjugated bilirubins (503). It is obvious that there is still much more to be learned about the binding of copper in bile and its possible reabsorbability.

Salivary excretion

Little or no attention had been given to the presence of copper in saliva until 1952 when Dreizen et al. (170) reported finding in the whole saliva of 14 normal humans (48 samples) a mean copper concentration of 25.6 μg/100 ml. In general agreement with these findings are those of De Jorge et al. (157) based on 40 normal, fasting subjects, giving a mean value of 31.7 μg/100 ml, and of Gollan et al. (264) based on 18 normal subjects and providing a mean value of 29 μg/100 ml. The copper of saliva is in the labile form, since reactions for ceruloplasmin are negative (157). If one considers the daily output of saliva to be 1.5 liters (range 1–2 liters), the total daily excretion of copper would amount to from 0.38 to 0.47 mg, on the basis of the data recorded above. There is also evidence that the copper-binding substances in saliva retain their activity after transit through the stomach to the site of absorption in the small intestine. De Jorge et al. (157) also report mean copper values of submaxillary, parotid and pancreas removed from 10 postmortem cases as 1.43, 0.55 and 0.85 mg/100 g dry weight of tissue, respectively.

Gastrointestinal excretion

In his pioneer studies on the metabolism of copper in man, Van Ravensteyn (805) found an average copper concentration of 0.023 mg/100 ml (range 0.01–0.04 mg/100 ml) in gastric juice of eight normal subjects. Some 27 years later, other data were provided by Gollan et al. (265) who, in four normal subjects, found a mean concentration of 0.034 mg/100 ml (range 0.02–0.96 mg/100 ml). In the latter studies gastric juice free of swallowed saliva and nasopharyngeal secretions was aspirated from fasting subjects, and particulate matter was removed by centrifugation at 2,000 $\times$ g for 20 minutes. Accepting the values reported by Gollan et al. (265), employing exacting collecting and analytical procedures, and considering current estimates that the daily volume of gastric secretions approximates 3 liters (range 2–4 liters), it can be calculated that the gastric mucosa secretes approximately 1.0 mg/day.

The only recorded study of duodenal secretion of copper is that of Gollan (263). Normal and secretin-stimulated aspirates of the duodenum, obtained from fasting normal subjects through a tube positioned such as to exclude gastric contents (and presumably to also exclude bile and pancreatic secretions) indicates the presence of copper-binding substances of low molecular weight such as also found in saliva and gastric juice. Gollan presents evidence that the latter binding substances retain their activity after transit through the stomach to the site of absorption in the small intestine. He also postulates that these secretions, through their capacity to solubilize the metal at an alkaline pH, may enhance the availability of copper for absorption.

Relatively little attention has been given to, or estimates made of, the amount of copper released into the feces via the extensive dehiscence of epithelial cells of the intestinal mucosa. In these cells there is a considerable amount of copper bound to metallothionein or metallothionein-like proteins, functioning in copper storage and in protection against excess copper intake. Considering that the absorptive cells lining intestinal villi are replaced every 5 to 6 days in man (475), this contribution of copper to the intestinal contents and to the fecal output may be quite significant, since it is thought to be nonabsorbable

(192). It may represent 17% of the daily fecal excretion (301). It certainly justifies more consideration as a factor in evaluating copper excretion and maintenance of copper balance in the human organism.

Questions arise concerning the fate of the large amount of copper bound to substances of low molecular weight (amino acids and peptides) which is excreted via the saliva, gastric juice and duodenal secretions. Unfortunately, studies presented record many data but make few predictions as to what the findings may mean with regard to copper absorption or metabolism. Some of this copper may be reabsorbed and some may be added to the feces, but the relative amounts are unknown. And, in addition, the physiological catabolism of ceruloplasmin may add about 0.1 mg to fecal excretion of copper per day (814).

Urinary excretion

Estimates of copper lost in the urine are somewhat variable, apparently due to differences in sensitivity and accuracy of methods used, and possible contamination from extraneous sources. Early reports are summarized by Butler and Newman (83) who, in a study of 12 healthy adults, reported mean excretion values of 18.0 μg/day, (range 3.9–29.6 μg/day). Values reported since that time are in reasonable accord with these results. If one selects from the literature those reports based upon 10 or more adult subjects, chronologically recording results in terms of μg/day excreted in the urine, the values are: 18 (113); 18 (765); 20 (253); 37 (398) and 52 (153). These values are all within the range of 10 to 60 μg/day proposed by Cartwright and Wintrobe (106). Thus, urinary excretion of copper, amounting to approximately 0.5 to 3.0% of the daily intake, places the main excretory responsibility on fecal excretion. There still remains the possibility that the human kidney possesses the capacity for tubular reabsorption of copper.

Sweat loss

The loss of copper through sweat has received limited consideration. The pioneer studies of Consolazio et al. (122) record that on a constant dietary intake of copper (3.5 mg) and in an environment of 37.8° and humidity of 50%, three normal subjects showed a significant negative copper balance. During 10 days of observation the sweat loss from the men averaged 1.6 mg/day, or about 45% of their total dietary intake. Consequently, the negative balance averaged 1.1 mg/day. Mitchell and Hamilton (528) found an average of 58 μg/liter in the sweat of four adult males under hot, humid conditions. Another report (343) records for 33 males after sauna bathing an average excretion of 550 ± 350 μg/liter in the sweat. In view of these data it appears that the loss of copper through sweat is much greater than heretofore recognized. In fact, Hohnadel et al. (343) and Sunderman et al. (764) extol the possible virtues of the sauna bath as a therapeutic method for increasing the excretion of toxic metals, such as copper in Wilson's disease. Technical methods defy measurements of copper loss through insensible perspiration.

Menstrual loss

Data on the loss of copper via menstrual flow is likewise meager. For four menstrual periods in three subjects values of 0.19, 0.24, 0.39 and 0.61 mg per period (aver. 0.47 mg) are given by Ohlson and Daum (572). Comparable average values of 0.32, 0.48, 0.65 and 0.74 mg copper for four consecutive periods in four different subjects are recorded by Leverton and Binkley (452), and a mean of 0.11 ± 0.07 mg per period for 12 adolescent girls is reported by Greger and Buckley (278).

COPPER IN THE DIET

Copper in foods

Copper is ubiquitous in plants and animals. Its widespread occurrence in food was demonstrated in the early reports of Lindow et al. (462) and of Hodges and Peterson (341) on the copper-content of samples of commonly used food in the USA, and that of Adolph and Chou (8) on Chinese foods. It is well recognized that the copper in foods varies greatly, depending upon the soils from which they have been obtained, and on contamination before and after reaching the market place.

The richest sources in human dietaries are liver (especially calf, lamb and beef), crustaceans and shell fish (especially oysters). Of somewhat lesser content, and roughly in descending order, are nuts and seeds, high-protein cereals, dried fruits, poultry, fish, meats, legumes, root vegetables, leafy vegetables, fresh fruits and non-leafy vegetables. One of the lowest of commonly used foods is cow's milk. The exceptionally high copper content of the Atlantic coast oyster, which may vary widely with the season and with degrees of contamination of environmental waters, is not true of the Pacific or the Australian oyster (290).

Throughout the literature one repeatedly finds the statement that the average North American diet provides 3 to 5 mg of copper per day. Because of the widespread presence of copper in foods and in drinking water, especially that obtained via copper pipes, it is difficult to devise a balanced diet composed of natural foodstuffs that contains less than 1 mg per day (50 μg/cal/day), according to Schroeder et al. (691) who give extensive data on copper in foods, beverages and water of many types. They also state that to provide such a diet the following foods must be avoided; most meats, shellfish, vegetables, phospholipids, legumes, fruits, nuts, some grains, gelatin, tea, coffee, soft drinks, beer and distilled liquors. Such a diet would be low in protein, monotonous and marginally deficient in several essential trace metals. In contrast, they estimate that a diet of only 1,200 calories, with 100 calories from each of the high copper foods (oysters, clams, pork, margarine, turnips, carrots, mushrooms, rhubarb, papaya, nuts, grapenuts and orange juice) would contain approximately 34 mg of copper.

There have been many other published lists giving the copper content of commonly used foods. A rather extensive list of copper and other inorganic elements in foods used in hospital menus has been presented by Gormican (273). A recent and complete compilation of data pertaining to the copper content of foods, as recorded by investigators worldwide, is that of Pennington and Calloway (595). Of the 222 references used in their literature survey only 104 specified the methods used, many of which represented individual modification of other methods. Methods of expressing values obtained were indeed numerous and often difficult to reduce to a common denominator. Aside from variable contamination of water, reagents and glassware in analytical procedures, factors such as copper content of soil, water source, season, and use of fertilizers, insecticides, pesticides and fungicides raised serious questions concerning the validity of values reported for the copper content of the vast list of food items recorded.

Hughes et al. (366) give analyses for copper in a great variety of commercially prepared baby foods. Highest levels were found in those containing beef liver and high protein cereals (2.64 and 1.85 mg/100 g, respectively). Next in order were other precooked cereal foods (range 0.78–0.26 mg/100 g), as compared to 0.04 to 0.30 mg/100 ml in human milk (pp. 2025–2026). Vegetables, fruits and desserts were variably lower. Cooked cereals, which frequently are the first non-milk foods offered to infants, if they are of high protein quality, will provide a large part of their requirement. It was their opinion that by the time infants reach 6 months of age the variety of supplementary foods normally offered should, in most cases, meet or exceed the generally accepted requirement of 0.05 mg/kg/day.

From what has been said, it is apparent that most populations appear to have an adequate dietary intake of copper, which well justifies previous opinions that a recognizable state of copper deficiency in adult man is not likely to be recognized. But this does not imply that some diets may not be decidedly marginal, as discussed in the following section. Such matters are constantly of concern in any review of reports on dietary intake and on balance studies which represent the basic information necessary for the determination of human copper requirements.

Dietary intake of copper

Before progressing to a discussion of human dietary needs of copper for adult man it may be pertinent to review what has been recorded concerning the usual dietary intake in various countries of the world. At the beginning it should be recognized that in the vast majority of such analyses copper has often been only one of many trace elements under investigation and often has been secondary compared to iron, zinc, and other elements. Unfortunately, there have been almost no studies in which copper has been the only, or even the primary, focus of attention.

On the basis of studies conducted in England, New Zealand and the United States, Underwood (798) estimates that most western-style mixed diets provide adults with 2 to 4 mg/day. Guthrie and Robinson (292) think that the copper status of some New Zealanders may be inadequate. In India, in adults consuming rice and wheat diets, the copper intake may be as much as 4.5 to 5.8 mg/day (154). Estimated daily intakes for adults in other countries have been reported as: 2.26 to 7.3 mg (mean 4.10) in Kiev and 11 other cities of the Ukraine (239); 1.29 to 6.39 mg for inmates of old people's homes in Switzerland (688); about 2.0 mg for New Zealanders (511); 1.5 mg for inhabitants of an isolated Polynesian island (510); 2 to 4 mg for Japanese (543) and about 2.0 mg for Taiwanese (793). In the latter study, a control subject maintained on a low copper diet for 2 weeks, providing a daily intake of 1.34 mg, maintained a positive copper balance of 0.12 mg. Unfortunately, the methods employed for analysis of copper were not stated. On the other hand, it is estimated that in 20 USDA diets examined the mean copper intake would provide 1.05 mg/day (419).

Recent and well planned studies based upon analyses of copper and zinc content of duplicate samples of daily diets of 22 subjects (14–64 years of age) over a 14-day period, provide valuable information (344, 860). Considering a 6-day average (after 8 days of adjustment) for each subject, the mean daily intake of copper was 1.01 mg day ± 0.4. This is considerably below estimates of 1.62 mg/day given by Hartley et al. (314), and 1.34 mg/day by Tu et al. (793), but in good agreement with the estimates of 1.05 mg by Klevay et al. (419).

There has also been an increasing awareness of an inadequacy of not only copper but also other trace elements and certain vitamins in the usual hospital diets (67, 273, 419). It is true that most patients are hospitalized over a sufficiently short period such that they can rely on liver and other tissue storage to compensate for inadequate intake. The problem of long term parenteral nutrition is a separate issue which will be discussed later (pp. 2028, 2034). However, it may be noted that a recent study of regular, vegetarian and renal diets in a hospital situation, based on diets collected over 7 consecutive days, indicate a mean daily copper intake of 0.90, 1.10 and 0.51 mg (67), respectively. For subjects with Wilson's disease such diets would be most desirable. For others, they may be marginal or inadequate.

Analyses of school lunches have given but rather fragmentary evidence of the copper content of the American diet for children and adolescents. A survey of such lunches served 6th grade children in 300 schools in 19 states of the USA (544, 545) indicates an average content of 0.34 mg/day (range 0.06–2.19 mg). Considering one-third of the daily intake represented, the average intake would amount to about 1.0 mg/day. These values are somewhat less than those reported in metabolic studies of 7 to 9 year-old children fed diets typical of low income groups in the southeastern USA, recording mean daily intakes of 1.67 mg/day (618). On the basis of mg/kg/food consumed, values given for institutionalized children in Samarkand are 0.46 to 1.62 (620), and for the same in 28 USA cities are 0.44 to 0.87 (548).

Waslein (830) reports that data collected on the copper content of the diet of 377 babies from the USA indicated a wide range of from 7 to 170 μg/kg body weight, or 0.18 to 0.92 mg/day. Total daily intakes of copper ranged from an average of 0.16 for 1-month old infants to 0.38 mg for 6-month old infants, 50 to 60% of the intake coming from milk. Furthermore, intakes of children participating in balance studies or living in institutions in the USA or USSR had mean copper intakes of 0.9 to 2.2 mg/day, and similar studies on adults in the United Kingdom and New Zealand gave values of 1.7 and 2.4 mg/day, respectively. However, the average copper intake of 5.8 mg/day from diets in India, determined on composites made from self-selected diets in a dozen locations throughout the country (154), is more than double the mean found for diets in developed countries, for which no explanation is given. In evaluating such reported data one must consider not only the differences in methods of assay and of care against contamination but also differences in sample preparation and differences in food preparation in different countries. There is also need to consider phytate and fiber content of diets, which may influence absorption or utilization of dietary copper. From what has been said, it is quite apparent that data based upon the daily intake of copper by peoples in different parts of the globe give relatively little guidance as to what the minimal or optimal level of intake may be.

COPPER METABOLISM IN PRENATAL AND POSTNATAL LIFE

A preceding section has dealt with the labile and the more firmly protein-bound types of copper in the blood cells and blood serum or plasma of normal adult man. Briefly stated, the labile pools represent about 40 and 7%, and the protein-bound pools (superoxide dismutase and ceruloplasmin) approximately 60 and 93%, of the copper present in blood cells and plasma, respectively. The ratio of cell to plasma copper is about 0.70 (100). The copper content of the red blood cells remains remarkably constant, little influenced by dietary intake or metabolic stresses (286, 435). That of the plasma is subject to rather remarkable changes during pregnancy, reflecting the influence of hormones, particularly estrogens, upon the synthesis and release of ceruloplasmin.

There exists a vast literature dealing with 1) the increase of maternal blood copper levels during pregnancy and the influence of estrogenic hormones; 2) the role of the placenta in transfer of copper to the fetus; 3) the role of fetal liver in storage of copper to meet inadequacies of mammary transfer during early lactation and 4) postnatal changes in blood copper levels in the infant and adolescent. Knowledge and interpretation of these processes are of importance not only in determining

the role of copper in reproductive physiology and neonatal development in man, but also in obtaining a better understanding of human requirements of copper for the infant and adolescent. It is the purpose of this section to review briefly what has been learned concerning the rather complex changes, not yet clearly understood, which occur in the pregnant mother, fetus and young infant.

Influence of pregnancy

It seems remarkable that the first investigators to demonstrate the presence of copper in human blood (827) should also have been the first to recognize not only normal sex differences but also increased levels of copper in the blood of pregnant women (426). These observations were soon verified by many other investigators (181, 184, 206, 294, 318, 345, 348, 434, 464, 556, 561, 577–579, 655, 660, 787). However, the significance of these findings remained obscure until evidence was presented that similar increases occur in infants receiving diethylstilbestrol therapeutically for treatment of hemophilia (794), and in adults of either sex receiving estrogens (183, 245, 368, 651) but not in those receiving progesterone or androgens (183). These investigations suggest that increased plasma copper levels in pregnancy could be explained by increased levels of estrogens, but this may not be the total story.

Beginning during the first trimester of pregnancy, there occurs a progressive increase in maternal plasma copper levels. In groups of pregnant women at successive lunar months of gestation, values have been reported to increase progressively from 146.1 to 277.6 μg/100 ml (181), and 131 to 213 μg/100 ml (757), and from 172 to 273 μg/100 ml (54). Similar data are presented by others (158, 524). The increased plasma copper levels of pregnancy have been well documented (23, 54, 77, 152, 231, 255, 318, 320, 324, 527, 574, 578, 686, 687, 847, 858, 878). The copper content of erythrocytes of mother and fetus remains remarkably constant (181, 345). Hence, the striking rise in plasma copper during pregnancy to about 2 to 3 × normal is attributable almost entirely to increased synthesis of ceruloplasmin (324, 491, 673).

Since there are no known alterations in absorption or excretion, the major source of the non-dietary copper for this synthesis is presumably the maternal liver. Direct evidence in support of this assumption is the much lower concentration of copper in the liver (as compared to other organs examined) in pregnant as compared to nonpregnant women, all victims of accidental death (524), and very low liver copper levels in women succumbing to late toxemia of pregnancy associated with unusually high serum ceruloplasmin levels (628). Assuming also increments of about 25% in plasma volume during gestation (166), maintenance of high plasma copper levels places special demands upon maternal tissue stores. Associated with increased plasma ceruloplasmin levels of copper there occurs a reciprocal decrease in plasma zinc levels both in states of pregnancy (152, 300, 324, 388, 843) and following use of oral contraceptives (297), although the latter statement has been questioned (579). Differences in competitive binding of these two elements under special circumstances may explain these inverse relationships of zinc and copper during gestation.

Richterich et al. (638), comparing their data with that of prior investigators (338, 491, 673), indicate general agreement that 1) ceruloplasmin blood levels in pregnant women are two to three times those of nonpregnant women, and that 2) the levels in mothers at term are approximately eight times those in umbilical cord blood. Ceruloplasmin values recorded are quite comparable, whether obtained by the enzymatic method of Ravin (629) or the immunological method of Hitzig (339). Maternal serum copper levels return to non-pregnant levels over a period of 4 weeks or more following legal abortion (54) and normal delivery (388, 561, 777). Since estrogen production and serum ceruloplasmin levels are not proportional during pregnancy, and since blood estrogens decrease rapidly after abortion or delivery compared to ceruloplasmin levels, questions are raised as to whether estrogenic stimuli alone are responsible for the increase of serum copper in pregnancy. A similar dilemma relates to the increase in serum copper levels, over and above those of normal pregnancy, observed in pre-eclampsia and eclampsia (205, 527, 552, 578, 628, 777, 847, 858, 868), and in a case of hydatidiform mole (318). Evidence that maternal serum copper levels show even greater increases with intervening infectious diseases and malignant processes has led to suggestions that increased serum copper levels in pregnancy reflect a resistance reaction of the maternal organism to continuous invasion of the fetus into the maternal circulation (181). Another concept relates these changes to a consequence of hormonal adaptation of the maternal organism to the increased metabolic and hormonal demands of pregnancy (167).

Influence of oral contraceptives

Reference has been made to early observations (183, 651, 794) of the therapeutic use of estrogens and the ensuing increase in plasma levels of ceruloplasmin which, in turn, suggested an explanation for the comparable phenomenon observed previously in pregnant women. To this may be added evidence (98) that in normal individuals oral contraceptives cause marked increases in serum copper levels involving increased synthesis of ceruloplasmin, often greater than that observed in the state of pregnancy. Since that time there has arisen a rather extensive literature on the effect of oral contraceptives and intrauterine copper devices in the human female.

Since this topic has been well reviewed in recent years (589, 723, 771), it will not be subject to further consideration here. However, it must be emphasized that the continued use of oral contraceptives has been, and will continue to be, an important factor in influencing copper homeostasis in women. Estrogens, whether endogenous or exogenous, have a remarkable capacity to stimulate synthesis of ceruloplasmin in the liver and to increase urinary excretion of copper. The extent to which prolonged use of oral contraceptives may decrease body copper storage and modify the daily copper requirement has not been examined. It does justify special study.

Placental transfer

Nonceruloplasmin copper readily crosses the placenta by passive diffusion, and its concentration in erythrocytes and plasma of mother and fetus is relatively constant throughout gestation (181, 673). Total copper in cord blood is about 1/4 to 1/5 that in maternal blood (181, 464, 552, 556, 561, 660, 673, 686). Studies in which blood of the umbilical vein (placenta to fetus) and umbilical artery (fetus to placenta) have been analyzed for copper give values of 53.4 to 40.0 μg/100 ml (556), 54.9 and 40.2 μg/100 ml (167) and 74.4 and 41.8 μg/100 ml (770), respectively. Such findings clearly indicate an important role of the placenta in transfer of copper from mother to fetus. The high copper concentration in the placenta (525, 605), liver and other fetal organs and tissues, referred to later, indicates the efficiency of this transfer.

Questions of placental transfer and of fetal synthesis of ceruloplasmin have never been satisfactorily clarified. It has been assumed that its large molecular size precludes placental transfer (673), although this may not be a valid conclusion (339). There are possibilities that with pronounced thinning of the hemoendothelial membrane of placental villi, and/or tiny breaks therein during late phases of gestation, some ceruloplasmin may be transferred to the fetal circulation (552). Also, one cannot exclude the possibility that ceruloplasmin may actually cross the placenta, and that its rate of utilization and breakdown may be equivalent to or greater than its rate of transfer (666). Although apoceruloplasmin can be identified immunologically in plasma of the newborn (496, 714), there is no evidence that ceruloplasmin can be synthesized by the fetus. It is assumed that synthesis by the fetal liver does not begin until shortly after birth. In the domestic pig neither apoceruloplasmin nor ceruloplasmin appear in the piglet serum until about 15 hours after birth (108, 109). In view of these facts, the presence of small amounts of ceruloplasmin in cord blood of the newborn (338, 606, 639, 673) suggests its transport from placenta to fetus. If this be so, the time over which this transfer may

take place and its magnitude is unknown, and almost impossible to determine. A question which naturally arises is whether the fetus has or needs a ferroxidase type of enzyme, as a substitute for lack of ceruloplasmin, to provide for the intensive hemopoietic activities of the fetal liver, spleen and bone marrow during fetal life. Somewhat ancillary to this discussion are observations of Widdowson et al. (842) that copper concentration in the liver of 30 fetuses representing the 20th to 41st weeks of gestation were consistently high (average 6.4, range 3.5–9.3 mg/100 g fresh tissue), as compared to values of 0.5 mg/100 g fresh tissue for adult human liver. Iyengar and Apte (377) give values of 4.76, 4.37, 4.38 and 4.23 mg/100 g fresh tissue for livers of 38 fetuses of gestational ages less than 28, 28 to 32, 33 to 36 and 37 to 40 weeks, respectively. On the other hand, Sultanova (761) reports that the more premature the infant the lower are the fetal liver reserves, while Butt et al. (85) find lower hepatic copper values in full term infants than in prematures. Neither study provides the firm data characterizing the first two studies (377, 842) mentioned. Significantly lower levels of total copper and ceruloplasmin in cord blood of neonates of undernourished mothers compared to those of well nourished mothers suggest that poor nutritional states of the mother are reflected in reduced capacity of the fetal liver to synthesize proteins in general, and ceruloplasmin in particular (429).

According to one investigator (526), amniotic fluid contains copper and other bioelements in about the same concentration as in the maternal plasma and, by virtue of its being swallowed in appreciable amounts, provides an additional supply to the developing fetus. However, other investigators report the presence of very small amounts or only traces of copper in this fluid (303, 321, 324, 564), which is in accord with the concept of the amniotic fluid as a protein-poor dialysate diluted with fetal urine.

Infancy and childhood

Following normal delivery a series of interesting and not fully explained events occur in mother and infant. Maternal levels of serum copper decrease to non-pregnant levels during the first 2 weeks postpartum (100, 206, 293, 294, 561). This is ascribed to the abrupt cessation of estrogenic stimuli for ceruloplasmin synthesis. At the same time, infant levels of serum copper, which are lower at birth than at any period of life, promptly increase until adult levels are attained between the 2nd and 3rd months of life (91, 293, 325, 690). This is due almost entirely to increased synthesis of ceruloplasmin by the infant's liver. In other studies, estimates of the age at which adult values are reached vary from about 3 to 6 months (338, 494, 638), to 9 to 12 months (411, 606). Several investigators report that after adult serum copper levels are attained during the first 2 or 3 months of life, these levels rise significantly above normal after the 4th month (758) or during the 2nd year of life (131, 362, 656), and then gradually decline to adult levels at puberty. Sass-Kortsak (666) gives mean values of 140, 129 and 117 μg/100 ml for 2-, 6- and 10-year old children. Hrgovic and Hrgovic (362) record mean values of 179, 151, 133 and 111 μg/100 ml for age groups 0 to 5, 5 to 10, 10 to 15 and 15 to 18 years. No sex differences are apparent until puberty, after which the effect of female estrogens on increased serum copper levels becomes manifest. Similar observations have been reported by other investigators (573, 776). Neither the reason for, nor the significance of these fluctuations in early life has been elucidated.

Immunological methods have identified an apoceruloplasmin in newborn infant plasma in concentrations similar to that of ceruloplasmin in the adult, thus indicating that only the inability to charge the apoprotein with its normal complement of copper is underdeveloped at birth (714). Similar observations have been made in studies with piglets (108, 109, 523).

On the other hand, remarkable changes occur in the liver of the newborn, which contains about one-half the copper in the body and a concentration, in terms of copper per unit weight, 5 to 10 times that of the adult liver (843, 846). A large component of this copper is bound to hepatic mitochondrocuprein, first isolated and described by Porter et al. (615). This copper-storage protein, found only in the fetus and newborn, is thought to represent a copper-rich polymerized form of metallothionein which sequesters copper prior to birth (611, 614). Liver copper rapidly disappears during the first few months of life (69, 627, 846), releasing copper for ceruloplasmin synthesis and the general needs of tissues of the rapidly growing infant. The ceruloplasmin synthesized by the neonate is identical to that of the adult (870). Thus there is a logical explanation for the early reports of Kleinman and Klinke (414) and Morrison and Nash (538) that the concentration of copper in the liver of newborn and young infants is 6- to 18-fold that of adults.

Although copper and ceruloplasmin blood levels are lower in the newborn than at any other period of life, the copper concentration in fetal and neonatal organs and tissues is much higher than in the adult (207, 248, 414, 565, 781). The studies of Fazekas (207), based upon analysis of 29 different organs and tissues of 109 fetuses and full-term infants of varied gestational age, indicate that in addition to liver, the concentration of copper in muscle, skin, adrenal glands and thyroid is particularly high compared to that of adults. The copper content of the placenta is also rather high (525, 605). The high concentrations of copper in organs and tissues of the newborn decrease gradually to normal levels during the first year of postnatal life (69, 248, 565).

The unusually high concentrations of copper in liver and other tissues of the neonate appear to represent a reserve to assure an adequacy of copper for synthesis of ceruloplasmin and other copper-containing proteins to meet metabolic needs for hematopoietic, maturational and other functions in the rapidly growing infant and adolescent prior to puberty. These changes naturally create difficulties in reaching definitive conclusions concerning the dietary requirements during these early years of human development. For other details concerning the role of copper in pregnancy, and in prenatal and postnatal development, the reader is referred to a number of informative reviews (461, 533, 666, 843).

DIETARY COPPER DEFICIENCY

There appear repeated statements in the literature that in view of the ubiquitous occurrence of copper in foods of every type, and lack of evidence of any recognized manifestations of copper deficiency such as commonly observed after dietary depletion of copper in experimental animals or under natural conditions in farm animals, man appears to be free of hazards of a state of copper deficiency. However, there has developed convincing evidence that a copper deficiency state can occur in man, even though it may be of rare occurrence and as the result of rather special types of situations.

A syndrome characterized by hypocupremia, hypoferremia, hypoproteinemia, edema and hypochromic anemia, responsive to oral copper but not to iron, has been observed in infants fed diets limited largely to milk (432, 437, 758, 796, 797, 874). In certain cases, especially those of Ulstrom et al. (796, 797), a fundamental defect in protein metabolism at the cellular level may have been a primary factor, rather than exhaustion of neonatal copper stores (874). The fact that infants 6 to 18 months of age usually have been involved suggests a relation to periods of life when initial liver storage of copper has been depleted, combined with prolonged maintenance on milk diets and increased demands for copper during a period of rapid growth. However, the possibility of degrees of protein depletion sufficient to impair retention of dietary copper deserved consideration.

Maintenance of two infants (one 8 days old with multiple congenital anomalies, and the other 10 months old) for 4 to 5 months on a milk diet identical to one which produced copper deficiency in piglets, caused neither anemia nor hypocupremia (101). Comparable results were obtained in the studies of Wilson and Lahey (854) involving seven premature infants with mean body weight of 1.24 kg fed a similar milk diet for 7 to 10 weeks. It was concluded that small premature infants fed a diet providing approximately

15 μg/kg/day of elemental copper over a 2 to 3-month period do not differ, by any of the criteria used, from prematures fed five or more times this amount. However, it should be recognized that at this period such infants could be utilizing liver stores of copper, and that the depletion period was much shorter than that required for production of a deficiency state in piglets with a relatively more rapid rate of growth.

Not until 1964 was a state of dietary copper deficiency documented in humans when Cordano et al. (126, 128) reported finding in infants, recovering from marasmus on exclusive milk diets, deficiency manifestations (anemia, decreased plasma copper and ceruloplasmin levels, intermittent neutropenia, severe osteoporosis and pathological fractures) quite comparable to those observed after experimental copper deficiency in pigs (436). Similar findings were observed in a 6-year old child with severe chronic intestinal malabsorption, who gave a dramatic response to copper therapy (127). In a later report, Graham and Cordano (276) state that in a series of 173 infants suffering from severe malnutrition and chronic diarrhea, admitted to the British American Hospital, Lima, Peru, over a period of 6 years, 62 instances of copper deficiency were identified, of which 44 were judged to have been depleted of copper prior to admission. The peak incidence was at 7 to 9 months of age. Responses to oral copper therapy indicated that repletion of total serum copper was more important than restoration of ceruloplasmin in correction of the deficiency state (352). Instances of copper depletion have also been observed in infants with chronic diarrhea in the United States (354).

There have also appeared more recent reports of neonatal copper deficiency in a premature infant 3 months old (17), in three very small premature infants during their third month of life (280), in a premature infant 3 months of age (700), and in a premature infant at 6 months of age (25). Neutropenia, low plasma ceruloplasmin and osteoporosis have been among the manifestations regularly observed. Favorable response to oral copper has usually been reported. Although none of the investigators make reference to it, the clinical and pathological findings reported bear striking resemblance to many of those characteristic of Menkes' steely-hair syndrome (p. 2007). A comparable picture has been observed in an infant maintained for some months on total parenteral nutrition following surgery for ileal atresia (394) and in others treated likewise for protracted diarrhea (463). Also, a state of copper deficiency has been described in a 12-year old child and an adult after prolonged total parenteral therapy following extensive bowel resection (177). In all cases there was a good response to copper therapy.

It is worthy of note that in all instances where a naturally occurring copper deficiency has been observed, as described above, only premature infants have been involved. This is in accord with the fact that premature infants do not benefit from the additional copper storage in the liver and other tissues acquired by the full-term infant, and are customarily maintained for longer periods on natural milk or milk formulae before having access to cereals and other foods. Furthermore, prematures have much lower copper reserves in the liver and spleen than do full-term infants, and show a negative copper balance during the first month of life which tends to become positive only after the second month of life (761). Suggestions that consideration should be given to special supplementation of the premature infant formula with copper (843) appears to be well justified.

The major manifestations of copper deficiency in infancy, and their relationship to decreased activity of copper-containing proteins, justify brief summarization.

1) Neutropenia and hypochromic anemia responsive to oral copper but not to oral iron are early manifestations of deficiency, in large part the result of lowered levels of ceruloplasmin and impaired release and transport of iron from body stores.

2) Osteoporosis, with enlargement of costochondral cartilages, is also an early phenomenon, followed by cupping and flaring of metaphyses of long bones with spur formation and submetaphyseal fracture, periosteal reactions and spontaneous

fractures, especially of the ribs. These are usually referred to as "scurvy-like" changes, and may also suggest the "battered child syndrome." Deficiency of copper-containing oxidases, essential for the cross-linking of bone collagen, adequately explains these manifestations.

3) Decreased pigmentation of the skin and general pallor of copper-deficient infants, can be attributed to decreased activity of tyrosinase, necessary for the production of melanin.

4) In later stages of deficiency there may be neurological abnormalities such as hypotonia, episodes of apnea and possible psychomotor retardation, generally attributed to decreased levels of cytochrome c oxidase.

MENKES' DISEASE

This progressive brain disease inherited as a sex-linked recessive trait was first recognized in five young boys (siblings), and its major clinical and pathological manifestations described in 1962 by Menkes et al. (513). Other cases were soon reported by Bray (59) and Aguilar et al. (11). While subsequently referred to as "kinky-hair" disease and "trichopoliodystrophy" (225), the currently accepted designation is "steely-hair" disease (or syndrome) proposed by Danks et al. who (145) in 1972, first recognized the disease as an inherited defect in copper absorption; in fact, a congenital copper deficiency. Since the term "kinky-hair" implied crimped hair like that of the black races, whereas that of affected infants more closely resembled depigmentation and loss of crimp in wool observed in copper-deficient sheep (252), "steely-hair" appears to be more appropriate (146). It is said to occur in 1 of 35,000 live births (145). As of 1977, Ahlgren and Vestermark (12) list 42 cases reported in the literature.

Manifestations

Symptoms of Menkes' disease usually appear between birth and 3 months of age, followed by death prior to the 4th or 5th year of life. The age of onset is somewhat earlier in prematures than in full-term infants. Occurrence as late as the 6th year has been reported (28). Characteristics of the disease, as originally recorded by Menkes et al. (513), are: short, broken, spirally twisted scalp hair (pili torti) with loss of pigment; frequent convulsive seizures, failure to thrive or poor weight gain, mental retardation and, at necropsy, widespread degenerative changes in the cerebrum and cerebellum. To these manifestations have since been added: hypothermia (56, 72, 145, 148, 168, 225, 530); marked tortuosity, associated with defects of the internal elastic lamina and hyperplasia of the overlying intima, of large muscular arteries, particularly those supplying the brain and its appendages (4, 12, 114, 145, 146, 422, 582, 713, 717, 808, 817); excessive Wormian bone formation (283, 645, 732, 835) and pronounced changes in certain long bones similar to those of scurvy and/or the battered child syndrome (56, 145, 168, 669, 713, 717, 732). Biochemically, there is increased copper content of the intestinal mucosa (145, 148, 470); greatly reduced levels of serum copper and ceruloplasmin (55, 72, 148, 168, 310, 530, 713, 817) despite normal copper levels in erythrocytes, and much reduced levels of copper in the liver (145, 148, 329, 817) and brain (145, 817).

Other reports have made reference to deficient visual functions and ocular abnormalities (49, 310, 453, 697, 717, 863) and to neurogenic bladders with diverticulum formation (306, 838), presumably due to defective innervation or vascular abnormalities. In the only known case of Menkes' disease in a black infant, Volpintesta (809) observed a remarkable light skin in contrast to the dark-skinned parents, an unusual mottled skin pigmentation in a 7-year old female sibling, and a small degree of pili torti in the mother and two female siblings. Manifestations typical of Menkes' syndrome, except for the absence of steely hair, have been reported in a Japanese infant by Osaka et al. (582) who question whether some cases of the disease may go unrecognized because of too great a reliance on the hair abnormality as a diagnostic feature.

Several new observations have special relevance to early diagnosis of Menkes' disease. A recently described method for measuring ceruloplasmin using a dried blood clot (21) may have value in screening for early diagnosis, but only when applied at 3 months of age or later (495). An intense metachromasia in primary tissue cultures of fibroblasts has interesting possibilities as a genetic marker in early diagnosis and in identification of homozygotes and heterozygotes in affected families (145, 147). This defective cellular metabolism of copper in fibroblasts is indicated by other observations that cultured skin fibroblasts from subjects with Menkes' disease have an abnormally high copper content (259) and also can incorporate much greater amounts of ^{64}Cu from the medium than do fibroblasts of unaffected subjects (358). The copper content of the culture medium may be critical in such evaluations. Regrettably, there exist rather limited prospects that improvements in early diagnosis will be parallelled by more effective therapeutic measures. Widespread degeneration of cerebral grey matter, secondary to degeneration of cerebral white matter and diffuse atrophy of the cerebral cortex, associated with bizarre changes in shape and arrangement of Purkinje cells, as first described by Menkes et al. (513), has been confirmed by later neuropathologic studies (11, 251, 336, 624, 802, 810). Nerve tracts of the spinal cord may sometimes be involved (11, 251). Peripheral nerves are not affected. It is proposed that these lesions reflect two types of change; viz., cerebral necrosis due to abnormalities of the extracranial arteries, and typical dystrophic lesions in the cerebellar cortex (810). Confirming and extending the original descriptions of the cerebellar lesions by Menkes et al. (513) and Aguilar et al. (11), ultrastructural studies of the bizarre elaboration of perisomatic dendrites of Purkinje cells suggest retarded development of the somal membrane of these cells (336, 624). Such evidence is cited in support of the concept that the disease process is operative in utero (340).

A careful light and electron microscopic study of the eye has revealed degeneration of retinal ganglion cells, loss of nerve fibers, optic atrophy, abnormal pigment epithelium and abnormal elastin in Bruch's membrane (863). A similar study of aorta and skin in Menkes' disease has demonstrated abnormalities of elastic fibers similar to those observed in animal studies on copper deficiency (566). Reported ultrastructural changes in skeletal muscle (251) have not been confirmed (717). Neurochemical studies on two infants whose neuropathology was described by Aguilar et al. (11) record abnormally low levels of polyunsaturated glycerophosphates, especially in the frontal gray matter, and accumulation of oxidized lipid products in the neurones, suggesting an interference with the molecular machinery of the cells (567). These observations have been both challenged (469) and confirmed (645). French et al. (224, 225) who proposed the term "trichopoliodystrophy" report much reduced levels of cytochrome a and a₃ in mitochondria of brain, muscle and liver, and conclude that deficient terminal respiration and failure of tissue energetics, secondary to diminished body copper content, may explain some of the neuropathology of Menkes' disease. Significantly reduced levels of erythrocyte superoxide dismutase and of dopamine β-hydroxylase may have bearing upon manifestations of the disease (645).

Metabolic abnormalities

Danks et al. (145, 147) propose that the primary defect in Menkes' disease is diminished ability to transfer copper across absorptive cells of the intestinal mucosa to the serosal side and the portal circulation. While considering this an important factor, Bucknall et al. (72), based upon studies on a 3-month old infant, speculate that neurological damage may occur in utero, perhaps as a result of defective placental transport of copper. This is supported by reports of the occurrence of one or more manifestations of Menkes' disease at term or within the week thereafter (283, 513, 530). However, defective placental transport may not provide the total answer. Heydorn et al. (329) and Horn et al. (359) consider that defective binding of copper in the fetal liver or atypical distribution in fetal tissues may be involved. The conclusions of Heydorn et al. (329) are based upon tissue analyses of a fetus suspected of Menkes' disease, obtained by

therapeutic abortion at 18 weeks gestation. Compared to four normal fetuses of 15 to 21 weeks gestation, copper concentrations in brain, lung, spleen, kidney, pancreas, muscle, skin and placenta were several times greater than, but liver copper was only about one-third, that of controls. Yet, the estimated total copper content of all fetuses was essentially the same. These findings, until substantiated, do not eliminate possibilities of defective placental transfer. However, they do raise questions regarding copper storage in fetal liver and atypical distribution of copper in other fetal tissues and organs in Menkes' disease (329, 635).

Menkes' disease and nutritional copper deficiency have certain features in common; 1) usual occurrence in infancy; 2) subnormal plasma levels of copper and ceruloplasmin; 3) tortuosity and defects in elastin of the aorta due to lack of lysyl oxidase; 4) scorbutic-like changes in costochondral junctions and epiphyses of long bones; and 5) decreased pigmentation of skin or hair. Menkes' disease differs from the state of dietary copper deficiency in the following respects: 1) alterations of hair structure and decreased pigmentation of hair, the latter attributable to lack of tyrosinase; 2) highly variable and often extensive lesions involving both white and gray matter of the cerebrum and cerebellum, usually ascribed to lack of cytochrome oxidase and superoxide dismutase which, in turn, may also be factors involved in 3) hypothermia, a frequently observed phenomenon; and 4) the almost routine occurrence of convulsive seizures and mental retardation. To these may be added 5) absence of anemia and neutropenia and 6) unresponsiveness to orally administered copper other than significant increases in plasma levels of copper and ceruloplasmin.

Separate oral and intravenous administration of ⁶⁷Cu, permitting calculation of the percentage of dose absorbed, indicates that children with Menkes' disease absorb only 11 to 13% of oral copper as compared to 46% by unaffected controls, suggesting a reduced absorption of copper as an important factor in the disorder (159). Also, most of the copper absorbed is retained by the liver for extended periods of time and excretory loss is reduced, thus increasing the biological half-life in the body by two to three times, as compared to normal controls (159, 160). Under similar circumstances subjects with Wilson's disease show normal absorption of copper but, because of reduced biliary excretion, the half-life is increased to about the same degree as in Menkes' disease (160). Hence, these two diseases have dissimilarities relating to intestinal absorption but similarities in inability to release copper acquired by the liver.

Although a defect in the intestinal transport of copper undoubtedly plays an important role in postnatal life, it does not provide an adequate explanation for the diverse manifestations of Menkes' disease. With impressive evidence that this disease begins in utero, it would appear that varying degrees of genetic expression may explain differences in postnatal age when manifestations, such as frequent seizures, make their appearance. There remain many important questions the answers to which will be difficult to obtain. For example, is there defective placental transfer of copper comparable to that proposed in the intestine? Is placental transfer normal, but the types of fetal protein to which copper becomes bound abnormal? For this or for other reasons, is the concentration of normally or abnormally bound copper in certain tissues and organs significantly deranged? Are there abnormalities in the production of copper-containing enzymes or in membrane receptors in certain cells and tissues? Obviously, knowledge of the underlying metabolic disturbances in Menkes' disease is in a state of immaturity, but offers many challenges for future research. For further details the reader is referred to some recent reviews (75, 143, 144, 272, 301, 351, 818).

Therapy

Oral administration of copper salts to infants with Menkes' disease has been reported to cause slight clinical improvement, such as reduced hypothermia and improved hair color, and slight increase in serum copper levels (148, 467, 468), but other investigators find no beneficial effect (72, 243, 566, 833, 849). Intramuscular injections of copper complexed with EDTA can cause a significant increase in serum copper and serum ceruloplasmin (146, 817, 838), as also can a slow subcutaneous drip of copper sulphate over a period of 2 hours every 3 to 4 days (161). In one case so treated for 5 months a moderately encouraging clinical response was obtained (161). However, Wheeler and Roberts (838) report that while intramuscular injections of a copper-EDTA complex maintained reasonably normal serum copper and ceruloplasmin levels for 8 months in one infant, no clinical improvement was apparent.

Intravenously administered copper in various forms (copper sulphate, copper acetate, copper-albumin, copper-EDTA complexes and human ceruloplasmin) has produced increases in serum copper and ceruloplasmin to values approaching normal (72) or essentially normal (146, 161, 282, 283, 833, 849), or no significant change (243, 244). Usually the period of treatment has been short (7–10 days) or intermittent over somewhat longer periods. In one instance normal serum copper levels and subnormal ceruloplasmin levels were maintained for more than 9 months by weekly intravenous infusions (833). A similar experience with 427 days of subcutaneously administered copper as a $CuCl_2$ + L-histidine complex, has also been reported (849). However, in all cases the disease has pursued its relentless course. But a faint gleam of hope comes from a report of Grover and Scrutton (282, 283) who, employing repeated infusions of copper sulphate once or twice weekly in an infant diagnosed as having Menkes' disease at 3 days of age, obtained mental functional levels equivalent to 4 months at 6 months of age. However, similar treatment of another infant beginning at 4 months of age and continued for 9 months provided no improvement. Hence, the answer is equivocal. Excessive urinary excretion of copper observed after parenteral therapy (242, 243, 849) is attributed to decreased hepatic uptake of copper, reflecting an abnormality of transport comparable to that in the intestinal mucosa. These observations suggest that a defect in membrane transport could explain both the in utero and postnatal deprivation of copper at multiple organ levels including placenta, intestine and liver; however, a favored alternative is that of a defect in intracellular transport in intestine, liver and kidney due to abnormalities in the transport and storage protein, metallothionein (242, 244).

From the information currently available, it seems questionable whether institution of any type of therapeutic measure during the period of gestation, if such were possible, would significantly alter the course of this genetically determined abnormality of copper metabolism.

Animal models

It seems obvious that there is still much to be learned regarding the metabolic defect in Menkes' disease. Challenging opportunities for future research are provided by several genetic animal models of this disease. One model is a recessive gene mutation (crinkled, CR) in mice. Such mice have a smooth coat with thin skin, delayed pigmentation, early mortality, and hair changes closely resembling those of Menkes' disease (374). In fact, all three types of hair abnormalities found in Menkes' disease are demonstrable (373). The observation that increased dietary intake of copper during pregnancy and lactation favorably altered the expression of the mutant gene (374) is certainly worthy of further exploration. Another model, a sex-linked "brindled" or "mottled" (MO^br) mutant in the mouse, is characterized by subnormal levels of lysyl oxidase (648), plasma ceruloplasmin, decreased copper levels in brain and liver, increased copper in the intestinal wall and virtual absence of hair pigmentation (371). Moreover, a recent study (200) indicates that in the affected homozygous male both intestinal absorption and hepatic uptake are impaired, and that in the heterozygous female they are intermediate between the affected male and normal mice. Danks (143, 144) and Holtzman (351) present excellent reviews of the literature and interesting comparisons of altered copper metabolism in the mottled mutant mouse and infants with Menkes' disease. A third mouse mutant called "quaking" manifests some of the neurological signs of copper-

deficient animals. Dietary copper decreases their tremors, indicating that copper metabolism is involved in expression of the gene (396).

Furthermore, Prohaska and Wells (621) describe striking similarities between biochemical abnormalities in the brain of suckling young of copper-deficient rats and those observed in Menkes' disease. These involve slow growth, abnormal behavior, decrease in myelin, reduction in cerebellar cytochrome c oxidase and superoxide dismutase and a 5-fold reduction in brain copper. Extensive lesions of the cerebral cortex and mid-brain have also been described in copper-deficient rats (92). In the guinea pig, which undergoes considerable myelination in utero, copper deficiency causes gross brain abnormalities, aneurisms, agenesis of the cerebellum, ataxia, wiry nature and depigmentation of hair, abnormal behavior patterns, and decreased liver copper (201). Morphologically, there is underdevelopment of myelin and cellular derangement and loss of neural elements in the cerebellum (202). Further study of the copper-deficient rat and guinea pig might well shed further light on the nature of Menkes' disease.

WILSON'S DISEASE

A vast literature has dealt with the nature, diagnosis and treatment of Wilson's disease. The findings have been well recorded in a number of reports and reviews (37, 38, 46, 137, 262, 267, 555, 666–668, 672, 678, 679, 683, 684, 737, 740, 744, 747, 756, 791, 821, 822). What follows is largely a summation of early observations concerning the nature of the disease, current concepts concerning the metabolic abnormalities involved and therapeutic measures.

Nature of the disease

The history of this disease, as well outlined by Goldstein and Owen (262), goes back to 1912 when Wilson (855) described a familial disease associated with cirrhosis of the liver and neurological manifestations, occurring predominantly during the first few decades of life. The term "hepatolenticular degeneration" was coined in 1921 by Hall (296), who also recognized the recessive mode of inheritance of the disease. This designation has since been largely replaced by the term "Wilson's disease." Not until 1953, through the more extensive studies of Bearn (36), was the autosomal recessive nature of this inborn error of metabolism clearly established; i.e., that both parents of an affected subject must be heterozygote carriers of the abnormal gene, and that their siblings have a one to four chance of receiving both genes; i.e., in being homozygous abnormal. For these reasons, the number of affected individuals is maintained at a relatively low level in the population, accentuated only by consanguinity. Other studies over the period (1912–1954) provided valid evidence that this disease represented a state of copper toxicosis characterized by 1) abnormally high levels of copper in the liver and brain (102, 134, 258, 316); 2) increased urinary excretion of copper (163, 485, 499, 609, 731, 873); 3) aminoaciduria (123, 136, 163, 499, 608, 735); 4) low serum levels of ceruloplasmin (674); 5) decreased fecal excretion of copper (41, 80, 581, 753, 873) and 6) the occurrence of Kayser-Fleischer rings (134, 258) which had been shown as early as 1934 to represent excessive accumulations of copper around the cornea (249).

Symptoms of the disease are decidedly variable in nature, time of onset and degree of severity. In the experience of some investigators the predominance of hepatic and neurological manifestations is about equally divided. In that of others, one or the other has been predominant. An excellent discussion of laboratory findings and clinical manifestations has been given by Strickland and Lev (756), Sass-Kortsak and Bearn (668) and Tu (791). How genetic determinants hold in check the metabolic and clinical expression of the disease for such variable periods of postnatal life, and often for many decades, is unexplained. Heterogeneity of the gene for Wilson's disease may be an important factor. One may consider the fact that while heterozygote carriers (parents of patients with Wilson's disease) cannot be identified clinically, they do differ from normal individuals in showing a prolonged biological turnover of ^{67}Cu (580, 753), reduced biliary excretion of copper (581), hyper-

cupriuresis after penicillamine loading (792) and certain renal dysfunctions (448).

Metabolic abnormalities

The classic form of this relatively rare inborn error of copper metabolism is characterized by: 1) usual, but not universal, low serum levels of copper, primarily of ceruloplasmin, suggesting defective synthesis of this cuproprotein by the liver; 2) abnormally high storage of copper in the liver, associated with decreased fecal excretion and chronic liver disease, reflecting impaired biliary excretion of copper and/or abnormal copper protein binding by the liver; 3) progressive accumulation of copper in the brain, leading to a wide variety of neurological disorders; 4) accumulation of copper in the kidney, associated with renal damage, cupruresis and aminoaciduria; 5) deposition of copper in the cornea, leading to the formation of Kayser-Fleischer rings and, occasionally, sunflower-type cataracts (87); and 6) episodes of hemolysis reflecting a rather sudden release of copper from a supersaturated and cirrhotic liver. Since in normal man concentration of copper is higher in the liver, central nervous system and kidney than in other organs and tissues (p. 1982) it might be expected that these levels would be significantly increased in a state of copper toxicosis. The report of a high concentration of copper in the skin of two patients with Wilson's disease (113) warrants verification.

Of particular interest is recent evidence that in subjects with this disease there is in the liver an abnormal metallothionein having a binding constant for copper about 4-fold that in normal liver (197). It is felt that the increased binding affinity of this protein alters normal homeostasis such that decreased biliary copper excretion and decreased ceruloplasmin synthesis result, and with saturation of binding sites in hepatocytes non-ceruloplasmin copper is released to the serum. Whether this protein, or the presence of an abnormal protein of similar nature, may explain copper accumulation in non-hepatic organs and tissues is an unresolved question.

In view of the fact that low serum ceruloplasmin levels are characteristic of young infants and subjects with Wilson's disease, it is not possible to diagnose this disease (other than perhaps by liver biopsy) and to institute therapeutic measures, prior to the 3rd month of life (638). Largely for this reason little has been learned about the presymptomatic manifestations of the disease during early and late infancy. However, the report of Scheinberg and Sternlieb (682) that copper concentrations in the liver of a 3½-year old child with Wilson's disease were at least 40-fold normal adult levels, does indicate progressive liver storage prior to clinical manifestation of the disease and supports the concept that the liver is the primary site of the disorder. The latter is characterized by a disruption of the normal homeostatic mechanisms for utilization and excretion of copper. Possibly at fault is the presence of either an abnormal protein with high avidity for copper, as proposed by Uzman et al. in 1956 (801), a similar protein unusually rich in sulfhydryl groups and given the designation L-6D (536) or a metallothionein-like protein with a protein-binding constant about 4-fold that of normal man (197). The concept that the metabolic defect in Wilson's disease is liver-based is supported by observations that in two teen-age boys with Wilson's disease treated with orthoptic liver transplantation the extrahepatic manifestations of the disease were significantly reduced (281). A similar response to the same procedure is reported in a 11-year old boy in whom there was strong but not incontrovertible evidence of Wilson's disease (172).

In the normal infant liver stores of copper are gradually decreased and serum copper levels increased during the first 3 or more months of life, until a close to zero copper balance is maintained. According to a recent evaluation of Wilson's disease (672), there may be an early arrest of these postnatal processes, especially abilities to synthesize normal amounts of ceruloplasmin and to excrete the normal fraction of dietary copper through hepatic lysosomes (normally an important function of lysosomes) into the biliary system. As a result, copper progressively accumulates in the liver, leading to inflammatory reactions, hepatic cell necrosis and post-necrotic cirrhosis. Meanwhile, excessive amounts of non-ceruloplasmin copper cause, in an unpredictable manner, accumulation and injury to different regions of the brain, the kidney and the cornea.

It is somewhat academic to ask whether administered estrogens or those of pregnancy can significantly influence the low serum ceruloplasmin levels in Wilson's disease. Bearn (37) finds that synthetic estrogens may have a significant effect in some patients but not in others, with no influence on urinary copper excretion. With somewhat larger oral doses of a different estrogen, German (250) reports improvement in some cases and accentuation of symptoms in others, and also notes a cupriuresis in some cases correlated with increased serum levels of direct reacting copper but not with ceruloplasmin. Subjects with Wilson's disease have been able to complete gestation with delivery of normal infants (14, 33, 47, 104, 155, 680). There is a report of one untreated case in which there was an appreciable increase in ceruloplasmin, reaching a maximum at delivery (104). Effects of pregnancy upon the clinical status of the mothers have been equivocal. In instances where penicillamine treatment was discontinued prior to gestation (155) and after the first trimester (680), neither ceruloplasmin levels nor clinical symptoms were improved. In fact, in one case occurrence of hemolytic anemia during the 5th month required restoration of therapy (155). In three other instances, where therapy was maintained throughout pregnancy, there is reported definite amelioration of clinical manifestations which continued postpartum for periods of a few weeks (14), 3 months (47) and 6 months (706). Data on serum ceruloplasmin are fragmentary. The ocurrence of several spontaneous abortions during therapy, both prior to (47) and following (14) pregnancies, raises questions concerning possible deleterious effects of penicillamine upon the fetus.

Although the copper-binding capacity of bile is not altered in Wilson's disease (233), there is increasing evidence that decreased biliary excretion of copper represents a major metabolic defect (234, 235, 581, 752, 753), and also that this defect may reside in the hepatic cell lysosomes (260, 261, 749, 755) whose catabolic functions and importance in transfer of copper to the bile canaliculi are well recognized. It appears that early in the disease copper is diffusely distributed in hepatocytes, later as more discrete granules, and that when hepatic damage is more widespread it becomes more localized in the lysosomes, where it may be less toxic (261). Delay in this uptake by lysosomes could be a key factor in the defective liver transport of copper in Wilson's disease (721). Questions still remain as to whether abnormal copper-binding proteins or lack of unknown cell enzymes involved in transfer of copper to, or in release of copper from, the lysosomes are responsible. The interesting observations of Goldfisher and Sternlieb (161) have raised the hypothesis that Wilson's disease may prove to be a "lysosomal disease," as discussed in some detail by Sternlieb et al. (749) and Strickland et al. (755).

Major results of reduced biliary excretion are increased copper accumulation in hepatocytes, varying degrees of pathology, jaundice and episodes of hemolytic anemia, the latter being secondary to release of copper from an overloaded and damaged liver into the blood stream. If this release is sudden, there can be severe damage to circulating erythrocytes, resulting in repetitive or fatal episodes of hemolytic anemia. A recent report (516) tabulates pertinent data on 18 reports involving 28 subjects. Of these, six presented hemolysis prior to any diagnosis of Wilson's disease and 20 showed evidence of hemolysis at the time of diagnosis. Evidence of hepatic dysfunction was noted in at least 22, whereas neurological dysfunction was recognized in only three or four. A more recent report of two cases of fulminating hemolysis in Wilson's disease calls attention to acute renal failure as well as hepatic failure (302). Hence, this hemolytic manifestation of Wilson's disease has become a more common phenomenon than previously recognized. In view of the fact that there is an associated marked increase in the copper content of erythrocytes and in the number of Heinz bodies during periods of crisis, hemolysis is attributed to increased

oxidative stress due to an excessive accumulation of copper in the cells (155, 508). Whether this is primarily a membrane defect is still an open question (516). It has been considered (102, 155, 508) a counterpart of the well known "enzootic jaundice" in sheep, the history and nature of which has been presented by Underwood (798). This concept is strongly supported by a recent study of controlled, experimental copper poisoning in sheep demonstrating extensive formation of Heinz bodies, predominantly membrane-attached, as the first morphological alteration observed (725). Hepatocellular and renal tubular necrosis were also noted.

Therapy

The chance observation of Mandelbrote et al. (485), in a study of copper mobilization in multiple sclerosis, that one of the control subjects who was later found to have Wilson's disease was greatly benefited by treatment with BAL (β,β-dimercaptopropanol), known to have properties of a chelator, provided the first therapeutic measure, introduced by Cumings in 1948 (135). While daily intramuscular injections proved effective in increasing the urinary output of copper (39, 46, 135, 163), there was no effect upon the aminoaciduria or other clinical manifestations. The same was true when BAL treatment was combined with intravenous casein hydrolysate and oral potassium sulfide, the latter forming an insoluble copper compound in the digestive tract (102); and also when EDTA (ethylenediamine-tetra-acetic acid, or "versene") was extensively tested (46). Nine weeks of estrogen treatment of an adult male with Wilson's disease failed to improve serum copper or ceruloplasmin levels (652). Intravenous use of a purified concentrate of human ceruloplasmin also proved ineffective (681). These discouraging results, together with the adverse side effects of BAL therapy, stimulated search for better measures.

In 1956 Walshe (820) described the remarkable effectiveness of oral DL-penicillamine as a chelating agent capable of markedly increasing the urinary output of copper. A few years later the less toxic D-penicillamine (β,β-dimethylcysteine) became available and has since been extensively used, often in combination with low-copper diets, in the treatment of Wilson's disease. If instituted during early phases of the disease, especially in asymptomatic patients, it can gradually reduce excessive tissue levels to reasonably normal levels and provide assurance of a normal life expectancy provided no adverse reactions occur (24, 156, 745, 746, 821). In such instances, which are rare, Walshe (823) proposes the use of tetraethylene tetramine dihydrochloride. This compound, which is cheap and easy to prepare, has not been found to be associated with toxic reactions. It is very effective as a chelating agent, and its mobilization of copper may differ from the action of penicillamine (823). It has not been produced commercially, but would seem to justify more thorough testing as an inexpensive therapeutic agent. Beneficial effects of L-dopa as an adjunct to a copper-deficient diet and oral penicillamine are reported (246) but not verified.

Despite disappearance of disease symptoms and remarkable improvement in liver function following penicillamine therapy for 2 to 7 years (277) and 9 to 13 years (156), hypocupremia, hypoceruloplasminenia and hypercupruria have persisted (156) and no more than limited improvement in liver morphology has been observed in most cases (277). One exception is that of a 10-year old girl in whom 27 months of penicillamine treatment not only abolished clinical symptoms but greatly improved liver morphology (204). Mitochondrial abnormalities of hepatocytes characteristic of Wilson's disease are less pronounced or absent after 3 to 5 years of therapy, which may have relevance to improved liver function, but liver structure is not significantly influenced (738).

Penicillamine has the properties of a lathyrogen, with ability to not only chelate copper but also to inhibit cross-linking in collagen (381, 560). Grand and Vawter (277) suggest that penicillamine may retard the formation of permanent scars if begun prior to the onset of the cirrhotic process, as it appears to do in the case of chronic active hepatitis (440). Once cirrhosis is established one might expect some thinning of fibrous scars with prolonged therapy (277). It is disappointing that morphological and ultrastructural studies on biopsies of liver exposed to many years of penicillamine therapy make no comment on changes observed in liver collagen (204, 738). Another feature of penicillamine action that justifies further exploration is the generalized loss of taste acuity in a variable number of subjects with scleroderma, rheumatoid arthritis, cystinuria and idiopathic pulmonary fibrosis given penicillamine treatment, and the restoration to normal after oral administration of copper (323). That only 4% of Wilson's disease subjects under the same treatment show hypogeusia is attributed to the fact that only rarely are their tissue stores of copper sufficiently reduced (323). A further complexity is presented by a case of hypogeusia in a patient with multiple myeloma which responded effectively to either oral copper or oral zinc (322). The role of copper in taste acuity is still questionable.

Low-copper diets often used in addition to penicillamine treatment of patients with Wilson's disease, usually providing 1.0 to 1.5 mg copper, not only exclude a number of generally consumed foods but also are monotonous and of low nutritional value (90). In predominantly rice-eating countries, such as Taiwan, preparation and acceptance of such diets present no great problem (754, 755, 793). A vegetarian diet is said to be highly effective in decreasing positive copper balance and in increasing fecal output, due perhaps to copper binding to some unabsorbed component of the diet (90). There appears to be no confirmation of these observations.

Related disorders

Two other abnormalities of copper metabolism, both associated with low serum levels of ceruloplasmin justify brief mention. Gahlot et al. (240) describe 15 cases of primary retinitis pigmentosa unresponsive to conventional treatment. Serum ceruloplasmin levels were very low and urinary copper excretion very high, although serum copper levels were normal or nearly normal. The investigators suggest that this retinal pigmentary disturbance, in certain cases at least, may not be an abiotrophy but a condition of chronic copper toxicity reflecting an inborn error in copper metabolism. The results of penicillamine treatment, said to be in progress, and further exploration of these observations by others, will be anticipated with much interest.

There has also been described, in three brothers, a hereditary disorder characterized by dementia, spastic dysarthria, vertical eye movement paresis, gait disturbance, splenomegaly and an abnormal metabolism of copper (851). The disorder is prepubertal in onset and progresses slowly over many years. Copper kinetic studies indicate similarities to those of heterozygote carriers of Wilson's disease. However, the unique combination of dementia, splenomegaly, and abnormalities of speech, vision and gait favor the view that this condition represents a new syndrome distinct from Wilson's disease. As far as can be determined, no comparable cases have since been reported. Both abnormalities may possibly prove to be variants of Wilson's disease.

Wilson's disease is not the only disorder in which high liver levels of copper occur. Chronic active liver disease closely resembles Wilson's disease in changes in hepatic function and morphology, but can be differentiated from the latter in that ceruloplasmin levels are elevated in about 50% of the cases and not below normal levels in others (442), and the cupriuria after penicillamine treatment is comparable to that of normal individuals (473).

One other liver disease requires special consideration. Levels of liver copper quite comparable to and even greater than those found in Wilson's disease occur in primarily biliary cirrhosis (215, 369, 721, 722, 862), a chronic, slowly progressive disease with evidence of extrahepatic biliary obstruction (223). Unlike the situation in Wilson's disease, plasma clearance and liver uptake of intravenous ^{64}Cu are normal (721). Similar conclusions were reached by Fleming et al. (215) on the basis of other evidence, including a new observation that patients with primary biliary cirrhosis also had significantly increased levels of copper in the renal cortex and spleen.

In a study involving an extensive evaluation of 81 patients with primary biliary cirrhosis, Kayser-Fleischer rings were found in three cases, and also in another patient with chronic active liver disease (216). In the three patients mentioned, copper in serum, urine and liver were significantly elevated, resembling conditions seen in Wilson's disease except for the high serum copper and capacity to incorporate radiocopper into ceruloplasmin. Concentration of liver copper above a specified level of 250 μg/g of dry tissue, previously considered as one of the four or five criteria for diagnosis of Wilson's disease, now appears to have limited value with accumulated evidence that such elevated concentrations occur in the two types of liver disease just mentioned. Furthermore, the presence of Kayser-Fleischer rings can no longer be considered pathognomonic of Wilson's disease.

HYPOCUPREMIA

Previous sections have dealt with Menkes' syndrome and states of copper deficiency in premature infants in which low blood levels of copper, especially of ceruloplasmin, are associated with various other manifestations of copper deficiency. States of hypocupremia without any evidence of dietary copper deficiency characterize Wilson's disease and occur, somewhat infrequently, in a variety of other metabolic and disease situations. Certain of these justify recording.

The terms "hypocupremia" and "hypercupremia" were introduced by Sachs et al. (655) whose excellent review of early studies on copper and iron in human blood, and their newer contributions, are worthy of note. Hypocupremia is defined as a serum copper level of 80 μg/100 ml or less (106). Since 93% of serum copper is normally bound to ceruloplasmin, hypocupremia must of necessity be synonymous with hypoceruloplasminemia, except in unusual circumstances. A syndrome characterized by hypocupremia, hypoferremia, hypoproteinemia, edema and hypochromatic anemia has been described in infants and children and attributed to either a dietary deficiency of copper and iron, with hypoproteinemia considered a secondary effect of iron depletion (432, 437, 759, 874), to a transient dysproteinemia (796, 797), or to inability to synthesize the apo-enzyme of ceruloplasmin (412). Other studies by Schubert and Lahey (692), based upon 14 infants with the above mentioned syndrome and 54 infants with iron-deficiency anemia but no hypocupremia, led to the hypothesis that an initial severe deficiency of iron results in marked anemia and consequent protein depletion which, in turn, causes impaired copper retention and resultant development of the complete syndrome.

Reduced serum levels of copper, ceruloplasmin, iron and protein are also characteristic of kwashiorkor (76, 180, 269, 305, 402, 433, 632, 664) and marasmus (305, 402, 532). Only one investigator reports no significant change in marasmus (269). There are other findings that in kwashiorkor and marasmus both plasma and erythrocyte copper levels are significantly reduced (402). There is general accord that the hypocupremia is not due to dietary insufficiency of copper but is secondary to a state of hypoproteinemia and inability to provide adequate amounts of the apoprotein for ceruloplasmin synthesis. Opinions differ as to whether in kwashiorkor the copper content of hair is significantly decreased (269, 474) or unaffected (76, 443). A report describing marked hypercupremia in Filipino children and attributed to states of malnutrition (750) may well be ascribed to faulty methodology and inadequate controls.

Hypocupremia has also been described in subjects with non-tropical sprue (78, 101, 284, 739), tropical sprue and macrocytic anemia (86, 106), malabsorption due to small bowel disease (739), and with both hyperchromic and hypochromic anemia (315). There are also isolated reports of hypocupremia associated with excessive gastrointestinal loss of protein (814, 869), celiac disease (27), cystic fibrosis of the pancreas (702) and the nephrotic syndrome (78, 101, 106, 491). In the latter disorder hypoceruloplasminemia comparable to that in Wilson's disease may occur, attributable primarily to high urinary loss of ceruloplasmin. In the other states of hypocupremia mentioned

above decreased levels of serum ceruloplasmin are characteristic, suggesting qualitative or quantitative abnormalities of protein metabolism rather than insufficient intake or absorption of copper.

HYPERCUPREMIA

Since the early observations of Krebs (426) that hypercupremia is associated not only with the state of pregnancy but also with many acute and chronic infections, there has accumulated an extensive literature on a wide variety of diseases and abnormal physiological states in which hypercupremia, predominantly due to hyperceruloplasminemia occurs. It is beyond the scope of this review to discuss these observations in detail, especially since there have been provided no well accepted hypotheses or explanations of the mechanisms involved in this apparent stimulus for increased synthesis and release of ceruloplasmin. However, comments will be made on certain disease states involving hypercupremia which appear relevant to the purpose of this review.

Infectious diseases. Hypercupremia has been recorded as a phenomenon commonly associated with chronic and acute infectious diseases of man. The lists recorded by various investigators are bewildering. There is general agreement that it is ceruloplasmin which is primarily increased and that during the recovery period, whether spontaneous or the result of therapy, normal levels are restored. This has been well demonstrated, for example, in cases of tuberculosis (61, 319, 542, 593, 655), leprosy (403), viral hepatitis, and pneumonia and chickenpox (413). In many instances there has also been recorded a decreased serum level of iron (61, 63, 103) and of zinc (718), reflecting differences in the proportions of circulating albumins and globulins to which these metals may be bound.

Hematologic disorders. Hypercupremia is commonly associated with iron deficiency anemia (100, 103, 319, 879) hemorrhagic, aplastic and pernicious anemias (100, 103, 237, 319) and sickle cell anemia (576). In most anemias there is an inverse relationship between serum copper and iron (100, 655, 657), but both may be increased in pernicious anemia, aplastic anemia and thalassemia major (103). It should be kept in mind that in view of decreased blood iron levels in anemia, the increased copper levels may be more apparent than real. In iron deficiency anemia, pernicious anemia and leukemia, as well as in chronic infections, there is an increased copper level in whole blood, red blood cells and plasma, and only in iron deficiency anemia is there an increase in the ratio of erythrocyte to plasma copper (100, 592). Aside from states of copper toxicity, blood cell copper remains quite constant. Since direct reacting copper of serum is only about 7% of the total, both hypo- and hypercupremic states reflect changes primarily in ceruloplasmin copper. To the present there have been proposed no acceptable explanations of the basic mechanisms involved, of the tissues from which the copper is mobilized, or the function(s) that hypercupremia serves. An extensive literature on this subject has been well reviewed elsewhere (7, 44, 100, 211, 319, 666).

Neoplasms. Hypercupremia is a common feature of acute and chronic leukemia (100, 162, 630, 773), lymphatic leukemia (255), Hodgkin's disease (100, 328, 363, 364, 386, 774, 775), malignant tumors (255) and of multiple and acute myeloma (255, 268, 456, 457). In leukemia of children plasma zinc levels are low, and the ratio of zinc to copper may prove useful in monitoring the response to treatment (162). In Hodgkin's disease blood copper levels are valuable in evaluating the disorder itself and the effects of therapy (363, 364, 774, 775, 778, 829).

Cases of multiple myeloma appear to present special abnormalities of copper metabolism. Goodman et al. (268) report a case in a 69-year old woman whose serum copper levels ranged from 20- to 40-fold normal, due entirely to a phenomenal increase in nonceruloplasmin copper. Evidence indicated its association with an abnormal monoclonal immunoglobulin. More recently, Lewis et al. (457) recorded a quite similar hypercupremia, with blood copper levels as much as 14-fold normal, in a 41-year old woman manifesting an early, clinically asymptomatic stage of multiple myeloma. Liver (biopsy) was normal

in structure and copper concentration. In both cases there was extensive copper infiltration of the cornea and of the anterior and posterior surface of the lens, not unlike that seen in the Kayser-Fleischer ring of Wilson's disease. These observations raise questions regarding the pathognomonic value of the latter and also the possible recognition of a unique variety of multpile myeloma, both of which justify further exploration.

Largely in the hope of finding an additional diagnostic criterion of value, attention has been given to serum levels of copper, and in some studies to zinc and iron, in subjects with varied types of neoplasia. In osteosarcoma, serum copper and copper-zinc ratios are increased in the primary phase, further increased following metastasis, and approach normal levels in patients whose tumor is amputated and show no clinical sign of the disease (212). Also, copper in the bone of osteogenic carcinoma is significantly greater than in normal bone (384). In lung and breast carcinoma the serum copper/iron ratio is high (602, 769). In gastric and pulmonary carcinoma serum copper levels are significantly increased, but not in cases of tumors of the large intestine (670). Only one study reports no differences between the serum copper content of healthy humans and those suffering from malignant tumors (22). Other reports indicate increased serum copper in lymphomas and certain other malignancies (539), and no change in prostatic carcinoma prior to or during radiation therapy (363). In Hodgkin's disease, leukemia and lymphomas, there is general agreement that serum copper levels have merit in diagnosis and in evaluation of therapy (162, 375, 386, 421, 539, 592, 773), as is also true of osteosarcomas (212). However, in none of the studies referred to above has a clear explanation, or even a challenging hypothesis, been provided toward explaining the possible mechanisms involved.

Neurological diseases. Recognition of low serum ceruloplasmin and copper levels as one criterion of Wilson's disease led to numerous studies on a wide variety of neurological diseases and disorders, many directed toward hopes of finding other conditions wherein increased or decreased levels of copper might provide a useful diagnostic measure of the disease state. On the whole, these efforts have proved rather unfruitful. Considerable controversy has arisen regarding schizophrenia and other psychotic states, following an early report of high serum copper levels in the majority of 27 cases of schizophrenia and in cases of manic depression and epilepsy (319). Subsequent studies have indicated a tendency toward significant increases in ceruloplasmin serum levels in schizophrenia (2, 675, 677), in manic depression and senile psychosis (13), but values obtained overlap with those of normal subjects to variable degrees. Since the activity of copper oxidase is reduced as serum ascorbic acid increases, it is felt that the increased levels observed in many states of mental illness may reflect low ascorbate intake in subjects institutionalized for prolonged periods (13, 20). Other investigators find no significant changes in serum copper in schizophrenia (30, 31, 360, 575), or in brain tissue (279). These differences might relate to the fact that schizophrenics are very heterogeneous biochemically, such as in serum levels of histamine, in serum levels of zinc and manganese, and in reactions to penicillamine and to contraceptive estrogens in particular (596, 597). In any case, serum copper levels have no diagnostic value (677).

In epilepsy there is said to be an increase in serum copper (70, 89) involving whole blood, serum and blood cell levels (800). Cerebrospinal fluid copper is reported to be decreased (89) and increased (800), and urinary and fecal copper increased (800). These unverified and somewhat variant observations probably have little relevance.

Cardiovascular diseases. More than 25 years ago Vallee (803) reported a pronounced hypercupremia during the acute phase of myocardial infarction, which subsided during recovery, and later Adelstein et al. (5) demonstrated a linear relationship between the serum copper, ceruloplasmin and copper oxidase activity. These findings have been well confirmed (405, 806, 831), and a reciprocal decrease in serum zinc has been noted (806, 831). In myocardial infarction, but not in angina, coronary insufficiency or myocardial ischemia, there is also a marked elevation in serum of the zinc-dependent enzymes, malic and lactic dehydrogenase (811), and in benzidine oxidase (760). Such findings naturally raise questions as to whether increases in serum ceruloplasmin represent anything other than a reaction to acute stress.

There are but a few unconfirmed reports indicating hypercupremia in atherosclerosis (53, 659), arteriosclerosis (81, 82) and hypertension (287); also, decreased levels of copper in the wall of larger arteries (404) and coronary arteries (836) of subjects with atherosclerosis. There is also described a linear decrease in the copper content of the wall of larger arteries with increase in degree of atherosclerosis (404), and a questionably significant lower level of copper in the coronary artery of subjects with atherosclerosis and myocardial infarction (836), which may reflect decreased metabolic activity of the altered arterial tissue.

Hemolysis associated with hypercupremia, usually transient and self-limiting, is a well recognized manifestation of Wilson's disease (see p. 2014). It may occur also as a fulminating event secondary to acute liver failure (643), sometimes combined with acute renal failure (302). It can be attributed to sudden release of nonceruloplasmic copper from a damaged liver and excessive accumulation in erythrocytes, resulting in acute oxidative stress upon the cells and cell membranes (155, 302, 643).

Liver diseases. Considering the key role of the liver in initial storage of absorbed copper, in the synthesis and release of ceruloplasmin, and in excretion of copper via the biliary system, it is to be expected that metabolic and pathologic dysfunctions of this organ might well be reflected in atypical levels of copper in the serum, and also perhaps in erythrocytes of the circulating blood. This has been well demonstrated. Serum copper levels are significantly elevated in portal cirrhosis, biliary tract disease and hepatitis (62, 245, 255, 271, 285, 600), possibly reflecting interference with the normal excretion of copper via the bile and consequent release of an excess into the circulation. Although states of hypocupremia are rare in liver disease, low serum copper levels are reported in hemolytic jaundice, hemochromatosis and some types of liver cirrhosis (255, 824), presumably the result of reduced capacity of the damaged liver to synthesize ceruloplasmin (824).

Liver biopsies from subjects of long-standing hepatic diseases due to biliary obstruction regularly show in periportal hepatocytes accumulations of coarse granules staining with the rubeanic acid method and the Mallory-Parker hematoxlin method for copper, and reacting positively to orcein, which indicates the presence of sulfhydryl groups, all of which suggest the binding of copper to a metallothionein type of protein (661, 719, 720). Rubeanic acid-staining granules of similar type have been described in the livers of vineyard sprayers exposed for many years to copper sulfate sprays (599), but this staining procedure is not a particularly reliable test for liver copper. In view of the role of copper as a hepatoxin in sheep (784), it is possible that copper may contribute to the development of liver cirrhosis in long-standing liver cholestasis (661). It should be of interest to explore the possible relation of these granules to hepatic lysosomes, and also to learn what effect penicillamine may have upon their histochemical picture.

Liver copper levels are not altered in extrahepatic biliary obstruction (862) or in acute hepatitis, steatosis of the liver, hepatic amyloidosis or hemochromatosis (640). In viral hepatitis, serum copper levels are said to be significantly increased during the acute phase according to one report (270) and during improvement of the clinical state according to another (326), but no change in liver copper levels has been reported. Patients with chronic active hepatitis respond favorably to 5 months or more of penicillamine therapy (440).

Rheumatic diseases. For many centuries copper amulets have been worn, hopefully, for relief from arthritis, rheumatism and many other afflictions of man, and copper has been a common component of folk remedies for arthritis in particular. There is reported (815) a recent correspondence and questionnaire type of study, involving 240 sufferers of arthritis/rheumatism, half of whom were previous wearers of copper bracelets and the other half not, randomly allocated to three treatment groups wearing copper bracelets or placebo (anodised aluminum) bracelets, or neither. Preliminary results of psychological analyses of the questionnaire responses indicate that "previous users seem to be significantly worse when not wearing their copper bracelets." However, convincing evidence of beneficial effects of copper bracelets does not yet exist. These studies did reveal that surprisingly large amounts of copper (average of 13 mg/month from a 14-g bracelet) can be absorbed through the dermis, which would give in 12 months more than the total amount estimated to be present in the human body. The rationale for copper therapy in rheumatic diseases is not at all clear, and little or no information exists concerning copper metabolism in such states other than in rheumatoid arthritis, and that is somewhat conflicting.

In rheumatoid arthritis, serum copper levels are said to be appreciably increased (133, 423, 559, 604, 622, 623) and in the synovial fluid there is an increased level of ceruloplasmin copper, as well as of iron and zinc (558, 559). On the other hand, mean values for the copper levels and superoxide dismutase activity of erythrocytes of male and female subjects with rheumatoid arthritis do not differ significantly from normal controls (696). A marked elevation of nonceruloplasmin serum copper reported by Lorber et al. (466) has not been substantiated (743), which may be due to differences in methodology (465). However, the more recent studies of Bajpayee (29) in which serum ceruloplasmin levels were significantly increased in rheumatoid arthritis patients on estrogens, but were normal in female patients not on estrogens and in male patients, raise serious questions concerning the validity of data previously reported. Bajpayee points out that in prior investigations no effort was made to segregate, from the populations studied, those females who were on estrogen treatment.

Nevertheless, copper has received much attention in the treatment of rheumatoid and other forms of arthritis. The claimed efficacy of intravenous administration of an organic salt of copper (221) is not substantiated (795). Penicillamine has been used with some response in about 80% of cases after 6 months or more of treatment (88, 380). Efforts have been made to enhance the effectiveness of aspirin, salicylates and penicillamine by forming with them copper coordination compounds. As tested only by the rat model for evaluating inflammatory and antiulcer potentials, these have given somewhat equivocal results (626, 728, 729) depending upon the route of administration and the degree of tissue irritation produced. The hypothesis of Sorenson (728, 729) that anti-inflammatory drugs might react in vivo with available copper to generate more effective complexes for regulation of inflammatory or non-inflammatory states certainly justifies further exploration. So also does the question of whether the higher serum copper levels in females as compared to males bears any relation to the high female to male ratio seen in rheumatoid arthritis. Spontaneous remissions of rheumatoid arthritis are associated with obstructive biliary/liver disease and with pregnancy, characterized by increased serum ceruloplasmin levels. These questions are raised by Whitehouse (841) in his review and critical discussion of the topics referred to above. Obviously, there are fertile fields for new explorations of the possible role of copper in arthritis and related diseases.

Pellagra. Krishnamachari (427) describes in pellagrins in India a hypercupremia uniquely due to increase in non-ceruloplasmin copper and associated with wide variation in urinary copper excretion, both of which return to normal levels after oral administrations of nicotinic acid. On the basis of evidence that the high leucine content of the millet *Sorghum vulgare*, a staple food of populations in India, is causally related to pellagra, healthy adult volunteers were given 5-g L-leucine for 6 consecutive days. They showed comparable degrees of hypercupremia and urinary loss both of which disappeared after leu-

cine withdrawal. This investigator suggests that leucine enhances the absorption of dietary copper in normal subjects. From the same area of India is the report of Deosthale and Gopalan (164) that certain varieties of sorghum also greatly increase serum copper levels and urinary copper excretion, attributable to the high molybdenum content of the sorghum samples. Unfortunately, serum levels of direct reacting copper and ceruloplasmin were not determined. Hence, there is need for more critical study of the possible role of leucine and/or molybdenum excesses in producing the hypercupremia and hypercupriuria described in pellagrins, and for confirmation that the hypercupremia is due primarily to increased nonceruloplasmin copper. Bantu pellagrins in South Africa are said to manifest a hypercupremia which is reduced rapidly after an intramuscular injection of pantothenic acid, but not after oral nicotinamide (210). The latter observations carried out 20 years ago, seem not to have been denied or confirmed.

Skin disorders. Elevated serum copper levels occur in psoriasis (400, 430, 531, 751, 859, 872, 875) but not in other dermatoses (872). Although these levels have been generally attributed to increased ceruloplasmin, as a reaction to disturbed keratinization (751, 876), several reports state that ceruloplasmin levels are normal (400, 438) unless associated with conditions of arthritis (423). The tissue copper levels of psoriatic lesions are no different from those of uninvolved skin, although zinc levels are increased (529, 531). After beneficial response to heliotherapy or thalassotherapy most patients show clinical improvement, with return of serum copper ceruloplasmin levels toward normal (875). The mechanisms involved are unknown. With regard to vitiligo, information is both limited and contradictory. This disorder is said to be characterized by hypercupremia, which is reduced in subjects responding favorably to heliotherapy (247, 876), whereas others find that in about 39% of subjects both albumin-bound and ceruloplasmin serum copper levels are below the normal range (372). Again the question of methodology arises.

The states of hypercupremia to which reference has been made clearly indicate the remarkable homeostatic mechanism in copper metabolism. These involve to a large degree the increased synthesis of ceruloplasmin in response to a variety of body stresses, including hormonal influences (44). Also, in body states involving inflammatory reactions, ceruloplasmin may function in the role of an "acute phase reactant" (48, 636, 637).

COPPER TOXICITY

Hemochromatosis. There is a long history of acute and chronic toxicity of copper in man. Some of this was recorded in 1891 by Lehmann (448) who was one of the earliest investigators to test the effects of various copper salts on experimental animals. He also states that two of his students showed no ill effects of additions of up to 10 to 20 mg of copper sulfate and up to 5 to 30 mg of copper acetate to their daily beer. This is somewhat greater than a current estimated toxic level of 10 to 15 mg of inorganic copper for adult man (75, 865). In 1898, Baum and Seeliger (35) described extensive deposition of blood pigments, then designated hematoidin and hemosiderin, in the liver cells of the goat, sheep, dog and cat fed copper salts. These observations were more extensively explored by Mallory et al. (480–484) who reported that chronic oral intake of copper acetate in the rabbit, sheep and monkey produces a condition comparable to hepatic hemosiderosis in man.

Mallory (481) described in detail the hepatic changes characteristic of human hemochromatosis (pigment cirrhosis) based upon 19 necropsies, presenting circumstantial evidence of copper toxicity as basically involved. These interpretations were supported by other pathologists reporting liver copper levels up to 10-fold normal in a large series of cases of hemochromatosis (295, 327, 586). Yet Mills (522) found no evidence of hemochromatosis in 100 necropsies of Korean people using copper and brass utensils routinely in daily life. Although the animal studies of Mallory and coworkers (480, 482, 484) on which their hypothesis of the cause of hemochromatosis was based were also confirmed by certain investigators (295, 519), others attempted in vain to duplicate their results (218, 587, 607). Differences in susceptibility and in levels and duration of exposure to copper salts were proposed (482) to explain the discrepancies in the experimental findings.

Copper poisoning in man The oral ingestion of excess copper produces a metallic taste in the mouth, nausea, vomiting, epigastric pain, diarrhea and, to variable degrees, jaundice, hemolysis, hemoglobinuria, hematuria and oliguria. The vomitus, stool and saliva may appear blue or green. In severe cases, anuria, hypotension and coma occur. The ingested copper is promptly absorbed from the upper gut and rapidly and dramatically increases the level of direct reacting copper in the blood, due in large part to its accumulation in the red blood cells. When this accumulation reaches a certain level, hemolysis occurs, whether it be the result of oral ingestion (120, 203, 641), absorption through denuded skin (353), dialysis procedures (51, 52, 376, 487) or exchange transfusions (50). This hemolysis is comparable to that commonly seen in Wilson's disease, which is attributed to a sudden release of copper into the blood stream from a liver damaged by an increasing load of copper unable to be utilized in ceruloplasmin synthesis or excreted via the biliary system (97, 155, 508, 516). This hemolysis may reflect, to variable degrees, inhibition of erythrocyte glycolysis and of glucose-6-phosphate dehydrogenase, oxidation of glutathione and denaturation of hemoglobin with Heinz body formation (203). A variety of other factors may be involved (588). Manifestations of slow copper poisoning of a non-fatal type as seen in copper and brass workers are well described by Chatterji and Ganguly (111). There are symptoms of laryngitis, bronchitis, intestinal colic with catarrh and diarrhea, general emaciation and anemia.

Since much of the information on copper toxicity comes from instances of accidental or intentional intake (mostly suicide), data concerning oral intake necessary to produce symptoms of toxicity are decidedly meager. Ingestion of 10 to 15 mg of inorganic copper will cause nausea, vomiting and diarrhea and, in larger doses, intravascular hemolysis (75, 865). It has also been stated (685) that in India, where copper sulfate is a frequent mechanism for suicide, such symptoms are seen when about 10 mg of cupric ion are ingested. Yet, Roberts (641), in reviewing cases of copper sulfate poisoning admitted to a large city hospital over 7 years, describes one individual who knowingly consumed an estimated 20 g of copper sulfate two to three times weekly over a period of 4 months (total of about 600 g of the crystals, or about 1.25 g of anionic copper per day). Aside from the usual symptoms of toxicity, there was an associated hemolytic anemia, possibly the earliest recorded as due to copper toxicity. There was reasonably rapid recovery under conventional procedures of that period. Two possible explanations for this unusually high degree of tolerance to copper are that the subject greatly overestimated his previous intake of copper sulfate or that he had adapted to a high copper intake similar to that occurring in pigs (767).

There are numerous reports of accidental and suicidal poisoning from oral intake of copper sulfate in India (111, 118, 120, 288, 813). In one hospital in India, of all cases of accidental poisoning admitted, copper sulfate poisoning represented 33.6% of 238 admissions in 1961 (120) and 26.5% of admissions in a 9-month period during 1969–1970 (112). In cases of acute copper poisoning, analyses of urine and feces for copper give exceedingly high values (111).

Under more normal circumstances of daily living, varied degrees of copper toxicity have been recorded, as for example: 1) in young infants presumably exposed via drinking water and cooked foods, to water derived from all-copper storage and conduit systems (662, 816); 2) in children given tablets containing sulfates of copper, iron and manganese (220) or accidentally consuming a solution of copper sulfate (819); 3) in workers imbibing tea made from water contaminated by corroded geysers (557, 701); 4) in consumers of carbonated beverages from post-mix type of vending machines with defective valves (356, 450), or from bottles with corroded pouring spouts (512); 5) in consumers of alcoholic beverages left in copper-lined containers (865) or brewed at home in metal containers (633); 6) in children given copper sulfate as an emetic (355); and 7) in subjects after exchange transfusions (50) and hemodialyses (51, 52, 376, 471, 472, 487, 497), due to copper present in tap-water used, or to copper-containing valves and stopcocks used, in the conduits. Copper can cross dialyzing membranes, even against a concentration gradient, and rather small traces of copper introduced intraveneously are highly toxic. Frequently, the result is hemolytic anemia. Hemodialysis has proved to be ineffective in treating acute copper poisoning, but this may have been due to a delay of 13 hours in instituting treatment (10). Bremner (60) reviews the toxicity of copper and other heavy metals and Cohen (121) discusses health hazards from industrial exposure to copper.

At times it may be difficult in young infants to determine whether a state of toxicosis is attributable to an early phase of Wilson's disease or to high levels of copper in the family drinking water from copper pipes (816). Ever since the development of metal conduits for potable water, man has been exposed to possibilities of zinc poisoning from galvanized pipes, and of copper poisoning from copper conduits and storage tanks. In certain city water supplies, copper salts are added to maintain a concentration of about 0.06 ppm to restrict the growth of algae in the reservoirs (550). It is also recognized that soft waters tend to leach copper conduits more than do hard waters. An impressive analysis of complexities involved in engineering design of copper conduit systems to reduce the corrosion process itself, and to minimize the retention time of water in small-bore tubes, has been presented by Page (591). Nevertheless, these problems are more or less controlled by cosmetic considerations, since water with high copper content develops a surface scum due to formation of insoluble copper compounds. It is generally accepted that a limit of 1 ppm of copper in supplies of drinking water is safe and acceptable.

Copper represents one of the earliest additives for enhancement of the appeal of foods such as green peas, beans and pickles. The early studies of Drummond (171) failed to demonstrate in experimental animals (dogs, cats) any deleterious effects from consumption of such "greened" vegetables. It is now generally accepted that in the processes of cooking, canning and storage of foods and beverages any increment in copper content is largely related to contact with copper in the vessels and conduits utilized. In present day societies hazards are reduced to a minimum. These and other aspects of copper toxicity are well reviewed by Lich (459).

INTERRELATIONSHIPS BETWEEN COPPER AND OTHER TRACE ELEMENTS

Studies on laboratory and farm animals have revealed numerous interrelationships between copper and other trace elements and substances (notably iron, zinc, molybdenum, cadmium and ascorbic acid) in mammalian metabolism (332, 333). On the basis of some of these reactions, Hill and Matrone (332) advanced the thesis that "those elements whose physical and chemical properties are similar will act antagonistically to each other biologically." This concept has since been well substantiated. Davies (149, 150) classifies interactions between trace elements as non-competitive, and multi-element reactions. The non-competitive type is exemplified by the requirement of dietary copper for mobilization of iron for hemoglobin synthesis, as discussed earlier (pp. 1985–1986), and by interactions between molybdenum, sulfur and copper in ruminants as recently reviewed by Suttle (766) and Pitt (603). Interactions of this type are not predictable from a knowledge of the chemistry of the elements in question, as are those of the competitive type. The latter type is evident in the mutually antagonistic effects of copper and zinc, such as the protective effect of copper in reducing toxicity resulting from high dietary intakes of zinc in chicks (332); and the effect of increased dietary intake of zinc in increasing the tolerance of pigs to excess intake of copper (767, 768). The multi-element type of interaction is seen in studies with chicks where dietary zinc induces or exacerbates a conditioned deficiency of copper which in turn restricts the utilization of iron (332).

Speaking in general terms, in non-ruminants interactions of copper with iron and zinc are of particular significance whereas in ruminants interactions of copper with molybdenum in the presence of sulfur take precedence, especially in terms of practical considerations in animal husbandry. Molybdenum toxicity, long recognized in grazing cattle in many parts of the world, causes biochemical and pathological changes closely resembling those of copper deficiency, as well recognized in the pioneer studies of Davis (150). They are readily prevented or cured by copper sulfate. Compared to cattle, sheep are less susceptible to high dietary intakes of molybdenum and more susceptible to low intake of molybdenum, which can lead to chronic copper poisoning (798). Species reactions vary greatly (603).

Non-ruminants are much more tolerant of excess molybdenum and of high copper intake than are ruminants. Moreover, effects of high dietary copper can be accentuated by low levels of zinc and iron, and low copper intake by ascorbic acid which is thought to interfere with the absorption of copper. An interesting difference is that in ruminants dietary sulfur potentiates a copper-molybdenum antagonism such that tissue copper levels are decreased, whereas in non-ruminants sulfur alleviates this antagonism. Moreover, the capacities of dietary sulfur to accentuate or ameliorate the toxic effects of molybdenum vary with the copper status of the animal. Among the proposals offered to explain the basic mechanisms involved have been: 1) formation in the rumen of unabsorbable complexes such as thiomolybdate, cupric sulfide or cupric molybdate; 2) interference of liver uptake of copper by molybdenum and sulfur; and 3) formation of stable complexes of copper and molybdenum in the plasma. Obviously, much remains to be clarified.

Copper is quite routinely incorporated in mineral mixtures added to commercial livestock feeds to increase rate of weight gain and food efficiency and is recognized as a safe ingredient (up to a level of 15 ppm), but regulations prohibit molybdenum additions. Under conditions in which both forage and feeds are naturally low in molybdenum, states of copper toxicity, often fatal, have occurred in flocks of sheep (798). This practice of adding excess copper without molybdenum to livestock and poultry feeds represents a potential hazard to the consuming public, especially to the young infant consuming baby foods made from liver (71). The practical as well as the purely scientific aspects of trace element interactions, complex as they may be, fully justify some consideration. For further information on the complex interrelationships between molybdenum, sulfate and copper, the reader is referred to a number of reviews on the subject (71, 110, 140, 165, 493, 517, 603, 766, 798) and to a series of recent research reports (110).

In man, there is but fragmentary evidence of significant interrelationships of copper and molybdenum, and of a role of molybdenum in human nutrition. By virtue of molybdenum being a component of xanthine oxidase, it may participate in the reduction of cellular ferric to ferrous ferritin such that high copper-molybdenum ratio may contribute to abnormalities of iron metabolism and utilization (698, 699). It is postulated that high copper-molybdenum ratios in the American diet may contribute to iron-deficiency anemias and may also have influence upon metabolic abnormalities of copper metabolism such as seen in Wilson's disease (699). From India come several interesting reports dealing with high molybdenum-copper ratios. Volunteers fed diets containing sorghum with increasing content of molybdenum showed increasing levels of urinary copper excretion, which appeared to reflect mobilization of copper from body stores (164). In regions where creation of large dams brings about marked changes in trace element balance in the soil, food grains and drinking water tend to acquire a high molybdenum-copper ratio as molybdenum is leached out by alkaline conditions and the ratio possibly increased further by high fluoride content of soils. As a result the poorest groups of the population whose staple food is sorghum, which accumulates more molybdenum than rice or wheat, become victims of genu valgum and osteoporosis of the long bones (9, 428). Genu valgum, previously considered the result of fluoride toxicosis, now appears to represent either a state of molybdenosis or one of copper deficiency induced by excess molybdenum, or a modification of either by high fluoride intake. In experimental and farm animals there are characteristic differences in osseous lesions in these two conditions, as well described by Asling and Hurley (26). In the studies discussed above no reference is made to the status of farm animals in the same localities, or to any plan to test effects of the sorghum versus other diets upon experimental animals. Returning to the capacity of molybdenum to reduce tissue copper levels and to increase urinary excretion of copper, Suttle (766) has questioned whether or not molybdenum might have therapeutic value in the treatment of Wilson's disease, apparently unaware of one report (74) of its ineffectiveness in four cases of the disease treated for 4 to 11 months.

In the case of trace elements occurring mainly in ionic form, such as molybdenum, selenium and iodine, deficiencies and excesses are readily reflected in components of the food chain and in not only grazing animals but also in man himself (515). An interesting example of this and of copper-molybdenum interactions may be cited. In mountainous areas of Russia where the soil is notoriously high in molybdenum, a high incidence of molybdenum toxicity, characterized not by genu valgum but by increased blood xanthine oxidase and uric acid, and urinary uric acid, leading to symptoms of gout, was observed in the population of one province but not in that of another where molybdenum intake was equally high; the difference was ascribed to significantly higher blood copper and resultant lower blood molybdenum levels in the non-affected population (424, 425). Data pertaining to these studies are summarized by Mertz (515). The explanation proposed is in accord with extensive knowledge of such interactions in experimental and farm animals.

Interactions between copper and zinc have long been recognized in animals and man. Excess of one is often associated with diminution of the other in body fluids and liver. Competition for binding sites on metallothionein or metallothionein-like proteins, complex as these interactions appear to be (518), provides the best explanation. These proteins are present in the liver, kidney, intestinal mucosa, pancreas and spleen. They play an important role in copper homeostasis. In man, these reciprocal interactions are less apparent than in animals where the intake and imbalance of the elements can be more specifically controlled. However, a striking example is the reported occurrence of typical copper deficiency, with microcytic hypochromic anemia and leukopenia, in one patient, and very low levels of serum copper in 7 of 13 others, receiving unusually high levels of zinc for the treatment of sickle cell anemia (64). All responded favorably to daily supplements of copper.

The question of the dietary ratio of zinc to copper has been given considerable attention by Kelvay (416–418, 420) in support of a hypothesis that high zinc to copper ratio and the associated hypercholesteremia increase the risk of ischemic heart disease, and may also play an important role in the genesis of arteriosclerosis. This hypothesis has received limited support (81, 82). Of some relevance are recent observations that myocardial lesions associated with hypercholesteremia occur in rats fed a copper-deficient diet for 7 to 9 weeks after weaning (16). Cardiac hypertrophy, subendocardial hemorrhage, necrosis of muscle fibers, abnormalities of elastic tissue of the aorta but not of the coronary arteries, and occasional heart rupture are described. In other studies with copper-deficient rats similar lesions have been observed and ascribed to a marked reduction in cytochrome c oxidase activity (3, 401). With repletion of copper, cytochrome c oxidase activity is normalized, after which cardiac hypertrophy and splenomegaly are greatly reduced (3). Unquestionably, interest has been stimulated, but there is need for specific research on man directed toward the possible role of zinc/copper ratios and cholesterol status in ischemic heart disease.

HUMAN REQUIREMENTS

In discussing requirements of any nutrient, a variety of terms are in common usage, such as "basic," "minimal" and "optimal" requirements; and "recommended" allowances. An excellent discussion and definition of these terms has been presented by Mertz (514). According to his interpretation, the "basic" requirement for a trace element represents that daily intake permitting absorption of an amount just sufficient to prevent a state of deficiency; whereas the "optimal" requirement represents that daily intake which will allow maintenance at a near-optimal level of all biological and physiological functions in which the element is involved, under the various stress conditions of life. The somewhat intermediate term "minimal," traditionally used in balance studies, is defined as that daily intake which equals the daily excretory loss from the body. This term best fits the nature of the data on which estimates of human requirements for copper are based. The term "optimal" is somewhat comparable to the term "recommended dietary allowance." According to Harper (307), the RDA represents estimates of the amount of an essential nutrient which "each person in a healthy population must consume in order to provide reasonable assurance that physiological needs will be met."

In the case of copper requirements, the problem is not as simple as it might appear. Most difficult to evaluate are the reported differences in the copper content of foods, diets, body fluids and tissues attributable to the great variety of analytical methods employed over the past half century, and to possible contamination of samples prior to or during analytical procedures. An excellent discussion and critical appraisal of methods in use up to 1965 for the determination of copper and ceruloplasmin in biological materials is presented by Sass-Kortsak (666). The methods described have been variably modified and newer ones introduced. In some instances there is rather remarkable agreement between early and later reports. In other instances there appear differences which, on inspection, might reflect variable sensitivity of the methods employed. Any effort to identify and evaluate methodologies used in particular studies would be rather futile.

What has been outlined in this conspectus, up to this point, has been an assessment of past and current knowledge regarding the role that copper may play in the metabolism of man, with occasional reference to ancillary information gained from observations on laboratory and farm animals. Attention has been called to the distribution of copper in the body; the vast array of cuproproteins and evidence as to their roles in maintaining functional and morphological integrity of specific tissues and organs; the absorption, transport and excretion of copper; its omnipresence in foods; its important roles in prenatal and postnatal life, and; the nature of states induced by naturally occurring, experimentally induced and congenitally determined copper deficiency. It is hoped that this digest of knowledge will provide an adequate basis for considerations of the minimal copper requirements of man.

In considering human requirements for copper there are many factors whose influence is exceedingly difficult to evaluate because of limited knowledge available. A few examples may be cited. That portion of dietary copper which is actually absorbed probably varies considerably, depending upon its chemical state in the foods consumed and the influence of other dietary components. Best estimates indicate an absorption of 40 to 60% of the oral intake (p. 1991). In addition to the unabsorbed copper and biliary copper components of the feces, inadequate consideration has been given to contributions provided by secretions of the salivary glands, gastric and intestinal mucosa and pancreas, and by dehiscence of epithelial cells of intestinal villi. At least, the extent of reabsorption of copper released via these various pathways has not been clearly determined. Despite frequent statements in the literature that some of the copper in bile may be reabsorbed, there exists other evidence that this copper is so firmly bound to proteins that it is not reabsorbed by the gall bladder or intestinal mucosa in any significant amounts (266).

Balance studies are limited by the precision with which intake and output can be measured. For an element such as copper which has a slow rate of turnover, a variable degree of intestinal absorption, strong homeostatic mechanisms and an almost exclusive output via the feces, interpretations of balance studies becomes very difficult. The sporadic nature of defecation and rather wide individual variation make balance studies of 7 to 14 days necessary for obtaining valid data. Replacement of carmine by polyethylene glycol 4000, as a fecal marker, should shorten this time period (848).

Biological availability is also an important but largely unknown factor. Little is known about the chemical nature of copper in foods, the extent to which it may react with chelating substances such as dietary fiber, or how its absorption may be influenced by the protein-binding potentialities of other trace elements such as zinc and molybdenum. To these factors must be added the inflence of acute and chronic infections, use of antimicrobial agents, dysfunction of the gastrointestinal tract and other stress states. Usually, in well conducted copper balance studies on man, healthy subjects are selected and as many as possible of the above mentioned influences are eliminated. The discussion to follow will focus on accumulated evidence from balance studies and from experiences with total parenteral nutrition as to what may represent the minimal requirements of man for copper during infancy, childhood and adulthood.

Infants

Specific requirements of healthy human infants for copper have been difficult to determine with any degree of accuracy. To provide a picture of the problem, it seems appropriate to review current information with respect to: 1) milk as a source of copper for the premature and full-term infant; 2) copper balance studies on infants; 3) naturally occurring states of copper deficiency; and 4) studies on infants largely or totally dependent upon total parenteral nutrition (hyperalimentation) for extended periods of time.

Milk as a source of copper. It has long been recognized that the copper content of human milk is two to three times higher than that of cow's milk, and that the content of human colostrum is two to three times that of later milk (437, 449, 541, 647, 877). Moreover, the somewhat lower ratio of zinc to copper (about 4:1) in human milk may significantly enhance copper absorption in breast-fed infants (843).

Cow's milk has a very low content of copper. Values recorded by different investigators have varied widely, and their documentation would serve no useful purpose. Suffice it to say that three of the more recent reports (546, 598, 843) give values within a range of 0.04 to 0.30 mg/liter. Difference in forage and in season of the year are largely responsible for variations in values obtained. Special attention may be called to analyses of commercial milk samples from 65 cities throughout the USA giving a national mean of 0.086 (range 0.04–0.19) mg/liter (547).

The first serious study of the copper content of human milk, by Zondek and Bandmann (877), indicated levels of 0.5 to 0.6 mg/liter in 85 samples obtained during the first 2 months of lactation. Munch-Peterson (541), who carried out 74 analyses of milk from 10 mothers during the first 8 days of lactation, recorded a mean content of 0.48 mg/liter. He also found that intravenous administration of a water-soluble compound containing 19% of copper given to seven other mothers had no influence on the copper content of the milk, even though serum copper levels were greatly increased. This confirmed the early report of Elvehjem et al. (189) that a 5 to 10-fold increase in dietary intake of copper had no demonstrable effect on its level in the milk of the cow or goat. This restriction in mammary transfer of copper might reflect a homeostatic mechanism for protection of the neonate. Rottger (647) reported a mean value of 0.44 (range 0.27–0.84) mg/liter for 15 samples of human milk during early phases of lactation. Munch-Peterson (541) and Rottger (647) independently estimated a daily intake of about 0.25 mg/Cu by young infants. In comparison, other investigators have reported higher values for early milk (107, 437, 449) and others give values approximately one-half or less than those recorded above, for mature human milk not identified as early milk (275, 546, 598, 843). A striking decrease in copper content of milk

at successive months of lactation (11.2, 7.3, 5.4, 4.6 and 1.5 µg/100 ml) is reported by Kleinbaum (410). Similar data are given by Hambidge (299).

Noteworthy is the recent and extensive study of Picciano and Guthrie (598), based on analyses of 350 milk samples from 50 lactating, healthy women (seven samples each). Copper content varied considerably among women and with the same woman. Several samples taken over periods of days or weeks were necessary to provide a reliable estimate of the copper content of milk from any individual. Their mean value of 0.24 (range 0.09–0.63) mg/liter is essentially the same as that reported by Murthy and Rhea (546); namely, about 0.24 ± 0.08 mg/kg, on analyses of 22 milk samples from lactating women.

Picciano and Guthrie (598) calculated that breastfed infants less than 3 months of age, with a body weight of 4 kg and a daily milk intake of 850 ml, would ingest approximately 0.2 mg/day (or 0.05 mg/kg/day). These estimates are in good agreement with the values of 0.25 mg/day of Munch-Peterson (541) and Rottger (647), also based upon human milk. They are also slightly less than estimates of 0.05 to 0.10 mg/kg/day based on balance studies with young children 3 to 6 years of age (142, 695), the estimate of 0.08 mg/kg/day by Cartwright (100), and the statement of the Committee on Recommended Dietary Allowances of the National Research Council (549) that "The requirements of infants and children have been estimated at between 0.05 and 0.1 mg/kg of body weight per day; an intake of 0.08 mg/kg/day appears to be adequate." The World Health Organization in its 1973 report (861) recommends 0.08 mg/kg per day for infants and young children and 0.04 mg/kg per day for older children. It would seem that under normal circumstances the copper provided by nature in human milk is, when supplemented by storage in the newborn liver, a reasonably good measure of optimal requirements during early life.

The premature infant presents special problems. According to Widdowson et al. (843) about ¾ of fetal copper is transferred during the last 10 to 12 weeks of gestation. As a consequence, premature infants of 28 to 30 weeks gestation, weighing about 1 kg, have much smaller reserves of copper in the liver, spleen and other tissues to be called upon postnatally than do full-term infants. Sultanova (761) has carried out copper analyses of livers and spleens from groups of premature infants with birth weights of 1.0 to 1.5, 1.5 to 2.0 and 2.0 to 2.5 kg, and term infants dying soon after birth. In successive groups there were definite increases in the copper levels per gram of tissue in both organs. Hence, the smaller the premature the lower the copper concentration in its tissues. As another handicap, the premature is usually obliged to subsist on an exclusive milk diet for much longer periods than the full-term infant. Although in newborn prematures copper deficiency is unknown, their status does place them in a more precarious situation than full-term infants when states of malnutrition intervene. To compensate for this, Widdowson et al. (843) have suggested that premature infants be provided a special milk formula which might assure a retention of at least 0.085 mg of copper per day. Cordano (124) feels that for prematures the recommended 0.06 mg/100 kcal for infants (18) should be increased to 0.09 mg/100 kcal (i.e., 0.1 mg/kg/day). This is the current recommendation of the American Academy of Pediatrics (19) for low-birth-rate infants.

Balance studies. A pioneer balance study of copper in infancy, to which relatively little has since been added, is that of Kleinbaum (409), who studied six breast-fed full-term infants over the 13th to 23rd days of life. Birth weights averaged 3.4 kg, but later weights are not given. Total copper intake and output for the 10-day period averaged 4.74 and 4.72 mg, respectively. Three infants showed a negative and three a positive copper balance. Hence, these data might be interpreted as indicating that healthy full-term infants during the first month of life require an intake of approximately 0.5 mg/Cu/day to keep in positive balance. The 10-day balance study of Priev (619) on two infants 8 and 3 months of age indicates requirements of 0.30 and 0.42 mg/day, respectively. Similar 10-day balance studies of Kleinbaum (409) on 31 premature infants initiated at ages of 2 to 82 days, and with average intakes of 0.28 mg reveal a slightly negative balance in all instances. Hence in the balance studies described there is reasonably good accord with a requirement of approximately 0.05 mg/kg/day for maintaining a positive copper balance in young infants of the six infants weighing in the range of 6 to 10 kg.

States of copper deficiency. In studies with experimental animals, while the daily intake necessary to prevent development of a deficiency of a nutrient provides the most reliable estimate of basic requirements, a determination of the smallest intake necessary to effect cure of an early stage of deficiency also provides the next best estimate of minimal requirements. Such procedures are, for many reasons, not applicable to man at any age. Even though an arbitrary level of therapy might prove to be marginal in effect, deficiencies or even excesses of other nutrients, together with malabsorption and diarrhea, are usually present and a simple deficiency state such as obtainable in experimental animals does not exist.

Such a situation characterizes the pioneer studies of Cordano et al. (126) on four malnourished infants manifesting anemia, neutropenia, scurvy-like bone changes and hypocupremia. Rehabilitation on high caloric diets supplemented with iron, ascorbic acid, folic acid and other vitamins was incomplete without the addition of elemental copper. In fact, it was later recognized that the increased growth rate resulting from the improved diet greatly decreased the protective effect of the low levels of copper provided by the milk diet (28–42 μg/kg body weight). On the basis of varied levels of copper supplementation it was estimated that for rapidly growing infants 6 to 9 months of age, with inadequate stores of copper and maintained exclusively on milk diets, the daily requirement for copper was greater than 0.042 mg but less than 0.135 mg/kg body weight. Since each of the children weighed approximately 10 kg at the beginning of supplementation, these values are slightly higher than those derived from balance studies but approximate the estimated requirements of 0.077 to 0.11 mg/kg body weight for growing pigs (772). In later studies on 21 similar infants 4 to 19 months of age (128), daily supplements of greater than 0.15 mg/kg proved quite adequate to correct for neutropenia, considered to be the earliest manifestation and most sensitive indicator of adequacy of treatment of copper deficiency in man. Subsequently, oral supplements of 2.5 mg/day were usually employed as a routine measure to assure much more than estimated requirements (276).

On the basis of his personal experiences, Cordano (124, 125) recommends that manufactured formulas for premature infants be supplemented with copper such as to provide 0.09 mg/100 kcal, rather than the 0.06 mg/100 kcal recommended by the Committee on Nutrition of the American Academy of Pediatrics (19) which, since then, has recognized this need. This provides approximately 0.1 mg/kg/day, and is somewhat less than the supplement of 0.1 to 0.5 mg/day proposed by Ashkenazi et al. (25) for prematures subsisting on milk only. In such considerations there has been recognized a need to make provision for such commonplace factors as intestinal interactions between copper and iron in iron-fortified formulas (700), regurgitation, prolonged diarrhea and infections. On the basis of the evidence presented, it seems that the daily requirement of copper for young and reasonably healthy infants may be met by daily intakes of 0.05 to 0.1 mg/kg/day.

Total parenteral nutrition. The development of a procedure for providing "total parenteral nutrition" by means of an infusate of nutrients introduced via an indwelling catheter inserted into a large central vein by Dudrick et al. (176)and Wilmore et al. (852, 853) ushered in a new era in therapeutic nutrition. Its original application in conjunction with surgical treatment of catastrophic gastrointestinal anomalies of infants has since been widely extended to the management of a variety of gastrointestinal disorders, burns, infections and other situations in which subjects are unable to meet nutritional needs by the oral route. By appropriate modifications, this procedure has been effectively ex-tended from its hospital applications to the prolonged maintenance of subjects in the home environment (66, 304, 385, 441, 711, 724). Total parenteral nutrition, especially when prolonged in infants and adults, has provided much new and helpful information concerning copper requirements of man.

However, problems arise in the interpretation of the results. One must first assume that copper introduced parenterally substitutes for that portion of orally ingested copper absorbed by the intestinal tract and transported to the liver and to the systemic vascular system. While, as discussed previously (p. 1991), it is generally accepted that roughly 40 to 60% of ingested copper is absorbed, wide individual variations exist, due to differences in gastrointestinal functions, nature of the diet, derangements of metabolism and states of stress.

It is noteworthy that in their classic studies with infants, Dudrick et al. (175, 176) and Wilmore et al. (853) took care to provide in their parenteral fluids both vitamins and minerals. The latter included zinc, copper, manganese, cobalt and iodine. Copper was provided at a level of 0.22 mg/kg body weight. This represents a rather generous supply when compared to estimated requirements of 0.05 to 0.10 mg/kg/day. In any case, failure to follow these guidelines resulted in occurrence of several cases of copper deficiency in infants (25, 394, 463) and in adults (177, 808).

Although traces of copper are present in fibrin and casein hydrolysates and in crystalline amino acid mixtures commonly used in parenteral solutions, direct analyses (57, 317, 342, 590) demonstrate their variability and inadequacy to meet nutritional needs for copper. The proposed use of plasma transfusions given twice weekly (209) does not compensate for this (704). What is said of copper is also true of zinc (57, 342, 590). Investigators now add trace elements to the basic hyperalimentation formulae (174, 214, 367, 382, 383, 709, 710, 712, 724) providing copper in approximately the amount (0.22 mg/kg body weight) originally proposed by Wilmore et al. (853). Essentially the same supplement is recommended by Ricour et al. (639), Wretling (864) and by Karpel and Peden

TABLE 1

Copper balance studies—children 3 to 10 years old

References	Subjects' age and sex	Type of diet	Period of study[1]	Copper intake	Copper loss	Copper balance	Estimated daily requirement	Method[2]
			day	mg/day	mg/day	mg/day	mg/kg/day	
Daniels and Wright (1934)	3–6 yr (5 M-3 F)	Meat + milk or cereal + milk	5	1.48	1.03	+0.45	0.1	COL
Scoular (1938)	3–6 yr (3 M)	Mixed, controlled, 3 types	5	1.36	0.60	+0.76	0.053–0.085	SPG
Macy (1944)	8–11 yr	Self-selected 8 yr / 11 yr		4.9 / 5.2		+2.7 / +3.1	0.08 / 0.05	Not given
Engel et al. (1967)	6–10 yr (12 F)	Liberal protein, controlled	4	1.18	1.19	+0.01	2.05	COL
Engel et al (1967)	6–10 yr (12 F)	Low animal protein, controlled	4	1.06	1.14	-0.08	(but with allowance of 1.25 for sweat loss and safety factor)	COL
Engel et al (1967)	6–10 yr (12 F)	Vegetarian type	4	3.35	2.33	+1.02		COL
Price et al (1970)	7–9 yr (15 F)	Representative of low income group, USA (5 diets)	6	1.67	1.01	+0.66	Similar	AASM
Price and Bunce (1972)	7–9 yr (15 F)	Same + supplements Ca and N. (4 diets)	6	0.99	0.95	+0.04	Similar	AASM

[1] After period of 3 to 8 days of adjustment to diet before balance study. [2] AASM-atomic absorption spectrometry; COL-colorimetric; SPG-spectrographic.

(394) after experiences in compensating for a copper deficiency state developing in an infant with ileal atresia and short bowel syndrome maintained on total parenteral nutrition for the first 6.75 months of life. In current practice for complete intravenous feeding of premature infants of less than 1,050 g birth weight, James and MacMahon (383) provide 50 μg/kg/day of copper. Quite in accord with these opinions are those of Ashkenazi et al. (25), recording copper deficiency in a premature infant 6 months old fed a diet of only whole milk and 5% cane sugar, and in a premature infant subjected to bowel surgery and maintained on parenteral feeding for 3 months. Both responded rapidly to oral copper, and investigators recommended that small premature infants be given supplements of 0.1 to 0.5 mg of copper daily while milk is their only food, or during prolonged intravenous feeding.

On the basis of the evidence cited above, it seems reasonable to assume that the daily requirement of intravenous copper for infants, beyond the age at which they can depend upon prenatal tissue reserves (about 2 months), may be in the range of 0.1 to 0.2 mg/day. On the assumption that approximately 40% of orally ingested copper is absorbed, this requirement would be the equivalent of 0.25 to 0.5 mg/day of oral copper. For a 10-kg infant this would represent 0.025 to 0.05 mg/kg/day. Thus, the information provided by parenteral nutrition is in general concordance with that from studies in milk intake, copper balance and recovery from deficiency states, which indicate requirements of about 0.025 to 0.05 mg/kg/day for healthy full-term infants during early years of life, with somewhat more generous allowances for premature and low-birth-rate infants.

Young children and adolescents

The basis for determining the minimal daily requirements of copper for young children and adolescents is decidedly limited, as is indicated in table 1. Two pioneer studies on 3- to 6-year old children (142, 695), although carried out 40 or more years ago, warrant special consideration. Daniels and Wright (142) studied five boys and three girls and employed two diets, one high in meat and cereals and the other high in cereals without meat, but similar in copper content. After 3 days of adjustment to the diet, 5-day balance studies were made. Mean copper intakes, fecal plus urinary excretions and balances were, respectively, 1.48, 1.03 and +0.45 mg/day. It was concluded that diets for children of pre-school age should include not less than 0.10 mg/kg/day of copper. Scoular (695) carried out similar balance studies on three boys of the same age, based upon three different but well controlled diets. On the average, copper intakes, fecal and urinary losses and retentions were, respectively, 1.36, 0.60, and +0.76 mg/kg/day. In their best judgment, the minimal requirement of boys of that age would be between 0.053 and 0.085 mg/kg/day. Similar conclusions were reached by Macy (477) in balance studies on school children 8 and 11 years of age. It may be noted that both of these estimates fall within the range of estimated copper requirements for infants (0.05–0.1 mg/kg/day) as discussed above.

Balance studies carried out by Engel et al. (190) on groups of 12 girls 6 to 10 years of age, during summer months of 1956, 1958 and 1962, employing liberal protein, low animal protein and vegetarian type diets, leave open questions concerning requirements. Calculations made (by writer) from the data given indicate that the first two of these diets provided average copper intakes of 0.04 and 0.037 mg/kg/day and copper balances of −0.01 and −0.08 mg/day, respectively. Comparable values for the vegetarian diet were 0.12 mg/kg/day and +1.02 mg/day. These data would suggest a minimal intake somewhat less than proposed in the two studies just described. However, Engel et al. (190) estimated, by regression analysis, that the daily intake in their studies was 1.3 mg/day, and that the suggested allowance be 2.5 mg/day. In this suggestion was included a sweat loss of 0.5 mg/day and a safety margin of 0.7 mg/day, added to the 1.3 mg/day intake. For matters of comparison, sweat loss was not incorporated in other balance studies recorded, and the estimated loss appears to be more than generous for the subjects. Furthermore, the

TABLE 2

Dietary copper intakes—human adults

Reference	Subjects	Type of diet	Period of collection (days)	Copper intake (mg/day)	Method[1]
Soman et al. (1969)	Not given	24-hour diet composites from 9 regions of India	—		AASP
		Ovovegetarian (4)		5.7	
		Nonvegetarian (5)		7.1	
White (1969)	College st. 21 F	33 diet composites	—	0.58±0.9	EMSP
	High sch. 15 F	Self-selected (24 hr diets)		0.34±0.23	
Gormican (1970)	Not given	5 diets highest in copper, out of hospital diets	—	0.53	EMSP
Guthrie (1973)	11 F	unrestricted (New Zealand)	3–21	2.4	AASM
Guthrie and Robinson (1977)	(19–21 yrs) 12 F	Dormitory diet (no liver)	3–21	1.5	AASM
	(20–50 yrs) 11 F	Self-selected, non-institutional (with liver)	3–21	7.6	
Brown et al. (1977)	Not given	Hospital diet (regular)	7	0.9 ±0.8	AASM
		Hospital diet (vegetarian)		1.1 ±0.09	AASP
Holden et al. (1978)	11 M, 11 F	Self-selected	14	1.0 ±0.4	AASP

[1] AASM—atomic absorption spectrometry; AASP—atomic absorption spectrophotometry; EMSP—emission spectroscopy.

margin of safety factor does not apply to estimates of minimal requirements. Considering evidence that in their first two studies intakes of about 0.04 mg/kg/day resulted in relatively small negative balances, and accepting small losses in sweat (largely dependent upon degrees of physical activity) but disregarding safety allowances, minimal requirements would be somewhat less than those proposed by Daniels and Wright (142), and in accord with those of Scoular (695). It is to be noted that the estimates for sweat and safety do bring up the unexpectedly low estimates of requirements to what was then the generally accepted level of 2.5 mg/day.

Later studies by Price et al. (618) at the same institution designed to test diets composed of foods consumed by low income groups in the Southeastern United States, varying in protein and calcium content (which had no influence on copper balances), involved 15 girls 7 to 9 years of age. All five diets used maintained good positive balances at intakes averaging 1.67 mg/day (from the range of body weights given, this represents about 0.05–0.07 mg/kg body weight). In other studies by Price and Bunce (617) on 16 girls of the same age, the average intake of copper was approximately 1 mg/day, yet sufficient to maintain positive balance. Not included in the table because of lack of comparable data, is a study on eight healthy children ranging in age from ¾ to 10 years, maintained on home diets, in whom mean intakes, excretions and balances were 0.035, 0.030 and +0.005 mg/kg/day, respectively, and intakes ranged from 0.2 mg/day at 3 months to 0.65 mg/day at about 8 years of age (15). The short balance period of 3 days in these studies may account for the rather low values obtained.

Despite difficulties in comparing results of the few balance studies recorded on young or preadolescent children, there is little reason to dispute the requirement estimates of 0.05 to 0.1 mg/kg/day made by Daniels and Wright (142) and Scoular (695). It may be noted that these are twice the estimated copper requirements of growing infants. Unfortunately, there are no data to indicate whether during puberty and post-pubertal adolescence any significant changes in copper requirements occur. Considering the rather bizarre food intakes and eating habits of this segment of populations, there is real need for copper balance studies on pre-college teenagers. Except for the inconclusive observations of Dawson et al. (152), no consideration has been given to the special nutritional requirements, including those of copper, in teen-age pregnancies. Considering that in such situations there is need to meet growth requirements of the adolescent mother as well as those of the developing fetus, it may be assumed that requirements are appreciably greater than in adult pregnant women.

Adults

Since adults are past the growing phase of life, copper requirements are expressed in terms of mg/day rather than as mg/kg/day, as in the case of infants and adolescents.

Dietary intake. An earlier section (pp. 1998–1999) deals with the wide variation in copper content of human diets in various countries and of individuals of different ages. Table 2 summarizes additional data from studies in which the daily dietary intake of copper (often as only one of many trace elements), exclusive of copper balance, was of primary concern. Indian diets, which are predominately vegetarian in composition, are notably high in copper content. Analyses of diets of ovovegetarian and nonvegetarian populations in India by Soman (727) indicate, by writers's calculation from the data given, intakes of about 5.7 and 7.1 mg/day, respectively. An exceptionally high content of copper in Indian diets is also reported by De (154) as shown in table 3. These values are considerably in excess of those reported from other countries. Only in the studies of Guthrie (289, 291) is mention made of the influence of liver, well known to be much higher in copper than other food constituents. In other studies in which composition of the diet employed is given, liver has not been listed as an ingredient. Somewhat surprising are the low copper levels found in student diets (White), hospital diets (Gormican; Brown et al.) and self-selected diets (Holden et al.). The values reported

are appreciably lower than those for comparable types of diets in the balance studies recorded in table 3. The studies summarized in table 2 merely give some picture of variations in the copper intake of small groups of individuals in several different countries. They provide no valid information concerning requirements for copper, since there is no evidence of their ability to maintain positive balance over long periods of time. To a certain extent the same may be said of traditional balance studies such as recorded in table 3, but the latter do provide data on copper retention, in terms of intake less fecal excretion. While they provide data over only a limited period of days or weeks, they do represent a measure of daily requirements somewhat equivalent to that provided by total parenteral nutrition.

Balance studies. Table 3 summarizes, in chronological sequence, data pertaining to balance studies on human adults. In 6 of the first 10 studies, extending from 1934 to 1954, the estimated requirement ranges from 2.0 to 2.6 mg/day. These data provided the basis for the wide acceptance of 2.0 or 2.0 to 2.5 mg as the daily requirement of copper for adult man. However, Cartwright and Wintrobe (106) later state that at lower levels of intake adjustments may be made to reduce copper excretion such that the daily requirement would be less than 2 mg and might even be negligible. Presumably, a major factor in this adjustment would be a call upon copper stores in the liver and other organs.

The levels of copper intake reported by Holt and Scoular (349) are truly excessive and the investigators, noting the much lower values recorded by Leverton and Binkley (452) for college students fed similar diets, somewhat naively attribute this difference to "a regional effect upon the composition of food." Considering also the unreasonably low fecal and urinary loss and high retention values (calculated from tabular data reported but not commented upon in the report) the atypical results recorded suggest unknown defects in methodology. The somewhat high copper content of Indian diets of De (154) is in accord with the observations of Soman (727), table 1. Whether the predominantly

TABLE 3

Copper balance—human adults

References	Subjects	Type of diet	Period of study	Average intake	Average loss	Balance	Daily require-ment	Method[1]
			days	mg/day	mg/day		mg/day	
Tompsett (1934)	14 adults	Hospital (presumably)	6–21	2.35	2.32	+0.02	ca 2.3	COL
Chou and Adolph (1935)	1 M 2 F	Simple diet, with increment amount Cu	2–3	Varied	Varied	Varied	ca 2.0	COL
Ohlson and Daum (1935)	3 F	Self-chosen	5–15	1.06	1.22	–0.02 av.	ca 1.2	COL
Kyer and Bethell (1936)	(preg) 1 F	Hospital (presumably)	90 pre- and 14 post	2.20	2.15	+0.05	ca 2.2	Not given
Leverton (1939)	24 F	Self-chosen	7	2.50	2.00	+0.56	ca 2.0	Not given
Kehoe, et al (1940)	1 M	Not given	14 consec.	2.32	2.00	+0.32	<2	SPG
Leverton and Binkley (1944)	65 F	Self-chosen	7	2.65	1.80	+0.85	<2.0	COL
	4 F	Adequate, constant,	75–140	2.37	2.14	+0.23		
Holt and Scoular (1948)	17 F	College dormitory diet	3–5	8.10	0.83	?	?	PLM
De (1949)	2 M	Indian sago diet	6	2.83	2.09	+0.74	ca 2.0	COL
	5 M	Indian veg.-rice diet	6–9	3.74	2.79	+0.95		
	17 M	Indian rice-fish diet	6–9	4.76	3.07	+1.67		
	8 M	Indian whole wheat diet	6–9	5.83	3.39	+2.44		
Cartwright et al. (1954)	3 M	Balance diet for metabolic ward	10	2.62	2.61	+0.01	ca 2.6	SPM
Tu, et al. (1965)	1 M	Low-Cu for Wilson's disease	14 consec.	1.34	1.22	+0.12	<2	Not given
Tipton et al. (1966)	1 F	Self-selected	30	1.04	1.04	0.00	ca 1	AESP
		Self-selected	30	0.91	1.34	–0.43		
Tipton et al. (1969)	1 M	Self-selected	347	0.95	1.30	–0.30	>1	AESP
	1 M	Self-selected	347	1.70	1.30	+0.40		
Strickland et al. (1971)	1 M	Low Cu for Wilson's disease	12	1.20	0.99	+0.21	<1.2	COL
White and Gynne (1971)	9 F	Mixed diet; same amt. all subjects	30	0.59	1.04	–0.45	?	EMS
Robinson et al. (1973)	4 F	Balance diet (N.Z.)	27	1.94	1.63	+0.31	<2	AASM
Butler and Daniel (1973)	10 F	Bal. with peanut flour[2]	10	4.35	2.62	+1.73	?	AASM
	10 F	Bal. w/casein-albumin[2]	10	3.90	2.11	+1.79		
Hartley, et al. (1974)	5 M 6 F	Metabolic ward diet	14	1.91	1.49	+0.42	<2	FAAS

[1] AASM—atomic absorption spectrometry; AESP—arc emission spectrography; COL—colorimetric; FAAS—flame atomic absorption spectrophotometry; PLM—photolometric; SPG—spectrographic; SPM—spectrophotometric. [2] Diet contained a mineral mixture providing an additional 2.37 mg copper per day.

vegetarian type of diet, differences in copper content of soil and/or water, contamination through common use of tinned-copper cooking utensils, or some combination of these factors can provide an explanation is speculative. The estimated minimal requirement of 2.0 mg is based upon statistical analyses of the balance data (154). The data of De (154) clearly support observations of others (100, 451, 452) that as dietary copper intake increases there is an increase in the amount retained, up to an intake of about 8 mg/day. It should also be noted that in the diets used by Butler and Daniel (84) a mineral and baking powder mix was added, providing at two meals a total of 2.37 mg of copper per day, thus explaining the high levels of intake and output. However, there is no valid basis for their concluding statement that "a copper allowance of 4.5 to 5.0 mg is needed to cover the requirements of all healthy young women, depending on climatic conditions."

The study of Kyer and Bethel (431) is the only known report on copper requirements of the pregnant woman. In view of a 2- to 3-fold increase in serum ceruloplasmin during gestation, presumably attained through calls upon storage depots of the liver and other organs and tissues, an increase in daily intake of copper to replace this tissue depletion would be anticipated. In this study a healthy young woman was maintained during the last 3 months of her pregnancy and for 2 weeks after delivery on a uniform diet providing a daily intake of about 2.2 mg of copper. At this level of intake she was able to meet normal needs for pregnancy and early lactation.

Balance studies carried out during the past 14 years, represented by the last eight listed in table 3, indicate that levels less than 2 mg and sometimes not greatly in excess of 1 mg may maintain positive copper balance. Such conclusions are in general accord with information provided by parenteral nutrition studies, as discussed in the following section. Nevertheless, it is important to bear in mind that at these low levels of intake there is, as yet, no means of determining to what extent body mechanisms of copper homeostasis may in-

volve decreases of copper stored in the liver and other tissues of the body.

Total parenteral nutrition. The advent of total parenteral nutrition (hyperalimentation) and its application to problems of post-surgical nutrition and gastrointestinal disorders has added greatly to knowledge of copper utilization and requirements. A number of observations which have particular relevance to adult human requirements for copper warrant consideration at this point.

Shils et al. (712) report the case of an adult male, with bowel resected from the third part of the duodenum to the ascending colon, who was maintained in good nutritional status solely on parenteral feeding for many months. The basic parenteral fluid was essentially devoid of copper, but was supplemented with various trace elements which included 0.40 mg copper/day. Bergstrom et al. (45) describe a 43-year old woman suffering from epilepsy and cerebral damage due to CO_2 intoxication from a fire, who was maintained for 7 months and 13 days on total parenteral nutrition, with an estimated daily intake of 0.10 mg/day of copper.

Perhaps more impressive is similar treatment of a 36-year old woman during a 10-month period in a hospital following resection of her intestinal tract between the duodenum and descending colon (790). During her hospitalization she gained 34 pounds. Subsequently, after mastering the technique of administering her parenteral fluids at home, she was able to carry out her household duties effectively. Throughout the postoperative period her parenteral solution provided 0.018 mg/day of copper. The only other source of copper, the 100 mg of protein hydrolysate, might have provided about 0.075 mg/day and accounted for a total intake of 0.093 mg/day. Essentially the same experience, with employment of a similar parenteral fluid supplemented with 0.06 mg/day is reported by Langer et al. (441) in the management of two women, 21 and 34 years of age, following extensive intestinal resection. These two reports (441, 790) appear to indicate that the minimal daily intravenous requirement for adult man may well be less than the proposed additions of 0.3 to 0.4 mg/day to solutions used for total parenteral nutrition for prolonged periods (177, 711, 712, 864). To these, of course, must be added the amount contributed by the casein hydrolysate or other protein components of the infusate. These vary considerably in their copper content. Somewhat contrary to these estimates is the report of McKenzie et al. (511) that in seven adult patients in a surgical intensive care unit a parenteral infusate providing 0.09 to 0.8 mg of copper resulted in a negative balance in all cases.

Some useful information has also come from studies concerned with copper levels required to compensate for states of copper deficiency resulting from an inadequacy in parenteral fluids. An excellent example is the study of Vilter et al. (808). In a 56-year old woman with malabsorption and severe systemic sclerosis of the intestine, maintained on total parenteral nutrition for 2.5 months, they observed typical manifestations of copper deficiency. For 4 months she had shown leucopenia, neutropenia and a hypocellular bone marrow, considered typical manifestations of copper deficiency. Serum copper was very low (0.02 μg/ml) and serum ceruloplasmin was not demonstrable. Intravenous administration of 1 mg/day for 7 days resulted in an excellent response, still evident 90 days later. Hence 7 mg of copper sulfate distributed over 90 days, equivalent to 0.077 mg of copper per day, represented more than minimal requirements for this woman. Here again, a reasonable estimate of copper acquired via the protein hydrolysate component might increase the uptake to approximately 0.1 mg/day.

Dunlap et al. (177) describe a state of copper deficiency in a 45-year old woman and a 12-year old girl receiving long-term parenteral nutrition following extensive bowel surgery. The older subject, after almost total dependence on parenteral feeding for about 17 months, developed anemia and neutropenia which responded rapidly to oral copper sulfate (5 mg $CuSO_4$ or 1.25 mg elemental copper) daily, which was continued for 45 days. With discontinuation of copper-therapy for about one month, deficiency symptoms were again apparent and responded well to 1.6 mg

copper sulfate (0.4 mg/day) given intravenously. After 2 weeks the daily dose was increased to 1 mg copper for 5 weeks. Subsequently, she was on a parenteral dose of 0.4 mg copper daily and showed no evidence of recurrence of hematologic abnormalities. The younger subject, who had been dependent entirely on parenteral nutrition for only 4 months, showed neutropenia (but no anemia) which also responded to oral copper therapy. The fact that oral copper was effectively absorbed by both subjects, in whom the duodenum had been anastomosed to the transverse colon, provides additional evidence that the stomach and duodenum play a major role in the absorption of copper in man. Of special interest are the data derived from studies on the older subject clearly indicating that a daily parenteral intake of 0.4 mg of elemental copper effected a rapid recovery from a deficiency state. The observations of Vilter et al. (808), also carried out on a single adult woman, are in close agreement with those of Dunlap et al. (177).

One conclusion that may be justified from these two studies is that the "uncomplicated" minimal intravenous requirement of copper for man may well be less than 0.4 mg per day. By "uncomplicated" is meant under situations where ingested copper is not being subjected to the influence of many other components of the diet (other trace elements which compete for binding sites, dietary fiber, phytates, etc.) or may otherwise interfere with maximal absorption. Assuming a 40 to 60% absorption of oral copper, this would represent an oral intake of approximately 1 mg/day.

Two recent examples of the inadequacy of parenteral infusates commonly in use in hospitals can be cited. Weekly serum copper determinations on eight adult patients receiving total parenteral nutrition for 3 to 13 weeks revealed a progressive decrease of serum copper and three patients showed severe hypocupremia. The infusate had no detectable copper. All responded rapidly to oral copper feeding (217). Another study (726) describes a progressive decline in plasma copper (and also zinc) in 13 subjects with active gastrointestinal disorders maintained on total parenteral nutrition for 8 days to 7.5 weeks (mean, 4.5 weeks). The infusate, providing nitrogen as crystalline L-amino acids, contained no copper detectable by a method sensitive to 20 μg/liter. Usually more than 2 months of total parenteral nutrition with unsupplemented infusates are required before clinical evidence of copper deficiency becomes apparent (590). The need for more general inclusion of trace elements, especially copper and zinc, in parenteral fluids is obvious.

Despite the widely recognized need for adequate provision of copper and other trace elements in intravenous solutions, recommendations and practices of different investigators reveal wide variations. According to the calculations presented by Jacobson and Wester (379), the recommendations for copper in trace element mixtures per 24 hours in total parenteral nutrition for 70 kg adults vary from 1.54 mg (173), 1.0 mg (709, 710), 0.11 mg (367), 0.3 mg (864) and 0.1 mg (379). It is the opinion of Jacobson and Wester (379) that a daily intake of 0.3 mg represents the best recommendation. This again represents an oral intake less than 1 mg/day.

It is of particular interest to find that data based upon milk intake in infants and upon balance studies and prolonged maintenance with total parenteral nutrition have shown remarkably good agreement. Briefly stated, the evidence suggests that copper requirements for the maintenance of good health lie within the range of 0.025 to 0.05 mg/kg for young infants, 0.05 to 0.1 mg/kg for older children and adolescents, and in the neighborhood of 1.0 to 1.5 mg/day for adult man.

RESUME

There has been presented a review of research findings relative to the distribution of copper in the human body: the nature and function of a large array of cuproproteins; the omnipresence of copper in foods; its absorption, transport and excretion; naturally occurring states of copper deficiency; dietary interrelationships and states of toxicity; the congenital disorders of Menkes' disease and Wilson's disease; copper metabolism of pregnancy,

neonatal and postnatal life; and copper requirements of infancy, adolescence and adulthood as determined by balance studies and data derived from experiences with parenteral nutrition.

The human body contains approximately 75 mg of copper, about one-third of which is present in the liver and brain. Lesser concentrations exist in the heart, kidney, pancreas, spleen, bone and skeletal muscle. In organs and tissues copper is bound to a wide variety of cuproproteins, most of which have properties of enzymes. Among the trace elements copper is unique in terms of the large number of metabolically important enzymes of which it is an essential component, and the wide variety of organs and tissues in the mammalian organism whose functional and structural integrity are dependent upon these enzymes. Of these, ceruloplasmin, superoxide dismutase, cytochrome c oxidase, lysyl oxidase, tyrosinase and neonatal mitochrondrocuprein are recognized as important in human metabolism. Metallothionein and similar low molecular weight cuproproteins, non-enzymatic in nature, have roles in copper storage and detoxification. Still awaiting further investigation are other cuproproteins some of which might well prove to have important but as yet unrecognized roles in human metabolism.

Ceruloplasmin, whose biological role has long been a mystery, is now recognized as a multifunctional cuproprotein possessing a broad spectrum of oxidase activity. Its role as feroxidase I in the mobilization of plasma iron provides a satisfying answer to questions raised 50 years ago concerning the role of copper in nutritional anemia. Its role as a cuproprotein transferring copper to tissues for the synthesis of vitally important enzymes, the most important of which is cytochrome c oxidase, has been relatively unexplored. The same may be said of the possible capacity of ceruloplasmin to maintain and control blood and tissue levels of biogenic amines. In view of the importance of these amines in normal brain functions and the neurological deficits found in both Wilson's and Menkes' disease, this will unquestionably be a fruitful area for future investigation, both experimental and clinical.

Cytochrome c oxidase, an enzyme vital to essentially all forms of life, has been clearly shown in experimental and farm animals to be involved in the myelination of nerve fibers and in maintaining structure and function of myocardial tissue. What relevance such observations may have to brain and cardiac functions in man offer challenging avenues for future research. Aside from lysyl oxidase, well recognized as essential for the cross-linking of elastin and collagen, are other monoamine oxidases in mammalian tissues which future research may well show to be of great importance in the metabolism of man.

Metallothionein, a nonenzymic cuproprotein, may well prove to be merely one of a family of cuproproteins of relatively low molecular weight playing important roles in the mechanisms of intestinal absorption and transport, and of liver storage and transfer. There is urgent need for better identification of such proteins and increased knowledge of their metabolic roles. New information of this nature may add greatly to understanding the nature and treatment of the two well recognized inborn errors of copper metabolism and possibly of other disorders not yet well recognized.

Copper is ubiquitous in nature and its relative amount in different foods is well established. Very little is known regarding the chemical forms in which it exists in foods or the influence which methods of processing and cooking may have upon its availability. In man, there is only limited knowledge of how absorption of available copper may be influenced by interactions in the gut between it and other trace elements, metallothionein-like proteins, dietary phytates, sulfates and ascorbic acid. Copper is absorbed chiefly by gastric and duodenal mucosa, and approximately 40 to 60% of that ingested is actually absorbed, bound to albumin and amino acids and transported to the liver. The liver serves as the control center for copper metabolism and homeostasis by virtue of its functions as a major storage depot, the major site of copper excretion via the bile and the only site of ceruloplasmin synthesis.

In blood, the ratio of copper in red cells to that in plasma is approximately 0.7. Of that in erythrocytes, which is remarkably constant in normal man, 40% is in a labile form bound to amino acids and 60% is more firmly bound in superoxide dismutase. Of the copper in blood serum, about 7% is labile, bound more to albumin than to amino acids, the remaining 93% being firmly bound as an important component of ceruloplasmin, synthesized only by the liver.

States of hypocupremia in man are relatively rare, occur usually in children and, except for high urinary loss of ceruloplasmin in the nephrotic syndrome, are generally due to hypoproteinemia and inability to provide adequate amounts of apoprotein for ceruloplasmin synthesis. On the other hand hypercupremia, due almost exclusively to hyperceruloplasminemia, is commonly observed in pregnancy, after oral intake of contraceptives and in association with innumerable disease states and disorders. Elevated serum ceruloplasmin in states where inflammation is involved reflects its function as an "acute phase reactant"; in non-inflammatory states reasons for its increase are shrouded in mystery.

There are unsettled questions concerning placental transfer of ceruloplasmin. But of far greater importance is the need for much more information on fetal copper metabolism, including the distribution and nature of protein binding of copper in different organs and tissues of the fetus. Such information is of particular relevance to a better understanding of the basic defect in Menkes' disease. Because of ethical and other restrictions, the answers may have to come from studies on lower primates which, to date, have not been utilized in studies on copper metabolism.

Menkes' steely-hair disease, first described in 1962, represents a state of copper deficiency induced in young infants by a sex-linked recessive defect in copper metabolism. The primary metabolic defect is unknown. Some findings suggest a block in the transfer of copper across absorptive cells of the intestinal mucosa, but there are possibilities of a defect in placental transfer of copper or the presence of an atypical protein-binding of copper in the liver and other organs of the fetus and infant. An intrauterine defect could explain why even in infants with early postnatal diagnosis, therapeutic measures of varied types have done little more than improve serum copper and ceruloplasmin levels, while the disease process continues unabated. The recent discovery and study of two genetic animal models in mice with striking similarities to Menkes' disease, combined with continued study of dietary copper deficiency in the rat and guinea pig, offer challenging opportunities for further investigation of the metabolic defect(s) underlying this disease and some remote possibility of more effective therapeutic measures than currently exist, even though intervention in utero may be the only recourse.

Mystery also still surrounds the primary defect in Wilson's disease (hepatolenticular degeneration), an autosomal recessive inborn error of metabolism first described in 1912 and characterized by the accumulation of excessive and often toxic amounts of copper in the liver, central nervous system, kidney and other tissues. Accumulating evidence points to the liver as the site of metabolic derangement, and decreased biliary excretion of copper the basic reason for the progressive increase of liver copper to toxic levels. Hypotheses proposed suggest: 1) the presence in the liver, and possibly in other affected tissues, of an intracellular protein having greatly increased affinity for the binding of copper; 2) defects in a liver protein or peptide serving in a specific "carrier mechanism" for copper or, 3) defective intracellular transport of copper secondary to dysfunction of hepatocyte lysosomes. The further pursuit of these concepts should open new vistas concerning the metabolic defect in Wilson's disease. As an example, recent evidence of dramatic improvement in extrahepatic manifestations of Wilson's disease following orthoptic liver transplantation also supports the concept that the metabolic defect in Wilson's disease is liver-based. For more than 20 years the therapeutic use of D-penicillamine, a copper chelator, has led to slow clinical improvement, especially when instituted in early states of the disease. A real need

exists for an improved method for diagnosis of asymptomatic cases of the disease, replacing liver biopsy and radiocopper studies, to permit earlier establishment of therapeutic measures. The possible existence of a more effective therapeutic agent seems not to have been given the attention deserved. There is recent evidence that at least two liver diseases, primary biliary cirrhosis and chronic active liver disease, resemble Wilson's disease with respect to elevated levels of liver copper. Whether in these disorders benefits may be derived from penicillamine therapy has not been established.

In the development and practical application of total parenteral nutrition over the past 10 years, isolated instances of states of copper deficiency occurring in children and adult man have emphasized the need for more serious attention to the content of copper and other trace elements in parenteral solutions. Information gained from experiences with parenteral nutrition have given strong support to conclusions reached by balance studies concerning the minimal requirements of copper for infants and adults. A much greater hazard has been created by copper-contaminated tap water or copper-containing valves and stopcocks in conduits employed in hemodialysis, due to the high toxicity of intravenous copper. There are sporadic reports of accidental and suicidal poisoning from oral intake of copper salts. There is little or no evidence of toxicity from industrial sources.

Extensive evidence based upon the copper content of human milk (approximately three times that of cow's milk), copper balance studies and experiences with total parenteral nutrition indicate that copper requirements for young full-term infants are 0.025 to 0.05 mg/kg/day, and that those for premature infants are somewhat greater. Rather limited data, based largely on balance studies, suggest requirements in the range of 0.05 to 0.10 mg/kg/day for young and adolescent children. There is a serious lack of information concerning copper requirements of teenagers, and especially pregnant teenagers. It has long been felt that an adult man requires 2.0 to 2.5 mg copper daily. Balance studies of the past 12 years suggest that a copper intake not much in excess of 1 mg/day may represent the minimal requirement.

There is recent evidence that interactions between zinc and copper, and between molybdenum and copper can seriously interfere with absorption and/or utilization of copper in man, as is well known to be true of domestic and laboratory animals.

ACKNOWLEDGMENTS

Preparation of this conspectus was carried out under Contract No. E-13357-ARS-76 with the Nutrition Institute, United States Department of Agriculture. This is the last of a series of conspectuses by the Nutrition Institute, USDA, Beltsville, MD on the nutritional requirements of man for protein, amino acids, vitamin A, calcium, zinc, vitamin C, iron and folacin. All have been published in previous issues of The Journal of Nutrition. The Nutrition Institute wishes to acknowledge the great assistance and cooperation of the Editors and reviewers of The Journal of Nutrition in making the publication of these conspectuses possible.

The writer wishes to thank Drs. Walter Mertz, Robert D. Reynolds and G. Thomas Strickland for their valued judgments and constructive criticism of the manuscript, and Mrs. Shirley Cress for her patience and painstaking preparation of the same. Tribute is also paid to the late Dr. Isabel Irwin who, prior to her death March 25, 1975, had collected an extensive literature on the subject of this conspectus.

LITERATURE CITED

1. Abderhalden, E. (1900) Die Beziehungen des Eisens zur Blutbildung. Ztschr. Biol. 39, 482–523.
2. Abood, L. G., Gibbs, F. A. & Gibbs, E. (1957) Comparative study of blood ceruloplasmin in schizophrenia and other disorders. A.M.A. Arch. Neurol. Psychiat. 77, 643–645.
3. Abraham, P. A. & Evans, J. L. (1972) Cytochrome oxidase activity and cardiac hypertrophy during copper depletion and repletion. In: Trace Substances and Environmental Health (Hemphill, D. D., ed.), vol. V, pp. 335–347, Univ. Missouri, Columbia.
4. Adams, P. C., Strand, R. D., Bresnan, M. J. & Lucky, A. W. (1974) Kinky hair syndrome: serial study of radiological findings with emphasis on the similarity to the battered child syndrome. Radiol. 112, 401–407.
5. Adelstein, S. J., Coombs, T. L. & Vallee, B. L. (1956) Metalloenzymes and myocardial infarction. I. The relation between serum copper and ceruloplasmin and its catalytic activity. New Engl. J. Med. 255, 105–109.
6. Adelstein, S. J. & Vallee, B. L. (1961) Copper metabolism, in man. New Engl. J. Med. 265, 892–897; 941–946.
7. Adelstein, S. J. & Vallee, B. L. (1962) Copper. In: Mineral Metabolism (Comar, C. L. & Bronner, F., eds.), vol. 2, part B, pp. 371–401, Academic Press, New York.
8. Adolph, W. H. & Chou, T. (1933) Copper in Chinese food materials. Chinese J. Physiol. 7, 185–188.
9. Agarwal, A. K. (1975) Crippling cost of India's big dam. New Scientist 65, 260–261.
10. Agarwal, B. N., Bray, S. H., Bercz, P., Plotzker, R. & Labovitz, E. (1975) Ineffectiveness of hemodialysis in copper sulphate poisoning. Nephron 15, 74–77.
11. Aguilar, M. J., Chadwick, D. L., Okuyama, K. & Kamoshita, S. (1966) Kinky hair disease. 1. Clinical and pathological features. J. Neuropath. & Exper. Neurol. 25, 507–522.
12. Ahlgren, P. & Vestermark, S. (1977) Menkes' kinky hair disease. Neuroradiol. 13, 159–163.
13. Akerfeldt, S. (1957) Oxidation of N,N-dimethyl-p-phenylenediamine by serum from patients with mental disease. Science 125, 117–119.
14. Albukerk, J. N. (1973) Wilson's disease and pregnancy. A case report. Fertil. Steril. 24, 494–497.
15. Alexander, F. W., Clayton, B. E. & Delves, H. T. (1974) Mineral and trace metal balances on children receiving normal and synthetic diets. Quart. J. Med. 43, 89–111.
16. Allen, K. G. D. & Klevay, L. M. (1978) Cholesterolemia and cardiovascular abnormalities in rats caused by copper deficiency. Atheroscler. 29, 81–93.
17. Al-Rashid, R. A. & Spangler, J. (1971) Neonatal copper deficiency. New Engl. J. Med. 285, 841–843.
18. American Academy of Pediatrics, Committee on Nutrition (1976) Commentary on breast feeding and infant formulas, including proposed standards for formulas. Pediatrics 57, 278–285.
19. American Academy of Pediatrics, Committee on Nutrition (1977) Nutritional needs of low-birth-weight infants. Pediatrics 60, 519–530.
20. Angel, C., Leach, B. E., Martens, S., Cohen, M. & Heath, R. G. (1957) Serum oxidation tests in schizophrenic and normal subjects. A.M.A. Arch. Neurol. Psychiat. 78, 500–504.
21. Aoki, T. & Nakahashi, M. (1977) New screening method for Wilson's disease and Menkes' kinky-hair disease. Lancet 2, 1140.
22. Arachi, H., Tomii, S. & Mega, T. (1974) Studies on the copper in the human serum and organs. J. Nara. Med. Assn. 25, 171–179.

23. Ardelt, W., Dehnhard, F. & Shussler, J. (1973) Serumkupfer und hitzestabile alkalische Phosphatase bei normaler und pathologischer Schwangerschaft. Ztschr. Geburtshilfe Perinatal. *177*, 188–192.

24. Arima, M. & Komiya, K. (1970) Prevention of Wilson's disease: a long term followup. Paediatr. Univ. Tokyo *18*, 22–24.

25. Ashkenazi, A., Levin, S., Djaldetti, M., Fishel, E. & Benvenisti, D. (1973) The syndrome of neonatal copper deficiency. Pediatrics *52*, 525–533.

26. Asling, C. W. & Hurley, L. S. (1963) The influence of trace elements on the skeleton. Clin. Orthop. Related Res. *27*, 213–262.

27. Axtrup, S. (1946) The Blood Copper in Anaemias of Children with Special Reference to Premature Cases. P. H. Lindstedts Universitets-Bokhandel, Lund.

28. Baerlocher, K., Nussbaumer, A., Werder, E. A. & Spycher, M. (1974) Menkes' kinky hair disease: confirmation of copper deficiency. Pediat. Res. *8*, 135.

29. Bajpayee, D. P. (1975) Significance of plasma copper and caeruloplasmin concentrations in rheumatoid arthritis. Ann. Rheum. Dis. *34*, 163–165.

30. Bakwin, R. M., Mosbach, E. H. & Bakwin, H. (1958) Ceruloplasmin activity in serum of children with schizophrenia. Pediatrics *22*, 905–909.

31. Bakwin, R. M., Mosbach, E. H. & Bakwin, H. (1961) Concentration of copper in serum of children with schizophrenia. Pediatrics *27*, 642–644.

32. Baldassi, G. (1940) Le funzioni biologiche del rame (Rassegna). Quad. Nutrizione *7*, 250–270.

33. Baldi, E. M. & Gonzales-Somoza, E. (1957) Enfermedad de Wilson y ciclo gravidopuerperal. Obst. Ginecol. Latino-Amer. *15*, 27–31.

34. Barrass, B. C., Coult, D. B. & Pinder, R. M. (1972) 3-Hydroxy-4-methoxyphenethylamine: the endogenous toxin of parkinsonism? J. Pharm. Pharmacol. *24*, 499–501.

35. Baum, & Seeliger (1898) Die chronische Kupfergiftung. Arch. Thierheilk. *24*, 80–127.

36. Bearn, A. G. (1953) Genetic and biochemical aspects of Wilson's disease. Am. J. Med. *15*, 442–449.

37. Bearn, A. G. (1957) Wilson's disease. An inborn error of metabolism with multiple manifestations. Amer. J. Med. *22*, 747–757.

38. Bearn, A. G. (1960) A genetical analysis of 30 families with Wilson's disease (hepatolenticular degeneration). Ann. Hum. Genet. *24*, 33–43.

39. Bearn, A. G. & Kunkel, H. G. (1952) Biochemical abnormalities in Wilson's disease. J. Clin. Invest. *31*, 616.

40. Bearn, A. G. & Kunkel, H. G. (1954) Localization of ⁶⁴Cu in serum fractions following oral administration: an alteration in Wilson's disease. Proc. Soc. Exp. Biol. & Med. *85*, 44–48.

41. Bearn, A. G. & Kunkel, H. G. (1955) Metabolism studies in Wilson's disease using ⁶⁴Cu. J. Lab. Clin. Med. *45*, 623–631.

42. Beckner, W. M., Strickland, G. T., Leu, M. L. & O'Reilly, S. (1969) External gamma scintillation counting of ⁶⁷Cu over the liver and other sites in patients with Wilson's disease, family members and controls. J. Nucl. Med. *10*, 320.

43. Beinert, H. (1966) Cytochrome c oxidase: present knowledge of the state and function of its copper components. In: The Biochemistry of Copper (Peisach, J., Aisen, P. & Blumberg, W. E., eds.), pp. 213–234, Academic Press, New York.

44. Beisel, W. R. & Pekarek, R. S. (1972) Acute stress and trace element metabolism. Internat. Rev. Neurobiol. Suppl. *1*, 53–82.

45. Bergstrom, K., Bloomstrand, R. & Jacobson, S. (1972) Long-term complete intravenous nutrition in man. Nutr. Metab. *14*, (Suppl.), 118–149.

46. Bickel, H., Neale, F. C. & Hall, G. (1957) A clinical and biochemical study of hepatolenticular degeneration (Wilson's disease). Quart. J. Med. *26*, 527–558.

47. Bihl, J. H. (1959) The effect of pregnancy on hepatolenticular degeneration (Wilson's disease). Report of a case. Amer. J. Obst. & Gynecol. *78*, 1182–1188.

48. Billingham, M. E. J. & Gordon, A. H. (1976) The role of the acute phase reactions in inflammation. Agents Actions *6*, 195–199.

49. Billings, D. M. & Degnan, M. (1971) Kinky hair syndrome. A new case and a review. Am. J. Dis. Child. *121*, 447–449.

50. Bloomfield, J. (1969) Copper contamination in exchange transfusions. Lancet *1*, 731–732.

51. Bloomfield, J., Dixon, S. R. & McCredie, D. A. (1971) Potential hepatotoxicity of copper in recurrent hemodialysis. Arch. Int. Med. *128*, 555–560.

52. Bloomfield, J., McPherson, J. & George, C. R. P. (1969) Active uptake of copper and zinc during haemodialysis. Brit. Med. J. *2*, 141–145.

53. Bober-Vandzhura, I. P. (1968) Copper metabolism in atherosclerotic patients. Terap. Arh. *40*, 64–66 (Russian).

54. Borglin, N. E. & Heijkenskjold, F. (1967) Studies on serum copper in pregnancy. Acta Obstet. Gynecol. Scand. *46*, 119–125.

55. Bourgeois, J., Galy, G., Baltassat, P. & Béthenod, M. (1974) Maladie de Menkes. Etude métabolisme du cuivre dans une observation personnelle. Pediatrie *29*, 573–594.

56. Bourgeois, J., Vittori, F., Collombel, C. & Béthenod, M. (1974) Maladie de Menkes. Présentation clinique d'une observation personelle. Pediatrie *29*, 561–572.

56a. Bowering, J., Sanchez, A. M. & Irwin, M. I. (1976) A conspectus of research on iron requirements of man. J. Nutr. *106*, 985–1074.

57. Bozian, R. C. & Shearer, C. (1976) Copper, zinc and manganese content of four

amino acid and protein hydrolysate preparations. Am. J. Clin. Nutr. 29, 1331–1332.

58. Brady, F. O., Monaco, M. E., Forman, H. J., Schutz, G. & Feigelson, P. (1972) On the role of copper in activation of and catalysis by tryptophane -2,3-dioxygenase. J. Biol. Chem. 247, 7915–7922.

59. Bray, P. F. (1965) Sex-linked neurodegenerative disease associated with monilethrix. Pediatrics 36, 417–420.

60. Bremner, I. (1974) Heavy metal toxicities. Quart. Rev. Biophys. 7, 75–124.

61. Brendstrup, P. (1953) Serum copper, serum iron and total iron-binding capacity of serum in acute and chronic infections. Acta Med. Scand. 145, 315–325.

62. Brendstrup, P. (1953) Serum iron, total iron-binding capacity of serum and serum copper in acute hepatitis. Acta Med. Scand. 146, 107–113.

63. Brenner, W. (1948) Beiträge zur Kenntris des Eisen-und Kupferstoffwechsels im Kindesalter. Serumeisen und Serumkupfer bei akuten und chronischen Infektionen. Ztschr. Kinderheil. 66, 14–35.

64. Brewer, G. J., Shoomaker, E. B., Leichtman, D. A., Kruckeberg, W. C., Brewer, L. F. & Meyers, N. (1977) The use of pharmacological doses of zinc in the treatment of sickle cell anemia. In: Zinc Metabolism: Current Aspects in Health and Disease (Brewer, G. J. & Prasad, A. A., eds.), pp. 241–258, A. R. Liss, Inc., New York.

65. Broman, L. (1964) Chromatographic and magnetic studies on human ceruloplasmin. Acta Soc. Med. Upsalien 69 (Suppl. 7), 1–85.

66. Broviac, J. W. & Scribner, B. H. (1974) Prolonged parenteral nutrition in the home. Surg. Gyn. Obst. 139, 24–28.

67. Brown, E. D., Howard, M. P. & Smith, J. C., Jr. (1977) The copper content of regular, vegetarian and renal diets. Federation Proc. 36, 1122.

68. Brown, F. C. & Ward, D. N. (1959) Studies on mammalian tyrosinase. II Chemical and physical properties of fractions purified by chromatography. Proc. Exp. Biol. Med. 100, 701–704.

69. Brückmann, G. & Zondek, S. G. (1939) Iron, copper and manganese in human organs at various ages. Biochem. J. 33, 1845–1857.

70. Brunia, C. H. M. & Buyze, G. (1972) Serum copper levels and epilepsy. Epilepsia. 13, 621–625.

71. Buck, W. A. & Ewan, R. C. (1973) Toxicology and adverse effects of mineral imbalance. Clin. Toxicol. 6, 459–485.

72. Bucknall, W. E., Haslam, R. H. A. & Holtzman, N. A. (1973) Kinky hair syndrome: response to copper therapy. Pediatrics 52, 653–657.

73. Buffoni, F. & Blaschko, H. (1964) Benzylamine oxidase and histaminase: purification and crystallization of an enzyme from pig plasma. Proc. R. Soc. London Ser. B 161, 153–167.

74. Bühler, H. O. & Kägi, H. R. (1974) Human hepatic metallothioneins. FEBS Letters 39, 229–234.

75. Burch, R. E., Hahn, H. K. J. & Sullivan, J. F. (1975) Newer aspects of the roles of zinc, manganese and copper in human nutrition. Clin. Chem. 21, 501–520.

76. Burger, F. J. (1974) Changes in the trace-element concentration in the sera and hair of kwashiorkor patients. In: Trace Element Metabolism in Animals—2 (Hoekstra, W. G., Suttie, J. W., Ganther, H. E. & Mertz, W., eds.), pp. 671–674, University Park Press, Baltimore.

77. Burrows, S. & Pekala, B. (1971) Serum copper and ceruloplasmin in pregnancy. Amer. J. Obstet. & Gynecol. 109, 907–909.

78. Bush, J. A. (1956) The role of trace elements in hemopoiesis and in the therapy of anemia. Pediatrics 17, 586–595.

79. Bush, J. A., Mahoney, J. P., Gubler, C. J., Cartwright, G. E. & Wintrobe, M. M. (1956) Studies on copper metabolism. XXI. The transfer of radiocopper between erythrocyte and plasma. J. Lab. Clin. Med. 47, 898–906.

80. Bush, J. A., Mahoney, J. P., Markowitz, H., Gubler, C. J., Cartwright, G. E. & Wintrobe, M. M. (1955) Studies on copper metabolism. XVI. Radioactive studies in normal subjects and in patients with hepatolenticular degeneration. J. Clin. Invest. 34, 1766–1778.

81. Bustamante Bustamante, J., Martin Mateo, M. C. & DeQuiros, F. B. (1975) Estudio del cobre, ceruloplasmina y cinc en relacion con el metabolismo de los lipidos en arterioscleroticos. Rev. Clin. Espanola 139, 243–246.

82. Bustamante Bustamante, J., Martin Mateo, M. C., DeQuiros, F. B. & Manchado, O. O. (1977) Valores séricos de cobre, ceruloplasmina y lipidos en ancianos: Estudio comparativo con enfermos arterioscleróticos. Rev. Clin. Espanol 146, 27–30.

83. Butler, E. J. & Newman, G. E. (1956) The urinary excretion of copper and its concentration in the blood of normal human adults. J. Clin. Pathol. 9, 157–161.

84. Butler, L. C. & Daniel, J. M. (1973) Copper metabolism in young women fed two levels of copper and two protein sources. Am. J. Clin. Nutr. 26, 744–749.

85. Butt, E. M., Nusbaum, R. E., Gilmour, T. C. & DiDio, S. L. (1958) Trace metal patterns in disease states. II. Copper storage diseases, with consideration of juvenile cirrhosis, Wilson's disease, and hepatic copper of the newborn. Am. J. Clin. Pathol. 30, 479–497.

86. Butterworth, C. E., Gubler, C. J., Cartwright, G. E. & Wintrobe, M. M. (1958) Studies on copper metabolism. XXVI Plasma copper in patients with tropical sprue. Proc. Soc. Exp. Biol. Med. 98, 594–597.

87. Cairns, J. E., Williams, H. P. & Walshe, J. M. (1969) "Sunflower cataract" in Wilson's disease. Brit. Med. J. 3, 95–96.

88. Camus, J. P., Bénichou, C., Guillien, P., Crouzet, J. & Lièvre, J. A. (1971) Traite-

ment de la polyarthrite rhumatoide commune par la D-pénicillamine. Rev. Rhum. Mal. Osteoartic. *38*, 809–820.

89. Canelas, H. M., Assis, L. M., De Jorge, F. B., Tolosa, A. P. M. & Cintra, A. B. U. (1964) Disorders of copper metabolism in epilepsy. Acta Neurol. Scand. *40*, 97–105.

90. Canelas, H. M., De Jorge, F. B. & Tognola, W. A. (1967) Metabolic balances of copper in patients with hepatolenticular degeneration submitted to vegetarian and mixed diets. J. Neurol. Neurosurg. Psychiat. *30*, 371–373.

91. Cantarutti, F. & Panzion, F. (1975) Le modificazioni della cupremia nal periodo postnatale. Lattente *25*, 721–723.

92. Carlton, W. W. & Kelly, W. A. (1969) Neural lesions in the offspring of female rats fed a copper-deficient diet. J. Nutr. *94*, 42–52.

93. Carnes, W. H. (1971) Role of copper in connective tissue metabolism. Federation Proc. *30*, 995–1000.

94. Carnes, W. H., Coulson, W. F., Smith, D. W. & Weissman, N. (1968) The role of copper in the circulatory system. In: Trace Substances in Environmental Health II (Hemphill, D. D., ed.), pp. 29–40, Univ. of Missouri, Columbia.

95. Carrico, R. J. & Deutsch, H. F. (1969) Isolation of human hematocuprein and cerebrocuprein. Their identity with erythrocuprein. J. Biol. Chem. *244*, 6087–6093.

96. Carrico, R. J. & Deutsch, H. F. (1970) The presence of zinc in human cytocuprein and some properties of the apoprotein. J. Biol. Chem. *245*, 723–727.

97. Carr-Saunders, E. & Laurence, B. M. (1965) Wilson's disease presenting as an acute hemolytic anemia. Proc. Roy. Soc. Med. *58*, 614–615.

98. Carruthers, M. E., Hobbs, C. B. & Warren, R. L. (1966) Raised serum copper and caeruloplasmin levels in subjects taking oral contraceptives. J. Clin. Pathol. *19*, 498–500.

99. Cartwright, G. E. (1947) Dietary factors concerned in erythropoiesis. IV. Minerals. Blood *2*, 256–298.

100. Cartwright, G. E. (1950) Copper metabolism in human subjects. In: A Symposium on Copper Metabolism (McElroy, W. D. & Glass, B., eds.), pp. 274–314, Johns Hopkins Press, Baltimore.

101. Cartwright, G. E. (1955) The relationship of copper, cobalt and other trace elements to hemopoiesis. Am. J. Clin. Nutr. *3*, 11–17.

102. Cartwright, G. E., Hodges, R. E., Gubler, C. J., Mahoney, J. P., Daum, K., Wintrobe, M. M. & Bean, W. B. (1954) Studies on copper metabolism. XIII Hepatolenticular degeneration. J. Clin. Invest. *33*, 1487–1501.

103. Cartwright, G. E., Huguley, C. M. Jr., Ashenbrucker, H., Fay, J. & Wintrobe, M. W. (1948) Studies on free erythrocyte protoporphyrin, plasma iron and plasma copper in normal and anemic subjects. Blood *3*, 501–528.

104. Cartwright, G. E., Markowitz, H., Shields, G. S. & Wintrobe, M. M. (1960) Studies on copper metabolism. XXIX. A critical analysis of serum copper and ceruloplasmin concentrations in normal subjects, patients with Wilson's disease and relatives of patients with Wilson's disease. Am. J. Med. *28*, 555–563.

105. Cartwright, G. E. & Wintrobe, M. M. (1964) Copper metabolism in normal subjects. Am. J. Clin. Nutr. *14*, 224–232.

106. Cartwright, G. E. & Wintrobe, M. M. (1964) The question of copper deficiency in man. Am. J. Clin. Nutr. *15*, 94–110.

107. Cavell, P. A. & Widdowson, E. M. (1964) Intakes and excretions of iron, copper, and zinc in the neonatal period. Arch. Dis. Child. *39*, 496–501.

108. Chang, I. C., Lee, T. P. & Matrone, G. (1975) Development of ceruloplasmin in pigs during the neonatal period. J. Nutr. *105*, 624–630.

109. Chang, I. C., Milholland, D. C. & Matrone, G. (1976) Controlling factors in the development of ceruloplasmin in pigs during the neonatal growth period. J. Nutr. *106*, 1343–1350.

110. Chappell, W. R. & Peterson, K. K. (1976) Molybdenum in the Environment, vol. 1, Dekker, New York.

111. Chatterji, S. K. & Ganguly, H. D. (1950) Copper in human urine and faeces. Indian J. Med. Res. *38*, 303–314.

112. Chawla, S. C. & Mehta, S. P. (1973) A study of host and environmental factors in cases of accidental poisoning admitted in Irwin hospital. Indian J. Med. Res. *61*, 724–731.

113. Ch'en, P. (1957) Abnormalities of copper metabolism in Wilson's disease. A preliminary report. Chinese Med. J. *75*, 917–924.

114. Chiossi, F. M., Bertolini, A. & Guarino, M. (1977) Aspetti angiografiei ed istologici della malattia di Menkes. Gaslini *9*, 65–70.

115. Chou, T. & Adolph, W. H. (1935) Copper metabolism in man. Biochem. J. *29*, 476–479.

116. Chou, W. S., Rucker, R. B., Savage, J. E. & O'Dell, B. L. (1970) Impairment of collagen and elastin crosslinking by an amine oxidase inhibitor. Proc. Soc. Exp. Biol. Med. *134*, 1078–1082.

117. Chou, W. S., Savage, J. E. & O'Dell, B. L. (1968) Relation of monoamine oxidase activity and collagen crosslinking in copper-deficient and control tissues. Proc. Soc. Exp. Biol. Med. *128*, 948–952.

118. Chowdhury, A. K. R., Ghosh, S. & Pal, D. (1961) Acute copper sulphate poisoning. J. Ind. Med. Assn. *36*, 330–336.

119. Chugh, T. D., Gulati, R. C. & Gupta, S. P. (1973) A study of serum copper and ceruloplasmin in normal healthy individuals. Indian J. Med. Sci. *27*, 309–312.

120. Chuttani, H. K., Gupta, P. S., Gulati, S. & Gupta, D. N. (1965) Acute copper sulfate poisoning. Am. J. Med. *39*, 849–854.

121. Cohen, S. R. (1974) A review of the health hazards from copper exposure. J. Occup. Med. *16*, 621–624.

122. Consolazio, C. F., Nelson, R. A., Matoush, L. O., Hughes, R. C. & Urone, P. (1964) The Trace Mineral Losses In Sweat, pp. 1–14, U.S. Army Med. Res. Nutr. Lab. Report No. 284.

123. Cooper, A. M., Eckhardt, R. D., Faloon, W. W. & Davidson, C. S. (1950) Investigation of the aminoaciduria in Wilson's disease (hepatolenticular degeneration): demonstration of a defect in renal function. J. Clin. Invest. 29, 265–278.

124. Cordano, A. (1974) The role played by copper in the physiopathology and nutrition of the infant and the child. Ann. Nestlé 33, 2–16.

125. Cordano, A. (1978) Copper deficiency in clinical medicine. In: Zinc and Copper in Clinical Medicine (Hambidge, K. M. & Nichols, B. F., Jr., eds.), pp. 119–126, Spectrum, New York.

126. Cordano, A., Baertl, J. M. & Graham, G. G. (1964) Copper deficiency in infancy. Pediatrics 34, 324–336.

127. Cordano, A. & Graham, G. G. (1966) Copper deficiency complicating severe chronic intestinal malabsorption. Pediatrics 38, 596–604.

128. Cordano, A., Placko, R. P. & Graham, G. G. (1966) Hypocupremia and neutropenia in copper deficiency. Blood 28, 280–283.

129. Coulson, W. F. & Carnes, W. H. (1963) Cardiovascular studies on copper-deficient swine. V. The histogenesis of the coronary artery lesions. Am. J. Pathol. 43, 945–954.

130. Coulson, W. F. (1972) Copper deficiency, with special reference to the cardiovascular system. In: Methods and Achievements in Experimental Pathology (Bajusz, E. & Jasmin, G., eds.), vol. 6, pp. 111–138, Karger, Basel.

131. Cox, D. W. (1966) Factors influencing serum ceruloplasmin levels in normal individuals. J. Lab. Clin. Med. 68, 893–904.

132. Crampton, R. F., Matthews, D. M. & Poisner, R. (1965) Observations on the mechanism of absorption of copper by the small intestine. J. Physiol. (London) 178, 111–126.

133. Crouzet, J., Nafziger, J., Guillien, P., Camus, J.-P. & Lièvre, J.-A. (1973) Étude du métabolisme du cuivre dans la polyarthrite rheumatoide et de l'influence du traitement par la D-pénicillamine. Rev. Rhuma. 40, 485–489.

134. Cumings, J. N. (1948) The copper and iron content of brain and liver in the normal and in hepato-lenticular degeneration. Brain 71, 410–415.

135. Cumings, J. N. (1951) The effects of B.A.L. in hepatolenticular degeneration. Brain 74, 10–22.

136. Cumings, J. N. (1954) Copper storage in hepatolenticular degeneration and allied diseases. Proc. Roy. Soc. Med. 47, 152–154.

137. Cumings, J. N. (1959) Heavy Metals and the Brain. Part 1: Copper: hepatolenticular degeneration, pp. 1–74, Blackwell Sci. Pub., Oxford.

138. Cumings, J. N. (1968) Trace metals in the brain and in Wilson's disease. J. Clin. Pathol. 21, 1–7.

139. Cunningham, I. J. (1931) Some biochemical and physiological aspects of copper in animal nutrition. Biochem. J. 25, 1267–1294.

140. Cunningham, I. J. (1950) Copper and molybdenum in relation to diseases of cattle and sheep in New Zealand. In: A Symposium on Copper Metabolism (McElroy, W. D. & Glass, B., eds.), pp. 246–272, Johns Hopkins Univ. Press, Baltimore.

141. Curzon, G. & O'Reilly, S. (1960) A coupled iron-caeruloplasmin oxidation system. Biochem. Biophys. Res. Comm. 2, 284–286.

142. Daniels, A. L. & Wright, O. E. (1934) Iron and copper retentions in young children. J. Nutr. 8, 125–138.

143. Danks, D. M. (1975) Steely hair, mottled mice and copper metabolism. New Engl. J. Med. 293, 1147–1149.

144. Danks, D. M. (1977) Copper transport and utilisation in Menkes' syndrome and in mottled mice. Inorgan. Persp. Biol. Med. 1, 73–100.

145. Danks, D. M., Campbell, P. E., Stevens, B. J., Mayne, V. & Cartwright, E. (1972) Menkes's kinky hair syndrome. An inherited defect in copper absorption with widespread effects. Pediatrics 50, 188–201.

146. Danks, D. M., Cartwright, E. & Stevens, B. J. (1973) Menkes' steely-hair (kinky hair) disease. Lancet 1, 891.

147. Danks, D. M., Cartwright, E., Stevens, B. J. & Townley, R. R. W. (1973) Menkes' kinky hair disease: further definition of the defect in copper transport. Science 179, 1140–1142.

148. Danks, D. M., Stevens, B. J., Campbell, P. E., Gillespie, J. M., Walker-Smith, J., Blomfield, J. & Turner, B. (1972) Menkes' kinky-hair syndrome. Lancet 1, 1100–1103.

149. Davies, N. T. (1974) Recent studies of antagonist interactions in the aetiology of trace element deficiency and excess. Proc. Nutr. Soc. 33, 293–298.

150. Davis, G. K. (1950) The influence of copper on the metabolism of phosphorus and molybdenum. In: A Symposium on Copper Metabolism (McElroy, W. D. & Glass, G., eds.), pp. 216–229, J. Hopkins Press, Baltimore.

151. Dawson, C. R., Strothkamp, K. G. & Krul, K. G. (1975) Ascorbate oxidase and related copper proteins. Ann. N.Y. Acad. Sci. 258, 209–220.

152. Dawson, E. B., Clark, R. R. & McGanity, W. J. (1969) Plasma vitamins and trace metal changes during teen-age pregnancy. Am. J. Obstet. Gynecol. 104, 953–958.

153. Dawson, J. B., Ellis, D. J. & Newton-John, H. (1968) Direct estimation of copper in serum and urine by atomic absorption spectroscopy. Clin. Chim. Act. 21, 33–42.

154. De, H. N. (1949) Copper and manganese metabolism with typical Indian dietaries and assessment of their requirement for

the Indian adult. Indian J. Med. Res. 37, 301–309.

155. Deiss, A., Lee, G. R. & Cartwright, G. E. (1970) Hemolytic anemia in Wilson's disease. Ann. Intern. Med. 73, 413–418.

156. Deiss, A., Lynch, R. E., Lee, G. R. & Cartwright, G. E. (1971) Long term therapy of Wilson's disease. Ann. Intern. Med. 75, 57–65.

157. De Jorge, F. B., Canelas, H. M., Dias, J. C. & Cury, L. (1964) Studies on copper metabolism. III. Copper contents of saliva of normal subjects and of salivary glands and pancreas of autopsy material. Clin. Chim. Acta 9, 148–150.

158. De Jorge, F. B., Delascio, D. & Antunes, M. L. (1965) Copper and copper oxidase concentrations in the blood of normal pregnant women. Obstet. Gynecol. 26, 225–227.

159. Dekaban, A. S., Aamodt, R., Rumble, W. F., Johnston, G. S. & O'Reilly, S. (1975) Kinky hair disease. Study of copper metabolism with use of ^{67}Cu. Arch. Neurol. 32, 672–675.

160. Dekaban, A. S., O'Reilly, S., Aamodt, R. & Rumble, W. F. (1974) Study of copper metabolism in kinky hair disease (Menkes' disease) and in hepatolenticular degeneration (Wilson's disease) utilizing ^{67}Cu and radioactivity counting in the total body and various tissues. Trans. Am. Neurol. Assoc. 99, 106–109.

161. Dekaban, A. S. & Steusing, J. K. (1974) Menkes' kinky hair disease treated with subcutaneous copper sulphate. Lancet 2, 1523.

162. Delves, H. T., Alexander, F. W. & Lay, H. (1973) Copper and zinc concentration in the plasma of leukaemic children. Brit. J. Haematol. 24, 525–531.

163. Denny-Brown, D. & Porter, H. (1951) The effect of BAL (2,3-dimercaptopropanol) on hepatolenticular degeneration (Wilson's disease). New Engl. J. Med. 245, 917–926.

164. Deosthale, Y. G. & Gopalan, C. (1974) The effect of molybdenum levels in sorghum (Sorghum vulgare Pers.) on uric acid and copper excretion in man. Brit. J. Nutr. 31, 351–355.

165. De Renzo, E. C. (1962) Molybdenum. In: Mineral Metabolism—An Advanced Treatise (Comar, C. L. & Bronner, F., eds.), vol. 2, part B, pp. 483–498, Academic Press, New York.

166. Dieckmann, W. J. & Wegner, C. R. (1934) The blood in normal pregnancy. 1. Blood and plasma volumes. Arch. Intern. Med. 53, 71–86.

167. Dokumov, S. I. (1968) Serum copper and pregnancy. Am. J. Obstet. Gynecol. 101, 217–222.

168. Dorn, G., Neuhäuser, G., Heye, D. & Kielhorn, A. (1973) Das Kinky-Hair Syndrom von Menkes. Klin. Paediatr. 185, 480–489.

169. Dowdy, R. P. (1969) Copper metabolism. Am. J. Clin. Nutr. 22, 887–892.

170. Dreizen, S., Spies, H. A., Jr. & Spies, T. D. (1952) The copper and cobalt levels of human saliva and dental caries activity. J. Dent. Res. 31, 137–142.

171. Drummond, J. C. (1925) The absorption of copper during the digestion of vegetables artificially coloured with copper salts. Analyst 50, 481–485.

172. Du Bois, R. S., Giles, G., Rodgerson, D. O., Lilly, J., Martineaux, G., Halgrimson, C. G., Shroter, G., Starzl, T. E., Sternlieb, I. & Scheinberg, I. H. (1971) Orthotopic liver transplantation for Wilson's disease. Lancet 1, 505–508.

173. Dudrick, S. J. & Rhoads, J. E. (1971) New horizons for intravenous feeding. J. Am. Med. Assn. 215, 939–949.

174. Dudrick, S. J. & Ruberg, R. L. (1971) Principles and practice of parenteral nutrition. Gastroenterology 61, 901–910.

175. Dudrick, S. J., Groff, B. & Wilmore, D. W. (1969) Long term venous catherization in infants. Surg. Gynecol. Obstet. 129, 805–808.

176. Dudrick, S. J., Wilmore, D. W., Vars, H. M. & Rhoades, J. E. (1968) Long-term total parenteral nutrition with growth, development and positive nitrogen balance. Surg. 64, 134–142.

177. Dunlap, W. M., James, G. W., III, & Hume, D. M. (1974) Anemia and neutropenia caused by copper deficiency. Ann. Intern. Med. 80, 470–476.

178. Earl, C. J. (1961) Anatomical distribution of copper in human brain. In: Wilson's Disease, Some Current Concepts, (Walshe, J. M. & Cumings, J. N., eds.), pp. 18–23, Blackwell, Oxford.

179. Earl, C. J., Moulton, M. J. & Selverstone, B. (1954) Metabolism of copper in Wilson's disease and in normal subjects: studies with Cu-64. Am. J. Med. 17, 205–213.

180. Edozien, J. C. & Udeozo, I. O. K. (1960) Serum copper, iron and iron binding capacity in kwashiorkor. J. Trop. Pediat. 6, 60–64.

181. Effkemann, G. & Röttger, H. (1950) Über den Kupferhaushalt während der Schwangerschaft. Klin. Wochenschr. 28, 216–220.

182. Eggleton, W. G. E. (1940) The zinc and copper contents of the organs and tissues of Chinese subjects. Biochem. J. 34, 991–997.

183. Elsner, P. & Hornykiewicz, O. (1954) Die beeinflussbarkeit der p-Polyphenoloxydaseaktivität des menschlichen Blutserums durch Sexualhormone. Archiv. Gynäkol. 185, 251–257.

184. Elsner, P., Hornykiewicz, O., Linder, A. & Niebauer, G. (1953) Über das vorkommen einer polyphenoloxydase in serum nicht gravider und gravider frau. Wien. Klin. Wochenschr. 65, 193–195.

185. Elvehjem, C. A. (1935) The biological significance of copper and its relation to iron metabolism. Physiol. Rev. 15, 471–507.

186. Elvehjem, C. A., Duckles, D. & Mendenhall, D. R. (1937) Iron versus iron and copper in the treatment of anemia in infants. Am. J. Dis. Child. 53, 758–793.

187. Elvehjem, C. A. & Hart, E. B. (1929) The relation of iron and copper to hemoglobin synthesis in the chick. J. Biol. Chem. 84, 131–141.

188. Elvehjem, C. A. & Hart, E. B. (1932) The necessity of copper as a supplement to iron for hemoglobin formation in the pig. J. Biol. Chem. 95, 363–370.

189. Elvehjem, C. A., Steenbock, H. & Hart, E. B. (1929) The effect of diet on the copper content of milk. J. Biol. Chem. 83, 27–34.

190. Engel, R. W., Price, N. O. & Miller, R. F. (1967) Copper, manganese, cobalt, and molybdenum balance in pre-adolescent girls. J. Nutr. 92, 197–204.

191. Evans, G. W. (1971) Function and nomenclature for two mammalian copper proteins. Nutr. Rev. 29, 195–197.

192. Evans, G. W. (1973) Copper homeostasis in the mammalian system. Physiol. Rev. 53, 535–570.

193. Evans, G. W. (1973) The biological regulation of copper homeostasis in the rat. World Rev. Nutr. Diet. 17, 225–249.

194. Evans, G. W. (1977) Metabolic disorders of copper metabolism. In: Advances in Nutritional Research, (Draper, H. H., Broquist, H. P., Henderson, L. M., Kritchevsky, D., Pitt, G. A. J., Sandstead, H. H. & Somogyi, J. C., eds.), vol. 1, pp. 167–187, Plenum, New York.

195. Evans, G. W. (1978) New aspects of the biochemistry and metabolism of copper. In: Zinc and Copper in Clinical Medicine (Hambidge, K. M. & Nichols, B. F., Jr., eds.), pp. 113–118, Spectrum, Jamaica, New York.

196. Evans, G. E. & Cornatzer, W. E. (1971) Biliary copper excretion in the rat. Proc. Soc. Exp. Biol. Med. 136, 719–721.

197. Evans, G. W., Dubois, R. S. & Hambidge, K. M. (1973) Wilson's disease: Identification of an abnormal copper binding protein. Science 181, 1175–1176.

198. Evans, G. W. & LeBlanc, F. N. (1976) Copper-binding protein in rat intestine: Amino acid composition and function. Nutr. Rep. Internat. 14, 281–288.

199. Evans, G. W., Majors, P. F. & Cornatzer, W. E. (1970) Ascorbic acid interactions with metallothionein. Biochem. Biophys. Res. Comm. 41, 1244–1247.

200. Evans, G. W. & Reis, B. L. (1978) Impaired copper homeostasis in neonatal male and adult female brindled (Mo^br) mice. J. Nutr. 108, 554–560.

201. Everson, G. J., Huang-Chan, C. T. & Wang, T. (1967) Copper deficiency in the guinea pig. J. Nutr. 43, 533–540.

202. Everson, G. J., Shrader, R. E. & Wang, T. (1968) Chemical and morphological changes in the brains of copper-deficient guinea pigs. J. Nutr. 96, 115–125.

203. Fairbanks, V. F. (1967) Copper sulphate-induced hemolytic anemia. Inhibition of glucose-6-phosphate dehydrogenase and other possible etiologic mechanisms. Ann. Intern. Med. 120, 428–432.

204. Falkmer, S., Samuelson, G. & Sjolin, S. (1970) Penicillamine-induced normalization of clinical signs, and liver morphology and histochemistry in a case of Wilson's disease. Pediatrics 45, 260–268.

205. Fattah, M. M. A., Ibrahim, F. K., Ramadan, M. A. & Sammour, M. B. (1976) Ceruloplasmin and copper level in maternal and cord blood and in the placenta in normal pregnancy and in pre-eclampsia. Acta Obstet. & Gynecol. Scand. 55, 383–385.

206. Fay, J., Cartwright, G. E. & Wintrobe, M. M. (1949) Studies on free erythrocyte protoporphyrin, serum iron, serum iron-binding capacity and plasma copper during normal pregnancy. J. Clin. Invest. 28, 487–491.

207. Fazekas, I. Gy., Romhányi, I. & Rengei, B. (1963) Copper content of fetal organs. Kiserl. Orvostud. 15, 230–238. (Hungarian)

208. Fell, G. S., Smith, H. & Howie, R. A. (1968) Neutron activation analysis for copper in biological material applied to Wilson's disease. J. Clin. Pathol. 21, 8–11.

209. Filler, R. M., Eraklis, A. J., Rubin, V. G. & Das, J. B. (1970) Long-term total parenteral nutrition in infants. New Engl. J. Med. 281, 589–594.

210. Findlay, G. H. & Venter, I. J. (1958) An effect of pantothenic acid on serum copper values in human pellagra. J. Invest. Dermatol. 31, 11.

211. Fisher, G. L. (1975) Function and homeostasis of copper and zinc in mammals. Sci. Total Environ. 4, 373–412.

212. Fisher, G. L., Byers, V. S., Shifrine, M. & Levin, A. S. (1976) Copper and zinc levels in serum from human patients with sarcomas. Cancer 37, 356–363.

213. Fitzpatrick, T. B., Seiji, M. & McGugan, A. D. (1961) Melanin pigmentation. New Engl. J. Med. 265, 328–332; 374–378; 430–432.

214. Flack, H. L., Gans, J. A., Serlick, S. E. & Dudrick, S. J. (1971) The current status of parenteral hyperalimentation. Am. J. Hosp. Pharm. 28, 326–335.

215. Fleming, C. R., Dickson, E. R., Baggenstoss, A. H. & McCall, J. T. (1974) Copper and primary biliary cirrhosis. Gastroenterology 67, 1182–1187.

216. Fleming, C. R., Dickson, E. R., Wahner, H. W., Hollenhorst, R. W. & McCall, J. T. (1977) Pigmented corneal rings in non-Wilsonian liver disease. Ann. Intern. Med. 86, 285–288.

217. Fleming, C. R., Hodges, R. E. & Hurley, L. S. (1976) A prospective study of serum copper and zinc levels in patients receiving total parenteral nutrition. Am. J. Clin. Nur. 29, 70–77.

218. Flinn, F. B. & Von Glahn, W. C. (1929) A chemical and pathologic study of the effects of copper on the liver. J. Exp. Med. 49, 5–20.

219. Flynn, A., Franzmann, A. W., Arneson, P. D. & Oldemeyer, J. L. (1977) Indications of copper deficiency in a subpopulation of Alaskan moose. J. Nutr. 107, 1182–1189.

220. Forbes, G. (1947) Poisoning with a preparation of iron, copper and manganese. Br. Med. J. 1, 367–370.

221. Forestier, J. & Certonciny, A. (1946) Le traitement des rhumatismes chroniques par

les sels organiques de cuivre. Presse Med. *54*, 884–885.

222. Forssen, A. (1972) Inorganic elements in the human body. 1. Occurrence of Ba, Br, Ca, Cd, Cs, Cu, K, Mn, Ni, Sn, Sr, Y and Zn in the human body. Ann. Med. Exp. Biol. Fenniae *50*, 99–162.

223. Foulk, W. T., Baggenstoss, A. H. & Butt, H. R. (1964) Primary biliary cirrhosis: re-evaluation by clinical and histologic study of 49 cases. Gastroenterology *47*, 354–374.

224. French, J. H., Moore, C. L., Ghatak, N. R., Sternlieb, I., Goldfischer, S. & Hirano, A. (1973) Trichopoliodystrophy (Menkes' kinky hair syndrome): A copper dependent deficiency of mitochondrial energetics. Pediat. Res. *7*, 386.

225. French, J. H., Sherard, E. S., Lubell, H., Brotz, M. & Moore, C. L. (1972) Trichopoliodystrophy. 1. Report of a case and biochemical studies. Arch. Neurol. *26*, 229–244.

226. Frieden, E. (1970) Ceruloplasmin, a link between copper and iron metabolism. Nutr. Rev. *28*, 87–91.

227. Frieden, E. (1971) Ceruloplasmin, a link between iron and copper metabolism. In: Bioinorganic Chemistry, Advances in Chemistry Series (Gould, R. F., ed.), pp. 292–321, American Chemical Society, Washington, D.C.

228. Frieden, E. (1973) The ferrous to ferric cycles in iron metabolism. Nutr. Rev. *31*, 41–44.

229. Frieden, E. (1974) The biochemical evolution of the iron and copper proteins. In: Trace Element Metabolism in Animals—2. (Hoekstra, W. G., Suttie, J. W., Ganther, H. E. & Mertz, W., eds.), pp. 105–118, University Park Press, Baltimore.

230. Frieden, E. & Hsieh, H. S. (1976) Ceruloplasmin: the copper transport protein with essential oxidase activity. In: Advances in Enzymology and Related Areas of Molecular Biology (Meister, A., ed.), vol. 44, pp. 187–236, Wiley, New York.

231. Friedman, S., Bahary, C., Eckerling, B. & Gans, B. (1969) Serum copper level as an index of placental function. Obstet. Gynecol. *33*, 189–193.

232. Friedman, S. & Kaufman, S. (1965) 3-4-dihydroxyphenylethylamine β-hydroxylase: a copper protein. J. Biol. Chem. *240*, 552–554.

233. Frommer, D. J. (1971) The binding of copper by bile and serum. Clin. Sci. *41*, 485–493.

234. Frommer, D. J. (1972) The measurements of biliary copper secretion in humans. Clin. Sci. *42*, 26P. (Abstract).

235. Frommer, D. J. (1974) Defective biliary excretion of copper in Wilson's disease. Gut *15*, 125–129.

236. Frommer, D. J. (1977) Biliary copper excretion in man and the rat. Digestion *15*, 390–396.

237. Fukushima, K., Senda, N., Uenoyama, T., Inui, H., Ishigami, S., Kariya, A., Naka, K., Iwasaki, T. & Sakao, K. (1951) Copper deficiency anemia in human adults. Med. J. Osaka Univ., English ed. 2, 157–170.

238. Fushimi, H., Hamison, C. R. & Ravin, H. A. (1971) Two new copper proteins from human brains. J. Biochem. *69*, 1041–1054.

239. Gabovich, R. D. (1966) Contents of some trace elements in the food in certain cities and towns of the USSR. Hygiene Sanitation *31* (7), 41–47.

240. Gahlot, D. K., Khosla, P. K., Makashir, P. D., Vasuki, K. & Basu, N. (1976) Copper metabolism in retinitis pigmentosa. Br. J. Ophthal. *60*, 770–774.

241. Gallagher, C. H. (1957) The pathology and biochemistry of copper deficiency. Austr. Vet. J. *33*, 311–317.

242. Garnica, A. D. & Fletcher, S. R. (1975) Parenteral copper in Menkes' kinky-hair syndrome. Lancet 2, 659–660.

243. Garnica, A. D., Frias, J. L., Easley, J. F. & Rennert, O. M. (1974) Menkes kinky hair disease. A defect in metallothionein metabolism? In: Birth Defects: Original Article Series (Bergama, D., ed.), vol. 10, pp. 149–155.

244. Garnica, A., Frias, J. & Rennert, O. (1973) Studies of ceruloplasmin in Menkes' kinky hair disease. Pediat. Res. *7*, 387 (Abstr.).

245. Gault, M. H., Stein, J. & Aronoff, A. (1966) Serum ceruloplasmin in hepatobiliary and other disorders: significance of abnormal values. Gastroenterology *50*, 8–18.

246. Gelmers, H. J., Troost, J. & Willemse, J. (1973) Wilson's disease: modification by L-dopa. Neuropaediatrie *4*, 453–457.

247. Genov, D., Bozhokov, B. & Zlatkov, N. B. (1972) Copper pathochemistry in vitiligo. Clin. Chem. Acta 37, 207–211.

248. Gerlach, W. (1934) Untersuchungen über den Kupfergehalt menschlicher (und tierischer) Organe. Virch. Arch. Pathol. Anat. Physiol. *294*, 171–197.

249. Gerlach, W. & Rohrschneider, W. (1934) Besteht das pigment des Kayser-Fleischerschen Hornhautringes aus Silber. Klin. Wochenschr. *13*, 48–49.

250. German, J. L., III. (1961) Induced variation in copper metabolism in Wilson's disease. In: Wilson's Disease, Some Current Concepts (Walshe, J. M. & Cumings, J. N., eds.), pp. 198–204, Blackwell, Oxford.

251. Ghatak, N. R., Hirano, A., Poon, T. P. & French, J. H. (1972) Trichopoliodystrophy. II Pathological changes in skeletal muscle and nervous system. Arch. Neurol. *26*, 60–72.

252. Gillespie, J. M. (1973) Keratin structure and changes with copper deficiency. Austr. J. Derm. *14*, 127–131.

253. Giorgio, A. J., Cartwright, G. E. & Wintrobe, M. M. (1964) Determination of urinary copper by means of direct extraction with zinc dibenzyl dithiocarbamate. Am. J. Clin. Pathol. *41*, 22–26.

254. Gipp, W. F., Pond, W. G., Kallfelz, F. A., Tasker, J. B., Van Campen, D. R., Krook, L. & Visek, W. J. (1974) Effect of dietary copper, iron and ascorbic acid levels on hematology, blood and tissue copper, iron

and zinc concentrations and ^{64}Cu and ^{59}Fe metabolism in young pigs. J. Nutr. *104*, 532–541.

255. Gisinger, E. (1955) Beiträge zum Kupferstoffwechsel. Wein Ztschr. Inn. Med. *36*, 168–183.

256. Gitlin, D., Hughes, W. L. & Janeway, C. A. (1960) Absorption and excretion of copper in mice. Nature *188*, 150–151.

257. Glass, B. (1950) A summary of the symposium on copper metabolism. In: A Symposium on Copper Metabolism, (McElroy, W. D. & Glass, B., eds.), pp. 7–36, J. Hopkins Press, Baltimore.

258. Glazebrook, A. J. (1945) Wilson's disease. Edinb. Med. J. *52*, 83–87.

259. Goka, T. J., Stevenson, R. E., Hefferan, P. M. & Howell, R. R. (1976) Menkes disease: A biochemical abnormality in cultured human fibroblasts. Proc. Nat. Acad. Sci. U.S.A. *73*, 604–606.

260. Goldfischer, S. (1965) The localization of copper in the pericanalicular granules (lysosomes) of liver in Wilson's disease (hepatolenticular degeneration). Am. J. Pathol. *46*, 977–983.

261. Goldfischer, S. & Sternlich, I. (1968) Changes in the distribution of hepatic copper in relation to the progression of Wilson's disease (hepatolenticular degeneration). Am. J. Pathol. *53*, 883–902.

262. Goldstein, N. P. & Owen, C. A. (1974) Introduction: Symposium on Copper Metabolism and Wilson's Disease. Mayo Clinic Proc. *49*, 363–367.

263. Gollan, J. L. (1975) Studies on the nature of complexes formed by copper with human alimentary secretions and their influence on copper absorption in the rat. Clin. Sci. Molec. Med. *49*, 237–245.

264. Gollan, J. L., Davis, P. S. & Deller, D. J. (1971) Binding of copper by human alimentary secretions. Am. J. Clin. Nutr. *24*, 1025–1027.

265. Gollan, J. L., Davis, P. S. & Deller, D. J. (1971) Copper content of human alimentary secretions. Clin. Biochem. *4*, 42–44.

266. Gollan, J. L. & Deller, D. J. (1973) Studies on the nature and excretion of biliary copper in man. Clin. Sci. *44*, 9–15.

267. Gollan, J. L., Stocks, J., Dormandy, T. L. & Sherlock, S. (1977) Reduced oxidase activity in the caeruloplasmin of two families with Wilson's disease. J. Clin. Pathol. *30*, 81–83.

268. Goodman, S. I., Rodgerson, D. O. & Kauffman, J. (1967) Hypercupremia in a patient with multiple myeloma. J. Lab. Clin. Med. *70*, 57–62.

269. Gopalan, C., Reddy, V. & Mohan, V. S. (1963) Some aspects of copper metabolism in protein-calorie malnutrition. J. Pediat. *63*, 646–649.

270. Gorczynska, Z. (1973) On the disturbances of the iron and copper metabolism in the course of viral hepatitis. Rocz. Akad. Bialymstoku, *18*, 93–112 (Polish).

271. Gordon, A. H. & Rabinowitch, I. M. (1933) Yellow atrophy of the liver. Report of a case, with particular reference to the metabolism of copper. Arch. Intern. Med. *51*, 143–151.

272. Gordon, N. (1974) Menkes' kinky-hair (steely-hair) syndrome. Devel. Med. Child. Neurol. *16*, 827–829.

273. Gormican, A. (1970) Inorganic elements in foods used in hospital menus. J. Am. Diet. Assn. *56*, 397–403.

274. Gorter, E. (1933) Copper and anemia. Am. J. Dis. Child. *46*, 1066–1075.

275. Gorter, E., Grendel, F. & Weyers, W. A. M. (1931) Le role du cuivre dans l'anémie infantile. Rev. Franc. Pediat. *7*, 747–765.

276. Graham, G. G. & Cordano, A. (1969) Copper depletion and deficiency in the malnourished infant. J. Hopkins Med. J. *124*, 139–150.

277. Grand, R. J. & Vawter, G. F. (1975) Juvenile Wilson's disease: Histologic and functional studies during penicillamine therapy. J. Pediatrics *87*, 1161–1170.

278. Greger, J. L. & Buckley, S. (1977) Menstrual loss of zinc, copper, magnesium and iron by adolescent girls. Nutr. Rep. Internat. *16*, 639–647.

279. Greiner, A. C., Chan, S. C. & Nicolson, G. A. (1975) Human brain contents of calcium, copper, magnesium and zinc in some neurological pathologies. Clin. Chim. Acta *64*, 211–213.

280. Griscom, N. T., Craig, J. N. & Neuhauser, E. B. D. (1971) Systemic bone disease developing in small premature infants. Pediatrics *48*, 883–895.

281. Groth, C. G., Dubois, R. S., Corman, J., Gustafsson, A., Iwatsuki, S., Rodgerson, D. O., Halgrimson, C. G. & Starzl, T. E. (1973) Metabolism effects of hepatic replacement in Wilson's disease. Transplant. Proc. *5*, 829–833.

282. Grover, W. D. & Scrutton, M. C. (1974) The effect of prolonged intravenous therapy on copper metabolism in trichopoliodystrophy. Pediat. Res. *8*, 389.

283. Grover, W. D. & Scrutton, M. C. (1975) Copper infusion therapy in trichopoliodystrophy. J. Pediat. *86*, 216–220.

284. Gubler, C. J. (1956) Copper metabolism in man. J. Am. Med. Assn. *161*, 530–535.

285. Gubler, C. J., Brown, H., Markowitz, H., Cartwright, G. E. & Wintrobe, M. M. (1957) Studies on copper metabolism. XXIII. Portal (Laennec's) cirrhosis of the liver. J. Clin. Invest. *36*, 1208–1216.

286. Gubler, C. J., Lahey, M. E., Cartwright, G. E. & Wintrobe, M. M. (1953) Studies of copper metabolism. IX. The transportation of copper in blood. J. Clin. Invest. *32*, 405–414.

287. Gumbatov, N. B. (1972) The content of cobalt, copper, zinc and iron in the blood of patients suffering from hypertension. Terap. Arkh. *44* (4), 65–68 (Russian).

288. Gupta, P. S., Bhargava, S. P. & Sharma, M. L. (1962) Acute copper sulphate poisoning with special reference to its management

with corticosteroid therapy. J. Assn. Phys. India 10, 287–292.

289. Guthrie, B. E. (1973) Daily dietary intakes of zinc, copper, manganese, chromium and cadmium by some New Zealand women. Proc. Univ. Otago Med. School. 51, 47–49.

290. Guthrie, B. E. (1975) Chromium, manganese, copper, zinc and cadmium content of New Zealand foods. N.Z. Med. J. 82, 418–424.

291. Guthrie, B. E. & Robinson, M. F. (1977) Dietary intakes of manganese, copper, zinc and cadmium by New Zealand women. Br. J. Nutr. 38, 55–63.

292. Guthrie, B. E. & Robinson, M. F. (1978) The nutritional status of New Zealanders with respect to manganese, copper, zinc and cadmium: a review. N.Z. Med. J. 87, 3–8.

293. Hagberg, B., Axtrup, S. & Berfenstam, R. (1953) Heavy metals (iron, copper, zinc) in the blood of the fetus and the infant. Études Néo-natal. 2, 81–90.

294. Hahn, N., Paschen, K. & Haller, J. (1972) Des Verhalten von Kupfer, Eisen, Magnesium, Calcium und Zink bei Frauen mit normalem Menstruationscyclus, unter Einnahme von Ovulationshemmern und in der Graviditat. Arch. Gynakol. 213, 176–186.

295. Hall, E. M. & Butt, E. M. (1928) Experimental pigment cirrhosis due to copper poisoning. Its relation to hemochromatosis. Arch. Pathol. 6, 1–25.

296. Hall, H. C. (1921) La dégénérescence hépato-lenticularie; maladie de Wilson-pseudo-sclérose, pp. 190–192, Masson, Paris.

297. Halsted, J. A., Hackley, B. M. & Smith, J. C., Jr. (1968) Plasma-zinc and copper in pregnancy and after oral contraceptives. Lancet 2, 278.

298. Hambidge, K. M. (1973) Increase in hair copper concentration with increase distance from the scalp. Am. J. Clin. Nutr. 26, 1212–1215.

299. Hambidge, K. M. (1976) The importance of trace elements in infant nutrition. Current Med. Res. Opin. 4 (Suppl. 1), 44–53.

300. Hambidge, K. M. & Droegemueller, W. (1974) Changes in plasma and hair concentrations of zinc, copper, chromium, and manganese during pregnancy. Obstet. & Gynecol. 44, 666–672.

301. Hambidge, K. M. & Walravens, P. (1975) Trace elements in nutrition. In: Practice of Pediatrics, vol. 1, chap. 29, pp. 1–40, Harper & Rowe, Hagerstown, Maryland.

302. Hamlyn, A. N., Gollan, J. L., Douglas, A. P. & Sherlock, S. (1977) Fulminating Wilson's disease with haemolysis and renal failure: copper studies and assessment of dialysis regimens. Br. Med. J. 2, 660–663.

303. Hankiewicz, J. & Sevećek, E. (1974) Untersuchungen über den Kupfer- und Zeruloplasmingehalt bei Frauen während der Schwangerschaft und bei solchen mit gewissen gynäkologischen Krankheiten. Zentralbl. Gynäk. 96, 905–909.

304. Hankins, D. A., Riella, M. C., Scribner, B. H. & Babb, A. L. (1976) Whole blood trace element concentrations during total parenteral nutrition. Surgery 79, 674–677.

305. Hansen, J. D. L. & Lehmann, B. H. (1969) Serum zinc and copper concentrations in children with protein-calorie malnutrition. S. African Med. J. 43, 1248–1251.

306. Harcke, H. T., Jr., Capitanio, M. A., Grover, W. D. & Valdes-Dapena, M. (1977) Bladder diverticula and Menkes' syndrome. Radiology 124, 459–461.

307. Harper, A. E. (1976) Basis of recommended dietary allowances for trace elements. In: Trace Elements in Human Health and Disease (Prasad, A. S. & Oberleas, D., eds.), vol. 2, pp. 371–378, Academic Press, New York.

308. Harris, E. D. & O'Dell, B. L. (1974) Copper and amine oxidases in connective tissue metabolism. In: Protein-Metal Interactions Friedman, M., ed.), pp. 267–284, Plenum, New York.

309. Harris, E. D., Rayton, J. K. & De Groot, J. E. (1977) A critical role for copper in aortic elastin structure and synthesis. Adv. Exp. Med. Biol. 79, 543–559.

310. Harris, W. O., Jr., Kopp, J. E., Rinaldi, I. & Peach, W. F., Jr. (1975) Menkes' kinky hair syndrome. Va. Med. Monthly 102, 725–728.

311. Hart, E. B., Elvehjem, C. A., Waddell, J. & Herrin, R. C. (1927) Iron in nutrition. IV. Nutritional anemia on whole milk diets and its correction with the ash of certain plant and animal tissues or with soluble iron salts. J. Biol. Chem. 72, 299–320.

312. Hart, E. B., Steenbock, H., Elvehjem, C. A. & Waddell, J. (1925) Iron in nutrition. I. Nutritional anemia on whole milk diets and the utilization of inorganic iron in hemoglobin building. J. Biol. Chem. 65, 67–80.

313. Hart, E. B., Steenbock, H., Waddell, J. & Elvehjem, C. A. (1928) Iron in Nutrition. VII. Copper as a supplement to iron for hemoglobin building in the rat. J. Biol. Chem. 77, 797–812.

314. Hartley, T. F., Dawson, J. B. & Hodgkinson, A. (1974) Simultaneous measurement of Na, K, Ca, Mg, Cu and Zn balances in man. Clin. Chim. Acta 52, 321–333.

315. Hasegawa, M. & Ito, S. (1954) The importance of copper in the treatment of anemia. Keio J. Med. 3, 25–34.

316. Haurowitz, F. (1930) Über eine Anomalie des Kupferstoffwechsels. Hoppe-Seyler's Ztschr. Physiol. Chem. 190, 72–74.

317. Hauer, E. C. & Kaminski, M. V. (1978) Trace metal profile of parenteral nutrition solutions. Am. J. Clin. Nutr. 31, 264–268.

318. Heijkenskjold, F. & Hedenstedt, S. (1962) Serum copper determinations in normal pregnancy and abortion. Acta Obstet. Gynecol. Scand. 41, 41–47.

319. Heilmeyer, L., Keiderling, W. & Stüwe, G. (1941) Kupfer und Eisen als Körperigene Wirkstoffe und ihre Bedeutung beim Krankheitsgeschehen. Fisher, Jena.

320. Hejduk, J. (1963) Untersuchunger uber das Verhalten von Eisen und Kupfer im

Blutserum der Frauen in der Schwangerschaft, unter der Geburt, im Wochenbett sowie bei Neugeborenen. Geburtsh. Gynaek. 160, 187–199.

321. Henkin, R. I. (1971) Newer aspects of copper and zinc metabolism. In: New Trace Metals and Nutrition (Mertz, W. & Cornatzer, W., eds.), pp. 255–312, Marcel Dekker, New York.

322. Henkin, R. I. & Bradley, D. F. (1969) Regulation of taste acuity by thiols and metal ions. Proc. Nat. Acad. Sci. U.S.A. 62, 30–37.

323. Henkin, R. I., Keiser, H. R., Jaffe, I. A., Sternlieb, I. & Scheinberg, I. H. (1967) Decreased taste sensitivity after D-penicillamine reversed by copper administration. Lancet 2, 1268–1271.

324. Henkin, R. I., Marshall, J. R. & Meret, S. (1971) Maternal-fetal metabolism of copper and zinc at term. Am. J. Obst. Gynecol. 110, 131–134.

325. Henkin, R. I., Schulman, J. D., Schulman, C. B. & Bronzert, D. A. (1973) Changes in total, nondiffusible and diffusible plasma zinc and copper during infancy. J. Pediat. 82, 831–837.

326. Henkin, R. I. & Smith, F. R. (1972) Zinc and copper metabolism in acute viral hepatitis. Am. J. Med. Sci. 264, 401–409.

327. Herkel, W. (1930) Über die Bedeutung des Kupfers (Zinks und Mangans) in der Biologie und Pathologie. Beitrag. Pathol. Anat. Allg. Pathol. 85, 513–551.

328. Herring, W. B., Leavell, B. S., Paixao, L. M. & Yoe, J. H. (1960) Trace metals in human plasma and red blood cells. A study of magnesium, chromium, nickel, copper and zinc. II. Observations of patients with some hematologic diseases. Am. J. Clin. Nutr. 8, 855–863.

329. Heydorn, K., Damsgaard, E., Horn, N., Mikkelsen, M., Tygstrup, I., Vestermark, S. & Weber, J. (1975) Extra-hepatic storage of copper. A male foetus suspected of Menkes' disease. Humangenetik. 29, 171–175.

330. Hill, C. H. (1969) A role of copper in elastin formation. Nutr. Rev. 27, 99–100.

331. Hill, C. H. & Matrone, G. (1961) Studies on copper and iron deficiencies in growing chickens. J. Nutr. 73, 425–431.

332. Hill, C. H. & Matrone, G. (1970) Chemical parameters in the study of in vivo and in vitro interactions of transition elements. Federation Proc. 29, 1474–1481.

333. Hill, C. H. & Starcher, B. (1965) Effect of reducing agents on copper deficiency in the chick. J. Nutr. 85, 271–274.

334. Hill, C. H., Starcher, B. & Kim, C. (1967) Role of copper in the formation of elastin. Federation Proc. 26, 129–133.

335. Hill, J. M. & Kim, C. S. (1967) The derangement of elastin synthesis in pyridoxine deficiency. Biochem. Biophys. Res. Comm. 27, 94–99.

336. Hirano, A., Liena, J. F., French, J. H. & Ghatak, N. R. (1977) Fine structure of the cerebellar cortex in Menkes' kinky-hair disease. X. Chromosome-linked copper malabsorption. Arch. Neurol. 34, 52–56.

337. Hitier, Y. (1976) Répercussions de la carence en acide ascorbique sur la céruloplasmine et le cuivre tissulaire. Internat. J. Vit. Nutr. Res. 46, 48–57.

338. Hitzig, W. H. (1960) Das Bluteiweissbild im Säuglingsalter. Habilitationsschrift, Zurich (cited by Richterich, ref. 638).

339. Hitzig, W. H. (1961) Das Bluteiweissbild beim gesunden Säugling. Spezifische Proteinbestimmungen mit besonderer Berücksichtigung immunochemischer Methoden. Helv. Paediat. Acta 16, 46–81.

340. Hockey, A. & Masters, C. L. (1977) Menkes' kinky (steely) hair disease. Aust. J. Dermatol. 18, 77–80.

341. Hodges, M. A. & Peterson, W. H. (1931) Manganese, copper and iron content of serving portions of common foods. J. Am. Diet. Assn. 7, 6–16.

342. Hoffmann, R. P. & Ashby, D. M. (1976) Trace element concentrations in commercially available solutions. Drug Intell. Clin. Pharmacol. 10, 74–76.

343. Hohnadel, D. C., Sunderman, F. W., Jr., Nechay, M. W. & McNeely, M. D. (1973) Atomic absorption spectrometry of nickel, copper, zinc, and lead in sweat collected from healthy subjects during sauna bathing. Clin. Chem. 19, 1288–1292.

344. Holden, J. M., Wolf, W. R. & Mertz, W. (1979) Dietary levels of zinc and copper in self selected diets. J. Am. Diet. Assn. 75, 23–28.

345. Holmberg, C. G. (1941) Über die Verteilung des Kupfers zwischen Plasma und roten Blutkörperchen bei extremen physiologischen Verschiebungen im Cu-Gehalt des Blutes. Acta Physiol. Scand. 2, 71–77.

346. Holmberg, C. G. & Laurell, C. B. (1948) Investigations in serum copper. II. Isolation of the copper containing protein, and a description of some of its properties. Acta Chem. Scand. 2, 550–556.

347. Holmberg, C. G. & Laurell, C. B. (1951) Investigations in serum copper. III. Coeruloplasmin as an enzyme. Acta Chem. Scand. 5, 476–480.

348. Holmberg, C. G. & Laurell, C. B. (1951) Oxidase reactions in human plasma caused by coeruloplasmin. Scand. J. Lab. Invest. 3, 103–107.

349. Holt, F. & Scoular, F. I. (1946) Iron and copper metabolism of young women on self-selected diets. J. Nutr. 35, 717–723.

350. Holtkamp, H. C. & Van Eijk, H. G. (1975) Over het voorkomen en de functie van koper in het menselijk lichaam. Maandschr. Kindergeneeskd. 43, 36–55.

351. Holtzman, N. A. (1976) Menkes' kinky hair syndrome: a genetic disease involving copper. Federation Proc. 35, 2276–2280.

352. Holtzman, N. A., Charache, P., Cordano, A. & Graham, G. G. (1970) Distribution of

serum copper in copper deficiency. Johns Hopkins Med. J. *126*, 34–42.

353. Holtzman, N. A., Elliot, D. A. & Heller, R. H. (1966) Copper intoxication: report of a case with observations on ceruloplasmin. New Engl. J. Med. *275*, 347–352.

354. Holtzman, N. A., Graham, G. G., Charache, P. & Haslam, R. (1967) Effect of copper on ceruloplasmin concentration. Pediat. Res. *1*, 219.

355. Holtzman, N. A. & Haslam, R. H. A. (1968) Elevation of serum copper following copper sulfate as an emetic. Pediat. *42*, 189–193.

356. Hopper, S. H. & Adams, H. S. (1958) Copper poisoning from vending machines. Pub. Health. Rep. *73*, 910–914.

357. Horčička, J., Borovansky, J. & Duchŏn, J. (1973) Verteilung von Zink und Kupfer in menschlichen Kopfhaar verschiedener Farbtöne. Dermatol. Monatsch. *159*, 206–209.

358. Horn, N. (1976) Copper incorporation studies on cultured cells for prenatal diagnosis of Menkes' disease. Lancet *1*, 1156–1158.

359. Horn, N., Mikkelsen, M., Heydorn, K., Damsgaard, E. & Tygstrup, I. (1975) Copper and steely hair. Lancet *1*, 1236.

360. Horwitt, M. K., Meyer, B. J., Meyer, A. C., Harvey, C. C. & Haffron, D. (1957) Serum copper and oxidase activity in schizophrenic patients. Arch. Neurol. Psychiat. *73*, 275–282.

361. Howell, J. McC. & Davison, A. N. (1959) The copper content and cytochrome oxidase activity of tissues from normal and swayback lambs. Biochem. J. *72*, 365–368.

362. Hrgovcic, R. & Hrgovcic, M. (1969) Normal serum copper levels during childhood. Jugoslav. Pedijat. *11*, 83–94 (Serbo-crotian).

363. Hrgovcic, M., Tessmer, C. F., Thomas, F. B., Fuller, L. M., Gamble, J. F. & Shullenberger, C. C. (1973) Significance of serum copper levels in adult patients with Hodgkin's disease. Cancer *31*, 1337–1345.

364. Hrgovcic, M., Tessmer, C. F., Thomas, F. B., Ong, P. S., Gamble, J. F. & Shullenberger, C. C. (1973) Serum copper observations in patients with malignant lymphoma. Cancer *32*, 1512–1524.

365. Hsieh, H. S. & Frieden, E. (1975) Evidence for ceruloplasmin as a copper transport protein. Biochem. Biophys. Res. Comm. *67*, 1326–1331.

366. Hughes, G., Kelley, V. J. & Stewart, R. A. (1960) The copper content of infant foods. Pediatrics *25*, 477–484.

367. Hull, R. L. (1974) Use of trace elements in intravenous hyperalimentation solutions. Am. J. Hosp. Pharm. *31*, 759–761.

368. Humoller, F. L., Mockler, M. P., Holthaus, J. M. & Mahler, D. L. (1960) Enzymatic properties of ceruloplasmin. J. Lab. Clin. Med. *56*, 222–234.

369. Hunt, A. H., Parr, R. M., Taylor, D. M. & Trott, G. G. (1963) Relation between cirrhosis and trace metal content of liver: with special reference to primary biliary cirrhosis and copper. Br. Med. J. *2*, 1498–1501.

370. Hunt, C. E., Carlton, W. W. & Newberne, P. M. (1970) Interrelationships between copper deficiency and dietary ascorbic acid in the rabbit. Br. J. Nutr. *24*, 61–69.

371. Hunt, D. M. (1974) Primary defect in copper transport underlies mottled mutants in the mouse. Nature *249*, 852–854.

372. Huriez, C., Bizerte, D. & Bialais, M. (1972) Les troubles du métabolisme du cuivre dans la vitiligo. Ann. Dermatol. Syphil. *49*, 29–40.

373. Hurley, L. S. (1976) Interaction of genes and metals in development. Federation Proc. *35*, 2271–2275.

374. Hurley, L. S. & Bell, L. T. (1975) Amelioration by copper supplementation of mutant gene effects in the crinkled mouse. Proc. Soc. Exp. Biol. Med. *149*, 830–834.

375. Ilicin, G. (1971) Serum copper and magnesium levels in leukemia and malignant lymphoma. Lancet *2*, 1036–1037.

376. Ivanovich, P., Manzler, A. & Drake, R. (1969) Acute hemolysis following hemodialysis. Trans. Am. Soc. Artif. Intern. Organs. *15*, 316–318.

377. Iyengar, L. & Apte, S. V. (1972) Nutrient stores in human fetal livers. Br. J. Nutr. *27*, 313–317.

378. Jacob, R. A., Klevay, L. M. & Logan, G. M. (1978) Hair as a biopsy material. V. Hair metal as an index of hepatic metal in rats: copper and zinc. Am. J. Clin. Nutr. *31*, 477–480.

379. Jacobson, S. & Wester, P. O. (1977) Balance study of twenty trace elements during total parenteral nutrition in man. Br. J. Nutr. *37*, 107–126.

380. Jaffe, I. A. (1968) Penicillamine in rheumatoid disease with particular reference to rheumatoid factor. Postgrad. Med. J. *44* (Suppl.), 34–40.

381. Jaffe, I. A., Merriman, P. & Jacobus, D. (1968) Copper: relation to penicillamine-induced defect in collagen. Science *161*, 1016–1017.

382. James, B. E. & MacMahon, R. A. (1970) Trace elements in intravenous fluids. Med. J. Australia *2*, 1161–1163.

383. James, B. E. & MacMahon, R. A. (1976) Balance studies of nine elements during complete intravenous feeding of small premature infants. Austr. Pediat. J. *12*, 154–162.

384. Janes, J. M., McCall, J. T. & Elveback, L. R. (1972) Trace metals in human osteogenic sarcoma. Mayo Clin. Proc. *47*, 476–478.

385. Jeejeebhoy, K. N., Zohrab, W. J., Langer, B., Phillips, M. J., Kuskis, A. & Anderson, G. H. (1973) Total parenteral nutrition at home for 23 months, without complication and with good rehabilitation. A study of technical and metabolic features. Gastroenterology *65*, 811–820.

386. Jensen, K. B., Thorling, E. B. & Andersen, C. J. (1964) Serum copper in Hodgkin's disease. Scand. J. Hematol. *1*, 63–74.

387. Jensen, W. N. & Kamin, H. (1957) Copper transport and excretion in normal subjects and in patients with Laennec's cir-

rhosis and Wilson's disease: A study with Cu[64]. J. Lab. Clin. Med. *49*, 200–210.

388. Johnson, N. C. (1961) Study of copper and zinc metabolism during pregnancy. Proc. Soc. Exp. Biol. Med. *108*, 518–519.

389. Josephs, H. (1931) Treatment of anaemia of infancy with iron and copper. Bull. J. Hopkins Hosp. *49*, 246–258.

390. Josephs, H. W. (1971) The effect of copper on iron metabolism: A clinical study. Johns Hopkins Med. J. *129*, 212–235.

391. Judd, E. S. & Dry, T. J. (1934) The significance of iron and copper in the bile of man. J. Lab. Clin. Med. *20*, 609–615.

392. Kagi, J. H. R. & Vallee, B. L. (1960) Metallothionein: a cadmium and zinc-containing protein from equine renal cortex. J. Biol. Chem. *235*, 3460–3465.

393. Kagi, J. H. R. & Vallee, B. L. (1961) Metallothionein: a cadmium and zinc-containing protein from equine renal cortex. II. Physico-chemical properties. J. Biol. Chem. *236*, 2435–2442.

394. Karpel, J. T. & Peden, V. H. (1972) Copper deficiency in long-term parenteral nutrition. J. Pediat. *80*, 32–36.

395. Kasper, C. B. & Deutsch, H. F. (1963) Physiochemical studies of human ceruloplasmin. J. Biol. Chem. *238*, 2325–2337.

396. Keen, C. L. & Hurley, L. S. (1976) Copper supplementation in quaking mutant mice: reduced tremors and increased brain copper. Science *193*, 244–246.

397. Kehoe, R. A., Cholak, J. & Story, R. V. (1940) A spectrochemical study of the normal ranges of the concentration of certain trace metals in biological materials. J. Nutr. *19*, 579–592.

398. Kehoe, R. A., Cholak, J. & Story, R. V. (1940) Manganese, lead, tin, aluminum, copper and silver in normal biological material. J. Nutr. *20*, 85–97.

399. Keil, H. L. & Nelson, V. E. (1931) The role of copper in hemoglobin regeneration and in reproduction. J. Biol. Chem. *93*, 49–57.

400. Kekki, M., Koskelo, P. & Lassus, A. (1966) Serum ceruloplasmin-bound copper and nonceruloplasmin-bound copper in uncomplicated psoriasis. J. Invest. Dermatol. *47*, 159–161.

401. Kelly, W. A., Kesterson, J. W. & Carlton, W. W. (1974) Myocardial lesions in the offspring of female rats fed a copper deficient diet. Exper. Molec. Pathol. *20*, 40–56.

402. Khalil, M., Kabiel, A., El-Khateeb, S., Aref, K., El Lozy, M., Jahin, S. & Nasr, F. (1974) Plasma and red cell water and elements in protein-caloric malnutrition. Am. J. Clin. Nutr. *27*, 260–267.

403. Khaire, D. S. & Magar, N. G. (1972) Copper in leprosy blood plasma concentration and urinary excretion. Indian J. Med. Res. *60*, 1697–1701.

404. Khandekar, J. D., Mukerji, D. P., Naik, G. D. & Sepaha, G. C. (1972) Regional variation in copper content of arterial wall. Experientia *28*, 917.

405. Khandekar, J. D., Mukerji, D. P. & Sepaha, G. C. (1972) Serum copper and iron in ischemic heart disease. Ind. J. Med. Sci. *26*, 813–818.

406. Kimmel, J. R., Markowitz, H. & Brown, D. M. (1959) Some chemical and physical properties of erythrocuprein. J. Biol. Chem. *234*, 46–50.

407. King, J. C., Raynolds, W. L. & Margen, S. (1978) Absorption of stable isotopes of iron, copper and zinc during oral contraceptive use. Am. J. Clin. Nutr. *31*, 1198–1203.

408. Kirchgessner, M., Weser, U. & Muller, H. L. (1967) Cu-Absorption bei Zulag von Glucon-, Citronen Salicyl- und Oxalsaure. 7. Zur Dynamik der Kupfer absorption. Ztschr. Tierphysiol. Tieremahrung Futtermittelk. *23*, 28–30.

409. Kleinbaum, H. (1962) Kupferstoffwechselbilanzen bei Sauglingen. Ztschr. Kinderheilk. *87*, 101–115.

410. Kleinbaum, H. (1962) Über den Kupfergehalt der Nahrungsmittel des Kindes. Ztschr. Kinderheilk. *86*, 655–666.

411. Kleinbaum, H. (1963) Über die Ceruloplasmin-oxydase-Aktivät im Serum bei gesunden Kindern verschiedener Atersklassen. Ztschr. Kinderkeilk. *88*, 11–21.

412. Kleinbaum, H. (1963) Vorübergehende Hypoproteinamine mit Hypocuprämie und Eisenmangelänemie bei dystrophen Säuglingen. Ztschr. Kinderheilk. *88*, 29–34.

413. Kleinbaum, H. (1968) Coeruloplasmin, direkt reagierendes Kupfer und Gesamptkupfergehalt bei verschiedenen Infectionskrankheiten und entzündlichen Zustandsbildern. Ztschr. Kinderheil. *102*, 84–94.

414. Kleinmann, H. & Klinke, J. (1929) Über den Kupfergehalt menschlicher Organe. Virch. Arch. Path. Anat. Physiol. *275*, 422–435.

415. Klevay, L. M. (1970) Hair as a biopsy material. II. Assessment of copper nutriture. Am. J. Clin. Nutr. *23*, 1194–1202.

416. Klevay, L. M. (1974) An association between the amount of fat and the ratio of zinc to copper in 71 foods: inferences about the epidemiology of coronary heart disease. Nutr. Rep. Internat. *9*, 393–399.

417. Klevay, L. M. (1975) Coronary heart disease: the zinc/copper hypothesis. Am. J. Clin. Nutr. *28*, 764–774.

418. Klevay, L. M. (1975) The ratio of zinc to copper of diets in the United States. Nutr. Rep. Internat. *11*, 237–242.

419. Klevay, L. M., Reck, S. & Barcome, D. F. (1977) United States diets and the copper requirement. Federation Proc. *36*, 1175.

420. Klevay, L. M., Vo-Khactu, K. P. & Jacob, R. A. (1975) The ratio of zinc to copper of cholesterol-lowering diets. In: Trace Substances in Environmental Health—IX. (Hemphill, D. D., ed.), pp. 131–138, Univ. of Missouri, Columbia.

421. Kolaric, K., Rogujić, A. & Fuss, V. (1975) Serum copper levels in patients with solid tumors. Tumori *61*, 173–177.

422. Kopp, N., Tommasi, M., Carrier, H., Pialat, J., Gilly, J. & Herve, C. (1975) Neuropathologie de la trichopoliodystrophie (Maladie de Menkes): une observation anatomoclinique. Rev. Neurol. (Paris) 131, 775–789.

423. Koskelo, P., Kekki, M., Virkunen, M., Lassus, A. & Somer, T. (1966) Serum ceruloplasmin concentration in rheumatoid arthritis, ankylosing spondylitis, psoriasis and sarcoidosis. Acta Rheum. Scand. 12, 261–266.

424. Kovalskiy, V. V. & Yarovaya, G. A. (1966) Molybdenum: infiltrated biochemical provinces. Agrokhimiya 8, 68–91 (Russian).

425. Kovalskiy, V. V., Yarovaya, G. A. & Shmavonyan, D. M. (1961) Changes in purine metabolism in man and animals under conditions of molybdenum biogeochemical provinces. Zh. Obsch. Biol. 22, 179–191 (Russian).

426. Krebs, H. A. (1928) Über das Kupfer im menschlichen Blutserum. Klin. Wochenschr. 7, 584–585.

427. Krishnamachari, K. A. V. R. (1974) Some aspects of copper metabolism in pellagra. Am. J. Clin. Nutr. 27, 108–111.

428. Krishnamachari, K. A. V. R. (1976) Further observations on the syndrome of endemic genu valgum of South India. Indian J. Med. Res. 64, 284–291.

429. Krishnamachari, K. A. V. R. & Rao, K. S. J. (1972) Ceruloplasmin activity in infants born to undernourished mothers. J. Obst. Gynaecol. Br. Commwlt. 79, 162–165.

430. Kushnir, M. P. (1972) The role of disorders of copper and vitamin C metabolism in the pathogenesis of psoriasis. Vestn. Derm. Vener. 46, (4), 23–26 (Roumanian) (cited in Nutr. Abstr. Rev. 43, 1026, 1971).

431. Kyer, J. L. & Bethell, F. H. (1936) The requirement of iron and copper and the influence of diet upon hemoglobin formation during normal pregnancy. J. Biol. Chem. 114, lx–lxi.

432. Lahey, M. E. (1957) Iron and copper in infant nutrition. Am. J. Clin. Nutr. 5, 516–526.

433. Lahey, M. E., Behar, M., Viteri, F. & Scrimshaw, N. S. (1958) Values for copper, iron and iron-binding capacity in the serum in kwashiorkor. Pediatrics 22, 72–78.

434. Lahey, M. E., Gubler, C. J., Cartwright, G. E. & Wintrobe, M. M. (1953) Studies on copper metabolism. VI. Blood copper in normal human subjects. J. Clin. Invest. 32, 322–328.

435. Lahey, M. E., Gubler, C. J., Cartwright, G. E. & Wintrobe, M. M. (1953) Studies on copper metabolism. VII. Blood copper in pregnancy and various pathologic states. J. Clin. Invest. 32, 329–339.

436. Lahey, M. E., Gubler, C. J., Chase, M. S., Cartwright, G. E. & Wintrobe, M. M. (1952) Studies on copper metabolism. II. Hematologic manifestations of copper deficiency in swine. Blood 7, 1053–1074.

437. Lahey, M. E. & Schubert, W. K. (1957) New deficiency syndrome occurring in infancy. Am. J. Dis. Child 93, 31–34.

438. Lal, S., Rajagopal, G. & Subrahmanyam, K. (1971) Serum caeruloplasmin in psoriasis. Indian J. Derm. 16, 103–104.

439. Lang, N. & Renschler, H. E. (1958) Untersuchungen zum Ort der Coeruloplasminbildung mit Radiokupfer (⁶⁴Cu). Ztschr. Exp. Med. 130, 203–214.

440. Lange, J., Schumacher, K. & Wischer, H. P. (1971) Die Behandlung des chronisch—aggressiven Hepatitis mit d-penicillamine. Deutsch. Med. Wochenschr. 96, 139–145.

441. Langer, B., McHattie, J. D., Zohrab, W. J. & Jeejeebhoy, K. N. (1973) Prolonged survival after complete bowel resection using intravenous alimentation at home. J. Surg. Res. 15, 226–233.

442. La Russo, N. F., Summerskill, W. H. J. & McCall, J. T. (1976) Abnormalities of chemical tests for copper metabolism in chronic active liver disease: differentiation from Wilson's disease. Gastroenterology, 70, 653–655.

443. Lea, C. M. & Luttrell, V. A. S. (1965) Copper content of hair in kwashiorkor. Nature 206, 413.

444. Lee, G. R., Nacht, S., Christensen, D., Hansen, S. P. & Cartwright, G. E. (1969) The contribution of citrate to the ferroxidase activity of serum. Proc. Soc. Exp. Biol. Med. 131, 918–923.

445. Lee, G. R., Nacht, S., Lukens, J. N. & Cartwright, G. E. (1968) Iron metabolism in copper deficient swine. J. Clin. Invest. 47, 2058–2069.

446. Lee, G. R., Williams, D. M. & Cartwright, G. E. (1976) Role of copper in iron metabolism and heme biosynthesis. In: Trace Elements in Human Health and Disease (Prasad, A. S. & Oberleas, D., eds.), vol 1, pp. 373–390, Academic Press, New York.

447. Lehmann, K. B. (1891) Kritische und experimentelle Studien uber die hygienishe Bedeutung des Kupfers. Munch. Med. Wochenschr. 38, 631–633.

448. Leu, M. L. & Strickland, G. T. (1971) Renal function in heterozygotes for Wilson's disease. Am. J. Med. Sci. 263, 19–24.

449. Leu, M. L., Strickland, G. T. & Gutman, R. A. (1970) Renal function in Wilson's disease: response to therapy. Am. J. Med. Sci. 260, 381–398.

450. Le Van, J. H. & Perry, E. I. (1961) Copper poisoning on shipboard. Pub. Health Rep. 76, 334.

451. Leverton, R. M. (1939) The copper metabolism of young women. J. Nutr. 17, 17.

452. Leverton, R. M. & Binkley, E. S. (1944) The copper metabolism and requirement of young women. J. Nutr. 27, 43–53.

453. Levy, N. S., Dawson, W. W., Rhodes, B. J. & Garnica, A. (1974) Ocular abnormalities in Menkes' kinky hair disease. Am. J. Ophthalmol. 77, 319–325.

454. Lewis, K. O. (1973) The nature of the copper complexes in bile and their relationship to the absorption and excretion of copper in normal subjects and in Wilson's disease. Gut 14, 221–232.

455. Lewis, M. S. (1931) Iron and copper in the treatment of anemia in children. J. Am. Med. Assn. 96, 1135–1138.
456. Lewis, R. A., Falls, H. F. & Troyer, D. O. (1975) Ocular manifestations of hypercupremia associated with multiple myeloma. Arch. Ophthamol. 93, 1050–1053.
457. Lewis, R. A., Hultquist, D. E., Baker, B. L., Falls, H. F., Gershowitz, H. & Penner, J. A. (1976) Hypercupremia associated with monoclonal immunoglobulin. J. Lab. Clin. Med. 88, 375–388.
458. Li, T. K. & Vallee, B. L. (1968) The biochemical and nutritional role of trace elements. In: Modern Nutrition in Health and Disease. (Wohl, M. G. & R. S. Goodhart, eds.), p. 377, Lea & Febiger, Philadelphia.
459. Lich, N. P. (1971) Effets toxiques de certains oligo-éléments. Aliment. Vie 59, 103–153.
460. Lifschitz, M. D. & Henkin, R. I. (1971) Circadian variation in copper and zinc in man. J. Appl. Physiol. 31, 88–92.
461. Linder, M. C. & Munro, H. N. (1973) Iron and copper metabolism during development. Enzyme 15, 111–138.
462. Lindow, C. W., Elvehjem, C. A. & Peterson, W. H. (1929) The copper content of plant and animal foods. J. Biol. Chem. 82, 465–471.
463. Lloyd-Still, J. D., Scwachman, H. & Filler, R. M. (1973) Protracted diarrhea of infancy treated by intravenous alimentation. 1. Clinical studies of 16 infants. Am. J. Dis. Child. 125, 358–364.
464. Locke, A., Main, E. R. & Rosbash, D. O. (1932) The copper and non-hemoglobinous iron contents of the blood serum in disease. J. Clin. Invest. 11, 527–542.
465. Lorber, A. (1969) Communication in response to Sternlieh et al. 1969. Arth. Rheum. 12, 459–460.
466. Lorber, A., Cutler, L. S. & Chang, C. C. (1968) Serum copper levels in rheumatoid arthritis: relationship of elevated copper to protein alterations. Arth. Rheum. 11, 65–71.
467. Lott, I. T., DiPaolo, R., Schwartz, D., Janowska, S. & Kanfer, J. N. (1975) Copper metabolism in the steely-hair syndrome. New Engl. J. Med. 292, 197–199.
468. Lott, I. T., DiPaola, R., Schwartz, D., Kanfer, J. N. & Moser, H. W. (1975) The pathogenesis and treatment of copper deficiency in steely-hair syndrome. Trans. Am. Neurol. Assn. 100, 151–154.
469. Lou, H. C., Holmer, G. K., Reske-Nielsen, E. & Vagn-Hansen, P. (1974) Lipid composition in gray and white matter of the brain in Menkes' disease. J. Neurochem. 22, 377–381.
470. Louis, J., Blanckaert, D., Desbonnets, P., Farriaux, J. P. & Fontaine, G. (1975) Anomalies originales dans une nouvelle observation de maladie de Menkes. Nouv. Presse Med. 15, 1138.
471. Lyle, W. H. (1967) Chronic dialysis and copper poisoning. New Engl. J. Med. 276, 1209–1210.
472. Lyle, W. H., Payton, J. E. & Hui, M. (1976) Haemodialysis and copper fever. Lancet 1, 1324–1325.
473. Lynch, R. E., Lee, G. R. & Cartwright, G. E. (1973) Penicillamine-induced cupriuria in normal subjects and in patients with active liver disease. Proc. Soc. Biol. Med. 142, 128–130.
474. MacDonald, I. & Warren, P. J. (1961) The copper content of the liver and hair of African children with kwashiorkor. Br. J. Nutr. 15, 593–596.
475. MacDonald, W. C., Trier, J. S. & Everett, N. B. (1964) Cell proliferation and migration in the stomach duodenum,. and rectum of man: radiographic studies. Gastroenterology 46, 405–417.
476. MacKay, H. M. M. (1933) Copper in the treatment of nutritional anemia in infancy. Arch. Dis. Childhood 8, 145–154.
477. Macy, I. B. (1944) Feeding school children to meet dietary needs. J. Am. Dietet. Assn. 20, 602–608.
478. Mahler, H. R. (1963) Uricase. In: The Enzymes (Boyer, P. D., Lardy, H. & Myrback, eds.), vol. 8, part B, pp. 285–296, Academic Press, New York.
479. Mallette, M. F. (1950) The nature of the copper enzymes involved in tyrosine oxidation. In: A Symposium on Copper Metabolism (McElroy, W. D. & Glass, B., eds.), pp. 48–75, J. Hopkins Press, Baltimore.
480. Mallory, F. B. (1925) The relation of chronic poisoning with copper to hemochromatosis. Am. J. Path. 1, 117–133.
481. Mallory, F. B. (1926) Hemochromatosis and chronic poisoning with copper. Arch. Intern. Med. 37, 336–362.
482. Mallory, F. B. & Parker, F., Jr. (1931) Experimental copper poisoning. Am. J. Pathol. 7, 351–364.
483. Mallory, F. B. & Parker, F., Jr. (1931) The microchemical demonstration of copper in pigment cirrhosis. Am. J. Pathol. 7, 365–371.
484. Mallory, F. B., Parker, F., Jr. & Nye, R. M. (1921) Experimental pigment cirrhosis due to copper and its relation to hemochromatosis. J. Med. Res. 42, 461–496.
485. Mandelbrote, B. M., Stanier, M. W., Thompson, R. H. S. & Thruston, M. N. (1948) Studies on copper metabolism in demyelinating diseases of the central nervous system. Brain 71, 212–228.
486. Mann, T. & Keilin, D. (1939) Haemocuprein and hepatocuprein, copper-protein compounds of blood and liver in mammals. Proc. Roy. Soc. Lond., Series B., 126, 303–315.
487. Manzler, A. D. & Schreiner, A. W. (1970) Copper-induced acute hemolytic anemia. A new complication of hemodialysis. Ann. Intern. Med. 73, 409–412.
488. Marceau, N. & Aspin, N. (1973) The intracellular distribution of the radiocopper derived from ceruloplasmin and from albumin. Biochim. Biophys. Acta 328, 338–350.
489. Marceau, N. & Aspin, N. (1973) The association of the copper derived from cerulo-

plasmin with cytocuprein. Biochim. Biophys. Acta *328*, 351–358.

490. Markowitz, H., Cartwright, G. E. & Wintrobe, M. M. (1959) Studies on copper metabolism. XXVII. Isolation and properties of erythrocyte cuproprotein (erythrocuprein). J. Biol. Chem. *234*, 40–45.

491. Markowitz, H., Gubler, C. J., Mahoney, J. P. Cartwright, G. E. & Wintrobe, M. M. (1955) Studies on copper metabolism. XIV. Copper, ceruloplasmin and oxidase activity in sera of normal human subjects, pregnant women, and patients with infection, hepatolenticular degeneration and the nephrotic syndrome. J. Clin. Invest. *34*, 1498–1508.

492. Markowitz, H., Shields, G. S., Klassen, W. H., Cartwright, G. E. & Wintrobe, M. M. (1961) Spectrophotometric determination of total erythrocyte copper. Anal. Chem. *33*, 1594–1598.

493. Marston, H. R. (1952) Cobalt, copper and molybdenum in the nutrition of animals and plants. Physiol. Rev. *32*, 62–111.

494. Masi, M., Paolucci, P., Vecchi, V. & Vivarelli, F. (1975) La ceruloplasminemia nel bambino normale. Minerva Pediat. *27*, 1175–1180.

495. Matsuda, I. (1978) Screening for Wilson's disease. Lancet *1*, 562.

496. Matsuda, I., Pearson, T. & Holtzman, N. A. (1974) Determination of apoceruloplasmin by radioimmunoassay in nutritional copper deficiency, Menkes' kinky hair syndrome, Wilson's disease, and umbilical cord blood. Pediat. Res. *8*, 821–824.

497. Matter, B. J., Pederson, J., Psimenos, G. & Lindeman, R. D. (1969) Lethal copper intoxication in hemodialysis. Trans. Soc. Artif. Intern. Organs *15*, 309–315.

498. Matthews, W. B. (1954) The absorption and excretion of radiocopper in hepatolenticular degeneration (Wilson's disease). J. Neurol. Neurosurg. Psychiat. *17*, 242–246.

499. Matthews, W. B., Milne, M. D. & Bell, M. (1952) The metabolic disorder in hepatolenticular degeneration. Quart. J. Med. *21*, 425–446.

500. McCord, J. M. & Fridovich, I. (1969) Superoxide dismutase. An enzymic function for erythrocuprein (hemocuprein). J. Biol. Chem. *244*, 6049–6055.

501. McCord, J. M. & Fridovich, I. (1970) The utility of superoxide dismutase in studying free radical reactions. II. The mechanism of the mediation of cytochrome c reduction by a variety of electron carriers. J. Biol. Chem. *245*, 1374–1377.

502. McCosker, P. J. (1961) Paraphenylenediamine oxidase activity and copper-levels in mammalian plasmas. Nature *190*, 887–889.

503. McCullars, G. M., O'Reilly, S. & Brennan, M. (1977) Pigment binding of copper in human bile. Clin. Chim. Acta *74*, 33–38.

504. McDermott, J. A., Huber, C. T., Osaki, S. & Frieden, E. (1968) Role of iron in the oxidase activity of ceruloplasmin. Biochem. Biophys. Acta *151*, 541–557.

505. McEwen, C. M., Jr. (1965) Human plasma monoamine oxidase. 1. Purification and identification. J. Biol. Chem. *240*, 2003–2010.

506. McEwen, C. M., Jr. & Harrison, D. C. (1965) Abnormalities of serum monoamine oxidase in chronic congestive heart failure. J. Lab. Clin. Med. *65*, 546–559.

507. McHargue, J. S. (1926) Further evidence that small quantities of copper, manganese and zinc are factors in the metabolism of animals. Am. J. Physiol. *77*, 245–255.

508. McIntyre, N., Clink, H. M., Levi, A. J., Cummings, J. N. & Sherlock, S. (1967) Hemolytic anemia in Wilson's disease. New Engl. J. Med. *276*, 439–444.

509. McKenzie, J. M. (1974) Tissue concentration of cadmium, zinc and copper from autopsy samples. N.Z. Med. J. *79*, 1016–1019.

510. McKenzie, J. M., Guthrie, B. E. & Prior, I. A. M. (1978) Zinc and copper status of Polynesian residents in the Tokelau Islands. Am. J. Clin. Nutr. *31*, 422–428.

511. McKenzie, J. M., Van Rij, A. M., Robinson, M. F. & Guthrie, B. E. (1976) Trace element balance studies during total parenteral nutrition. In: Trace Substances in Environmental Health, X. University of Missouri, Columbia.

512. McMullen, W. (1971) Copper contamination in soft drinks from bottle pourers. Health Bulletin (Scotland) *29*, 94–96.

513. Menkes, J. H., Alter, M., Steigleder, G. K., Weakley, D. R. & Sung, J. H. (1962) A sex-linked recessive disorder with retardation of growth, peculiar hair, and focal cerebral and cerebellar degeneration. Pediatrics *29*, 764–779.

514. Mertz, W. (1972) Human requirements: basic and optimal. Ann. N.Y. Acad. Sci. *199*, 191–201.

515. Mertz, W. (1976) Defining trace element deficiencies and toxicities in man. In: Molybdenum in the Environment. The Biology of Molybdenum. (Chapell, W. R. & Peterson, K. K., eds.), vol. I, pp. 267–286, Marcel Dekker, New York.

516. Meyer, R. J. & Zalusky, R. (1977) The mechanisms of hemolysis in Wilson's disease: study of a case and review of the literature. Mt. Sinai J. Med. *44*, 530–538.

517. Miller, R. F. & Engel, R. W. (1960) Interrelations of copper, molybdenum and sulfate sulfur in nutrition. Federation Proc. *19*, 666–677.

518. Mills, C. F. (1974) Trace-element interactions: effects of dietary composition on the development of imbalance and toxicity. In: Trace Element Metabolism in Animals—2 (Hoekstra, W. G., Suttie, J. W., Ganther, H. E. & Mertz, W., eds.), pp. 79–90, University Park Press, Baltimore.

519. Mills, E. S. (1924) Hemochromatosis with special reference to its frequency and to its occurrence in women. Arch. Intern. Med. *34*, 292–300.

520. Mills, E. S. (1930) The treatment of idiopathic (hypochromic) anaemia with iron and copper. Canad. Med. Assn. J. 22, 175–178.

521. Mills, E. S. (1931) Idiopathic hypochromemia. Am. J. Med. Sci. 182, 554–565.

522. Mills, R. G. (1925) The possible relation of copper to disease among the Korean people. J. Am. Med. Assn. 84, 1326–1327.

523. Milne, D. B. & Matrone, G. (1970) Forms of ceruloplasmin in developing piglets. Biochem. Biophys. Acta 212, 43–49.

524. Mirzakarimov, M. G. (1957) Blood copper of women during pregnancy. Akush. Ginekol. 1, 55–85 (Russian).

525. Mischel, W. (1958) Die anorganischen Bestandteile der Placenta. VII. Der Kupfergehalt der reifen und unreifen, normalen und pathologischen menschlichen Placenta. Arch. Gynakol. 191, 1–7.

526. Mischel, W. (1960) Die anorganischen Bestandteile des menschlichen Fruchtwassers. Geburtsh. Frauenheilk. 20, 584–594.

527. Mischel, W. (1961) Über das Verhalten des Serumkupfers bei der Frau in der normalen und gestörten Schwangerschaft, im Wochenbett, in der Nabelschnur sowie bei verschiedenen gynäkologischen Erkrankungen. Ztschr. Geburtsch. Gyn. 155, 197–215.

528. Mitchell, H. H. & Hamilton, T. S. (1949) The dermal excretion under controlled environmental conditions of nitrogen and minerals in human subjects, with particular reference to calcium and iron. J. Biol. Chem. 178, 345–361.

529. Molin, L. & Wester, P. O. (1973) Cobalt, copper and zinc in normal psoriatic epidermis. Acta Dermatol. Venereol. 53, 477–480.

530. Møllekaer, A. M. (1974) Case report. Kinky hair syndrome. Acta Paediat. Skand. 63, 289–296.

531. Molokhia, M. M. & Portnoy, B. (1970) Neutron activation analysis of trace elements in skin. V. Copper and zinc in psoriasis. Br. J. Dermatol. 83, 376–381.

532. Mönckeberg, F., Vildósola, J., Figueroa, M., Oxman, S. & Meneghello, J. (1962) Hematologic disturbances in infantile malnutrition. Values for copper, iron, paraphenelene diamine oxidase and iron-binding capacity in the serum. Am. J. Clin. Nutr. 11, 525–529.

533. Mondorf, A. W., Mackenrodt, G. & Halberstadt, E. (1971) Coeruloplasmin. Teil I: Die Biochemie des Coeruloplasmins. Teil II: Der Einfluss von Östrogenen auf den Coeruloplasmingehalt des Serums. Klin. Wochnschr. 49, 61–70.

534. Mondovi, B., Rotilio, G., Finazzi, A. & Scioscia-Santoro, A. (1964) Purification of pig-kidney diamine oxidase and its identity with histaminase. Biochem. J. 91, 408–415.

535. Morell, A. G. & Scheinberg, I. H. (1960) Heterogeneity of human ceruloplasmin. Science 131, 930–932.

536. Morell, A. G., Shapiro, J. R. & Scheinberg, I. H. (1961) Copper binding protein from human liver. In: Wilson's Disease, Some Current Concepts. (Walshe, J. M. & Cumings, J. N., eds.), p. 36–42, Blackwell, Oxford.

537. Morell, A. G., Van Den Hamer, C. J. A. & Scheinberg, I. H. (1969) Physical and chemical studies on ceruloplasmin. VI. Preparation of human ceruloplasmin crystals. J. Biol. Chem. 244, 3494–3496.

538. Morrison, D. B. & Nash, T. P., Jr. (1930) The copper content of infant livers. J. Biol. Chem. 88, 479–483.

539. Mortazavi, S. H., Bani-Hashemi, A., Mozafari, M. & Raffi, A. (1972) Value of serum copper measurement in lymphomas and several other malignancies. Cancer 29, 1193–1198.

540. Müller, A. H. (1935) Die Rolle des Kupfers im Organismus mit besonderer Berücksichtigung seiner Beziehungen zum Blut. Ergebn. Inn. Med. 48, 444–469.

541. Munch-Petersen, S. (1950) On the copper content of mother's milk before and after intravenous copper administration. Acta Paediat. 39, 378–388.

542. Munch-Petersen, S. (1950) On serum copper in patients with pulmonary tuberculosis. Acta Tuberc. Scand. 24, 132–153.

543. Murakami, Y. (1973) A study on the copper content in daily food consumption in Japan. Osaka Shiritsu Daiagku Igaku Zasshi, 22, 13–48 (Japanese).

544. Murphy, E. W., Page, L. & Watt, K. B. (1971) Trace minerals in type A school lunches. J. Am. Diet. Assn. 58, 115–122.

545. Murphy, E. W., Watt, B. K. & Page, L. (1971) Regional variations in vitamin and trace element content of type A school lunches. In: Trace Substances in Environmental Health, IV. (Hemphill, D. D., ed.), pp. 194–205, University of Missouri, Columbia.

546. Murthy, G. K. & Rhea, U. S. (1971) Cadmium, copper, iron, lead, manganese, and zinc in evaporated milk, infant products, and human milk. J. Dairy Sci. 54, 1001–1005.

547. Murthy, G. K., Rhea, U. S. & Peeler, J. T. (1972) Copper, iron, manganese, strontium and zinc content of market milk. J. Dairy Sci. 55, 1666–1674.

548. Murthy, G. K., Rhea, U. S. & Peeler, J. T. (1973) Levels of copper, nickel, rubidium, and strontium in institutional total diets. Environ. Sci. Technol. 7, 1042–1045.

549. National Research Council (1974) Recommended Dietary Allowances, 8th rev. ed., 128 pp., Food and Nutrition Board, National Academy of Sciences, Washington, D.C.

550. National Research Council (1977) Copper. Committee on Medical and Biological Effects of Environmental Pollutants, 115 pp., National Academy of Sciences, Washington, D.C.

551. Neale, F. C. & Fischer-Williams, M. (1958) Copper metabolism in normal adults and in clinically normal relatives of patients with Wilson's disease. J. Clin. Pathol. 11, 441–447.

552. Neri, A., Eckerling, B. & Bahary, C. (1969) The copper and copperoxidase content of maternal and infant umbilical arterial and venous blood serum at delivery. Gynaecologia 138, 40–48.

553. Neumann, P. Z. & Sass-Kortsak, A. (1963) Binding of copper by serum proteins. Vox Sang. 8, 111–112.

554. Neumann, P. Z. & Sass-Kortsak, A. (1967) The state of copper in human serum: Evidence for an amino acid-bound fraction. J. Clin. Invest. 46, 646–658.

555. Neumann, P. Z. & Silverberg, M. (1967) Metabolic pathways of red blood cell copper in normal humans and in Wilson's disease. Nature 213, 775–779.

556. Neuweiler, W. (1942) Über die fetale Resorption von Kupfer aus der Placenta. Klin. Wochenschr. 21, 521–522.

557. Nicholas, P. O. (1968) Food-poisoning due to copper in the morning tea. Lancet 2, 40–42.

558. Niedermeier, W., Creitz, E. E. & Holley, H. L. (1962) Trace metal composition of synovial fluid from patients with rheumatoid arthritis. Arthr. Rheum. 5, 439–444.

559. Niedermeier, W. & Griggs, J. H. (1971) Trace metal composition of synovial fluid and blood serum of patients with rheumatoid arthritis. J. Chron. Dis. 23, 527–536.

560. Nimni, M. E. & Bavetta, L. A. (1965) Collagen defect induced by pencillamine. Science 150, 905–907.

560. Nielsen, A. L. (1944) On serum copper. IV. Pregnancy and parturition. Acta Med. Scand. 118, 92–96.

562. Nordberg, G. F., Nordberg, M., Piscator, M. & Vesterberg, O. (1972) Separation of two forms of rabbit metallothionein by isoelectric focusing. Biochem. J. 126, 491–498.

563. Norstrand, I. F. & Glantz, M. D. (1973) Purification and properties of human liver monoamine oxidase. Arch. Bioch. Biophys. 158, 1–11.

564. Nusbaum, M. J. & Zettner, A. (1973) The content of calcium, magnesium, copper, iron, sodium, and potassium in amniotic fluid from eleven to nineteen weeks' gestation. Am. J. Obstet. Gynecol. 115, 219–226.

565. Nusbaum, R. E., Alexander, G. V., Butt, E. M., Gilmour, T. C. & Didio, S. L. (1958) Some spectrographic studies of trace element storage in human tissues. Soil Sci. 85, 95–99.

566. Oakes, B. W., Danks, D. M. & Campbell, P. E. (1976) Human copper deficiency: ultrastructural studies of the aorta and skin in a child with Menkes' syndrome. Exp. Mol. Pathol. 25, 82–98.

567. O'Brien, J. S. & Sampson, E. L. (1966) Kinky hair disease. II. Biochemical studies. J. Neuropath. Exp. Neurol. 25, 523–530.

568. O'Dell, B. L. (1976) Biochemistry of copper. Med. Clin. N. Am. 60, 687–703.

569. O'Dell, B. L. (1976) Biochemistry and physiology of copper in vertebrates. In: Trace Elements in Human Health and Disease (Prasad, A. S. & Oberleas, D., eds.),

vol. 1, pp. 391–413, Academic Press, New York.

570. O'Dell, B. L. (1976) Copper. In: Nutrition Reviews. Present Knowledge in Nutrition, 4th ed., pp. 302–309, The Nutrition Foundation, New York.

571. O'Dell, B. L., Hardwick, B. C., Reynolds, G. & Savage, J. E. (1961) Connective tissue defect in the chick resulting from copper deficiency. Proc. Soc. Exp. Biol. Med. 108, 402–405.

572. Ohlson, M. A. & Daum, K. (1935) A study of the iron metabolism of normal women. J. Nutr. 9, 75–89.

573. Ohtake, M. & Tamura, T. (1976) Serum zinc and copper levels in healthy Japanese children. Tohoku J. Exp. Med. 120, 99–103.

574. Olatunbosun, D. A., Adadevoh, B. K. & Adeniyi, F. A. (1974) Serum copper in normal pregnancy in Nigerians. J. Obst. Gynaecol. Br. Commonw. 81, 475–478.

575. Olatunbosun, D. A., Akindele, M. O., Adadevoh, B. K. & Asuni, T. (1975) Serum copper in schizophrenia in Nigerians. Br. J. Psychiat. 127, 119–121.

576. Olatunbosun, D. A., Isaacs-Sodeye, W. A., Adeniyi, F. A. & Adadeovh, B. K. (1975) Serum-copper in sickle-cell anaemia. Lancet 1, 285–286.

577. O'Leary, J. A. (1969) Serum copper levels as a measure of placental function. Am. J. Obstet. Gynecol. 105, 636–637.

578. O'Leary, J. A., Novalis, G. S. & Vosburgh, G. J. (1966) Maternal serum copper concentrations in normal and abnormal gestations. Obstet. Gynecol. 28, 112–117.

579. O'Leary, J. A. & Spellacy, W. N. (1969) Zinc and copper levels in pregnant women and those taking oral contraceptives. Am. J. Obstet. Gynecol. 103, 131–132.

580. O'Reilly, S., Strickland, G. T., Weber, P. M., Beckner, W. M. & Shipley, L. (1971) Abnormalities of the physiology of copper in Wilson's disease. I. The whole body turnover of copper. Arch. Neurol. 24, 385–390.

581. O'Reilly, S., Weber, P. M., Oswald, M. & Shipley, L. (1971) Abnormalities of the physiology of copper in Wilson's disease. III. The excretion of copper. Arch. Neurol. 25, 28–32.

582. Osaka, K., Sato, N., Matsumoto, S., Ogino, H., Kodama, S., Yokoyama, S. & Sugiyama, T. (1977) Congenital hypocupraemia syndrome with and without steely hair: Report of two Japanese infants. Develop. Med. Child. Neurol. 19, 62–68.

583. Osaki, S., Johnson, D. A. & Frieden, E. (1966) The possible significance of the ferrous oxidase activity of ceruloplasmin in normal human serum. J. Biol. Chem. 241, 2746–2751.

584. Osaki, S., Johnson, D. A. & Frieden, E. (1971) The mobilization of iron from the perfused mammalian liver by a serum copper enzyme, ferroxidase I. J. Biol. Chem. 246, 3018–3023.

585. Osaki, S., McDermott, J. A. & Frieden, E. (1964) Proof for the ascorbate activity of

ceruloplasmin. J. Biol. Chem. *239*, 3570–3575.

586. Oshima, F. & Schönheimer, R. (1929) Über den Kupfergehalt der normalen Leber und der Leber bein Hämochromatose, sowie von Gallensteinen und Gesamptblut. Ztschr. Physiol. Chem. *180*, 254–258.

587. Oshima, F. & Siebert, P. (1930) Experimentelle chronische Kupfergiftung, ein Beitrag zur Frage der Pathogenese der Hämochromatose. Beitrag. Path. Anat. Pathol. *84*, 106–111.

588. Oski, F. A. (1970) Chickee, the copper. Ann. Int. Med. *73*, 485–486.

589. Oster, G. & Salgo, M. P. (1977) Copper in mammalian reproduction. Adv. Pharmacol. Chemotherapy *14*, 327–409.

590. Ota, D. M., Macfadyen, B. V. Jr., Gum, E. T. & Dudrick, S. J. (1978) Zinc and copper deficiencies in man during intravenous hyperalimentation. In: Zinc and Copper in Clinical Medicine, (Hambidge, K. M. & Nichols, B. L., eds.), pp. 99–112, Spectrum, New York.

591. Page, G. G. (1973) Contamination of drinking water by corrosion of copper tubes. N.Z.J. Sci. *16*, 349–388.

592. Pagliardi, E., Giangrandi, E. & Vinti, A. (1958) Erythrocyte copper in iron deficiency anemia. Acta Hematol. *19*, 231–240.

593. Panvalkar, R. S., Kalgi, V. H. & Hegiste, M. D. (1961) Serum copper level in normal human subjects and in tuberculosis. Preliminary report. Indian J. Med. Sci. *15*, 456–459.

594. Partridge, S. M., Elsden, D. F., Thomas, J., Dorfman, A., Telser, A. & Ho, P-L. (1964) Biosynthesis of the demosine and isodesmonsine cross-bridges in elastin. Biochem. J. *93*, 30c.

595. Pennington, J. T. & Calloway, D. H. (1974) Copper content of foods. J. Am. Diet. Assn. *63*, 143–153.

596. Pfeiffer, C. C. & Cott, A. (1974) A study of zinc and manganese dietary supplements in the copper loaded schizophrenic. In: Clinical Applications of Zinc Metabolism (Pories, J., Strain, W. H., Hsu, J. M. & R. L. Woosley, eds.), pp. 260–278, Thomas, Springfield, Illinois.

597. Pfeiffer, C. C. & Iliev, V. (1972) A study of zinc deficiency and copper excess in the schrizophrenias. Internat. Rev. Neurobiol. *1* (Suppl), 141–165.

598. Picciano, M. F. & Guthrie, H. A. (1976) Copper, iron and zinc contents of mature human milk. Am. J. Clin. Nutr. *29*, 242–254.

599. Pimentel, J. C. & Menezes, A. P. (1977) Liver disease in vineyard sprayers. Gastroenterology *72*, 275–283.

600. Pineda, E. P., Ravin, H. A. & Rutenberg, A. M. (1962) Serum ceruloplasmin: observations in patients with cancer, obstructive jaundice, and other diseases. Gastroenterology *43*, 266–270.

601. Pinnell, S. R. & Martin, G. R. (1968) The cross-linking of collagen and elastin: enzymatic conversion of lysine in peptide linkage to α-amino-adipic-δ-semialdehyde (allysine) by an extract from bone. Proc. Nat. Acad. Sci. U.S.A. *61*, 708–716.

602. Pirrie, R. (1952) Serum copper and its relationship to serum iron in patients with neoplastic disease. J. Clin. Pathol. *5*, 190–193.

603. Pitt, M. A. (1976) Molybdenum toxicity: interactions between copper, molybdenum and sulphate. Agents Actions *6*, 758–769.

604. Plantin, L. O. & Standberg, P. O. (1965) Whole-blood concentrations of copper and zinc in rheumatoid arthritis studied by activation analysis. Acta Rheum. Scand. *11*, 30–34.

605. Poczekaj, J., Hejduk, J. & Chodera, A. (1963) Behaviour of copper in trophoblast and in placenta at term. Gynaecologia *155*, 155–159.

606. Pojerová, A. & Továrek, J. (1960) Ceruloplasmin in early childhood. Acta Paediat. *49*, 113–120.

607. Polson, C. J. (1929) Chronic copper poisoning. Br. J. Exp. Pathol. *10*, 241–245.

608. Porter, H. (1949) Amino acid excretion in degenerative diseases of the nervous system. J. Lab. Clin. Med. *34*, 1623–1626.

609. Porter, H. (1951) Copper excretion in the urine of normal individuals and of patients with hepatolenticular degeneration (Wilson's disease). Arch. Biochem. Biophys. *31*, 262–265.

610. Porter, H. (1966) The tissue copper proteins: cerebrocuprein, erythrocuprein, hepatocuprein, and neonatal hepatic mitochondrocuprein. In: The Biochemistry of Copper, (Peisach, J., Aisen, P. & Blumberg, W. E., eds.), pp. 159–174, Academic Press, New York.

611. Porter, H. (1974) The particulate half-cystine-rich copper protein of newborn liver. Relationship to metallothionein and subcellular localization in non-mitochondrial particles possibly representing heavy lysosomes. Biochem. Biophys. Res. Comm. *56*, 661–668.

612. Porter, H. & Ainsworth, S. (1959) The isolation of the copper-containing protein cerebrocuprein I from normal human brain. J. Neurochem. *5*, 91–98.

613. Porter, H. & Folch, J. (1957) Brain copper-protein fractions in the normal and in Wilson's disease. A.M.A. Arch. Neurol. Psychiat. *77*, 8–16.

614. Porter, H. & Hills, J. R. (1974) The half-cystine-rich copper protein of newborn liver, probable relationship to metallothionein and subcellular localization in non-mitochondrial particles possibly representing heavy lysosomes. In: Trace Element Metabolism in Animals—2 (Hoekstra, W. G., Suttie, J. W., Ganther, H. E. & Mertz, W., eds.), pp. 482–485, University Park Press, Baltimore.

615. Porter, H., Sweeney, M. & Porter, E. M. (1964) Neonatal hepatic mitochondrocuprein. II. Isolation of the copper-containing subfraction from mitochondria of newborn human liver. Arch. Biochem. Biophys. *104*, 97–101.

616. Porter, H., Sweeney, M. & Porter, E. M. (1964) Human hepatocuprein. Isolation of a copper protein from the subcellular soluble fraction of adult human liver. Arch. Biochem. Biophys. 105, 319–325.

617. Price, N. O. & Bunce, G. E. (1972) Effect of nitrogen and calcium on balance of copper, manganese, and zinc in preadolescent girls. Nutr. Rep. Internat. 5, 275–280.

618. Price, N. O., Bunce, G. E. & Engel, R. W. (1970) Copper, manganese, and zinc balance in preadolescent girls. Am. J. Clin. Nutr. 23, 258–260.

619. Priev, I. G. (1966) Daily copper requirements of children and adults. Vopr. Pitan. 25 (3), 61–63 (Russian).

620. Priev, I. G. & Krasny, B. A. (1966) Copper and iron content in the ready-to-eat dishes at children's institutions and in nutritional treatment dishes of some in-patient departments of the city of Samarkand. Vop. Pitan. 25, (5), 22–26 (Russian).

621. Prohaska, J. R. & Wells, W. W. (1974) Copper deficiency in the developing rat brain: a possible model for Menkes' steely-hair disease. J. Neurochem. 23, 91–98.

622. Pshetakovsky, I. L. (1972) Clinical value of studying trace elements (Cu, Ni, Mn) and their pathogenetic role in rheumatoid arthritis. Terapeut. Arkhiv (Moscow) 44, (6), 23–27 (Russian).

623. Pshetakovsky, I. L. (1973) Pathogenetic role of trace elements (Cu, Ni, Mn) and their diagnostic value in ankylosing spondyloarthritis (Bechterew's disease). Vop. Rheum. 13 (2), 17–20 (Russian).

624. Purpura, D. P., Hirano, A. & French, J. H. (1976) Polydendritic Purkinge cells in X-chromosome linked copper malabsorption: a Golgi study. Brain Res. 117, 125–129.

625. Ragan, H. A., Nacht, S., Lee, G. R., Bishop, C. R. & Cartwright, G. E. (1969) Effect of ceruloplasmin on plasma iron in copper-deficient swine. Am. J. Physiol. 217, 1320–1323.

626. Rainsford, K. D. & Whitehouse, M. W. (1976) Concerning the merits of copper aspirin as a potential anti-inflammatory drug. J. Pharm. Pharmacol. 28, 83–86.

627. Ramage, H., Sheldon, J. H. & Sheldon, W. (1933) A spectrographic investigation of the metallic content of the liver in childhood. Proc. Roy. Soc. London, Series B, 113, 308–327.

628. Rasuli, Z. M. (1963) Copper metabolism in toxemia of late pregnancy. Akush. Ginek 39, 63–66 (Russian).

629. Ravin, H. A. (1961) An improved colorimetric enzymatic assay of ceruloplasmin. J. Lab. Clin. Med. 58, 161–168.

630. Rechenberger, J. (1957) Serumeisen und Serumkupfer bei akuten und chromischen Leukamien sowie bei Morbus Hodgkin. Deut. Ztschr. Verdann. Stoffwech. 17, 78–85.

631. Reed, D. W., Passon, P. G. & Hultquist, D. E. (1970) Purification and properties of a pink copper protein from human erythrocytes. J. Biol. Chem. 245, 2954–2961.

632. Reiff, B. & Schnieden, H. (1959) Plasma copper and iron levels and plasma paraphenylene diamine oxidase activity (plasma copper oxidase activity) in kwashiorkor. Blood 14, 967–971.

633. Reilly, C. (1972) Zinc, iron and copper contamination in home-produced alcoholic drinks. J. Sci. Food Agric. 23, 1143–1144.

634. Reinhold, J. G. (1975) Trace elements: a Selective Survey. Clin. Chem. 21, 476–500.

635. Reske-Nielsen, E., Lou, H. O. C., Anderson, P. & Vagn-Hansen, P. (1973) Brain-copper concentration in Menkes' disease. Lancet 1, 613.

636. Rice, E. W. (1960) Correlation between serum copper, ceruloplasmin activity and C-reactive protein. Clin. Chim. Acta 5, 632–636.

637. Rice, E. W. (1961) Evaluation of the role of ceruloplasmin as an acute-phase reactant. Clin. Chim. Acta 6, 652–655.

638. Richterich, R., Rossi, E., Stillhart, H. & Gautier, H. (1961) The heterogeneity of caeruloplasmin in the newborn. In: Wilson's Disease. Some Current Concepts (Walshe, J. M. & Cummings, J. N., eds.), pp. 81–95, Blackwell Sci. Pub., Oxford.

639. Ricour, C., Dunhamel, J. F., Gross, J., Mazihère, B. & Comar, D. (1977) Oligoelements chez l'enfant en nutrition parenterale exclusive: estimation des besoins. Arch. Franc. Pediat. 34, (Suppl. 7), xcii-c.

640. Ritland, S., Steinnes, E. & Skrede, S. (1977) Hepatic copper content, urinary copper excretion, and serum ceruloplasmin in liver disease. Scand. J. Gastroent. 12, 81–88.

641. Roberts, R. H. (1956) Hemolytic anemia associated with copper sulfate poisoning. Mississippi Doctor 33, 292–294.

642. Robinson, M. F., McKenzie, J. M., Thomson, C. D. & van Rij, A. L. (1973) Metabolic balance of zinc, copper, cadmium, iron, molybdenum and selenium in young New Zealand women. Br. J. Nutr. 30, 195–205.

643. Roche-Sicot, J. & Benhamou, J. P. (1977) Acute intravascular hemolysis and acute liver failure associated as a first manifestation of Wilson's disease. Ann. Intern. Med. 86, 301–303.

644. Rosenberg, E. B., Strickland, G. T., Feng, Y. S. & Blackwell, R. Q. (1971) Comparison of immunologic and enzymatic methods for ceruloplasmin quantitation in Wilson's disease. J. Formosan Med. Assn. 70, 49–53.

645. Rohmer, A., Krug, J. P., Mennesson, M., Mandel, P., Mack, G. & Zawislak, R. (1977) Maladie de Menkes: Etude de deux enzymes cupro-dependantes. Pediatrie 32, 447–456.

646. Rosenthal, R. W. & Blackburn, A. (1974) Higher copper concentrations in serum than in plasma. Clin. Chem. 20, 1233–1234.

647. Rottger, H. (1950) Kupfer bei Mutter und Kind. Arch. Gynakol. 177, 650–660.

648. Rowe, D. W., McGoodwin, E. B., Martin, G. R., Sussman, M. D., Grahn, D., Faris, B.

& Franzblau, C. (1974) A sex-linked defect in the cross-linking of collagen and elastin associated with the mottled locus in mice. J. Exp. Med. *139*, 180–192.

648a. Rucker, R. B. & Murray, J. (1978) Cross-linking amino acids in collagen and elastin. Am. J. Clin. Nutr. *31*, 1221–1236.

649. Rucker, R. B. & O'Dell, B. L. (1971) Connective tissue amine oxidase. I. Purification of bovine aorta amine oxidase and its comparison with plasma amine oxidase. Biochem. Biophys. Acta *235*, 32–43.

650. Rucker, R. B. & Tom, K. (1976) Arterial elastin. Am. J. Clin. Nutr. *29*, 1021–1034.

651. Russ, E. M. & Raymunt, J. (1956) Influence of estrogens on total serum copper and caeruloplasmin. Proc. Soc. Exp. Biol. Med. *92*, 465–466.

652. Russ, E. M., Raymunt, J. & Pillar, S. (1957) Effect of estrogen therapy on ceruloplasmin concentration in a man with Wilson's disease. J. Clin. Endocrinol. & Metab. *17*, 908–909.

653. Rydén, L. & Björk, I. (1976) Reinvestigation of some physico-chemical and chemical properties of human ceruloplasmin (ferroxidase). Biochem. *15*, 3411–3417.

654. Rydén, L. & Deutsch, H. F. (1978) Preparation and properties of the major copper-binding component in human fetal liver. Its identification as metallothionein. J. Biol. Chem. *253*, 519–524.

655. Sachs, A., Levine, V. E. & Fabian, A. A. (1935) Copper and iron in human blood. Arch. Intern. Med. *55*, 227–253.

656. Sachs, A., Levine, V. E. & Fabian, A. A. (1936) Copper and iron in human blood. IV. Normal children. Arch. Intern. Med. *58*, 523–530.

657. Sachs, A., Levine, V. E., Hill, F. C. & Hughes, R. (1943) Copper and iron in human blood. Arch. Intern. Med. *71*, 489–501.

658. Sakar, B. & Kruck, T. P. A. (1966) Copper-amino acid complexes in human serum. In: Biochemistry of Copper (Peisach, J., Aison, P. & Blumberg, W. E., eds.), pp. 183–196, Academic Press, New York.

659. Sakharchuk, V. M., Yatsula, G. S. & Rakitskaya, N. V. (1972) Clinico-experimental studies of the content of some trace elements in atherosclerosis. Kardiologiya *12* (1), 131–133 (Russian).

660. Sala, I. & Gambara, L. (1957) Contenuto in rame e attivita ossidasica del plasma materno e funiculare. Lattante *28*, 458–470.

661. Salaspuro, M. P. & Sipponen, P. (1976) Demonstration of an intracellular copper-binding protein by orcein staining in long-standing cholestatic liver diseases. Gut *17*, 787–790.

662. Salmon, M. A. & Wright, T. (1971) Chronic copper poisoning presenting as pink disease. Arch. Dis. Child. *46*, 108–110.

663. Sandstead, H. H. (1975) Some trace elements which are essential for human nutrition: zinc, copper, manganese and chromium. Prog. Food Nutr. Sci. *1*, 371–391.

664. Sandstead, H. H., Shukry, A. S., Prasad, A. S., Gabr, M. K., Hifney, A. E., Mokhtar, N. & Darby, W. J. (1965) Kwashiorkor in Egypt. I. Clinical and biochemical studies, with special reference to plasma zinc and serum lactic dehydrogenase. Am. J. Clin. Nutr. *17*, 15–26.

665. Sarzeau, A. (1830) Sur la présence du cuivre dans les végétaux et dans le sang. J. Pharm. Sci. Accessoires *16*, 505–518.

666. Sass-Kortsak, A. (1965) Copper metabolism. Adv. Clin. Chem. *8*, 1–67.

667. Sass-Kortsak, A. (1975) Wilson's disease. A treatable liver disease in children. Pediat. Clin. North. Amer. *22*. 963–984.

668. Sass-Kortsak, A. & Bern, A. G. (1978) Hereditary disorder of copper metabolism. [Wilson's disease (hepatolenticular degeneration) and Menkes' disease (kinky-hair or steely-hair syndrome)]. In: The Metabolic Basis of Inherited Disease (Standbury, J. B., Wyngaarden, J. B. & Fredrickson, D. S., eds.), pp. 1098–1126, McGraw-Hill, New York.

669. Sato, F., Shimura, Y., Yokota, J., Suzuki, M., Takita, S., Yabuta, K. & Fukuyama, Y. (1975) Menkes' kinky hair disease. A report of the first Japanese case and review of literature. No To Hattatsu (Brain & Develop.) *7*, 132–145.

670. Scanni, A., Licciardello, L., Trovato, M., Tomirotti, M. & Biraghi, M. (1977) Serum copper and ceruloplasmin levels in patients with neoplasias localized in the stomach, large intestine or lung. Tumori *63*, 175–180.

671. Scheinberg, I. H. (1966) Ceruloplasmin. A review. In: The Biochemistry of Copper (Peisach, J., Aisen, P. & Blumberg, W. E., eds.), pp. 513–524, Academic Press, New York.

672. Scheinberg, I. H. (1976) The effects of heredity and environment on copper metabolism. Med. Clin. N. Amer. *60*, 705–712.

673. Scheinberg, I. H., Cook, C. D. & Murphy, J. A. (1954) The concentration of copper and ceruloplasmin in maternal and infant plasma at delivery. J. Clin. Invest. *33*, 963.

674. Scheinberg, I. H. & Gitlin, D. (1952) Deficiency of ceruloplasmin in patients with hepatolenticular degeneration (Wilson's disease). Science *116*, 484–485.

675. Scheinberg, I. H., Harris, R. S., Morell, A. G. & Dubin, D. (1958) Some aspects of the relation of ceruloplasmin to Wilson's disease. Neurol. *8* (Suppl. 1), 44–51.

676. Scheinberg, I. H. & Morell, H. G. (1973) Ceruloplasmin. Inorganic Biochem. *1*, 306–319.

677. Scheinberg, I. H., Morell, A. G., Harris, R. S. & Berger, A. (1957) Concentration of ceruloplasmin in plasma of schizophrenic patients. Science *126*, 925–926.

678. Scheinberg, I. H. & Sternlieb, I. (1959) The liver in Wilson's disaese. Gastroenterology *37*, 550–564.

679. Scheinberg, I. H. & Sternlieb, I. (1960) Copper metabolism. Pharmacol. Rev. *12*, 355–381.

680. Scheinberg, I. H. & Sternlieb, I. (1960) The long term management of hepatolen-

ticular degeneration (Wilson's disease). Am. J. Med. *29*, 316–333.

681. Scheinberg, I. H. & Sternlieb, I. (1960) Environmental treatment of a hereditary illness: Wilson's disease. Ann. Intern. Med. *53*, 1151–1161.

682. Scheinberg, I. H. & Sternlieb, I. (1960) The pathogenesis and clinical significance of the liver disease in hepatolenticular degeneration (Wilson's disease). Med. Clin. N. Amer. *44*, 665–679.

683. Scheinberg, I. H. & Sternlieb, I. (1963) The dual role of the liver in Wilson's disease. Med. Clin. N. Amer. *47*, 815–824.

684. Scheinberg, I. H. & Sternlieb, I. (1975) Wilson's disease. In: Biology of Brain Dysfunction (Gaull, G. E., ed.), vol. 3, p. 247–264, Plenum, Pub., New York.

685. Scheinberg, I. H. & Sternlieb, I. (1976) Copper toxicity and Wilson's disease. In: Trace Elements in Human Health and Disease (Prasad, A. S. & Oberleas, D., eds.), vol. 1, pp. 415–438, Academic Press, New York.

686. Schenker, J. G., Jungreis, E. & Polishuk, W. Z. (1969) Serum copper levels in normal and pathological pregnancies. Am. J. Obst. Gynecol. *105*, 933–937.

687. Schenker, J. G., Jungreis, E. & Polishuk, W. Z. (1972) Maternal and fetal serum copper levels at delivery. Biol. Neonate. *20*, 189–195.

688. Schlettwein-Gsell, D. & Seiler, H. (1972) Analysen und Berechnungen des Gehalts der Nahrung an Kalium, Natrium, Calcium, Eisen, Magnesium, Kupfer, Zink, Nickel, Cobalt, Chrom, Mangan und Vanadium in Altersheimen und Familien. Mitteil Gebiete Lebensmittel. Hyg. *63*, 188–206.

689. Schonheimer, R. & Herkel, W. (1931) Uber das Vorkommen von Schwermetallen in menschlichen Gallensteinen. Klin. Wchnschr. *10*, 345–346.

690. Schorr, J. B., Morell, A. G. & Scheinberg, I. H. (1958) Studies of serum ceruloplasmin during early infancy. Am. J. Dis. Child. *96*, 541.

691. Schroeder, H. A., Nason, A. P., Tipton, I. H. & Balassa, J. J. (1966) Essential trace metals in man: Copper. J. Chron. Dis. *19*, 1007–1034.

692. Schubert, W. K. & Lahey, M. E. (1959) Copper and protein depletion complicating hypoferric anemia of infancy. Pediatrics *24*, 710–733.

693. Schultze, M. (1940) Metallic elements and blood formation. Physiol. Rev. *20*, 37–67.

694. Schutz, G. & Feigelson, P. (1972) Purification and properties of rat liver tryptophan oxygenase. J. Biol. Chem. *247*, 5327–5332.

695. Scoular, F. I. (1938) A quantitative study, by means of spectrographic analysis, of copper in nutrition. J. Nutr. *16*, 437–450.

696. Scudder, P., Stocks, J. & Dormandy, T. L. (1976) The relationship between erythrocyte superoxide dismutase activity and erythrocyte copper levels in normal subjects

and in patients with rheumatoid arthritis. Clin. Chim. Acta *69*, 397–403.

697. Seelenfreund, M. H., Gartner, S. & Vinger, P. F. (1968) The ocular pathology of Menkes' disease (kinky hair disease). Arch. Opthalm. *80*, 718–720.

698. Seelig, M. S. (1972) Review: relationships of copper and molybdenum to iron metabolism. Am. J. Clin. Nutr. *25*, 1022–1037.

699. Seelig, M. S. (1973) Proposed role of copper-molybdenum interaction in iron-deficiency anemia and iron-storage diseases. Am. J. Clin. Nutr. *26*, 657–672.

700. Seely, J. R., Humphrey, G. B. & Matter, B. J. (1972) Copper deficiency in a premature infant fed an iron-fortified formula. New Engl. J. Med. *286*, 109–110.

701. Semple, A. B., Parry, W. H. & Phillips, D. E. (1960) Acute copper poisoning. An outbreak traced to contaminated water from corroded geyser. Lancet *2*, 700–701.

702. Shahidi, N. T., Diamond, L. K. & Schwachman, H. (1961) Anemia associated with protein deficiency. A study of two cases with cystic fibrosis. J. Pediat. *59*, 533–542.

703. Shapiro, J., Morell, A. G. & Scheinberg, I. H. (1961) A copper-protein of human liver. J. Clin. Invest. *40*, 1081.

704. Shaw, J. C. L. (1973) Parenteral nutrition in the management of sick low birthrate infants. Pediatric Clin. N. Amer. *20*, 333–358.

705. Sheldon, J. H. & Ramage, H. (1931) A spectrographic analysis of human tissues. J. Biochem. *25*, 1608–1627.

706. Sherwin, A. L., Beck, I. T. & McKenna, R. D. (1960) The cause of Wilson's disease (hepatolenticular degeneration) during pregnancy and after delivery. Canad. Med. Assn. J. *83*, 160–163.

707. Shields, G. S., Coulson, W. F., Kimball, D. A., Carnes, W. H., Cartwright, G. E. & Wintrobe, M. M. (1962) Studies on copper metabolism. XXXII. Cardiovascular lesions in copper-deficient swine. Am. J. Pathol. *41*, 603–621.

708. Shields, G. S., Markowitz, H., Klassen, W. H., Cartwright, G. E. & Wintrobe, M. M. (1961) Studies on copper metabolism. XXXI. Erythrocyte copper. J. Clin. Invest. *40*, 2007–2015.

709. Shils, M. E. (1972) Guide lines for total parenteral nutrition. J. Am. Med. Assn. *220*, 1721–1729.

710. Shils, M. E. (1972) Minerals in total parenteral nutrition. Drug Intel. Clin. Pharm. *6*, 385–393.

711. Shils, M. E. (1975) A program for total parenteral nutrition at home. Am. J. Clin. Nutr. *28*, 1429–1435.

712. Shils, M. E., Wright, W. L., Turnbull, A. & Brescia, F. (1970) Long-term parenteral nutrition through an external arteriovenous shunt. Report of a case. N. Engl. J. Med. *283*, 341–344.

713. Shinomiya, N., Yasuda, T., Arimura, A., Aoki, T., Haraoka, K., Niwa, N. & Matsu-

shima, Y. (1977) Menkes' kinky hair disease—two cases report. No To Shinkei (Brain & Nerve) 29, 331–339.

714. Shokeir, M. H. K. (1971) Investigations in the nature of ceruloplasmin deficiency in the newborn. J. Clin. Genet. 2, 223–227.

715. Shokeir, M. H. K. & Schreffler, D. C. (1969) Cytochrome oxidase deficiency in Wilson's disease: A suggested ceruloplasmin function. Proc. Nat. Acad. Sci. U.S.A. 62, 867–872.

716. Siegel, R. C., Pinnell, S. R. & Martin, G. R. (1970) Cross-linking of collagen and elastin. Properties of lysyl oxidase. Biochemistry 9, 4486–4492.

717. Singh, S. & Bresnan, M. J. (1973) Menkes' kinky-hair syndrome (trichopoliodystrophy). Low copper levels in the blood, hair, and urine. Am. J. Dis. Child 125, 572–578.

718. Sinha, S. N. & Gabrieli, E. R. (1970) Serum copper and zinc levels in various pathologic conditions. Am. J. Clin. Pathol. 54, 570–577.

719. Sipponen, P. (1976) Orcein positive hepatocellular material in long-standing biliary diseases. I. Histochemical characteristics. II. Ultrastructural studies. Scand J. Gastroent. 11, 553–557.

720. Sipponen, P., Hjelt, L., Törnkvist, T. & Salaspuro, M. (1976) X-ray microanalysis of copper accumulation in liver in secondary biliary cirrhosis. Arch. Pathol. 100, 664–666.

721. Smallwood, R. A., McIlveen, G., Rosenoer, V. M. & Sherlock, S. (1971) Copper kinetics in liver disease. Gut 12, 139–144.

722. Smallwood, R. A., Williams, H. A., Rosenoer, V. M. & Sherlock, S. (1968) Liver-copper levels in liver disease. Studies using neutron activation analysis. Lancet 2, 1310–1313.

723. Smith, J. C., Jr. & Brown, E. D. (1976) Effects of oral contraceptive agents on trace element metabolism: a review. In: Trace Elements in Human Health and Disease (Prasad, A. S. & Oberleas, D., eds.), vol. II, pp. 315–345, Academic Press, New York.

724. Solassol, Cl., Joyeux, H., Etco, L., Pujol, H. & Romieu, Cl. (1974) New techniques for long-term intravenous feeding: an artificial gut in 75 patients. Ann. Surg. 179, 519–522.

725. Søli, N. E. & Nafstad, I. (1976) Chronic copper poisoning in sheep. Structural changes in erythrocytes and organs. Acta Vet. Scand. 17, 316–327.

726. Solomons, N. W., Layden, T. J., Rosenberg, I. H., Vo-Khactu, K. & Sandstead, H. H. (1976) Plasma trace metals during total parenteral alimentation. Gastroenterology 70, 1022–1025.

727. Soman, S. D., Panday, V. K., Joseph, K. T. & Raut, S. J. (1969) Daily intake of some major and trace elements. Health Physics 17, 35–40.

728. Sorenson, J. R. J. (1976) Copper chelates as possible active forms of the antiarthritic agents. J. Med. Chem. 19, 135–148.

729. Sorensen, J. R. J. (1977) Evaluation of copper complexes as potential anti-arthritic drugs. J. Pharm. Pharmacol. 29, 450–452.

730. Sourkes, T. L. (1972) Influence of specific nutrients on catecholamine synthesis and metabolism. Pharmacol. Rev. 24, 349–359.

731. Spillane, J. D., Keyser, J. W. & Parker, R. A. (1952) Amino-aciduria and copper metabolism in hepatolenticular degeneration. J. Clin. Pathol. 5, 16–24.

732. Stanley, P., Gwinn, J. L. & Sutcliffe, J. (1976) The osseous abnormalities in Menkes' syndrome. Ann. Radiol. 19, 167–172.

733. Starcher, B. C. (1969) Studies on the mechanism of copper absorption in the chick. J. Nutr. 97, 321–326.

734. Starcher, B., Hill, C. H. & Matrone, G. (1964) Importance of dietary copper in the formation of aortic elastin. J. Nutr. 82, 318–322.

735. Stein, W. H., Bearn, A. G. & Moore, S. (1954) The amino acid content of the blood and urine in Wilson's disease. J. Clin. Invest. 33, 410–419.

736. Sternlieb, I. (1967) Gastrointestinal copper absorption in man. Gastroenterology 52, 1038–1041.

737. Sternlieb, I. (1972) Evolution of the hepatic lesion in Wilson's disease (hepatolenticular degeneration). In: Progress in Liver Disease, (Popper, H. & Schaffner, F., eds.), vol. 4, pp. 511–525, Grune and Stratton, New York.

738. Sternlieb, I. & Feldmann, G. (1976) Effects of anticopper therapy on hepatocellular mitochondria in patients with Wilson's disease. An ultrastructural and stereological study. Gastroenterology 71, 457–461.

739. Sternlieb, J. & Janowitz, H. D. (1964) Absorption of copper in malabsorption syndromes. J. Clin. Invest. 43, 1049–1055.

740. Sternlieb, I., Morell, A. G., Bauer, C. D., Combes, B., de Bobes-Sternberg, S. & Scheinberg, I. H. (1961) Detection of the heterozygous carrier of the Wilson's disease gene. J. Clin. Invest. 40, 707–715.

741. Sternlieb, I., Morell, A. G. & Scheinberg, I. H. (1962) The uniqueness of ceruloplasmin in the study of plasma protein synthesis. Trans. Assoc. Amer. Physicians 75, 228–234.

742. Sternlieb, I., Morell, A. G., Tucker, W. D., Greene, M. W. & Scheinberg, I. H. (1961) The incorporation of copper into ceruloplasmin in vivo: Studies with copper⁶⁴ and copper⁶⁷. J. Clin. Invest. 40, 1834–1840.

743. Sternlieb, I., Sandson, J. I., Morell, A. G., Korotkin, E. & Scheinberg, I. H. (1969) Nonceruloplasmin copper in rheumatoid arthritis. Arth. Rheum. 12, 458–459.

744. Sternlieb, I. & Scheinberg, I. H. (1961) Ceruloplasmin in health and disease. Ann. N.Y. Acad. Sci. 94, 71–76.

745. Sternlieb, I. & Scheinberg, I. H. (1964) Penicillamine therapy for hepatolenticular degeneration. J. Am. Med. Assn. 189, 748–754.

746. Sternlieb, I. & Scheinberg, I. H. (1968) Prevention of Wilson's disease in asymptomatic patients. N. Engl. J. Med. *278*, 352–359.

747. Sternlieb, I. & Scheinberg, I. H. (1974) Wilson's disease. In: The Liver and Its Diseases (Schaffner, F., Sherlock, S. & Leevy, C. M., eds.), pp. 328–336, Intercontinental Medical Book Corp., New York.

748. Sternlieb, I., van den Hamer, C. J. A. & Alpert, S. (1967) Role of intestinal lymphatics in copper absorption. Nature *216*, 824.

749. Sternlieb, I., van den Hamer, C. J. A., Morell, A. G., Alpert, S., Gregoriadis, G. & Scheinberg, I. H. (1973) Lysosomal defect of hepatic copper excretion in Wilson's disease (hepatolenticular degeneration). Gastroenterology *64*, 99–105.

750. Stransky, E., Dauis-Lawas, D. T. & Lawas, I. L. (1952) On serum copper level and its importance in childhood. Ann. Paediat. *179*, 1–11.

751. Stratigos, J., Kasimatis, B., Panas, E. & Capetanakis, J. (1976) Le cuivre et la céruléoplasmine dans le serum des psoriasiques. Ann. Dermatol. Syphil. *103*, 584–587.

752. Strickland, G. T., Beckner, W. M. & Leu, M-L. (1972) Absorption of copper in homozygotes and heterozygotes for Wilson's disease and controls: Isotope tracer studies with ⁶⁷Cu and ⁶⁴Cu. Clin. Sci. *43*, 617–625.

753. Strickland, G. T., Beckner, W. M., Leu, M-L. & O'Reilly, S. (1972) Turnover studies of copper in homozygotes and heterozygotes for Wilson's disease and controls: Isotope tracer studies with ⁶⁷copper. Clin. Sci. *43*, 605–615.

754. Strickland, G. T., Blackwell, R. Q. & Watten, R. H. (1971) Metabolic studies in Wilson's disease. Evaluation of efficacy of chelation therapy in respect to copper balance. Am. J. Med. *51*, 31–40.

755. Strickland, G. T., Frommer, D., Leu, M-L., Pollard, R., Sherlock, S. & Comings, J. N. (1973) Wilson's Disease in the United Kingdom and Taiwan. Quart. J. Med. *42*, 619–638.

756. Strickland, G. T. & Leu, M-L. (1975) Wilson's disease: Clinical and laboratory manifestations in 40 patients. Medicine *54*, 113–137.

757. Studnitz, W. von & Berezin, D. (1958) Studies on serum copper during pregnancy, during the menstrual cycle, and after administration of oestrogens. Acta Endocrinol. *27*, 245–252.

758. Sturgeon, P. (1954) Studies on iron requirements in infants and children: 1. Normal values for serum iron, copper and free erythrocyte protoporphyrin. Pediatrics *13*, 107–125.

759. Sturgeon, P. & Brubaker, C. (1956) Copper deficiency in infants: a syndrome characterized by hypocupremia, iron deficiency anemia, and hypoproteinemia. Am. J. Dis. Child. *92*, 254–265.

760. Sullivan, J. F. & Hart, K. T. (1960) Serum benzidine oxidase. J. Lab. Clin. Med. *55*, 260–267.

761. Sultanova, G. F. (1970) Peculiarities in copper metabolism in the prematurely born infants of the first months of life. Pediatrija *49* (10), 14–18 (Russian).

762. Sumino, K., Hayakawa, K., Shibata, T. & Kitamura, S. (1975) Heavy metals in normal Japanese tissues. Amounts of 15 heavy metals in 30 subjects. Arch. Environ. Health *30*, 487–494.

763. Sunderman, F. W., Jr. (1973) Atomic absorption spectrometry of trace metals in clinical pathology. Hum. Pathol. *4*, 549–582.

764. Sunderman, F. W., Jr., Hohnadel, D. C., Evenson, M. A., Wannamaker, B. B. & Dahl, D. S. (1974) Excretion of copper in sweat of patients with Wilson's disease during sauna bathing. Ann. Clin. Lab. Sci. *4*, 407–412.

765. Sunderman, F. W., Jr. & Roszel, N. O. (1967) Measurements of copper in biological materials by atomic absorption spectrometry. Am. J. Clin. Pathol. *48*, 286–294.

766. Suttle, N. F. (1974) Recent studies of the copper-molybdenum antagonism. Proc. Nutr. Soc. *33*, 299–305.

767. Suttle, N. F. & Mills, C. F. (1966) Studies of the toxicity of copper to pigs. 1. Effects of oral supplements of zinc and iron salts on the development of copper toxicosis. Br. J. Nutr. *20*, 135–137.

768. Suttle, N. F. & Mills, C. F. (1966) Studies of the toxicity of copper to pigs. 2. Effect of protein source and other dietary components on the response to high and moderate intakes of copper. Br. J. Nutr. *20*, 149–161.

769. Tani, P. & Kokkola, K. (1972) Serum iron, copper, and iron-binding capacity in bronchogenic pulmonary carcinoma. Scand. J. Resp. Dis. (Suppl. 80), 121–128.

770. Taradaiko, Y. V. (1963) The content of copper in the organism of the mother and fetus. Akush. Ginek. *39*, 59–63 (Russian).

771. Tatum, H. J. (1974) Copper-bearing intrauterine devices. Clin. Obst. & Gynecol. *17*, 93–119.

772. Teague, H. S. & Carpenter, L. E. (1951) The demonstration of a copper deficiency in growing pigs. J. Nutr. *43*, 389–399.

773. Tessmer, C. F., Hrgovcic, M., Brown, B. W., Wilbur, J. & Thomas, F. B. (1972) Serum copper correlations with bone marrow. Cancer *29*, 173–179.

774. Tessmer, C. F., Hrgovcic, M., Thomas, F. B., Fuller, L. M. & Castro, J. R. (1973) Serum copper as an index of tumor response to radiotherapy. Radiol. *106*, 635–639.

775. Tessmer, C. F., Hrgovcic, M. & Wilbur, J. (1973) Serum copper in Hodgkin's disease in children. Cancer *31*, 303–315.

776. Tessmer, C. F., Krohn, W., Johnston, D., Thomas, F. B., Hrgovcic, M. & Brown, B. (1973) Serum copper in children (6–12 years old): An age-correction factor. Am. J. Clin. Path. *60*, 870–878.

777. Thompson, R. H. S. & Watson, D. (1949) Serum copper levels in pregnancy and in pre-eclampsia. J. Clin. Pathol. 2, 193–196.

778. Thorling, E. B. & Thorling, K. (1976) The clinical usefulness of serum copper determinations in Hodgkin's disease. A retrospective study of 241 patients from 1963–1973. Cancer 38, 225–231.

779. Thornton, I. & Alloway, B. J. (1974) Geochemical aspects of the soil-plant-animal relationship in the development of trace element deficiency and excess. Proc. Nutr. Soc. 33, 257–274.

780. Tingey, A. H. (1957) The iron, copper and manganese content of the human brain. J. Mental Sci. 83, 452–460.

781. Tipton, I. H. & Cook, M. J. (1963) Trace elements in human tissue. Part II. Adult subjects from the United States. Health Phys. 9, 103–145.

782. Tipton, I. H., Stewart, P. L. & Dickson, J. (1969) Patterns of elemental excretion in long term balance studies. Health Phys. 16, 455–462.

783. Tipton, I. H., Stewart, P. L. & Martin, P. G. (1966) Trace elements in diets and excreta. Health Phys. 12, 1683–1689.

784. Todd, J. R., Gracey, J. F. & Thompson, R. H. (1962) Studies on chronic copper poisoning. I. Toxicity of copper sulphate and copper acetate in sheep. Br. Vet. J. 118, 482–491.

785. Tompsett, S. L. (1934) The excretion of copper in urine and faeces and its relation to the copper content of the diet. Biochem. J. 28, 2088–2091.

786. Tompsett, S. L. (1935) The copper and "inorganic" iron contents of human tissues. Biochem. J. 29, 480–486.

787. Tompsett, S. L. & Anderson, D. F. (1935) The copper content of the blood in pregnancy. Br. J. Exp. Pathol. 16, 67–69.

788. Topham, R. W. & Frieden, E. (1970) Identification and purification of a non-ceruloplasmin ferroxidase of human serum. J. Biol. Chem. 245, 6698–6705.

789. Trip, J. A., Que, G. S., Botterweg-Span, Y. & Mandema, E. (1969) The state of copper in human lymph. Clin. Chim. Acta 26, 371–372.

790. Tsallas, G. & Baun, D. C. (1972) Home care total parenteral alimentation. Am. J. Hosp. Pharm. 29, 840–846.

791. Tu, J-B. (1963) A genetic, biochemical and clinical study of Wilson's disease among Chinese in Taiwan. Acta Paediat. Sinica 4, 81–104.

792. Tu, J-B. & Blackwell, R. Q. (1967) Studies on levels of penicillamine-induced cupriuresis in heterozygotes of Wilson's disease. Metabolism 16, 507–513.

793. Tu, J-B., Blackwell, R. Q. & Watten, R. H. (1965) Copper balance studies during the treatment of patients with Wilson's disease. Metabolism 14, 653–666.

794. Turpin, R., Schmitt-Jubeau, H. & Jerome, H. (1950) Action du diéthylstilboestrol sur la cuprémie. C.R. Soc. Biol. 144, 352–355.

795. Tyson, T. L., Holmes, H. H. & Ragan, C. (1950) Copper therapy of rheumatoid arthritis. Am. J. Med. Sci. 220, 418–420.

796. Ulstrom, R. A., Smith, N. J. & Heimlich, E. M. (1956) Transient dysproteinemia in infants, a new syndrome: I. clinical studies. A.M.A. J. Dis. Child. 92, 219–253.

797. Ulstrom, R. A., Smith, N. J., Nakamura, K. & Heimlich, E. (1957) Transient dysproteinemia in infants. II. Studies of protein metabolism using amino acid isotopes. A.M.A. J. Dis. Child. 93, 536–547.

798. Underwood, E. J. (1977) Trace Elements in Human and Animal Nutrition, 4th ed., Academic Press, New York.

799. Usher, S. J., MacDermot, P. N. & Lozinski, E. (1935) Prophylaxis of simple anemia in infancy with iron and copper. Am. J. Dis. Child. 49, 642–657.

800. Utin, A. V. (1970) Copper metabolism and its significance in epilepsy. Zn. Nevropatol. Psikhiat. S.S. Korsakova 70, 721–727 (Russian) (cited in Nutr. Abstr. rev. 41, 662, 1971).

801. Uzman, L. L., Iber, F. L., Chalmers, T. C. & Knowlton, M. (1956) The mechanism of copper deposition in the liver in hepatolenticular degeneration (Wilson's disease). M. J. Med. Sci. 231, 511–518.

802. Vagn-Hansen, P. L., Reske-Nielsen, E. & Lou, H. C. (1973) Menkes' Disease: a new leucodystrophy (?). A clinical and neuropathological review together with a new case. Acta Neuropathol. 25, 103–119.

803. Vallee, B. L. (1952) The time course of serum copper concentrations of patients with myocardial infarctions. I. Metabolism 1, 420–434.

804. Van Campen, D. R. (1971) Absorption of copper from the gastrointestinal tract. In: Intestinal Absorption of Metal Ions, Trace Elements and Radionucleotides (Skoryna, S. C. & Waldron-Edward, D., eds.), pp. 211–227, Pergamon Press, Oxford.

805. Van Ravesteyn, A. H. (1944) Metabolism of copper in man. Acta Med. Scand. 118, 163–196.

806. Versieck, J., Barbier, F., Speecke, A. & Hoste, J. (1975) Influence of myocardial infarction on serum manganese, copper, and zinc concentrations. Clin. Chem. 21, 578–581.

807. Vidal, G. P., Shieh, J. J. & Yasunobu, K. T. (1975) Immunological studies of bovine aorta lysyl oxidase: evidence for two forms of the enzyme. Biochem. Biophys. Res. Commun. 64, 989–995.

808. Vilter, R. W., Bozian, R. C., Hess, E. V., Zellner, D. C. & Petering, H. G. (1974) Manifestations of copper deficiency with systemic sclerosis on intravenous hyperalimentation. New Engl. J. Med. 291, 188–191.

809. Volpintesta, E. J. (1974) Menkes' kinky hair syndrome in a black infant. Am. J. Dis. Child. 128, 244–246.

810. Vuia, O. & Heye, D. (1974) Neuropathologic aspects in Menkes' kinky hair disease (trichopoliodystrophy). Neuropadiarie. 5, 329–339.

811. Wacker, W. E. C., Ulmer, D. D. & Vallee, B. L. (1956) Metalloenzymes and myocardial infarction. II. Malic and lactic dehydrogenase activities and zinc concentrations in serum. N. Eng. J. Med. 255, 449–456.

812. Waddell, J., Elvehjem, C. A., Steenbock, H. & Hart, E. B. (1928) Iron in nutrition. VI. Iron salts and iron-containing ash extracts in the correction of anemia. J. Biol. Chem. 77, 777–795.

813. Wahl, P. K., Mittal, V. P. & Bansal, O. P. (1965) Renal complications in acute copper sulphate poisoning. Indian Pract. 18, 807–812.

814. Waldman, T. A., Morell, A. G., Wochner, R. D., Strober, W. & Sternlieb, I. (1967) Measurement of gastrointestinal protein loss using ceruloplasmin labeled with ⁶⁷copper. J. Clin. Invest. 46, 10–20.

815. Walker, W. R. & Keats, D. M. (1976) An investigation of the therapeutic value of the "copper bracelet:" dermal assimilation of copper in arthritic/rheumatoid conditions. Agents Actions 6, 454–459.

816. Walker-Smith, J. & Blomfield, J. (1973) Wilson's disease or chronic copper poisoning? Arch. Dis. Child. 48, 476–479.

817. Walker-Smith, J. A., Turner, B., Blomfield, J. & Wise, G. (1973) Therapeutic implications of copper deficiency in Menkes's steely-hair syndrome. Arch. Dis. Child. 48, 958–962.

818. Walravens, P. A. (1977) Trace element nutrition and brain development. In: Proc. 4th Internat. Congress, Internat. Assn. Sci. Study Mental Deficiency (Mittler, P., ed.), vol. III, pp. 355–364, University Park, Baltimore.

819. Walsh, F. M., Crosson, F. J., Bayley, M., McReynolds, J. & Pearson, B. J. (1977) Acute copper intoxication. Pathophysiology and therapy with a case report. Am. J. Dis. Child. 131, 149–151.

820. Walshe, J. M. (1956) Penicillamine, a new oral therapy for Wilson's disease. Am. J. Med. 21, 487–495.

821. Walshe, J. M. (1967) The physiology of copper in man and its relation to Wilson's disease. Brain 90, 149–176.

822. Walshe, J. M. (1972) The biochemistry of copper in man and its role in the pathogenesis of Wilson's disease (hepatolenticular degeneration). In: Biochemical Aspects of Nervous Diseases (Cumings, J. N., ed.), pp. 111–150, Plenum, New York.

823. Walshe, J. M. (1973) Copper chelation in patients with Wilson's disease, a comparison of penicillamine and tetraethylene tetramine dihydrochloride. Quart. J. Med. 42, 441–452.

824. Walshe, J. M. & Briggs, J. (1962) Caeruloplasmin in liver disease. A diagnostic pitfall. Lancet 2, 263–265.

826. Walshe, J. M. & Potter, G. (1977) The pattern of the whole body distribution of radioactive copper (⁶⁷Cu, ⁶⁴Cu) in Wilson's disease and various control groups. Quart. J. Med. (New Series) 46, 445–462.

827. Warburg, O. & Krebs, H. A. (1927) Uber locker gebundenes Kupfer und Eisen in Blutserum. Biochem. Ztschr. 190, 143–149.

828. Warren, P. J., Earl, C. J. & Thompson, R. H. S. (1960) The distribution of copper in human brain. Brain 83, 709–717.

829. Warren, R. L., Jelliffe, A. M., Watson, J. V. & Hobbs, C. B. (1969) Prolonged observations on variations in the serum copper in Hodgkin's disease. Clin. Radiol. 20, 247–256.

830. Waslein, C. I. (1976) Human intake of trace elements. In: Trace Elements in Human Health and Disease, (Prasad, A. S. & Oberleas, D., eds.), vol. 2, pp. 347–370, Academic Press, New York.

831. Webb, J., Kirk, K. A., Jackson, D. H., Niedermeier, W., Turner, M. E., Rackley, C. E. & Russell, R. O. (1976) Analysis by pattern recognition techniques of changes in serum levels of 14 trace metals after acute myocardial infarction. Exp. Molec. Pathol. 25, 322–331.

832. Weber, P. M., O'Reilly, S., Pollycove, M. & Shipley, L. (1969) Gastrointestinal absorption of copper: studies with ⁶⁴Cu, ⁹⁵Zr, a wholebody counter and the scintillation camera. J. Nuclear. Med. 10, 591–596.

833. Wehinger, H., Witt, I., Losel, I., Denz-Seibert, G. & Sander, C. (1975) Intravenous copper in Menkes' kinky-hair syndrome. Lancet 1, 1143–1144.

834. Wertime, T. A. (1964) Man's first encounter with metallurgy. Science 146, 1257–1267.

835. Wesenberg, R. L., Gwinn, J. L. & Barnes, G. R., Jr. (1969) Radiological findings in the kinky-hair syndrome. Radiology 92, 500–506.

836. Wester, P. O. (1971) Trace elements in the coronary arteries in the presence and absence of atherosclerosis. Atherosclerosis 13 (3), 395–412.

837. Wharton, D. C. & Gibson, Q. H. (1966) Spectrophotometric characterization and function of copper in cytochrome c oxidase. In: The Biochemistry of Copper (Peisach, J., Aisen, P. & Blumberg, W. E., eds.), pp. 235–244, Academic Press, New York.

838. Wheeler, E. M. & Roberts, P. F. (1976) Menkes' steely hair syndrome. Arch. Dis. Child. 51, 269–274.

839. White, H. S. (1969) Inorganic elements in weighed diets of girls and young women. J. Am. Diet. Assn. 55, 38–43.

840. White, H. S. & Gynne, T. N. (1971) Utilization of inorganic elements by young women eating iron-fortified foods. J. Am. Diet. Assn. 59, 27–33.

841. Whitehouse, M. W. (1976) Ambivalent role of copper in inflammatory disorders. Agents Actions 6, 201–206.

842. Widdowson, E. M., Chan, H., Harrison, G. E. & Milner, R. D. G. (1972) Accumulation of Cu, Zn, Mn, Cr and Co in the human liver before birth. Biol. Neonate. 20, 360–367.

843. Widdowson, E. M., Dauncey, J. & Shaw, J. C. L. (1974) Trace elements in foetal and early postnatal development. Proc. Nutr. Soc. 33, 275–284.

844. Widdowson, E. M. & Dickerson, J. W. T. (1964) Chemical composition of the body. In: Mineral Metabolism, an Advanced Treatise, (Comar, C. L. & Bronner, F., eds.), chap. 17, pp. 1–247, Academic Press, New York.

845. Widdowson, E. M., McCance, R. A. & Spray, C. M. (1951) The chemical composition of the human body. Clin. Sci. 10, 113–125.

846. Widdowson, E. M. & Spray, C. M. (1951) Chemical development in utero. Arch. Dis. Child. 26, 205–214.

847. Wilken, H. (1960) Serumkupfer bei Spätschwangerschaftstoxikosen. Arch. Gynäkol. 194, 158–164.

848. Wilkinson, R. (1971) Polyethylene glycol 4000 as a continuously administered non-absorbable faecal marker for metabolic balance studies in human subjects. Gut 12, 654–660.

849. Williams, D. M., Atkin, C. L., Frens, D. B. & Bray, P. F. (1977) Menkes' kinky hair syndrome: studies of copper metabolism and long term therapy. Pediat. Res. 11, 823–826.

850. Williams, D. M., Lee, G. R. & Cartwright, G. E. (1974) Ferroxidase activity of rat ceruloplasmin. Am. J. Physiol. 227, 1094–1097.

851. Willvonseder, R., Goldstein, N. P., McCall, J. T., Yoss, R. E. & Tauxe, W. N. (1973) A hereditary disorder with dementia, spastic dysarthria, vertical eye movement paresis, gait disturbance, splenomegaly and abnormal copper metabolism. Neurology 23, 1039–1049.

852. Wilmore, D. W. & Dudrick, S. J. (1968) Growth and development of an infant receiving all nutrients exclusively by vein. J.A.M.A. 203, 860–864.

853. Wilmore, D. W., Groff, D. B., Bishop, H. C. & Dudrick, S. J. (1969) Total parenteral nutrition in infants with catastrophic gastrointestinal anomalies. J. Pediat. Surg. 4, 181–189.

854. Wilson, J. F. & Lahey, M. E. (1960) Failure to induce dietary deficiency of copper in premature infants. Pediatrics 25, 40–49.

855. Wilson, S. A. K. (1912) Progressive lenticular degeneration: a familial nervous disease associated with cirrhosis of the liver. Brain 34, 295–309.

856. Winge, D. R., Premakumar, R., Wiley, R. D. & Rajagopalan, K. V. (1975) Copperchelatin: purification and properties of a copper-binding protein from rat liver. Arch. Biochem. Biophys. 170, 253–266.

857. Wintrobe, M. M., Cartwright, G. E. & Gubler, C. J. (1953) Studies on the function and metabolism of copper. J. Nutr. 50, 395–419.

858. Wojcicka, J. & Zapalowski, Z. (1963) The serum-copper level in the blood of pregnant women in cases of normal and complicated pregnancies. Ginek. Polska 34, 693–697 (Polish).

859. Wolf, P. I. (1975) An investigation of serum copper in dermatologic conditions. Lab. Invest. 32, 461.

860. Wolf, W. R., Holden, J. & Greene, F. E. (1977) Daily intake of zinc and copper from self selected diets. Federation Proc. 36, 1175.

861. World Health Organization. Technical Report Series No. 532 (1973) Trace elements in human nutrition. Report of a WHO Expert Committee, 65 pp., World Health Organization, Geneva.

862. Worwood, M., Taylor, D. M. & Hunt, A. H. (1968) Copper and manganese concentrations in biliary cirrhosis of liver. Br. Med. J. 3, 344–346.

863. Wray, S. H., Kuwabara, T. & Sanderson, P. (1976) Menkes' kinky hair disease: a light and electron microscopic study of the eye. Invest. Ophthalmol. 15, 128–138.

864. Wretlind, A. (1972) Complete intravenous nutrition. Theoretical and experimental background. Nutr. Metabol. 14, (Suppl.), 1–57.

865. Wylie, J. (1957) Copper poisoning at a cocktail party. Am. J. Pub. Health 47, 617.

866. Yamada, H., Kumagai, H., Kawasaki, H., Matsui, H. & Ogata, K. (1967) Crystallization and properties of diamine oxidase from pig kidney. Biochem. Biophys. Res. Commun. 29, 723–727.

867. Yamada, H. & Yasunobu, K. T. (1962) Monoamine oxidase. II. Copper, one of the prosthetic groups of plasma monoamine oxidase. J. Biol. Chem. 237, 3077–3082.

868. Ylostalo, P. & Reinila, M. (1973) Serum copper in normal and complicated pregnancies compared with urinary estrogens. Ann. Chirurg. Gynaecol. Fenniae 62, 117–120.

869. Yoshida, T., Konno, T. & Arakawa, T. (1969) Hypocupremic infant associated with mental retardation and hepatic cirrhosis: probably a copper malabsorption syndrome. Tohoku J. Exp. Med. 98, 229–239.

870. Young, S. N. & Curzon, G. (1974) Neonatal human caeruloplasmin. Biochim. Biophys. Acta 336, 306–308.

871. Yunice, A. A., Lindeman, R. D., Czerwinski, A. W. & Clark, M. (1974) Influence of age and sex on serum copper and ceruloplasmin levels. J. Gerontol. 29, 277–281.

872. Zackhcim, H. S. & Wolf, P. (1972) Serum copper in psoriasis and other dermatoses. J. Invest. Dermatol. 58, 28–32.

873. Zimdahl, W. T., Hyman, I. & Cook, E. D. (1953) Metabolism of copper in hepatolenticular degeneration. Neurology 3, 569–578.

874. Zipursky, A., Dempsey, H., Markowitz, H., Cartwright, G. & Wintrobe, M. M. (1958) Studies on copper metabolism. XXIV. Hypocupremia in infancy. A.M.A.J. Dis. Child. 96, 148–158.

875. Zlatkov, N. B., Bozhkov, B. & Genov. D. (1973) Serum copper and ceruloplasmin in patients with psoriasis after helio- and thalassotherapy. Arch. Derm. Forsch. 247, 289–294.

876. Zlatkov, N. B., Petkov, I., Genov, D. & Bozhkov, B. (1971) Kupferstoffwechael bei Kranken mit Vitiligo nach Heliotherapie. Dermatologica (Basel) 143, 115–120.

877. Zondek, S. G. & Bandmann, M. (1931) Kupfer in Frauenmilch und Kuhmilch. Klin. Wochenschr. 10, 1528–1531.

878. Zudikova, S. I. (1967) Copper in blood of pregnant women with late toxicosis. Vop. Omrany Mater. Det. 12 (12), 69–70 (Russian).

879. Zurukzoglu-Sklavounou, S. (1953) Hypochrome Anämie im Kindesalter: Studie auf Grund von 373 Fallen. Helvet. Paediat. Acta 8, 251–275.

Index